T3-BPX-011

ONCOGENIC VIRUSES

SECOND EDITION

ONCOGENIC VIRUSES

SECOND EDITION
COMPLETELY REVISED AND ENLARGED

by

LUDWIK GROSS, M.D., F.A.C.P.

Chief, Cancer Research Unit
Veterans Administration Hospital
Bronx, New York

PERGAMON PRESS

OXFORD · LONDON · EDINBURGH · NEW YORK
TORONTO · SYDNEY · PARIS · BRAUNSCHWEIG

Pergamon Press Ltd., Headington Hill Hall, Oxford
4 & 5 Fitzroy Square, London W.1
Pergamon Press (Scotland) Ltd., 2 & 3 Teviot Place, Edinburgh 1
Pergamon Press Inc., Maxwell House, Fairview Park, Elmsford, New York 10523
Pergamon of Canada Ltd., 207 Queen's Quay West, Toronto 1
Pergamon Press (Aust.) Pty. Ltd., 19a Boundary Street, Rushcutters Bay, N.S.W. 2011, Australia
Pergamon Press S.A.R.L., 24 rue des Écoles, Paris 5e
Vieweg & Sohn GmbH, Burgplatz 1, Braunschweig

First edition 1961
Second revised edition 1970

Library of Congress Catalog Card Number 68-57887

PRINTED IN GREAT BRITAIN BY PURNELL AND SONS LTD.
PAULTON (SOMERSET) AND LONDON

08 013236 7

Contents

List of Illustrations

List of Tables

Introduction

THIS monograph was written with the purpose of reviewing animal tumors caused by oncogenic viruses. It would be difficult to define precisely a virus-caused neoplasm. With only few exceptions, however, such a definition would refer to tumors that can be transmitted in the laboratory by inoculation of filtrates.

At first, only very few tumors could be transmitted by filtrates. More recently, however, the number of tumors transmissible by cell-free extracts has been increasing at an accelerated pace. It is now quite apparent that most of the chicken tumors, and the great majority of mouse tumors, are of viral origin.

It would be rather difficult to assume that malignant tumors in other species are of different origin. It is thus quite possible, perhaps even probable, that malignant tumors in various animal species, including humans, are also caused by viruses.

It is immediately realized that objections will be raised at this point. It is true that cell-free transmission of many fowl and murine neoplasms has been demonstrated. Such tumors are unquestionably caused by transmissible, submicroscopic agents. This does not necessarily imply, however, that all other tumors are caused by similar submicroscopic agents, or that oncogenic viruses are indispensable causative factors in the induction of tumors.

Sufficient experimental data are not yet available to answer many of the fundamental questions referring to the etiology of tumors in animals and in man. It is helpful, however, to be guided by a working hypothesis, provided that facts are used as guideposts.

The interest in oncogenic viruses has increased considerably during the past few decades, and particularly during the last ten years. Many new and unexpected observations have been made, particularly in the fowl leukosis complex and in the field of murine tumors.

The use of newborn animals for inoculation of oncogenic viruses, the propagation of some of such viruses in tissue culture, the visualization of oncogenic agents with the aid of the electron microscope, have contributed considerably to the acceleration of the pace of progress in experimental cancer research. These are fascinating times in tumor research. New observations are being reported almost every few months.

The information concerning filterable, transmissible, oncogenic agents is scattered, however, in different journals, and printed in different languages. The bibliography has been accumulating at such a rapid rate that it becomes difficult to keep abreast of latest developments.

In this monograph an attempt has been made to review the known oncogenic viruses, to discuss the current status of experimental approach to virus-caused neoplasms, and to list the most important bibliographical references.

It would be beyond the means of a single author to review adequately all data referring to oncogenic viruses as a group. With even best intentions, the author is obviously better informed on some aspects of this problem, than in other fields. Furthermore, limitation of space precludes entering into greater detail.

This monograph could be compared with a sketchbook, outlining in general terms the problem of tumor viruses in experimental cancer research. The reader interested in a particular field should be able to find more detailed information in references which are included at the end of each chapter. An effort was made to include the most important references; each was checked individually from the original publication.

* * *

The second edition of this monograph has been completely revised. There have been many changes and advances in experimental cancer research since the first edition was prepared. Most of the chapters have been rewritten in order to include new and additional data.

The information about many known oncogenic viruses has been considerably enlarged; as an example, the Rous sarcoma virus was found to be oncogenic not only for chickens and related species, but also for mice, rats, and hamsters. Other oncogenic agents, such as the bovine papilloma virus, also revealed an unsuspected pathogenic potential and ability to induce malignant tumors in other animal species. This additional information required a revision of the respective chapters, and a review of a large number of pertinent and recent publications.

Similar, although not necessarily such striking, changes and additional new data had to be incorporated in other chapters. The chapters on chicken leukosis and on mouse leukemia have been completely revised and considerably enlarged. New chapters dealing with recently isolated oncogenic viruses, such as the mouse osteosarcoma virus, the murine sarcoma virus, and viruses causing leukemia and lymphosarcomas in cats, dogs, and guinea pigs, have been added.

An important chapter on the oncogenic potency of the recently isolated simian virus 40 (SV 40) has also been added. Another new and significant chapter deals with the oncogenic potency of human adenoviruses. Bovine leukosis and Burkitt lymphoma in African children have been reviewed in separate chapters, although experimental documentation of the viral nature of these two diseases has not yet been established. Finally, information concerning the possible viral nature of human neoplasms, and in particular human leukemia, has been reviewed, enlarged, and brought up-to-date; this chapter includes the discussion of recently published data on the presence of polyoma-like virus particles in human demyelinating brain disease.

* * *

Most of the electron micrographs printed in the first edition have been replaced, and a substantial number of additional photographs has been added. New techniques in electron microscopy, including improved methods in the process of embedding, cutting, and staining of ultrathin sections, as well as technical advances in the construction and performance capacity of electron microscopes, made it possible to improve the quality and resolution of electron micrographs. As a result of a better and more realistic interpretation of electron micrographs, our knowledge of the formation and morphology of viruses and their relation to cell components has advanced considerably.

An effort has been made to make the second edition more comprehensive than the first printing; revision of previous chapters and addition of new chapters necessitated a review of several hundred additional references. As in the first edition, in the preparation of the second edition also, each new reference has been reviewed individually by the author from the original publication.

L.G.

Acknowledgments

THE task of preparing the original and the second revised edition of this monograph was facilitated by the very kind cooperation of a large number of friends, colleagues, and other distinguished workers in the field of oncogenic viruses and related areas, who discussed with the author various aspects of problems related to their personal experience, exchanged correspondence in this matter, or read through drafts of chapters, or parts of chapters, referring to their particular fields of interest, and gave the benefit of their impressions. It should not be inferred, however, that these scientists endorsed all the views or statements expressed in this book.

It would be difficult to list the names of all those who very kindly assisted the author, replied to inquiries, and provided reprints of their publications, or manuscripts of papers prepared for publication. In addition to the names listed in the Acknowledgments of the first edition of this monograph, the following were particularly helpful in assisting the author in obtaining the necessary information for the preparation of the respective chapters of the second revised edition: Drs. C. G. Ahlström, Joseph W. Beard, H. J. Bendixen, Wilhelm Bernhard, Marcel Bessis, Michel Boiron, W. Ray Bryan, Austin M. Brues, Denis P. Burkitt, Ben R. Burmester, F. C. Chesterman, Leon Dmochowski, Wm. R. Duryee, Bernice E. Eddy, Miriam P. Finkel, T. N. Fredrickson, Charlotte Friend, Jacob Furth, Arnold Graffi, Françoise Haguenau, N. Haran-Ghera, R. J. C. Harris, J. J. Harvey, Maurice R. Hilleman, Robert J. Huebner, W. F. H. Jarrett, C. W. Jungeblut, Henry S. Kaplan, Werner H. Kirsten, John B. Moloney, Raymond Latarjet, Pierre Lépine, J. F. Loutit, Robert R. Marshak, Joseph L. Melnick, Carl Olson, J. H. Pope, G. Rabotti, Peyton Rous, Wallace P. Rowe, Albert B. Sabin, B. Thorell, John J. Trentin, Arthur C. Upton, G. Winqvist, and Gabriele M. Zu Rhein.

Most of the electron micrographs used in the second edition were supplied by Dr. Dorothy G. Feldman of our laboratory. In addition, electron micrographs were generously provided by Drs. June D. Almeida, E. L. Benedetti, Wilhelm Bernhard, H. S. Di Stefano, Leon Dmochowski, M. A. Epstein, Nicole Granboulan, Françoise Haguenau, A. F. Howatson, Helen M. Laird, Philip D. Lunger, H. D. Mayor, D. H. Moore, C. Olson, Charles G. Rickard, R. Scherrer, R. S. Stone, M. Tajima, John J. Trentin, Gabriele Zu Rhein, and others.

Miss Ethel Tanzer in particular, as well as Miss Margaret M. Kinney and other members of the Medical Library staff of the Veterans Administration Hospital, Bronx, N.Y., were very helpful and resourceful, searching for references, checking authors' names, the titles of publications, and securing the original publications or photostatic copies of the references quoted; many of these papers were printed in foreign and not readily accessible journals; some publications were very old, a few had been printed over a century ago.

The tedious task of typing the manuscript and checking references was accomplished very efficiently by my secretary, Mrs. Mitzi Rinkle Trivisani.

The photographs of mice, rats and tumors, and photomicrographs of tumor sections were prepared by the Medical Illustration Service at this hospital.

Most of the portrait photographs were obtained directly from the scientists, or from their immediate families. The photographs of Prof. V. Ellermann and Prof. O. Bang were received from Prof. H. Gormsen, Copenhagen, through the courtesy of Col. Frank, M. Townsend and Prof. H. C. Bendixen. The photograph of Dr. B. Lucké was obtained from the U.S. Armed Forces Institute of Pathology in Washington, D.C. The photograph of Prof. A. Borrel was received through the courtesy of the Library of the Pasteur Institute in Paris. The photographs of Drs. M. Bessis and H. Rubin were obtained from O.R.T.F., Robert Siegler, Paris, and Barry Evans Studio in Berkeley, respectively. The portrait of Dr. W. M. Stanley was received from photographer Fritz Esohen, Berlin-Wilmersdorf.

My wife, Dorothy, assisted in editing the early drafts, and also the final form of the manuscript, gave the benefit of her suggestions, checked references, and later also assisted in reading the galley proofs.

Dr. Dorothy G. Feldman reviewed with the author those parts of the chapters which refer to electron microscopic studies of oncogenic viruses. Miss Yolande Dreyfuss of our laboratory tabulated experimental data forming the basis of our studies on murine leukemia; in addition, she also read and checked the manuscript and assisted in searching for references. Dr. T. E. Ehrenreich, Miss Lorraine A. Moore and other members of our research staff have been also very helpful in carrying out our research program over a long period of years at this hospital.

I am very grateful to the Publisher of Pergamon Press, I. R. Maxwell, M.C., M.P., and also to E. J. Buckley, Deputy Managing Director, for their cooperation and generosity in giving the author complete freedom in the preparation of the manuscript, in the selection of the type of print and headings, and in planning the general layout and organization of the monograph, in the inclusion of all necessary photographs and electron micrographs, and in accepting the many changes, alterations, and additions submitted by the author, making it possible to include the most recent developments in the field of oncogenic viruses.

Finally, a word about the U.S. Government Agency and private Foundations, without whose assistance the author would not have had the opportunity to carry out his work. The U.S. Veterans Administration has generously supported the work of the author for the past 23 years. The author has also had an excellent understanding and cooperation of the administrative officers, as well as his colleagues and other members of the professional staff, at this hospital.

The Damon Runyon Memorial Fund and the American Cancer Society have generously contributed to the support of the studies of the author, and have thus, indirectly, contributed to the preparation of this monograph. Sincere gratitude is expressed for this support.

CHAPTER 1

General Considerations

THE EXPERIMENTAL INOCULATION OF COMMUNICABLE DISEASES

The question whether or not a disease is communicable is obviously of fundamental importance, and should be clarified, if possible, before any further study of the disease has been made. There are, however, no particular criteria to indicate, *a priori*, that a disease is caused by a transmissible agent. In fact, in many instances, when studying a new and obscure disease, the investigator may be confronted with symptoms that appear to develop "spontaneously" in one individual or another. At first, it may be very difficult, if not impossible, to trace the mode of transmission of the hypothetical pathogenic agent. And yet, the disease may be communicable.

Whenever the communicability of an obscure disease was suspected, one of the first experiments in the laboratory consisted of an attempt to transmit such a condition by artificial inoculation to other hosts. Actually, this was an attempt to duplicate experimentally, at will, the suspected natural transmission of the obscure disease.

It was common knowledge a long time before the microscope and the world of microbes were discovered, that smallpox, and probably also some other diseases of man, could be transmitted by artificial inoculation. The same was known of certain communicable diseases of animals, such as foot-and-mouth disease of cattle. Gradually it has been learned that the great majority of the known communicable diseases could be transmitted by inoculation, from one host to another.

Successful transmission of a communicable disease from one host to another was possible only when certain experimental conditions were met. These conditions varied for different diseases. Until such requirements were determined, some of the infectious diseases could not be transmitted in the laboratory.

Many difficulties may confront the investigator. In principle, the causative agent is to be transmitted to a susceptible host. It may not be an easy task, however, to recover the pathogenic agent in sufficient quantity from the diseased host, unless the epidemiology of the particular agent is known. The causative agent may be present in the blood of the diseased host or in the diseased tissues at certain periods of the disease only; in some instances difficulties may be encountered when attempts are made to recover the agent at the time when the disease is already fully developed.

In order to reproduce the disease, the causative agent must be introduced into a susceptible host. This may be readily accomplished in cases where the pathogenic agent has a broad range of infectivity, such as the virus of hydrophobia, which can infect a large variety of species. Many pathogenic agents, however, have a narrow range of hosts. Thus, in the study of certain obscure diseases, hosts of the same species must be employed for the initial inoculation. Furthermore, certain pathogenic agents have to be inoculated into very young, perhaps only into newborn hosts.*

THE FILTERABLE VIRUSES

With the progress of bacteriology, the identification, isolation, and selective, *in vitro*, propagation of various pathogenic microorganisms became a laboratory routine. It was soon realized, however, that in the case of many obviously communicable diseases, such as smallpox, hydrophobia, or foot-and-mouth disease, no microbes could be visualized in the diseased tissues with the aid of a microscope; yet, inoculation of extracts prepared from such tissues into susceptible hosts reproduced characteristic symptoms of the same disease. It was quite apparent that such extracts may contain microorganisms so small as to be invisible to the human eye, even when examined with a powerful optical microscope. Only the recent advent of the electron microscope made it possible to visualize the smallest pathogenic agents, the viruses.

Pasteur tried vainly to find the microbe of hydrophobia in the brain or spinal cord of infected dogs (Pasteur *et al.*, 1884). When asked by an apparently impatient member of the Academy of Sciences† in Paris (who must have been impressed by Pasteur's successive and rapid discoveries of various microbes) " ... will there ever be a microbe of hydrophobia?", Pasteur replied in 1884: " ... one is tempted to believe, that ... this is a microorganism infinitesimally small."

The existence of such infinitesimally small microorganisms, invisible to the human eye under the optical microscope and suspected by Pasteur already in 1881 (Roux, 1903), was substantiated some ten years later, in 1892, by Iwanowski.

The mosaic disease of tobacco plants causes mottling of leaves with a

* It is quite apparent that such limitations may cause almost insurmountable difficulties in attempts to transmit experimentally certain obscure, progressive, and generally fatal human diseases, such as pemphigus, malignant neoplasms, and leukemias.

† Dr. Bouley, vice-president of the French Academy of Sciences (Pasteur *et al.*, 1884).

brown discoloration; the leaves become brittle and damaged. In 1892, Iwanowski, in St. Petersburg, Russia, reported (1894*, 1898) that the juice obtained from leaves of tobacco plants afflicted with this disease could be passed through porcelain filters, which retained all visible microbes, and that such filtrates were fully capable of reproducing mosaic disease when inoculated into healthy plants. A few drops of the infectious fluid placed on leaves of a new plant, or instilled into the ground on which such a plant was growing, transmitted the disease.

In 1898, Beijerinck, in Delft, the Netherlands, made a similar observation. Since he was able to transmit the mosaic disease in tobacco plants by filtrates which did not contain any visible microbes, he assumed that this disease is caused by a "contagium vivum fluidum" (Beijerinck, 1898). Although his experiments were reported four years later than those of Iwanowski (1894), Beijerinck claimed (1899) that he had no knowledge of Iwanowski's studies when he wrote his report.

At about the same time, similar observations were made with pathogenic agents causing certain diseases in animals and in man. In 1898, G. Sanarelli in Montevideo, Uruguay, described a contagious and fatal disease afflicting rabbits and causing multiple myxomatous swellings in the subcutaneous tissue around the nostrils, mouth, ears, anus, and vagina. The causative agent was found to be so small that it could not be detected under a microscope. Thus, curiously enough, a tumor was one of the first diseases recognized to be transmissible by a submicroscopic agent. Sanarelli, however, did not filter his agent. Filtration experiments were carried out later.†

That same year, in 1898, Loeffler and Frosch, in Berlin, Germany, reported that the "foot-and-mouth disease" of cattle, a highly contagious disease of cloven-footed animals, could be transmitted by filtrates. It was thus evident that this disease is caused by a submicroscopic, invisible agent.

Gradually, many other communicable diseases of animals and man, for which no specific causative microbes could be detected under the microscope, were found to be transmissible by filtrates. Blood, or pathologically altered tissues, removed from hosts suffering from such communicable diseases as smallpox, hydrophobia, infantile paralysis, herpes, encephalitis, etc., were found to contain invisible and filterable pathogenic agents. These agents could be transferred indefinitely from one host to another; hence, it was evident that they reproduced themselves in their hosts.

It thus became apparent that among transmissible diseases some were caused by agents so small that they could not be detected with an ordinary

* The paper was read at the Academy of Sciences in St. Petersburg on February 12, 1892, but was published (in German) in the Bulletin of the Academy in 1894 (Iwanowski, 1894).

† See Rabbit Myxomatosis in this monograph.

optical microscope. The term "viruses" which had been previously employed on a more general basis, and which at first included a broad group of pathogenic microorganisms, gradually became restricted to very small, submicroscopic pathogenic agents.*

Filtration

Most of the larger microbes are retained by bacterial filters, whereas viruses generally pass through. There exists a large variety of filters employed in the laboratory. The filter pads, filter membranes, or filter candles vary in porosity and can be selected according to needs. Most of the filters employed, such as Chamberland, Berkefeld, or Selas filter candles, or Seitz filter pads, retain the larger microbes, but allow the smaller viruses to pass through. A certain quantity of virus particles is lost during filtration procedure, because of absorption of the particles by filter pads or filter candles. This is particularly true when Seitz asbestos filter pads, and to a lesser extent when infusorial earth filter candles (Berkefeld) or unglazed porcelain filter candles (Chamberland or Selas), are employed. Sinter glass filter candles are also available, as well as graded collodion membranes; the latter allow most of the virus particles to pass with relatively minimal loss due to filtration procedure.

A filtrate passed under good technical conditions through bacterial filters of proper porosity, such as Berkefeld N, Chamberland L 3, or Selas O2, or O3, may contain viruses, but is considered "bacteriologically sterile", i.e. free from the larger microbes. Minute defects may occur,

* Émile Roux, a close associate of Pasteur, reviewed the problem of "invisible" microbes in 1903. He noted that although all microbes are very small, as their name implies, and require a microscope to be seen, their size actually varies to a considerable extent. The Schaudin's *Bacillus Bütschlii* (a very large microbe found in the intestine of cockroaches) has a diameter of 3 to 6 μ. This is a real giant as compared with Pfeiffer's bacillus; the latter (*Hemophilus influenzae*) has a diameter of only 0.5 μ. Since, for all practical purposes, using transmitted light, the limit of visibility is about 0.2 μ, a microbe only four or five times smaller than Pfeiffer's bacillus could not be seen even under the best optical microscope.

What justification do we have, asked Roux, to assume that the world of microbes ceases to exist at the level of 0.1 or 0.2 μ? It is only logical to assume, Roux noted, that there exist microorganisms much smaller, and therefore invisible to the human eye.

Roux quoted Pasteur who suspected as early as 1881 that rabies is caused by a virus so small that it cannot be seen under the microscope. At that time the invisible viruses were only "beings of reason" ("êtres de raison").

Since it was established, however, that tobacco mosaic disease in plants (1892) and foot-and-mouth disease in cattle (1898) could be transmitted by filtrates, the "beings of reason" became "beings of reality."

A short half of a century later, electrons, employed instead of light waves, opened the world of viruses to the human eye.

however, in the filter candles, and for that reason filtrates should always be tested for bacterial sterility.

* * *

Filtration thus became a very convenient tool in the study of virus diseases. Whenever an investigator was confronted with an obscure, and possibly infectious disease, one of the initial experiments consisted usually of an attempt to transmit such a disease from one host to another by means of a filtrate. If an extract prepared from diseased tissues could be filtered without losing its pathogenic potential, i.e. when the filtrate reproduced symptoms of the same disease following inoculation into a susceptible host, it was generally assumed that such a disease was caused by a virus.

The term "filterable viruses" was employed to designate very small pathogenic agents capable of passing through bacteria-tight filters and responsible for many transmissible diseases in humans, animals, and plants.

Some Fundamental Properties of Viruses

Viruses are generally smaller than ordinary microbes. As a rule, they are less than 400 mμ in longest diameter. Some viruses are very small, about 20 mμ or even less in particle diameter. Others exceed 200 mμ in diameter. Their shapes vary from round or spheroidal particles to rods, filaments, or brick-shaped crystals.

Although our knowledge of the biochemical structure of viruses is still very fragmentary, it is quite probable that most viruses consist of a central core of nucleic acid, which is the genetic material responsible for infectivity, and of an outside protein shell.

Viruses are specific pathogenic agents. They cause symptoms of characteristic diseases. Some have a wide range of hosts. Other viruses have a narrow host range and infect only a single species. Some are transmitted directly from host to host, whereas others require intermediary hosts, such as insect vectors, for transmission. In certain instances man may be only an accidental, occasional host of a virus which usually may be maintained in nature primarily in other species.

Many viruses have a preference to invade and multiply in certain cells of particular organs. This selectivity of a virus for a particular cell type may be quite strict. Yet, most viruses may adapt themselves to various types of tissues and may thus be able to infect, under proper conditions, a broad spectrum of cells.

In a group of virus particles of the same kind produced in a multiplication cycle, a certain proportion may contain genetic material slightly different from the rest. This altered genetic constitution may then be retained in successive virus generations. Such spontaneous mutations occur now and then among viruses.

Viruses may frequently remain latent, causing only occasionally symptoms of disease. In this respect they do not differ from many bacterial infections. Latent carriers of viruses and pathogenic microbes are by far more frequent than those with frank symptoms of disease.

Viruses are obligate cell parasites. After entering a susceptible cell, the virus loses its identity and disappears within the cell. The virus may then become latent and completely incorporated in the genetic material of the host's cell. The cells may later multiply and carry along the invisible virus through successive cell generations.

The virus may, on the other hand, induce fundamental changes in the metabolism and morphology of the cell, which may lead to degeneration and eventually to cell destruction, with a concurrent liberation of a large number of newly formed virus particles.

The reproduction of viruses differs fundamentally from that of the ordinary microbes. Some of the larger microbes, such as gonococci or brucella organisms, also grow intracellularly. The ordinary microbes multiply, however, by binary fission. From one microbe, two are formed; the two now split, and four are formed; under ideal conditions, the number increases in geometrical progression, to eight, sixteen, thirty-two, sixty-four, and so forth.

The reproduction of viruses is quite different. Actually, what happens in the cell following the entry of an infective virus particle is poorly understood. It is apparent, however, that the virus particle disintegrates and ceases to be infective on bio-assay, or to be detectable in the electron microscope. After a latency period (eclipse phase) which varies for different viruses, a large number of newly formed, reconstituted virus particles, as many as two hundred or more, reappear in groups (inclusion bodies), or scattered, and at about the same time in the nucleus or in the cytoplasm.

The cell's genetic material serves as a ready source for the replication of the genetic cores of the newly formed virus particles. The cell's cytoplasm then serves to complete the formation of virus particles providing the outer protein shell for the virus. Degeneration and eventual destruction of the cell follows, with the liberation of a large number of newly formed virus particles.

The virus particles can now infect new cells and either remain latent, or proceed, after a brief eclipse phase, with their reproductive cycle, which ends again with the destruction of the cell and the liberation of newly formed virus particles.

As an alternate possibility, the infected cell may remain apparently unharmed, but individual virus particles are formed by the process of budding, usually at the edge of plasma membrane, and are then released into the intercellular space. The virus particles may also bud into the vacuolar membrane, and later be released, with the cell remaining again apparently unharmed.

Finally, the virus particles may enter susceptible cells, and disappear; the infected cells may, or may not, alter their morphology, and the virus particles which entered such cells may remain undetected.

* * *

It is thus quite apparent that viruses differ in several respects from the larger microbes. The viruses are not only submicroscopic, filterable micro-organisms. They are obligate cell parasites; they differ from microbes fundamentally in their method of reproduction, and in their relationship to the harboring cells.

The limit of visibility, in an optical microscope, using transmitted light, is for all practical purposes approximately 0.2 μ, or 200 mμ, since the object viewed must have the size of about one-half of the wave length of the light used.

The electron microscope, in which a stream of electrons is employed, instead of the beam of light used in the optical microscope, makes it possible to visualize and study the structure of the smallest virus particles, less than 20 mμ or even 10 mμ in diameter.

THE TRANSPLANTATION OF TUMORS IN ANIMALS BY CELL-GRAFT

M. Novinsky (1876), in Russia, was probably the first to report successful transplantation of a malignant tumor from one animal to another. Novinsky removed a cancerous growth (medullary carcinoma)* from the nose of a 4-year-old female dog and transplanted fragments of this tumor under the skin of several dogs; in one of the inoculated dogs a small tumor appeared after only a few weeks at the site of inoculation; a metastatic tumor also developed in the adjoining lymph nodes. The tumor was removed and transplanted successfully into a $1\frac{1}{2}$-month-old puppy. In 1884, Wehr, in Lwów, also succeeded in transplanting a tumor from dog to dog† (Wehr, 1888).

In 1889, A. Hanau, at the Institute of Pathological Anatomy in Zurich, Switzerland, reported the first successful transplantation of a cancerous tumor in the rat. He implanted a small piece of tumor tissue removed from a female rat into the testicles of 2 male rats: tumor nodules developed in both rats after 2 to 3 months.

In 1890, v. Eiselsberg, at the Surgical Clinic of the University of Vienna, found a spontaneous tumor (spindle-cell sarcoma) in an adult rat. He

* In 1877 Novinsky also transplanted the venereal dog sarcoma. See chapter on the transmissible dog tumor in this monograph and also reviews of Shimkin (1955) and Stewart *et al.* (1959).

† See also page 96.

removed a fragment of this tumor and implanted it into the mesenteric folds of 2 half-grown rats. In one of these animals a tumor developed at the site of implantation after a latency of less than 2 months. The microscopic structure of this tumor was identical with that of the spontaneous growth.

One year later, in 1891, a young French investigator, H. Morau, published in Paris a paper relating his experimental transmission of a spontaneous mouse mammary carcinoma through several successive hosts. The inoculations consisted of implantations of small pieces of tumor tissue under the skin of mice by means of a trocar. The tumors grew slowly, and the implantations did not always succeed. In several cases, however, the carcinomatous tumors could be successfully transplanted from one mouse to another through several successive animal passages.

In 1892, Firket, in Liège, Belgium, transplanted successfully a spindle-cell sarcoma from rat to rat and carried it through threc successive rat passages.

In 1898, Velich, in Austria, also reported successful transplantation of a rat sarcoma through eight successive generations.

To none of these communications was any special attention devoted. Several years elapsed before similar work began in various other laboratories on a more extensive scale, in the United States (Loeb, 1901, 1902), France (Borrel, 1903), Denmark (Jensen, 1903), England (Bashford *et al.*, 1904, 1905), Germany (Ehrlich and Apolant, 1905), etc., and the findings of Hanau, Morau, and others were fully confirmed.*

It was evident that tumors in rats and mice could be transplanted from host to host, provided that undamaged tumor cells were transferred from the tumor-bearing animal into another animal of the same species and race. Transplantations of tumors from mice to guinea pigs, or to rabbits, failed, and it was generally recognized that tumors could be transferred only within the same species. After a successful transplantation, the tumor grew in the new host and, in most instances, eventually killed the animal. Often, however, the transplantation did not succeed: even large amounts of the tumor tissue implanted under the skin, or in the muscles of the new host, failed to proliferate, and no new growth appeared. In other instances, an implanted tumor grew only temporarily and then gradually regressed.

Paul Ehrlich (1905, 1907), in Germany, was able to obtain from various dealers 278 female mice with spontaneous breast tumors. One hundred and eight were excised and implanted into new mice, but only 14 transplantations were successful.

Initial Difficulties. Thus, in the initial transplantation experiments,

* It would be beyond the scope of this monograph to consider in more detail the initial experiments dealing with transplantation of tumors in mice and rats. The interested reader will find additional information and references in the early reviews of this subject by Woglom (1913, 1929).

difficulties were encountered. This was true not only for mouse tumors, but also for tumor transplantations in other species. In some instances, such as in the case of Rous chicken sarcoma, blood relatives of the original host, in which the tumors had originally developed, had to be employed for the initial inoculations. Gradually, however, in the course of successive transplantations, some of the tumors became more potent and grew with less difficulty in hosts of the same species.

Many factors affected the outcome of tumor transplantation. Younger hosts were found to be substantially more susceptible to tumor inoculation than older animals. Newborn animals were most susceptible. In some instances, strain and occasionally even species barriers could be crossed by inoculating newborn animals. Certain sites of inoculation were also found to be more sensitive than others. The intracerebral or intraperitoneal routes of inoculation were more sensitive than the subcutaneous route.

Transplantations were performed routinely by implanting, with the aid of a trocar, small fragments of tumor tissue, under the skin, or in the muscles, of new hosts. Later on, however, tumor cell suspensions were found more suitable, permitting, under sterile conditions, a more accurate dosage.

Heterologous transplantations succeeded when tumor fragments were implanted into the anterior chamber of the eye (Smirnova, 1937. Greene, 1938–1943).

Treatment of the host with cortisone, or by total body X-ray irradiation, was frequently found to lower the host's resistance sufficiently to allow successful implantation of heterologous tumors in such pre-treated hosts (Toolan, 1951–1953).

Some of the mouse tumors, which initially grew only with difficulty on transplantation, gradually increased in their potency. After a large number of successive transplantations, some of these tumors acquired such a growth potential that they now could be successfully implanted into mice of almost any breed. Eventually, strains of highly malignant, transplantable mouse tumors have been obtained, such as "Ehrlich mouse sarcoma," "Ehrlich mouse carcinoma," or "Sarcoma 37," which grew indiscriminately in almost any commercially available laboratory mice and were for that reason extensively used in various laboratories for experimental studies on cancer.*

Other tumors, however, which developed spontaneously, or were induced with carcinogenic chemicals, or by other means, in mice or other species of animals, could be transplanted only with difficulty, if at all, into hosts of the same species.

The development of inbred strains of mice greatly facilitated cell

* The interested reader is referred to the excellent review "Transplantable and Transmissible Tumors of Animals" by H. L. Stewart *et al.* (1959).

transplantation of tumors. Mice which were uniformly susceptible to the implantation of certain tumors now became available; generally, tumors developing in a mouse of a given inbred strain could be transplanted without difficulty to other mice of the same inbred line. Mice of other genetically unrelated inbred strains were generally resistant to the implantation of such tumors, unless newborn mice were used for inoculation. With successive transplantations, many tumors, however, gradually became sufficiently potent to grow in mice of genetically unrelated strains.

TRANSMISSION OF TUMORS BY FILTRATES

Transplantation of tumors by cell-graft became a useful tool in experimental cancer research. It was not considered to be similar, however, to the experimental transmission of communicable diseases. The development of a tumor resulting from the implantation of tumor cells into a susceptible host was not compared with the induction of a disease by a pathogenic agent. It was rather considered to be similar to a graft of a normal tissue from one host to another. Tumor cells removed from one host and transplanted into another continued to multiply, the new host furnishing only shelter and supplying food for the implanted, but actually extraneous, new growth. The participation of the host was thus considered to be only indirect.

These considerations did not apply to those instances in which malignant tumors could be transmitted from one host to another by inoculation of filtrates. No cell-graft was involved in these cases. Experimental cell-free transmission of a tumor implied that an agent sufficiently small to pass through bacteria-tight filters was able to reproduce a malignant neoplasm following inoculation into a new host. This was comparable to the transmission of common communicable diseases by inoculation of submicroscopic viruses.

It was thus necessary to conclude that those tumors which could be transmitted by filtrates were caused by submicroscopic, filterable viruses. This concept, however, has been accepted only gradually.

The following is a chronologic list of isolations of some of the more important oncogenic viruses.

In 1898, G. Sanarelli, in Montevideo, recognized the viral nature of a highly contagious disease, the rabbit myxomatosis. This is a tumor-like condition caused by a transmissible agent; the actual filtration experiments, however, were carried out only in 1911 by A. Moses. The virus causes fibromas in wild, cottontail rabbits, and fatal myxomatosis in domestic rabbits.

In 1908, V. Ellermann and O. Bang, in Copenhagen, succeeded in transmitting by filtrates the erythro-myeloblastic form of chicken leukemia.

In 1911, Peyton Rous, at the Rockefeller Institute in New York, succeeded in transmitting the first solid tumor, a chicken sarcoma, by a filtrate.

There followed a long interval of time during which no additional tumors could be transmitted by filtrates. Some 20 years later, Richard E. Shope, at the Rockefeller Institute in Princeton, New Jersey, succeeded in transmitting the rabbit fibroma (1932) and shortly thereafter the rabbit papilloma (1933) by filtrates.

In 1933, Jacob Furth transmitted chicken lymphomatosis by filtrate.

In 1936, John J. Bittner, at the Jackson Memorial Laboratory in Bar Harbor, Maine, reported that the mouse mammary carcinoma agent is transmitted through the milk of nursing female mice.

In 1938, Baldwin Lucké, in Philadelphia, reported evidence that frog kidney carcinoma is caused by a transmissible virus.

In 1946, B. R. Burmester, C. O. Prickett, and T. C. Belding, at the Regional Poultry Research Laboratory in East Lansing, Michigan, succeeded in transmitting chicken lymphomatosis and osteopetrosis by filtrates.

In 1951, mouse leukemia was transmitted by filtrates in our laboratory (Gross, 1951). The mouse leukemia virus was later found to be also pathogenic for rats and capable of inducing a variety of leukemias and lymphomas in both species of animals. In 1956, Graffi and his associates in Berlin observed the development of leukemia following inoculation into newborn mice of cell-free extracts prepared from transplanted mouse tumors. It was thus determined that the mouse leukemia virus can be carried in a latent form in transplanted mouse tumors.

In 1953, the mouse parotid tumor virus was isolated in our laboratory from leukemic mouse tissues (Gross, 1953). Some of the newborn mice inoculated with the parotid tumor virus developed not only salivary gland tumors, but also subcutaneous sarcomas, mammary carcinomas and medullary adrenal tumors (Gross, 1953, 1955). In 1957, Stewart and Eddy at the National Institute of Health reported that the parotid tumor virus could be propagated in tissue culture on mouse embryo cells and in other cell lines, and that the tissue-culture-grown parotid tumor virus, which they designated "polyoma virus," has an increased potency and could induce tumors not only in mice, but also in rats and hamsters.

In 1957, Charlotte Friend, at the Sloan-Kettering Institute in New York, isolated a filterable agent which could be passed serially in young, weanling mice, inducing an erythroblastosis-like syndrome characterized by considerable enlargement of spleen and liver, and a rapidly progressing anemia.

Eddy and her coworkers at the National Institute of Health (1961, 1962) and, at about the same time, Girardi and his colleagues (1962) at the Merck Institute in West Point, Pa., observed that Simian Virus 40, a latent virus present in normal rhesus monkey kidney cells, can induce progressively growing sarcomas following inoculation into newborn hamsters.

In 1962, Trentin and his coworkers at Baylor University in Houston reported that human adenovirus type 12 induced sarcomas following inoculation into newborn hamsters. Several other types of human adenoviruses were later also found to have oncogenic potential.

Recently, cell-free transmission of mast-cell leukemia (mastocytoma) in dogs (Lombard *et al.*, 1963. Rickard and Post, 1968), and lymphosarcoma in cats (Jarrett *et al.*, 1964. Rickard *et al.*, 1968) have also been reported.

In 1966, Finkel and her coworkers isolated from a spontaneous mouse bone sarcoma a filterable virus which reproduced osteosarcomas following inoculation into newborn mice.

TABLE 1. SOME OF THE MORE IMPORTANT ONCOGENIC VIRUSES

1908	Chicken Leukemia	Ellermann & Bang
1911	Chicken Sarcoma	Rous
1932	Rabbit Fibroma	Shope
1933	Rabbit Papilloma	Shope
1934	Frog Kidney Carcinoma	Lucké
1936	Mouse Mammary Carcinoma	Bittner
1951	Mouse Leukemia	Gross
1953–1957	Mouse Parotid Tumor (i.e. Polyoma) Virus	Gross, Stewart & Eddy
1960–1962	Vacuolating Simian Virus 40	Sweet & Hilleman, Eddy *et al.*, Girardi *et al.*
1962	Human Adenovirus Type 12	Trentin *et al.*
1964	Cat Leukemia	Jarrett *et al.*
1966	Mouse Osteosarcoma	Finkel *et al.*

This is a very incomplete list. No reference is made here to the transmission by filtrates of human warts and papillomas, and of oral papillomas in dogs or rabbits, of cutaneous papillomas in horses and cattle, etc.

It is obvious that the list of tumors transmissible by filtrates has been growing at an accelerated pace. At the present time practically all fowl tumors, including the various forms of chicken leukosis complex, are transmissible by filtrates. With some reservations, a similar statement could be made in reference to mouse and rat tumors. It can already be stated that, with only some exceptions, most of the mouse and rat tumors, including various forms of leukemias and lymphomas, can be transmitted by filtrates.

Thus, most of the tumors and leukemias in chickens, mice, and rats are now known to be caused by transmissible viruses, even though it is not yet quite clear how some of these oncogenic viruses are naturally transmitted under normal life conditions in these animals.

Host Spectrum of Some of the Oncogenic Viruses

Some 20 years ago the general opinion was prevalent that oncogenic viruses have a rather narrow host spectrum, and that they may be pathogenic either for a single species, or at best for a few related species or families of hosts. However, a gradual change in this opinion has developed, particularly during the preceding decade. On the basis of accumulated experimental data it now appears that some oncogenic viruses may have a rather broad pathogenic potential. Here are a few examples:

The Rous sarcoma virus was found to be pathogenic not only for chickens, ducks, pigeons, turkeys, and pheasants, but also for mice, rats, hamsters, *Mastomys*,* and to some extent also for rabbits and monkeys.

The parotid tumor, i.e. polyoma virus, was found to be pathogenic not only for mice, but also for rats, hamsters, and *Mastomys*.

Human adenovirus type 12 was found to be pathogenic for hamsters, mice, rats, and *Mastomys*.

The bovine cutaneous papilloma virus was found to be pathogenic for cattle, horses, hamsters, and mice.

Accordingly, it is now quite apparent that oncogenic viruses are not limited in their pathogenic potential to a single species, genus, family, or even class of animals; at least some of these viruses have a relatively broad host range.

REFERENCES

Bashford, E. F., and Murray, J. A., The significance of the zoological distribution, the nature of the mitoses, and the transmissibility of cancer. *Brit. Med. J.*, **1**: 269–271, 1904.

Bashford, E. F., Murray, J. A., and Cramer, W., The growth of cancer under natural and experimental conditions. *Scientific Report, Imperial Cancer Research Fund.* Part II. pp. 1–96. Taylor & Francis, London, 1905.

Bashford, E. F., Murray, J. A., and Cramer, W., Einige Ergebnisse der experimentellen Krebsforschung. *Berliner klin. Wochenschr.*, **42**: (No. 46) 1433–1435, 1905.

Beijerinck, M. W., Ueber ein Contagium vivum fluidum als Ursache der Fleckenkrankheit der Tabaksblätter. *Verhandl. Koninkl. Akad. Wetenschappen te Amsterdam*, **6**: 3–22, 1898.

Beijerinck, M. W., Ueber ein Contagium vivum fluidum als Ursache der Fleckenkrankheit der Tabaksblätter. *Centralbl. f. Bakt.*, Abt. II, **5**: 27–33, 1899.

Beijerinck, M. W., Bemerkung zu dem Aufsatz von Herrn Iwanowski über die Mosaikkrankheit der Tabakspflanze. *Centralbl. f. Bakt.*, Abt. II, **5**: 310–311, 1899.

* *Rattus* (*Mastomys*) *natalensis*, an African rodent intermediate in size between the rat and the mouse.

BITTNER, J. J., Some possible effects of nursing on the mammary gland tumor incidence in mice. *Science*, **84**: 162, 1936.

BORREL, A., Épithelioses infectieuses et épitheliomas. *Ann. Inst. Pasteur*, **17**: 81–122, 1903.

BURMESTER, B. R., PRICKETT, C. O., and BELDING, T. C., A filtrable agent producing lymphoid tumors and osteopetrosis in chickens. *Cancer Research*, **6**: 189–196, 1946.

BURNET, F. M., *Principles of Animal Virology*, p. 486. Academic Press, New York, 1955.

BURNET, F. M., and STANLEY, W. M., *The Viruses*: Vol. 1, *General Virology*, p. 609. Vol. 2, *Plant and Bacterial Viruses*, p. 408. Vol. 3, *Animal Viruses*, p. 428. Academic Press, New York, 1959.

CLUNET, J., Recherches expérimentales sur les tumeurs malignes. p. 336. Thèse de Paris. G. Steinhal, 1910.

EDDY, B. E., BORMAN, G. S., BERKELEY, W. H., and YOUNG, R. D., Tumors induced in hamsters by injection of rhesus monkey kidney cell extracts. *Proc. Soc. Exp. Biol. & Med.*, **107**: 191–197, 1961.

EDDY, B. E., BORMAN, G. S., GRUBBS, G. E., and YOUNG, R. D., Identification of the oncogenic substance in rhesus monkey kidney cell cultures as Simian Virus 40. *Virology*, **17**: 65–75, 1962.

EDDY, B. E., STEWART, S. E., YOUNG, R., and MIDER, G. B., Neoplasms in hamsters induced by mouse tumor agent passed in tissue culture. *J. Nat. Cancer Inst.*, **20**: 747–761, 1958.

EDDY, B. E., STEWART, S. E., STANTON, M. F., and MARCOTTE, J. M., Induction of tumors in rats by tissue-culture preparations of SE polyoma virus. *J. Nat. Cancer Inst.*, **22**: 161–171, 1959.

EHRLICH, P., Experimentelle Studien an Mäusetumoren. *Zeitschr. f. Krebsforsch.*, **5**: 59–81, 1907.

EHRLICH, P., and APOLANT, H., Beobachtungen über maligne Mäusetumoren. *Berliner klin. Wochenschr.*, **62**: 871–874, 1905.

v. EISELSBERG, A., Ueber einen Fall von erfolgreicher Transplantation eines Fibrosarkoms bei Ratten. *Wiener klin. Wochenschr.*, **3**: 927–928, 1890.

ELLERMANN, V., and BANG, O., Experimentelle Leukämie bei Hühnern. *Centralbl. f. Bakt.*, Abt. I, (Orig.), **46**: 595–609, 1908.

FINKEL, M. P., BISKIS, B. O., and JINKINS, P. B., Virus induction of osteosarcomas in mice. *Science*, **151**: 698–700, 1966.

FIRKET, C., De la réussite de greffes sarcomateuses en série.—Note préliminaire. *Bull. de l'Acad. Royale de Med. de Belgique*, (IV series), **6**: 1147–1148, 1892.

FRIEND, C., Cell-free transmission in adult Swiss mice of a disease having the character of a leukemia. *J. Exp. Med.*, **105**: 307–318, 1957.

FURTH, J., Lymphomatosis, myelomatosis, and endothelioma of chickens caused by a filterable agent. I. Transmission experiments. *J. Exp. Med.*, **58**: 253–275, 1933.

GIRARDI, A. J., SWEET, B. H., SLOTNICK, V. B., and HILLEMAN, M. R., Development of tumors in hamsters inoculated in the neonatal period with vacuolating virus, SV 40. *Proc. Soc. Exp. Biol. & Med.*, **109**: 649–660, 1962.

GRAFFI, A., BIELKA, H., and FEY, F., Leukämieerzeugung durch ein filtrierbares Agens aus malignen Tumoren. *Acta Haemat.*, **15**: 145–174, 1956.

GREENE, H. S. N., Heterologous transplantation of human and other mammalian tumors. *Science*, **88**: 357–358, 1938.

GREENE, H. S. N., Heterologous transplantation of mammalian tumors. I. The transfer of rabbit tumors to alien species. II. The transfer of human tumors to alien species. *J. Exp. Med.*, **73**: 461–486, 1941.

GREENE, H. S. N., Heterologous transplantation of a human fibrosarcoma. *Cancer Research*, **2**: 649–654, 1942.

GREENE, H. S. N., and LUND, P. K., The heterologous transplantation of human cancers. *Cancer Research*, **4**: 352–363, 1944.

GROSS, L., "Spontaneous" leukemia developing in C3H mice following inoculation, in infancy, with Ak-leukemic extracts, or Ak-embryos. *Proc. Soc. Exp. Biol. & Med.*, **78**: 27–32, 1951.

GROSS, L., A filterable agent, recovered from Ak-leukemic extracts, causing salivary gland carcinomas in C3H mice. *Proc. Soc. Exp. Biol. & Med.*, **83**: 414–421, 1953.

GROSS, L., Induction of parotid carcinomas and/or subcutaneous sarcomas in C3H mice with normal C3H organ extracts. *Proc. Soc. Exp. Biol. & Med.*, **88**: 362–368, 1955.

HABEL, K., The nature of viruses and viral diseases. *Med. Clin. N. America*, **43**: 1275–1290, 1959.

HANAU, A., Erfolgreiche experimentelle Übertragung von Carcinom. *Fortschr. d. Med.*, **7**: 321–339, 1889.

IWANOWSKI, D., Über die Mosaikkrankheit der Tabakspflanze. *Bull. Acad. Imp. Sci., St. Petersbourg*, n.s. **3** (35): 67–70, 1894.

IWANOWSKI, D., Über die Mosaikkrankheit der Tabakspflanze. *Centralbl. f. Bakt.*, Abt. II, **5**: 250–254, 1899.

JARRETT, W. F. H., MARTIN, W. B., CRIGHTON, G. W., DALTON, R. G., and STEWART, M. F., Leukemia in the cat. Transmission experiments with leukemia (lymphosarcoma). *Nature*, **202**: 566–567, 1964.

JENSEN, C. O., Experimentelle Untersuchungen über Krebs bei Mäusen. *Centralbl. f. Bakt.*, Abt. I, (Orig.), **34**: 28–34, 1903, and **34**: 122–143, 1903.

JUNGEBLUT, C. W., and KODZA, H., Studies of leukemia L_2C in guinea pigs. *Arch. Ges. Virusforsch.*, **12**: 537–551, 1962.

LÉPINE, P., *Aspects de la reproduction des virus dans ses rapports avec les structures cellulaires*. Chapter IX, pp. 333–380 in: Problèmes d'organisation et de fonctions chez les bactéries et les virus. Masson & Cie, Paris, 1958.

LOEB, L., On transplantation of tumors. *J. Med. Research*, **1**: 28–38, 1901.

LOEB, L., Further investigations in transplantation of tumors. *J. Med. Research*, **3**: 44–73, 1902.

LOEFFLER, (F.), and FROSCH, (P.)*, Berichte der Kommission zur Erforschung der Maul und Klauenseuche bei dem Institut für Infektionskrankheiten in Berlin. *Centralbl. f. Bakt.*, Abt. I., **23**: 371–391, 1898.

LOMBARD, L. S., MOLONEY, J. B., and RICKARD, C. G., Transmissible canine mastocytoma. *Ann. N.Y. Acad. Sci.*, **108**: 1086–1105, 1963.

LUCKÉ, B., Carcinoma in the leopard frog: Its probable causation by a virus. *J. Exp. Med.*, **68**: 457–468, 1938.

MORAU, H., Inoculation en série d'une tumeur épitheliale de la souris blanche. *Compt. Rend. Soc. Biol.*, **43**: 289–290, 1891.

MORAU, H., Note complémentaire sur les inoculations en série d'un épithelioma cylindrique spontané de la souris blanche. *Compt. Rend. Soc. Biol.*, **43**: 721–722, 1891.

MOSES, A., O virus do mixoma does coelhos. Untersuchungen ueber das Virus myxomatosum der Kaninchen. *Mem. Inst. Oswaldo Cruz*, **3**: 46–53, 1911.

NOWINSKY, M., Zur Frage über die Impfung der krebsigen Geschwülste. *Centralbl. f. med. Wissensch.*, **14**: 790–791, 1876.

OBERLING, C., *Le Cancer*. 7th Edition, p. 381. Gallimard, Paris, 1954.

* No first name initials in the original paper.

PASTEUR, CHAMBERLAND, and ROUX*, Nouvelle communication sur la rage. *Compt. Rend. Acad. Sci. (Paris)*, **98**: 457–463, 1884.

RICKARD, C. G., and POST, J. E., Cellular and cell-free transmission of a canine mast cell leukemia. *Proc. 3rd Internat. Symp. Comp. Leuk. Res., July 11–13, 1967, Paris*, pp. 279–281, S. Karger, Basel and New York, 1968.†

RICKARD, C. G., GILLESPIE, J. H., LEE, K. M., NORONHA, F., POST, J. E., and SALVAGE, E. L., Transmission and electron microscopy of lymphocytic leukemia in the cat. *Proc. 3rd Internat. Symp. Comp. Leuk. Res., July 11–13, 1967, Paris*, pp. 282–284, S. Karger, Basel and New York, 1968.†

ROUS, P., Transmission of a malignant new growth by means of a cell-free filtrate. *J. Am. Med. Assoc.*, **56**: 198, 1911.

ROUX, E., Sur les microbes dits "invisibles". *Revue. Bull. Inst. Pasteur*, **1**: 7–12, and **1**: 49–56, 1903.

SANARELLI, G., Das myxomatogene Virus. Beitrag zum Studium der Krankheitserreger ausserhalb des Sichtbaren. *Centralbl. f. Bakt.*, Abt. I., **23**: 865–873, 1898.

SHIMKIN, M. B., M. A. Novinsky. A note on the history of transplantation of tumors. *Cancer*, **8**: 653–655, 1955.

SHOPE, R. E., A filterable virus causing tumor-like condition in rabbits and its relationship to virus myxomatosum. *J. Exp. Med.*, **56**: 803–822, 1932.

SHOPE, R. E., Infectious papillomatosis of rabbits. *J. Exp. Med.*, **58**: 607–624, 1933.

SMIRNOVA, E., La greffe hétérogène des tumeurs malignes. *Bull. de Biol. et de Méd. Expér., USSR*, **4**: 6–10, 1937.

STEWART, H. L., SNELL, K. C., DUNHAM, L. J., and SCHLYEN, S. M., Transplantable and transmissible tumors of animals. *Atlas of Tumor Pathology*, Sect. 12, Fasc. 40, p. 378, Am. Reg. Path., Armed Forces Inst. of Path., Washington, D.C., 1959.

STEWART, S. E., EDDY, B. E., GOCHENOUR, A. M., BORGESE, N. G., and GRUBBS, G. E., The induction of neoplasms with a substance released from mouse tumors by tissue culture. *Virology*, **3**: 380–400, 1957.

TOOLAN, H. W., Successful subcutaneous growth and transplantation of human tumors in X-irradiated laboratory animals. *Proc. Soc. Exp. Biol. & Med.*, **77**: 572–578, 1951.

TOOLAN, H. W., Growth of human tumors in the subcutaneous tissues of X-radiated laboratory animals: Their practical use for experimental purposes. (Abstract.) *Cancer Research*, **12**: 302, 1952.

TOOLAN, H. W., Growth of human tumors in cortisone-treated laboratory animals: The possibility of obtaining permanently transplantable human tumors. *Cancer Research*, **13**: 389–394, 1953.

TOOLAN, H. W., Conditioning of the host. *J. Nat. Cancer Inst.*, **14**: 745–765, 1953.

TRENTIN, J. J., YABE, Y., and TAYLOR, G., Tumor induction in hamsters by human adenovirus. (Abstract.) *Proc. Am. Assoc. Cancer Research*, **3**: 369, 1962.

VELICH, A., Beitrag zur Frage nach der Uebertragbarkeit des Sarcoms. *Wien. med. Blätter*, **21**: 711–712, and **21**: 729–731, 1898.

WEHR, (W.)*, Demonstration der durch Impfung von Hund auf Hund erzeugten Carcinomknötchen. *Centralbl. f. Chirurgie*, **15** (Suppl. to No. 24): 8–9, 1888.

WOGLOM, W. H., *Studies in Cancer and Allied Subjects: The Study of Experimental Cancer, A review*, Vol. I, Columbia University Press, N.Y., p. 288, 1913.

WOGLOM, W. H., Immunity to transplantable tumours. *Cancer Rev.*, **4**: 129–214, 1929.

* No first name initials in the original paper.

† Bibliotheca Haematologica No. 30.

CHAPTER 2

Rabbit Myxomatosis and Shope Rabbit Fibroma

RABBIT MYXOMATOSIS

In 1895 the Government of Uruguay invited Professor Giuseppe Sanarelli, Director of the Hygiene Institute of the University of Siena, to set up a Hygiene Institute in Montevideo. While organizing the new Institute, Sanarelli acquired some domestic European rabbits for the routine production of immune sera.

The Unexpected Outbreak of a Devastating Disease Among Domestic Rabbits. In 1896 a mysterious, highly contagious, and rapidly fatal disease occurred in these rabbits. This devastating disease, quite unlike anything that Sanarelli or anyone else had previously seen in Europe, was characterized by inflammation and swelling of the skin around the eyes, with accompanying blepharo-conjunctivitis, and the development of numerous mucinous tumor nodules in the skin in the neighborhood of nose, mouth, ears and genital organs. On sections, the tumors revealed a gelatinous consistency. Under the microscope, they resembled certain myxomatous tumors found in man. The rabbits died within one to two weeks after the development of first symptoms of disease. The disease spread rapidly from one animal to another, apparently by contact, and could also be transmitted by inoculation of a drop of an extract prepared from secretions of the eyes, from tumors, blood, or various organs of diseased animals. Many species of animals were inoculated in the initial study, including man; the domestic rabbit, however, was the only host susceptible to the induction of the generalized, uniformly fatal disease.

Sanarelli recognized the viral nature of rabbit myxomatosis and suspected that the causative agent was too small to be seen under the microscope. He designated it "the myxomatogenous virus." Sanarelli wrote an account of his investigations (1898) in which he named the disease "infectious myxomatosis of rabbits." The actual filtration experiments, however, which demonstrated that the causative agent could pass through filters impervious to ordinary bacteria, were carried out only in 1911 by Moses, and later on also by Hobbs in 1928, and others.

Outbreaks of this devastating disease among domestic European rabbits occurred sporadically from time to time in several places in Brazil, and also in Argentina. However, nearly half a century passed before the explanation of "spontaneous" outbreaks of myxomatosis in various parts of South America was provided by H. Aragão (1942, 1943).

The Brazilian Tropical Forest Rabbit: A Natural Carrier of the Virus of Myxomatosis. It was obvious that the virus of myxomatosis could not have been carried in domestic rabbits, since the disease induced in that species was uniformly fatal. It was also known from preliminary experiments that the disease had a narrow host range apparently limited to the family of rabbits (*Leporidae*). Aragão suspecting a local virus-carrier examined extensively the wild tropical forest rabbit (*Sylvilagus brasiliensis*), called also *tapeti* (a transcription of the Tupi Indian name). The susceptibility of these animals had been tested previously by Moses (1911) who reported that they were more resistant and only rarely became infected. However, Aragão found that 40 per cent of wild "*Sylvilagus brasiliensis*" could be easily infected with the myxoma virus. Furthermore, a wild tropical forest rabbit was caught in the State of Rio with an ocular lesion from which myxomatosis could be transmitted to domestic rabbits. This observation established beyond doubt that the tropical forest rabbit is a natural reservoir of the virus of myxomatosis.

It became apparent, therefore, that the virus of myxomatosis is harbored as a chronic, indigenous infection by the native, wild tropical forest rabbit (*Sylvilagus brasiliensis*) which is common in certain parts of South America, particularly in certain areas of Brazil and Uruguay. In these wild animals, the virus causes only a harmless disease in the form of fibromatous tumors developing at the site of infection. These tumors serve as virus reservoirs for mosquitoes and other arthropod vectors which subsequently transfer the virus mechanically to other rabbits. The European or domestic rabbit (*Oryctolagus cuniculus*), however, is highly susceptible, and when brought into contact with the virus under natural life conditions, or when inoculated in the laboratory, develops a rapidly fatal disease.

Outbreaks of Myxomatosis Among Domestic Rabbits in California. Myxomatosis was unknown in North America, except in the laboratory, until 1930 when the disease was observed to occur in domestic European rabbits in San Diego (Kessel *et al.*, 1931). This outbreak was thought to have originated in a shipment of diseased domestic rabbits from Baja California, Mexico, to San Diego. Subsequent outbreaks of local epizootics have been recorded. The origin of these apparently "spontaneous" outbreaks of rapidly spreading and fatal disease among domestic rabbits was obscure until rather recently when the investigations by Marshall and Regnery (1960, 1963) revealed that the local wild brush rabbit (*Sylvilagus bachmani*) is a reservoir host of the virus of myxomatosis. Several brush rabbits trapped near the outbreak area of myxomatosis in Palo Alto, California, were found to have fibromatous tumors which contained the myxoma virus. The virus isolated from brush rabbits in California produced fatal disease in domestic rabbits, and again reproduced small fibromatous lesions when inoculated back into its native Californian host, the brush rabbit (*Sylvilagus bachmani*). The skin lesions of *Sylvilagus bachmani* were usually infectious in mosquitoes for about 30 days, but in some instances they remained infectious for several months. The wild brush rabbit has a fairly extensive range on the West Coast of the United States.

The Californian strain of the myxoma virus is slightly different from the South American strain in its antigenic characteristics and in certain other properties, such as type of pocks induced when grown on the chorioallantoic membrane, as well as in severity and symptoms of disease induced in domestic rabbits.

The Leporidae Family: Hares, Domestic Rabbits, Cottontails, Tropical Forest and Brush Rabbits

In order to understand the pattern of natural transmission of the virus of myxomatosis and its ability to induce either generalized myxomatosis or other related forms of disease, such as localized fibromas, it is necessary to have basic information concerning the different genera and species of rabbits. These different species vary considerably in their susceptibility to infection with this virus.

The natural hosts of the myxoma virus are species of the New World genus *Sylvilagus*, belonging to the family *Leporidae*.

The genus *Lepus* comprises the hares and jackrabbits. They are country animals, quite resistant to the myxomatosis virus.

The genus *Oryctolagus cuniculus* is the European domesticated rabbit, highly susceptible to the virus of myxomatosis and developing, upon infection, a rapidly fatal disease.

The American genus *Sylvilagus*, which has a close resemblance to the European rabbit, comprises three species:

Sylvilagus floridanus, commonly called the Eastern cottontail rabbit and prevalent in North America.

Sylvilagus brasiliensis, commonly called tropical forest rabbit, or *tapeti*, and prevalent in South America, particularly in Brazil.

Sylvilagus bachmani, commonly called the brush rabbit, prevalent in the western part of North America from Oregon in the north, to Mexico including the State of California.

There exist many other species and genera of the family of *Leporidae*; however, we have mentioned among the *Leporidae* only those that are known to play a dominant role as natural hosts of the virus of myxomatosis, or as animals susceptible to the pathogenic potency of this virus.

Properties of the Virus of Myxomatosis

The virus of myxomatosis and the Shope fibroma virus are so similar in their properties that at least some of their characteristics will be discussed together here and also on subsequent pages dealing with the description of the Shope rabbit fibroma.

Myxomatosis is caused by a rather large virus which belongs to the poxvirus group. The virus is ovoid, approximately 230×280 mμ in diameter. On electron microscopic examination it is found in the cytoplasm of infected cells. The myxomatosis virus belongs to the same group as the viruses of vaccinia, variola (smallpox), ectromelia (mouse pox), cow pox, fowlpox, and molluscum contagiosum. The Shope rabbit fibroma and the squirrel fibroma virus, which will be discussed in the next part of this chapter, also belong to this group.

The myxoma and the fibroma viruses are inactivated following exposure *in vitro* to ethyl ether (Andrewes and Horstmann, 1949. Kilham *et al.*, 1958). The myxoma virus and the virus of Shope fibroma are sensitive to heat and can be readily inactivated by heating to 50°C for 30 minutes (Hobbs, 1928), to 55°C for 10 to 15 minutes (Hyde, 1936), and to 60°C for only a few minutes (Bronson and Parker, 1943).

Neither the myxoma nor the fibroma virus is capable of agglutinating red blood cells *in vitro* (Fenner, 1953).

Electron Microscopic Studies. Although some preliminary electron microscopic studies of the myxoma virus and related poxviruses have been reported, the information thus far available on the morphology of the myxomatosis virus, its formation, and location in different cells, is still incomplete and requires further studies.

The early electron micrographs of shadowed myxoma and vaccinia virus particles (Farrant and Fenner, 1953) showed that they were indistinguishable in size and morphology, a conclusion consistent with results of more recent electron microscopic studies of specimens prepared by the negative staining technique with phosphotungstic acid (Nagington and Horne, 1962. Chapple and Westwood, 1963. Padgett *et al.*, 1964). In an electron microscopic study of shadowed preparations, myxoma virus particles were found morphologically indistinguishable from the rabbit fibroma virus (Lloyd and Kahler, 1955).

The results of electron microscopic studies of the myxomatosis virus thus far performed, incomplete as they are at the moment, suggest, nevertheless, that this is a rather large, ovoid or brick-shaped virus, approximately 220 to 280 mμ in diameter. This virus appears to be morphologically indistinguishable from the vaccinia virus, or from the virus of Shope rabbit fibroma (Bernhard, 1958. Chapple and Westwood, 1963. Padgett *et al.*, 1964. Fenner, 1965. Woodroofe and Fenner, 1965. Takehara and Schwerdt, 1967. Scherrer, 1968).

Propagation of the Myxoma and Fibroma Viruses in Tissue Culture. Propagation of the myxoma and fibroma viruses in tissue culture had been reported in the early years by Benjamin and Rivers (1931) and Plotz

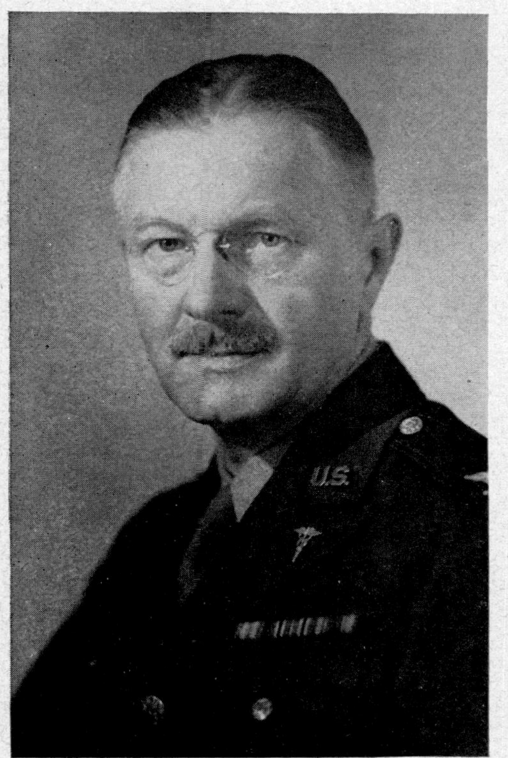

Baldwin Lucké

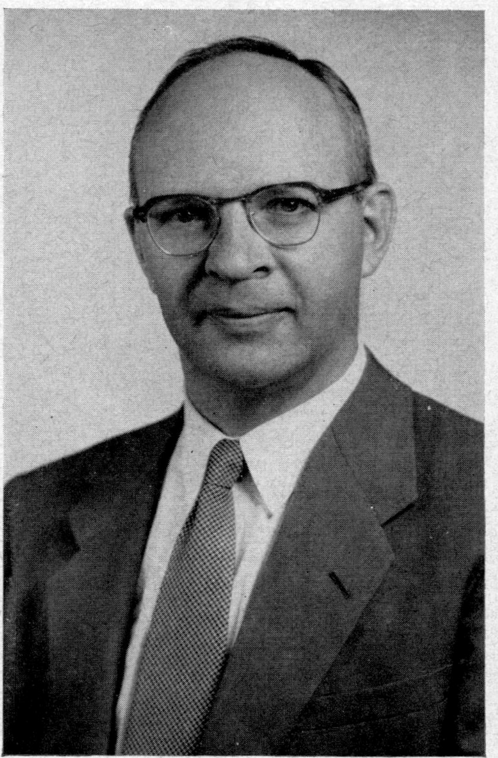

Carl Olson

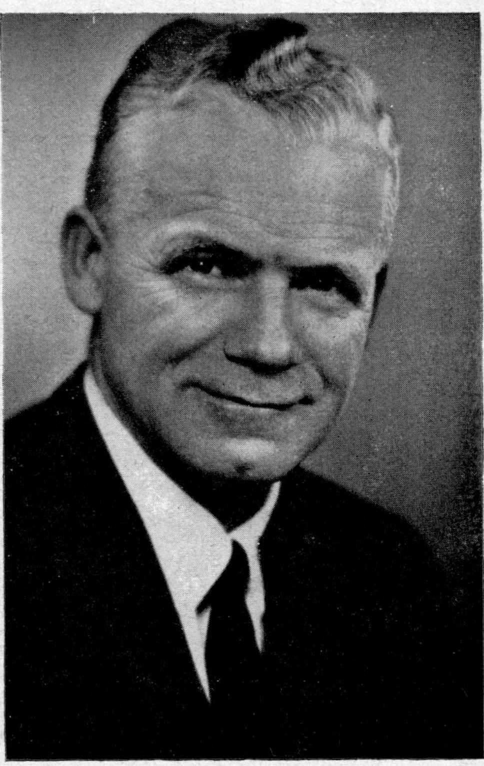

Jerome T. Syverton

FIG. 1

(1932). More recently it was found that myxoma virus multiplied in both rabbit kidney epithelial cells, and also in heart fibroblasts (Chaproniere, 1956). In rabbit kidney cells the virus induces eosinophilic cytoplasmic inclusions, and vacuolation of the nucleus. In the rabbit heart fibroblasts it induces large stellate cells with basophilic granules in the nucleus, and little inclusion material in the cytoplasm.

More recently methods of plaque induction by myxoma or fibroma viruses have been reported in primary rabbit kidney cells (Schwerdt and Schwerdt, 1962. Verna and Eylar, 1962. Moore and Walker, 1962. Woodroofe and Fenner, 1965). Plaque counts offer a sensitive and accurate method of assay of both myxoma and fibroma viruses especially in rabbit kidney cell monolayers.

Propagation of the Myxoma and Fibroma Viruses in Developing Chick Embryo. The myxoma virus could be propagated serially on the chorioallantoic membrane of developing chicken embryos (Lush, 1937. Haagen and Du Dscheng-Hsing, 1938. Hoffstadt and Pilcher, 1938. Fenner and McIntyre, 1956). As a result of virus infection small pocks developed on the surface of the chorioallantoic membrane. Pock counting is a useful method of assay, although not as reproducible as plaque counting. Pock size can be used to characterize certain strains of myxoma virus.

Host Range. The pathogenic potency of the myxoma virus appears to be limited to the family of rabbits. It produces a devastating, generalized, and almost consistently fatal disease in domestic European rabbits (*Oryctolagus cuniculus*). In that species the spread of the virus through the body follows the same general pattern as other generalized poxvirus infections. The spread is accompanied by the formation of multiple swellings on the skin, especially at the muco-cutaneous junctions, such as eyelids, nose, anogenital region, and to a lesser extent on the legs and on the general body. The swellings are due largely to the accumulation of mucinous material together with cellular proliferation.

In its natural host, *Sylvilagus brasiliensis*, the myxomatosis virus produces only a localized lesion. There are exceptions, since in very young animals it can produce also a generalized disease; however, as a rule, in adult animals only a localized lesion develops at the site of infection in the form of a fibromatous tumor; the lesion contains the virus and may serve as a source of virus infection for mosquito vectors.

The European hare is as a rule resistant, although occasionally it may develop generalized myxomatosis following inoculation of a large dose of virus.

The North American *Sylvilagus floridanus* (Eastern cottontail) is resistant, and following inoculation of the virus reacts only by the development of a transient local lesion.

The Californian *Sylvilagus bachmani* is also relatively resistant and is a natural carrier of a strain of myxoma virus. It develops only a local fibromatous lesion following infection with the virus; however, the same virus will produce a fatal general myxomatosis when transmitted to domestic rabbits.

Both the South American and Californian strains of myxoma virus cause in their natural hosts, *Sylvilagus brasiliensis* and *Sylvilagus bachmani*, respectively, local lesions very similar to those produced by the Shope fibroma virus in the cottontail rabbits (*Sylvilagus floridanus*). However, whereas the myxoma virus causes a highly lethal generalized infection when transferred from native carrier hosts to domestic rabbit *Oryctolagus cuniculus*, the Shope fibroma virus produces in most instances only a benign and localized tumor not only in the cottontail, but in the domestic rabbit also.

Under certain limited experimental conditions, such as following inoculation into newborn domestic rabbits, the Shope fibroma virus can also produce a generalized disease; generalization of fibroma in domestic rabbits can also be induced in rabbits following treatment with cortisone or tar. This is discussed in more detail in the second part of this chapter.

Natural Transmission of Myxomatosis. The Importance of the Arthropod Vector. We have already indicated that in their natural carriers, *Sylvilagus brasiliensis* and *Sylvilagus bachmani*, the myxomatosis virus produces a local fibromatous lesion which may last several weeks or a few months. In mature, susceptible animals the lesions appear 7 to 8 days after infection, reach their maximum size 2 weeks later, and may persist from 3 to 5 months before crusting and regressing. These lesions contain live virus in considerable quantities. Mosquitoes or fleas which feed on such lesions transmit the virus to other rabbits. In the arthropod vector the virus is invariably associated with the head and mouth parts, and mechanical transmission of virus occurs. Whether the virus multiplies in its insect-vector is still open to question.

It is of interest that transmission by mosquitoes of the virus of fowlpox, which is related to the myxoma virus, had been known since the studies of Kligler, Muckenfuss and Rivers (1929) in the United States.

The importance of insect transmission of myxomatosis was first appreciated by Aragão who showed as early as 1920 that the disease could be transmitted in domestic rabbits by cat fleas. Torres (1936) first showed that mosquitoes could act as vectors. The natural transmission of the virus of rabbit myxomatosis by mosquitoes (*Aedes scapularis* and *Aedes aegypti*) was demonstrated in Brazil by Aragão (1943). The mechanism of virus transmission by the *Aedes aegypti* and other arthropod vectors was later studied by Fenner and his associates (1952) in Australia. Among other arthropod vectors in Australia, the mosquito *Anopheles annulipes* developed the habit of harboring in rabbit burrows and was thus in a position to become a major intermediary in the spread of myxomatosis. By biting through the skin lesions, which in rabbits suffering from myxomatosis are usually rich in the virus, the biting parts of the mosquitoes are contaminated and small amounts of virus can thus be transmitted mechanically to any rabbits subsequently bitten. This can be imitated by sticking a point of a needle into a myxomatous lesion and testing its infectivity by pricking the skin of a normal rabbit. Actually, myxoma can thus be readily transmitted. The mosquitoes which spread myxomatosis could be compared, therefore, to "flying pins," as Fenner suggested. Others feel, however, that transmission of the virus of myxomatosis through mosquitoes is not entirely mechanical. The mosquitoes can retain the virus for prolonged periods of time, at least 25 days after feeding on skin lesions of domestic rabbits infected with myxomatosis.

Transmission of the Virus of Myxomatosis is not Limited to One or a Few Particular Mosquito Species or Varieties. A large number of arthropods has been tested in the laboratory. Every mosquito species tested was found to be capable of transmitting myxomatosis in domestic rabbits, as have been certain flies, fleas, ticks, mites, and lice. The lack of specificity and the fact that interrupted feeding is effective, as well as absence of an incubation period for the mosquito and other insect vectors, indicate that transmission is mechanical, at least in the early stages; however, the possibility of the virus multiplying in the mosquito vectors has not yet been entirely excluded. Such an assumption has been strengthened by the very prolonged infectivity of some mosquitoes, present even after hibernation, and the finding that positive results are often obtained during the third, fourth, and fifth week after the infective feeding.

Immunity to Myxomatosis Following Infection with Shope Fibroma Virus

Infection of domestic rabbits with fibroma virus rapidly induces active immunity to myxomatosis; however, complete resistance is of short duration, lasting only several weeks, or at best a few months. Challenge infection after several months results in the development of local lesions, or of a generalized and fatal disease.

Vaccine Against Myxomatosis. A vaccine consisting of the fibroma virus was used on a very large scale some years ago and is still used on a more moderate scale, primarily to protect breeding animals. The vaccine has been quite effective protecting some 70 per cent of the vaccinated animals from mortality due to myxomatosis

Attenuated strains of myxomatosis virus, which were found in naturally infected rabbits, have been also used as a vaccine.

The European Domestic Rabbit: A Source of Food, and Also of Destruction to Native Vegetation

Rabbits must have been hunted and trapped by man as a source of food since early time. The European domesticated rabbits were brought to North and South America, and later to New Zealand, Australia, and to many oceanic islands. They have multiplied rapidly and spread all over the continents.

The average doe is ready to breed when 6 to 10 months old, occasionally earlier. The oestrus occurs at intervals of 7 days. Ovulation is induced in the rabbit normally by coitus. The gestation period is about 30 days (Myers and Poole, 1962). The majority of litters contain 3 to 7 young.

Bucks wait for the does at the mouth of the resting burrows, and mate with them immediately after they emerge following dropping of their litters. It is therefore quite usual for the doe to nurse her offspring and at the same time become pregnant again.

Under favorable conditions, with sexual activity starting in March or April and the last litters dropped at the end of November, an average doe may produce and wean some 24 offspring. Taking into consideration the mortality among the newborn, and other adverse factors, an eight-fold, or at least a five-fold population increase can be anticipated in a year. This would permit the rabbits in an area to recover from an 80 per cent mortality within 12 months (Fenner and Ratcliffe, 1965).

Within 20 years following introduction of wild rabbits into Australia (1859), they had become the country's major pest. In 1887 the Government of New South Wales offered a prize of £25,000 for the eradication of rabbits from the colony. The swarms of rabbits overran continental Australia to such an extent, and were so destructive to vegetation, that at the beginning of this century a barrier fence was built over an area of several thousand miles in an effort to protect regions that were still free from an invasion by these fast multiplying animals. This fence built at a tremendous cost and effort was not a success, and other methods were considered in order to limit the spread of rabbits in Australia and also on other continents.

Among the methods proposed for biological control of rabbits in Australia was the introduction of the virus of myxomatosis. Such a project was feasible because the Australian wild rabbits are descendants of European domestic rabbits originally imported to Australia; the Australian rabbit (*Oryctolagus cuniculus*) is therefore highly susceptible to the virus of myxomatosis.

Attempts to Control the Rabbit Population in Australia by Introduction of the Virus of Myxomatosis

The first suggestion to introduce myxomatosis in Australia in order to deplete the rabbit population was made by Aragão in 1919. This suggestion was not favorably acted upon at the time. A similar suggestion was made again in 1924 by Dr. R. H. Seddon and more recently by Dr. J. Macnamara (1934) and others (reviewed by Fenner and Ratcliffe, 1965). Following a favorable report from the Institute of Animal Pathology in Cambridge (Martin, 1936), and after additional field experiments which extended over a period of several years, the Australian Commonwealth Scientific and Industrial Research Organization decided in 1949 to introduce the virus of myxomatosis in extensive field trials for the biological control of the rabbit population. After a series of trial releases of the virus in the coastal regions of Australia, and later on also in the interior parts of the continent, the myxomatosis virus was introduced by massive inoculations, and subsequent release of infected rabbits in suitable areas in Australia. Severe and widespread epizootics of this disease resulted among the wild rabbits during the summer seasons of 1951 and 1952, and very large numbers of rabbits perished, particularly in the south-eastern part of the continent. In other areas the results were less successful.

After the initial introduction of the virus, epidemic myxomatosis flared up in one or another trial site; at first the disease spread sometimes with dramatic speed, then gradually subsided; however, the disappearance of the disease was only apparent, since it was followed by occasional outbreaks of epizootic disease developing now and then periodically in association with local or seasonal arthropod activities. Success depended on favorable weather, which facilitated transmission of the disease by insect vectors; this was particularly possible in areas rich in flies and mosquitoes, along the rivers and marshes. Transmission did not occur readily in dry or semi-arid interior parts of the country.

Following its introduction on the Australian continent, myxomatosis gradually became established as an enzootic disease of the Australian wild rabbit, with epidemic outbreaks developing periodically in association with local and seasonal arthropod activities.

Attempts to Introduce Myxomatosis for the Biological Control of Rabbits in Europe

Following the favorable report of Martin (1936), several attempts were made to introduce the virus of myxomatosis for the biological control of wild rabbits in Europe. On the Danish island of Vejro (Schmit-Jensen, 1939) groups of about 150 rabbits were caught, marked, inoculated with the myxomatosis virus, and released. About twice as many uninoculated rabbits died as the number of released animals. This experiment was repeated in three successive years with similar results. It appeared that myxomatosis introduced in this manner did not persist for more than two or three months.

In another attempt carried out in 1938 on the Dufeke Estate in southern Sweden, 18 rabbits inoculated with the virus of myxomatosis were released. This caused an extensive spread of disease all over the large estate in which this field trial was carried out. However, the disease did not become established, and next year only one infected rabbit was seen in this area.

A similar attempt was made to establish myxomatosis on the island of Skokholm (Lockley, 1940). However, the induced disease spread only slightly and soon died out.

Successful Introduction of the Myxomatosis Virus in France. On June 14, 1952, Dr. P. F. Armand-Delille, apparently annoyed by the presence of rabbits damaging flowers and vegetation on his large estate at Maillebois (Eure-et-Loire) in France, inoculated and released on his estate two wild rabbits with myxoma virus which he obtained from his friend Professor Hauduroy of the Bacteriological Laboratory in Lausanne, Switzerland. The virus which Delille obtained originated in Brazil. Following this initial inoculation, myxomatosis spread not only on the 600-acre country estate at Maillebois, but all over Europe. Within a month of the introduction of the virus all the rabbits on Delille's estate had died, and cases of myxomatosis had been reported among wild rabbits in villages up to 30 miles distant from Maillebois. The following year violent and destructive outbreaks of myxomatosis occurred in both wild and domestic *Oryctolagus* rabbits; gradually myxomatosis spread to almost every part of France, and later also to Spain, Holland, Belgium, Germany and England. Cases of myxomatosis were subsequently also reported in Switzerland, Italy and Austria.

> The following is an excerpt from a letter written to the author on May 6, 1960, by Dr. P. Lépine of the Pasteur Institute in Paris:
>
> "The spread of the disease resulted in complete eradication of rabbits in wide areas of France.
>
> Practically only a few zones of the West (Bretagne) and in the South (Provence) remained free from myxomatosis. The central regions of France (Île-de-France, Orléanais, Sologne), which were by tradition the hunting grounds for rabbit shooting, are now almost totally devoid of rabbits.
>
> In some places rabbits have reappeared in small numbers, but as soon as such numbers increased there was noted a reappearance of myxomatosis. Thus it seems that a certain type of balance has established itself between the presence of the virus and the rabbit population.
>
> The geographical situation of Maillebois is in Eure-et-Loire, a region roughly west of Paris. The epidemic has spread from Maillebois within six months and took more than one year to reach the borders. From France the epidemic has extended in neighboring countries: Belgium, Netherlands and England, but it seems that the results in these countries were not so devastating as they have been in France."

Both wild and domestic *Oryctolagus* were of considerable commercial importance in France as a source of food consumption and also as game animals for hunters. Before the introduction of myxomatosis, some 140 million domestic rabbits were produced and consumed annually in France, and many retired workers were dependent upon rabbit raising for their livelihood. In 1954 it was estimated that 30 to 40 per cent of the domestic rabbit population was destroyed by the spread of myxomatosis. At the same time it was estimated that up to 90 per cent of the wild rabbits in France had been killed by myxomatosis. Accordingly, the rabbit ceased to be a game animal in many parts of France, and its place has been taken by hares, partridges, and pheasants.

Myxomatosis in Britain

Following the outbreak of epizootics of myxomatosis in Australia, attempts were also made to introduce myxomatosis in Britain. When the sheep farmers in Scotland requested that the myxomatosis virus should be tried in their rabbit-infested areas, Shanks and his coworkers (1955) introduced myxomatosis by releasing groups of virus-infected laboratory rabbits on the rabbit-infested Heisker Islands of the Hebrides in Scotland in July, 1952, and again in May, 1955. Although myxomatosis caused considerable mortality in 1953 among the rabbit population on the islands, it did not become enzootic, and the following year the rabbit population was again as large as it had been before the introduction of the virus. However, in spite of this and a few other similar unsuccessful attempts to introduce myxomatosis deliberately to Britain, the virus gradually gained foothold on the island reaching England from France by unknown means in August or September, 1953. The proximity of the considerable epizootic outbreaks of myxomatosis in France in 1953 led to the inevitable spread of myxomatosis from France to England. The first case was reported near Edenbridge, Kent, in October, 1953. The virus isolated from this outbreak was found to be indistinguishable from the Lausanne strain introduced by Dr. Delille in France (Fenner and Marshall, 1957). As soon as the disease was recognized, attempts were made to contain or eradicate it, but without success. The disease spread gradually in a centrifugal manner with establishment of several hundred separate foci in different counties (Armour and Thompson, 1955). After another year myxomatosis became an enzootic disease in Britain.

The spread of myxomatosis in Britain has shown certain epidemiological differences from that which was found in France and Australia. The seasonal incidence has been much less pronounced, suggesting a different mode of transmission in England from that found in France where mosquitoes cause some epidemics. It appears that the rabbit flea (*Spilopsyllus cuniculi*) is an efficient vector of myxomatosis, and British investigators believe that it has been the most important factor transmitting myxomatosis in Britain (Andrewes *et al.*, 1959).

By the end of 1955 there were few areas of Britain unaffected by the disease, and at this time it was calculated that over 90 per cent of the wild rabbits on the island had died from myxomatosis. There were, of course, small pockets of rabbits which escaped infection and continued to breed. In the following years, 1956–1960, myxomatosis was less common and there was a slow increase in the number of rabbits; however, there was another flare-up of myxomatosis in 1961 and 1962.

Myxomatosis has remained an enzootic disease throughout England, Scotland, and Wales, and since 1958 cases have occurred in most counties each month of the year. Temporary freedom from myxomatosis has led to local increases in the number of rabbits; frequently, under such circumstances, myxomatosis has then been again introduced into the increased rabbit population usually by the deliberate (though illegal) release of infected rabbits. The overall rabbit population has remained relatively low when compared with the numbers present in 1952.

* * *

Myxomatosis is therefore a highly contagious, rapidly fatal disease in the domestic rabbit, and it can be readily understood that many students of cancer have been reluctant to incorporate this condition into the group of true neoplasms, even though microscopic appearance of myxomatous nodules seems to warrant their classification as true tumors.

It would be beyond the scope of this monograph to review in more detail the fascinating studies on the spread and control of myxomatosis, and on the properties of the virus of this disease. The interested reader is referred to the excellent monograph on "Myxomatosis" by Fenner and Ratcliffe (1965).

THE SHOPE RABBIT FIBROMA

In 1932, Richard E. Shope of the Rockefeller Institute in Princeton shot a wild cottontail rabbit near Princeton, New Jersey. Under the skin of the front and hind feet of this rabbit there were small nodules, which proved to be fibromatous tumors when examined under a microscope.

FIG. 2. THE SHOPE RABBIT FIBROMA VIRUS.

(A). Shope fibroma virus particles in the cytoplasm of rabbit kidney cells grown in tissue culture. The virus particles (arrow) are in their early phase of development. The nucleus (N) is on the right side of the electron micrograph. Magnification 30,000×. (B). A group of Shope fibroma virus particles, in a more advanced phase of development, in the cytoplasm of rabbit kidney cells grown in tissue-culture. Magnification 75,000×. Electron micrographs prepared by R. Scherrer, Institut de Recherches Scientifiques sur le Cancer, Villejuif (Seine), France.

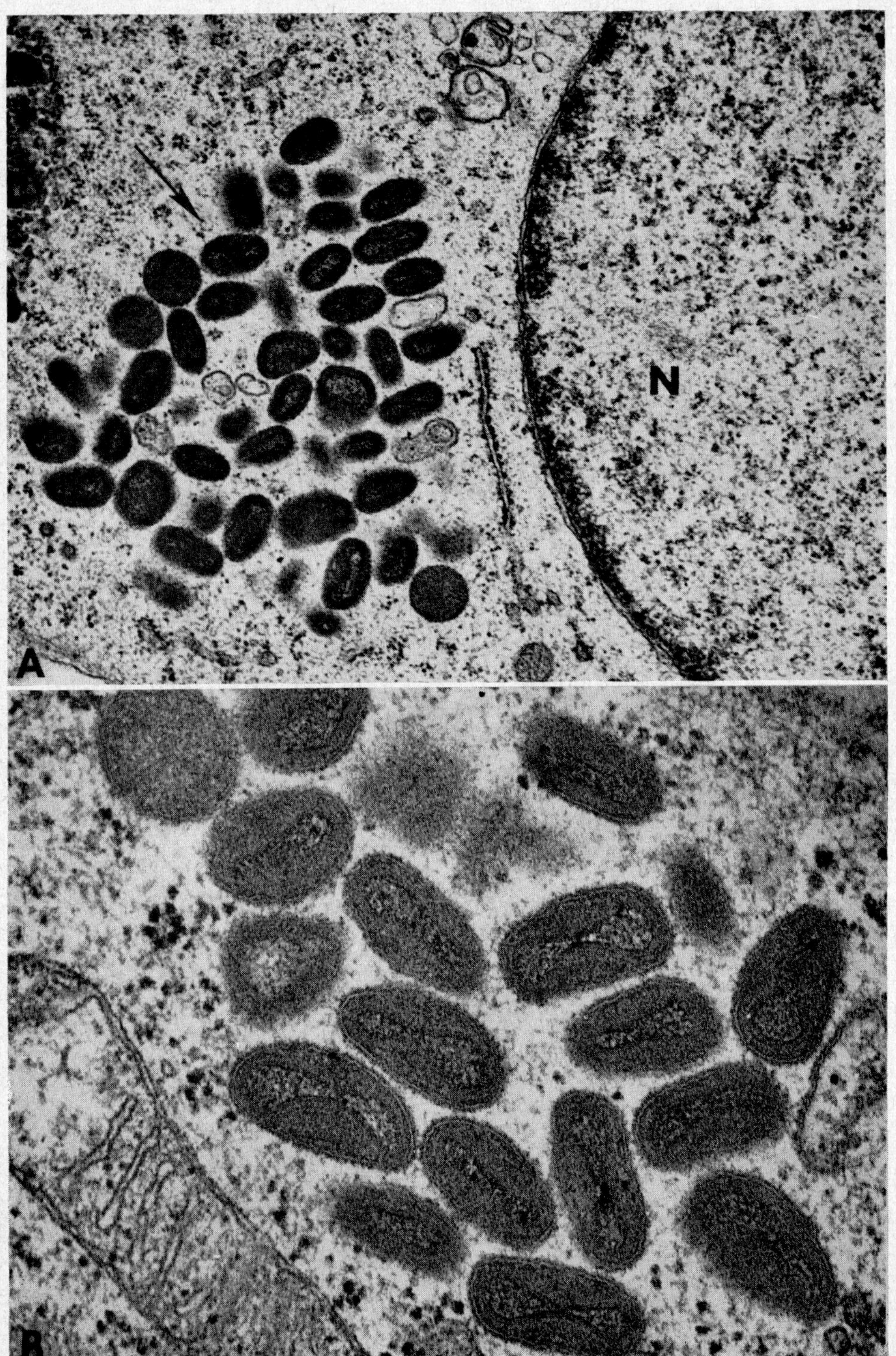

FIG. 2. THE SHOPE RABBIT FIBROMA VIRUS

The tumor could be transmitted by inoculation of filtrates to both cottontail and domestic rabbits. The inoculation of tumor filtrates was found to cause in domestic rabbits fibromatous tumors similar to those occurring naturally in many cottontail rabbits over a wide section of the United States, particularly in parts of New Jersey, in northern New York State, and in certain areas in the Middle West. In wild rabbits these tumors can usually be found on the feet. When transmitted by inoculation to either domestic or cottontail rabbits, these tumors grow fairly rapidly in the beginning; later, however, they remain stationary and eventually most of them regress.

Transmission of Rabbit Fibroma Virus by Mosquitoes

The rabbit fibroma virus, although readily transmissible by filtrates in the laboratory, is not contagious. It appears, however, that this virus, like the closely related myxomatosis agent, is transmitted in nature from host to host by insect vectors. Kilham and Woke (1953) carried out a series of experiments at the National Institute of Health, in Bethesda, Md., in which they demonstrated that the rabbit fibroma virus could be transmitted through the intermediary of fleas (which are frequently found on the cottontail rabbits) and also through *Aedes aegypti* mosquitoes. These experiments were carried out on cottontail rabbits which are the natural carriers of the fibroma virus. When either fleas or *Aedes aegypti* mosquitoes, after feeding on fibromatous tumors, were released and allowed to feed on healthy cottontail rabbits, typical fibromas, similar in appearance to those of natural occurrence, developed on the feet and legs of such animals. The mosquitoes could transmit the virus even 2 weeks after they had their blood meal on the fibromas.

Later on Kilham and Dalmat (1955) found that three species of native mosquitoes (*Anopheles quadrimaculatus*, *Culex pipiens*, and *Aedes triseriatus*) could transmit the rabbit fibroma virus among cottontail rabbits as readily as do *Aedes aegypti*.

Further studies demonstrated that the infected mosquitoes carried the virus for several weeks, and that the fibroma virus was localized in such insects entirely in head parts.

The cottontail rabbits which carried fibromas remained infective for mosquitoes for up to 10 months, suggesting that cottontails could serve as effective reservoirs of the rabbit fibroma virus in nature.

Dr. Shope also observed natural transmission of fibroma from cottontail to domestic rabbits in an area of southern New Jersey, where this disease is endemic in cottontails. Domestic rabbits were placed in cages on the ground and developed fibromas. Transmission occurred presumably through the intermediary of mosquitoes. (Personal communication to the author from Dr. R. E. Shope, 1960).

Immunological Relationship between Rabbit Myxoma and Fibroma

Myxoma and fibroma of rabbits appeared to be two entirely distinct diseases: myxoma is a disease contagious and regularly fatal for the domestic rabbit, whereas fibroma is not transmitted by direct contact and is not fatal to either the cottontail or domestic rabbits. The initial lesions, however, developing at the site of inoculation of either the myxoma or fibroma virus, have a superficial resemblance. The myxoma virus, which induces an acute and lethal disease in domestic rabbits, is much less pathogenic for the cottontail; it induces in the cottontail rabbit a transient, localized disease in which the only manifestation of infection is a fibromatous tumor developing at the site of infection and very similar in appearance to naturally occurring cottontail fibromas caused in that species by the fibroma virus.

This similarity of the initial lesions led Shope (1932) to study a possible immunological relationship between these two diseases. The surprising discovery was made that infection of rabbits with the fibroma virus rendered them refractory to myxoma. Rabbits that recovered from fibromas and were subsequently inoculated with the myxoma virus came down with a myxomatosis showing only little generalization, and, what was most remarkable, such animals almost never died from this disease. Thus, previous fibroma virus infection gave such rabbits sufficient protection against the myxoma virus to prevent a fatal outcome. The immune response in the reverse direction was very difficult to determine, because almost all domestic rabbits inoculated with myxoma develop a fatal disease. The very rare rabbit, however, that survived a primary myxoma virus infection proved to be resistant to both the myxoma and also fibroma viruses.

It was thus established that there exists a cross-immunity between the fibroma and myxoma viruses, and that these two viruses are probably closely related (Shope, 1936).

Fibroma-Myxoma Virus Transformation

Stimulated by the work of Griffith (1928) and Avery (reviewed by Avery *et al.*, 1944) on the pneumococcus transformation, and impressed by the apparent close immunological relationship between the fibroma and myxoma viruses, Berry and Dedrick (1936) attempted to transform the fibroma virus into a virus causing myxomatosis. They succeeded in a series of brilliant experiments in which they demonstrated that if the myxoma virus, which had been inactivated by heating to either 60°C or 75°C, was mixed with live fibroma virus and then administered to domestic rabbits, the inoculated animals, instead of developing fibromas, frequently developed generalized myxomatosis leading to death of the inoculated animals. Heated myxoma virus alone did not produce disease in control animals.

After many initial difficulties, these experiments were later confirmed in several other laboratories, suggesting that some component of the myxoma virus, not destroyed at 75°C, was capable of combining with the fibroma virus, converting it to the virus of myxomatosis (Hurst, 1937. Shope, 1950. Smith, 1952).

More recently, Kilham reported (1957, 1958) that transformation of the fibroma virus into the virus of myxomatosis could be accomplished in the test tube by adding heated (67°C for 40 minutes) myxoma virus to live fibroma virus grown in tissue culture on rabbit kidney, or on rabbit testes cells.

It is apparent, therefore, that the myxoma and fibroma viruses are closely related. Heating of the myxoma virus to 67°C for 40 minutes inactivates its infectivity; the virus can be "revived," however, and its full infectivity restored if the destroyed part of the virus is "replaced" by an apparently similar part furnished by the fibroma virus. Actually, what happens by mixing these two components may be less simple, involving an exchange of complicated virus components. The fact remains, however, that an inactivated myxoma virus can be reactivated and returned to its full vitality and infectivity by bringing it, under proper experimental conditions, into contact with live fibroma virus.

Some Characteristics of the Myxoma and Fibroma Viruses

Some of the properties of the fibroma and myxoma viruses have already been discussed on preceding pages of this chapter dealing with rabbit myxomatosis. To recapitulate, the viruses of myxoma and fibroma appear to be closely related. Neither of them appears to be capable of agglutinating red blood cells (Fenner, 1953). Both the myxoma and fibroma viruses are sensitive to ethyl ether, and they both produce acidophylic intracytoplasmic inclusion bodies in the epithelial cells of the infected skin lesions and in the ectodermal cells of the chorioallantoic membrane of the chicken embryo. The diameter of virus particles, which have an ovoid shape, was thought to be somewhere around 175 mμ, as determined by filtration and centrifugation experiments (Schlesinger and Andrewes, 1937). On the basis of electron microscopic examinations, however, the fibroma virus particles, which are indistinguishable from the virus of myxomatosis, appear much larger, about 230 by 280 mμ in diameter.

The myxoma and fibroma viruses also appear to be closely related to the virus of vaccinia, and to that of fowlpox and ectromelia (Fenner, 1953. Gaylord and Melnick, 1953). The latter three viruses, however, are resistant to ethyl ether, whereas myxoma and fibroma viruses are sensitive to ether (Andrewes and Horstman, 1949. Kilham *et al.*, 1958).

Electron Microscopy

On electron microscopic studies, the rabbit myxoma virus was found to be quite similar to the virus of rabbit fibroma (Bernhard *et al.*, 1954. Lloyd and Kahler, 1955. Scherrer, 1968) and also to that of the poxviruses in general (Farrant and Fenner, 1953. Gaylord and Melnick, 1953. Morgan *et al.*, 1954. Bernhard, 1958).

On ultrathin sections (Bernhard *et al.*, 1954), the fibroma virus appears as an ovoid particle about 230 mμ in diameter. The particles are usually located in the cytoplasm, in the vicinity of nucleus, in agglomerations which are visible as Feulgen-positive inclusion bodies in the light microscope (Constantin and Febvre, 1956, 1958). Some of the particles are surrounded by a single membrane; at a more advanced stage the virus particles have a double membrane. Outside of cells the particles may have a brick-shaped morphology (Scherrer, 1968).

The cytoplasmic lesions found in rabbit fibroma are very similar to those observed in vaccinia, ectromelia, and molluscum-contagiosum virus infections (Morgan *et al.*, 1954. Bernhard, 1958. Dourmashkin and Duperrat, 1958).

Generalized Fibromatosis in Rabbits Inoculated with the Fibroma Virus, Following Treatment with Tar, X-Rays, or Cortisone. Andrewes and Ahlström (1938) in England attempted to influence the pathogenic potency of the fibroma virus by treatment of domestic rabbits with tar. They observed that rabbits which had been injected intramuscularly with tar responded in an abnormal way to the subsequent inoculation with the fibroma virus. Regression of lesions produced by intradermal or subcutaneous inoculation of the virus was delayed in tarred animals; some of the subcutaneous tumors grew progressively and invasively. After intravenous inoculation of the fibroma virus into tarred rabbits, generalized fibromatosis commonly developed and was in some instances fatal. A single dose of tar given on the same day as the virus also produced the effects described; a series of inoculations was unnecessary. Benzpyrene and other carcinogenic hydrocarbons produced a similar effect to that of tar, but it was not certain how far the effect was specific for carcinogenic substances.

In a rabbit which had received 2 intramuscular tar injections 4 months apart, followed by intravenous injection of fibroma virus, the virus became localized at the tarred site and later a fibrosarcoma developed there. This tumor proved transplantable in a series through 12 rabbits. At first regression was the rule, but later many of the rabbits showed progressive growth and in some metastatic tumors developed. All attempts to demonstrate fibroma virus in the sarcoma by direct and indirect means failed. In 2 rabbits transplants of the sarcoma regressed, but showed renewed growth following intravenous inoculation of fibroma virus.

Clemmesen (1939) demonstrated that following intravenous inoculation of the fibroma virus into rabbits that had been irradiated with X-rays (300 to 700 R, total body, 24 hours prior to virus inoculation), generalized fibromatosis developed. Massive treatment with cortisone of virus-injected rabbits had a similar effect, leading to generalized fibromatosis (Harel and Constantin, 1954).

Generalized Disease Following Inoculation of the Fibroma Virus into Newborn Rabbits. Duran-Reynals inoculated the fibroma virus into newborn domestic rabbits and observed (1940, 1945) that either a generalized, fatal, inflammatory disease, or local or generalized fibromas or, finally, fatal, metastasizing sarcomas could be induced. The inoculated dose and the age of the suckling rabbits at the time of inoculation were the principal factors determining the response of the inoculated hosts.

Propagation of the Fibroma Virus in Tissue Culture

Initial attempts to grow an "inflammatory strain" of the rabbit fibroma virus on normal rabbit cells in tissue culture were carried out by Faulkner and Andrewes in 1935. Recently Kilham (1956) succeeded in propagating a fully active fibroma virus on normal rabbit cells in tissue culture. Similar results were also reported by Constantin (1956), Bauer (1956), and their associates. In Kilham's experiments (1956), the Shope fibroma virus could be propagated through at least 14 successive serial passages in tissue culture on normal cottontail (*Sylvilagus*) rabbit testes. Multiplication of virus occurred, and titers up to 10^{-4} could be obtained. Increase in virus titer was evident in each individual passage, the maximum being reached about 2 weeks after inoculation of the tissue culture cells; later on, when the tissue culture cells were degenerating, the titer gradually declined. Such degeneration of cells was also observed in non-inoculated control cultures. There was no evidence of cell-destruction resulting from infection.

Growth of virus in tissue culture cells was accompanied by the formation of acidophylic intra-cytoplasmic inclusions (Kilham, 1956. Constantin and Febvre, 1956, 1958. Constantin *et al.*, 1956) similar to those reported by Shope (1932) in the natural host of the virus, the cottontail rabbit. These cytoplasmic inclusion bodies studied also by Herzberg and Thelen (1938) closely resembled those described by Feller and his associates (1940) in their study of vaccinia virus on chick fibroblasts. This resemblance further emphasized the possible relationship of poxviruses to those of fibroma and myxoma (Fenner, 1953).

Rabbit fibroma virus was shown to cause consistent destruction in primary kidney and skin cell cultures prepared from newborn rabbits, as well as in established rabbit cell lines (Verna and Eylar, 1962). Virus adsorption and multiplication in cell monolayers resulted in formation of plaques 1 to 2 mm in diameter on the fourth or fifth day. There was a linear relation between relative virus concentration and average plaque counts. Approximately 90 per cent of the virus was adsorbed in $2\frac{1}{2}$ to 3 hours at 37°C. Virus titers determined by *in vitro* assay were comparable with titers obtained by rabbit inoculation.

More recently Hinze and Walker (1964) also reported propagation of the Shope fibroma virus on primary and serially cultured rabbit kidney cells. Characteristic changes were observed in cell morphology and growth pattern in the infected cultures. Cells showing such alterations had the ability to form tumors following inoculation into hamster cheek pouch.

The Myxoma and Fibroma Viruses and Their Pathogenic Effect on Their Natural, Wild Leporidae Carriers, and on the Domestic Rabbit

We can recognize, in geographically separated parts of the Americas, three related poxviruses which have evolved in association with three different species of *Sylvilagus*. They are Californian myxoma virus in *Sylvilagus bachmani*, South American myxoma virus in *Sylvilagus brasiliensis*, and Shope's fibroma virus in *Sylvilagus floridanus*. Each virus produces a localized benign fibroma in the host in which it has evolved and produces either slightly more severe, or, more commonly, quite trivial lesions in related species of *Sylvilagus*. In *Oryctolagus cuniculus*, the European domestic rabbit, two of these viruses cause a lethal generalized disease, whereas the virus carried by *Sylvilagus floridanus* (Shope's fibroma virus) produces a benign localized fibroma in *Oryctolagus* also.

In almost all *Leporidae* tested, both the South American and Californian types of myxoma virus and Shope's fibroma virus produce lesions which

---

FIG. 3. DEER FIBROMA VIRUS.

(A). Spontaneous deer fibroma. Section of a cell in a parakeratotic area. The nucleus contains multiple crystals of viral particles. Average size of virus particles about 34 mμ. Magnification 21,000×. This deer, about $1\frac{1}{2}$ years old, was shot in Wisconsin; it had extensive fibromas on the head, the trunk, and on upper parts of the extremities. (B). Deer fibroma virus particles (extracted from the case described above) negatively stained with potassium phosphotungstate. Average diameter of negatively stained virus particles about 53 mμ. Magnification 156,000×. Electron micrographs prepared by M. Tajima, D. E. Gordon and C. Olson, Department of Veterinary Science, College of Agriculture, University of Wisconsin, Madison. (From: *Am. J. Vet. Research*, 29: 1185, 1968.)

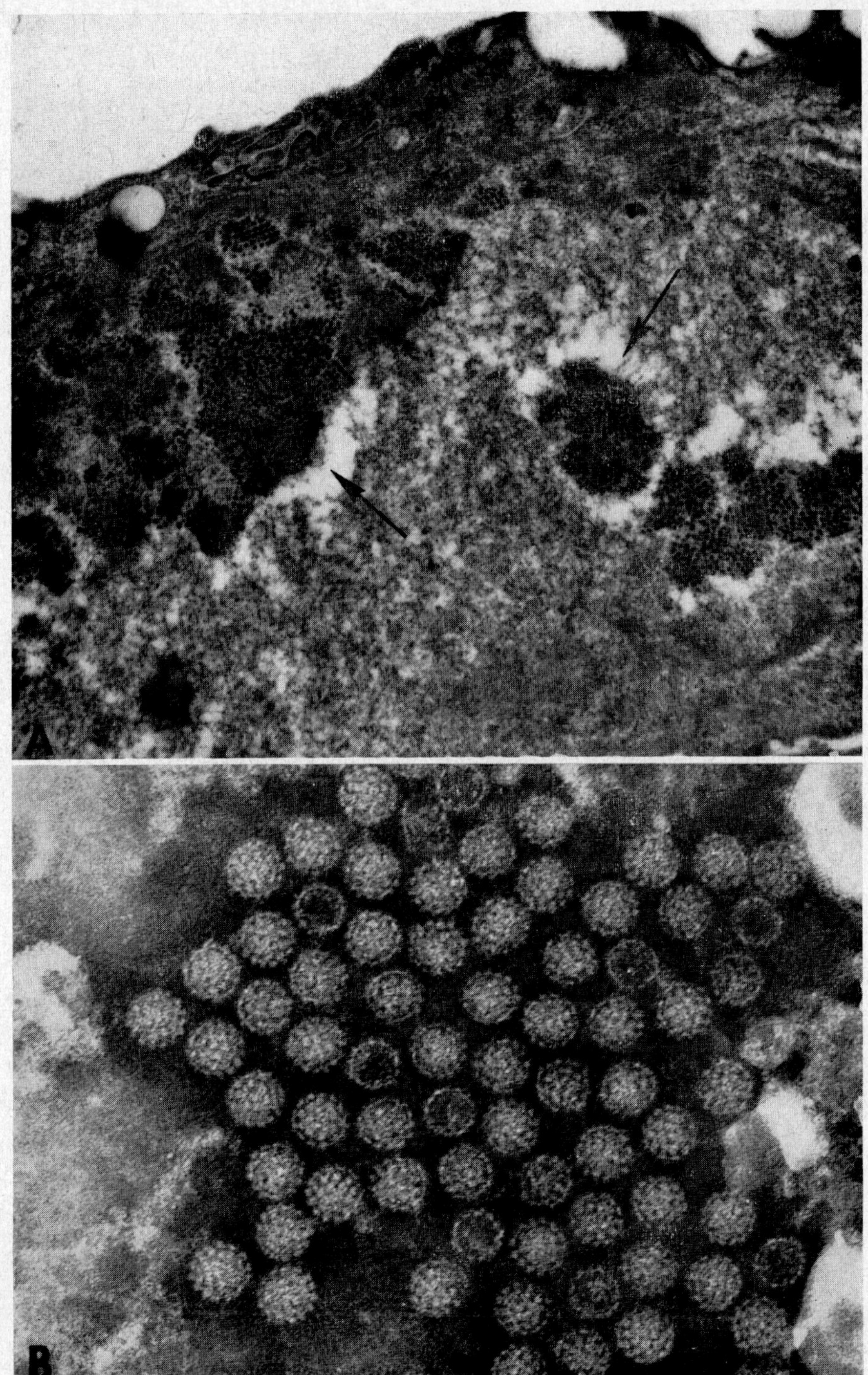

Fig. 3 Deer Fibroma Virus

can best be described as fibromas. Only in *Oryctolagus cuniculus* is a generalized and usually lethal disease produced by myxoma virus. Shope's fibroma virus produces a fibroma in this host also. Two other related viruses, squirrel fibroma and hare fibroma virus, produce small tumors in *Oryctolagus*, no lesions in *Sylvilagus*, and large fibromas in their natural hosts.

The epidemiology of the benign fibromas of *Sylvilagus* is not fully understood, but extensive spread of the disease during the summer and autumn months is apparently due to the activity of arthropod vectors which acquire virus when they probe through the fibromas and transmit it mechanically to other susceptible rabbits. The mechanism of over-wintering may be similar in many of the virus-induced skin tumors of wild animals; it implies the persistence of virus in tumors remaining infectious for biting arthropods for long periods of time.

TRANSMISSIBLE FIBROMA OF GREY SQUIRRELS

In 1953, L. Kilham and his co-workers at the National Institute of Health in Bethesda, Md., described a virus-caused, transmissible fibroma of grey squirrels (*Sciurus carolinensis*). Multiple fibromatous tumors were found on the skin of 6 grey squirrels trapped in Maryland counties adjacent to the District of Columbia. These tumors were located on all parts of animals, from eyelids to tail and toes, measured from a few millimeters to 2.5 cm in diameter, and varied in numbers from 5 on one squirrel to between 50 and 100 on others. The tumors could be transmitted by inoculation of cell-free centrifuged extracts into suckling squirrels; adult squirrels were found to be relatively resistant. There was considerable difficulty in obtaining a sufficient number of animals for inoculation. Squirrels were trapped in the vicinity of Bethesda, Md., as a part of a wild-life management program; females found to be pregnant by palpation under ether anesthesia were kept in small cages, and after the litters were born, suckling squirrels were inoculated. Approximately 2 weeks after intracutaneous inoculation of the extracts, small tumors developed at the site of inoculation. In most instances the induced fibromas enlarged at first, then remained stationary, and finally regressed. In some animals, however, the tumors continued to grow, and later metastatic tumors developed in the skin and also in the lungs. Young woodchucks (*Marmota monax*) were also found to be susceptible and developed skin tumors following intracutaneous inoculation of the squirrel fibroma extracts.

The virus could be transmitted from one squirrel to another by mosquito vectors (*Aedes aegypti* and *Anopheles quadrimaculatus*). The mosquitoes were able to transmit the virus as long as 16 days after feeding on fibroma-carrying squirrels.

On microscopic sections the squirrel fibroma resembles the Shope rabbit fibroma. Cytoplasmic acidophilic inclusion bodies can be found in islands of epidermal cells located in the tumors. That the virus of squirrel fibroma is also immunologically related to the Shope rabbit fibroma was evident from serum neutralization tests: the squirrel fibroma virus could be completely neutralized *in vitro* by mixing the virus-containing extracts with equal amounts of Shope fibroma immune rabbit serum; the inoculation of such mixtures resulted in no lesions, whereas normal serum had no neutralizing effect.

When inoculated into domestic rabbits, the squirrel fibroma virus induced tumors that regressed promptly; no virus could be recovered from such tumors. On the other hand, the Shope rabbit fibroma virus did not induce tumors when inoculated into squirrels. Although immunologically related, these are therefore two distinct viruses.

It has been previously stated that the Shope rabbit fibroma virus could induce transformation of the heat-inactivated myxoma virus into a live and pathogenic myxoma agent (Berry and Dedrick, 1936). A similar transformation, in tissue culture, could be induced by mixing the heat-inactivated myxoma virus with either a live rabbit fibroma virus (Kilham, 1957) or with a live squirrel fibroma virus (Kilham, 1958). This experiment suggested a rather close relationship between the squirrel fibroma virus and that of the rabbit fibroma.

Pulmonary Adenomatosis Induced with Squirrel Fibroma Virus

Kirschstein, Rabson, and Kilham (1958) reported that following intratracheal inoculation of the squirrel fibroma virus into suckling squirrels, multiple, small, pearl-like, gray-white, glistening lesions, 3 to 4 mm in diameter, developed in the lungs of some of the inoculated animals. Histologically, there was in such areas a marked papillary proliferation of bronchial epithelium, with eosinophilic inclusion bodies present in epithelial cells. These lesions were similar to pulmonary adenomatosis previously observed in sheep (Borrel, 1903. Cowdry, 1925. Duran-Reynals *et al.*, 1958), mice (Horn *et al.*, 1952), and other animal species, including man (Swan, 1949).

THE INFECTIOUS FIBROMA OF DEER

In 1955, R. E. Shope of the Rockefeller Institute in New York described fibromatous tumors in deer, transmissible by filtrates. Six deer killed in New Jersey by the Division of Fish and Game, N. J. Department of Conservation and Economic Development, had multiple tumors on the head and neck. The individual nodules ranged from 0.5 to 10 cm in diameter. On cut sections they were firm, white, and fleshy. Microscopically, they were fibromas.

Tumors from several deer were pooled and kept in 50 per cent glycerin-saline for up to 22 months. Extracts were then made, centrifuged, passed through Berkefeld N filter candles, and inoculated into the skin of two young adult deer. After an incubation period of approximately 7 to 8 weeks, small multiple fibromatous tumors, identical with the naturally occurring fibromas, appeared in both animals at the site of inoculation. Under the microscope these tumors had the same uniform cellular pattern as had been seen in the original naturally-occurring fibromas in the deer.

REFERENCES

Ahlström, C. G., and Andrewes, C. H., Fibroma virus infection in tarred rabbits. *J. Path. & Bact.*, **47**: 65–86, 1938.

Andrewes, C. H., Change in rabbit-fibroma virus suggesting mutation; I. Experiments on domestic rabbits. *J. Exp. Med.*, **63**: 157–172, 1936.

Andrewes, C. H., and Ahlström, C. G., A transplantable sarcoma occurring in a rabbit inoculated with tar and infectious fibroma virus. *J. Path. & Bact.*, **47**: 87–99, 1938.

Andrewes, C. H., and Horstmann, D. M., The susceptibility of viruses to ethyl ether. *J. Gen. Microbiol.*, **3**: 290–297, 1949.

Andrewes, C. H., Thompson, H. V., and Mansi, W., Myxomatosis: Present position and future prospects in Great Britain. *Nature*, **184**: 1179–1180, 1959.

Aragão, H. B., Transmissão do virus do myxoma dos coelhos pelas pulgas. *Brasil-Medico*, **34**: 753–754, 1920.

Aragão, H. B., Sensibilidade do coelho do mato ao virus do mixoma; transmissão pelo *Aedes scapularis* e pelo *Stegomyia*. *Brasil-Medico*, **56**: 207–209, 1942.

Aragão, H. B., O virus do mixoma no coelho do mato (*Sylvilagus minenses*), sua transmissão pelos *Aedes scapularis e aegypti*. *Mem. Inst. Oswaldo Cruz*, **38**: 93–99, 1943.

Armand-Delille, P. F., Une méthode nouvelle permettant à l'agriculture de lutter efficacement contre la pullulation du lapin. *Compt. Rend. Acad. Agric. de France*, **39**: 638–642, 1953.

Armour, C. J., and Thompson, H. V., Spread of myxomatosis in the first outbreak in Great Britain. *Ann. Appl. Biol.*, **43**: 511–518, 1955.

Avery, O. T., MacLeod, C. M., and McCarty, M., Studies on the chemical nature of the substance inducing transformation of pneumococcal types. *J. Exp. Med.*, **79**: 137–158, 1944.

Bauer, A., and Constantin, T., Multiplication du virus de Shope dans les cellules en culture. Étude au microscope électronique. *Compt. Rend. Soc. Biol.*, **150**: 246–249, 1956.

Benjamin, B., and Rivers, T. M., Regeneration of virus myxomatosum (Sanarelli) in the presence of cells of exudates surviving *in vitro*. *Proc. Soc. Exp. Biol. & Med.*, **28**: 791–792, 1931.

Bernhard, W., Electron microscopy of human cells and tumor viruses. A review. *Cancer Research*, **18**: 491–509, 1958.

Bernhard, W., Bauer, A., Harel, J., and Oberling, C., Les formes intracytoplasmiques du virus fibromateux de Shope. Étude de coupes ultrafines au microscope électronique. *Bull. du Cancer*, **41**: 423–444, 1954.

Berry, G. P., The transformation of the virus of rabbit fibroma (Shope) into that of infectious myxomatosis (Sanarelli). (Abstract). *Proc. Am. Philosophical Soc.*, **77**: 473–476, 1937.

Berry, G. P., and Dedrick, H. M., A method for changing the virus of rabbit fibroma (Shope) into that of infectious myxomatosis (Sanarelli). *J. Bact.*, **31**: 50–51, 1936.

Berry, G. P., and Dedrick, H. M., Further observations on the transformation of the virus of rabbit fibroma (Shope) into that of infectious myxomatosis (Sanarelli). (Abstract). *J. Bact.*, **32**: 356, 1936.

Borrel, A., Epithelioses infectieuses et epitheliomas. *Ann. Inst. Pasteur*, **17**: 81–122, 1903.

Bronson, L. H., and Parker, R. F., The inactivation of the virus of infectious myxomatosis by heat. *J. Bact.*, **45**: 177–181, 1943.

Chapple, P. J., and Westwood, J. C. N., Electron microscopy of myxoma virus. *Nature*, **199**: 199–200, 1963.

Chaproniere, D. M., The effect of myxoma virus on cultures of rabbit tissues. *Virology*, **2**: 599–610, 1956.

Clemmesen, J., The influence of Roentgen radiation on immunity to Shope fibroma virus. *Am. J. Cancer*, **35**: 378–385, 1939.

Constantin, T., and Febvre, H., Les corps d'inclusion observés dans les cultures de tissus infectées par le virus du fibrome de Shope du lapin. *Compt. Rend. Soc. Biol.*, **150**: 114–116, 1956.

Constantin, T., and Febvre, H., Évolution des acides nucléiques dans les corps d'inclusions provoqués par le virus du fibrome de Shope. *Compt. Rend. Acad. Sci.* (*Paris*), **246**: 332–334, 1958.

Constantin, T., Febvre, H., and Harel, J., Cycle de multiplication du virus du fibrome de Shope *in vitro* (souche OA). *Compt. Rend. Soc. Biol.*, **150**: 347–348, 1956.

Cowdry, E. V., Studies on the etiology of Jagziekte. I. The primary lesions. *J. Exp. Med.*, **42**: 323–333, 1925.

Day, M. F., Fenner, F., and Woodroofe, G. M., Further studies on the mechanism of mosquito transmission of myxomatosis in the European rabbit. *J. Hyg.* (*Cambridge*), **54**: 258–283, 1956.

Dourmashkin, R., and Duperrat, B., Observation au microscope électronique du virus du *Molluscum Contagiosum*. *Compt. Rend. Acad. Sci.* (*Paris*), **246**: 3133–3136, 1958.

Duran-Reynals, F., Production of degenerative inflammatory or neoplastic effects in the newborn rabbit by the Shope fibroma virus. *Yale J. Biol. & Med.*, **13**: 99–110, 1940.

Duran-Reynals, F., Immunological factors that influence the neoplastic effects of the rabbit fibroma virus. *Cancer Research*, **5**: 25–39, 1945.

Duran-Reynals, F., Jungherr, E., Cuba-Caparó, A., Rafferty, K. A., Jr., and Helmboldt, C., The pulmonary adenomatosis complex in sheep. *Ann. N.Y. Acad. Sci.*, **70**: 726–742, 1958.

Epstein, M. A., An investigation into the purifying effect of a fluorocarbon on vaccinia virus. *Brit. J. Exp. Path.*, **39**: 436–446, 1958.

Epstein, M. A., Observations on the mode of release of Herpes virus from infected HeLa cells. *J. Cell Biol.*, **12**: 589–597, 1962.

Epstein, B., Reissig, M., and de Robertis, E., Studies by electron microscopy of thin sections of infectious myxomatosis in rabbits. *J. Exp. Med.*, **96**: 347–354, 1952.

FARRANT, J. L., and FENNER, F., A comparison of the morphology of vaccinia and myxoma viruses. *Australian J. Exp. Biol. & Med. Sci.*, **31**: 121–125, 1953.

FAULKNER, G. H., and ANDREWES, C. H., Propagation of a strain of rabbit fibroma virus in tissue culture. *Brit. J. Exp. Path.*, **16**: 271–275, 1935.

FELLER, A. E., ENDERS, J. F., and WELLER, T. H., The prolonged coexistence of vaccinia virus in high titer and living cells in roller tube cultures of chick embryonic tissues. *J. Exp. Med.*, **72**: 367–388, 1940.

FENNER, F., Classification of myxoma and fibroma viruses. *Nature*, **171**: 562–563, 1953.

FENNER, F., Viruses of the myxoma-fibroma subgroup of the poxviruses. II. Comparison of soluble antigens by gel diffusion tests, and a general discussion of the subgroup. *Australian J. Exp. Biol. & Med. Sci.*, **43**: 143–156, 1965.

FENNER, F., and MCINTYRE, G. A., Infectivity titrations of myxoma virus in the rabbit and the developing chick embryo. *J. Hyg.* (*Cambridge*), **54**: 246–257, 1956.

FENNER, F., and MARSHALL, I. D., A comparison of the virulence for European rabbits (*Oryctolagus cuniculus*) of strains of myxoma virus recovered in the field in Australia, Europe and America. *J. Hyg.* (*Cambridge*), **55**: 149–191, 1957.

FENNER, F., and RATCLIFFE, F. N., *Myxomatosis*. pp. 379. Cambridge Univ. Press, London, 1965.

FENNER, F., DAY, M. F., and WOODROOFE, G. M., The mechanism of the transmission of myxomatosis in the European rabbit (*Oryctolagus cuniculus*) by the mosquito *Aedes aegypti*. *Australian J. Exp. Biol. & Med. Sci.*, **30**: 139–152, 1952.

FENNER, F., DAY, M. F., and WOODROOFE, G. M., Epidemiological consequences of the mechanical transmission of myxomatosis by mosquitoes. *J. Hyg.* (*Cambridge*), **54**: 284–303, 1956.

FENNER, F., POOLE, W. E., MARSHALL, I. D., and DYCE, A. L., Studies in the epidemiology of infectious myxomatosis of rabbits. VI. The experimental introduction of the European strain of myxoma virus into Australian wild rabbit populations. *J. Hyg.* (*Cambridge*), **55**: 192–206, 1957.

GAYLORD, W. H., JR., and MELNICK, J. L., Intracellular forms of pox viruses as shown by the electron microscope (vaccinia, ectromelia, molluscum contagiosum). *J. Exp. Med.*, **98**: 157–172, 1953.

GRIFFITH, F., The significance of pneumococcal types. *J. Hyg.*, **27**: 113-159, 1928.

GRODHAUS, G., REGNERY, D. C., and MARSHALL, I. D., Studies in the epidemiology of myxomatosis in California. II. The experimental transmission of myxomatosis in brush rabbits (*Sylvilagus bachmani*) by several species of mosquitoes. *Am. J. Hyg.*, **77**: 205–212, 1963.

HAAGEN, E., and DU, DSCHENG-HSING, Weitere Untersuchungen über das Verhalten des Kaninchenmyxomvirus *in vitro*. *Zentralbl. f. Bakt.*, Abt. I, (Orig.), **143**: 23–31, 1938.

HAREL, J., and CONSTANTIN, T., Sur la malignité des tumeurs provoquées par le virus fibromateux de Shope chez le lapin nouveau-né et le lapin adulte traité par des doses massives de cortisone. *Bull. du Cancer*, **41**: 482–497, 1954.

HERZBERG, K., and THELEN, A., Über den Nachweis und den Vermehrungsvorgang des Virus de Shopeschen Kaninchenfibroms. *Virchow Arch. Path. Anat.*, **303**: 81–89, 1936.

HINZE, H. C., and Walker, D. L., Response of cultured rabbit cells to infection with the Shope fibroma virus. I. Proliferation and morphological alteration of the infected cells. *J. Bact.*, **88**: 1185–1194, 1964.

HOBBS, J. R., Studies on the nature of the infectious myxoma virus of rabbits. *Am. J. Hyg.*, **8**: 800–839, 1928.

HOFFSTADT, R. E., and PILCHER, K. S., The use of the chorio-allantoic membrane of the developing chick embryo as a medium in the study of virus myxomatosum. *J. Bact.*, **35**: 353–367, 1938.

HORN, H. A., CONGDON, C. C., ESCHENBRENNER, A. B., ANDERVONT, H. B., and STEWART, H. L., Pulmonary adenomatosis in mice. *J. Nat. Cancer Inst.*, **12**: 1297–1315, 1952.

HURST, E. W., Myxoma and Shope fibroma. III. Miscellaneous observations bearing on the relationship between myxoma, neuromyxoma and fibroma viruses. *Brit. J. Exp. Path.*, **18**: 23–30, 1937.

HYDE, K. E., The relationship between the viruses of infectious myxoma and the Shope fibroma of rabbits. *Am. J. Hyg.*, **23**: 278–297, 1936.

KESSEL, J. F., PROUTY, C. C., and MEYER, J. W., Occurrence of infectious myxomatosis in southern California. *Proc. Soc. Exp. Biol. & Med.*, **28**: 413–414, 1931.

KILHAM, L., Metastasizing viral fibromas of gray squirrels: Pathogenesis and mosquito transmission. *Am. J. Hyg.*, **61**: 55–63, 1955.

KILHAM, L., Propagation of fibroma virus in tissue cultures of cottontail testes. *Proc. Soc. Exp. Biol. & Med.*, **92**: 739–742, 1956.

KILHAM, L., Transformation of fibroma into myxoma virus in tissue culture. *Proc. Soc. Exp. Biol. & Med.*, **95**: 59–62, 1957.

KILHAM, L., Fibroma-myxoma virus transformations in different types of tissue culture. *J. Nat. Cancer Inst.*, **20**: 729–739, 1958.

KILHAM, L., and DALMAT, H. T., Host-virus-mosquito relations of Shope fibromas in cottontail rabbits. *Am. J. Hyg.*, **61**: 45–54, 1955.

KILHAM, L., and FISHER, E. R., Pathogenesis of fibromas in cottontail rabbits. *Am. J. Hyg.*, **59**: 104–112, 1954.

KILHAM, L., HERMAN, C. M., and FISHER, E. R., Naturally occurring fibromas of gray squirrels related to Shope's rabbit fibroma. *Proc. Soc. Exp. Biol. & Med.*, **82**: 298–301, 1953.

KILHAM, L., and WOKE, P. A., Laboratory transmission of fibromas (Shope) in cottontail rabbits by means of fleas and mosquitoes. *Proc. Soc. Exp. Biol. & Med.*, **83**: 296–301, 1953.

KILHAM, L., LERNER, E., HIATT, C., and SHACK, J., Properties of myxoma virus transforming agent. *Proc. Soc. Exp. Biol. & Med.*, **98**: 689–692, 1958.

KIRSCHSTEIN, R. L., RABSON, A. S., and KILHAM, L., Pulmonary lesions produced by fibroma viruses in squirrels and rabbits. *Cancer Research*, **18**: 1340–1344, 1958.

KLIGLER, I. J., MUCKENFUSS, R. S., and RIVERS, T. M., Transmission of fowlpox by mosquitoes. *J. Exp. Med.*, **49**: 649–660, 1929.

LLOYD, B. J., and KAHLER, H., Electron microscopy of the virus of rabbit fibroma. *J. Nat. Cancer Inst.*, **15**: 991–999, 1955.

LOCKLEY, R. M., Some experiments in rabbit control. *Nature*, **145**: 767–769, 1940.

LUSH, D., The virus of infectious myxomatosis of rabbits on the chorioallantoic membrane of the developing egg. *Australian J. Exp. Biol. & Med. Sci.*, **15**: 131–139, 1937.

MARSHALL, I. D., and REGNERY, D. C., Myxomatosis in a Californian brush rabbit (*Sylvilagus bachmani*). *Nature*, **188**: 73–74, 1960.

MARSHALL, I. D., and REGNERY, D. C., Studies in the epidemiology of myxomatosis in California. III. The response of brush rabbits (*Sylvilagus bachmani*) to infection with exotic and enzootic strains of myxoma virus, and the relative infectivity of the tumors for mosquitoes. *Am. J. Hyg.*, **77**: 213–219, 1963.

MARSHALL, I. D., REGNERY, D. C., and GRODHAUS, G., Studies in the epidemiology of myxomatosis in California. I. Observations on two outbreaks of myxomatosis in coastal California and the recovery of myxoma virus from a brush rabbit (*Sylvilagus bachmani*). *Am. J. Hyg.*, **77**: 195–204, 1963.

MARTIN, C. J., Observations on *Myxomatosis cuniculi* (Sanarelli) made with a view to the use of the virus in the control of rabbit plagues. *Bull. Coun. Sci. Industr. Research Australia*, No. 96, 1936.

MOORE, M. S., and WALKER, D. L., Accentuation of plaques of myxoma and fibroma viruses by immune serum. *Proc. Soc. Exp. Biol. & Med.*, **111**: 493–497, 1962.

MORGAN, C., ELLISON, S. A., ROSE, H. M., and MOORE, D. H., Structure and development of viruses observed in the electron microscope. II. Vaccinia and fowl pox viruses. *J. Exp. Med.*, **100**: 301–310, 1954.

MORGAN, C., ROSE, H. M., HOLDEN, M., and JONES, E. P., Electron microscopic observations on the development of herpes simplex virus. *J. Exp. Med.*, **110**: 643–656, 1959.

MOSES, A., O virus do mixoma dos coelhos. Untersuchungen ueber das Virus myxomatosum der Kaninchen. *Mem. Inst. Oswaldo Cruz*, **3**: 46–53, 1911.

MYERS, K., and POOLE, W. E., A study of the biology of the wild rabbit, *Oryctolagus cuniculus* (L.) in confined populations. *Aust. J. Zool.*, **10**: 225–267, 1962.

NAGINGTON, J., and HORNE, R. W., Morphological studies of orf and vaccinia viruses. *Virology*, **16**: 248–260, 1962.

PADGETT, B. L., WRIGHT, M. J., JAYNE, A., and WALKER, D. L., Electron microscopic structure of myxoma virus and some reactivable derivatives. *J. Bact.*, **87**: 454–460, 1964.

PLOTZ, H., Culture du virus myxomatosum (Sanarelli) en présence de cellules vivantes. *Compt. Rend. Soc. Biol.*, **109**: 1327–1329, 1932.

SANARELLI, G., Das myxomatogene Virus. Beitrag zum Studium der Krankheitserreger ausserhalb des Sichtbaren. *Centralbl. f. Bakt.*, Abt. I., **23**: 865–873, 1898.

SCHERRER, R., Morphogénèse et ultrastructure du virus fibromateux de Shope. *Path. Microbiol. (Basel)*, **31**: 129–146, 1968.

SCHLESINGER, M., and ANDREWES, C. H., The filtration and centrifugation of the viruses of rabbit fibroma and rabbit papilloma. *J. Hyg.*, **37**: 521–526, 1937.

SCHMIT-JENSEN, H. O., Summary of the experiments carried out in Vejrø by the State Veterinary Serum Laboratory on the extermination of rabbits by myxomatosis virus. Report to Danish Ministry for Agriculture and Fisheries, 1939. (Quoted by FENNER and RATCLIFFE, *Myxomatosis*, 1964.)

SCHWERDT, P. R., and SCHWERDT, C. E., A plaque assay for myxoma virus infectivity. *Proc. Soc. Exp. Biol. & Med.*, **109**: 717–721, 1962.

SHANKS, P. L., SHARMAN, G. A. M., ALLAN, R., DONALD, L. G., YOUNG, S., and MARR, T. G., Experiments with myxomatosis in the Hebrides. *Brit. Vet. J.*, **111**: 25–34, 1955.

SHOPE, R. E., A filterable virus causing tumor-like condition in rabbits and its relationship to virus myxomatosum. *J. Exp. Med.*, **56**: 803–822, 1932.

SHOPE, R. E., Infectious fibroma of rabbits. IV. The infection with virus myxomatosum of rabbits recovered from fibroma. *J. Exp. Med.*, **63**: 43–57, 1936.

SHOPE, R. E., *"Masking," transformation, and interepidemic survival of animal viruses.* pp. 79–92 in Viruses 1950, California Inst. of Technol. Press, Pasadena, Calif., 1950.

SHOPE, R. E., An infectious fibroma of deer. *Proc. Soc. Exp. Biol. & Med.*, **88**: 533–535, 1955.

SMITH, M. H. D., The Berry-Dedrick transformation of fibroma into myxoma in the rabbit. *Ann. N.Y. Acad. Sci.*, **54**: 1141–1152, 1952.

SWAN, L. L., Pulmonary adenomatosis of man. *Arch. Path.*, **47**: 517–544, 1949.

TAKEHARA, M., and SCHWERDT, C. E., Infective subviral particles from cell cultures infected with myxoma and fibroma viruses. *Virology*, **31**: 163–166, 1967.

TORRES, S., Transmissão da mixomatose dos coelhos pelo *Culex quinquefasciatus. Bol. Soc. Bras. Med. Vet.*, **6**: 4, 1936.

VERNA, J. E., and EYLAR, O. R., Rabbit fibroma virus plaque assay and *in vitro* studies. *Virology*, **18**: 266–273, 1962.

WOODROOFE, G. M., and FENNER, F., Viruses of the myxoma-fibroma subgroup of the poxviruses. I. Plaque production in cultured cells, plaque-reduction tests, and cross-protection tests in rabbits. *Australian J. Exp. Biol. & Med. Sci.*, **43**: 123–142, 1965.

CHAPTER 3

Papillomas, Warts, and Related Neoplasms in Rabbits, Dogs, Horses, Cattle, and Man

THE SHOPE RABBIT PAPILLOMA

Wild cottontail rabbits in Kansas and Iowa frequently carry tumors of the skin on the abdomen, and particularly around the neck and shoulders. These tumors resemble large, horny warts, with irregular, fissured surfaces. Richard E. Shope of the Rockefeller Institute in Princeton, New Jersey, found in 1933 that this tumor, a papilloma, is caused by a filterable agent and that it could be transmitted without difficulty by rubbing the filtrate into the scarified skin of either domestic or wild (cottontail) rabbits. The rabbit was found to be the only susceptible host. Mice, rats, guinea pigs, cats, dogs, pigs, and goats were inoculated without success. The causative agent was found to be very specific and induced typical papillomas only when inoculated into the scarified skin. When the filtrate was introduced (without touching the skin) directly into the muscles, or when internal organs were inoculated, no papillomas resulted. Similarly, no papillomas resulted when the filtrate was introduced under surface of the tongue, cheeks, gums, lips, eyelids, or genital organs of rabbits.

The following is the description of the discovery of the rabbit papilloma virus in Dr. R. E. Shope's own words, reprinted with his permission from unpublished notes:

> "The father of the wife of one of our staff members was visiting his daughter in Princeton shortly after I had started my experiments with the rabbit fibroma. This old gentleman was from Iowa and was quite a hunter out there. Because of this, his daughter had asked me if I would show her father the tumor that I had gotten from one of our New Jersey rabbits. I showed him what I considered a good example. He looked at it disdainfully and said that this was nothing compared with the sort of things that they had in the Iowa rabbits. He said he had shot rabbits with horns out of the side of their heads like Texas steers, or out of the top of their noses like a rhinoceros. Naturally, I was intrigued by this colorful description and speculated as to what the character of these growths might be. It seemed entirely likely from the old gentleman's description that they must be papillomata. I asked him how prevalent they were and he said that up there where he lived around Cherokee, almost every other rabbit

shot had them; so I made arrangements to go back to Cherokee with him when he returned to Iowa, and we put in about four days of hunting there. It was in September and the underbrush was still pretty heavy for rabbit shooting. However, we did kill a few animals, but, unfortunately, none had these horns that he had spoken of. We had a young boy by the name of Cliff Peck hunting with us, so when at the end of four days I had to return to New Jersey empty-handed, I left a bottle of glycerol and a five dollar bill with Cliff and told him that if he would get me the horns of one of these rabbits and send them to me in glycerol, I would give him another five dollars. Needless to say, Cliff really scoured the underbrush for rabbits and within the course of a week I had my bottle of glycerol back and in it were several so-called horns from a cottontail rabbit shot near Cherokee. Examination of the horns in the glycerol bottle indicated clearly that they were papillomas and, of course, I was immediately interested to learn whether or not they could be transmitted. The skin of several laboratory rabbits was scarified by needle and a suspension prepared from the warts was rubbed into the scarifications. After about a week, examination of the experimental animals revealed the presence of tiny red elevations along the scarifications. These increased in size until by the end of another week, or two, it became evident that they were tiny papillomas. Histologically they were benign papillomas. The causative agent proved to be filterable, and capable of prolonged storage in glycerol. Furthermore, it withstood heating to as much as 65°C for a half hour at a time and, therefore, appeared to be one of the more stable viruses. I thought that I was all set to work with the thing in a leisurely manner. However, this thought was short-lived because when I harvested warts from my first domestic rabbit passage, ground them up as I had the wild rabbit papillomas, and applied the suspension to the scarified skin of the second passage rabbit, nothing at all happened. It appeared that though the papillomas in the first passage domestic rabbit had undoubtedly been induced by a virus, no virus could be demonstrated in them. Subsequent work has indicated that though virus cannot be demonstrated directly in the domestic rabbit warts, it is present there in a masked or non-infectious form. The domestic rabbit tumor, therefore, partook of the character of a spontaneous tumor in which no extrinsic infective agent could be demonstrated. By this I mean that were I to give a papillomatous domestic rabbit to an investigator experienced in the study of tumors, he would have had to conclude that this papilloma was a growth of unknown etiology and fell, therefore, into the category of most spontaneous neoplasms. He would have been unable to transmit the growth by any other means than grafting and certainly would not have suspected that it originated as a result of infection with a virus. Proof that the virus was present in the growth could only be effected when one had access to infective wild rabbit virus. This proof was of an indirect character and entailed serological tests. Thus, a suspension of domestic rabbit warts, though incapable of inducing papillomas when applied to the scarified skin of other domestic rabbits, did immunize them solidly, when given subcutaneously, against the effect of the wild rabbit virus, and the serum from such immunized domestic rabbits was capable of neutralizing wild rabbit virus."

The remarkable fact was therefore observed that the virus could be recovered without difficulty from papillomas growing in cottontail rabbits, whereas it was in most instances impossible to recover it from apparently identical papillomas growing in domestic rabbits, even though such papillomas had been induced by inoculation of the same filtrates. Only in isolated instances was it possible to recover the virus from papillomas growing in domestic rabbits.

Factors Influencing the Yield of Infective Virus in Rabbit Papilloma. The "Immature," and the "Infective" Virus

The presence of infective virus in cottontail papillomas, and the considerable difficulty in recovering infective virus from similar papillomas grown on domestic rabbits presented a challenging problem to the investigator. This difference in the yield of infective virus among apparently similar tumors grown in two different rabbit species could be explained by a difference in the quantity of virus present in such papillomas, assuming that otherwise the same type of virus is present in both instances. Another explanation, however, could also be considered.

A few years ago Noyes and Mellors (1957) observed by means of fluorescent antibody technique that most of the papilloma virus could be found in the nuclei of the differentiated keratinizing cells on the top of the papillomas in the cottontail rabbit. In subsequent experiments, Noyes demonstrated by means of microcautery technique that the papilloma virus could be extracted from the keratinized layers of cells and not from the actively proliferating cells at the base of the papillomas. Subsequent electron microscopic studies (Stone *et al.*, 1959) in which the distribution of the virus was investigated on ultrathin sections of papillomas, and which will be discussed in more detail later in this chapter, also suggested that spherical virus particles, presumably representing the fully infective virus, could be found only in the nuclei of the differentiated cells of the upper part of rabbit papillomas. Thus, the work of Noyes (1957, 1959),

Stone (1959) and their associates suggested that the virus of rabbit papilloma exists in two forms: one of these is mature, fully infective virus, visible with the electron microscope as a spherical particle in the nuclei of differentiated keratinized cells in the upper portion of rabbit papillomas; the other is immature, non-infective virus, not visible in the electron microscope except as granular material within the nucleoli of the cells in the basal germinal layers of the papillomas. The mature, infective virus, present in the upper keratinized part of the cottontail's papillomas, has presumably completed its developmental cycle and is then ready to infect new hosts, but has otherwise no other function or influence on its own host's cells.

The immature virus, on the other hand, present in the basal layers of the papillomas, although not infectious from one animal to another, may nevertheless infect cells within the same animal, maintaining the neoplastic proliferation of the papillomatous growth.

In the wild cottontail rabbit the virus proceeds through its successive forms of maturation and ends as an infective particle localized in the upper parts of the papillomas. It can then be recovered from such papillomas and passed by inoculation into new hosts. The domestic rabbit, on the other hand, differs from the wild cottontail in that it seems to possess no mechanism for forcing the neoplastic non-infective "masked" virus to maturation as infective papilloma virus. However, in both the wild and the domestic rabbit, the non-infective virus is responsible for the tumor formation.

More recent experiments of Shope* demonstrated that when the papilloma virus is inoculated into the skin of either cottontail or domestic rabbits, it "disappears" after only about 8 hours. In other words, after this interval of time no presence of the virus can be demonstrated by infectivity tests: the virus enters into eclipse. In the cottontail, the virus reappears as soon as the papillomas develop. In the domestic rabbit, on

* Personal communication to the author from Dr. R. E. Shope (October, 1960).

FIG. 4. THE SHOPE RABBIT PAPILLOMA VIRUS.

(A). Ultrathin sections of a Shope papilloma taken from a New Jersey cottontail rabbit which had been inoculated with the papilloma virus harvested from a Kansas rabbit. Arrays of small virus particles of uniform size are shown in remnants of keratinized cells of the cornified skin layer. Magnification 21,200×. Electron micrograph (unpublished) from a study by R. S. Stone, R. E. Shope and D. H. Moore, Rockefeller Institute for Medical Research, New York. (B). Negatively stained Shope papilloma virus particles in a preparation treated by potassium phosphotungstate. Magnification 200,000×. Electron micrograph prepared by A. F. Howatson, Ontario Cancer Institute, Toronto, Canada. (From: *Advances in Cancer Research*, 8: 1, 1964.)

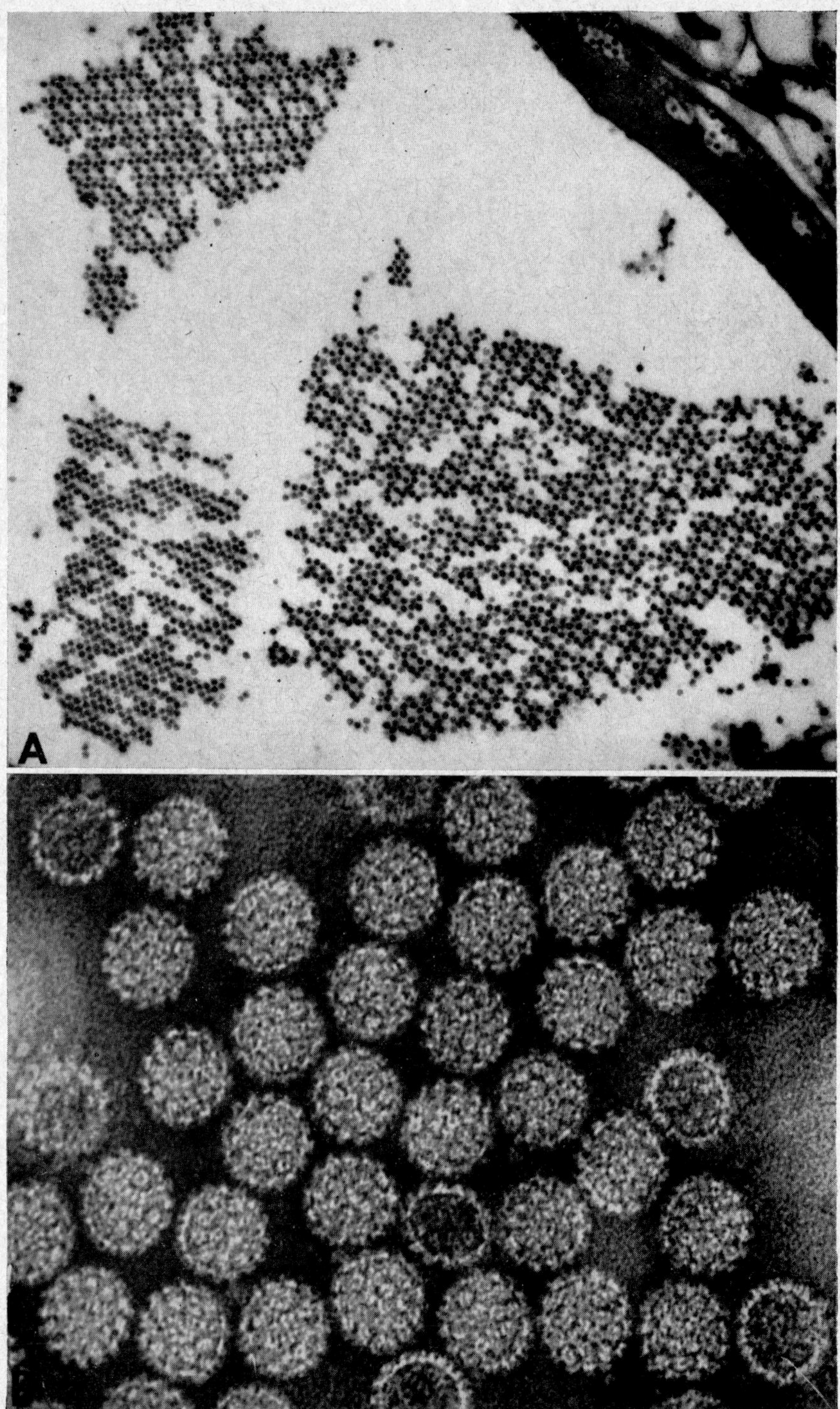

FIG. 4. THE SHOPE RABBIT PAPILLOMA VIRUS

the other hand, even though morphologically similar papillomas develop some 7 to 21 days after inoculation, the virus remains undetectable by either infectivity tests or electron microscopy. Its presence, however, can be demonstrated by serological tests; it apparently exists in domestic rabbit papillomas in its immature, non-infective form; in this form it fully retains its antigenic potency when employed for immunization of rabbits against the infective papilloma virus.

The factors which determine the maturation of the virus in the papillomas are obscure. The host influence is obviously of considerable importance, but other factors must also exist, although they have not yet been fully determined. The quantity of infective virus that can be recovered from papillomas grown in cottontail rabbits is considerably higher when Kansas cottontails are used instead of wild rabbits maintained in the open or in cages in New Jersey.*

Even domestic rabbits, which in the United States usually do not yield papilloma virus, behave differently in this respect in Russian laboratories (Nartsissov, 1959. Shope, 1960*). Shope furnished the papilloma virus to Russia in 1939. Through successive years the papilloma virus has been maintained in Russian laboratories without difficulty through serial passage performed on domestic rabbits. The papillomas grown on domestic rabbits in Russian laboratories apparently yield infective papilloma virus, not unlike those grown in our Kansas cottontails. It is therefore apparent that the maturation of the virus does not depend entirely on the genetic susceptibility of the host. The geographical location in which the host is infected and the related environmental factors are of prime importance. It is of interest, therefore, that among cottontails in the United States, the geographical belt where papillomas occur in high frequency is relatively narrow, extending from north-eastern Oklahoma up through eastern Kansas, western Missouri, eastern Nebraska, and probably South Dakota, western Iowa, and up into Minnesota.† The virus has been repeatedly introduced into the East, without becoming established. Among other speculations, the presence of some trace elements essential in biological processes assuring maturation of virus in certain geographical areas should be considered (Shope, 1960*).

The Change from Papilloma to Carcinoma

The cutaneous papillomas induced with the filtrates grew rather fast in the domestic and more slowly in the cottontail rabbits; at a certain point,

* Personal communication to the author from Dr. R. E. Shope (October, 1960).

† In general, papillomas do not appear in rabbits in the Western Hemisphere, east of the Mississippi River. On the other hand, fibromas do not occur in rabbits west of Illinois (personal communication to the author from Dr. R. E. Shope, 1960).

which varied in individual animals, they remained stationary, and some of them eventually regressed. Although they were at first considered to be "benign" papillomas, they had a malignant potential. This was soon discovered by Rous and Beard (1934); they removed small fragments of cutaneous papillomas and implanted them into the muscles or internal organs of the rabbits. The papillomas thus implanted acquired invasive properties, grew into the surrounding tissues, and some of them changed into squamous cell carcinomas. Further observations by Rous and Beard (1935) revealed that in some of the domestic rabbits inoculated with the papilloma virus, the resulting cutaneous papillomas changed spontaneously into squamous cell carcinomas. This change occurred in some of those papillomas that persisted for 4 to 9 months. At first the impression was prevalent that such a papilloma-to-carcinoma change occurred only in the domestic rabbit, and that in the cottontails the cutaneous papillomas either remained stationary, or eventually regressed. This opinion could not be maintained for very long, since Syverton and Berry (1935) reported a papilloma-to-carcinoma change in a spontaneous papilloma found in a wild cottontail rabbit received from southern Kansas. Later on, Syverton and his colleagues (1950, 1952) reported in a comprehensive study that the change of cutaneous papillomas into carcinomas was not unusual in wild cottontail rabbits, provided that these animals were kept under observation for a sufficiently long period of time. In Syverton's experiments, after the sixth month of observation, more than a third of the naturally induced papillomas disappeared spontaneously in the cottontail rabbits, whereas none of the experimentally induced lesions in either variety of hosts underwent regression (Syverton, 1952). The most significant observation, however, concerned the change of papillomas into cancers in the cottontails. Over 25 per cent of the cottontail rabbits, whether naturally or experimentally infected with the papilloma virus, developed cancerous skin lesions, when kept for more than 6 months. Among domestic rabbits infected with the papilloma virus, and kept for more than 6 months, 75 per cent terminated in developing cancer. No papilloma virus could be recovered from the cancerous tumors. This was no surprise in the case of the domestic rabbits, since no virus could be recovered in these hosts from the virus-induced papillomas. There was no difficulty, however, in recovering the virus from papillomas grown in cottontails, and for that reason it was a surprise to find that as soon as the papillomas in these wild rabbits changed into carcinomas, no virus could be recovered any more from such tumors. That the virus was still present in such tumors, although in a masked, not infective form, could be demonstrated only by serological methods determining the presence of specific antibodies.

It would be of fundamental importance, of course, to determine whether the papilloma virus actually induces cancer in the rabbit, or whether it induces only papillomas, the subsequent papilloma-to-carcinoma sequence occurring independently.* Such a concept appeared logical to some investigators, since no infective virus could be recovered from the papilloma-derived cancerous tumors. On the other hand, it would be possible to speculate that the virus was responsible not only for the induction of papillomas, but also for the second step in the papilloma-to-carcinoma sequence. The fact that no infective virus could be recovered from the cancerous tumors does not necessarily imply that the virus was not the initiating cause; many obviously virus-caused papillomas, such as practically all those induced in the domestic rabbits, and very occasionally also those in the cottontails, do not yield infective virus on extraction procedure. One could further speculate that the papilloma virus which, as we now realize, is a rather small, spherical particle averaging about 40 mμ in diameter, requires special environmental and biochemical conditions for its full development into an infective virus, and that in very fast growing tumors, or in papillomas changed into cancer, conditions necessary for the complete synthesis of the infective virus particle may not be present. Under such circumstances, the virus synthesis could reach only an incomplete phase of development. Accordingly, no infective virus particles could be recovered from such growths, but the presence of the virus could still be detected by immunological methods. This is pure speculation, however.

Electron Microscopic Studies of the Shope Papilloma Virus

In earlier studies (Sharp *et al.*, 1946. Beard, 1948. Kahler and Lloyd, 1952) the Shope rabbit papilloma virus was studied on metal-shadowed drop preparations. No internal structure could be revealed in such studies and the particles examined could not be readily distinguished from other

* The following comment by Dr. J. T. Syverton, University of Minn., Minneapolis (personal communication to the author, December 3, 1958) may be of interest: "Normal rabbits upon parenteral injection of large amounts of metastatic carcinomatous tissue from rabbits with primary epidermoid carcinomas failed to develop antibodies for papilloma virus. On the other hand, normal rabbits injected with extracts from papillomas in the proliferative, stationary or regressive stages, or from primary epidermoid carcinomas, did develop papilloma antibodies. I interpreted these findings to indicate that Shope papilloma virus did not serve as the actuating carcinogenic agent, but that it did operate as a provocative agent. I should like to have concluded otherwise, but our data did not permit such an assumption. Our subsequent studies suggested that nucleic acid or other virus constituents may be responsible for the cancer that results in 25 per cent of the cottontail rabbits and 75 per cent of domestic rabbits as sequelae of primary infection by Shope papilloma virus. In other words, we are continuing to seek conclusive evidence that Shope papilloma virus is responsible for the terminal stage of the virus-induced Shope papilloma-to-carcinoma sequence."

unrelated biological material of similar size and morphology. In these preliminary studies the papilloma virus was found to be a spherical particle with a diameter of 40 to 47 mμ.

More recently, electron microscopic studies of ultrathin sections of cottontail rabbit papillomas (Moore *et al.*, 1959. Stone *et al.*, 1959) revealed that the virus is a spherical particle about 33 mμ in diameter, located mostly in the nuclei of epidermal cells. The papilloma virus was found to begin its proliferation in the nucleoli of the infected cells. Aggregates of fine, closely packed granules of virus were found in the nucleolar area, in cells of the lower, germinal layer of the papilloma. In the upper portion of the papilloma, in the nuclei of the keratinized cells, the virus was found later to fill the nucleus and spread into the whole cell.

At the papilloma surface some tumor cells contained nuclei which were densely packed with virus particles. In some instances the viral particles were arranged in orderly arrays, forming rows, squares, pentagons, or hexagons. Often the nuclear membranes were no longer recognizable and the cells consisted of thick wall shells containing very large quantities of virus. The individual virus particle was about 33 mμ in diameter, consisting of a circular dark area surrounded by a concentric paler zone.

In a recent study by Haguenau and her associates (1960), ultrathin sections of ultracentrifuged pellets of sedimented rabbit (cottontail) papilloma virus revealed on electron microscopic examination the presence of innumerable spherical particles 26 to 29 mμ in diameter with a dense internal structure.

It is quite apparent that the diameters of particles measured on ultrathin sections were smaller than those reported in previous studies (Sharp *et al.*, 1946. Kahler and Lloyd, 1952) in which measurements were made on air-dried drop preparations. A similar discrepancy, however, has been observed in studies of other viruses. The average size of viruses on ultrathin sections is usually smaller than that on air-dried drop preparations. This is due to the technique of the preparation of samples for electron microscopy. The drop preparations may appear larger because of flattening, and because of a coat of protein adhering to such particles; metallic coating in metal-shadowed drop preparations may further increase the size of such particles. On the other hand, the alcohol-dehydration and methacrylate embedding employed in preparations of specimens for ultrathin sections may cause appreciable shrinkage of the virus particles.

The Shope rabbit papilloma virus is therefore a very small particle and develops in the nuclei of the infected cells. In this respect this virus is similar to the parotid tumor (polyoma) virus; the latter will be discussed in a separate chapter of this monograph.

Immunization of Rabbits to the Virus of Shope Papilloma

Rabbits in which papillomas developed following inoculation of the papilloma virus were found to be partially or completely resistant to reinoculation of the virus. Serum from such rabbits was found to contain antibodies capable of neutralizing the virus.

In earlier experiments it was also found that the virus had to be inoculated into the skin in order to induce tumors. Injected intravenously, intraperitoneally, or intracerebrally into an animal with normal skin, the virus caused no clinically recognizable illness and no tumors. Some of these rabbits were then tested for resistance to the virus applied to the scarified skin and were found to be completely immune. These findings suggested that multiple injections of the papilloma virus by other routes than those inducing tumors might prove to be an efficient immunizing procedure.

That rabbits could be immunized, at will, against papillomatosis, was demonstrated by Shope (1937). Two intraperitoneal injections of either infectious or non-infectious glycerinated rabbit papilloma suspensions actively immunized either domestic or cottontail rabbits against this disease.

ORAL PAPILLOMATOSIS OF RABBITS

Small, benign papillomas develop occasionally in the mouth, particularly on the inferior surface of the tongue, in domestic rabbits. Robert J. Parsons and John G. Kidd found in 1936, at the Rockefeller Institute for Medical Research in New York City, that these papillomas are caused by a filterable virus. Over 17 per cent of 385 domestic rabbits obtained from various local sources were found by these investigators to carry in the mouth, usually on the under surface of the tongue, small, pedunculated, or filiform papillomatous tumors, about 4 to 5 mm in diameter. No similar tumors were found, however, to occur spontaneously in wild cottontail rabbits. Under the microscope these tumors were diagnosed as benign papillomas. Filtrates prepared from these tumors, and inoculated by tattooing or scarification into the inferior surface of the tongue, reproduced the same tumors in either domestic or cottontail rabbits. The virus was found to be remarkably specific. The inferior surface of the tongue was most susceptible. When the filtrate was introduced into the mucous membrane covering the dorsum of the tongue, or the floor of the mouth, papillomas could also be induced, but less frequently. No papillomas resulted, however, when the filtrate was inoculated into the mucous membranes of the nose, eye conjunctiva, or genital organs. The lips and the abdominal skin were also tested and found to be completely resistant. The domestic and wild cottontail rabbits were the only susceptible hosts found. Inoculation of the filtrates into the mucous membranes of the mouth of dogs, guinea pigs, rats, or mice was without effect and did not induce lesions.

Following inoculation of the filtrate into the mouth of domestic or cottontail rabbits, small papillomatous growths appeared within 2 to 4 weeks; they slowly increased in size and then persisted, sometimes for several months or even longer, but eventually they regressed and disappeared spontaneously. Those rabbits in which the papillomas regressed were found to be resistant to the reinoculation of the same virus.

The rabbit oral papilloma virus was found to be distinct from the Shope papilloma virus. Animals immune to one were susceptible to the other; one virus induced lesions when inoculated into the mucous membrane of the mouth, the other when inoculated into the skin.

The virus of rabbit oral papilloma could be washed out of the mouth of rabbits carrying the growths. In some instances the virus could also be recovered from the mouths of apparently normal animals. Natural infection occurs most probably from rabbit to rabbit. The disease is therefore contagious.

The virus was found to be quite resistant; it could be preserved in 50 per cent glycerin solution, and it could withstand heating to 65°C for 30 minutes. A temperature of 75° to 80°C was needed to inactivate it completely.

ORAL PAPILLOMATOSIS OF DOGS

In 1898 Penberthy described an epizootic outbreak of mouth warts in otherwise healthy foxhound puppies. Only 3 out of 40 puppies in a kennel escaped the disease. M'Fadyean and Hobday (1898) obtained two wart-bearing puppies from Penberthy and were able to transfer the warts by tissue extracts applied to scarified buccal mucosa of healthy puppies. The incubation period was approximately 4 to 6 weeks. In most cases the warts disappeared spontaneously after about 6 weeks.

That the dog oral papillomas are actually caused by a filterable virus was demonstrated in 1932 by W. A. DeMonbreun and E. W. Goodpasture at the Department of Pathology, Vanderbilt Medical School, in Nashville, Tenn. In England, G. M. Findlay mentioned in 1930 that these tumors could be transmitted by a filtrate, but he did not indicate details of his transmission experiments.

The virus of dog oral papilloma was found to be readily filterable and could be serially transmitted, particularly in young puppies. Older dogs were found more resistant to inoculation. The virus was remarkably specific and induced papillomas only when inoculated into the mucous membrane of the mouth. Inoculation of the virus into the mucous membrane of vagina, into the conjunctiva, into or under the skin, did not induce papillomas. Only the dog was found to be susceptible. Inoculations of kittens, mice, rats, guinea pigs, rabbits, or monkeys remained without results.

In young puppies the filtrate induced in about 30 to 33 days small oral papillomas, resembling in appearance human warts. These lesions remained stationary for several weeks, but eventually regressed. The dogs which recovered from papillomas were without exception resistant to the reinoculation of the virus. That the virus could spread spontaneously from one dog to another became evident when mouth warts developed in healthy, non-injected, young adult dogs, following contact with infected puppies.

The virus could be preserved in equal parts of glycerin and physiological saline solution. Heating to 58°C for 30 minutes inactivated the virus.

Microscopically, the induced tumors were benign papillomata, resembling human warts. Basophilic intranuclear inclusion bodies were found in some of the large wart cells of the older lesions.

Recently, Cheville and Olson (1964) investigated the microscopic morphology of canine oral papilloma. They observed that the first tissue reaction to viral infection was hyperplasia of keratin-producing cells with no detectable virus present. As the lesion grew, large vesicular cells appeared which contained Feulgen positive inclusion material in the nucleus. There was no evidence of virus in the proliferating keratogenic cells which were responsible to a large extent for the general tissue reaction to virus infection.

Virus particles first appeared in cells of the upper stratum spinosum. In the stratum granulosum intranuclear virus particles were seen in diffuse and in linear patterns. The formation of virus arrays as seen with the electron microscope correlated with the development of basophilic inclusions seen by light microscopy.

Electron microscopy of negatively stained preparations revealed that the virus particles were spherical and measured 40 to 50 mμ in diameter, and that they were composed of a capsid consisting of an inner core and of well defined capsomeres. Further studies revealed that the canine papilloma virus is relatively stable, that it could be stored indefinitely in 50 per cent glycerin, and that it is not ether sensitive.

CUTANEOUS PAPILLOMA OF THE HORSE

Cutaneous papillomas are rather common in horses 1 to 2 years old. The papillomas, or warts, appear on the nose and around the lips, as small, elevated, circumscribed, horny masses from 2 to 10 mm in diameter; occasionally, when only a few appear, they may reach a diameter of 15 to

20 mm. They may number only a few or as many as 100 or more, and occasionally may cover the entire muzzle. As a rule these warts cause the animal little inconvenience and eventually disappear without leaving scars.

Cadeac (1901) was first to transmit experimentally a skin papilloma from one horse to another, by applying the ground papillomatous material to a scarified area of the neck. More recently, R. H. Cook and C. Olson (1951) at the Department of Animal Pathology and Hygiene, University of Nebraska, in Lincoln, transmitted horse papilloma by filtrates and thereby demonstrated that, as in other species, in the horse also, cutaneous papilloma is caused by a transmissible virus. Equine cutaneous papilloma was at that time enzootic in young horses raised at the University of Nebraska. The tumors were removed from several donors by excision, ground to a suspension with physiological saline solution, centrifuged, and filtered through Mandler filters. The bacteriologically sterile filtrates were then inoculated into scarified skin, or injected intradermally or subcutaneously in shaved areas of the neck of several young horses. Non-filtered supernatant fluid and resuspended sediment from centrifuged extracts were also used in parallel experiments. All extracts tested, including the filtrates, were infectious and induced papillomas after a latency of about two months. The largest papillomas developed following inoculation of supernatant fluid. The induced papillomas remained stationary or temporarily increased in size, but later, after 6 to 8 weeks, they gradually scaled off and eventually all regressed. Those horses in which the papillomas regressed spontaneously were found to be resistant to reinoculation of the papilloma virus.

The active agent present in the papilloma extracts was inactivated after heating to 55°C for 30 minutes. It could be stored for at least 2 months in 50 per cent glycerin at 4°C and in a suspension frozen at −35°C for 6 months.

Attempts to transmit the horse cutaneous papilloma to calves, lambs, dogs, rabbits, and guinea pigs did not succeed.

FIG. 5. BOVINE PAPILLOMA VIRUS.

(A). Section of a portion of nucleus of a cell from the upper stratum granulosum of a cutaneous bovine fibropapilloma. Virus particles about 35 mμ in diameter having a distinct hexagonal profile in crystalline formations. Magnification 78,000 ×. This fibropapilloma was induced by intradermal inoculation of finely minced cell suspension prepared from a spontaneous bovine fibropapilloma; the inoculation was made into a one-week-old calf; the wart appeared at the site of inoculation after a latency of about 3½ months, and continued to grow after the biopsy was made; however, all warts induced in cattle eventually disappear. (B). Bovine papilloma virus negatively stained with potassium phosphotungstate. Average diameter of negatively stained virus particles about 54 mμ. Magnification 156,000 ×. Electron micrographs prepared by M. Tajima, D. E. Gordon and C. Olson, Department of Veterinary Science, College of Agriculture, University of Wisconsin, Madison. (From: *Am. J. Vet. Research*, 29: 1185, 1968.)

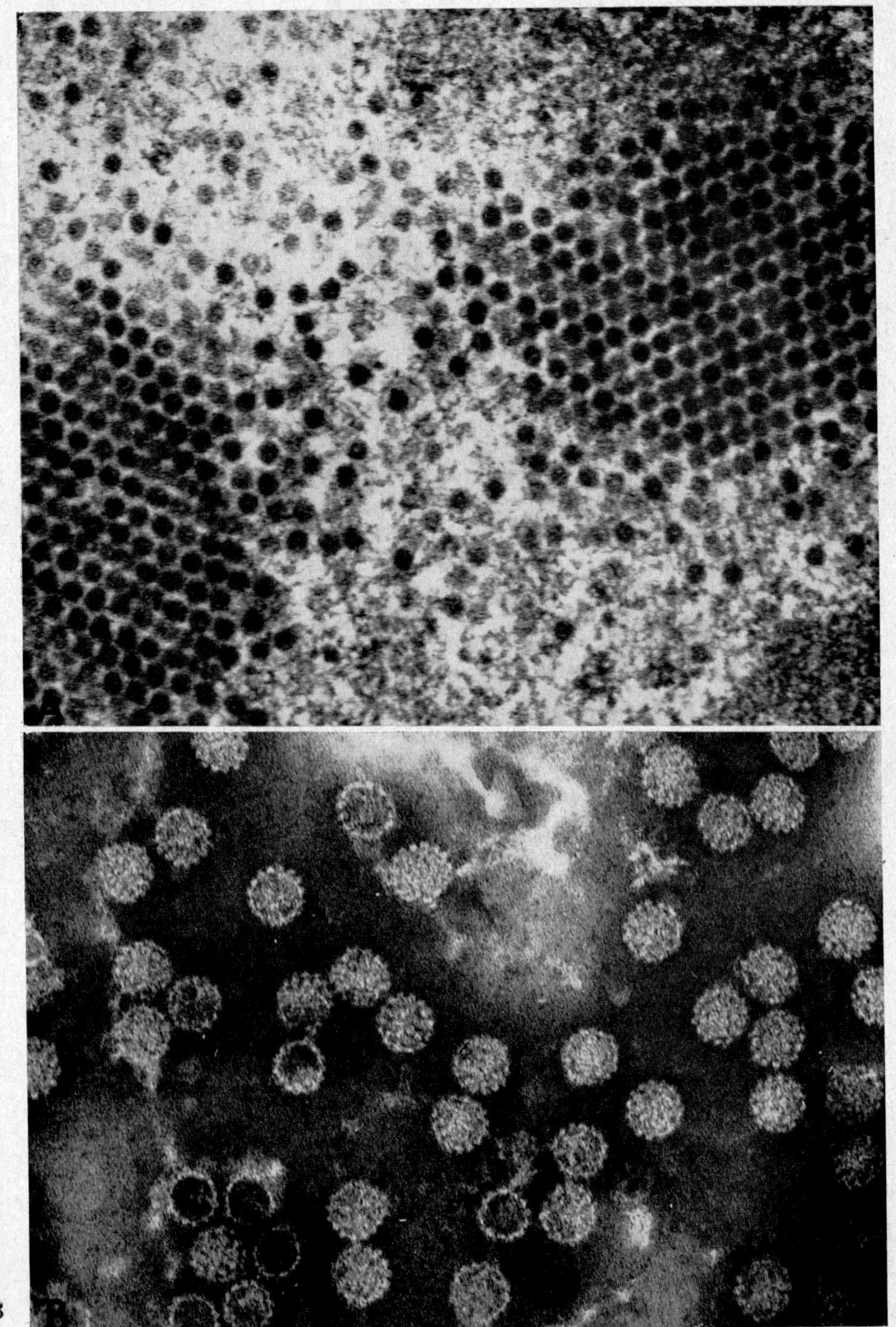

Fig. 5. Bovine Papilloma Virus

BOVINE PAPILLOMAS

Warts have long been observed in cattle. In adult cows these growths are frequently located on the udders. In young calves the warts are often located on the head, on the sides of the neck, or on the shoulders; they may spread over large areas of the skin. As the animals become older, the warts usually disappear spontaneously. In some instances, however, the warts may gradually become large and pedunculated, or they may become large cauliflowerlike tumors, several inches in diameter; they may then show a tendency to bleed and give off offensive odors, sapping the strength of the animals. Their chief damage, from an economical point of view, is observed in calfskins and cattle hides after tanning; weak spots or even holes may be found in tanned hides where the warts occurred, giving a moth-eaten appearance to the finished leather.

Warts may occur on any part of the skin in cattle, but the more likely places appear to be those parts of the body subject to abrasions of the skin. Sometimes warts develop at man-made wounds, as in the ears of young calves that have been tagged or tattooed for identification, or in some animals at the site of venipuncture or dehorning. The source of infection in such cases is not known. The virus might have existed in such animals in a latent form, or could have been introduced by contaminated instruments, or by accidental contact infection. Occasionally in certain cattle, massive growth of warts may cover large areas of the skin. Such massive infection can develop as a result of the animal scratching its back on an object contaminated with wart virus.

Cutaneous papillomatosis has been reported in cattle of most parts of the world. Warts may be quite common among cattle in some areas (U.S. Dept. Agricult., 1946. Bagdonas and Olson, 1953. Olson, 1963). In one survey (Olson *et al.*, 1962), about 1,000 beef cattle 10 to 21 months old, assembled from approximately 130 farms of Wisconsin, were examined for the presence and location of warts. About one-fourth of the cattle were or had been affected with warts. However, except for a few individual animals, the disease was not regarded as a serious problem.

As the papilloma in the dog, in the rabbit, and in the horse, and as human warts, the bovine warts could also be transmitted by inoculation of filtrates. The first successful transmission of a bovine wart by inoculation of filtrate was reported in 1920 by Magalhães in Rio de Janeiro, Brazil. A comprehensive series of experiments dealing with experimental transmission of cattle warts was carried out in 1929 by G. T. Creech in the laboratories of the U.S. Department of Agriculture, in Washington, D.C. Specimens of warts of bovine origin were obtained from cattle-slaughtering establishments in Chicago, Illinois, and in Fort Worth, Texas. The specimens were cut with scissors, ground with sterile physiological saline solution, and the extracts thus obtained were passed through Berkefeld N filter candles. The filtrates were inoculated intracutaneously on the side of neck and shoulders of young calves. A few animals were also inoculated with unfiltered extracts. As a result, 15 out of 22 inoculated cattle developed typical warty tumors 1 to 2 months after inoculation. Eight calves developed warts following inoculation of unfiltered extracts, and 7 calves developed warts following inoculation of the filtrates. In their appearance the warts induced by inoculation of either unfiltered or filtered extracts were indistinguishable from those occurring naturally. Microscopic examination revealed a structure characteristic of papillomatous growth. The induced warty tumors gradually increased in size, but later on most of them became stationary and eventually regressed spontaneously.

Immunity Following Spontaneous Regression. Cutaneous papillomatosis in cattle is nearly always a self-limiting disease and usually lasts from one to twelve months. There is considerable variation in the natural resistance of cattle to the bovine papilloma virus. Some cattle are quite resistant and may be refractory to experimental exposure. On the other hand, a few cattle are extremely susceptible. In highly susceptible animals the warts may grow to a large size, may spread to various parts of the skin, and may last for more than a year. Regarding the ultimate fate of warts in cattle, the consensus of opinion appears to be that they are likely to regress eventually.* Whether this would always happen is open to question, however, since comparatively few cattle are permitted to live out their normal life span.

Most calves in which the warts regressed were found to be immune to either natural exposure to papilloma infection or to experimental inoculation of the virus; furthermore, at least some of the calves with actively growing warts were also found to be resistant to reinoculation of the virus. The immunity which follows spontaneous regression of warts may last several years, but does not seem to be permanent. A significant number of cattle was observed to develop warts following exposure to reinfection two years after an initial episode of papillomatosis (Bagdonas and Olson, 1953, 1954. Olson *et al.*, 1960).

Electron Microscopic Studies. Spherical particles, approximately 40 $m\mu$ in diameter, presumably representing the bovine papilloma virus, were found on electron microscopic examination of ultrathin sections of bovine cutaneous fibropapillomas in the nuclei of keratinized epithelial cells, and in some instances also in the nuclei of degenerating fibroblasts (Brobst and Hinsman, 1966. Fujimoto and Olson, 1966). Virus particles were found in naturally occurring and also in experimentally induced bovine

* Wayne A. Anderson, U.S. Dept. of Agriculture, Animal Disease Research Laboratory, Denver, Col., and Carl Olson, Dept. of Veterinary Science, University of Wisconsin, Madison. Personal communications to the author.

cutaneous warts. In general, the number of virus particles was rather small. The particles were most numerous in the stratum granulosum and in the corneal layer. In this respect these observations were similar to those previously reported in studies dealing with electron microscopy of papillomas in rabbits and in other species.

The ultrastructure of the normal bovine skin is similar to that of human skin. The layers of bovine epidermis are the stratum germinativum, stratum spinosum, stratum granulosum, and stratum corneum.

In electron microscopic studies of bovine papilloma extracts employing the negative staining method, the virus particles were found to have a diameter of approximately 47 mμ, and to be formed of 42 capsomeres. Accordingly, the bovine papilloma virus would appear to belong to the same group as the viruses of human warts, Shope papilloma, and S.V. 40 (Lévy *et al.*, 1963).

Both degenerative and proliferative changes were found in the infected cells. The degenerative changes were aggregation and margination of chromatin in the nucleus; in addition, epithelial cells had cytoplasmic vacuolization, focal necrosis, increased electron-opaque globules, and dilatation of intercellular spaces. When these changes were marked, the cells could be recognized as "pale cells" by light microscopy, and usually occurred in groups. Viral multiplication appeared confined to these degenerating cells, and no viral particles could be found in the proliferating cells (Fujimoto and Olson, 1966).

Bladder Tumors, and Chronic Enzootic Hematuria in Cattle. Tumors of the urinary bladder in cattle are common in certain parts of the world. One of the characteristic manifestations of this disease is presence of blood in the urine of the affected animals; for that reason the common designation of this disease is "chronic enzootic hematuria." In certain endemic areas, usually in wooded regions in mountainous country, the incidence of bladder tumors in cattle may be very high; up to 90 per cent of animals over 2 years old may be affected. The disease has been observed in the Pacific Northwest coastal areas of the United States and Canada, also in France, Germany, Italy, Yugoslavia, Turkey, India, and Formosa. The etiology of the naturally occurring bladder tumors in cattle is not known.

The presence of a high incidence of these tumors in so-called "hematuria farms" and in certain wooded mountainous areas could be related to the ingestion of bracken fern (*Pteris aquilina*) by cattle feeding on pastures in which this plant is growing. This plant may contain carcinogenic components which may induce bladder tumors after prolonged oral ingestion (Rosenberger and Heeschen, 1960. Pamukcu, 1962, 1963. Pamukcu *et al.*, 1966, 1967. Döbereiner *et al.*, 1966).

This explanation of endemic occurrence of bladder tumors in certain areas where bracken fern is growing may represent one factor contributing to the development of this disease and would not necessarily exclude the possible viral etiology of this neoplasm. Bladder tumors, and hematuria resulting from the presence of such neoplasms, have also been observed in cattle that had not been exposed to bracken fern.

Development of Urinary Bladder Tumors in Cattle Following Submucosal Inoculation of Bovine Cutaneous Papilloma. Olson and his coworkers (1959) at the Department of Veterinary Science, University of Wisconsin, in Madison, induced polyps of the mucosa and fibroma-like tumors in the urinary bladder of calves, following injection of extracts prepared from bovine cutaneous papilloma. The extracts, which consisted of suspensions of bovine wart tissue stored in 50 per cent glycerin, were inoculated in the submucosa of urinary bladder either by suprapubic cystostomy or, in females, transurethrally. Thirteen out of 15 calves which received bovine papilloma extracts developed tumors of urinary bladders. The tumors and polyps thus induced in the urinary bladder persisted, some for prolonged periods of time, but eventually they regressed; at certain stages, however, they were similar in their morphology to naturally occurring bladder tumors (Brobst and Olson, 1965).

In more recent experiments, the presence of a transmissible oncogenic virus could be demonstrated in naturally-occurring bovine urinary bladder tumors; this virus was found to be capable of inducing not only polypoid tumors in the bladder, but also fibropapillomas of the skin and vagina. In experiments performed by Olson, Pamukcu and Brobst (1965) suspensions of 6 field cases of bovine urinary bladder tumors induced fibropapillomas of the skin and vagina, as well as polypoid tumors and fibromas in the urinary bladders of test calves. The bladder tumors used for the transmission experiments came from cattle raised in areas where chronic enzootic hematuria was common; these tumors were naturally occurring hemagiomas, papillomas, and carcinomas. The extracts were inoculated intradermally in the skin and vaginal wall, or rubbed into scarified skin. The inoculation into the bladder was made into the submucosa either through a cystoscope, or following suprapubic cystostomy. The incubation period ranged from 25 to 111 days. Three serial passages of an isolate were made. The infective agent, which was filterable, resembled the bovine wart virus in its behavior in test calves. In experiments carried out by Pamukcu (1962, 1963), inoculation of extracts prepared from naturally occurring bladder tumors, obtained from cattle in Turkey, also induced fibropapillomas in the skin and vaginal mucosa of test calves.

Transmission of Bovine Papilloma to Horses. Bovine papilloma extracts were found to induce sarcoma-like growth following inoculation into the skin of the horse (Olson and Cook, 1951). Centrifuged, fresh, or glycerinated extracts, prepared from field cases of bovine cutaneous papillomas, were inoculated intradermally or placed on scarified skin in young horses. Small firm nodules appeared at the site of inoculation after 2 to 4 weeks and gradually attained a size of 2 to 3 cm in diameter after 1 to 2 months. In most horses the induced nodules disappeared 3 to 5 months after their initial appearance. In one horse the induced tumor grew rapidly, recurred after excision, attaining a diameter of about 5 cm, and persisted for over 18 months. The tumor was eventually excised; microscopic examination revealed a sarcoma-like morphology resembling naturally occurring equine sarcoid (Olson, 1948). In another experiment, glycerinated material from one field case of equine sarcoid was placed on 4 susceptible horses; growth similar to that resulting from inoculation of bovine papilloma extracts developed in one horse at 2 sites of intradermal inoculation.

Although the horse appears quite susceptible to the bovine papilloma virus, recovery of the virus from the tumors induced in the horse, and transmission back to the cattle did not always succeed. Twelve calves were inoculated with extracts prepared from the sarcoma-like growth induced in the horse with bovine papilloma extracts, and only 4 of the 12 inoculated cattle developed warts (Olson *et al.*, 1960).

Transmission of Bovine Papilloma to Hamsters. Inoculation of extracts prepared from bovine papillomas into newborn hamsters caused the development of progressively growing fibromas in most of the inoculated animals. In experiments carried out by Friedmann and his colleagues (1963) in the Laboratories of Experimental Hematology at Saint-Louis Hospital in Paris, extracts prepared from bovine papillomas were inoculated intradermally, by superficial scarification, into the skin of 16 suckling, less than 2-day-old, hamsters. As a result, 15 hamsters developed tumors at the site of inoculation after a latency varying from 2 to $5\frac{1}{2}$ months. Microscopic examination revealed that these tumors were fibromas. The tumors grew progressively and none of them regressed during an observation period extending from 3 to 6 months.

In another study carried out in the same laboratories (Lasneret *et al.*, 1965), centrifuged cell-free bovine papilloma extracts were inoculated into suckling, less than 8-day-old, hamsters. In one experimental group, the extracts were inoculated by superficial skin scarification into 34 suckling hamsters, and 33 animals developed single or multiple nodules at the site of inoculation after a latency of 2 months. Most of these tumors grew progressively; only 4 regressed. In another group, the extracts were inoculated subcutaneously into 9 suckling hamsters, and all animals developed progressively growing tumors after 4 months. Following intraperitoneal inoculation, 2 out of 6 inoculated hamsters developed disseminated papillomas on the eyelids, on the muzzle, and also on the feet. Following intracerebral inoculation, two animals developed intracranial fibrosarcomas, and several other hamsters developed disseminated fibro-papillomas after a latency of 4 months.

Adult animals were much less susceptible. When 10 young adult, 2-month-old, hamsters were inoculated subcutaneously, only one developed a tumor after a latency of $4\frac{1}{2}$ months.

Except for the two fibrosarcomas induced by intracerebral inoculation, all other tumors induced in hamsters had the morphology of fibromas; however, many of them grew progressively infiltrating the surrounding tissues, and often attained considerable volume, in some instances becoming almost as large as the tumor-carrying animals. Robl and Olson (1967) observed a case in which the tumor induced by the bovine papilloma extract weighed 150 grams, whereas the rest of the hamster weighed only 100 grams.

The tumors induced in hamsters could not be transmitted to other hamsters by filtrates; however, they could be transplanted from hamster to hamster by cell-graft, particularly when newborn animals were inoculated. Newborn hamsters were uniformly susceptible to the implantation of tumor cell suspensions or fragments of tumor tissue; adult hamsters were more resistant. The latency was long and lasted up to 6 months when the initial tumor implantation was made; however, on second, third, and subsequent serial hamster-to-hamster tumor transplantations, the latency became much shorter and did not usually exceed one month; furthermore, after the second or third serial passage in hamsters, adult animals could also be used for tumor transplantation.

Similar results were observed in other laboratories (Wooding, 1964. Robl and Olson, 1967). In experiments performed at the Department of Veterinary Science, University of Wisconsin, in Madison, by Robl and Olson (1967), hamsters of any age, including adult animals, were found to be susceptible to subcutaneous inoculation of bovine papilloma extracts. Up to 90 per cent of inoculated hamsters developed tumors after a rather long latency of about 9 months. Microscopic examination revealed that the induced tumors were fibromas. About 10 per cent of the inoculated animals developed metastatic tumors in the lungs and in the liver; in addition, some animals developed papillomas on their paws.

The tumors induced in hamsters with bovine papilloma extracts could be transplanted to other hamsters by cell-graft; however, hamster tumors could not be transmitted back to cattle.

Inoculation of Bovine Papilloma Extracts into Newborn Mice. Bovine papilloma extracts were also inoculated into newborn mice of strains C57 Black and C3H (Boiron *et al.*, 1964. Friedmann *et al.*, 1965). Mice of strain C57 Black were found to be resistant; a few tumors could be induced in mice of strain C3H. The tumors appeared at the site of inoculation, gradually increased in size, and did not regress. Microscopic examination revealed that these tumors were fibromas, very similar in their morphology to neoplasms induced in hamsters with the same bovine papilloma extracts. However, mice were much less susceptible than hamsters, and only a few of them developed tumors following inoculation of bovine papilloma extracts.

Transformation of Mouse and Calf Cells in Tissue Culture Following Inoculation of Bovine Papilloma Extracts. Bovine papilloma extracts were inoculated into embryonic mouse cells, and also into fetal bovine conjunctiva and embryonic calf cells grown in tissue culture. Distinct morphologic transformation of the inoculated cells resulted (Thomas *et al.*, 1963, 1964). These experiments suggested that the bovine papilloma virus may induce transformation of fetal mouse and calf cells *in vitro*.

WARTS AND PAPILLOMAS IN MAN

Warts and papillomas are common in humans. It appears that, as in other animal species, in humans also these growths are caused by transmissible viruses. In this group belong the common human wart (*verruca vulgaris* and *verruca plana*), the condyloma acuminatum ("venereal wart") growing usually on the skin and mucous membranes in the vicinity of genital organs, as well as the papillomas, including those growing on mucous membranes, such as laryngeal papilloma.

Transmission by Filtrates. The transmission by experimental inoculation of warts and papillomatous tumors in man has long been observed (Blank *et al.*, 1955. Blank, 1959). Variot, in 1894, and two years later Jadassohn, found that common warts, so often observed in man and especially in children, can readily be transmitted from man to man by inoculation. Ciuffo observed in 1907 that human warts are transmissible from man to man by inoculation of cell-free filtrates that had been passed through infusorial earth filters retaining all visible cells and microbes.

The experiments on the transmission of human warts by filtrates were confirmed and extended in 1919 by Wile and Kingery in the United States. These authors were able to transmit human warts successively, through several human volunteers, by inoculating intradermally cell-free filtrates prepared from freshly removed warts. Typical warts, clinically indistinguishable from those occurring naturally, developed at the site of inoculation after periods of latency varying from 3 weeks to 6 months.

At about the same time, E. V. Ullman, in Vienna, was able to transmit a human papilloma by transplantation of a cell suspension, and later on by a cell-free filtrate. On June 2, 1921, Ullman operated upon a 6-year-old boy whose larynx and windpipe were almost filled with papillomatous tumors; the larynx was therefore excochleated; a tumor fragment was removed and ground with physiological saline solution; the resulting suspension was then aspirated into a small syringe and immediately inoculated into the skin of the left arm of Dr. Ullman. After 3 months typical warts appeared at the site of inoculation, slightly elevated over the surface of the skin. These warts were excised, again ground with saline solution, and inoculated into the skin of the left arm of Dr. Adler, a colleague of Dr. Ullman. This time, after 5 weeks only, papillomatous tumors developed at the site of inoculation; these papillomas grew so rapidly, spreading beyond the inoculation area, that it was decided to remove them promptly. The excised papillomatous tumors were again ground with saline solution, but this time the resulting cell suspension was passed through a bacteria-tight filter, retaining all cells and visible microbes. The filtrate was now inoculated into the skin of the arm and buttock of Dr. Ullman, and also into the skin of one of his assistants. As a result, one papilloma appeared on the arm after 5 weeks, and another, 3 weeks later, on the buttock. In the meantime, the boy from whom the tumor had been originally removed, developed a typical wart on the skin of his cheek, where the patient was scratched during the operation by an instrument used for the removal of the tumor.

Other common papillomatous tumors of man were, in the meantime, also found to be readily transmissible by inoculation. Thus, in 1917, Waelsch transplanted into human volunteers condyloma acuminatum, a common papillomatous growth developing quite often in the moist skin on the edge of the mucous membranes of the external genital organs of young men and women. Waelsch removed the tumor from the genital organs of a medical student, prepared a cell suspension, and inoculated it into the skin of his own arm, as well as that of one of his colleagues; the third volunteer was a young girl who was inoculated with the same suspension into the mucous membrane adjacent to the external orifice of vagina. After a period of latency of 3 months, Waelsch developed a flat wart on the skin of his arm at the site of inoculation. This wart was of a brown color and it increased slowly in size; after 2 years, however, the wart regressed spontaneously, leaving only a slight discoloration of the skin locally. The colleague of Dr. Waelsch developed a similar flat wart which also disappeared after 2 years approximately. The girl developed at the site of inoculation a typical papillomatous condyloma acuminatum. Thus, the transplantation of condyloma acuminatum from man to man appeared to result in the development of either a flat wart or that of a typical condyloma acuminatum, according to the inoculated site.

A few years later, in 1924, Serra demonstrated that condyloma acuminatum in man is readily transmissible from one person to another by cell-free filtrates. This observation was later confirmed by other investigators.

More recently, Goldschmidt and Kligman (1958) confirmed the work of earlier investigators and observed that inoculation of extracts prepared from moist genital warts (condylomata acuminata) into the skin of adult humans resulted in the development of typical common warts.

Inclusion bodies have been observed in human warts examined with the light microscope (Bloch and Godman, 1957).

Electron Microscopic Studies. Preliminary electron microscopic studies of shadowed drop preparations of centrifuged extracts from human warts and papillomas were made by Strauss (1949, 1950), Melnick (1952), and their colleagues. These studies revealed the presence of innumerable spherical particles which were frequently arranged in crystalline arrays forming rows of hexagonal figures. When packed tightly, the particles had an average diameter of about 52 mμ. Bunting (1953), using the newly introduced technique of ultrathin sections, examined 3 human papillomas. Although the preservation of tissues and the quality of electron micrographs were not yet quite satisfactory in these initial studies, the presence of intranuclear arrays of closely packed virus particles having a diameter of approximately 38 mμ could be recognized. The smaller size of particles observed on ultrathin sections as compared with larger size previously reported on the basis of studies dealing with examination of shadowed drop preparations could be attributed to differences in preparative procedures. More recently Charles (1960) published electron microscopic studies of ultrathin sections of 2 human warts and observed convincing evidence of the presence of intranuclear virus particles having a diameter of about 33 mμ. In similar electron microscopic studies of ultrathin sections of human warts removed from the heel and finger, and carried out by Chapman and his coworkers (1963), virus particles were found in both the nucleus and cytoplasm. Extraordinarily dense aggregates of desmosomes were associated with the cells, and these persisted as long as the cells could be distinguished. The virus particles had a maximum diameter of approximately 38 mμ. Nonviral intranuclear inclusions were identified and were probably distinct from the nucleolus.

Williams and his colleagues (1961) examined 4 human warts using the technique of ultrathin sections. The nuclei of some of the cells in the anular layer, close to the keratin layer, contained uniform particles of a mean diameter of 56 mμ. In another series prepared from several human warts, either shadowed preparations were made, or specimens were prepared by the negative staining method. In shadowed preparations the average diameter of particles in closely packed arrays was 55 mμ. Electron microscopic examinations of specimens prepared by the negative staining method revealed that the surface of the particles is composed of symmetrically arranged capsomeres; it appeared that the shell, or capsid, of the particles consists of 42 capsomeres arranged in 5:3:2 axial symmetry. The overall diameter of the particles had an average value of 55 mμ, the same as that observed in shadowed preparations. The number and arrangement of the capsomeres on the wart virus was the same as that established by Wildy and his colleagues (1960) for the polyoma virus; however, the polyoma virus is smaller, having an average diameter of 45 mμ.

A detailed electron microscopic study of ultrathin sections of human warts and of the sites of virus production was carried out by Almeida, Howatson, and Williams (1962). These studies revealed that human wart virus is formed in the nucleoli of cells in the stratum spinosum. Virus particles subsequently spread throughout the nuclei of cells in the stratum granulosum and persist as closely packed aggregates embedded in the substance of the stratum corneum. The formation and development of virus arrays as seen in the electron microscope is correlated with the development of the basophilic inclusions as seen in the light microscope. Osmiophilic intranuclear inclusions corresponding to the eosinophilic inclusions of light microscopy consist of keratin-like material and are not directly related to the virus.

The sequence of development of virus in the human wart resembles very closely that described for Shope papilloma virus in rabbit papillomas (Stone *et al.*, 1959). In humans and in rabbits specific particles are first seen in association with the nucleoli of cells in the stratum spinosum. The subsequent spread of the particles throughout the nuclei in the stratum granulosum, and eventual dissolution of all cell constituents leaving only aggregates of virus embedded in keratin in the stratum corneum at the surface of the skin and warts, is the same in both species. A further point of resemblance between the human wart and the rabbit papilloma is that no specific particles are detectable in proliferating cells, but they are apparent, and multiply, in cells that are undergoing degeneration and necrosis (Noyes, 1959). Similar observations have been made recently in electron microscopic studies of bovine cutaneous papilloma (Brobst and Hinsman, 1966. Fujimoto and Olson, 1966).

FIG. 6. HUMAN WART VIRUS.

(A). Section of a cell from granular layer of a human wart, showing intranuclear arrays of spherical virus particles (arrow); average diameter of virus particles on ultrathin sections about 40 to 54 mμ. Magnification 20,000 ×. (B). Human wart virus particles in a negatively stained preparation treated with sodium phosphotungstate. Average diameter of virus particles in negatively stained preparations about 55 mμ. Magnification 240,000 ×. Electron micrographs prepared by A. F. Howatson, Ontario Cancer Institute, Toronto, Canada.

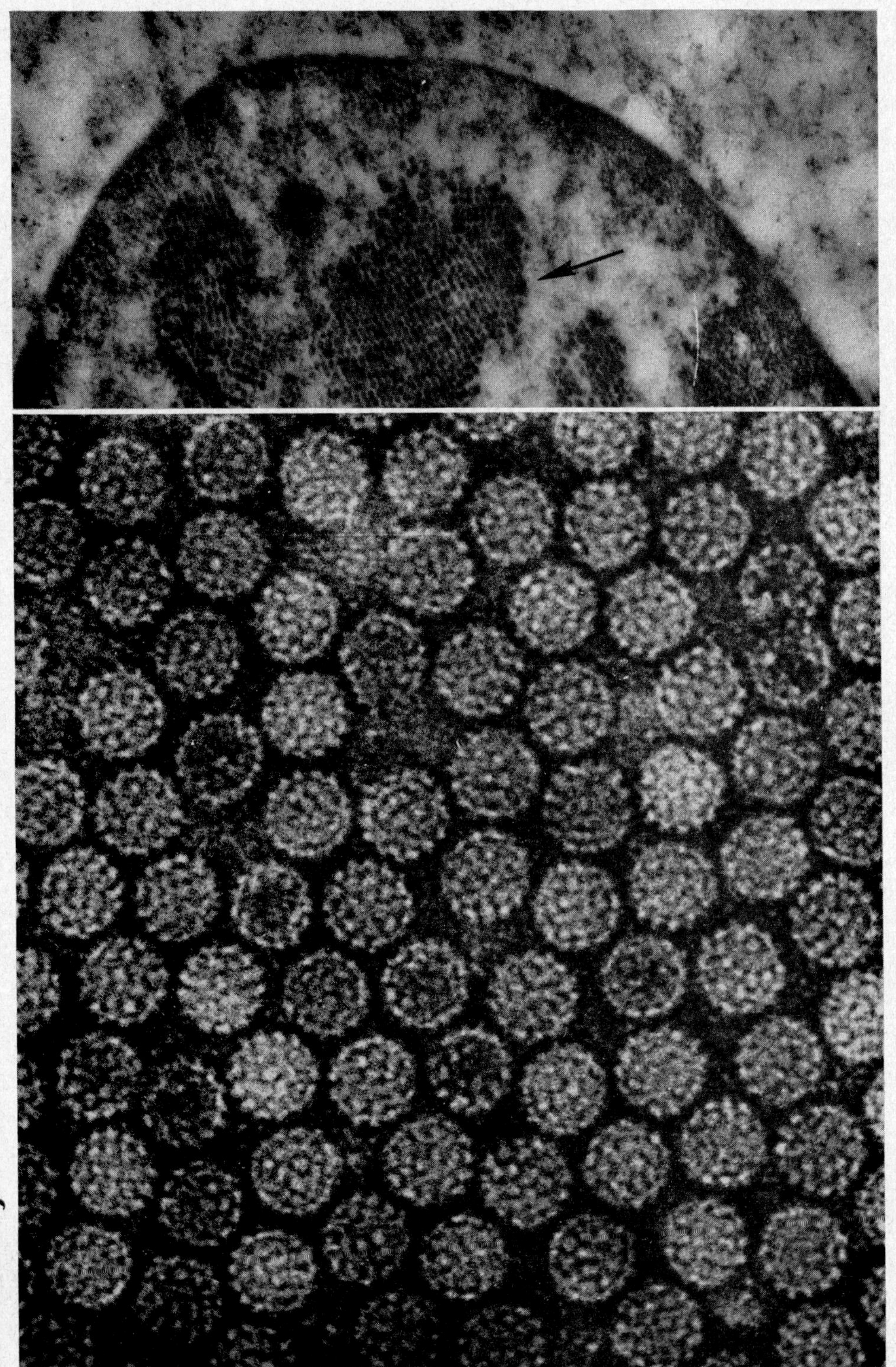

D

Fig. 6. Human Wart Virus

REFERENCES

ALMEIDA, J. D., HOWATSON, A. F., and WILLIAMS, M. G., Electron microscope study of human warts; Sites of virus production and nature of the inclusion bodies. *J. Invest. Dermat.*, **38**: 337–345, 1962.

BAGDONAS, V., and OLSON, C., JR., Observations on the epizootiology of cutaneous papillomatosis (warts) of cattle. *J. Am. Vet. Med. Assoc.*, **122**: 393–397, 1953.

BAGDONAS, V., and OLSON, C., JR., Observations on immunity in cutaneous bovine papillomatosis. *Am. J. Vet. Research*, **15**: 240–245, 1954.

BEARD, J. W., Review. Purified animal viruses. *J. Immunol.*, **58**: 49–108, 1948.

BEARD, J. W., and ROUS, P., A virus-induced mammalian growth with the characters of a tumor (The Shope rabbit papilloma). II. Experimental alterations of the growth on the skin: Morphological considerations: The phenomena of retrogression. *J. Exp. Med.*, **60**: 723–740, 1934.

BLANK, H., Common viral diseases of the skin. *Med. Clin. N. America*, **43**: 1401–1418, 1959.

BLANK, H., and RAKE, G., *Viral and Rickettsial Diseases of the Skin, Eye and Mucous Membranes of Man*, p. 285, Little, Brown & Co., Boston, 1955.

BLOCH, D. P., and GODMAN, G. C., A cytological and cytochemical investigation of development of the viral papilloma of human skin. *J. Exp. Med.*, **105**: 161–176, 1957.

BOIRON, M., LÉVY, J.-P., THOMAS, M., FRIEDMANN, J.-C., and BERNARD, J., Some properties of bovine papilloma virus. *Nature*, **201**: 423–424, 1964.

BROBST, D., and HINSMAN, E. J., Electron microscopy of the bovine cutaneous papilloma. *Path. Vet.*, **3**: 193–207, 1966.

BROBST, D. F., and OLSON, C., Histopathology of urinary bladder tumors induced by bovine cutaneous papilloma agent. *Cancer Research*, **25**: 12–19, 1965.

BUNTING, H., Close-packed array of virus-like particles within cells of a human skin papilloma. *Proc. Soc. Exp. Biol. & Med.*, **84**: 327–332, 1953.

CADEAC, *., Sur la transmission expérimentale des papillomes des diverses espèces. *Bull. Soc. sc. vet. d. Lyon*, **4**: 280–286, 1901.

CHAPMAN, G. B., DRUSIN, L. M., and TODD, J. E., Fine structure of the human wart. *Am. J. Path.*, **42**: 619–642, 1963.

CHARLES, A., Electron microscope observations on the human wart. *Dermatologica*, **121**: 193–203, 1960.

CHEVILLE, N. F., and OLSON, C., Epithelial and fibroblastic proliferation in bovine cutaneous papillomatosis. *Path. Vet.*, **1**: 248–257, 1964.

CHEVILLE, N. F., and OLSON, C., Cytology of the canine oral papilloma. *Am. J. Path.*, **45**: 849–872, 1964.

CIUFFO, G., Innesto positivo con filtrate di verruca vulgare. *Giornale Italiano delle Malattie Veneree*, **42**: 12–17, 1907.

COOK, R. H., and OLSON, C., JR., Experimental transmission of cutaneous papilloma of the horse. *Am. J. Path.*, **27**: 1087–1097, 1951.

CREECH, G. T., Experimental studies of the etiology of common warts in cattle. *J. Agr. Research*, **39**: 723–737, 1929.

DEMONBREUN, W. A., and GOODPASTURE, E. W., Infectious oral papillomatosis of dogs. *Am. J. Path.*, **8**: 43–55, 1932.

DÖBEREINER, J., OLSON, C., BROWN, R. R., PRICE, J. M., and YESS, N., Metabolites in urine of cattle with experimental bladder lesions and fed bracken fern. *Pesq. Agropec. Brasil.*, **1**: 189–199, 1966.

* No first name initial in original publication.

FINDLAY, G. M., Warts. Chapter XVIII, **7**: 252–258, in *A System of Bacteriology in Relation to Medicine*, Great Britain Medical Research Council, London, 1930.

FRIEDMANN, J.-C., LÉVY, J.-P., LASNERET, J., THOMAS, M., BOIRON, M., and BERNARD, J., Induction de fibromes sous-cutanés chez le hamster doré par inoculation d'extraits acellulaires de papillomes bovins. *Compt. Rend. Acad. Sci. (Paris)*, **257**: 2328–2331, 1963.

FRIEDMANN, J.-C., LASNERET, J., GIBEAUX, L., and BOIRON, M., Développement de fibromes prolifératifs chez la souris à l'aide d'extraits acellulaires de papillomes bovins et leur transformation maligne par greffes isologues. *Rec. Med. Vet.*, **141**: 115–122, 1965.

FUJIMOTO, Y., and OLSON, C., The fine structure of the bovine wart. *Path. Vet.*, **3**: 659–684, 1966.

GOLDSCHMIDT, H., and KLIGMAN, A. M., Experimental inoculation of humans with ectodermotropic viruses. *J. Invest. Dermat.*, **31**: 175–182, 1958.

HAGUENAU, F., BONAR, R. A., BEARD, D., and BEARD, J. W., Ultrastructure of the rabbit papilloma virus. *J. Nat. Cancer Inst.*, **24**: 873–881, 1960.

HOWATSON, A. F., Viruses connected with tumours and warts. *Brit. Med. Bull.*, **18**: 193–198, 1962.

JADASSOHN, (J.),* Sind die *Verrucae vulgares* übertragbar? *Verhandl. d. deutsch. derm. Gesellsch.*, **5**: 497–512, 1896.

KAHLER, H., and LLOYD, B. J., Electron microscopic study of the Shope papilloma virus. *J. Nat. Cancer Inst.*, **12**: 1167–1175, 1952.

LASNERET, J., CHUAT, J.-C., LÉVY, J.-P., and BOIRON, M., Étude des tumeurs provoquées chez le hamster par le virus de la papillomatose bovine. *Path. Biol.*, **13**: 1174–1179, 1965.

LÉVY, J.-P., BOIRON, M., HOLLMANN, K. H., HAGUENAU, F., THOMAS, M., and FRIEDMANN, J.-C., Étude au microscope électronique par coloration négative du virus de la papillomatose bovine. *J. Microscopie*, **2**: 175–182, 1963.

LUCKÉ, B., RATCLIFFE, H., and BREEDIS, C., Transmissible papilloma in monkeys. (Abstract). *Fed. Proc.*, **9**: 337, 1950.

M'FADYEAN, J., and HOBDAY, F., Note on the experimental transmission of warts in the dog. *J. Comp. Path. & Therap.*, **11**: 341–344, 1898.

MAGALHÃES, O., Verruga dos bovideos. *Brasil-Medico*, **34**: 430–431, 1920.

MELNICK, J. L., BUNTING, H., BANFIELD, W. G., STRAUSS, M. J., and GAYLORD, W. H., Electron microscopy of viruses of human papilloma, molluscum contagiosum, and vaccinia, including observations on the formation of virus within the cell. *Ann. N.Y. Acad. Sci.*, **54**: 1214–1225, 1952.

MOORE, D. H., STONE, R. S., SHOPE, R. E., and GELBER, D., Ultrastructure and site of formation of rabbit papilloma virus. *Proc. Soc. Exp. Biol. & Med.*, **101**: 575–578, 1959.

NARTSISSOV, N. V., The complement fixation reaction in relation to rabbit papilloma. pp. 220–225, in: *Pathogenesis and Immunology of Tumours*, Edit. by G. V. Vygodchikov (translated from Russian), p. 258, Pergamon Press, New York and London, 1959.

NOYES, W. F., Studies on the Shope rabbit papilloma virus. II. The location of infective virus in papillomas of the cottontail rabbit. *J. Exp. Med.*, **109**: 423–428, 1959.

NOYES, W. F., and MELLORS, R. C., Fluorescent antibody detection of the antigens of the Shope papilloma virus in papillomas of the wild and domestic rabbit. *J. Exp. Med.*, **106**: 555–562, 1957.

* No first name initial in original publication.

OLSON, C., JR., Equine sarcoid, a cutaneous neoplasm. *Am. J. Vet. Research*, **9**: 333–341, 1948.

OLSON, C., Cutaneous papillomatosis in cattle and other animals. *Ann. N.Y. Acad. Sci.*, **108**: 1042–1056, 1963.

OLSON, C., JR., and COOK, R. H., Cutaneous sarcoma-like lesions of the horse caused by the agent of bovine papilloma. *Proc. Soc. Exp. Biol. & Med.*, **77**: 281–284, 1951.

OLSON, C., JR., and PALIONIS, T., The transmission of proliferative stomatitis of cattle. *J. Am. Vet. Med. Assoc.*, **123**: 419–426, 1953.

OLSON, C., LUEDKE, A. J., and BROBST, D. F., Incidence of bovine cutaneous papillomatosis in beef cattle. *J. Am. Vet. Med. Assoc.*, **140**: 50–52, 1962.

OLSON, C., PAMUKCU, A. M., BROBST, D. F., KOWALCZYK, T., SATTER, E. J., and PRICE, J. M., A urinary bladder tumor induced by a bovine cutaneous papilloma agent. *Cancer Research*, **19**: 779–782, 1959.

OLSON, C., PAMUKCU, A. M., and BROBST, D. F., Papilloma-like virus from bovine urinary bladder tumors. *Cancer Research*, **25**: 840–849, 1965.

OLSON, C., SEGRE, D., and SKIDMORE, L. V., Cutaneous papillomatosis (warts) of cattle. pp. 219–226 in: *Proc. U.S. Livestock Sanitary Assoc., 58th Ann. Meeting*, Nov., 1954.

OLSON, C., SEGRE, D., and SKIDMORE, L. V., Further observations on immunity to bovine cutaneous papillomatosis. *Am. J. Vet. Research*, **21**: 233–242, 1960.

PAMUKCU, A. M., Tumors of the urinary bladder in cattle, with special reference to etiology and histogenesis. *Acta Internat. Union Against Cancer*, **18**: 625–638, 1962.

PAMUKCU, A. M., Epidemiologic studies on urinary bladder tumors in Turkish cattle. *Ann. N.Y. Acad. Sci.*, **108**: 938–947, 1963.

PAMUKCU, A. M., GÖKSOY, S. K., and PRICE, J. M., Urinary bladder neoplasms induced by feeding bracken fern (*Pteris aquilina*) to cows. *Cancer Research*, **27**: 917–924, 1967.

PAMUKCU, A. M., OLSON, C., and PRICE, J. M., Assay of fractions of bovine urine for carcinogenic activity after feeding bracken fern (*Pteris aquilina*). *Cancer Research*, **26**: 1745–1753, 1966.

PARISH, W. E., A transmissible genital papilloma of the pig resembling condyloma acuminatum of man. *J. Path. & Bact.*, **81**: 331–345, 1961.

PARSONS, R. J., and KIDD, J. G., Tissue affinity of Shope papilloma virus. *Proc. Soc. Exp. Biol. & Med.*, **35**: 438–441, 1936.

PARSONS, R. J., and KIDD, J. G., A virus causing oral papillomatosis in rabbits. *Proc. Soc. Exp. Biol. & Med.*, **35**: 441–443, 1936.

PARSONS, R. J., and KIDD, J. G., Oral papillomatosis of rabbits: A virus disease. *J. Exp. Med.*, **77**: 233–250, 1943.

PENBERTHY, J., Contagious warty tumours in dogs. *J. Comp. Path. & Therap.*, **11**: 363–365, 1898.

RICHTER, W. R., SHIPKOWITZ, N. L., and RDZOK, E. J., Oral papillomatosis of the rabbit. An electron microscope study. *Lab. Invest.*, **13**: 430–438, 1964.

ROBL, M. G., and OLSON, C., Oncogenic action of bovine papilloma virus in hamsters. *Cancer Research*, **28**: 1596–1604, 1968.

ROSENBERGER, G., and HEESCHEN, W., Adlerfarn (Pteris aquilina)—die Ursache des sog. Stallrotes der Rinder (Haematuria vesicalis bovis chronica). *Deutsche tierärztl. Wochenschr.*, **67**: 201–208, 1960.

ROUS, P., and BEARD, J. W., Carcinomatous changes in virus-induced papillomas of the skin of the rabbit. *Proc. Soc. Exp. Biol. & Med.*, **32**: 578–580, 1934.

ROUS, P., and BEARD, J. W., A virus-induced mammalian growth with the characters of a tumor (The Shope rabbit papilloma). I. The growth on implantation within favorable hosts. *J. Exp. Med.*, **60**: 701–722, 1934.

ROUS, P., and BEARD, J. W., A virus-induced mammalian growth with the characters of a tumor (The Shope rabbit papilloma). III. Further characters of the growth. General discussion. *J. Exp. Med.*, **60**: 741–766, 1934.

ROUS, P., and BEARD, J. W., The progression to carcinoma of virus-induced rabbit papillomas (Shope). *J. Exp. Med.*, **62**: 523–548, 1935.

SCHLESINGER, M., and ANDREWES, C. H., The filtration and centrifugation of the viruses of rabbit fibroma and rabbit papilloma. *J. Hyg.*, **37**: 521–526, 1937.

SERRA, A., Studi sul virus della verruca, del papilloma, del condiloma acuminato. Etiologia, patogenesi, filtrabilita. *Giornale Italiano delle Malattie Veneree e della Pelle*, **65**: 1808–1814, 1924.

SHARP, D. G., TAYLOR, A. R., HOOK, A. E., and BEARD, J. W., Rabbit papilloma and vaccinia viruses and T_2 bacteriophage of *E. coli* in "shadow" electron micrographs. *Proc. Soc. Exp. Biol. & Med.*, **61**: 259–265, 1946.

SHOPE, R. E., Infectious papillomatosis of rabbits. *J. Exp. Med.*, **58**: 607–624, 1933.

SHOPE, R. E., Immunization of rabbits to infectious papillomatosis. *J. Exp. Med.*, **65**: 219–231, 1937.

SHOPE, R. E., Comments (in "Symposium on the possible role of viruses in cancer"). *Cancer Research*, **20**: 742–743, 1960.

STONE, R. S., SHOPE, R. E., and MOORE, D. H., Electron microscope study of the development of the papilloma virus in the skin of the rabbit. *J. Exp. Med.*, **110**: 543–546, 1959.

STRAUSS, M. J., BUNTING, H., and MELNICK, J. L., Virus-like particles and inclusion bodies in skin papillomas. *J. Invest. Dermat.*, **15**: 433–444, 1950.

STRAUSS, M. J., SHAW, E. W., BUNTING, H., and MELNICK, J. L., "Crystalline" virus-like particles from skin papillomas characterized by intranuclear inclusion bodies. *Proc. Soc. Exp. Biol. & Med.*, **72**: 46–50, 1949.

SYVERTON, J. T., The pathogenesis of the rabbit papilloma-to-carcinoma sequence. *Ann. N.Y. Acad. Sci.*, **54**: 1126–1140, 1952.

SYVERTON, J. T., and BERRY, G. P., Carcinoma in the cottontail rabbit following spontaneous virus papilloma (Shope). *Proc. Soc. Exp. Biol. & Med.*, **33**: 399–400, 1935.

SYVERTON, J. T., DASCOMB, H. E., WELLS, E. B., KOOMEN, J., JR., and BERRY, G. P., The virus-induced papilloma-to-carcinoma sequence. II. Carcinomas in the natural host, the cottontail rabbit. *Cancer Research*, **10**: 440–444, 1950.

TAJIMA, M., GORDON, D. E., and OLSON, C., Electron microscopy of bovine papilloma and deer fibroma viruses. *Am. J. Vet. Research*, **29**: 1185–1194, 1968.

THOMAS, M., BOIRON, M., TANZER, J., LÉVY, J.-P., and BERNARD, J., *In vitro* transformation of mice cells by bovine papilloma virus. *Nature*, **202**: 709–710, 1964.

THOMAS, M., LÉVY, J.-P., TANZER, J., BOIRON, M., and BERNARD, J., Transformation *in vitro* de cellules de peau de veau embryonnaire sous l'action d'extraits acellulaires de papillomes bovins. *Compt. Rend. Acad. Sci.* (*Paris*), **257**: 2155–2158, 1963.

ULLMANN, E. V., On the aetiology of the laryngeal papilloma. *Acta Oto-Laryng.*, **5**: 317–334, 1923.

U.S. DEPT. OF AGRICULTURE, Warts on Cattle. U.S. Dept. Agr., Leaflet No. 75, pp. 1–4, U.S. Gov't Printing Office, 1946.

VARIOT, G., Un cas d'inoculation expérimentale des verrues de l'enfant à l'homme. *J. Clin. Thérap. Infant.*, **2**: 529–531, 1894.

WAELSCH, L., Übertragungversuche mit spitzem Kondylom. *Arch. f. Dermat. u. Syph.*, **124**: 625–646, 1917.

WILDY, P., STOKER, M. G. P., MACPHERSON, I. A., and HORNE, R. W., The fine structure of polyoma virus. *Virology*, **11**: 444–457, 1960.

WILE, U. J., and KINGERY, L. B., The etiology of common warts: Their production in the second generation. *J. Am. Med. Assoc.*, **73**: 970–973, 1919.

WILLIAMS, M. G., HOWATSON, A. F., and ALMEIDA, J. D., Morphological characterization of the virus of the human common wart (*Verruca vulgaris*). *Nature*, **189**: 895–897, 1961.

WOODING, W. L., Susceptibility of various animals to bovine cutaneous papilloma materials. Thesis, M.S., Univ. of Wisconsin, Madison, 1964.

CHAPTER 4

The Lucké Frog Kidney Carcinoma

Baldwin Lucké of the Laboratory of Pathology, University of Pennsylvania, in Philadelphia, reported in 1934–1938 that carcinoma of the kidney, apparently caused by a transmissible virus, is rather frequent in the leopard frog (*Rana pipiens*), particularly in the northern New England states, primarily the Lake Champlain region of northern Vermont and bordering areas of Quebec Province, Canada (Lucké, 1934, 1938, 1952).

Occurrence and Geographical Distribution. In a survey of over 10,000 frogs from Vermont and the adjacent parts of Quebec, about 2.7 per cent of full grown, mature frogs, particularly males, were found to have kidney tumors. According to Lucké, tumor-bearing frogs have also been observed in North Dakota, Indiana, and the Mississippi Valley. A relatively high incidence of similar kidney tumors has been found recently also in the leopard frog from the Minnesota and Wisconsin areas of the North Central United States (McKinnell, 1965).

In a recent study, McKinnell found a relatively high incidence of renal tumors in frogs from North Central States ranging from Wisconsin to eastern South Dakota. Out of 884 primarily wild-type *Rana pipiens* frogs examined, 79 or 8.9 per cent had histologically confirmed renal carcinomas; among these 8.8 per cent were in females and 9.6 per cent in males. In another series, 204 *burnsi* mutant frogs from the same region were examined and 13 had renal tumors: five were found in males (5.7 per cent) and 8 in females (6.8 per cent).

Thus out of a total of 1,088 frogs in both groups examined, 92, or 8.5 per cent, had renal tumors. The frog populations from which these sample groups were obtained were located approximately 1,000 miles west of Lake Champlain in Vermont.

Appearance and General Morphology of the Kidney Tumors. The tumors occur in one or both kidneys as solitary or frequently multiple, ivory-white growths, contrasting with the brownish renal tissue, and are somewhat firmer in consistency than the surrounding normal kidney. They range in size from very small nodules to large irregular masses several times the size of the kidney which they may eventually replace; the mean size is approximately 4 to 6 mm in diameter, that is about one-third to one-half the size of the normal frog kidney. In about 50 per cent of the tumor-bearing frogs, the neoplastic nodules develop in multiple centers arising from several independent points of origin in the same kidney. Microscopically, these tumors have the appearance of typical adenocarcinomas.

Intranuclear Inclusion Bodies and Their Possible Relation to Virus Production. The outstanding characteristic of the frog kidney tumor is the frequent presence of acidophilic intranuclear inclusion bodies which in their general appearance are similar to those found in herpes and certain other diseases known to be caused by viruses. Lucké found such inclusion bodies in more than one-half of the frog kidney tumors observed. They were invariably confined to the tumor cells and were never found in normal epithelium of the kidneys, or in the cells of other organs examined. On electron microscopic examination (Fawcett, 1956), which will be discussed in more detail later in this chapter, the nuclear inclusion bodies were found to contain mature virus particles, as well as empty vesicles of the same size as virus particles, presumably representing virus precursors. It is quite possible, therefore, that the intranuclear inclusion bodies, so characteristic for the Lucké kidney carcinoma cells, may be related to the production of mature virus particles.

Lucké observed that there appeared to be seasonal variations: the inclusions could be observed more often in winter and spring than in summer and autumn. This observation and other related data suggest that prolonged low temperature may be one of the factors favoring formation of the inclusion bodies, and presumably also virus production.

The intranuclear inclusion bodies were classified by some observers (Rafferty, 1964) as "type A" in Cowdry's terminology (1934), a designation disputed by others (Duryee, 1964).

Cytoplasmic Inclusions. In addition to the nuclear inclusions, cytoplasmic inclusions, either filamentous or in forms of peculiar clusters of membranous vacuoles, were also described. These inclusion bodies also seem to be related to the presence of virus particles, but their origin and significance remain obscure. At least some of these cytoplasmic inclusion bodies were found to be Feulgen-positive (Duryee and Doherty, 1954. Fawcett, 1956. Tweedell, 1965. Freed and Rosenfeld, 1965. Rafferty, 1965).

Progressive Growth of the Tumors. The frog kidney tumors were found to grow progressively and eventually kill their hosts. At first they may remain localized in their early stages, but gradually they increase in size; eventually many of these tumors spread through the blood stream, forming metastatic tumors in distant organs. Lucké observed over 100 frogs in which the kidney tumors disseminated, most frequently to the lungs and to the liver.

Factors Influencing Tumor Formation. Environmental temperature seems to exert a significant influence on the formation and growth of tumors. Formation of tumors was retarded at environmental temperatures of

13.5°C, whereas temperatures of 23°C or 26°C lead to the development of an incidence of 25 to 50 per cent of spontaneous tumors (Rafferty, 1964). It is quite possible, therefore, that warm climate promotes tumor growth at the expense of virus production.*

Transplantation of Tumors by Cell-Graft. Regression of Primary Tumor Implants Followed by Development of Kidney Tumors. The kidney tumors could be transplanted by cell-graft from one frog to another. Following implantation into the anterior chamber of the eye, which was found to be the most suitable site for that purpose, they grew progressively, forming large tumor masses, and could then be transplanted to other frogs. If left undisturbed, the implanted tumors eventually regressed in most animals; however, solitary or multiple kidney tumors developed in such frogs either simultaneously, or after a delay of a few weeks or months; the renal tumors did not regress, but grew progressively. Similarly, if the tumor cells were implanted either as small fragments of tumor tissue, or as tumor cell suspensions, by different routes of inoculation, such as under the skin, into the muscles of the thigh, into the abdominal cavity, or into the brain, no significant local growth resulted at any of the inoculation sites, and the implanted material eventually disappeared. In more than 20 per cent of those animals, however, that survived for more than six months, tumors identical with the naturally occurring neoplasms developed in the kidneys.

Transmission by Desiccated or Glycerinated Tumor Extracts. In another series of experiments carried out by Lucké, kidney tumors that had been either desiccated, or placed in 50 per cent glycerin, and had been kept at refrigerator temperature for about three weeks, were used for inoculation. Among frogs that survived for more than six months, following the inoculation of either desiccated or glycerinated tumor extracts, 21 per cent developed typical kidney tumors.

In the control group, 6.7 per cent of frogs surviving for more than 6 months developed renal tumors. This incidence was higher than the 2.7 per cent observed among frogs living under natural conditions, but far below the incidence observed in the group that had been inoculated with either desiccated or glycerinated tumor extracts.

Lucké concluded that the causative agent responsible for the development of renal carcinomas is a virus. Such a conclusion was consistent with the fact that following inoculation of either viable tumor cells, or desiccated or glycerinated tumor extracts (which in all probability did not contain viable tumor cells), no growth resulted at the site of injection, but tumors were induced in the kidneys. The presence of the characteristic inclusion bodies in the tumor cells also suggested that the causative agent is a virus.

* In recent electron microscopic studies, induction of virus production was observed following prolonged low temperature (7° to 8°C) treatment of frogs bearing "virus-free" renal adenocarcinomas (Mizell, *et al.*, 1968).

Transmission by Filtrates. That the frog carcinoma agent is actually a filterable virus was demonstrated in a series of experiments carried out by W. R. Duryee (1956, 1965). The frog renal tumors were ground up, centrifuged, and then passed through Selas 02 filter candles. The filtrates were then injected directly into the kidneys of healthy frogs; as a result, in the initial study 17 per cent of the inoculated frogs developed kidney carcinomas (Duryee, 1956). In more recent experiments (Duryee, 1965) out of 106 injected frogs, 37 per cent developed kidney carcinomas after a latency of 3 to 7 months.

Host Specificity. That the frog kidney carcinoma agent is species specific was evident from a series of experiments carried out by Lucké, in which either desiccated or live, fresh tumor cells from *Rana pipiens* kidney tumors were inoculated into over 100 green frogs (*Rana clamitans*), or half-grown bullfrogs (*Rana catesbiana*), or into frogs of a subspecies of *R. pipiens*. None of the frogs of foreign species, or of alien race, developed renal tumors. Similarly, Lucké found that the kidney tumor agent from Vermont frogs did not induce tumors in *Rana pipiens* frogs of New Jersey. Others have shown that intraocular grafts of the Vermont frog tumors did not induce renal tumors in the more distant *Rana pipiens* of Wisconsin, Illinois, or Kentucky.

Transplantation to Tadpoles. Briggs (1942) implanted small tumor fragments of the kidney adenocarcinoma of adult frogs into a total of 163 tadpoles. The transplantations were made into different sites of the tadpole, and typical growing tumors developed in the subcutaneous tissue of trunk (7 cases), in the mesenchyme of dorsal tail fin (27 cases), in an area adjacent to the kidney (2 cases), in the liver (1 case), and in the body cavity (1 case). The tumors in the trunk subcutaneous tissue grew well, and in two cases survived metamorphosis of the host. The tumors in the tail ceased to grow and eventually regressed during later stages in the development of the host tadpoles. Typical tumors developed in a small number of cases from implants in the liver and body cavity, and in the area adjacent to the kidney. However, the majority of implants in these sites were eventually resolved and regressed completely. Six of the hosts which failed to develop tumors at the implantation site were found to have multiple tumors in their kidneys. These occurred only in hosts which had completed metamorphosis.

In a control series, 180 tadpoles received implants of normal kidney tissues, and none developed tumors.

Electron Microscopic Studies. In the initial studies carried out by D. W. Fawcett (1956) electron microscopic examination of ultrathin sections of frog kidney carcinoma cells revealed that approximately one-third of the tumors examined contained spheroidal particles of uniform size and distinctive morphology which in all probability represented the virus. These particles consisted of hollow spheres 90 to 100 mμ in diameter, having a thick capsule and a dense inner core about 35 to 40 mμ in diameter eccentrically placed within the central cavity. Virus particles of this kind were found principally in the cytoplasm, but occasionally also in the nuclei, and in the extracellular spaces of the tumors. No similar particles were found in normal kidney cells.

Electron microscopic study of the intranuclear inclusion bodies has shown that they contain numerous spherical vesicles with thin limiting membranes, embedded in a finely granular matrix. Some of the thin walled vesicles were found to contain a dense inner body like that of the cytoplasmic virus particles; this suggested that they may represent mature virus particles (Fawcett, 1956).

More recently the frog kidney carcinoma virus particles and their formation were studied in more detail on ultrathin sections, employing improved embedding and staining technique (Lunger, 1964. Came and Lunger, 1966).

Ultrastructure and Formation of the Frog Kidney Carcinoma Virus. On the basis of electron microscopic studies thus far performed it now appears that the frog kidney carcinoma virus is formed in the cell nucleus. As stated before, the virus particles are round, or oval, and approximately 100 mμ in diameter. The virus particles acquire additional membranes by entering nuclear vacuoles from which they are extruded into the cell cytoplasm. They apparently acquire an additional layer, or layers, of membranes when they are in the cytoplasm, and later leave the cell by rupture of virus-containing vacuoles at the cell surface. This sequence is quite reminiscent of the herpes virus (Morgan *et al.*, 1959. Epstein, 1962. Lunger, 1964).

Ultrastructure of the Virus Studied by Negative Staining Technique. In

---

FIG. 7. THE LUCKÉ FROG KIDNEY CARCINOMA VIRUS.

(A). Intranuclear inclusion body from a tissue fragment of a spontaneous renal adenocarcinoma from an adult Vermont male frog (*Rana pipiens*). A crystalline array of virus particles. The hexagonal profile of the particles is apparent; occasional nucleoids can be observed in a few particles. Average particle diameter 100 mμ. Magnification 52,000×. (From: P. D. Lunger, *Advances in Virus Research*, **12**: 1, 1966.) (B). Section of a fragment from a spontaneous kidney tumor of an adult Vermont male frog (*Rana pipiens*). A cluster of "herpes-like" mature virus particles in the lumen of proximal convoluted tubule. The particles are spheroidal and are surrounded by a loose-fitting envelope; the average total diameter of the virus particles is approximately 140 mμ. Most of the virus particles contain electron-dense nucleoids about 80 mμ in diameter. Magnification 50,000×. This tumor contained virus particles also in the nucleus and in the cytoplasm. Electron micrographs prepared by P. D. Lunger, Department of Biological Sciences, University of Delaware, Newark.

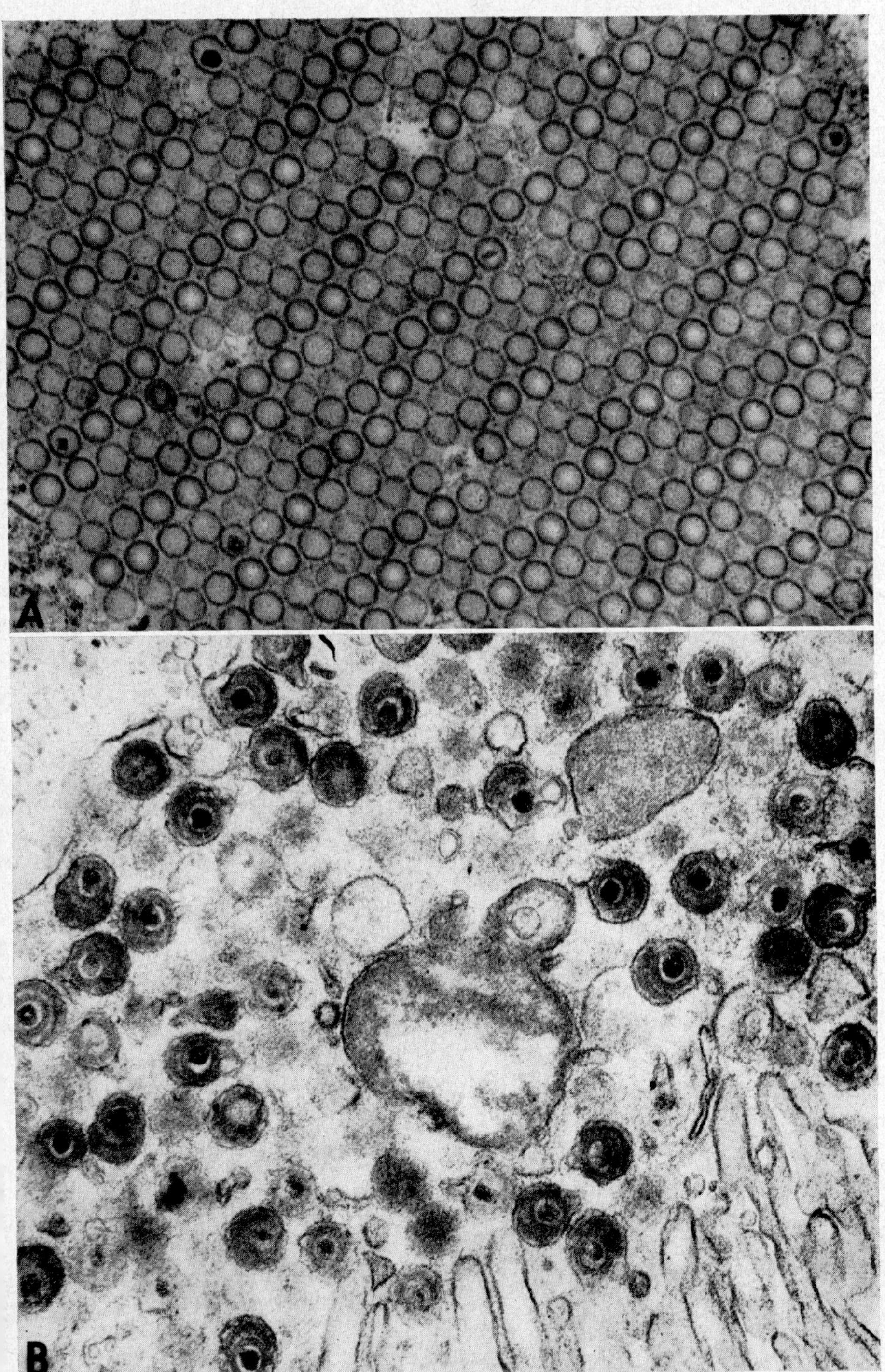

Fig. 7. The Lucké Frog Kidney Carcinoma Virus

a recent study (Lunger, 1964) the frog kidney carcinoma virus was isolated from spontaneous renal tumors removed from 9 leopard frogs obtained from Vermont and Wisconsin. The virus was purified and concentrated by differential centrifugation, and the pellets containing sedimented virus particles were studied in the electron microscope. Both ultrathin sections and negative staining technique were employed for the preparation of specimens for electron microscopy. The particles studied by negative staining contrast were found to consist of either "empty" or "full" capsids approximately 100 mμ in diameter, occasionally surrounded by a loose fitting envelope 160 to 240 mμ in diameter. On ultrathin sections, the capsid could be seen to enclose a dense core, or nucleoid, about 55 to 80 mμ in diameter. The capsids contained 162 hollow, elongated capsomeres arranged in an ordered architecture suggestive of icosahedral symmetry. Again, as in previous studies, there appeared to be a morphological similarity between the Lucké virus and those of the herpes group.

Cytochemical Studies. Zambernard and Vatter (1966) carried out a cytochemical study of the Lucké frog kidney carcinoma. Small pieces of leopard frog tumors with known viral inclusions were fixed and embedded. Ultrathin sections were then subjected to solutions of trypsin, pepsin, RNase, and DNase. Electron microscopic studies revealed that neither trypsin nor RNase had any visible effect on the viral nucleoids or capsids. Pepsin removed the viral capsid after one-half hour. The DNase digested the viral nucleoid within two hours.

On the basis of the results of this study, the authors concluded that the nucleoids of the nuclear, cytoplasmic, and extracellular particles found in the renal frog tumors examined are composed of DNA.

Transmission of Frog Kidney Carcinoma to Salamanders and the Unexpected Induction of Bone Tumors. S. Meryl Rose and Florence Rose (1952) at the Department of Zoology, University of Illinois, in Urbana, carried out a series of significant experiments suggesting that, under certain experimental conditions, the agent causing frog kidney carcinoma may change its specificity for the host, and perhaps also its affinity for certain cells. Small fragments of fresh frog kidney tumors from *Rana pipiens* of the Lake Champlain region were implanted into young salamanders (*Triturus viridescens*). The tumor grafts had to be chilled during the operation, and the salamanders had to be placed in a refrigerator at +6°C for a short period afterwards, or the operation could be carried out at room temperature provided that the salamanders were kept in a diluted pyribenzamine solution. Some of the implanted tumors grew progressively, others regressed. The most significant and unexpected result of these experiments, however, was the development of multiple bone chondrosarcomas in the limbs of the inoculated salamanders. When fragments of these bone tumors were then implanted into either Vermont or Wisconsin frogs, both bone tumors and typical kidney carcinomas developed in the inoculated frogs. The bone tumors invariably regressed in the frogs, but renal tumors grew progressively. Fragments of frog bone tumors, transplanted to other frogs, again induced bone and renal tumors. It was thus possible to transfer the renal tumor from the Vermont frog, through the salamander, to the Wisconsin frog (which is otherwise resistant to the direct inoculation of the Vermont kidney tumor agent). Rose concluded that the frog kidney carcinoma agent changed its cell-affinity after passage through a foreign host, i.e. salamander. When returned to its original host, the agent was able to induce tumors not only in the kidney, but also in the skeletal tissue.

Mutation or transformation of the frog renal carcinoma agent could be responsible for this remarkable change in its cell-affinity. Additional observations are needed, however, to determine whether such an assumption is correct, and whether another explanation should not be considered. Theoretically, it would be possible to speculate that several oncogenic agents may be carried in the cells of the frog renal carcinoma; under certain experimental conditions, a hitherto unsuspected and latent oncogenic agent present in the frog tumor may assert itself, inducing bone tumors. Another possibility would be that of a multipotent oncogenic agent, capable of inducing a variety of tumors, depending on the type of cells affected, and conditioning of the host.

Other Tumors and Viruses in Frogs. The Lucké frog kidney carcinoma is not the only malignant tumor observed in that species. Other tumors have also been observed in frogs and frog kidneys (Stewart *et al.*, 1959. Duryee, 1964). Furthermore, several viruses have been recently isolated from normal, and from tumor tissues of frogs (Rafferty, 1965. Granoff *et al.*, 1966. Darlington *et al.*, 1966), or observed in frog tumor cells (Lunger and Came, 1968). The relation, if any, of these viruses to the Lucké tumor is not clear.

How Is the Virus of Frog Kidney Carcinoma Transmitted from Host to Host Under Natural Life Conditions? It is necessary to emphasize that at the present time no sufficient data are yet available to determine the actual mechanism of transmission, under natural life conditions, of the virus of frog kidney carcinoma. A possibility which should be considered is that of vertical transmission of the virus from one generation to another directly through the germinal cells, i.e. through the fertilized ovum. This would be similar to the transmission of the leukemia virus in chickens and mice. Such a concept would be consistent with the observation that a relatively high incidence of kidney tumors remains limited to a particular species of frogs, living in a limited geographic area, in which the virus could be transmitted through successive generations of animals.

Vertical transmission of the virus through germinal cells would not necessarily exclude the possibility that additional "horizontal" virus transmission may occasionally occur also through other routes, particularly among newborn animals during larval stages, either through infected water, or by other means of contact transmission.

A limited "horizontal" transmission of the leukemic virus among newly hatched chicks or newborn mice has been also observed, even though the principal route of natural transmission of the leukemic virus in chickens and mice occurs through the infected sperm or ovum.

The two known areas of occurrence of kidney carcinomas in the frogs include large lake systems in Vermont and Wisconsin which have extraordinarily dense frog populations. During the active months spent on land, from May through October in Vermont and also in the Lake Champlain area, the leopard frog leads an essentially solitary life in the field. Late in the fall, around November 1, as the weather approaches freezing, the frogs migrate to the lake in large numbers to hibernate. According to Rafferty (1964) near Alburg, Vermont, 35,000 frogs have been collected in a single night. After entering the water the frogs lie on the bottom of the lake for the winter. McKinnell by cutting through the ice exposed hundreds of frogs huddled together on the muddy bottom of frozen ponds of Minnesota; it would seem likely that Lake Champlain frogs are similarly crowded during winter hibernation. Emergence and spawning then occur at the first melting of the ice in late March or April.

The very large density of the frog population and the extreme crowding could be contributing factors in the possible transmission of the tumors, although it is quite possible that actual transmission of the causative virus may rather occur during either pre-embryonic or larval phase.

Under natural life conditions, kidney tumors develop in the frogs in the summer, when these animals are 2 or 3 years old; a small proportion of these animals, less than 3 per cent, have small kidney tumors when they enter hibernation. Formation of the inclusion bodies in the tumor cells starts soon after the tumors are established, possibly in response to cold weather; at least half of the tumors of winter frogs contain inclusion bodies. During this phase, growth of the tumor virtually ceases, but virus production increases. By the time the frogs emerge from their hibernation, both the tumor cells and the intercellular spaces contain considerable amounts of virus, which presumably finds its way into the urine, and hence into the water at the time of spawning. Infection of the young may then occur at the moment of fertilization; it is possible also that tadpoles may be infected after hatching. The original infection would then be latent, the tumor formation beginning more than two years later. With the onset of warm weather the growth of the tumors would become accelerated, and eventually the afflicted frogs would die with large tumors during the summer or early fall.

It should be emphasized, however, that this description (Rafferty, 1964) of the sequence of events in the development of frog kidney carcinoma, and the possible manner of virus transmission under field conditions, are not yet sufficiently supported by experimental data and must be considered purely speculative at the present time.

* * *

Studies on the Transmission of Lymphosarcoma in the South African Clawed Toad, Xenopus laevis

It was observed recently that a lymphosarcoma found in the South African clawed toad (*Xenopus laevis laevis*) was found to be readily transferable to other *Xenopus laevis* subspecies, to another Xenopus species, and to certain other anuran amphibian species (Balls, 1964, 1965). Xenopus lymphosarcoma agent was found to be resistant to freeze-drying, but sensitive to heat (40 minutes at 56°C) and ethyl ether; it passed through a 100 mμ filter and remained in the supernatant fluid following centrifugation at 30,000 $\times g$ for 1 hour. Filtered extracts were infectious. It was also observed that the agent is passed from toad to toad in water in which the Xenopus live. Horizontal transmission was demonstrated in newts, and urine collected from lymphosarcoma-bearing frogs was used to transmit the tumor to young adult Xenopus (Balls and Ruben, 1967. Ruben and Balls, 1967). Newts thymectomized prior to injection with tumor homogenate developed lymphosarcomas, which demonstrated that this lymphoid disease does not depend on the presence or absence of thymus.

REFERENCES

Balls, M., Lymphoid tumor transfers from *Xenopus laevis laevis* to alien subspecies and species, including *Rana pipiens*. *Cancer Research*, **24**: 1261–1267, 1964.

Balls, M., Lymphosarcoma in the South African Clawed Toad, *Xenopus laevis:* A virus tumor. *Ann. N.Y. Acad. Sci.*, **126**: 256–273, 1965.

Balls, M., and Ruben, L. N., The transmission of lymphosarcoma in *Xenopus laevis*, the South African Clawed Toad. *Cancer Research*, **27**: 654–659, 1967.

Briggs, R., Transplantation of kidney carcinoma from adult frogs to tadpoles. *Cancer Research*, **2**: 309–323, 1942.

Came, P. E., and Lunger, P. D., Viruses isolated from frogs and their relationship to the Lucké tumor. *Arch. Ges. Virusforsch.*, **19**: 464–468, 1966.

Cowdry, E. V., The problem of intranuclear inclusions in virus diseases. *Arch. Path.*, **18**: 527–542, 1934.

Darlington, R. W., Granoff, A., and Breeze, D. C., Viruses and renal carcinoma of *Rana pipiens*. II. Ultrastructural studies and sequential development of virus isolated from normal and tumor tissue. *Virology*, **29**: 149–156, 1966.

DURYEE, W. R., Seminar on transmission studies on renal adenocarcinoma of the frog. *J. Franklin Inst.*, **261**: 377–379, 1956.

DURYEE, W. R., Precancer cells in amphibian adenocarcinoma. *Ann. N.Y. Acad. Sci.*, **63**: 1280–1302, 1956.

DURYEE, W. R., Comments on frog kidney tumor review by Dr. Rafferty. *Cancer Research*, **24**: 518–519, 1964.

DURYEE, W. R., Factors influencing development of tumors in frogs. *Ann. N.Y. Acad. Sci.*, **126**: 59–84, 1965.

DURYEE, W. R., and DOHERTY, J. K., Nuclear and cytoplasmic organoids in the living cell. *Ann. N.Y. Acad Sci.*, **58**: 1210–1230, 1954.

EPSTEIN, M. A., Observations on the mode of release of herpes virus from infected HeLa cells. *J. Cell Biol.*, **12**: 589–597, 1962.

FAWCETT, D. W., Electron microscope observations on intracellular virus-like particles associated with the cells of the Lucké renal adenocarcinoma. *J. Biophys. & Biochem. Cytol.*, **2**: 725–742, 1956.

FREED, J. J., and ROSENFELD, S. J., Frog renal adenosarcoma: Cytological studies *in situ* and *in vitro*. *Ann. N.Y. Acad. Sci.*, **126**: 99–114, 1965.

GRANOFF, A., CAME, P. E., and RAFFERTY, K. A., Jr., The isolation and properties of viruses from *Rana pipiens*: Their possible relationship to the renal adeno-carcinoma of the leopard frog. *Ann. N.Y. Acad. Sci.*, **126**: 237–255, 1965.

GRANOFF, A., CAME, P. E., and BREEZE, D. C., Viruses and renal carcinoma of *Rana pipiens*. I. The isolation and properties of virus from normal and tumor tissue. *Virology*, **29**: 133–148, 1966.

LUCKÉ, B., A neoplastic disease of the kidney of the frog, *Rana pipiens*. *Am. J. Cancer*, **20**: 352–379, 1934.

LUCKÉ, B., A neoplastic disease of the kidney of the frog, *Rana pipiens*. II. On the occurrence of metastasis. *Am. J. Cancer*, **22**: 326–334, 1934.

LUCKÉ, B., Carcinoma of the kidney in the leopard frog: The occurrence and significance of metastasis. *Am. J. Cancer*, **34**: 15–30, 1938.

LUCKÉ, B., Carcinoma in the leopard frog. Its probable causation by a virus. *J. Exp. Med.*, **68**: 457–468, 1938.

LUCKÉ, B., Characteristics of frog carcinoma in tissue culture. *J. Exp. Med.*, **70**: 269–276, 1939.

LUCKÉ, B., Kidney carcinoma in the leopard frog: A virus tumor. *Ann. N.Y. Acad. Sci.*, **54**: 1093–1109, 1952.

LUCKÉ, B., and SCHLUMBERGER, H., The manner of growth of frog carcinoma studied by direct microscopic examination of living intraocular transplants. *J. Exp. Med.*, **70**: 257–268, 1939.

LUNGER, P. D., Thin-section electron microscopy of the mature Lucké frog kidney tumor virus. *Virology*, **22**: 285–286, 1964.

LUNGER, P. D., The isolation and morphology of the Lucké frog kidney tumor virus. *Virology*, **24**: 138–145, 1964.

LUNGER, P. D., Amphibia-related viruses. *Advances in Virus Research*, **12** : 1–33, Academic Press, New York and London, 1966.

LUNGER, P. D., and CAME, P. E., Cytoplasmic viruses associated with Lucké tumor cells. *Virology*, **30**: 116–126, 1966.

LUNGER, P. D., DARLINGTON, R. W., and GRANOFF, A., Cell-virus relationships in the Lucké renal adenocarcinoma: An ultrastructure study. *Ann. N.Y. Acad. Sci.*, **126**: 289–314, 1965.

MCKINNELL, R. G., Incidence and histology of renal tumors of leopard frogs from the North Central states. *Ann. N.Y. Acad. Sci.*, **126**: 85–98, 1965.

McKinnell, R. G., and Zambernard, J., Virus particles in renal tumors obtained from spring *Rana pipiens* of known geographic origin. *Cancer Research*, **28**: 684–688, 1968.

Mateyko, G. M., and Kopac, M. J., Studies on the cytophysiology of frog renal adenocarcinoma. *Ann. N.Y. Acad. Sci.*, **126**: 22–58, 1965.

Mizell, M., Stackpole, C. W., and Halperen, S., Herpes-type virus recovery from "virus-free" frog kidney tumors. *Proc. Soc. Exp. Biol. & Med.*, **127**: 808–814, 1968.

Mizell, M., and Zambernard, J., Viral particles of the frog renal adenocarcinoma: Causative agent or passenger virus? II. A promising model system for the demonstration of a "lysogenic" state in a metazoan tumor. *Ann. N.Y. Acad. Sci.*, **126**: 146–169, 1965.

Morgan, C., Rose, H. M., Holden, M., and Jones, E. P., Electron-microscopic observations on the development of herpes simplex virus. *J. Exp. Med.*, **110**: 643–656, 1959.

Rafferty, K. A., Jr., Kidney tumors of the leopard frog: A review. *Cancer Research*, **24**: 169–185, 1964.

Rafferty, K. A., Jr., The cultivation of inclusion-associated viruses from Lucké tumor frogs. *Ann. N.Y. Acad. Sci.*, **126**: 3–21, 1965.

Rose, S. M., Interaction of tumor agents and normal cellular components in amphibia. *Ann. N.Y. Acad. Sci.*, **54**: 1110–1119, 1952.

Rose, S. M., and Rose, F. C., Tumor agent transformation in amphibia. *Cancer Research*, **12**: 1–12, 1952.

Ruben, L. N., and Balls, M., Further studies of a transmissible amphibian lymphosarcoma. *Cancer Research*, **27**: 293–296, 1967.

Stewart, H. L., Snell, K. C., Dunham, L. C., and Schlyen, S. M., Transplantable and transmissible tumors of animals. Tumors of the kidney. Renal adenocarcinoma. Frog, pp. 208–213 in: *Atlas of Tumor Pathology*. Sect. 12, Fasc. 40, Am. Reg. Path., Armed Forces Inst. of Path., Washington, D.C., 1959.

Tweedell, K. S., Cytopathology of a frog renal adenocarcinoma *in vitro* with fluorescence microscopy. *Ann. N.Y. Acad. Sci.*, **126**: 170–187, 1965.

Zambernard, J., and Mizell, M., Viral particles of the frog renal adenocarcinoma: Causative agent or passenger virus? I. Fine structure of primary tumors and subsequent intraocular transplants. *Ann. N.Y. Acad. Sci.*, **126**: 127–145, 1965.

Zambernard, J., and Vatter, A. E., The fine structural cytochemistry of virus particles found in renal tumors of leopard frogs. I. An enzymatic study of the viral nucleoid. *Virology*, **28**: 318–324, 1966.

CHAPTER 5

The Contagious Venereal Dog Sarcoma

No experimental evidence is available in support of an assumption that the venereal dog tumor is actually caused by a filterable oncogenic virus. This unusual neoplasm is nevertheless included in this monograph because it is one of the few naturally transmissible, contagious tumors known.

This transmissible tumor of dogs is of considerable interest, since it is one of the very few "contagious" tumors known. Most often the growth is found on the penis of the male dog, or in the vulva or vagina of the female. The tumor is transmitted naturally by coitus. During the early part of the twentieth century, this tumor, called the infectious or contagious dog lymphosarcoma, attracted considerable attention of investigators; it has been reported not only in European countries, but also in North and South America, in Japan, China, Java, even in New Guinea, and in Ceylon.

At the turn of the century, Smith and Washbourn (1898, 1899) in England demonstrated the venereal, natural transmission, by allowing a dog with a tumor on the penis to serve 12 bitches; as a result, about a month after they gave birth to puppies, 11 of them developed raspberry-like tumors in the vaginal wall. A second male dog that served three of the infected bitches subsequently developed a tumor on the penis; this dog, in turn, was allowed to serve two bitches, and transmitted the tumor to one of them.

Under natural life conditions, the venereal dog sarcoma is found most frequently, as its name implies, on genital organs of either males or females, i.e. on the penis or in the vagina. The tumors grow progressively and frequently ulcerate, allowing secondary infection to develop. They may form metastatic tumors in the adjoining lymph nodes, and in some animals they may eventually disseminate, forming distant metastatic nodules in the liver and spleen, or in other organs. Many of the spontaneously occurring tumors remain stationary for long periods of time, then may have periods of partial regression, followed by renewed growth. Some of them may regress completely.

The venereal dog sarcoma is a grayish-white, firm tumor, difficult to cut. Microscopically, it is composed of large, round cells containing large vesicular nuclei and abundant cytoplasm (see also Stewart *et al.*, 1959).

This tumor was first described as a carcinoma, but subsequently it was considered a round cell sarcoma; it has often been described as a lymphosarcoma, although there is not sufficient evidence for such terminology.

The following excerpt from a letter received by the author (Dec. 16, 1958) from Dr. A. S. Karlson, Section of Bacteriology, Mayo Clinic, Rochester, Minn., may be of interest to the reader:

"I know of no additional work on this tumor which may clarify the many peculiar aspects of its cytology, origin, and whether or not there is a viral agent involved. The microscopic appearance is that of a highly malignant neoplasm. Actually it is quite benign. Veterinarians reported uniformly good results following excision.

Since writing our paper (Karlson and Mann, 1952), I have talked with veterinary pathologists who see this tumor in their practice. It is the general consensus that it may be preferable to use the term "transmissible venereal tumor" than to call it a "lymphosarcoma."

The dog sarcoma can be readily transplanted, by inoculation, to other dogs, also to foxes, but not to other species. There appears to be no significant difference in susceptibility among the various breeds of dogs inoculated. Novinsky in Russia was the first, in 1877, to succeed in transplanting the dog sarcoma. Fragments of a tumor removed from the vagina of a 6-year-old female dog were transplanted under the skin of 2 puppies; about one month later, small nodules appeared at the site of implantation and grew progressively. Wehr, in Lwów, also reported in 1884 successful transplantation of a vaginal tumor in dogs. Wehr designated the tumor as a "sarcoma."

The interested reader is referred to Shimkin's recent review (1955) of Novinsky's historical tumor transplantation experiments, the first recorded in experimental cancer research (see also Stewart *et al.*, 1959). The transplantation by Novinsky of an alveolar carcinoma of dog in 1876 was discussed on page 7 in this monograph.

Wehr (1884, 1888, 1889) carried out his transplantation experiments with Professor Kadyj at the Veterinary School in Lwów (Lemberg), which was at that time the capital of Austrian Galicja, a province of southern Poland, and part of the Austro-Hungarian Monarchy. Wehr presented preliminary results of his transplantation experiments on June 3, 1884, at the IVth Convention of Polish Physicians and Biologists in Poznań and published his paper that same year in the Polish medical journal *Przegląd lekarski* (1884) in Kraków.

Smith and Washbourn (1899), in England, reported a few years later results of their experiments dealing with transplantation of the venereal dog tumor. Out of 17 dogs inoculated subcutaneously with small fragments of tumors, 13 developed tumor nodules at the site of implantation. Sticker*

* In some publications, the venereal dog sarcoma is referred to as "the Sticker tumor," although it had been reported and described in detail in earlier studies by other investigators.

(1904), in Germany, succeeded in transplanting the tumor to dogs and also to foxes, but failed in attempts to transmit it to cats, rabbits, guinea pigs, mice, or rats. Many other investigators have later transmitted the tumor in dogs (Stubbs and Furth, 1934. Karlson and Mann, 1952). In all transplantation experiments, live tumor cells had to be used. Inoculation of glycerinated or desiccated tumor extracts, or injection of tumor filtrates, did not transmit the disease. It appeared, therefore, that the dog venereal sarcoma, even though contagious and naturally transmissible, can be transmitted only by transplantation of live tumor cells.

Ajello reported (1960) that he was able to transmit the venereal dog sarcoma by inoculation of an extract, prepared from tumor tissues that had been passed through a paper filter and was then in addition centrifuged (3000 r.p.m. for 10 minutes) after filtration. The supernate was inoculated into two young puppies and induced in both animals tumors at the site of inoculation after a latency of 3 to 3½ months. This experiment is interesting, but does not entirely exclude the possibility of transmission by cells. In order to prove that the transmission was accomplished by a cell-free agent, the extract would have had to be passed through bacterial filters.

In view of recent experiments dealing with cell-free transmission of mouse leukemia, or the induction of tumors following inoculation of the polyoma virus in mice, rats, or hamsters, it is possible to speculate that particular experimental conditions may be needed to transmit dog sarcoma by filtrates. Newborn animals, perhaps puppies only a few hours old, and of a particular breed related to the donor host, may have to be employed for inoculation of the tumor filtrates. If proper experimental conditions are not met, the tumor may appear to be transmissible by cell-graft only.

The dog sarcoma, when transmitted by inoculation of tumor fragments or tumor cell suspensions, develops at the site of inoculation in the form of small nodules after a latency of about 2 to 3 weeks. The transplanted tumors then grow progressively for a period of time, but as a rule they later diminish in size and eventually disappear.

The rapidity with which even large tumors may regress, and disappear spontaneously, may be striking. In certain cases large tumors may completely disappear in the course of 10 to 15 days. Not all implanted tumors disappear, however. DeMonbreun and Goodpasture (1934) observed that tumors which developed following multiple, 6 to 10, subcutaneous inoculations, usually showed no tendency to regress. Instead, their growth was rapid, and the dogs bearing them usually died with widespread metastatic tumors within 3 to 4 months following inoculation.

Under normal conditions, however, tumors developing as a result of a single inoculation of tumor fragments, or of tumor cell suspensions, grow only temporarily and eventually regress. Dogs in which the tumors disappeared spontaneously were found to be immune to reinoculation of the dog sarcoma. This immunity is a most interesting phenomenon; it has been observed and confirmed by several investigators.

REFERENCES

AJELLO, P., Transmissione del tumore di Sticker con materiale acellulare. *Nuova Veterinaria*, **36**: 180–183, 1960.

DEMONBREUN, W. A., and GOODPASTURE, E. W., An experimental investigation concerning the nature of contagious lymphosarcoma of dogs. *Am. J. Cancer*, **21**: 295–321, 1934.

KARLSON, A. G., and MANN, F. C., The transmissible venereal tumor of dogs: Observations on forty generations of experimental transfers. *Ann. N.Y. Acad. Sci.*, **54**: 1197–1213, 1952.

NOWINSKY, M., Zur Frage über die Impfung der krebsigen Geschwülste. *Centralbl. f. med. Wissensch.*, **14**: 790–791, 1876.

NOWINSKY, M., On the question of the inoculation of malignant neoplasms (experimental investigations). Thesis. St. Petersburg, 1877.

SHIMKIN, M. B.,* M. A. Novinsky: A note on the history of transplantation of tumors. *Cancer*, **8**: 653–655, 1955.

SMITH, G. B., and WASHBOURN, J. W., Infective venereal tumours in dogs. *J. Comp. Path. & Therap.*, **11**: 41–51, 1898.

SMITH, G. B., and WASHBOURN, J. W., Infective sarcoma in dogs. *Brit. Med. J.*, **2**: 1346–1347, 1899.

STEWART, H. L., SNELL, K. C., DUNHAM, L. J., and SCHLYEN, S. M., Transplantable and transmissible tumors of animals. *Atlas of Tumor Pathology*, Sect. 12, Fasc. 40, pp. 378, Am. Reg. Path., Armed Forces Inst. of Path., Washington, D.C., 1959.

STICKER, A., Transplantables Lymphosarkom des Hundes: ein Beitrag zur Lehre der Krebsübertragbarkeit. *Zeitschr. f. Krebsforsch.*, **1**: 413–444, 1904.

STUBBS, E. L., and FURTH, J., Experimental studies on venereal sarcoma of the dog. *Am. J. Path.*, **10**: 275–286, 1934.

WEHR, W., O przeszczepianiu raka. *Przegląd lekarski*, **23** (No.27): 365–367, 1884.

WEHR, (W.),† Demonstration der durch Impfung von Hund auf Hund erzeugten Carcinomknötchen. *Centralbl. f. Chir.*, **15** (Suppl. to No. 24): 8–9, 1888.

WEHR, (W.),† Weitere Mittheilungen über die positiven Ergebnisse der Carcinom-Ueberimpfungen von Hund auf Hund. *Arch. f. klin, Chir.*, **39**: 226–228, 1889.

* This is a historical study by M. B. Shimkin entitled: "M. A. Novinsky: A note on the history of transplantation of tumors." Note that the name "Novinsky" is also spelled "Nowinsky" in other publications.

† No first name initial in the original paper.

CHAPTER 6

The Rous Chicken Sarcoma

In 1910, Peyton Rous, at the Rockefeller Institute in New York, became interested in investigating the nature of a tumor found in a barred Plymouth Rock hen. This tumor had existed for some 2 months before the fowl, then about a year-and-a-half old, was brought to the laboratory; the growth presented itself as a large, irregularly globular mass projecting sharply from the right breast. This growth was shown to resemble a classical tumor in all obvious ways. Microscopically, it proved to be a spindle-cell sarcoma, with a wide-spread necrotic center. Bits of the tumor were inoculated, by means of a trocar, into 2 hens of the same stock; as a result, a large nodule developed about a month later in one of them. Several successive transplantations of this tumor were accomplished; chickens of pure blood from the same, small, intimately related stock in which the growth occurred were used for implantations of fragments of tumor tissue. Young chickens were more susceptible than adults. Market-bought chickens of similar variety, and fowls of mixed breed, were found to be insusceptible in the initial studies, in which tumors of relatively low potency were used for inoculation. Within a few years, however, after successive transplantation, the tumor gained the ability to grow in chickens of all sorts. Rous designated this tumor "Chicken Tumor No. 1."

Transmission by Filtrate of Chicken Tumor No. 1

In a further study of this tumor, tests were made to determine whether it could be transmitted by filtrates. Since previous attempts to transmit rat, mouse, and dog tumors by cell-free extracts had not succeeded, it was anticipated that sarcoma of the fowl would not be different in this regard. It was a surprise, therefore, to find in preliminary experiments that a watery tumor filtrate passed through ordinary filter paper, or supernate resulting from centrifugation of the tumor cell suspension, induced characteristic growths when inoculated into young fowls of the variety in which the tumor originally occurred. Experiments were at once instituted to determine whether the tumor could be transmitted by cell-free filtrates prepared under strictly controlled experimental conditions. Accordingly, bits of tumor were mixed with sand, and ground with Ringer solution, then centrifuged at about 3000 r.p.m. for 5 to 15 minutes; the supernate was then passed through Berkefeld filter candles (No. 5, medium). The filter candles were tested both before and after the filtration, with *Bacillus prodigiosus*, and were found to hold back the microbes. The grinding, centrifugation, and filtration were carried out at approximately 39°C temperature. In the first experiment, 4 to 10 chickens inoculated with the filtrate developed tumors after several weeks. In a second experiment carried out under similar experimental conditions, one out of 10 fowls inoculated with the filtrate developed a tumor after only 11 days, and 7 more chickens among those inoculated with the filtrate had tumors 3 weeks later (Rous, 1911).

Chicken Tumor No. 7 (*Osteochondrosarcoma*) *Transmissible by Filtrate*. The fact that a chicken sarcoma could be transmitted by filtrate was obviously of fundamental importance, and led Rous to a further study of tumors of the fowl. Spontaneous chicken tumors are far from rare, and some 45 of them were obtained and investigated by Rous and his associates. The various tumors studied were given successive numbers. None of the growths was quite similar histologically to the Chicken Tumor No. 1, first transmitted by filtrates, and only a few of them proved to be transplantable by cell-grafts. One of these, Chicken Tumor No. 7, an osteochondrosarcoma producing a true cartilage and bone, could also be transmitted by filtrates in experiments carried out by Rous, Murphy and Tytler (1912).

Thus, two filterable agents were now available, both causing tumors in the fowl. The induced tumors were, however, quite different. The agent causing spindle-cell sarcoma could hardly be identical with that causing an osteochondrosarcoma. The latter did not change its peculiarity even when injected into connective tissue or into the voluntary muscles, the resulting growth elaborating cartilage and bone. Thus, it appeared that the histologic character of the osteochondrosarcoma was due to a peculiarity of the causative agent, which was retained when that agent was separated from the cells.

A Third Filterable Chicken Tumor. A new filterable tumor was soon added by Rous and his associates to the rapidly growing list of filterable fowl tumors. This new tumor was a spindle-cell sarcoma of a peculiar intracanalicular pattern, fissured by blood sinuses, quite different histologically and in its general behavior from either the Chicken Tumor No. 1 or from the filterable osteochondrosarcoma. The latency time was considerably longer, extending to several months after the injection of filtrate, and the growth of filtrate-induced tumors was slow (Rous *et al.*, 1913, 1914).

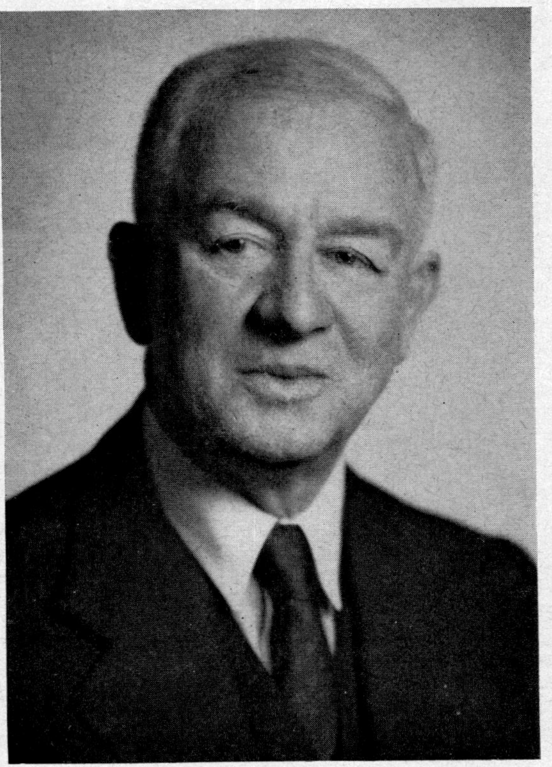

Peyton Rous

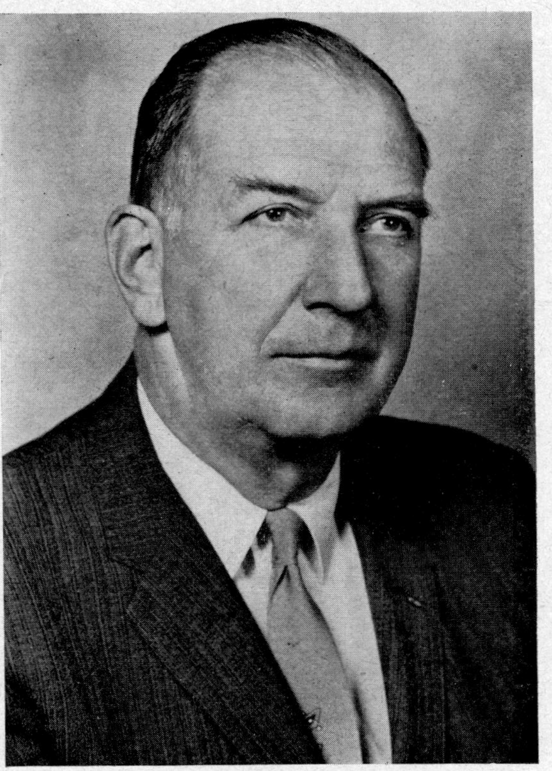

Richard E. Shope

FIG. 8

How Many Different Tumor Agents?

Causative agents have thus been separated from three different chicken tumors. This was accomplished after the tumors had been transplanted repeatedly and their malignancy enhanced. Each of the tumor agents gave rise only to the growth of the precise kind from which it had been derived.

There was good reason to suppose that other tumors of the fowl, besides those already studied, were also caused by filterable agents. Several additional chicken tumors had been studied by Rous and his associates. Some were entirely distinct. Thus the spindle-cell sarcoma first filtered (Chicken Tumor No. 1) was fundamentally different from the osteochondrosarcoma elaborating cartilage and bone (Chicken Tumor No. 7). Other tumors were less different, and at least a few tumors were practically indistinguishable in their appearance and general behavior.

In certain instances, spontaneous chicken tumors, such as No. 18 and 38, unlike in several important respects, gave rise on transplantation to neoplasms of identical character. Tumor No. 18, found in the gizzard, was a spindle-cell sarcoma rifted with blood sinuses, that could also be described as having a canalicular pattern. Tumor No. 38, originally found in the subcutaneous tissue of the groin, was a solid spindle-cell sarcoma of a close texture. After several transplantations, both tumors were characterized by slow growth, a tendency to metastasize to the skeletal muscles, and the morphology of a spindle-cell sarcoma; eventually, both became practically indistinguishable in appearance and general behavior. They seemed to be caused by different strains of a single agent.

Among some 45 fowl tumors studied, a few were from the beginning indistinguishable in appearance and general behavior. It was quite apparent, therefore, that chicken tumors of different types may have different filterable agents as their cause, but that, within certain limits, other tumors of rather various characters may at the same time be dependent upon a single agent (Rous, 1914).

Transmissible Myxosarcoma in Chicken Reported by Fujinami and Inamoto in Japan

At about the same time, in 1910, A. Fujinami and K. Inamoto at the Pathological Institute of the Imperial University in Kyoto, Japan, reported experiments dealing with the transplantation of a chicken myxosarcoma; the tumor reported in Japan was quite similar morphologically to the Rous sarcoma. The primary tumor reported by the Japanese investigators appeared in the neighborhood of the right wing of a mature hen. It could be transplanted by cell-graft to other chickens with remarkable success. Initial attempts to filter this tumor failed. Later on, however, Fujinami and

Inamoto (1914) also succeeded in transmitting their chicken tumor by Chamberland filtrates. The tumor could also be desiccated, retaining its ability to reproduce neoplasms when inoculated into susceptible birds. At the request of Professor Aschoff in Freiburg, the tumor was shipped to Europe, transplanted successfully and used for experimental studies first by F. Pentimalli, and later also by other workers on the Continent.

Heterotransplantation to Ducks of the Fujinami Chicken Sarcoma. One of the remarkable features of this chicken sarcoma described in the early Japanese publications (Fujinami and Suzue, 1928. Fujinami, 1930) was its ability to grow, on transplantation, without difficulty in ducks. Its growth in the duck was fairly rapid, the tumor attaining the size of a goose's egg in about three weeks; the tumors grew progressively in the ducks, killing these birds. Over 70 successive transplantations of this tumor in ducks were made by the Japanese investigators. After many successive transfers in the duck, the tumor could be transplanted without difficulty back to the chicken, growing again vigorously in the fowl.

It was later determined that the Rous sarcoma could also be propagated in ducks and other species. This is discussed on subsequent pages of this chapter.

The Importance of the Breed and Age of the Host Used for Inoculation of Filtrates

The genetic constitution and the age of the chickens used for the inoculation of the tumor filtrates were of considerable importance in determining the susceptibility to the tumor-inducing potency of the agent. Although certain breeds or strains of chickens have been found to be relatively, or almost completely, resistant to the virus, it was usually not difficult to locate highly susceptible strains for serial transmission of the tumor agent. The New Hampshire Red breed has been used extensively in the laboratory of Dr. W. Ray Bryan at the National Cancer Institute, whereas Carr (1947, 1953) and Harris (1953), in England, have used the Brown Leghorn breed (Edinburgh strain). White Leghorn chickens have been employed in many laboratories. However, even within particular breeds significant genetic variations in susceptibility to the virus have been reported among individual families (Waters and Fontes, 1960).

The age at which the chickens were inoculated was of considerable importance. Younger chicks were more susceptible than older birds. Four-week-old birds have been used routinely by Bryan and his coworkers for inoculation of the chicken tumor virus. Other investigators, including Carr and Harris, preferred to use younger birds, ranging in age from newly hatched chicks to 7-day-old pullets, which are very susceptible. However, it should be kept in mind that newly hatched chicks may respond to the inoculation of the virus with a hemorrhagic type of lesion rather than by a recognizable neoplastic growth (Duran-Reynals, 1940). As a rule, young chickens 2 to 3, or up to 4, weeks old have been found generally more suitable for routine passage transmission of Rous sarcoma.

Some Properties of the Rous Sarcoma Virus

The Rous sarcoma virus is a spherical particle which could be sedimented after centrifugation at $60{,}000 \times g$ for 60 minutes. The ultracentrifugation studies as well as experiments dealing with ultrafiltration of the tumor extracts through gradocol membranes (Elford and Andrewes, 1935) and also electron microscopic studies suggested that the approximate size of the agent is less than 100 $m\mu$ in diameter, probably somewhere between 70 and 100 $m\mu$.

The chicken tumor virus was found to be inactivated when heated to 55°C for only 15 minutes. In sarcomatous tissue autolyzing at the temperature of the chicken's body (41°C), the agent remained active for less than 48 hours. It was also found to be rapidly destroyed *in vitro* by bile, or by ordinary antiseptic solutions, such as 0.5 per cent phenol.

Most of the filtrates lost their activity within several hours when kept at a temperature of 37°C; it was later found, however, that the addition of a small amount (2 per cent) of horse or rabbit serum had a stabilizing effect on the extract. Bryan and his coworkers found that partially purified preparations of the virus were relatively stable in citrate buffers.

As early as 1911 James B. Murphy, in Peyton Rous' laboratory, demonstrated that the virus could be preserved in dried and powdered neoplastic tissue kept at room temperature for several months (Rous, 1911). Rous and Murphy also demonstrated that the agent survived when tumor tissue was placed in 50 per cent glycerin. In both instances, however, when either dried or preserved in glycerin, the agent was found to undergo gradual attenuation. In a study of the preservation of the chicken tumor virus by freeze-drying, very good recovery of infectivity, after dehydration, with highly purified virus extracts was obtained with media containing broth (Harris, 1953). The agent could be preserved without loss of infectivity for up to 2 years when kept in sealed ampoules, at −70°C, in carbon dioxide dry ice.

A technical procedure during the early work with the chicken tumor virus was the addition to filtrates of sterile infusorial earth, or some other substance capable of producing a non-specific tissue irritation at the site of the inoculation of the filtrate. By this procedure, the incidence of the induced tumors could be increased. After the virus had been propagated for a number of years, however, its potency increased sufficiently to induce tumors without the addition of tissue irritating substances.

Centrifuged extracts prepared from tumors were found to be substantially more potent than filtrates; a considerable amount of the virus was lost during the filtration procedure; frequently some 90 per cent of the amount of the virus present in the extract was retained by the filters.

The agent was found to be remarkably resistant to X-ray irradiation. According to Lacassagne and Nyka (1938), six million roentgens are required to inactivate the virus *in vitro*, although the sarcoma tissue is destroyed by less than 6,000 R, usually employed in the treatment of tumors. When Peacock (1946) treated the chicken sarcoma with doses varying from 4,000 to 10,000 R, the tumor disappeared, but the virus was not destroyed; it remained active around the edges of the tumor, at a certain distance from the zone of irradiation, eventually giving rise to the secondary development of sarcomatous nodules in that area.

Electron Microscopic Studies of the Rous Sarcoma Virus

Claude, Porter, and Pickels were first, in 1947, to find small, dense particles in the cytoplasm of the cultured Rous sarcoma cells. These particles were of round shape, quite uniform in appearance, about 70 to 80 mμ in diameter and had a tendency to occur in pairs or clusters. Initial attempts to confirm these observations by Bernhard and Oberling (1953) did not meet with success; later on, however, Bernhard and his associates at the Cancer Institute in Villejuif, in France, were able to confirm these findings (Bernhard, Dontcheff, Oberling and Vigier, 1953).

The electron microscopic study of the chicken sarcoma was considerably improved with the advent of the new technique of ultrathin sections of tumor cells, making it possible to visualize the internal structure of the particles. Gaylord (1955) at Yale University, in New Haven, Conn., first examined ultrathin sections of chicken sarcoma cells and reported the presence of characteristic virus-like particles occurring either in pairs, or in small clusters, usually on the outer surface of the cell membranes. The particles were round, about 50 mμ in diameter; they had an external membrane and a very dense center.

FIG. 9a. ROUS SARCOMA VIRUS PARTICLES GROWN ON CHORIOALLANTOIC MEMBRANE OF A CHICK EMBRYO.

(A). Ultrathin section of a cell fragment from chorioallantoic membrane of a chick embryo infected with the Bryan strain of Rous sarcoma virus. Virus particles are found characteristically at the surface of the plasma membrane. The dense nucleoids and the internal membranes are well visible. Magnification 90,000 ×.

(B). Ultrathin section of a fragment of a pock induced on the chorioallantoic membrane of a chick embryo by the Bryan strain of Rous sarcoma virus. Groups of characteristic virus particles in intercellular spaces. Magnification 30,000 ×. Electron micrographs (unpublished) prepared by F. Haguenau, Laboratoire de Médecine Expérimentale, Collège de France, Paris.

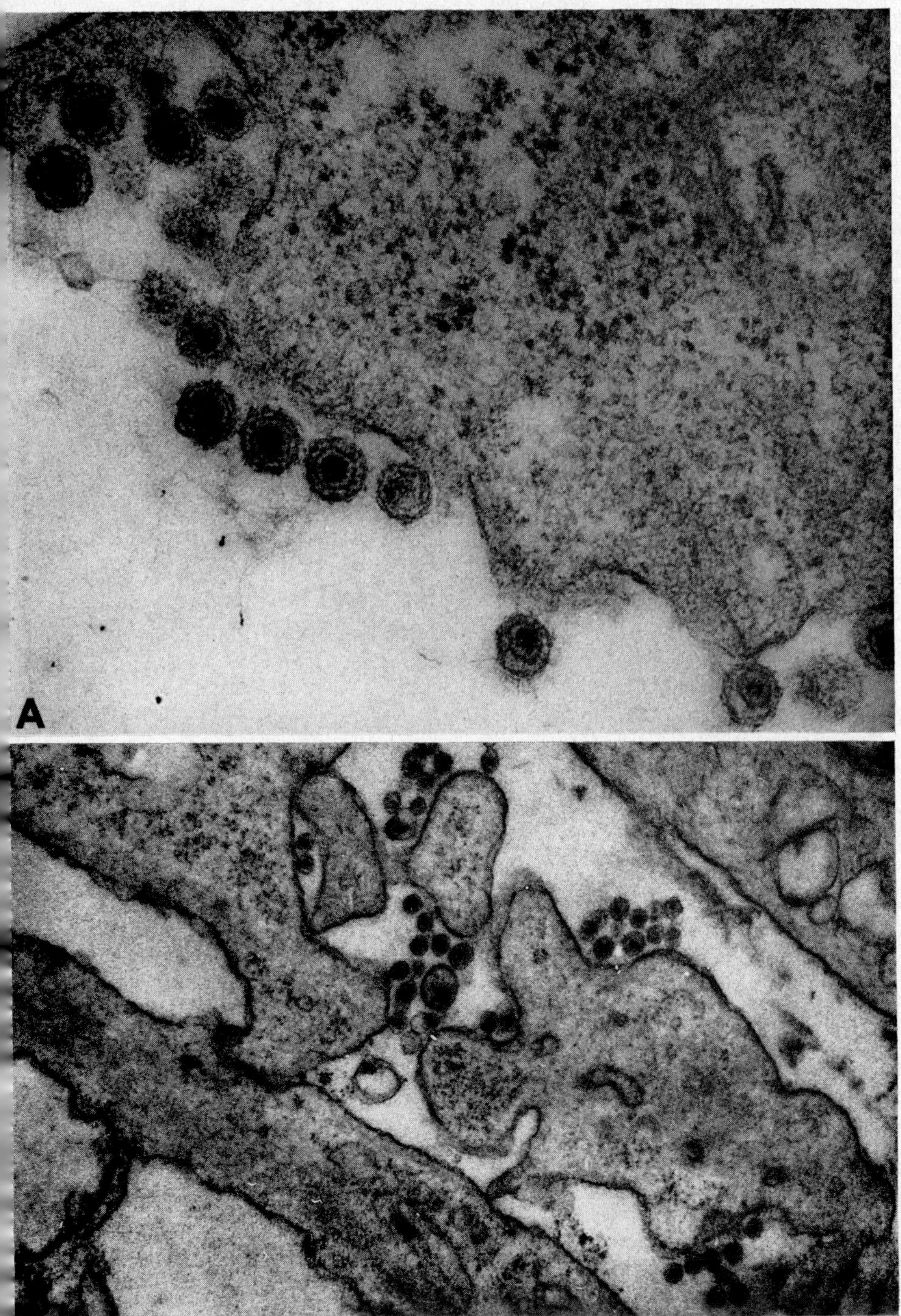

Fig. 9a. Rous Sarcoma Virus Particles Grown on Chorioallantoic Membrane of a Chick Embryo.

E

Bernhard, Oberling, and Vigier reported in an extensive study in 1956 that about two-thirds of 75 chicken tumors studied in the electron microscope contained typical spherical particles 70 to 80 mμ in diameter, average 75 mμ. The particles were surrounded by a distinct external membrane and had an internal, centrally located, electron-dense, nucleoid about 30 to 40 mμ in diameter. On electron micrographs with good resolution, and at high magnification, another internal concentric membrane could be seen surrounding the internal core.*

The particles were found in cytoplasm, quite frequently in agglomerations within cytoplasmic vacuoles. They were found in considerable numbers on the surface of cells, outside the cytoplasm, and also in the intercellular spaces. No particles were found in the nuclei.

Even in active tumors, however, the particles could not always be found. In some tumors a relatively large number of cells had to be examined in order to find a few containing the characteristic virus particles. In other tumors numerous virus particles could be found more readily on electron microscopic examination of cell sections. The tumor-inducing activity of extracts prepared from certain sarcomas could be correlated quantitatively with the number of particles observed in such tumors in the electron microscope (Epstein, 1956). This observation was of considerable interest, since it suggested that the particles observed in Rous sarcoma cells actually represent the Rous sarcoma virus.

Identical virus-like particles have also been shown on thin sections of centrifugation pellets prepared from very active tumor extracts. Again, a striking relationship between the number of virus particles present in pellets, and the ability of the same material to induce tumors on bio-assay, could be established (Haguenau *et al.*, 1958).

Examination of ultrathin sections in the electron microscope makes it possible to survey only an infinitesimally small area of the tumor. It is quite apparent that if the particles are not very numerous, they may be readily missed. Infectivity tests seem more reliable in revealing the presence, or absence, of infective virus particles in a sample examined, provided that uniformly susceptible animals are available, and are employed for the bio-assay tests. Epstein (1956, 1958) at the Middlesex Hospital in London carried out infectivity tests correlated with simultaneous electron microscopic studies and concluded tentatively that approximately 50 individual virus particles are needed to induce a tumor on inoculation tests.

In earlier studies Carr in Edinburgh (1947) attempted to determine the

* In size and morphology, the spherical particles observed in Rous sarcoma were for all practical purposes indistinguishable from those found in myeloblastosis, erythroblastosis, and lymphomatosis of chickens. (See chapter on the Chicken Leukosis Complex in this monograph.)

presumable infective dose per gram of tumor tissue on the basis of inoculation tests. He concluded that only very few individual virus particles could be expected to be present in an average cell examined. Such particles may be scattered only here and there; they may be frequently missed on electron microscopic examination, unless they are present in very large numbers in a particular area examined. Furthermore it is quite possible that oncogenic viruses present in tumor cells exist most frequently in a masked state and not in the form of particles, and cannot be detected in the electron microscope.

* * *

Spherical particles about 70 to 80 mμ in diameter and with the characteristic dense centers could be found not only in Rous sarcoma cells, but also in other chicken tumors. On electron microscopic examination, Mannweiler and Bernhard (1958) found in the Fujinami sarcoma cells characteristic spherical particles, indistinguishable morphologically from those found in the Rous sarcoma. Somewhat larger particles were found by Haguenau and her associates (1955) on ultrathin sections of Murray-Begg endothelioma examined in electron microscope.

* * *

Electron microscopic studies of the chicken tumors included also examination of presumably "normal" chicken tissues. It was *a priori* difficult, however, to assume that no virus-like particles at all would be found in such tissues, since tumor viruses may well be present in a latent, asymptomatic form in many normal, healthy animals. Many chickens are susceptible to the development of "spontaneous" leukosis, and most of them will develop sarcomas following treatment with carcinogenic chemicals. Chicken leukosis is known to be caused by a virus. The possibility is at hand that carcinogen-induced tumors may also be caused by latent viruses, and that the chemicals act only as triggers. Such chickens, when young and in good health, may already carry masked, but potentially pathogenic viruses.

It was not surprising, therefore, that spherical particles, similar to those observed in the Rous and Fujinami sarcomas, could also occasionally be found in presumably "normal" chicken tissues, i.e. in the cells of normal, healthy chickens. Benedetti (1957), in Bernhard's laboratory, studied 84 specimens from 25 normal chicken embryos and from 50 pullets. Out of 84 samples studied, 9 (10 per cent) have shown the presence of particles on electron microscopic examination. The possibility must be considered that the particles found in presumably normal animals belong to the group of viruses responsible for such "spontaneous" neoplastic diseases of the chicken as leukosis or sarcomas.

Antigenic Properties

Serological studies of the chicken tumors encountered considerable difficulties due to the fact that the tumor virus, when inoculated into heterologous hosts, such as rabbits, induced the formation of two types of antibodies, those directed against the virus itself, and others directed against the chicken proteins. It appears that avian sarcomas contain two types of antigen, one being the virus proper, the other of fowl origin. The serological studies established, nevertheless, that the various sarcoma viruses of the fowl are related, but that most of them are individually distinct.

Intracerebral Passage of the Chicken Sarcoma Virus. Groupé and his associates (1956), at Rutgers University, in New Brunswick, N.J., found that the agent of Chicken Tumor No. 1 could be propagated serially in brains of newly hatched, less than 7-day-old chicks. No tumor lesions resulted in the brain, but the agent propagated, as evidenced by titration tests. Within only a few minutes after intracerebral inoculation of the virus, there followed a period of time during which only a very small amount of the virus could be recovered from the brains of the inoculated animals. Beginning with the 4th day after inoculation, however, the content of virus in the brain increased considerably, and gradually reached its maximum in moribund chicks. When newly hatched, less than one-day-old chicks were inoculated, typical hemorrhagic disease, similar to that described by Duran-Reynals, frequently resulted; some of the chicks developed also hepatic lesions; the liver was small, and friable, and of a vividly yellow color. The hemorrhagic disease and the hepatic lesions were both associated with the presence of large quantities of the virus.

Growth of the Rous Chicken Sarcoma Virus in Embryonated Eggs

Rous and Murphy were first to utilize chick embryo for the propagation of tumors and as a medium for virus cultivation. In 1911 they inoculated successfully chicken embryos with the avian sarcoma virus; the most suitable time for inoculation was between the 7th and 10th day of the development of the embryo. They showed that the Rous sarcoma could be grown successfully in various parts of the chicken embryo and its membranes. Tumors could be induced with either tumor cells or with filtrates, in the chorioallontoic or allantoic membrane, or in the embryo itself. Most of these experiments were performed on embryonated chicken eggs, but similar tumors could also be induced in pigeon and duck embryos. Later on Murphy showed that tumors of foreign species would also grow in the chicken embryo. Embryonated chicken eggs are now used in considerable numbers for the cultivation of a large assortment of viruses.

More recently, Keogh (1938), in England, tried to apply the method of inoculating embryonated chicken eggs to quantitative studies on the Rous sarcoma virus. The virus concentration in a sample was estimated by the number of tumors induced by plating the sample on the chorioallantoic membrane of the developing chick embryo. As a result, characteristic small tumors developed, which, curiously, involved not only the mesodermal, but also ectodermal cells. This method was later employed for quantitative studies (Groupé *et al.*, 1957. Rubin, 1957. Prince, 1958). The Rous sarcoma virus induced ectodermal and mesodermal cell proliferations in the form of characteristic pustules on the chorioallantoic membrane of the chicken embryo. The type of growth induced depended apparently not on variation of the virus, but on the type of cell infected. It must be taken into consideration, however, that the ectodermal and mesodermal cells of the embryonic membranes of the developing chick embryo are not as completely differentiated from one another as are adult tissues.

The tumor cells thus induced were then assayed for the presence of liberated virus. From a series of quantitative studies it was concluded that an average sarcoma virus particle stays within the cell for half an hour after its completion. Further calculation showed that each sarcoma cell produces and releases only one to five tumor-forming units within 24 hours. The release of the tumor virus from the infected cell is continuous, but proceeds at a slow trickle.

Are all Chicken Sarcomas Caused by Filterable Agents? Filterability of Chicken Tumors Induced by Carcinogenic Chemicals

Nebenzahl, in 1934, reviewed about 30 spontaneous chicken tumors, examined in various parts of the world, and concluded that all sarcomas of the fowl that could be transplanted by graft for a sufficient number of passages would eventually also become filterable. It is true that only some of the spontaneous tumors could be transplanted successfully; it should be kept in mind, however, that transplantation experiments have often been carried out under unfavorable conditions. Most spontaneous tumors are of relatively low potency; for successful transplantation, in initial experiments,

---

FIG. 9b. ROUS SARCOMA VIRUS PARTICLES GROWN ON CHORIOALLANTOIC MEMBRANE OF A CHICK EMBRYO.

(A). Ultrathin section of a cell fragment from chorioallantoic membrane of a chick embryo infected with the Rous sarcoma virus. Characteristic row of virus particles on the surface of plasma membrane. Magnification 56,000 ×. (B). Ultrathin section of a fragment of chorioallantoic membrane of a chick embryo infected with the Rous sarcoma virus. Virus particles on the surface of plasma membrane and also in the intercellular space. Magnification 66,000 ×. Electron micrographs prepared by F. Haguenau, H. Febvre and J. Arnoult. (From: *J. Microscopie*, **1**: 445, 1962.)

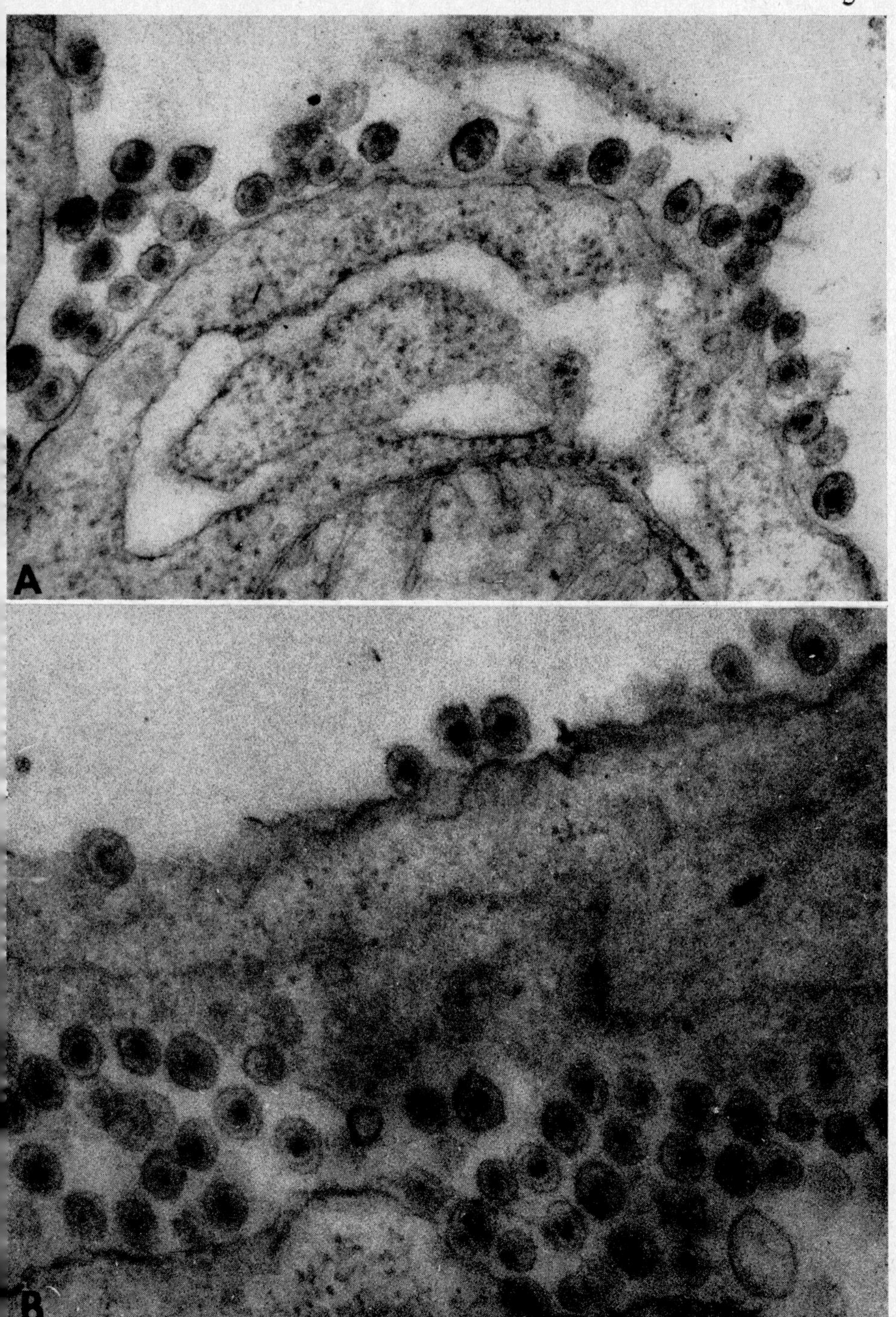

FIG. 9b. ROUS SARCOMA VIRUS PARTICLES GROWN ON CHORIOALLANTOIC MEMBRANE OF A CHICK EMBRYO.

these tumors often require highly susceptible hosts from intimately related stocks in which the growth occurred. Such tumors only gradually acquire sufficient potency to grow in chickens of any sort. Since susceptible hosts from intimately related stocks were not often available for the initial experiments, many spontaneous tumors could not be transplanted.

It gradually became apparent, nevertheless, to most of the investigators dealing with chicken tumors, that all spontaneous sarcomas which have been transplanted successfully have sooner or later also become filterable. In 1941 Murphy and Sturm also concluded that all spontaneous chicken tumors that could be transplanted, if properly investigated, have given evidence of containing a transmissible agent. It is quite possible to speculate, therefore, that essentially all chicken sarcomas are caused by viruses. It may be quite difficult, nevertheless, to actually transmit all such tumors by filtrates in the laboratory. The main difficulty may be related to the low quantity of infective particles present in most of the spontaneous tumors.

This may apply also to the various sarcomas that can be induced in the chickens by the injection of tar, or certain purified carcinogenic chemicals, such as methylcholanthrene or dibenzanthracene. Carrel was first to report (1925) that a chemically induced tumor of the fowl could be transmitted by filtrate. This report stirred a considerable controversy. Most investigators could not confirm Carrel's important observation. Peacock (1933) reported extensive studies in which tumors induced with chemicals were used for the preparation of filtrates; none of these filtrates proved active on inoculation tests. Others claimed, however, that they were able to transmit such tumors by filtrates. McIntosh (1933), who obtained 13 tumors in 21 hens injected with tar, was able to transmit three of these tumors by filtrates. Later on (1935) he added two additional, chemically induced tumors which he could also transmit by filtrates. His results were questioned, but additional incontestable evidence was reported in 1950 by Oberling and Guérin. The French authors described a sarcoma that appeared on the foot of a hen 32 months after injection of an oily solution of methylcholanthrene. This tumor, which grew slowly, could be transmitted by grafts, and attempts at transmission by filtrate were negative at the second and third passages. At the fourth passage, grafts made with glycerinated material were negative, but a month later, in the following passage, positive results were obtained with fragments kept for 7 to 27 days in glycerin in a refrigerator. At the fifth passage, 20 months after the appearance of the primary tumor, transmission by filtrate was positive, as it was also at the sixth passage.

It is apparent that under proper experimental conditions not only spontaneous avian tumors, but also at least some among those induced by chemicals, can be transmitted by filtrates. It is quite probable, however, that a great majority of these tumors contain only very small quantities of infective particles; the tumor virus may be present in most of these neoplasms in a masked form; this may account for the difficulty in transmitting such tumors by filtrates.

The Problem of Inactive Tumor Filtrates

Of the many fowl tumors investigated and transmitted by filtrates in the original study of Rous and his associates, the first tumor studied and designated "Chicken Tumor No. 1" (now generally referred to as "Rous sarcoma") has been used extensively in many laboratories. In the course of successive cell-free transmissions, the tumor gradually gained in virulence; some of the basic experimental conditions necessary for the successful transmission of this tumor have been determined. When removing a tumor for the preparation of extracts, actively growing healthy parts of the sarcomatous tissues had to be used, avoiding necrotic tissues frequently found in the center of the tumors. Rapidly growing tumors in young animals yielded more active filtrates than those growing slowly in old hens.

Even under apparently similar conditions, however, using for the preparation of filtrates rapidly growing tumors from young donors, the activity of the extracts still varied to a considerable degree. Some tumors, even though morphologically not different from those yielding active filtrates, could not be transmitted by cell-free extracts.

Even during the initial experiments the important observation was made by Rous that not infrequently filtrates prepared from malignant tissues under apparently best conditions proved entirely innocuous. Chicken tumor No. 1 contained abundantly mucinous substances which could possibly be blamed for clogging the filters during the filtration procedure, and thus retaining the virus. Extracts prepared from some of the other tumors, however, did not contain any conspicuous amount of mucine and ran rapidly through the filters; yet many of them were also inactive on inoculation tests.

Although Rous and others had long recognized the appearance after longer latent intervals, and the slower growth, of tumors induced with weak preparations of the sarcoma virus, it was W. Ray Bryan and his associates at the National Cancer Institute in Bethesda, Md., who studied this fundamental problem on a quantitative basis (Bryan, 1955, 1956. Bryan *et al.*, 1954, 1955. Moloney, 1956. Riley *et al.*, 1946) and determined that the amount of extractable virus from a tumor depends essentially on the amount of virus used in the initiating dose. Most spontaneous tumors found in the field contain very small quantities of infective and transmissible virus. Among tumors induced in the laboratory by inoculation of tumor filtrates, those induced with large amounts of virus appeared after a relatively short latency and yielded, in Bryan's studies, sizeable amounts of virus on extraction procedure. On the other hand, tumors induced with very small amounts of virus developed only after a relatively long latency. Some of the tumors that had been induced with low doses of virus grew relatively fast, once they had appeared. They were also grossly indistinguishable from those tumors that had been induced with high doses of virus. Yet, they yielded little or no virus on extraction procedure and could only occasionally be passed by filtrates to other hosts.

Another puzzling phenomenon reported during the early studies by many investigators, and probably related to the lower potency of the earlier tumors, was the temporary disappearance of filterability of a chicken sarcoma maintained in a given laboratory. For a period of several months, no virus could be extracted from a tumor; the sarcoma could be maintained, nevertheless, during that time by serial transplantation of tumor tissue; eventually, however, the tumor would again become filterable. The lower relative potencies of the earlier tumors were also responsible for the fact that not infrequently, among small test groups of chickens inoculated, one or two would fail to develop tumors. After many years of successive serial cell-free passages of the virus, we now have tumor material at hand which induces tumors in 100 per cent of inoculated chickens even when dilutions 10^{-4} of the cell-free extracts are used for inoculations. Dilutions 10^{-5} or 10^{-6} give 75 to 90 per cent takes, and such dilutions most probably correspond to the tumor extracts available under the best experimental conditions in earlier studies on the chicken sarcoma.

The strongest doses of this virus now induce grossly detectable tumors within 5 to 6 days, and microscopic evidence of the presence of the tumor is detectable as early as the 3rd or 4th day following inoculation of the cell-free extracts into young, 2 to 6-week-old, susceptible chicks.

Difficulties in Extracting Infective Virus from Chicken Sarcomas

The difficulties encountered in extracting infectious virus from chicken tumors, often so troublesome in the laboratory, represented, nevertheless, an interesting experimental challenge; the causes of such difficulties have been studied by a number of investigators. The age of the host in which the tumor had grown, and particularly the age of the tumor itself, exerted an influence on the amount of virus that could be extracted from the tumor. It was easier to recover infective virus from Rous sarcoma growing in younger hosts, as compared with tumors growing in older animals (Duran-Reynals and Freire, 1953). Moreover, the age of the tumor, i.e. the length of time the tumor had grown in the host, had a considerable influence on the amount of virus that could be extracted from such a tumor. In general, more infectious virus could be extracted from very young tumors (Carr, 1943. Duran-Reynals and Freire, 1953). Carr obtained maximum yields of virus and found no correlation with tumor age during the first 13 days of tumor growth. Tumors that had been grown 14 to 22 days yielded slightly less virus on extraction; those which had grown for 22 to 40 days showed a striking inverse correlation between tumor age and amount of extractable virus; the rate of this decrease depended also on the genetic background of the chicken. Tumors that had grown for more than 40 days, even in young susceptible hosts, yielded no virus at all on extraction. More recently Rubin (1962) observed that most tumors become non-infective at 30 days.

In general, tumors in this group were induced with relatively high doses of virus. Furthermore, such tumors were usually induced in young adult, immunologically competent chickens, and the gradual decrease, and eventual disappearance, of virus yield from such tumors could be interpreted as a result of an immunological reaction of the host (Rubin, 1962. Rubin and Hanafusa, 1963. Shimizu and Rubin, 1964). The fact that some of the tumors, induced in adult birds and growing for prolonged periods of time, eventually regressed spontaneously was consistent with such an assumption.

Freire, Bryan and Duran-Reynals (1953) observed no regression of tumors induced in chickens inoculated at 15 days of age, whereas spontaneous tumor regression occurred in 15 per cent of older birds. A considerably higher incidence of spontaneous regression of tumors induced in adult animals was observed by Rubin and Hanafusa (1963).

It must be stressed, however, that the susceptibility to tumor induction, and the incidence of spontaneous regression of the induced tumors, depended not only on the age, but also on genetic susceptibility of the hosts employed.

The Concept of a "Defective" Rous Sarcoma Virus and the Presumable Role of a "Helper Virus"

Another group of tumors, yielding small quantities of infective virus or no virus at all on extraction procedures, consisted of sarcomas that had been induced with very small doses of Rous sarcoma virus (Bryan *et al.*, 1955. Prince, 1959). The possibility that non-infective clones or tumors consisted of cells producing an incomplete or defective virus was considered (Prince, 1959). On the basis of extensive experiments, Rubin, Hanafusa, and their coworkers at the Virus Laboratory, University of California, in Berkeley, suggested that the Bryan high-titer strain of Rous sarcoma contains a "defective virus," which cannot reproduce infective virus particles in the absence of a "helper virus" (Rubin and Vogt, 1962. Hanafusa *et al.*, 1963). The "helper virus" was designated "Rous associated virus" or RAV. When chicken embryo cells are infected in tissue culture with the Rous sarcoma virus alone, under strict precautions to prevent contamination with a "helper virus," they become transformed into typical Rous sarcoma cells, but do not produce infectious virus. It is only when a "helper virus" is added that infectious Rous sarcoma virus is produced.

Further studies demonstrated that the "helper virus," or "Rous associated virus," can induce leukosis in chickens and is a virus of the avian leukosis complex.

It appears that the "helper virus," i.e. the chicken leukosis virus, is necessary to provide a protein coat for the Rous sarcoma virus and thus enable it to produce infective particles. Without the assistance of such a "helper virus," the Rous sarcoma virus is unable to form infectious virus particles, even though it retains its ability to induce malignant cell transformation, and thereby form tumors.

Propagation of the Rous Sarcoma Virus in Tissue Culture and Interference between the Chicken Leukosis Virus and Rous Sarcoma

It was reported in 1941 that when chicken fibroblasts growing *in vitro* were infected by the Rous sarcoma virus, they became altered in appearance and resembled typical sarcoma cells (Halberstaedter *et al.*, 1941). More recently it was observed (Manaker and Groupé, 1956) that following infection *in vitro* of chick embryo cells with Rous sarcoma virus derived from genetically susceptible chicken lines, altered cells appeared in discrete foci, and that the number of these foci was proportional to the concentration of infecting virus. The enumeration of these foci served as an accurate assay for the infectious titer of a Rous sarcoma virus preparation. In occasional sets of chick embryo cultures, however, up to 50 per cent of the embryo cells showed resistance to the inoculation of the virus.

The sporadic resistance to infection *in vitro* with Rous sarcoma virus was observed among pools of cells obtained from several chick embryos. Rubin observed (1960) that resistance encountered in such cell pools was always associated with the presence of one or more chicken embryos, serving as one of the donors of the cells, which were resistant when cultivated separately. An agent could be isolated from the medium of resistant cultures, which induced resistance to Rous sarcoma virus when added to susceptible cultures (Rubin, 1960). This "resistance-inducing factor," designated "RIF," multiplied extensively in infected cultures without causing a cytopathic effect.

The resistance-inducing factor could be sedimented in an ultracentrifuge under conditions similar to those required to sediment the Rous sarcoma virus, and could be neutralized by an immune anti-Rous sarcoma serum. These characteristics, added to the widespread occurrence of this agent in eggs, suggested that it is a virus of the avian leukosis complex (Rubin, 1960). Later on it was found that the "resistance-inducing factor" could actually induce leukosis in chickens, and that it is identical with congenitally transmitted virus of avian lymphomatosis (Rubin *et al.*, 1961. Rubin and Vogt, 1962. Hanafusa *et al.*, 1963).

The resistance induced by the chicken leukosis virus was not absolute; the cells infected with the leukosis virus were found to have reduced susceptibility to infection with the Rous sarcoma. In the resistant cultures infected with the leukosis virus only a fraction of the foci was formed as compared with unaffected control cultures.

The interference, in tissue culture, between the virus of chicken lymphomatosis and the Rous sarcoma virus offers an excellent, prompt, and quantitative *in vitro* assay system in studying the distribution of the avian leukosis virus in nature.

Experimental Contact Transmission of Rous Sarcoma

At the Regional Poultry Research Laboratory in East Lansing, Michigan, Burmester and his colleagues (1960) reported transmission of the Rous sarcoma virus by contact from inoculated to non-inoculated chicks.

A highly potent Rous sarcoma virus obtained from Dr. W. R. Bryan's laboratory was employed in these experiments. The chickens were of the very susceptible White Leghorn line 15-I. This particular strain of chickens was originally selected for its susceptibility to lymphomatosis and had been maintained in isolation for the preceding 18 years. More recently this line of chickens was also found to be quite susceptible to the Rous sarcoma virus (Burmester *et al.*, 1960).

In Burmester's experiments, 9-day-old chicks were inoculated subcutaneously with the Rous sarcoma virus, and over 94 per cent of them developed tumors in from 14 to 19 days. Non-inoculated birds of the same age were simultaneously placed in the same cubicles with the injected chicks and allowed to intermingle freely. In the first experiment, of 45 such non-inoculated birds, 35 (78 per cent) developed multiple tumors after a latency varying from 37 to 128 days. Some of the tumors involved

---

FIG. 10. ROUS SARCOMA VIRUS PARTICLES IN TUMOR CELLS.

(A). Ultrathin section of a chicken wing tumor induced with the Bryan strain of Rous sarcoma virus. A group of mature virus particles in an intercellular space, and also in a cytoplasmic vacuole. The particles are spherical, about 80 mμ in diameter, and have centrally located electron-dense nucleoids. Magnification 60,000 ×. (B). (Inset). Ultrathin section of a tumor cell from a fragment of chicken sarcoma induced with the Bryan strain of Rous sarcoma virus. Virus particle budding (arrow) from the edge of a cell membrane. Magnification 80,000 ×. Electron micrographs prepared by L. Dmochowski and K. E. Muse, Department of Virology, University of Texas, M. D. Anderson Hospital and Tumor Institute, Houston.

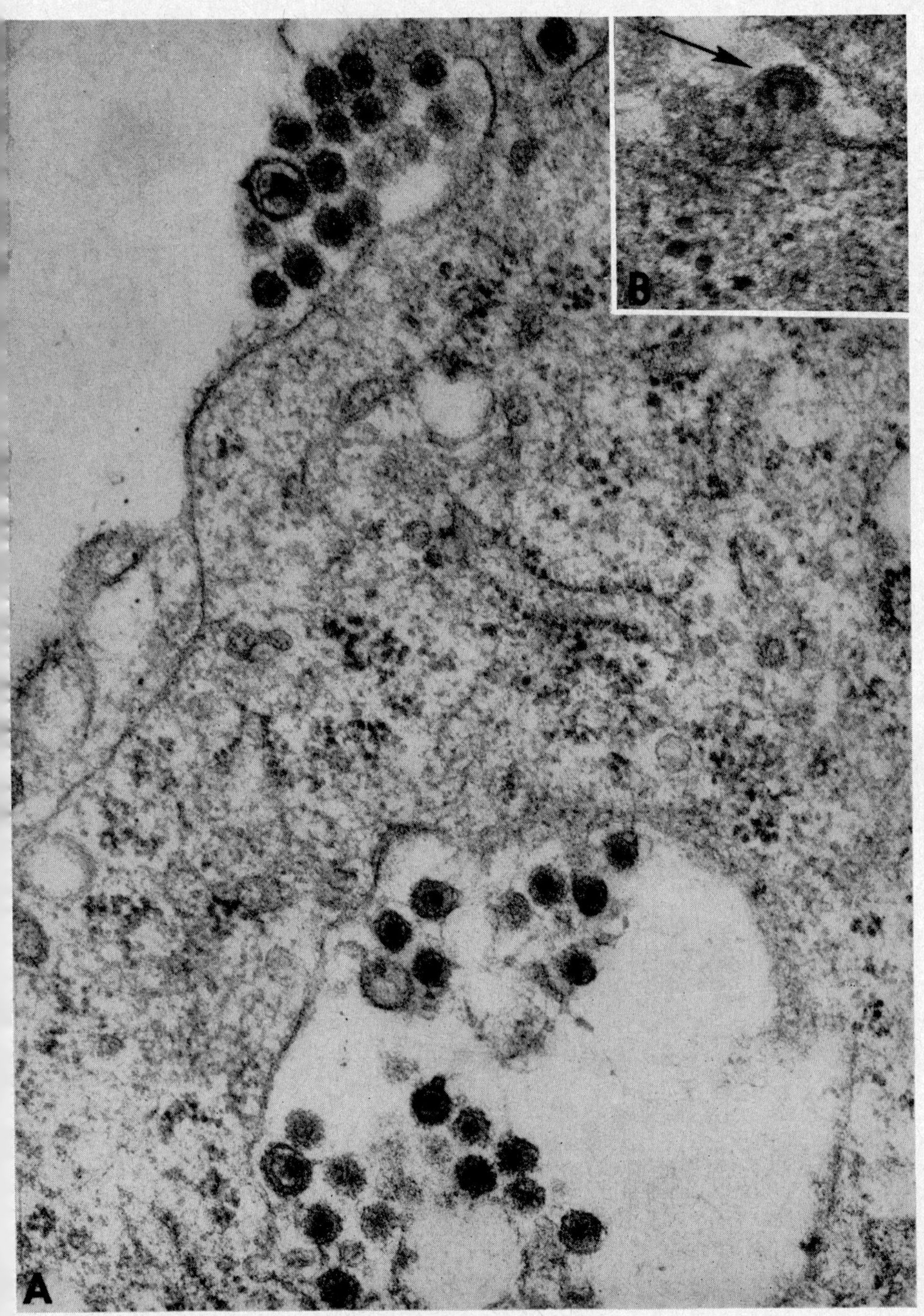

FIG. 10. ROUS SARCOMA VIRUS PARTICLES IN TUMOR CELLS.

developed in the skin or in the subcutaneous tissue and infiltrated the underlying muscles; they appeared on head, neck, wings, breast, legs, etc. More than one-half of the birds, however, had multiple visceral sarcomas without any skin involvement.

In another similar experiment, of 58 non-inoculated birds that had been in contact with inoculated chickens, 23 (40 per cent) developed multiple tumors after a latency varying from 42 to 104 days. Again, some of these tumors involved head, neck, wings, and legs. Other birds had only visceral sarcomas in the lungs, mesentery, liver, spleen and kidneys.

Curiously, of 50 birds that had been separated only by a double screen from the inoculated chickens, but had been kept otherwise in the same pen, none developed tumors. No tumors developed among 49 isolated controls kept in a separate cubicle.

These experiments suggested that under certain experimental conditions the Rous sarcoma virus could be transmitted from bird to bird by direct contact. The actual manner of such natural virus transmission remained unknown, however.

It is rather surprising that no similar observation had previously been made, even though the Rous sarcoma virus has been known and studied for half a century. It is possible that the high potency of the currently available Rous sarcoma strain, the high susceptibility of White Leghorn line 15-I chickens employed as test animals, and the long observation period, were directly related to the striking results observed by Burmester and his colleagues.

Hemorrhagic Disease Induced in Newly Hatched Chickens by the Rous Sarcoma Virus

F. Duran-Reynals at Yale University in New Haven, Conn., observed (1940) that newly hatched chicks may respond to the inoculation of the Rous sarcoma virus by diffuse hemorrhagic manifestations, instead of developing tumors. This hemorrhagic disease induced with the tumor agent in newly hatched chicks was a curious manifestation quite different from the effect of inoculation of the same tumor agent into fully grown birds.

Duran-Reynals (1940) described in the following manner the hemorrhagic lesions induced following inoculation of the Rous virus into newly hatched chicks:

"The blood in the peritoneal cavity was present in comparatively large amounts, fluid or clotted, the latter always adherent to one or several viscera. After the blood was washed away the organs were pale with numerous darker hemorrhagic lesions. Such lesions were of three types: (a) circumscribed, raised blebs; (b) more diffuse, flat, small, petechial spots; and (c) similar but larger extravasations of blood. The blebs varied in size from a fraction of a millimeter to several millimeters; they were constantly present in the liver and spleen, less frequently in gonads, intestines, pancreas, and kidneys. In the liver they often protruded from the surface of the organ: evidently they can easily rupture and the subsequent hemorrhage is the obvious cause of death. Extravasations of varying size, sometimes involving half the organ, and petechial spots were frequently observed in the lungs and kidneys, occasionally in the skin, heart, muscles, periosteum, and serous membranes. Pericardial exudate was present in some instances. Most affected of all the viscera was the spleen, which appeared greatly enlarged and showed numerous central or peripheral blebs."

The foregoing description corresponded to the pure form of the hemorrhagic disease in which no generalized neoplastic lesions were grossly visible. Such form was observed following inoculation of newly hatched chicks. Under such conditions, the disease revealed itself by the exclusive development of hemorrhagic lesions, usually confined to the viscera and causing death in a few days. When pullets were inoculated, a combined form of disease was often induced. Small, white nodules, easily recognizable as tumors, could be observed in such animals side by side with the hemorrhagic lesions.

That the hemorrhagic lesions were actually induced by the virus was determined in an experiment in which 8 successive intravenous passages of the virus were made through chicks in which only gross hemorrhagic lesions were induced without any evidence of tumors. When, after several serial hemorrhagic passages, extracts were prepared from such lesions and inoculated back into chickens, typical sarcomas were induced.

In further studies carried out by Milford and Duran-Reynals (1943) the Rous sarcoma virus was injected into chick embryos. Out of a total of 132 chick embryos injected intracelomically or intravenously, the virus produced hemorrhagic lesions in 64 hosts without inducing any tumors. The hemorrhagic lesions could be transmitted through 6 successive passages into other chick embryos, again without induction of tumors. The injection of extracts prepared from such hemorrhagic lesions into chicks and pullets resulted in the development of typical sarcomas.

Duran-Reynals designated this syndrome as "hemorrhagic disease," realized its importance, and demonstrated for the first time that an oncogenic virus can induce a non-neoplastic infectious disease without inducing tumors at the same time.

In their early studies Rous and Murphy had also observed (1913) that the Rous sarcoma virus may induce internal hemorrhages in association with tumors. In their studies in which they employed adult chickens for the inoculation of the virus, they occasionally observed visceral hemorrhages, particularly in the liver and in retroperitoneal space, but only in association with concurrent development of tumors. It was not realized at that time that the hemorrhages represented a particular manifestation of virus infection, and that they may occur in the absence of tumors.

Early Attempts to Transplant Chicken Tumors to Animals of Other Species, Order or Class

In the early studies, some thirty or forty years ago, it was common practice in many laboratories engaged in experimental cancer research to study heterotransplantation of tumors. Mouse tumors in particular, but chicken tumors also, were transplanted to animals of different species, or order, with varying success. As a rule, the implanted tumor fragments, or cell suspensions, either did not grow at all in foreign species, or grew only temporarily and later on regressed. Some of these transplantations were made into conditioned hosts, such as after preliminary or concomitant treatment with X-rays or cortisone. Tumor fragments or cell suspensions were also implanted into the brain, or in the anterior chamber of the eye.

Roskin (1926) reported growth of the Rous sarcoma in white mice in which the reticulo-endothelial system had been blocked with saccharated iron oxide. The growth was sustained as long as the blockade persisted, but eventually all tumors disappeared. Milone (1928) described "zig-zag" transplantation of Rous sarcoma in fowls and rats, but the grafts did not survive more than 12 days in rats. Shrigley, Greene, and Duran-Reynals (1945) transplanted Rous sarcoma cells to the anterior chamber of the eye of guinea pigs; these transplants initially increased in size and then persisted unchanged for several months. Greene (1951) transplanted Rous sarcoma to the brains of mice, guinea pigs, and rabbits. The incidence of takes was high, and growth was rapid, but only temporary, and terminated in regression of the tumors within 2 weeks. The tumors could be maintained by consecutive passages from brain to brain. Ageenko (1957) also succeeded in transplanting Rous sarcoma to the brains of mice and guinea pigs. The tumors attained maximum size 10 to 12 days after inoculation, but later regressed. In mice, the tumor was carried through 6 generations; in guinea pigs, through 3, and then transferred back to chickens with unchanged biological character.

Rous sarcoma was transplanted to cortisone-treated hamsters and maintained its size for more than 3 weeks (Kuwata *et al.*, 1958. Kuwata, 1960). When normal chick embryonic tissue was added to the hamster-grown tumors, they could be transplanted serially to conditioned hamsters for 9 generations. In non-treated hamsters the tumors regressed within 10 days.

Transmission of Chicken Tumors to Ducks, Pheasants, Turkeys, and Pigeons

It has been known since the early studies that chicken tumors could be transmitted, either by minced cell suspensions or by cell-free filtrate, to ducks, pheasants, turkeys, and pigeons.

Successful transmission of the Fujinami chicken sarcoma to ducks was reported by Fujinami and his coworkers in Japan (Fujinami and Suzue, 1928. Fujinami and Hatano, 1929. Fujinami, 1930). This transplantable chicken tumor was first described by Fujinami and Inamoto in 1914, and was later found by the Japanese authors to be readily transmissible, presumably by cell transplantation, to ducks also, growing progressively in both chickens and ducks. Gye (1931, 1932) confirmed these observations and was able to transmit the Fujinami sarcoma through 18 serial generations of tumor transfers by means of either filtrates or cell suspensions in ducklings.

Purdy (1932) propagated the Rous chicken sarcoma through 5 serial transplant generations in ducklings by injecting large amounts of minced tumor tissue. In 1-day-old and also in 4-day-old ducklings transplantation was consistently successful. The susceptibility decreased rapidly in older birds. Only some of the 11 to 14-day-old ducklings were found to be susceptible, while adult ducks were resistant.

Transmission of Rous sarcoma from chickens to ducklings by means of filtrates was accomplished in 1942 by F. Duran-Reynals. In this important study Duran-Reynals demonstrated that the Rous sarcoma virus could induce a variety of malignant tumors in ducks, provided that newly hatched, less than 24-hour-old, ducklings were inoculated, preferably by the intravenous route, with the virus filtrates.

There was a significant and rapid increase in resistance of the ducks to the virus, the greatest susceptibility being found at hatching. Newborn ducklings were also susceptible to the implantation of the chicken tumor cells.

The lesions induced with the chicken tumor in the ducks were either immediate or late. The immediate lesions appeared within some 30 days after inoculation and consisted of solitary spindle-cell sarcomas very similar to the original chicken tumor. The late lesions appeared generally several months after inoculation and consisted essentially of different types of sarcomas, giant-cell sarcomas of the bone, and lymphoblastomas developing in various locations. Extracts from the immediate tumors were ineffective in ducks, but induced typical tumors in chicks. On the other hand, extracts from the late sarcomatous duck tumors lost their power to induce sarcomas in adult chickens, but were able to induce in other ducks multiple tumors, particularly periosteal sarcomas; the latter had occasionally also been seen in chickens injected with the Rous sarcoma virus, attesting to some possible modification of the virus occurring also in the fowl. Practically all these tumors in ducks and chickens grew progressively until they killed their hosts.

The Rous sarcoma virus could therefore be transmitted to ducks by means of filtrates, and induced a wide spectrum of tumors, but only under particular experimental conditions; newly hatched ducklings had to be inoculated, preferably by the intravenous route.

Andrewes (1932) succeeded in transmitting the chicken sarcoma to

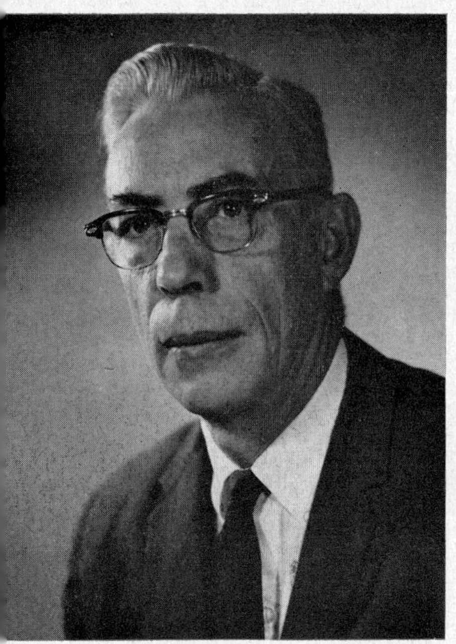

W. Ray Bryan

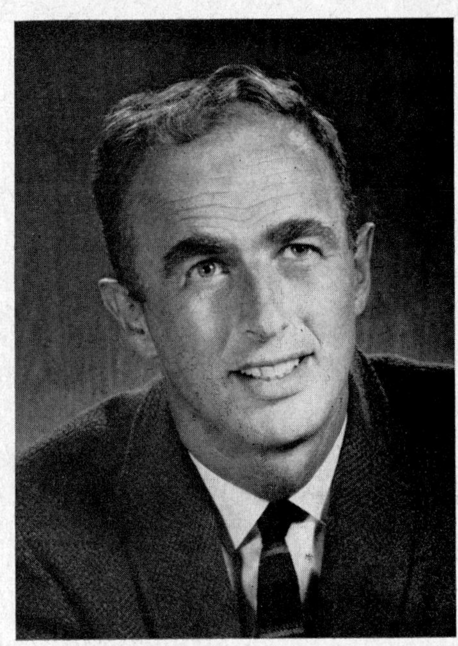

Harry Rubin

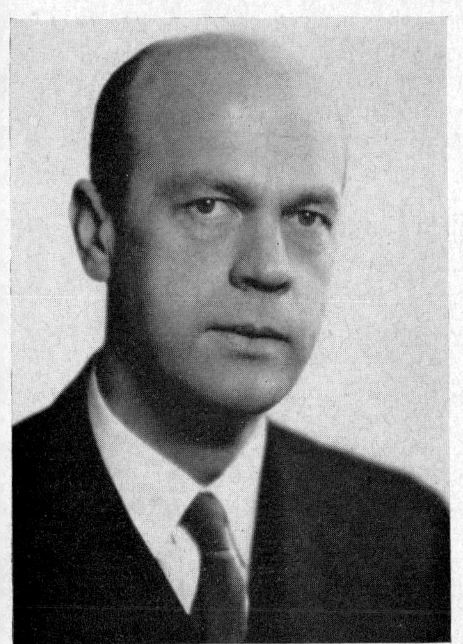

C. G. Ahlström

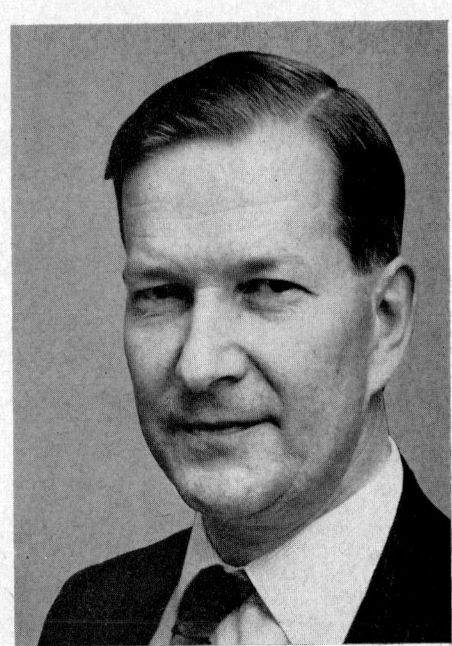

R. J. C. Harris

FIG. 11.

pheasants not only by cells, but also by filtrates. Des Ligneris (1932) transplanted Rous sarcoma by cell transplantation to turkeys and guinea fowls. Transmission of the chicken sarcoma to turkeys and guinea fowls by cell-free extracts was accomplished by Duran-Reynals (1943) who used very young birds for the inoculation of filtrates; the resulting tumors were slow-growing fibrosarcomas, producing massive metastatic growths in the Fver and spleen of the guinea fowls, and in the periosteal tissue of the turkeys.

It was also demonstrated that Rous sarcoma, after passage through ducklings, could successfully be transplanted by cell-graft (Duran-Reynals, 1947) or by filtrates (Borges and Duran-Reynals, 1952) to pigeons. Filtrates, effective both in chickens and ducks, induced tumors in 9 out of 17 pigeons inoculated. Cell suspensions produced tumors in all 12 pigeons inoculated (Borges and Duran-Reynals, 1952). Metastases were observed only in 3 cases, and spontaneous regression occurred in 11 birds. The tumors could not be maintained by further cell passages in pigeons.

INDUCTION OF HEMORRHAGIC MANIFESTATIONS, CYSTS, AND SARCOMAS IN MAMMALS FOLLOWING INOCULATION OF ROUS SARCOMA

One of the most striking developments in experimental cancer research in recent years was the observation that the Rous chicken sarcoma virus can induce tumors not only in chickens, ducks, pheasants, turkeys, and pigeons, but also in rats, mice, hamsters, guinea pigs, rabbits, and monkeys. Furthermore, the same virus was found to induce not necessarily tumors, but, under certain experimental conditions, and in some species, particularly in rats, also cysts and hemorrhagic manifestations; in certain instances the development of cysts was only a preliminary manifestation which was followed later by the development of sarcomas.

Our classical concept of an oncogenic virus limited in its pathogenic potential to its ability to induce only tumors of certain type and morphology, and in one or in a few related species only, had to be revised fundamentally.

The Various Strains of the Rous Sarcoma Virus and Significant Variations in Their Host Range and Pathogenic Potential

In order to review recent observations on successful transmission of the Rous chicken sarcoma to mammals, it is necessary to discuss several different strains of the Rous sarcoma virus employed in these studies. Most of these strains are sublines of the original virus isolated from Chicken Tumor No. 1 by Peyton Rous (1911). These strains have been carried for many years in several laboratories by serial virus passage in chickens. Gradually certain differences became apparent among several of those strains which have been widely employed in some of the more prominent laboratories in the United States and abroad. These differences included variations in potency, in antigenic and certain biological properties, such as the character of growth pattern on the chorioallantoic membranes, in embryonated eggs, etc. Most important of all, rather striking differences in oncogenic potential and host range became apparent among a few virus strains. Some of them could be transmitted consistently to mammals, inducing cysts, hemorrhagic disease, and eventually also malignant tumors. Other strains were pathogenic for mammals only very occasionally, or not at all.

Among the strains more prominently employed in experiments dealing with transmission of the Rous sarcoma virus into mammals are the following:

The Carr-Zilber Strain of the Rous Sarcoma Virus. One of the first Rous sarcoma strains successfully tested for its pathogenic potency in mammals was that employed by Dr. L. A. Zilber and his coworkers at the Gamaleya Institute of Microbiology in Moscow. This strain had originally been received from Dr. J. G. Carr of Edinburgh by Dr. B. I. Zbarsky, who in turn passed it on to Dr. Zilber in 1945. This strain, designated as the "Carr-Zilber" strain, was later sent to Dr. G. J. Svet-Moldavsky in Moscow, also to Dr. C. M. Southam in New York, and to other laboratories.

The Prague Strain. Another strain which proved to be pathogenic for mammals was the "Prague" strain. This virus strain was received by Dr. J. Svoboda at the Institute of Biology in Prague, from Dr. J. Englebreth-Holm of Copenhagen.

The Schmidt-Ruppin Strain. A virus strain of the Rous sarcoma which proved to be highly pathogenic for mammals was the "Schmidt-Ruppin" strain. This strain was received in 1953 from Dr. Charles Oberling of Paris by Dr. K. H. Schmidt-Ruppin who was at that time in the Laboratories of the Hoechst Company in Frankfurt, Germany, and later moved to the Geigy Company in Basel, Switzerland. The same strain was subsequently sent to, and was employed in experimental studies by, Dr. C. G. Ahlström at the Institute of Pathology, University of Lund, in Sweden, and later also in several other laboratories.

Other Strains of the Rous Sarcoma Virus. Among other strains employed in various laboratories, with a less pronounced oncogenic potential for mammals, are the following:

The Bryan Strain of the Rous sarcoma virus has been maintained by serial passages in chickens in Dr. Bryan's laboratory at the National Cancer Institute in Bethesda, Md.

The following personal communication was received by the author (1967) from Dr. W. Ray Bryan in reference to this strain:

"I received a lyophilized sample from Dr. Albert Claude in 1942, while he was still at the Rockefeller Institute. The vial was labeled: 'CTI 2755, 12-13-41.' All of my work was with virus propagated from this original sample.

"For many years the virus has been passed by usual procedures. When it was found that biological results varied significantly from virus-batch to virus-batch, but that the results were quantitatively reproducible in different experiments on the same virus-batch, and on the same strain of chickens, we started making large batches of virus and freezing numerous aliquots for use over long periods of time. Aliquots of such 'standard lots' were also supplied to various other investigators, who referred to them in publications as 'standard RSV, lot #, etc.' In this way the designation 'standard strain' came into being.

"The 'high titer strain' was developed by over 50 serial passages selecting for each successive virus passage the most rapidly growing tumor in individual groups of inoculated chickens."

The Harris Strain has been maintained for a number of years by Dr. R. J. C. Harris, first at the Chester Beatty Research Institute in London, and later in the laboratories of the Imperial Cancer Research Fund. Dr. Harris received this strain from Dr. J. G. Carr of Edinburgh.

The following personal communication was received by the author (1967) from Dr. R. J. C. Harris of the Imperial Cancer Research Fund in London concerning the origin and routine passage of this virus strain:

"My strain of Rous virus was given to me by Dr. J. G. Carr of Edinburgh in the late 1940's, when he and I were working together on the virus at the Chester Beatty Research Institute in London. Dr. Carr received it from Dr. C. R. Amies at the Lister Institute, where it was in use before the Second World War.

"The Mill Hill strain is not the same as the Harris strain. I have now been in touch with C. H. Andrewes about the Mill Hill strain of Rous sarcoma virus. He told me that he received his strain from W. E. Gye of this laboratory in 1927. Dr. Gye, in turn, must have certainly received his strain directly from Peyton Rous a few years earlier, since he began his work on this virus in 1923. So both Rous sarcoma virus Harris strain and Mill Hill strain originally appear to have come from Gye, and thus from Rous, in about 1923.

"The Carr strain is the same as the Harris strain, so far as the British material is concerned. The Carr-Zilber strain is quite different from the Harris strain, and probably reflects its stay in the U.S.S.R.

"Carr and I have only used the susceptible Edinburgh strain of Brown Leghorn chickens for virus passage. My virus has never been passed in any other fowl since 1947. For routine passage and tumor harvesting for virus production the chicks were used when 1 to 7 days old; we used for inoculation 'cell-free supernatants' routinely (not filtrates and not cell suspensions)."

The Mill Hill Strain. Dr. C. G. Ahlström in Lund, Sweden, received from Dr. C. H. Andrewes of the National Institute for Medical Research in Mill Hill, London, a Rous sarcoma strain which he designated the Mill Hill strain (Ahlström and Jonsson, 1962a). This chicken tumor material had been kept in a freeze-dried state in London and had been derived from the virus strain which Dr. W. E. Gye used in his experiments. Dr. Gye, in turn, had received it from Dr. Peyton Rous, probably in 1923.

All strains of Rous sarcoma virus are obviously interrelated and were derived from the original strain that had been isolated by Dr. Peyton Rous in 1911 from Chicken Tumor No. 1. Simons and Dougherty (1963) have drawn up a chart summarizing data on the origin of some of the Rous sarcoma virus strains.

In addition, there have been original isolations of avian tumor viruses from spontaneous chicken tumors. Rous and Murphy isolated filterable agents from several chicken tumors. Fujinami and Inamoto also isolated a filterable agent from a chicken sarcoma in Japan (Fujinami and Inamoto, 1914. Fujinami, 1930). Several subsequent isolations of avian tumor viruses from spontaneous chicken tumors have been made by different investigators (reviewed by Foulds, 1934. Nebenzahl, 1934. Vogt, 1965). Among the more recent isolations were those reported by Carr and Campbell (1958), Thurzo and coworkers (1963),* and others. Most of these virus strains have very similar characteristics to those of the Rous sarcoma virus, and presumably represent either the same virus prototype, or a closely related oncogenic agent.

Induction of Cysts and Hemorrhagic Disease in Rats Following Inoculation of the Carr-Zilber Strain of Rous Sarcoma into Rat Embryos, or into Newborn Rats

The curious observation that multiple cysts and diffuse hemorrhagic manifestations can be induced in rats following inoculation of Rous sarcoma extracts was reported in 1957 by L. A. Zilber and I. N. Kryukova, and independently at about the same time by Svet-Moldavsky in Moscow.

In experiments carried out by Zilber and Kryukova (1957) at the Gamaleya Institute of Epidemiology and Microbiology in Moscow, extracts were prepared from the Carr-Zilber strain of Rous chicken sarcoma; the extracts were centrifuged and the supernate was injected into rat embryos through the uterine wall, after dissection of the abdominal

* Thurzo and his coworkers (1963) found a spontaneous tumor in the liver of a White Leghorn hen. The tumor, a fibrosarcoma, was designated B77. It could be transplanted not only to hens, but also to pigeons, turkeys, pheasants, and ducks. Moreover, this tumor could also be successfully transplanted to cortisone-treated hamsters. Filtrates prepared from this tumor induced sarcomas in chickens, pigeons, and ducks.

wall of pregnant female rats on the 16th to 18th day of gestation. The same material was then injected again subcutaneously one week after birth, in some cases repeatedly. Within 2 to 3 weeks after the last injection, large cysts appeared in the cervical, axillary, and inguinal regions of the injected rats. In a first experiment 2 out of 15 rats, and in a second experiment 7 out of 8 inoculated rats developed multiple cysts and hemorrhages. In most cases there followed a gradual enlargement of such cysts causing their distension first with serous, later with hemorrhagic fluid. In addition, small cysts and either punctate or diffuse hemorrhages appeared in various tissues and organs, particularly in pleura, pericardium, and lungs, and also in the abdominal cavity, in the mesentery of these animals. In a few animals the lungs resembled clusters of vesicles filled with a sterile hemorrhagic transudate.

At about the same time, and in an independent study, Svet-Moldavsky at the L. A. Tarasevich State Control Institute of Sera and Vaccines, in Moscow, made a similar observation. The Rous sarcoma strain employed in his studies was obtained from Dr. Zilber's laboratory. In an attempt to transmit this tumor to rats, a heavy (about 50 per cent) and thoroughly minced cell suspension, prepared from Rous chicken sarcoma, was inoculated subcutaneously into embryos of white pregnant female rats (Svet-Moldavsky, 1957, 1958. Svet-Moldavsky and Skorikova, 1957, 1960). Out of a total of 123 inoculated rats, 74 (60 per cent) developed multiple cysts when they were about 2 to 3 weeks old. The susceptibility of rats to inoculation of the Rous sarcoma decreased rapidly with age. Inoculation of Rous sarcoma cell suspensions either subcutaneously or intraperitoneally into newborn, less than 2-day-old rats, also resulted in the development of multiple cysts; however, such cysts appeared later and in a smaller number of animals as compared with those which received the tumor extracts during the embryonic stage.

In many animals the cysts filled with hemorrhagic transudate increased in size progressively. Furthermore, some of the rats inoculated with the chicken tumor extracts either during the embryonic period, or when newborn, developed characteristic vesicular changes in the lungs with a hemorrhagic exudate in pleural cavity; often similar hemorrhages were observed in the liver, leading sometimes to the development of jaundice. In some animals the hemorrhagic manifestations developed at the same time as the cysts. In other animals the cysts developed without hemorrhagic manifestations, or only hemorrhagic manifestations developed without concurrent development of cysts. In general, the hemorrhagic manifestations were less common than the development of cysts.

The causal relationship between the development of these cysts and the inoculated virus became evident when a homogenized extract prepared from the cyst walls, and injected back into 1-month-old chicks reproduced typical Rous sarcoma within 30 to 40 days after inoculation (Svet-Moldavsky and Skorikova, 1957, 1960).

It was unexpected and rather surprising to observe the development of cysts in rats following inoculation of tumor extracts. However, the hemorrhagic manifestations observed in the inoculated rats were very similar to the hemorrhagic disease observed by Duran-Reynals (1940) following inoculation of the Rous sarcoma virus into chick embryos, or into 1-day-old chicks. The early experiments of Duran-Reynals established the fact that the Rous sarcoma virus can induce as a disease entity diffuse and generalized hemorrhagic manifestations with absence of tumors.

Confirmation of the Original Experiments, and Induction of Cysts and Hemorrhagic Disease with the Prague and Schmidt-Ruppin Strains of Rous Sarcoma. The development of cysts and characteristic diffuse hemorrhagic lesions in visceral organs could also be induced in rats with other strains of Rous sarcoma. At the Institute of Biology in Prague, Svoboda and Grozdanovič (1959), employing the Prague strain of Rous sarcoma which they had received from Dr. Engelbreth-Holm, confirmed the original observations of Zilber, Svet-Moldavsky and their coworkers. They reported that multiple cysts and characteristic diffuse hemorrhagic manifestations could readily be induced following a single intraperitoneal injection of fresh chicken tumor cell suspensions into suckling, 2 to 4-day-old, rats. No preliminary injection of this material into embryos was necessary in order to induce the characteristic pathological manifestations. Thirty-three rats were inoculated, and all developed multiple cysts situated chiefly in the inguinal region. In almost every case hemorrhagic nodes of varying size were also found mainly in the abdominal region below the sternum, and on the interior walls of the thoracic cavity. All these rats died when they were 4 to 5 weeks old from hemorrhages into the thoracic cavity or into the cysts. Development of cysts and hemorrhagic disease could also be induced following inoculation of the chicken tumor extracts into rat embryos. Of the 8 animals inoculated as embryos, only 4 per cent later developed, and died from, cysts and hemorrhages; however, these animals had received as inoculum homogenate crushed with sand, and not fresh tumor cell suspensions.

Multiple cysts with or without concomitant development of hemorrhagic manifestations could also be induced following inoculation of newborn rats with minced cell suspensions prepared from the Schmidt-Ruppin strain of Rous sarcoma (Ahlström and Jonsson, 1962a, b. Harris and Chesterman, 1964).

At the Sloan-Kettering Institute in New York, Munroe and Southam (1964) also inoculated newborn and less than 7-day-old Wistar or Sprague-Dawley rats with tumor cell extracts prepared from the Carr-Zilber strain of the Rous sarcoma. Out of 162 inoculated animals, 73 developed hemorrhagic cysts in cervical, axillary, and inguinal regions, after a latency varying from one to 16 weeks.

Induction of Sarcomas in Rats Following Inoculation of the Carr-Zilber Strain of Rous Sarcoma

In 1958 the surprising observation was reported by Svet-Moldavsky in Moscow that sarcomas could be induced following inoculation of extracts of the Carr-Zilber strain of Rous sarcoma into newborn rats. In the initial experiment a heavy suspension of tumor cells prepared from chicken sarcomas was inoculated into rat embryos of 4 laparotomized pregnant white female rats. Concurrently, serum of rabbits immunized with the Rous sarcoma virus was injected intraperitoneally into the same embryos. Of the four pregnant rats, two aborted, one gave birth to and destroyed its litter, and only one female bore successfully five infant rats of which three survived.

In two of the three surviving rats, small and very slowly growing cysts developed one month after inoculation and later regressed; however, 6 to 7 months later pleomorphic spindle-cell sarcomas developed, in one rat on the dorsal side of the neck, and in the other in the facial region, on the cheek. These sarcomas could be transplanted successfully by cell-graft to newborn rats.

In the initial experiment, serum of rabbits immunized with the Rous sarcoma virus was injected into the same embryos concurrently with the inoculation of chicken tumor cell suspensions; later on it was found, however, that the injection of immune serum in addition to tumor extract was not necessary in order to produce tumors. This was evident from an experiment in which a rat that had been inoculated as an embryo with Rous sarcoma extract, without a simultaneous injection of immune serum, developed a progressively growing spindle-cell sarcoma at 7 months of age.

The initial experiment was repeated (Svet-Moldavsky, 1961). Rat embryos were again inoculated with Rous sarcoma homogenate. Twenty-two pregnant female rats were employed for this experiment, but only 9 young rats survived. In 8 rats cysts developed in cervical or axillary regions at 4 to 6 weeks of age. One animal died, and in the 7 remaining rats the cysts later disappeared. However, in 4 rats, when these animals were 6 to 10 months old, progressively growing spindle-cell sarcomas developed near the regions where the Rous sarcoma extracts had been inoculated during the intrauterine period.

At about the same time Zilber and Kryukova (1958) reported that extracts of the Carr-Zilber strain of Rous sarcoma could induce fibromatous tumors in rabbits.

Successful transmission of Rous chicken sarcoma to mice and rats was reported in an apparently independent observation only one year later in Germany. In a discussion which followed a lecture on viruses and cancer ("Virus und Krebs") given at a German Cancer Congress in Berlin on March 12, 1959, by Professor Charles Oberling, Dr. K. H. Schmidt-Ruppin, of Frankfurt (1959), mentioned very briefly that he had transmitted Rous chicken sarcoma to mice and rats. In his initial communication no details were given of these experiments. Only a brief statement was made that either fresh or freeze-dried chicken tumor extracts were inoculated and induced polymorphous sarcomas in mice, or spindle-cell sarcomas in rats, and that the induced tumors could later be transplanted serially by cell-graft from mice to mice, or from rats to rats. The particular strain of Rous sarcoma employed in these studies had been obtained by Dr. Schmidt-Ruppin from Dr. Oberling in 1953.

The following personal communication was received by the author (1967) from Dr. K. H. Schmidt-Ruppin in reference to his heterotransplantation experiments:

"Since 1952 I was interested in the problem of heterotransplantation and resistance to tumor growth. In the initial experiments I transplanted tumors of humans, rats, mice, and also Rous sarcoma into the rabbit eye. Because it was fairly easy to obtain 'takes' in this test system with most of these tumors, in the following years I added other methods and I injected tumors subcutaneously, intramuscularly, and intraperitoneally into normal or pretreated (by irradiation or cortisone) adult rabbits, mice, and rats.

"At the time of my early systematic heterotransplantation experiments with our Rous sarcoma strain on mice and rats I was not familiar with the Russian experiments along similar lines. However, as we obtained a surprisingly high percentage of positive results in these experiments, I reviewed the entire literature on current research on heterotransplantation of Rous sarcoma, and I found the publications of Svet-Moldavsky and Zilber dealing with that subject. Accordingly, these studies had begun, and were performed, independently from each other."

* * *

These observations marked a turning point in the study of the oncogenic potential of the Rous sarcoma virus. It had been observed in previous experiments that inoculation of either rat embryos or newborn rats with Rous sarcoma tumor extracts, particularly with Rous sarcoma tumor cell suspensions, may result in the development of cysts and hemorrhagic manifestations in the inoculated animals. The observation, however, that chicken tumor extracts can induce in rats not only cysts and hemorrhagic manifestations, but also progressively growing sarcomas, was new and striking and opened a new chapter in experimental cancer research. These initial and preliminary experiments were soon repeated, confirmed, and extended in several laboratories, and it was thereby established for the

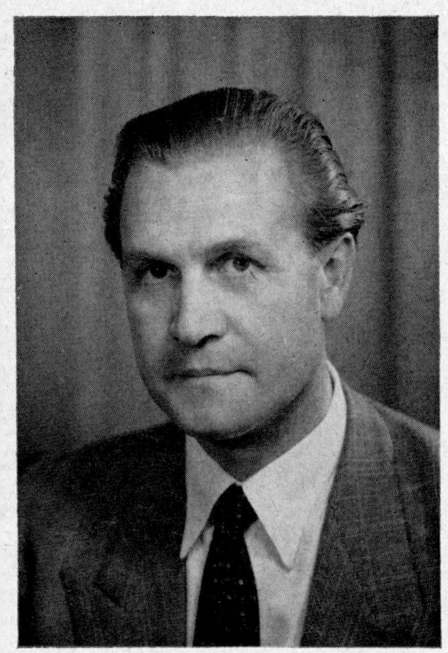

K. H. Schmidt-Ruppin

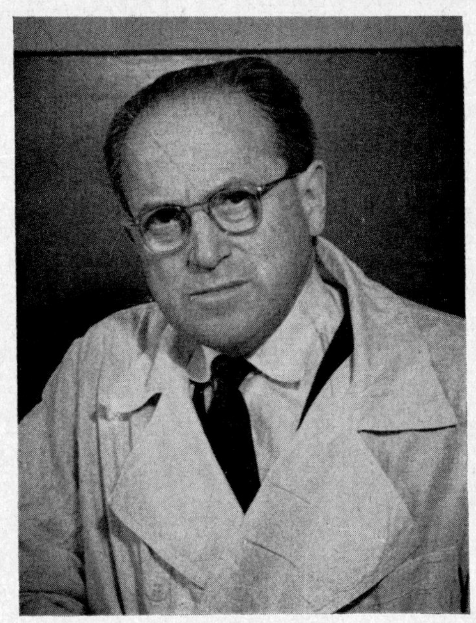

L. A. Zilber

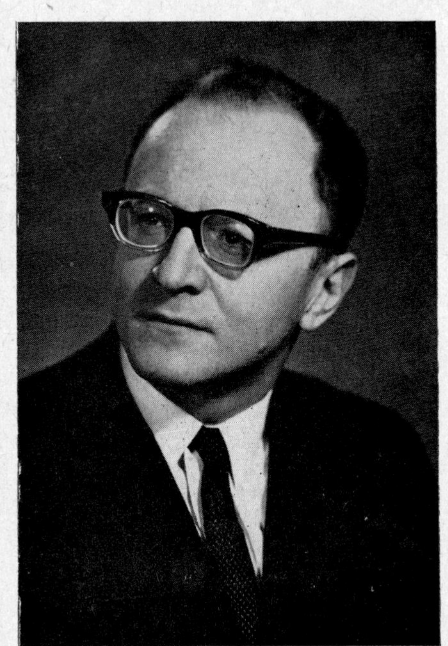

G. J. Svet-Moldavsky

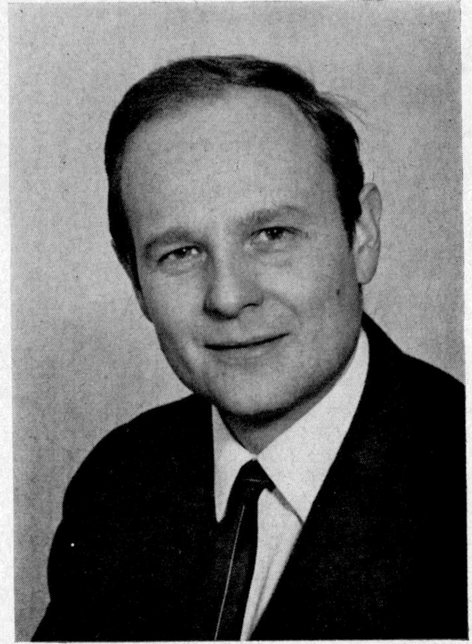

J. Svoboda

Fig. 12.

first time that a chicken sarcoma virus can cross not only species, or order, but also class of animals, and that it can induce malignant tumors in mammals.

Confirmation of the Preliminary Experiments. Induction of Sarcomas in Rats with the Carr-Zilber and Prague Strains of Rous Sarcoma Virus. The initial and preliminary reports on the transmission of the chicken tumor to mammals were at first accepted with skepticism; soon, however, they were confirmed and extended by several investigators. Zilber (1961), employing his strain of Rous sarcoma, inoculated supernatant, presumably cell-free fluid, obtained after centrifugation of chicken tumor extracts, into rat embryos, on the 16th to 18th day of gestation. One week after birth the animals received another dose of the same virus. Many of these animals developed subcutaneous cysts and hemorrhagic disease. However, most important of all, among the 151 inoculated rats, 8 developed progressively growing spindle-cell sarcomas.

Svoboda (1961), employing the Prague strain of Rous sarcoma, inoculated newborn and less than 7-day-old suckling rats with chicken tumor cell suspensions. Among the 87 inoculated rats several developed hemorrhagic cysts, and 2 rats developed sarcomas after a latency of $4\frac{1}{2}$ and 7 months.

Induction of Tumors in Rats and Mice with the Schmidt-Ruppin Strain of Rous Sarcoma. Schmidt-Ruppin reported at first very briefly in 1959 that sarcomas could be induced in mice and rats following inoculation of freeze-dried and also of fresh Rous chicken sarcoma tumor extracts. In a more recent publication (1964) Schmidt-Ruppin gave more details of his studies. He specified that either freshly minced chicken sarcoma suspensions or freeze-dried extracts were inoculated intramuscularly, subcutaneously, or intraperitoneally into mice which were about 6 weeks old at the beginning of the experiment, and also into 8 to 10-week-old Wistar strain rats. Several successive inoculations were made. A high incidence of progressively growing sarcomas was induced in mice and rats. Repeated intramuscular inoculations were most suitable for the induction of tumors. Intraperitoneal inoculations produced ascites tumors. Freeze-dried material proved more effective than fresh sarcoma material. The induced tumors could be transplanted serially by cell-graft in mice, or rats, respectively. Supernatant fluid resulting from centrifugation of a fresh chicken tumor extract also induced tumors in mice and rats, but the centrifuged extracts proved less active than either cell suspensions or freeze-dried extracts.

Ising-Iversen (1960) in Dr. Ahlström's laboratory, in Lund, repeated these experiments employing the Rous sarcoma strain obtained from Dr. Schmidt-Ruppin. Twelve rats were inoculated when less than 3 days old with the chicken tumor material, and two animals developed progressively growing sarcomas. The rat sarcoma could be transplanted back to chickens in which it induced a typical sarcoma; it could then be again transplanted back to young rats.

In a preliminary experiment, Ahlström and Jonsson (1962a) at the Institute of Pathology, University of Lund, Sweden, tried to reproduce this experiment employing a strain of the Rous sarcoma virus which they obtained from Dr. C. H. Andrewes of the Mill Hill Institute for Medical Research in London, and which they designated as the "Mill Hill" strain of Rous sarcoma. Tumor cell suspensions were inoculated into newborn and less than 3-day-old mice and rats. Within the first week after inoculation, about 20 per cent of the inoculated animals of both species developed slight swellings at the site of implantation. The swellings, which showed a histological morphology similar to that of a Rous chicken sarcoma, increased in size for a short time, but later on regressed and disappeared in all animals. None of the animals developed either cysts, hemorrhagic disease, or tumors. Ahlström and Jonsson concluded that failure to induce tumors in rats with the Mill Hill strain, as compared with previous successful induction of tumors in rats by Ising-Iversen with the Schmidt-Ruppin strain of Rous sarcoma in his laboratory, was probably due to differences in the strains of virus used since all other experimental conditions in these experiments were the same.

In a subsequent series of experiments Ahlström and Jonsson (1962b) employed the Schmidt-Ruppin strain of Rous sarcoma for their studies. The results were quite different from their previous preliminary studies. When suckling, 1 to 4-day-old rats were inoculated subcutaneously with finely minced tumor cell suspensions prepared from the Schmidt-Ruppin strain of Rous chicken sarcoma, subcutaneous cysts and also progressively growing sarcomas developed in over 70 per cent of the inoculated animals. At first some of the animals developed subcutaneous swellings within the first week after inoculation. These swellings appeared on the back at the site of inoculation and regressed after several days. However, after about 4 to 5 weeks subcutaneous cysts or progressively growing spindle-cell sarcomas began to develop in some of the inoculated animals. Several animals developed both sarcomas and cysts. A few of the sarcomas developed from the cyst wall. The tumors grew progressively and metastasized, usually to the lungs.

Of a total of 33 rats inoculated when 1 to 3 days old with a finely minced tumor cell suspension, 15 rats developed progressively growing sarcomas, 9 developed sarcomas and cysts, and 4 rats developed cysts only. Accordingly, a total of 24 out of 33 rats developed sarcomas.

Influence of Age at Inoculation on Susceptibility to the Induction of Cysts or Tumors. Ahlström and Jonsson (1962b) studied the relative susceptibility of suckling rats of several age groups, and of fully grown animals, to the pathogenic potency of Rous sarcoma cell suspensions. When the inoculations were made into suckling rats less than 4 days old, the animals were found to be highly susceptible to the induction of both cysts and sarcomas. Older rats were also relatively susceptible, but up to a certain age, and to the induction of sarcomas only.

It was of interest that the cysts developed only in the first experimental series in which newborn, and less than 4-day-old rats were inoculated. When 12-day-old rats were inoculated with tumor cell suspensions, 10 out of 11 animals developed tumors; however, in some animals of this group the tumors were smaller as compared with those resulting from inoculation of newborn rats.

The susceptibility to tumor induction diminished rapidly with increasing age. When 23-day-old rats were inoculated, only 3 out of 11 animals developed tumors. None of the 5 full-grown adult rats developed tumors during the 5 months observation time following inoculation of minced tumor material.

Induction of Tumors with Cell-free Extracts. Sarcomas could be induced in rats also following inoculation of centrifuged cell-free extracts.

The tumor cell suspension was centrifuged at 4,000 r.p.m. for 15 minutes; the supernate was then removed and centrifuged at 13,800 r.p.m. for 30 minutes; the supernate was again removed and centrifuged at the same speed for 30 minutes. This procedure was repeated once more, and the final supernate was employed for inoculation.

However, the incidence of the induced tumors was lower, and the latency period was longer, when cell-free extracts were employed. Only 15 out of 27 animals (56 per cent) developed tumors following inoculation of supernatant fluid resulting from centrifugation of tumor extracts. The latency was 2 to 4 months, as compared with one month in experiments in which cell suspensions were inoculated.

Transplantation of the Induced Tumors from Rats to Rats, and from Rats back to Chickens. The tumors induced in rats could be transplanted serially in young rats by cell-graft. After a few passages in newborn rats they could also be transplanted to one-month-old rats. However, all attempts to transfer the induced tumors from rats to rats by cell-free centrifuged extracts failed.

The rat tumors could be successfully transplanted back to chickens. Following inoculation of cell suspensions prepared from the rat tumors into 3-week-old chickens, typical progressively growing sarcomas having the morphology of Rous sarcoma developed after 2 to 3 weeks at the site of inoculation. Similar tumors could be induced in chickens with rat tumor material obtained from second and ninth rat tumor passages.

Induction of Tumors in Cotton Rats. Svet-Moldavsky and Svet-Moldavskaya (1964) inoculated cotton rats (*Sigmodon hispidus hispidus*) with a homogenate of Carr strain of Rous sarcoma. The rats were inoculated subcutaneously when they were less than 12 hours old. Sarcomas developed in 12 out of 23 inoculated rats.

Malignant Transformation of Rat Embryonic Cells Infected with Rous Sarcoma Virus. Rat embryo cells could be infected in tissue culture with the Rous sarcoma virus and transformed *in vitro* into tumor cells (Svoboda and Chýle, 1963. Febvre *et al.*, 1964). Svoboda and Chýle used the Prague strain of Rous sarcoma for their experiments; Febvre and his colleagues in Paris employed the Bryan strain.

> In Febvre's experiments, the rat embryo cell-lines infected *in vitro* with the high-titer Bryan strain of Rous sarcoma virus were changed into malignant cells in approximately 6 to 8 weeks. When such cells were inoculated into newborn rats, they produced tumors in 88 per cent of the inoculated animals. The induced tumors could be transplanted by cell-graft from rat to rat, and under certain experimental conditions they could also be grafted back to chickens. However, the tumors could not be transmitted by cell-free extracts. No virus could be detected on electron microscopic examination of the tumor cells.

In a similar experiment, malignant transformation *in vitro* of Chinese hamster embryonic fibroblasts with the Schmidt-Ruppin strain of Rous sarcoma virus was reported by Hložánek, Donner, and Svoboda (1966).

Induction of Tumors in Mice with Rous Sarcoma Extracts

Sarcomas could also be induced in mice with three different strains of the Rous sarcoma virus. In the experiments of Ahlström and his colleagues (1963, 1964), newborn mice were injected with the Schmidt-Ruppin strain of the Rous sarcoma virus; 25 per cent of them developed sarcomas after a latency varying from 14 days to 9 months after inoculation. The tumors developed at the site of inoculation infiltrating the surrounding tissues, and induced metastases in adjacent lymph nodes and in lungs. Most of the induced tumors were spindle-cell sarcomas. Newborn and less than 2-day-old mice were most susceptible, but tumors could also be induced in suckling, less than 10-day-old, animals. Older animals were resistant to the inoculation of tumor extracts.

The induced tumors could be transplanted by cell-graft in suckling mice. Transfer back to chicks by cell-graft was successful up to the 17th mouse generation. Neither cysts nor hemorrhagic lesions were observed in these experiments.

Schmidt-Ruppin (1959, 1964), employing his strain for his study, was able to induce sarcomas following 6 to 7 intramuscular injections of chicken tumor cell suspensions or of freeze-dried tumor extracts into 6-week-old mice. Intraperitoneal injection of chicken tumor extracts produced ascites tumors.

Sarcomas could also be induced in mice following inoculation of tumor cell suspensions of either the Carr strain (Morgunova and Kryukova, 1962), or of the Prague strain (Koldovský and Bubeník, 1964), of Rous sarcoma. Most of the tumors induced in mice grew progressively, but some regressed. The tumors could be transplanted by cell-graft from mice back to chickens.

Induction of Tumors in Syrian Hamsters

The pathogenic potency of Rous sarcoma extracts for Syrian hamsters (*Cricetulus aureus*) was established by Ahlström and Forsby (1962). Newborn hamsters were inoculated with finely minced cell suspensions prepared from the Schmidt-Ruppin strain of Rous chicken sarcoma; in 23 of 26 animals progressively growing sarcomas developed after 2 to 3 weeks following inoculation. In older animals sarcomas could also be induced, but the latency was considerably prolonged; the tumors developed in such animals within 2 to 4 months after inoculation of the tumor extracts. Sarcomas could also be induced following inoculation of either newborn or 2-month-old hamsters with supernatant fluid obtained by repeated centrifugations of chicken sarcoma cell suspensions. Secondary tumors appeared on the peritoneal surface, in the retroperitoneal and mediastinal lymph nodes, and in the lungs. The induced tumors were pleomorphic, had certain resemblance to rhabdomyosarcomas, but often had the character of spindle-cell sarcomas.

The tumors induced in hamsters could be transplanted by cell-graft to other hamsters, and also from the hamsters back to the chickens. However, all attempts to transfer the induced sarcomas from one hamster to another with cell-free extracts failed.

In general, the hamster proved to be more susceptible than the rat to inoculation of the chicken tumor extracts. Adult hamsters were susceptible, whereas full-grown rats were resistant; furthermore, the tumors appeared in the inoculated hamsters after a shorter latency than in rats.

Tumors could also be induced in hamsters with other strains of Rous sarcoma. Klement and Svoboda (1963) reported that sarcomas developed following inoculation of newborn hamsters with either the Schmidt-Ruppin or with the Prague strain of Rous sarcoma. The latter was slightly less oncogenic than the Schmidt-Ruppin strain.

The Carr strain of the Rous sarcoma also proved to be oncogenic for hamsters. Shevljaghin (1963, 1964) inoculated a tumor cell suspension of the Carr strain of Rous sarcoma into 2 hamsters 7 days old, and in both animals polymorphocellular sarcomas were induced. The induced tumors could be transplanted by cell-graft to newborn, and later to adult hamsters. One of the hamster tumors was also transplanted back into chickens, inducing a typical Rous sarcoma,

Eidinoff and his colleagues (1965) observed that the Bryan strain of the Rous sarcoma virus could also induce tumors following subcutaneous inoculation into hamsters, provided that large doses of the virus were injected. Cell-free centrifuged extracts were injected subcutaneously into 122 newborn hamsters; as a result, progressively growing sarcomas developed in 26 animals after a latency varying from 2 weeks to $6\frac{1}{2}$ months. The induced tumors were usually undifferentiated sarcomas, in some instances rhabdomyosarcomas.

Induction of Brain Tumors (Gliomas) in Hamsters Following Inoculation of Harris and Bryan Strains of Rous Sarcomas. Rabotti and his coworkers (1965a) induced tumors in hamsters with the Harris strain of Rous sarcoma. Newborn Syrian hamsters were inoculated intracerebrally when less than one-day-old with supernatant fluid resulting from differential centrifugation of the Harris strain of the Rous sarcoma chicken tumor. In the first experiment, after a latency of 4 to 5 weeks, 41 of 59 inoculated animals developed brain tumors, which on microscopic examination proved to be glioblastomas.

In another experiment, Rabotti and his colleagues (1965b) induced gliomas and choroid plexus papillomas following intracerebral inoculation of newborn hamsters with cell-free centrifuged extracts of the Bryan strain of Rous sarcoma. However, relatively high doses of the virus were required in order to induce tumors.

Similar results were obtained when newborn hamsters were inoculated intracerebrally with centrifuged extracts of the Schmidt-Ruppin strain of Rous sarcoma; multiple brain tumors, which had the microscopic morphology of gliomas, developed in most of the inoculated animals after an average latency varying from 3 to 8 weeks (Rabotti and Raine, 1964).

Induction of Sarcomas in Chinese Hamsters. Tumors could be induced with the Schmidt-Ruppin strain of Rous sarcoma in Chinese hamsters (*Cricelutus griseus*). The Chinese hamsters were less susceptible than Syrian hamsters and reacted in a different way (Ahlström *et al.*, 1964). Following inoculation of either homogenized or freshly prepared and finely minced chicken sarcoma cell suspensions into 1 to 2-day-old Chinese hamsters, tumors developed at the site of inoculation in 11 out of 15 inoculated animals after a latency of 2 to 8 weeks. The induced tumors grew slowly, infiltrating the surrounding tissues. Microscopically, the tumors showed the picture of spindle-cell sarcomas, or polymorphous sarcomas, occasionally also angiosarcomas or giant-cell sarcomas. Metastases appeared rather late and in some animals only, and were seen only in the lungs. The tumors induced in the Chinese hamsters could be transplanted by cell-graft back to chickens, inducing in the inoculated birds typical sarcomas. In general, the Chinese hamster appeared to be somewhat less susceptible than the Syrian hamster to the induction of tumors with the Rous chicken sarcoma.

Induction of Tumors in Guinea Pigs

Ahlström and his coworkers (1963) inoculated newborn guinea pigs with a suspension of finely minced Rous chicken sarcoma (Schmidt-Ruppin strain), or with presumably cell-free supernatant fluid obtained from repeated centrifugations of suspensions of homogenized chicken tumor extracts. Of 23 animals that received a single injection of chicken tumor cells, 18 developed tumors. Of 10 animals that received repeated inoculations of chicken tumor cell suspensions, 9 developed tumors. Cell-free centrifuged chicken tumor extracts induced neoplasms in 36 of 43 injected animals. However, when 6 newborn guinea pigs were inoculated with chicken sarcoma extract that had been passed through a Seitz filter, none developed tumors.

Firm, fibrous, and fairly well outlined tumors developed within 3 to 4 weeks, and appeared invariably at the site of inoculation. The tumors gradually increased in size; some of them later became soft and ulcerated. Microscopic examination revealed that the tumors had the morphology of spindle-cell sarcomas; some, however, were pleomorphic or resembled rhabdomyosarcomas. In a few cases metastases were seen in the lymph nodes adjacent to the tumors; in 4 guinea pigs there were numerous secondary nodules in the lungs. Although some of the guinea pigs with tumors died from secondary infection, in other animals the tumors gradually became harder and smaller, and eventually regressed.

The guinea pig sarcoma was successfully transplanted, by cell-graft, to newborn guinea pigs, and could be passed serially through three successive transplant generations. However, attempts to transfer the tumors in guinea pigs by means of cell-free extracts did not succeed.

Under certain experimental conditions the tumors induced in guinea pigs could be transplanted back into chickens. This was possible only when the tumor cell extracts were prepared from a guinea pig sarcoma that was only about 2 weeks old, actually one month old if the date was calculated from the time of inoculation of the virus into the guinea pig donor. Such early guinea pig tumors could be transplanted successfully into chickens and induced typical progressively growing sarcomas at the site of inoculation. Attempts to transplant the tumors to chickens, using as donors older guinea pig tumors, did not succeed.

In another experiment, 12 newborn guinea pigs were inoculated with a cell suspension of the Mill Hill strain of Rous chicken sarcoma, but none developed a tumor during an observation period of 4 months.

Induction of Fibromatous Tumors and Cysts in Rabbits

Zilber and Kryukova (1958) inoculated extracts prepared from the Carr-Zilber strain of Rous sarcoma into newborn rabbits. Either uncentrifuged cell suspensions or supernatant fluid after a single centrifugation at 2000 r.p.m. for 20 minutes was employed. The rabbits received four successive inoculations, one every other day.

The induced tumors had the microscopic morphology of fibromas; they increased gradually in size and persisted for a certain period of time; eventually, however, most of them regressed. Some of the inoculated rabbits developed also fibrous nodules in the liver; others developed petechial hemorrhages in various organs. In addition to fibrous nodules, cysts filled with a clear exudate developed in some of the animals.

Ahlström and his coworkers (1963) reproduced these experiments employing the Schmidt-Ruppin strain of Rous sarcoma; they also observed the development of fibrosarcoma-like tumors, which spontaneously regressed. Cysts also developed in some of the inoculated animals.

Transmission of Rous Sarcoma to Dogs

Rabotti and his coworkers (1966) reported that malignant brain tumors could be induced in dogs following intracerebral inoculation of centrifuged extracts prepared from the Bryan strain of Rous sarcoma. The extracts were inoculated intracerebrally into newborn Beagles. As a result, most of the inoculated dogs developed gliomas and leptomeningeal sarcomas after a latency varying from 1 to 3 months after inoculation.

Induction of Tumors in Monkeys

Tumors could also be induced in monkeys with the Carr strain of Rous sarcoma. In experiments reported by Munroe and Windle (1963) 4 adult and 7 newborn *Macaca mulatta* monkeys were injected with minced chicken tumor cell suspensions. None of the adult monkeys developed tumors after 11 weeks of observation; the other 7 monkeys developed tumors 2 to 6 weeks after inoculation. Three of the induced tumors were fibrosarcomas. Two monkeys were sacrificed one month after inoculation; the remaining 5 monkeys were reported to be under observation. It would have been of interest to learn whether the induced tumors grew progressively and killed their hosts, or whether all these tumors eventually regressed.

In a subsequent experiment, Munroe and his coworkers (1964) injected chicken tumor cell suspensions into 5 adult monkeys, 7 to 20 months old. Only one animal developed subcutaneous tumors at the site of inoculation;

however, both these tumors regressed spontaneously and disappeared after 4 weeks.

Similar experiments were carried out by Zilber and his associates (1965). They injected cell suspensions of the Carr-Zilber strain of Rous chicken sarcoma into 4 newborn monkeys (2 *Macacus rhesus*, 1 *Macacus nemestrinus*, and 1 *Papio hamadryas*). Tumors developed in all 4 animals after 2 to 5 weeks. Histologically, all these tumors were fibrosarcomas. The induced tumors grew progressively for 2 to 3 months. The *Macacus nemestrinus* monkey developed a very large tumor and died 81 days after injection. In the other three animals the tumors began to decrease in size during the third and fourth months after injection and eventually regressed spontaneously. The inoculation of cellular tumor extracts from two monkeys back into chickens reproduced typical sarcomas (Zilber *et al.*, 1965).

Rabotti and his colleagues reported recently (1967) that *in vitro* infection of cells from dura leptomeninges and cerebrum of rhesus (*Macaca mulatta*) monkeys with the Schmidt-Ruppin strain of the Rous sarcoma virus led to discrete foci of morphologically converted cells. These converted cells maintained their morphology on serial transfers *in vitro*. Inoculation of the converted leptomeningeal cells by different routes into 3 newborn rhesus monkeys resulted in malignant, infiltrating, metastasizing sarcomas in these hosts.

Induction of Metastasizing Sarcomas in Marmosets. Deinhardt (1966) inoculated five newborn marmosets (*Saguinus* sp.), small South American primates, with centrifuged cell-free extracts prepared from the Schmidt-Ruppin strain of Rous sarcoma virus. After a latency of 3 to 9 months, the five inoculated monkeys developed sarcomas which metastasized to the lymph nodes, lungs, kidneys and brain; all inoculated monkeys died from progressively growing tumors. Young adult marmosets, up to 5 months of age, were also found to be susceptible (F. Deinhardt, 1969, in press).

Implications of the Recent Experiments Dealing with Successful Transmission of Chicken Sarcoma to Mammals

Experiments reviewed on the preceding pages demonstrated that a chicken tumor could be transmitted not only to ducks, pheasants, turkeys, or pigeons, but also to rats, mice, hamsters, monkeys, and certain other mammals. Accordingly, our classical concept of an oncogenic virus limited in its pathogenic potential to its ability to induce only tumors of certain type and morphology, and in one or in a few related species only, had to be revised fundamentally.

The experiments dealing with transmission of the chicken sarcoma to mammals are of relatively recent date and several points may require further clarification. It appears that the chicken tumor could be transmitted to mammals either by cell suspension, by centrifuged cell-free extracts, or by homogenates, including freeze-dried tumor material. There is no clear evidence that the tumor virus could be transmitted to mammals in the form of filtrates. It seems that either cells or fragments of cells may be required to assure the transmission of the tumor.

The tumors induced with the chicken sarcoma in rats, mice, hamsters, and other mammals could be later transferred from one host to another within the new class and species, i.e. from rats to rats, from mice to mice, or from hamsters to hamsters, by inoculation of freshly prepared tumor cell suspensions, but not by filtrates or centrifuged cell-free extracts. Again, living, intact tumor cells seem to be necessary for successful transmission of the mammalian tumors, i.e. of the tumors induced in rats, mice, or hamsters, back to the chickens.

Inoculation of such tumor cell suspensions from the mammalian tumors into young chickens induced in most instances, but not always, typical sarcomas developing at the site of inoculation. Attempts to induce tumors in chickens with cell-free extracts or with homogenized extracts prepared from the mammalian tumors have thus far failed. However, once the tumors were again induced in the chickens, they could then be transmitted in their host of origin, i.e. from chickens to chickens, by filtrates.

The diversified host range, which includes animals of different species, order, or even class of the animal kingdom, susceptible to the oncogenic potential of Rous chicken sarcoma is most impressive, and emphasizes the recently recognized fact that at least some oncogenic viruses may have a relatively wide host range, and that they do not have to be limited in their oncogenic potential to one, or a few related species only. Similar, although less extensive, observations have been obtained recently with certain other oncogenic viruses, such as the papilloma, and also the polyoma viruses. These observations are discussed in more detail in other chapters of this monograph.

REFERENCES

Ageenko, A. I., Heterotransplantation of Rous chicken sarcoma in the brain. *Probl. Oncol.*, **3**: 170–175, 1957.

Ahlström, C. G., Neoplasms in mammals induced by Rous chicken sarcoma material, pp. 299–319, in: *Internat. Conference on Avian Tumor Viruses, Nat. Cancer Inst. Monograph No.* 17. U.S. Publ. Health Service, Bethesda, Md., 1964.

Ahlström, C. G., and Forsby, N., Sarcomas in hamsters after injection with Rous chicken tumor material. *J. Exp. Med.*, **115**: 839–852, 1962.

Ahlström, C. G., and Jonsson, N., Temporary growth of Rous sarcoma (strain Mill Hill) in new-born rats and mice. *Acta Path. & Microbiol. Scand.*, **54**: 136-144, 1962a.

Ahlström, C. G., and Jonsson, N., Induction of sarcoma in rats by a variant of Rous virus. *Acta Path. & Microbiol. Scand.*, **54**: 145–172, 1962b.

AHLSTRÖM, C. G., BERGMAN, S., and EHRENBERG, B., Neoplasms in guinea pigs induced by an agent in Rous chicken sarcoma. *Acta Path. & Microbiol. Scand.*, **58**: 177–190, 1963.

AHLSTRÖM, C. G., BERGMAN, S., FORSBY, N., and JONSSON, N., Rous sarcoma in mammals. *Acta Internat. Union Against Cancer*, **19**: 294–298, 1963.

AHLSTRÖM, C. G., KATO, R., and LEVAN, A., Rous sarcoma in Chinese hamsters. *Science*, **144**: 1232–1233, 1964.

ANDREWES, C. H., The immunological relationships of fowl tumors with different histological structure. *J. Path. & Bact.*, **34**: 91–107, 1931.

ANDREWES, C. H., Some properties of immune sera active against fowl-tumour viruses. *J. Path. & Bact.*, **35**: 243–249, 1932.

ANDREWES, C. H., The transmission of fowl-tumors to pheasants. *J. Path. & Bact.*, **35**: 407–413, 1932.

BENEDETTI, E. L., Présence de corpuscules identiques à ceux du virus de l'érythroblastose aviaire chez l'embryon du poulet et les poussins normaux. *Bull. du Cancer*, **44**: 473–482, 1957.

BERNHARD, W., and OBERLING, C., Échec de la mise en évidence de corpuscules-virus dans les cellules du sarcome de Rous examinées au microscope électronique. *Bull. du Cancer*, **40**: 178–185, 1953.

BERNHARD, W., DONTCHEFF, A., OBERLING, C., and VIGIER, P., Corpuscules-d'aspect virusal dans les cellules du sarcome de Rous. *Bull. du Cancer*, **40**: 311–321, 1953.

BERNHARD, W., OBERLING, C., and VIGIER, P. Ultrastructure de virus dans le sarcome de Rous, leur rapport avec le cytoplasme des cellules tumorales. *Bull. du Cancer*, **43**: 407–422, 1956.

BORGES, P. R. F., and DURAN-REYNALS, F., On the induction of malignant tumors in pigeons by a chicken sarcoma virus after previous adaptation of the virus to ducks. *Cancer Research*, **12**: 55–58, 1952.

BRYAN, W. R., Biological studies on the Rous sarcoma virus. I. General introduction. II. Review of sources of experimental variation and of methods for their control. *J. Nat. Cancer Inst.*, **16**: 285–315, 1955.

BRYAN, W. R., Biological studies on the Rous sarcoma virus. IV. Interpretation of tumor-response data involving one inoculation site per chicken. *J. Nat. Cancer Inst.*, **16**: 843–863, 1956.

BRYAN, W. R., CALNAN, D., and MOLONEY, J. B., Biological studies on the Rous sarcoma virus. III. The recovery of virus from experimental tumors in relation to initiating dose. *J. Nat. Cancer Inst.*, **16**: 317–335, 1955.

BRYAN, W. R., MOLONEY, J. B., and CALNAN, D., Stable standard preparations of the Rous sarcoma virus preserved by freezing and storage at low temperatures. *J. Nat. Cancer Inst.*, **15**: 315–329, 1954.

BUBENÍK, J., KOLDOVSKÝ, P., SVOBODA, J., KLEMENT, V., and DVOŘÁK, R., Induction of tumours in mice with three variants of Rous sarcoma virus and studies on the immunobiology of these tumours. *Folia Biol.*, **13**: 29–39, 1967.

BURMESTER, B. R., FONTES, A. K., and WALTER, W. G., Contact transmission of Rous sarcoma. *J. Nat. Cancer Inst.*, **25**: 307–313, 1960.

CARR, J. G., The relation between age, structure, and agent content of Rous No. 1 sarcomas. *Brit. J. Exp. Path.*, **24**: 133–137, 1943.

CARR, J. G., An unexplained discrepancy between the actual and expected yield of virus from avian tumours and its implications. *Proc. Roy. Soc. Edinb.*, **62**: 243–247, 1947.

CARR, J. G., Contribution à l'épidémiologie des sarcomes aviaires. *Bull. du Cancer*, **40**: 407–412, 1953.

CARR, J. G., Observation on the haemorrhagic disease induced by fowl tumour viruses. *Brit. J. Cancer*, **16**: 626–633, 1962.

CARR, J. G., and CAMPBELL, J. G., Three new virus-induced fowl sarcomata. *Brit. J. Cancer*, **12**: 631–635, 1958.

CARREL, A., Le principe filtrant des sarcomes de la poule produits par l'arsenic. *Compt. Rend. Soc. Biol.*, **93**: 1083–1085, 1925.

CARREL, A., Un sarcome fusocellulaire produit par l'indol et transmissible par un agent filtrant. *Compt. Rend. Soc. Biol.*, **93**: 1278–1280, 1925.

CLAUDE, A., PORTER, K. R., and PICKELS, E. G., Electron microscope study of chicken tumor cells. *Cancer Research*, **7**: 421–430, 1947.

DEINHARDT, F., Neoplasms induced by Rous sarcoma virus in New World monkeys. *Nature*, **210**: 443, 1966.

DES LIGNERIS, M. J. A., On the transplantation of Rous' fowl sarcoma No. 1 into guinea-fowls and turkeys. *Am. J. Cancer*, **16**: 307–321, 1932.

DOUGHERTY, R. M., SIMONS, P. J., and CHESTERMAN, F. C. Biological properties of three variants of Rous sarcoma virus. *J. Nat. Cancer Inst.*, **31**: 1285–1307, 1963.

DURAN-REYNALS, F., A hemorrhagic disease occurring in chicks inoculated with the Rous and Fuginami viruses. *Yale J. Biol. & Med.*, **13**: 77–98, 1940.

DURAN-REYNALS, F., The reciprocal infection of ducks and chickens with tumor-inducing viruses. *Cancer Research*, **2**: 343–369, 1942.

DURAN-REYNALS, F., The infection of turkeys and guinea fowls by the Rous sarcoma virus and the accompanying variations of the virus. *Cancer Research*, **3**: 569–577, 1943.

DURAN-REYNALS, F., A study of three new duck variants of the Rous chicken sarcoma. *Cancer Research*, **7**: 99–102, 1947.

DURAN-REYNALS, F., Transmission to adult pigeons of several variants of the Rous sarcoma of chickens. *Cancer Research*, **7**: 103–106, 1947.

DURAN-REYNALS, F., and ESTRADA, E., Protection of chick against Rous sarcoma virus by serum from adult chickens. *Proc. Soc. Exp. Biol. & Med.*, **45**: 367–372, 1940.

DURAN-REYNALS, F., and FREIRE, P. M., The age of the tumor-bearing hosts as a factor conditioning the transmissibility of the Rous sarcoma by filtrates and cells. *Cancer Research*, **13**: 376–382, 1953.

EIDINOFF, M. L., BATES, B., STEINGLASS, M., and HADDAD, J. R., Subcutaneous sarcomata in hamsters induced by Rous sarcoma virus (Bryan). *Nature*, **208**: 336–338, 1965.

ELFORD, W. J., and ANDREWES, C. H., Estimation of the size of a fowl tumour virus by filtration through graded membranes. *Brit. J. Exp. Path.*, **16**: 61–66, 1935.

EPSTEIN, M. A., The identification of the Rous virus; a morphological and biological study. *Brit. J. Cancer*, **10**: 33–48, 1956.

EPSTEIN, M. A., Intra-cellular identification of the Rous virus. *Nature*, **178**: 45–46, 1956.

EPSTEIN, M. A., Observations on the Rous virus; purification and identification of the particles from solid tumours. *Brit. J. Cancer*, **12**: 248–255, 1958.

EPSTEIN, M. A., and HOLT, S. J., Observations on the Rous virus; integrated electron microscopical and cytochemical studies of fluorocarbon purified preparations. *Brit. J. Cancer*, **12**: 363–369, 1958.

FEBVRE, H., ROTHSCHILD, L., ARNOULT, J., and HAGUENAU, F., *In vitro* malignant conversion of rat embryonic cell lines with the Bryan strain of Rous sarcoma virus. pp. 459–477, in: *Internat. Conference on Avian Tumor Viruses, Nat. Cancer Inst. Monograph No.* 17. U.S. Publ. Health Service, Bethesda, Md., 1964.

FOULDS, L., The growth and spread of six filterable tumours of the fowl, transmitted by grafts. *Eleventh Scientific Report. Imperial Cancer Research Fund.* pp. 1–13, Taylor and Francis, London, 1934.

FOULDS, L., The filterable tumours of fowls: A critical review. *Eleventh Scientific Report. Imperial Cancer Research Fund. Supplement.* pp. 1–41, Taylor and Francis, London, 1934.

FREIRE, P. M., BRYAN, E., and DURAN-REYNALS, F., Growth and regression of the Rous sarcoma as a function of the age of the host. *Cancer Research*, **13**: 386–388, 1953.

FUJINAMI, A., Special report: A pathological study in chicken sarcoma. *Trans. Japan. Path. Soc.*, **20**: 3–38, 1930.

FUJINAMI, A., and HATANO, S., Contribution to the pathology of heterotransplantation of tumours. A duck sarcoma from chicken sarcoma. *Gann*, **23**: 67–75, 1929.

FUJINAMI, A., and HATANO, S., Contribution to the pathology of heterotransplantation of tumor: A duck sarcoma from chicken sarcoma. *Trans. Japan. Path. Soc.*, **19**: 646–653, 1929.

FUJINAMI, A., and INAMOTO, K., Ueber Geschwülste bei japanischen Haushühnern insbesondere über einen transplantablen Turnor. *Zeitschr. f. Krebsfor*sch., **14**: 94–119, 1914.

FUJINAMI, A., and SUZUE, K., Contribution to the pathology of tumor growth. Experiments on transplantable chicken sarcoma. *Trans. Japan. Path. Soc.*, **15**: 281–282, 1925.

FUJINAMI, A., and SUZUE, K., Contribution to the pathology of tumor growth. Experiments on the growth of chicken sarcoma in the case of heterotransplantation. *Trans. Japan. Path. Soc.*, **18**: 616–622, 1928.

FURTH, J., Studies on the nature of the agent transmitting leukosis of fowls. I. Its concentration in blood cells and plasma and relation to the incubation period. *J. Exp. Med.*, **55**: 465–478, 1932.

GAYLORD, W. H., Virus-like particles associated with the Rous sarcoma as seen in sections of the tumor. *Cancer Research*, **15**: 80–83, 1955.

GREENE, H. S. N., The transplantation of tumors to the brains of heterologous species. *Cancer Research*, **11**: 529–534, 1951.

GREENWOOD, A. W., BLYTH, J. S. S., and CARR, J. G., Indications of the heritable nature of non-susceptibility to Rous sarcoma in fowls. *Brit. J. Cancer*, **2**: 135–143, 1948.

GROUPÉ, V., and RAUSCHER, F. J., "Nonviral" tumors produced in turkeys by Rous sarcoma virus. *Science*, **125**: 694–695, 1957.

GROUPÉ, V., and RAUSCHER, F. J., Growth curve of Rous sarcoma virus and relationship of infecting dose to yield of virus in chick brain. *J. Nat. Cancer Inst.*, **18**: 507–514, 1957.

GROUPÉ, V., DUNKEL, V. C., and MANAKER, R. A., Improved pock counting method for the titration of Rous sarcoma virus in embryonated eggs. *J. Bact.*, **74**: 409–410, 1957.

GROUPÉ, V., RAUSCHER, F. J., LEVINE, A. S., and BRYAN, W. R., The brain of newly-hatched chicks as a host-virus system for biological studies on the Rcus sarcoma virus (RSV). *J. Nat. Cancer Inst.*, **16**: 865–875, 1956.

GROUPÉ, V., RAUSCHER, F. J., and BRYAN, W. R., Hemorrhagic disease and unusual hepatic lesions associated with intracerebral passage of Rous sarcoma virus in chicks. *J. Nat. Cancer Inst.*, **19**: 37–47, 1957.

GYE, W. E., A note on the propagation of Fujinami's fowl myxo-sarcoma in ducks. *Brit. J. Exp. Path.*, **12**: 93–97, 1931.

GYE, W. E., The propagation of Fujinami's fowl myxo-sarcoma in ducklings. *Brit. J. Exp. Path.*, **13**: 458–460, 1932.

HAGUENAU, F., DALTON, A. J., and MOLONEY, J. B., A preliminary report of electron microscopic and bio-assay studies on the Rous sarcoma I virus. *J. Nat. Cancer Inst.*, **20**: 633–649, 1958.

HAGUENAU, F., FEBVRE, H., and ARNOULT, J., Mode de formation intra-cellulaire du virus du sarcome de Rous. Étude ultrastructurale. *J. Microscopie*, **1**: 445–454, 1962.

HAGUENAU, F., ROUILLER, C., and LACOUR, F., Corpuscules d'aspect virusal dans l'endothéliome de Murray-Begg. Étude au microscope électronique (Note préliminaire). *Bull. du Cancer*, **42**: 350–357, 1955.

HALBERSTAEDTER, L., DOLJANSKI, L., and TENENBAUM, E., Experiments on the cancerization of cells *in vitro* by means of Rous sarcoma agent. *Brit. J. Exp. Path.*, **22**: 179–187, 1941.

HANAFUSA, H., HANAFUSA, T., and RUBIN, H., The defectiveness of Rous sarcoma virus. *Proc. Nat. Acad. Sci., USA*, **49**: 572–580, 1963.

HANAFUSA, H., HANAFUSA, T., and RUBIN, H., Analysis of the defectiveness of Rous sarcoma virus. II. Specification of RSV antigenicity by helper virus. *Proc. Nat. Acad. Sci., USA*, **51**: 41–48, 1964.

HARRIS, R. J. C., Properties of the agent of Rous No. 1 sarcoma. *Advances in Cancer Research*, **1**: 233–271, Academic Press, New York, 1953.

HARRIS, R. J. C., and CHESTERMAN, M. B., Growth of Rous sarcoma in rats, ferrets, and hamsters. pp. 321–335, in: *Internat. Conference on Avian Tumor Viruses, Nat. Cancer Inst. Monograph No. 17*, U.S. Publ. Health Service, Bethesda, Md., 1964.

HAYASHI, N., Experimenteller Beitrag zu Myxosarkoma von Hühnern. *Verh. jap. path. Ges.*, **3**: 123, 1913.

HAYASHI, N., Einige experimentelle Untersuchungen von Hühnergeschwülsten. *Verh. jap. path. Ges.*, **5**: 130, 1915.

HLOŽÁNEK, I., DONNER, L., and SVOBODA, J., Malignant transformation *in vitro* of Chinese hamster embryonic fibroblasts with the Schmidt-Ruppin strain of Rous sarcoma virus and karyological analysis of this process. *J. Cell. Physiol.*, **68**: 221–236, 1966.

ISING-IVERSEN, U., Heterologous growth of Rous sarcoma. *Acta Path. & Microbiol. Scand.*, **50**: 145–155, 1960.

JONSSON, N., Sarcomas in albino mice inoculated with Rous chicken tumor material. *Acta Path. & Microbiol. Scand.*, **62**: 539–556, 1964.

KABAT, E. A., and FURTH, J., Chemical and immunological studies on the agent producing leukosis and sarcoma of fowls. *J. Exp. Med.*, **71**: 55–70, 1940.

KABAT, E. A., and FURTH, J., Neutralization of the agent causing leukosis and sarcoma of fowls by rabbit antisera. *J. Exp. Med.*, **74**: 257–261, 1941.

KEOGH, E. V., Ectodenmal lesions produced by the virus of Rous sarcoma. *Brit. J. Exp. Path.*, **19**: 1–9, 1938.

KLEMENT, V., and SVOBODA, J., Induction of tumors in Syrian hamsters by two variants of Rous sarcoma virus. *Folia Biol.*, **9**: 181–187, 1963.

KOLDOVSKÝ, P., and BUBENÍK, J., Occurrence of tumours in mice after inoculation of Rous sarcoma and antigenic changes in these tumours. *Folia Biol.*, **10**: 81–89, 1964.

KUWATA, T., Studies on the growth of Rous sarcoma and its variant strain in cortisone-treated hamsters. *Cancer Research*, **20**: 170–177, 1960.

KUWATA, T., YASUMURA, Y., and KANISAWA, M., Effect of viral infection and cortisone upon tumour growth in homologous and heterologous hosts. *Nature*, **182**: 1678–1679, 1958.

Kriukova, I. N., Observations on the haemorrhagic disease of rats caused by Rous virus—III. *Problems of Virology*, **5**: 656–666, 1960. (*Vopr. virusol.*, **5**: 602–611, 1960).

Lacassagne, A., and Nyka, W., Sur les conditions de stérilisation des virus par les rayons X: le virus vaccinal. *Compt. Rend. Soc. Biol.*, **128**: 1038–1040, 1938.

McIntosh, J., On the nature of the tumours induced in fowls by injections of tar. *Brit. J. Exp. Path.*, **14**: 422–434, 1933.

McIntosh, J., The sedimentation of the virus of Rous sarcoma and the bacteriophage by a high-speed centrifuge. *J. Path. & Bact.*, **41**: 215–217, 1935.

Manaker, R. A., and Groupé, V., Discrete foci of altered chicken embryo cells associated with Rous sarcoma virus in tissue culture. *Virology*, **2**: 838–840, 1956.

Mannweiler, K., and Bernhard, W., L'ultrastructure du myxosarcome de Fujinami. *Bull. du Cancer*, **45**: 223–236, 1958.

Milford, J. J., and Duran-Reynals, F., Growth of a chicken sarcoma virus in the chick embryo in the absence of neoplasia. *Cancer Research*, **3**: 578–584, 1943.

Milone, S., Innesti a zig-zag di sarcoma di Peyton Rous fra pollo e ratto. *Arch. Sci. Med.*, **52**: 362–368, 1928.

Moloney, J. B., Biological studies on the Rous sarcoma virus. V. Preparation of improved standard lots of the virus for use in quantitative investigations. *J. Nat. Cancer Inst.*, **16**: 877–888, 1956.

Morgunova, T. D., and Kryukova, I. N., Mouse sarcoma induced by Rous virus. *Vopr. virusol.*, **7**: 367–370, 1962.

Munroe, J. S., and Southam, C. M., Oncogenicity of two strains of chicken sarcoma virus for rats. *J. Nat. Cancer Inst.*, **32**: 591–623, 1964.

Munroe, J. S., and Windle, W. F., Tumors induced in primates by chicken sarcoma virus. *Science*, **140**: 1415–1416, 1963.

Munroe, J. S., Shipkey, F., Erlandson, R. A., and Windle, W. F., Tumors induced in juvenile and adult primates by chicken sarcoma virus. pp. 365–390 in: *Internat. Conference on Avian Tumor Viruses, Nat. Cancer Inst. Monograph No. 17*, U.S. Publ. Health Service, Bethesda, Md., 1964.

Murphy, J. B., Transplantability of malignant tumors to the embryos of a foreign species. *J. Am. Med. Assoc.*, **59**: 874–875, 1912.

Murphy, J. B., Transplantability of tissues to the embryos of foreign species. Its bearing on questions of tissue specificity and tumor immunity. *J. Exp. Med.*, **17**: 482–493, 1913.

Murphy, J. B., Studies in tissue specificity. The ultimate fate of mammalian tissue implanted in the chick embryo. *J. Exp. Med.*, **19**: 181–186, 1914.

Murphy, J. B., and Sturm, E., Further investigation of induced tumors in fowls. *Cancer Research*, **1**: 477–483, 1941.

Murphy, J. B., and Sturm, E., Further investigation on the transmission of induced tumors in fowls. *Cancer Research*, **1**: 609–613, 1941.

Nebenzahl, H., Étude expérimentale des tumeurs de la poule. p. 165. Thèse, Librairie E. le François, Paris, 1934.

Oberling, C., and Guérin, M., Sarcome de la poule par méthylcholantrène devenu filtrable. *Bull. du Cancer*, **37**: 5–14, 1950.

Oberling, C., Bernhard, W., Guérin, M., and Harel, J., Images de cellules cancéreuses au microscope électronique. *Bull. du Cancer*, **37**: 97–109, 1950.

Oberling, C., Bernhard, W., Dontcheff, A., and Vigier, P., Observation et étude quantitative de corpuscules d'aspect virusal dans des cultures de sarcome de Rous. *Experientia*, **10**: 138–140, 1954.

Peacock, P. R., Production of tumours in the fowl by carcinogenic agents: (1) Tar; (2) 1 : 2 : 5 : 6 Dibenzanthracene-lard. *J. Path. & Bact.*, **36**: 141–152, 1933.

Peacock, P. R., The etiology of fowl tumors. *Cancer Research*, **6**: 311–328, 1946.

Pentimalli, F., Über Metastasenbildung beim Hühnersarkom. *Zeitschr. f. Krebsforsch.*, **22**: 62–73, 1924.

Pentimalli, F., Über die elektive Wirkung des Virus des Hühnersarkoms. *Zeitschr. f. Krebsforsch.*, **22**: 74–78, 1924.

Prince, A. M., Quantitative studies on Rous sarcoma virus. I. The titration of Rous sarcoma virus on the chorio-allantoic membrane of the chick embryo. *J. Nat. Cancer Inst.*, **20**: 147–159, 1958.

Prince, A. M., Quantitative studies on Rous sarcoma virus. II. Mechanism of resistance of chick embryos to chorio-allantoic inoculation of Rous sarcoma virus. *J. Nat. Cancer Inst.*, **20**: 843–850, 1958.

Prince, A. M., Quantitative studies on Rous sarcoma virus. III. Virus multiplication and cellular response following infection of the chorio-allantoic membrane of the chick embryo. *Virology*, **5**: 435–457, 1958.

Prince, A. M., Quantitative studies on Rous sarcoma virus. IV. An investigation of the nature of "noninfective" tumors induced by low doses of virus. *J. Nat. Cancer Inst.*, **23**: 1361–1381, 1959.

Purdy, W. J., The propagation of the Fujinami fowl-myxosarcoma in adult ducks. *Brit. J. Exp. Med.*, **13**: 467–472, 1932.

Purdy, W. J., The propagation of the Rous sarcoma No. 1 in ducklings. *Brit. J. Exp. Path.*, **13**: 473–479, 1932.

Rabotti, G. F., Oncogenic effects of Rous sarcoma virus, strain CT559, in dogs. pp. 363–370 in: Some Recent Developments in Comparative Medicine. *Symposia of the Zoological Society of London*, No. 17. Academic Press, London and New York, 1966.

Rabotti, G. F., and Raine, W. A., Brain tumours induced in hamsters inoculated intracerebrally at birth with Rous sarcoma virus. *Nature*, **204**: 898–899, 1964.

Rabotti, G. F., Anderson, W. R., and Sellers, R. L., Oncogenic activity of Mill Hill (Harris) strain of Rous sarcoma virus for hamsters. *Nature*, **206**: 946–947, 1965a.

Rabotti, G. F., Grove, A. S., jun., Sellers, R. L., and Anderson, W. R., Induction of multiple brain tumours (gliomata and leptomeningeal sarcomata) in dogs by Rous sarcoma virus. *Nature*, **209**: 884–886, 1966.

Rabotti, G. F., Landon, J. C., Pry, T. W., Beadle, L., Doll, J., Fabrizio, D. P., and Dalton, A. J., Tumors in Rhesus monkeys inoculated at birth with homologous cells converted *in vitro* by Rous sarcoma virus, Schmidt-Ruppin strain. *J. Nat. Cancer Inst.*, **38**: 821–837, 1967.

Rabotti, G. F., Raine, W. A., and Sellers, R. L., Brain tumors (gliomas) induced in hamsters by Bryan's strain of Rous sarcoma virus. *Science*, **147**: 504–506, 1965b.

Riley, V. T., Calnan, D., and Bryan, W. R., Studies on the influence of age on the latent period response of chickens to the agent of chicken tumor I. *J. Nat. Cancer Inst.*, **7**: 93–98, 1946.

Roskin, G., Versuche mit heteroplastischer Überpflanzung der bösartigen Geschwülste. *Zeitschr. f. Krebsforsch.*, **24**: 122–125, 1926.

Rous, P., A transmissible avian neoplasm. (Sarcoma of the common fowl.) *J. Exp. Med.*, **12**: 696–705, 1910.

Rous, P., A sarcoma of the fowl transmissible by an agent separable from the tumor cells. *J. Exp. Med.*, **13**: 397–411, 1911.

Rous, P., Resistance to a tumor-producing agent as distinct from resistance to the implanted tumor cells. Observations with a sarcoma of the fowl. *J. Exp. Med.*, **18**: 416–427, 1913.

Rous, P., On certain spontaneous chicken tumors as manifestations of a single disease. I. Spindle-celled sarcomata rifted with blood sinuses. *J. Exp. Med.*, **19**: 570–576, 1914.

Rous, P., and Lange, L. B., The characters of a third transplantable chicken tumor due to a filterable cause. A sarcoma of intracanalicular pattern. *J. Exp. Med.*, **18**: 651–664, 1913.

Rous, P., and Murphy, J. B., Tumor implantations in the developing embryo. Experiments with a transmissible sarcoma of the fowl. *J. Am. Med. Assoc.*, **56**: 741–742, 1911.

Rous, P., and Murphy, J. B., The nature of the filterable agent causing a sarcoma of the fowl. *J. Am. Med. Assoc.*, **58**: 1938, 1912.

Rous, P., and Murphy, J. B., Variations in a chicken sarcoma caused by a filterable agent. *J. Exp. Med.*, **17**: 219–231, 1913.

Rous, P., and Murphy, J. B., On the causation by filterable agents of three distinct chicken tumors. *J. Exp. Med.*, **19**: 52–69, 1914.

Rous, P., and Murphy, J. B., On immunity to transplantable chicken tumors. *J. Exp. Med.*, **20**: 419–432, 1914.

Rous, P., Murphy, J. B., and Tytler, W. H., The role of injury in the production of a chicken sarcoma by a filterable agent. *J. Am. Med. Assoc.*, **58**: 1751, 1912.

Rous, P., Murphy, J. B., and Tytler, W. H., A filterable agent the cause of a second chicken-tumor, an osteochondrosarcoma. *J. Am. Med. Assoc.*, **59**: 1793–1794, 1912.

Rous, P., Murphy, J. B., and Tytler, W. H., The relation between a chicken sarcoma's behavior and the growth's filterable cause. *J. Am. Med. Assoc.*, **58**: 1840–1841, 1912.

Rous, P., Robertson, O. H., and Oliver, J., Experiments on the production of specific antisera for infections of unknown cause. II. The production of a serum effective against the agent causing a chicken sarcoma. *J. Exp. Med.*, **29**: 305–320, 1919.

Rubin, H., The production of virus by Rous sarcoma cells. *Ann. N.Y. Acad. Sci.*, **68**: 459–472, 1957.

Rubin, H., A virus in chick embryos which induces resistance *in vitro* to infection with Rous sarcoma virus. *Proc. Nat. Acad. Sci., USA*, **46**: 1105–1119, 1960.

Rubin, H., The nature of a virus-induced cellular resistance to Rous sarcoma virus. *Virology*, **13**: 200–206, 1961.

Rubin, H., The immunological basis for non-infective Rous sarcomas. *Cold Spring Harbor Symposia on Quantitative Biology*, **27**: 441–452, 1962.

Rubin, H., and Hanafusa, H., Significance of the absence of infectious virus in virus-induced tumors. pp. 508–525 in: Viruses, Nucleic Acids, and Cancer. *17th Ann. Symp. on Fundamental Cancer Research, Univ. of Texas, M. D. Anderson Hospital and Tumor Institute*, Williams & Wilkins, Baltimore, Md., 1963.

Rubin, H., and Vogt, P. K., An avian leukosis virus associated with stocks of Rous sarcoma virus. *Virology*, **17**: 184–194, 1962.

Rubin, H., Cornelius, A., and Fanshier, L., The pattern of congenital transmission of an avian leukosis virus. *Proc. Nat. Acad. Sci., USA*, **47**: 1058–1069, 1961.

Schmidt-Ruppin, K. H.,* Diskussion zum Vortrag Oberling. *Sonderbânde zur Strahlentherapie*, **41**: 26–27, 1959.

Schmidt-Ruppin, K. H., Heterotransplantation of Rous sarcoma and Rous sarcoma virus to mammals. *Oncologia*, **17**: 247–272, 1964.

Shevljaghin, V. J., Hamster tumors induced by Rous sarcoma virus (Carr strain). *Vopr. virusol.*, **8**: 617–619, 1963.

Shevljaghin, V. J., The study of golden hamster tumors induced by RSV. *Vopr. virusol.*, **9**: 533–538, 1964.

Shimizu, T., and Rubin, H., The dual origin of noninfective Rous sarcomas. *J. Nat. Cancer Inst.*, **33**: 79–91, 1964.

Shrigley, E. W., Greene, H. S. N., and Duran-Reynals, F., Studies on the variation of the Rous sarcoma virus following growth of the tumor in the anterior chamber of the guinea pig eye. *Cancer Research*, **5**: 356–364, 1945.

Simons, P. J., and Dougherty, R. M., Antigenic characteristics of three variants of Rous sarcoma virus. *J. Nat. Cancer Inst.*, **31**: 1275–1283, 1963.

Svec, F., Altaner, C., and Hlavay, E., Pathogenicity for rats of a strain of chicken sarcoma virus. *J. Nat. Cancer Inst.*, **36**: 389–404, 1966.

Svet-Moldavsky, G. J., Development of multiple cysts and of haemorrhagic affections of internal organs in albino rats treated during the embryonic or new-born period with Rous sarcoma virus. *Nature*, **180**: 1299–1300, 1957.

Svet-Moldavsky, G. J., Sarcoma in albino rats treated during the embryonic stage with Rous virus. *Nature*, **182**: 1452–1453, 1958.

Svet-Moldavsky, G. J., The pathogenicity of Rous sarcoma virus for mammals. Multiple cysts and haemorrhagic lesions of internal organs in white rats after inoculation with Rous virus during the embryonic or newborn period. *Acta Virologica* (English Edition), **2**: 1–6, 1958.

Svet-Moldavsky, G. J., Pathogenicity of Rous sarcoma virus for mammals. Sarcomas in rats, further studies on cyst-haemorrhagic disease and an attempt at isolating infectious ribonucleic acid from Rous sarcoma. *Acta Virologica* (English Edition), **5**: 167–177, 1961.

Svet-Moldavsky, G. J., and Skoreekova,† A. S., The development of multiple cysts in white rats after inoculating them in the embryonic period with Rous sarcoma virus. *Vopr. Oncologii*, **3**: 673–677, 1957.

Svet-Moldavsky, G. J., and Skorikova, A. S., The pathogenicity of Rous sarcoma virus for mammals. Detection of virus and of antigenic substances of Rous sarcoma in the cyst-haemorrhagic disease of albino rats. *Acta Virologica* (English Edition), **4**: 47–51, 1960.

Svet-Moldavsky, G. J., and Svet-Moldavskaja, I. A., Sarcoma in cotton rats inoculated with Rous virus. *Science*, **143**: 54–55, 1964.

Svoboda, J., The tumorigenic action of Rous sarcoma in rats and the permanent production of Rous virus by the induced rat sarcoma XC. *Folia Biol.*, **7**: 46–60, 1961.

Svoboda, J., Further findings on the induction of tumors by Rous sarcoma in rats and on the Rous virus-producing capacity of one of the induced tumors (XC) in chicks. *Folia Biol.*, **8**: 215–219, 1962.

* One of the participants of an informal discussion which followed a lecture entitled "Virus und Krebs" given by Prof. Charles Oberling at the 6th German Cancer Congress, on March 12, 1959, in Berlin.

† The same name is spelled in a different manner in two successive publications here quoted. We have followed the spelling exactly as the name was printed in the original publications.

Svoboda, J., and Chýle, P., Malignization of rat embryonic cells by Rous sarcoma virus *in vitro*. *Folia Biol.*, **9**: 329–342, 1963.

Svoboda, J., and Grozdanovič, J., Heterotransplantation of Rous sarcoma in young rats. *Folia Biol.*, **5**: 46–50, 1959.

Thorell, B., Induktion av njurtumör med leukämivirus. *Nord. Med.*, **59**: 762–763, 1958.

Thorell, B., Virusinducerad njurtumör hos höns. *Nord. Med.*, **62**: 1687, 1959.

Thurzo, V., Smida, J., Smidova-Kovarova, V., and Simkovic, D., Some properties of the fowl virus tumor B 77. *Acta Internat. Union Against Cancer*, **19**: 304–305, 1963.

Tytler, W. H., A transplantable new growth of the fowl, producing cartilage and bone. *J. Exp. Med.*, **17**: 466–481, 1913.

Vogt, P. K., Avian tumor viruses. *Advances in Virus Research*, **11**: 293–385, Academic Press, New York and London, 1965.

Vogt, P. K., A virus released by "nonproducing" Rous sarcoma cells. *Proc. Nat. Acad. Sci.*, USA, **58**: 801–808, 1967.

Waters, N. F., and Fontes, A. K., Genetic response of inbred lines of chickens to Rous sarcoma virus. *J. Nat. Cancer Inst.*, **25**: 351–357, 1960.

Zilber, L. A., Pathogenicity of Rous sarcoma virus for rats and rabbits. *J. Nat. Cancer Inst.*, **26**: 1295–1309, 1961.

Zilber, L. A., and Kriukova,* I. N., Haemorrhagic disease of rats caused by Rous sarcoma virus. *Vopr. virusol.*, **2**: 239–243, 1957.

Zilber, L. A., and Kryukova, I. N., Fibromatosis in rabbits caused by Rous sarcoma virus. *Vopr. virusol.*, **3**: 166–170, 1958.

Zilber, L. A., Lapin, B. A., and Adgighytov, F. I., Pathogenicity of Rous sarcoma virus for monkeys. *Nature*, **205**: 1123–1124, 1965.

* The same name is spelled in a different manner in two successive publications here quoted. We have followed the spelling exactly as the name was printed in the original publications.

CHAPTER 7

The Chicken Leukosis Complex

THE VARIOUS FORMS OF CHICKEN LEUKEMIA AND DIFFICULTIES IN THEIR CLASSIFICATION

Leukemia in chickens is a complex, neoplastic disease of many forms, involving blood cells, their precursors, and the reticular cells lining the circulatory system. Moreover, in some as yet not fully understood manner, fowl leukemias are associated with various forms of sarcomas and with renal carcinomas (nephroblastomas).

There exist several different forms of the chicken leukosis complex. The proper classification of these conditions is difficult; two or more forms may be found simultaneously in the same bird; animals afflicted with one form may subsequently develop another form of the chicken leukosis complex, or related neoplasms. Furthermore, filtrates prepared from one form of leukemia and inoculated into susceptible birds may, under certain not yet fully defined conditions, induce another form of the chicken leukosis complex, or related tumors.

The Transmission of Chicken Leukemia by Filtrates

The first avian leukemias studied experimentally were those in which erythroblasts and myeloblasts formed the predominant picture in the peripheral blood circulation. The erythro-myeloblastic chicken leukemia was actually the first true neoplastic condition transmitted by filtrates.

Erythroblastosis and Myeloblastosis

Erythroblastosis is a peculiar highly malignant form of chicken leukemia, manifested by the appearance of very large numbers of primitive erythroblasts in the peripheral blood circulation. Myeloblastosis, also designated "granuloblastosis," involves myeloid cells and is characterized by the appearance in peripheral blood circulation of large numbers of myeloblasts. Actually, pure erythroblastic or myeloblastic leukemias are rare in nature. More frequently, both types of primitive cells can be found in peripheral blood circulation in the leukemic chickens, although one type is usually predominant. Such leukemias represent a combination of myeloblastosis and erythroblastosis, and can be designated as erythro-myeloblastosis.

It was Ellermann and Bang, in Copenhagen, who in 1908 transmitted erythro-myeloblastic leukemia in chickens by inoculation of cell-free filtrates. This fundamental observation (Ellermann and Bang, 1908, 1909) did not at the time attract sufficient attention; neither was its importance immediately realized. Amply confirmed, and soon accepted as a fact, this unexpected discovery was considered as indicative of the infectious nature of chicken leukemia, thus classifying this disease of the fowl apart from leukemias and related tumors in other species. Only gradually it became apparent that transmission of chicken leukemia by filtrates was the first break in the fundamental approach to the problem of tumors.

The Early Important Observations and the Introduction of the Term "Aleukemic Leukemia." Ellermann and Bang noticed in their studies that some of the chickens inoculated with the leukemic extracts developed typical generalized leukemia, with large numbers of primitive blood cells appearing in peripheral blood; other birds, even though inoculated with the same extracts and under apparently identical conditions, developed leukemic changes in internal organs, such as infiltration with leukemic cells, slight swelling of spleen and liver, weakness, loss of weight, etc., and eventually died from the disease, but their blood picture remained essentially non-leukemic, i.e. "aleukemic." Ellermann and Bang designated this form of disease "pseudoleukemia," but they also used the term "aleukemic" leukemia; they realized, however, that actually the birds suffered from the same disease, even though leukemic cells did not appear in the blood circulation. That "pseudoleukemia" was only a form of true leukemia was evident from experiments in which extracts prepared from birds with "pseudoleukemia" were inoculated into other chickens and induced typical generalized leukemia. Ellermann and Bang suggested the term "leukosis" to designate both the leukemic and pseudoleukemic forms of chicken leukemia.

Even in cases of typical generalized leukemia there exist periods of time during which, temporarily at least, the peripheral blood picture returns to almost normal limits. This is true not only for cases under treatment, but also for untreated leukemias. Ellermann and Bang also recognized this fluctuation in the blood picture of leukemic birds, and the appearance of spontaneous, temporary remissions.

The term "pseudoleukemia" was replaced by the currently used designation "aleukemic leukemia," indicating that form of the disease in which there are essentially no leukemic cells in peripheral blood. It should be stressed, however, that true forms of aleukemic leukemia are quite rare, since even in the typical aleukemic forms some changes in the differential white cell count, in the number of platelets and in the morphology of peripheral blood picture, can usually be detected; as a rule, there is also anemia. Thus, the blood picture is only relatively "normal."

The Relation of Avian Leukemia to Sarcomas and Other Tumors

The problem of experimental chicken leukemia was complicated by the fact that in certain instances injection of leukemic filtrates into susceptible chickens resulted in the development of sarcomas. Oberling and Guérin (1933, 1934) studied extensively this aspect of chicken leukosis, and reported that the induction of various types of sarcomas with leukemic material is possible under certain conditions. When fragments of organs or blood removed from leukemic donors were preserved for some time in glycerin, in a refrigerator, and were then inoculated into chickens, various types of sarcomas could be induced. In turn, grafts of such sarcomas again induced leukemias. In two cases, epithelial proliferations, having an appearance resembling certain human epitheliomas, were found in close contact with the sarcoma.

Engelbreth-Holm (1932), Furth (1931–1936), and their associates have confirmed and extended these observations. Actually, it was not necessary to preserve the leukemic material in glycerin or in the refrigerator prior to injection. In experiments carried out by Furth and other investigators, fresh material prepared from leukemic donors and inoculated into susceptible chickens was able to induce various forms of sarcomas and leukemias. In certain instances, leukemias, particularly of the erythroblastic type, were found to be associated with a concurrent development of soft tissue sarcomas.

More recently, Carr (1956), in Edinburgh, observed that a virus of erythroblastic leukemia (strain ES 4) induced multiple adenocarcinomas of the kidneys, following inoculation into very young, less than 2-week-old, Brown Leghorn chicks. When older birds were inoculated, only leukemia resulted.

The Problem: One or Several Distinct Oncogenic Viruses? These and similar observations could be interpreted by assuming that a single oncogenic virus may be able to induce erythroblastic or myeloblastic leukemia, various forms of sarcomas, and possibly also carcinomas. Mutation of such a virus also had to be considered. On the other hand, it was also possible to assume that the material used for inoculation contained a mixture of distinct, though possibly related, oncogenic agents. This important problem will again be discussed in more detail in the latter part of this chapter.

A Survey of Diseases of the Avian Leukosis Complex

Provided that certain reservations are kept in mind, an arbitrary classification of diseases of the chicken leukosis complex is convenient; such a classification facilitates the review of chicken leukemias and allied neoplasms in a comprehensive manner.

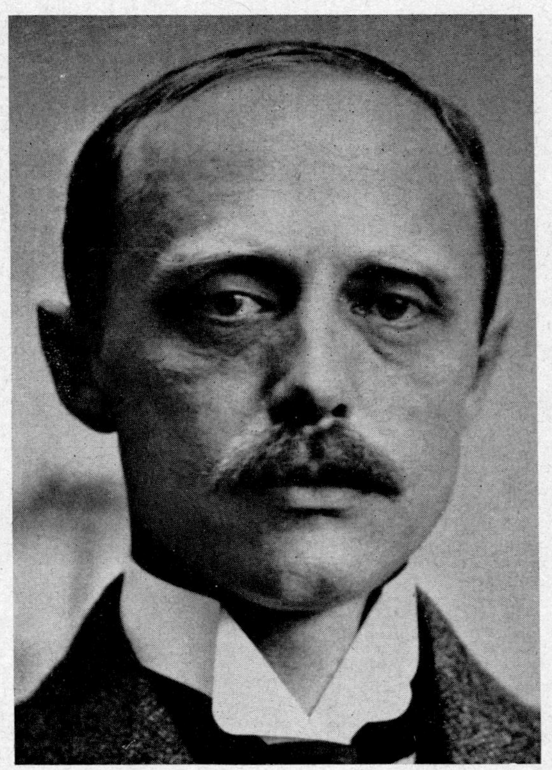

Vilhelm Ellermann

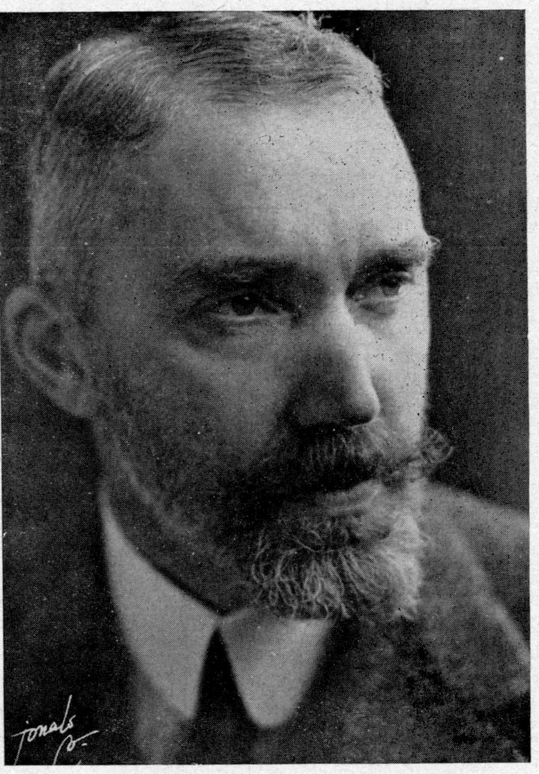

Oluf Bang

FIG. 13.

Essentially, the avian leukosis complex can be divided into two principal groups:

The Leukemic Group

"*Myeloblastosis*" *and* "*Erythroblastosis.*" This group includes the myeloblastic and erythroblastic leukemias, manifested in typical cases by the appearance of large numbers of myeloblasts and/or erythroblasts in the circulating blood. Pure myeloblastic or pure erythroblastic leukemias are rare in nature, but they have been developed, passed serially, and studied individually in the laboratory. Myeloblastosis occurs only rarely in field cases. Erythroblastosis occurs sporadically.

The "Extravascular" Group

This rather heterogenous group of diseases of the chicken leukosis complex consists of usually aleukemic forms in which primitive blood cells only occasionally reach the circulating blood.

"*Lymphoid Leukosis*" *or* "*Visceral Lymphomatosis.*" The most frequent form among diseases in this group is "lymphoid leukosis" or "visceral lymphomatosis" (called also "big liver disease"), a form of leukosis very common in commercial flocks in the United States, and responsible for a yearly loss exceeding $60,000,000 to the U.S. poultry industry (U.S. Dept. Agricult., 1955). Visceral lymphomatosis is characterized by involvement of lymphoid cells which infiltrate in large numbers the liver, lungs, and other internal organs. The pathologic picture in this disease is in effect similar to disseminated lymphosarcomatosis.

"*Neural Lymphomatosis.*" A rather endemic form of the chicken leukosis complex called "neural lymphomatosis," "range paralysis," or "Marek's disease," in which the infiltration with lymphoid cells is particularly prominent in the nerve trunks, causing paralysis.

"*Ocular Lymphomatosis.*" Another form called "ocular lymphomatosis," or "gray eye disease," is caused by infiltration of the eyes with lymphoid cells.

"*Osteopetrosis.*" A different form which involves the periosteum and results in excessive deposition of bone, as, for example, in the tibia, is called "osteopetrosis."

Sarcomas and Nephroblastomas. The various forms of reticular tumors and sarcomas, as well as renal carcinomas (nephroblastomas), form a distinct group.

The true relationship of osteopetrosis and the various sarcomas, as well as of renal carcinomas, to the chicken leukosis complex is still obscure and will be discussed again at the end of this chapter.

AVIAN MYELOBLASTIC AND ERYTHROBLASTIC LEUKEMIAS

We have already indicated in the preliminary introduction to this chapter that myeloblastosis occurs only rarely in field cases. Erythroblastosis is also very uncommon in the field, but may occur sporadically. Both forms of leukemia have been studied extensively in the laboratory, since virus strains inducing either of these forms were developed and have been passed serially, affording an excellent opportunity for the study of these interesting forms of the avian leukosis complex.

General Symptoms

On a farm, in a flock of chickens, the first indication that a bird is affected with leukemia may be a pronounced paleness of the comb, loss of weight, and muscular weakness. Some of the chickens may gradually exhibit ruffled feathers, a retracted neck, closed eyes, and a general dullness: when disturbed, they arouse sluggishly. When blood is obtained by puncture of the wing vein, it is frequently relatively pale and watery, and clots with difficulty. The disease may run a protracted, chronic course, with transitory periods of apparent recovery; loss of weight and gradual development of anemia usually can be observed in such birds. On the other hand, the disease may run an acute course, developing suddenly in otherwise apparently normal birds; such chickens may die within a few days.

The liver and spleen are usually enlarged, of a reddish-brown color. Hemorrhages into the subcutaneous tissue and into the mucosa of the intestinal tract are common; the bone marrow is pulpy and of reddish color.

Blood Picture

The fundamental manifestations of the intravascular leukemias concern the blood picture. There are two principal forms of avian leukemias, the erythroblastosis and the myeloblastosis. The relatively pure erythroblastic form occurs more frequently than relatively pure myeloblastosis.

Erythroblastosis is characterized by the appearance, in peripheral blood circulation, of large numbers of primitive erythroblasts. Myeloblastosis, also called granuloblastosis, is characterized by the appearance in peripheral blood of primitive cells of the granulocytic series, the myeloblasts. Since pure forms of either leukemia are rare, usually both types of primitive cells in varying proportions can be found in blood circulation. Anemia, as a rule, develops in both forms of leukemia, and the red blood cells, their shape, color, and numbers, are affected. The platelets diminish considerably in numbers. The thrombopenia probably accounts for poor clotting of blood collected from leukemic donors.

Although erythroblastosis and myeloblastosis may occur in the same host, experimental studies of this disease in chickens resulted in the recognition that each condition is probably a distinct pathological entity, which may occur individually.

It has not yet been determined how closely interrelated are the agents of myeloblastic and erythroblastic leukemias, and whether under certain conditions they may not mutate, and possibly change, one into another. At the present time it appears that these are distinct, though related, agents, each capable of causing a distinct disease in a susceptible bird. It is also apparent, however, that frequently a mixture of symptoms, characteristic for both disease entities, may occur in the same bird.

EXPERIMENTAL STUDIES ON AVIAN MYELOBLASTOSIS

Comprehensive studies on myeloblastic chicken leukemia were carried out by Dr. Joseph W. Beard and his colleagues (1952–1960), at Duke University in Durham, N.C., with a strain of myeloblastosis virus obtained initially from a single chicken brought to Duke University in 1949 by Dr. E. P. Johnson. This material was derived originally from two cases of neurolymphomatosis and was associated from time to time not only with lymphomatosis but also with erythroblastosis.

This virus, passed with filtered material alone, continued, however, as a pure myeloblastic strain, and remained as such for 10 years. In the examination of a very large number of blood smears from chicks with virus-induced myeloblastosis over a period of several years, there has been no evidence of change in the blood picture: neither was there a change in the host response to the virus. During all this time, since 1949, the virus has been passed from one chicken host to another, in over 150 successive passages, involving a total of over 100,000 birds. All inoculations were made with filtered blood plasma, or with virus obtained from filtered plasma by ultracentrifugation.

Myeloblastosis has long been known to be transmissible by cell-free filtrates prepared from blood plasma of diseased chickens; extreme variations, nevertheless, have been observed in the infectious capacity of such plasma. Only 10 to 20 per cent of leukemic chickens provided sufficiently high amounts of the virus in their plasma for successful transmission to other birds. In some instances, however, the virus was found to occur in very high concentrations in the plasma of infected birds.

The concentration of virus particles in the circulating plasma could be determined in Beard's laboratory by direct particle counts in the electron microscope. A special procedure was devised by Sharp and Beard (1952) for the estimation of virus amount by means of direct counts of the virus particles. A thin agar square was placed at the bottom of a 1 cm^3 ultracentrifuge cell filled with the appropriate dilution of plasma or extract containing the virus particles, and the virus was spun down on to the agar. The supernatant fluid was poured off, and time allowed for the agar to take up the residual fluid. The virus was then fixed on the agar surface with osmic acid vapor, removed in a collodion film, and shadowed for electron micrography. An estimate of the number of particles was obtained by counting those in a measured area of film.

Counts of up to 2,000,000,000 particles per one cm^3 of plasma were not unusual in chickens with myeloblastosis. In a few leukemic birds, the concentration of the virus reached a level as high as two trillion (2×10^{12}) particles per cm^3 of plasma. Such enormous concentration of virus particles reaching approximately 1.5 mg of hydrated or 0.3 mg of dry virus per cm^3 of plasma caused a visible turbidity of the fluid. These were extreme cases, however; more frequently the plasma showed a concentration in the order varying from 10 billion (10^{10}) to 100 billion (10^{11}) of particles per one cm^3; many birds showed a concentration of less than one billion (10^9) per one cm^3, actually the lower limit of concentration adequate for accurate particle counts. In those instances where still lower levels of virus were present, the plasma had no infectious potency on inoculation tests, even though the donor birds obviously died from myeloblastosis. Considerable numbers of particles were required to transmit the disease. Studies carried out in Beard's laboratory on a large number of chickens indicated that the median effective dose required to induce disease in 50 per cent of 3-day-old chicks of a highly susceptible strain varied from 4 million to 100 million particles, depending on the strain of chickens used for inoculation. Considerable differences in susceptibility were found, however, among the individual birds. As few as 6000 particles sufficed to induce the disease in an occasional bird (about 5 per cent), while up to 145 billion particles were required to induce myeloblastosis in practically all (95 per cent) of the injected chicks. The difference in the injected dose required to induce the disease varied from 10,000 to one millionfold. This difference suggested an impressive range of individual variations in natural resistance among hosts of a presumably susceptible breed to the inoculated virus (Beard, 1956, 1957).

Enzymatic Properties of the Virus of Myeloblastosis

An outstanding enzymatic property of the virus of avian myeloblastosis was discovered at Duke University by Mommaerts, Eckert, Beard, and their associates (Mommaerts *et al.*, 1952–1954): the virus of myeloblastosis was found to dephosphorylate adenosine triphosphate and inosine triphosphate. Based on this enzymatic activity, a colorimetric method was devised, which permitted the determination of the content of myeloblastosis virus in a given plasma within a few minutes.

A colorimetric micro-method was devised in Beard's laboratory by Mommaerts (Mommaerts *et al.*, 1952–1954), Green (Green *et al.*, 1954–1955) and their colleagues for the estimation of the enzyme activity, employing, as a basis for the test, measurements of change in pH associated with the liberation of phosphate. Blood was drawn into melting point tubes from a needle prick of the wing vein; the tubes were sealed at one end and centrifuged to sediment the cells. A volume of 3 lambda of cell-free plasma was taken off, and mixed with adenosine triphosphate in balanced salt solution in the presence of bromthymol blue. The rate of progress to acid reaction was followed by color change to a standard level. Under proper conditions, this required from thirty seconds to several minutes with the best plasmas.

Systematic studies provided substantial evidence that this enzymatic activity is quantitatively related to the virus particle and inseparable from it by the methods employed. It could be demonstrated in the plasma of many birds suffering from myeloblastosis, appearing only with the onset of the disease and remaining closely proportional to the number of virus particles. The activity could be concentrated following sedimentation of the particles by ultracentrifugation. These and other findings were consistent with the view that the enzyme is an integral constituent of the virus.

The enzymatic ability of the virus of myeloblastosis to dephosphorylate adenosine triphosphate proved to be of inestimable practical value, providing a rapidly applicable micro-screening test for selecting birds with high plasma content of infective particles.

It has been observed repeatedly that the plasma content of the virus of myeloblastosis varies over an extremely broad range in diseased chickens. Among birds suffering from myeloblastosis, only a few, not more than 10 to 20 per cent, contain adequate quantities of virus in their plasma to provide amounts sufficient for extensive transmission experiments.

Employing the micro-screening test, it was possible to select in advance leukemic donors with blood plasma rich in virus content. Instead of working with plasma of unknown potency, it was thus possible to provide, as source of the agent, plasmas of known infective potential, collected from selected donors. Time consuming and tedious experiments, such as titrations, could thus be carried out with a good and dependable source of virus material.

It is of considerable interest that the enzymatic ability to dephosphorylate adenosine triphosphate, found to be connected with the virus of chicken myeloblastosis, could not be established either for the virus of avian erythroblastosis, or, in fact, thus far, for any other oncogenic agents.

Difference in Susceptibility

Different strains and breeds of chickens vary greatly in their response to the inoculation of the virus of myeloblastosis. Several lines of inbred White Leghorns, notably line 15, developed at the Regional Poultry Research Laboratory in East Lansing, Michigan, were found to be highly susceptible to experimental inoculation with the virus. Commercial New Hampshire Red chicks were highly resistant, and so were several other commercial strains of White Leghorns.

The age of the host at the time of inoculation was of great importance. Very young chicks only a few days old were found most susceptible. For practical reasons, 3-day-old chicks, rather than newly hatched chicks, were used for inoculation. The susceptibility of the birds to the inoculation of the virus decreased rapidly with age. Ten-day-old chicks were 5 times, and those 21 days old were about 40 times, more resistant than 3-day-old chicks.

The route of inoculation was also of importance. The virus inoculated intravenously was about 15 times as effective in the induction of the disease as that inoculated into the muscle or in the peritoneum, and over 60 times more effective than that inoculated subcutaneously.

Course of the Disease in Inoculated Chicks. Following inoculation of the virus of myeloblastosis, primitive blood cells could be seen in the peripheral blood circulation in 9 days. The number of myeloblasts in the blood increased rapidly, reaching, in some birds at least, the figure of up to 2,000,000 per mm^3. A pronounced anemia usually developed. Some of the birds died as early as 12 days after inoculation of large doses of the virus; on the average, however, they died about 17 days after inoculation.

Titration of the Virus. Latency and its Relation to the Initiating Dose

In Beard's laboratory, good results could be obtained with three successive 10-fold dilutions of the virus of myeloblastosis inoculated intravenously into 3-day-old White Leghorn chicks of the highly susceptible line 15. It was found that the number of chicks developing leukemia, and the latency period, elapsing between the time of inoculation and the appearance of the disease, depended on the inoculated dose.

Actually, the latency period was a more consistent and convenient indicator related to the injected dose of the virus, than the percentage of chicks developing disease. With smaller doses of the virus injected, variations in natural susceptibility of the hosts interfered substantially with the expected incidence of birds developing disease. Higher concentrations of the virus induced disease after a shorter latency period. Inoculation of the more diluted virus filtrates was followed by a longer latency period preceding the development of disease.

FIG. 14. CHICKEN VISCERAL LYMPHOMATOSIS VIRUS.

(A). Ultrathin section of spleen of a chicken with visceral lymphomatosis. Mature virus particles, about 80 mμ in diameter in an intercellular space. Magnification 45,000 ×. (B). (Inset). Budding virus particle (arrow) in the spleen of a chicken with visceral lymphomatosis. Magnification 90,000 ×. (C). Mature virus particles about 80 mμ in diameter in a cytoplasmic inclusion in the spleen of a chicken with visceral lymphomatosis. Magnification 68,000 ×. Electron micrographs prepared by L. Dmochowski and P. L. Langford, Department of Virology, University of Texas, M. D. Anderson Hospital and Tumor Institute, Houston.

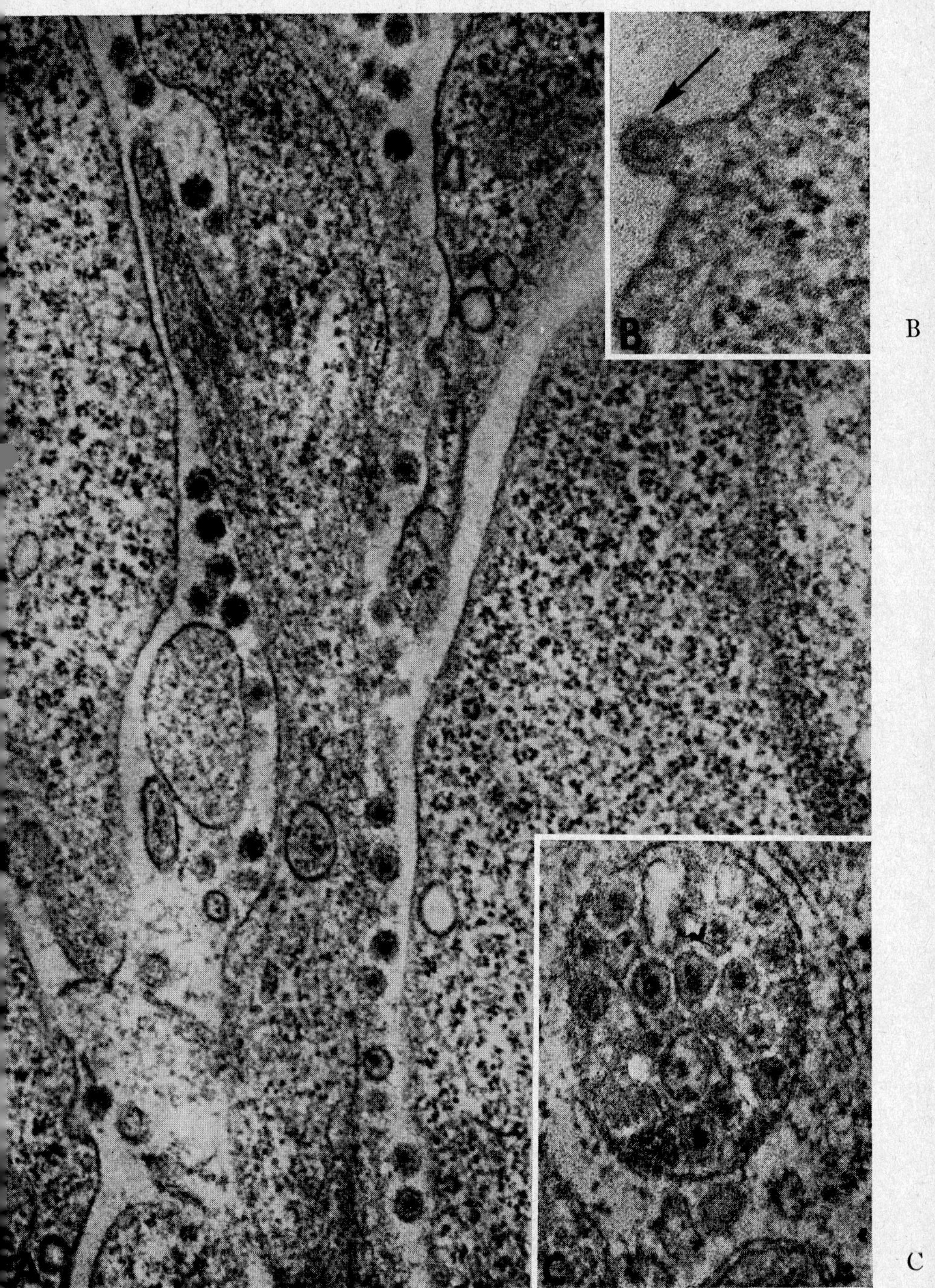

B

C

Fig. 14. Chicken Visceral Lymphomatosis Virus.

The close relation between the latency period and the initiating dose constituted, in the experiments of Beard and his coworkers, the basis for titration and bio-assay of the virus of myeloblastosis. In this respect the virus of myeloblastosis did not differ from the agent of chicken sarcoma. At the National Cancer Institute, W. Ray Bryan and his coworkers (1955) studied this problem on a quantitative basis in experiments dealing with the Rous sarcoma. They determined that the amount of extractable virus from a tumor, as well as latency in bio-assay experiments, depended essentially on the amount of virus used in the initiating dose.

EXPERIMENTAL STUDIES ON AVIAN ERYTHROBLASTOSIS

Avian erythroblastosis is a highly malignant form of leukemia, peculiar to chickens; it has no exact parallel in mammals. The cell involved is the erythroblast which proliferates in the bone marrow. The onset of erythroblastosis is detectable first by the increase in the number of polychrome erythrocytes. The change in color of the red blood cells is soon accompanied by the development of abnormalities in their shape, size, and nuclear structure. Characteristic, very large erythroblasts, pathognomonic for erythroblastosis, appear in peripheral blood. In its terminal phase, the number of erythroblasts in the peripheral blood circulation may reach 600,000 per mm^3.

The disease may kill the birds before pronounced symptoms develop. Some chickens may die suddenly without premonitory symptoms of illness, with relatively insignificant blood changes; in such instances, the cause may be related to a toxic response, or to a paralysis of the respiratory or circulatory center. In other instances, the birds exhibit weakness of wings, legs, are unable to stand, and may die after a brief period of respiratory difficulty.

The onset of virus-induced erythroblastosis can be recognized in susceptible chicks within 48 hours; some of the chicks may die as soon as 6 days after inoculation; the average, however, die from the virus-induced disease after 9 days.

Even though the avian erythroblastic leukemia is a highly malignant disease, animals with unquestionable clinical signs of erythroblastosis, and whose blood could transmit this condition on inoculation to other chickens, have been reported to recover occasionally.

A relatively pure strain of erythroblastosis has been studied extensively in the laboratory of Dr. Joseph W. Beard at Duke University, N.C. (Beard *et al.*, 1952, 1957). This strain of erythroblastosis was obtained from Dr. Astrid Fagraeus of the State Pathological Laboratory in Stockholm. Dr. Fagraeus, in turn, originally obtained this strain from Dr. Julius Engelbreth-Holm, Department of Pathological Anatomy, University of Copenhagen. It is of interest that this particular strain of erythroblastosis initially developed from myeloblastic leukemia.

A leukemic spleen from a chicken with virus-induced erythroblastosis, frozen in dry ice, was shipped from Stockholm to Duke University in January, 1955. Upon its arrival, 4 days later, the Thermos jug was found to be broken and thawed out. The virus, nevertheless, survived, since extracts immediately prepared, and inoculated into about 30 chicks, induced typical erythroblastic leukemia. Further transmission of the virus was accomplished with filtered blood plasma. Under the conditions of the study in Beard's laboratory, this form of leukemia has been maintained as relatively pure erythroblastosis without any evidence of mixture with, or transformation into, another form of leukemia.

The virus of erythroblastosis, like that of myeloblastosis, is present in the plasma of diseased chickens. There is a striking difference, however, in the concentration of the virus of erythroblastosis as compared with that of myeloblastosis. The concentration of virus particles in plasma of chickens with virus-induced erythroblastosis is only approximately one per cent of that in myeloblastosis, reaching in some birds about 10 billion virus particles per 1 cm^3. Variations occur, however, in the contents of the virus in plasma. Actually not many plasmas contain as many as 10^{10} particles per 1 cm^3 of plasma.

The infective potency of the virus, its ability to induce disease is greater, however, in erythroblastosis than in myeloblastosis. The number of particles of the virus of erythroblastosis required to induce disease is only about one hundredth of that necessary to induce myeloblastosis with the latter virus. In every respect, erythroblastosis is a more virulent disease, inducing symptoms and killing the birds after a shorter latency period, and within a shorter time, than myeloblastosis.

Lack of Enzymatic Activity of the Virus of Erythroblastosis

A fundamental difference between the virus of myeloblastosis and that of erythroblastosis was found in reference to their enzymatic activity. Whereas the virus of myeloblastosis was found to dephosphorylate adenosine triphosphate, such activity could not be demonstrated in any appreciable amount for the virus of erythroblastosis. Examination showed that the adenosinetriphosphatase activity of the erythroblastosis plasma was only slightly greater than that of plasma from normal birds (Bonar *et al.*, 1957).

From a practical point of view, this was a disadvantage to the investigator, since a very convenient tool for the selection of potent plasma, so useful in experiments with myeloblastosis, was not available in studies with erythroblastosis. In fact, birds to be used as donors for the virus of erythroblastosis had to be selected on the basis of hematological picture, i.e. on the basis of the presence of erythroblasts in the peripheral blood. Such donors were chosen in

Beard's laboratory on the basis of the concentration of erythroblasts seen in routine blood smears taken at daily intervals. Bleeding was postponed until the birds were practically moribund. It is not known, however, whether this was the best method for obtaining the agent in highest concentration. Selection of the donors could be made only in this manner, however, since the adenosine-triphosphatase reaction, so useful in the studies on myeloblastosis, could not be applied for preliminary estimation of virus concentration in the plasma in erythroblastosis.

Very frequently the amount of virus in donors with erythroblastosis varied considerably, even though the donors obviously had erythroblastic leukemia. Some donors had high numbers of virus particles in their peripheral blood, whereas in other donors there were far fewer numbers of particles present. No tests for the number of particles, except direct electron microscopy, precipitation with specific serum, or bio-assay, were available.

Host Response

The same inbred line 15 of White Leghorns, developed at the U.S. Department of Agriculture's Regional Research Laboratory in East Lansing, Michigan, and employed for experiments with the virus of myeloblastosis, also proved to be susceptible to inoculation with the virus of erythroblastosis.

Because of the apparently high infective potency of the virus for the inbred line 15 of White Leghorns, it was thought possible that another strain of hosts, preferably one readily obtained from commercial hatcheries, might be employed instead. Accordingly, the White Plymouth Rock, of the Arbor Acre strain, Glastonbury, Connecticut, was tested in three titration experiments. The results obtained were negative, suggesting that the White Plymouth Rock chicks were highly resistant and entirely unsuitable for the inoculation of the agent. Several other strains, such as line 6 and 7 of White Leghorns, bred at the Regional Poultry Research Laboratory in East Lansing, Michigan, were also found to be almost completely resistant to the virus of erythroblastosis. This strong genetic effect of the host response to the virus of erythroblastosis parallels that observed in experiments with myeloblastosis (Eckert *et al.*, 1956).

The Influence of Age at Inoculation

The principal and striking difference, however, between the host response to these two viruses was that related to the age of the host at the time of inoculation. Whereas 3-day-old chicks were most susceptible to the inoculation with the virus of myeloblastosis, and the resistance of these birds to the inoculation with that virus increased rapidly with age, the reverse was found to be true in experiments dealing with the virus of erythroblastosis. When, in a series of experiments carried out by Eckert and his colleagues (1955), chicks ranging in age from 7 to 77 days of the White Leghorn line 15 were inoculated with the same dose of the virus of erythroblastosis, the susceptibility was found to increase gradually with the age of the chicks inoculated.

Chicks 2 to 3 weeks old were found to be very suitable for inoculation and were used routinely; such birds were obviously more suitable for handling and housing, and were more readily injected intravenously than 3-day-old chicks used for the inoculation of the virus of myeloblastosis.

The most effective route of inoculation was directly into the blood stream. Intramuscular injection was about 20 times less sensitive. Subcutaneous injection of the virus was 1400 times less effective than that performed by the intravenous route.

The Relationship between the Antigenic Properties of the Virus of Myeloblastosis and that of Erythroblastosis

In studies carried out by Eckert, Beard, and their associates at Duke University, a specific anti-virus immune serum was prepared from chickens immunized with the myeloblastosis virus. The chickens were first treated with formalin-inactivated virus, and subsequently with filtered plasma containing untreated virus in high concentration. The serum was heated to 56°C for half an hour before use. The immune serum thus obtained not only neutralized the virus, but precipitated it quantitatively either from plasma or from virus concentrates. Under certain conditions, when the virus was concentrated, and the immune serum highly potent, the precipitation was essentially complete, and a visibly turbid virus-serum suspension became water-clear. The precipitation, and clumping of the virus particles occurring within minutes under the influence of a specific immune serum, could be observed in the electron microscope by Eckert and his coworkers in Beard's laboratory (1955).

Experimental studies have indicated a close antigenic relationship between the agents of erythroblastosis and myeloblastosis. Anti-myeloblastosis immune serum prepared from the chicken was found to neutralize *in vitro* not only the virus of myeloblastosis but also the agent of erythroblastosis. The reverse was also true. An anti-erythroblastosis chicken immune serum neutralized both the virus of erythroblastosis and that of myeloblastosis.

Although there was no apparent difference between myeloblastosis and erythroblastosis in the neutralization tests with chicken immune serum, a definite distinction was evident in cross-precipitin reactions studied by electron micrography. Anti-myeloblastosis immune serum from one chicken quantitatively precipitated the homologous virus but, under the same conditions, produced only partial precipitation of the virus of erythroblastosis. Anti-erythroblastosis chicken immune serum, on the other hand, precipitated only partially the virus of erythroblastosis, and had little, if any, precipitating effect against the myeloblastosis virus (Beard, 1957. Beard *et al.*, 1957).

Propagation of the Virus of Avian Erythroblastic and Myeloblastic Leukemia in Tissue Culture

In 1934, Furth and Stubbs grew sarcoma cells *in vitro*; during 67 days of observation these cells released a virus capable of inducing both sarcoma and erythroleukosis. In 1936, Verne, Oberling, and Guérin reported that the leukemic virus could be maintained in active state in culture of fowl bone marrow for 15 days. In 1937, Furth and Breedis maintained a strain of leukemic virus in culture of sarcoma cells for 158 days. When reinoculated, it still induced both leukemia and sarcoma. In 1938, Ruffilli succeeded in maintaining the OG strain of leukemic virus for 122 days by cultivating it in the myocardium of a leukemic fowl.

In 1939, van den Berghe and d'Ursel maintained strain OG of erythroblastic leukemia in tissue culture, consisting of chick embryo cells in Tyrode solution, for 11 successive passages, through approximately 6 weeks. Chickens inoculated with fluids collected from 5th and 11th passages developed typical erythroblastic leukemia. Doljanski and Pikovski (1942) reported continuous production of virus in normal chicken cells infected *in vitro* with a strain of avian leukosis virus; using for cultures the myocardium of a normal fowl explanted in leukemic plasma for 4 weeks, they were able to maintain the virus, and reproduce leukemia on inoculation tests. They also succeeded in conserving the virus for 178 days in culture of fibroblasts. They did not observe any morphological changes in the appearance of the cells concomitant with virus production.

More recently, Beaudreau and his associates in Beard's laboratory (1958, 1960) succeeded in growing avian myeloblastic cells in tissue culture. The myeloblasts were collected from peripheral blood of chicken donors with virus-induced myeloblastosis. The cells were then cultured *in vitro* with the medium changed at 1 to 6 day intervals. The myeloblastic cells could be maintained for at least 6 months. During that time the virus was found to be liberated continuously into the culture fluid. It could be shown in some groups of cultures from the cells of a single bird that as many as 40 particles per cell, per hour, reached the culture fluid, a total of almost 2000 particles per cell in the initial 48 hour period. The rate of virus liberation was greatest during the early periods of culture from 2 to 12 days, during which the average output was about 31 particles per cell, per hour (1500 particles per cell in 48 hours). Later, the process slowed somewhat, but in some cases, after a period of relative quiescence, it was again resumed at a high level. Cultures carried for long periods showed a decreasing rate of virus liberation after about 6 weeks.

The presence of the virus in culture fluid was determined by: (a) enzymatic activity, i.e. its ability to dephosphorylate adenosine triphosphate, (b) direct particle count in the electron microscope, and (c) titration of virus infectivity determined on bio-assay by inoculating susceptible chicks. A critical requirement for the stabilization of the growth of avian myeloblasts in tissue culture, and for the consistent release of virus particles under such conditions, was the addition to the medium employed of serum in high concentration (50 per cent chicken serum in medium 199), supplemented by B vitamins and folic acid (Beaudreau *et al.*, 1960a). Exposure of bone marrow cells, taken from normal chickens and grown in tissue culture, to avian myeloblastosis virus resulted in the appearance of cells which resembled leukemic myeloblasts (Beaudreau *et al.*, 1960b). These cells released new virus and showed in the electron microscope the same ultrastructure associated with virus production as that described for myeloblasts in leukemic chicks. The transformed cultures multiplied indefinitely whereas the non-infected cells did not increase in number. Lagerlöf (1960) also found production of new virus by bone marrow cells infected *in vitro* with erythroblastosis virus. There was no net increase in cell number, and no morphological malignant transformation; however, transplantation experiments suggested that the cells so infected became neoplastic.

Morphologic Transformation In Vitro of Cell Cultures Following Infection with Virus of Avian Myeloblastosis. Baluda and his coworkers observed that the avian myeloblastosis virus induces differentiation and proliferation of certain cells in cultures of explanted chick embryonic hematopoietic tissues (Baluda and Goetz, 1961. Baluda *et al.*, 1963). Avian myeloblastosis virus induces the formation of at least two new and stable, probably neoplastic types of cells, namely myeloblasts and osteo-

---

FIG. 15. CHICKEN VISCERAL LYMPHOMATOSIS. MATURE AND BUDDING VIRUS PARTICLES.

(A). Ultrathin section of fragments of two parathyroid epithelium cells from a chicken congenitally infected with avian lymphomatosis virus. This virus strain (ALV-F42) was originally isolated in tissue culture from the liver of a chicken with a field case of visceral lymphomatosis. Virus particles in an intercellular space. The particles are spherical, about 75 to 100 mμ in diameter (average approximately 80 mμ). Most of them have a centrally located internal electron-dense nucleoid. Magnification 105,500 ×. (B). Virus particle (arrow) budding from an ovarian medullary cord cell of a congenitally infected chick embryo (avian visceral lymphomatosis strain ALV-F42). Magnification 199,500 ×. Electron micrographs prepared by H. S. Di Stefano and R. M. Dougherty, Departments of Anatomy and Microbiology, State University of New York, Upstate Medical Center, Syracuse.

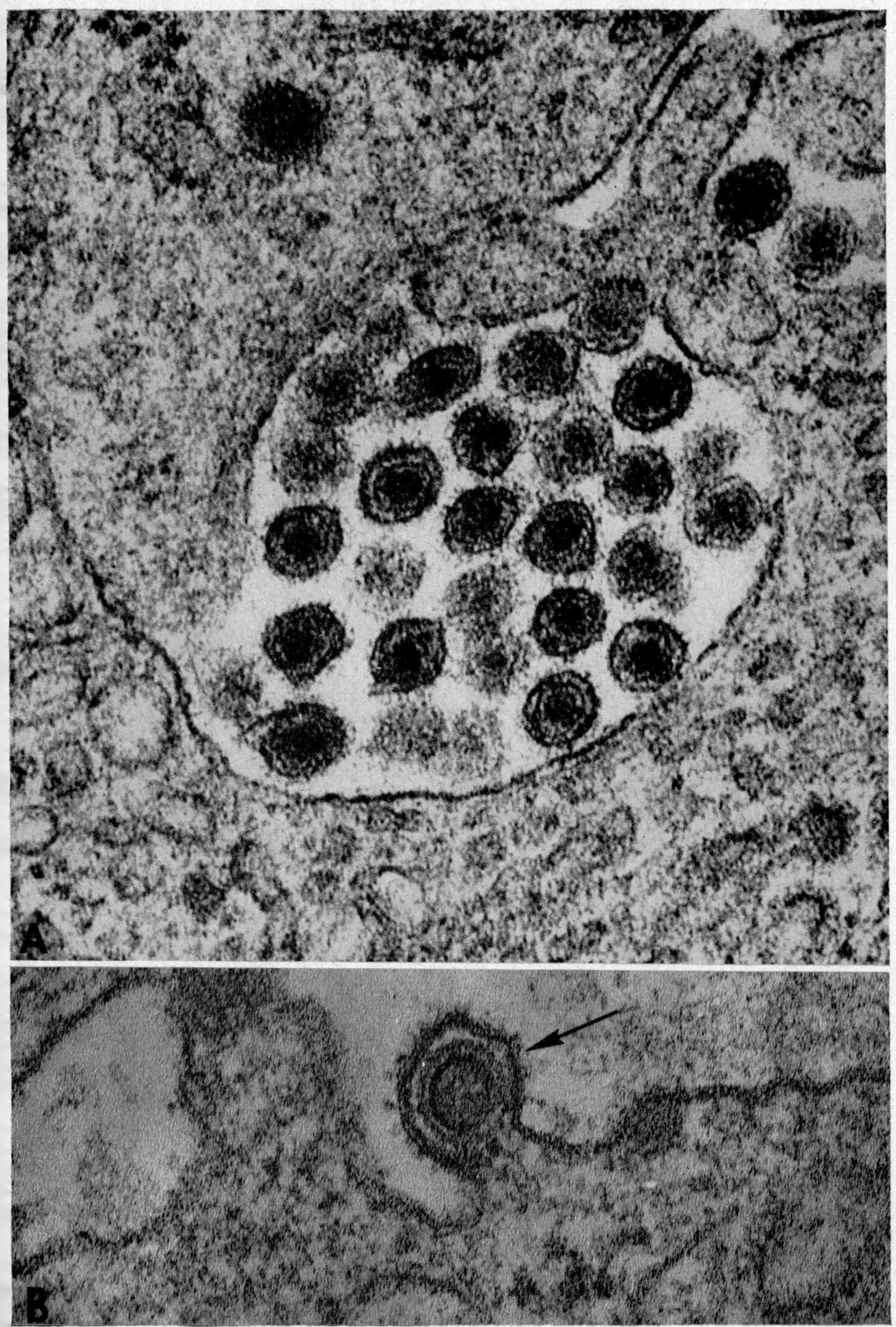

Fig. 15. Chicken Visceral Lymphomatosis. Mature and Budding Virus Particles.

blasts. The transforming effect of avian myeloblastosis virus upon cell cultures appears to be similar to the oncogenic effect of the virus *in vivo*. Transformation depends on the presence of susceptible target cells, which are presumably mesenchymal precursors of myeloblasts (Baluda and Goetz, 1961). When other cells become infected, they retain their normal morphology and multiply, but become virus producers. The formation of discrete foci of converted cells in monolayer cultures infected with avian myeloblastosis virus may provide an *in vitro* assay system.

In more recent experiments (Baluda *et al.*, 1964), several virus strains of avian lymphomatosis were tested and none induced differentiation and proliferation of myeloid or lymphoid precursor cells, although these viruses multiplied in cell cultures, as shown on bio-assay tests. Development of typical tumors in chickens resulted from inoculation of supernatant fluids of the infected cultures. Strain R of erythroblastosis was also tested and gave erratic results; the virus induced differentiation and a short-lived proliferation of erythroblasts, but only on the highest dose of infection employed. Baluda and his coworkers concluded that among the avian leukosis viruses only the avian myeloblastosis virus has the ability to induce *in vitro* maturation and proliferation of some myeloid and lymphoid precursor cells. Other leukosis viruses are unable to do so, although each one seems to possess the capacity to induce a distinct type of cellular transformation *in vitro*.

Transformation of chick fibroblast cultures by avian leukosis strain MC29 was described by Langlois and Beard (1967). This strain of avian leukosis virus, originally isolated from a Rhode Island Red chicken with spontaneous disease, produced a spectrum of neoplasms such as myelocytomatosis, myelocytomas, endotheliomas and renal tumors, following inoculation into 3-day-old Line 15 White Leghorn chicks (Mladenov *et al.*, 1967).

Electron Microscopic Studies of the Viruses of Myeloblastosis and Erythroblastosis

Preliminary Studies and Examination of Shadowed Virus Particles. In the initial experiments carried out in Beard's laboratory (Sharp *et al.*, 1952–1955. Beard, 1957) the virus particles were deposited in drop preparations on very thin and transparent formvar membranes, and were then examined with the electron microscope. This method required drying of the virus particles. When deposited on formvar membranes, the salt concentration increased to saturation and precipitation, resulting in distortion and flattening of the virus particles. To eliminate distortion, the virus preparations were placed on an agar block, so that the salts could diffuse into the block and leave no salt deposit on the surface. The virus particles were then fixed with osmic acid fumes, stripped from the agar and examined in the electron microscope.

Micrographs of unshadowed preparations of plasma concentrates obtained from either myeloblastosis or erythroblastosis showed circular images of an appearance suggesting that the particles consisted predominantly of a watery, gel-like material, surrounding a small, relatively dense internal structure. Such electron micrographs were not sufficiently clear, however. In order to bring out the three-dimensional effect, shadow-casting was then applied with metal vapor. When examined in the electron microscope under proper magnification, such particles could then be photographed as spherical, opaque bodies. No inner structure could be revealed, however, since only the surface of the particles, covered by a metal deposit, was accessible to the electron beam.

These preliminary electron microscopic studies carried out on blood plasma containing large quantities of virus of myeloblastosis revealed the presence of innumerable spheroidal particles varying widely in size, but averaging about 120 mμ in diameter (Sharp and Beard, 1954). These particles had a tendency to form aggregates when examined in drop preparations on formvar membranes. A correlation existed between the quantity of particles in a given sample of virus concentrate and the infectivity potential of the extract. The identification of particles representing the virus strain of avian myeloblastosis, and the correlation of their presence with their infectious ability to induce the disease, was established in Beard's laboratory by direct particle counts, by bio-assay, and also by specific precipitation with anti-viral, immune serum (Eckert *et al.*, 1952, 1955).

Electron microscopic studies were carried out in Beard's laboratory also on the virus of erythroblastosis. In this disease, the concentration of virus in the plasma of diseased chicks is about one hundredfold lower than in myeloblastosis. Ultracentrifugation of plasma filtrates resulted in only very small pellets. On electron microscopy, spherical particles also could be observed in such pellets, essentially similar to those observed in studies with myeloblastosis, except that they were somewhat smaller. The average diameter of particles observed in erythroblastosis was about 102 mμ (Sharp *et al.*, 1955), whereas the particles found in myeloblastosis had a diameter of about 120 mμ (Sharp *et al.*, 1954). In both diseases, the particles have been identified by correlations of the results obtained with physical, chemical and biological methods (Eckert *et al.*, 1955).

The introduction of the technique of ultrathin sections in electron microscopy, developed by Porter, Blum, and Palade in 1953, brought a fundamental change in the study of the morphology of viruses. The ultrathin sections, only 20 to 40 mμ in thickness, cut not only through the cells, but also through individual virus particles, and revealed their internal morphology. Electron microscopy could now be developed as a more useful and reliable tool in experimental cancer research. In studies of ultrathin sections, oncogenic, as well as other, viruses were found to have a morphology distinct from non-viral cell components, and from other material of similar size and shape.

The technique of ultrathin sections was first applied successfully to the study of chicken leukemias in 1956 at the Institut de Recherches sur le Cancer in Villejuif, Seine, France. Ultrathin sections were prepared by E. L. Benedetti, W. Bernhard, and C. Oberling from spleens and bone marrow of chicks with virus-induced erythroblastosis. The electron microscope revealed in the cytoplasm of the cells examined the presence of inclusion-like bodies some of which were most probably altered mitochondria, filled with large numbers of spherical particles. The external diameter of these particles varied, on average, from 75 to 80 mμ; surrounded by an external membrane, they had an inner, dense, nucleus-like center of a diameter varying from 30 to 40 mμ. These characteristic virus-like particles could be detected in the bone marrow or in the spleen of 12 out of 24 chicks examined.

When similar ultrathin sections were prepared from young, normal, healthy chicks, 3 out of 24 birds revealed on electron microscopic examination the presence of a small number of similar virus-like particles. Six normal, healthy chicken embryos were also examined, and no particles could be detected in their tissues. When, however, later on, Benedetti (1957) examined additional normal chickens and normal chicken embryos, he was able to find similar virus-like particles in 9 out of 84 hosts examined. It is well known that the virus of chicken leukosis is widely prevalent in the fowl, without necessarily causing symptoms of disease; accordingly, latent virus particles may be present occasionally also in healthy birds and in normal chick embryos.

In a cooperative study reported in 1958 by W. Bernhard from Villejuif, France, and J. W. Beard and his colleagues of Duke University in Durham, N.C., ultrathin sections were prepared from pellets obtained by ultracentrifugation of plasma from chicken donors with either myeloblastic or erythroblastic leukemia. The particles were very numerous in pellets from myeloblastosis. On the other hand, pellets from the plasma of chickens infected with erythroblastosis were much smaller and contained fewer particles. The morphology of particles found in either myeloblastosis or erythroblastosis preparations was the same, however. Spherical particles with a diameter varying from 60 to 110 mμ, with an average of about 80 mμ, could be found in myeloblastosis plasma preparations. The size of particles observed in erythroblastosis plasma was very similar, and varied from 75 to 80 mμ. The particles were surrounded by a membrane, which appeared single at low magnification, but was often double in pictures of high resolution. There was a central core, of a high electron absorbing property, about 35 to 40 mμ in diameter. Neither with respect to size, nor to ultrastructure, was there a clear difference in morphology between particles of myeloblastosis and those of erythroblastosis. No particles of similar morphology could be observed in pellets from plasmas of healthy chickens.

The ultrastructure of the agents of chicken myeloblastosis or erythroblastosis was morphologically not distinguishable from that of the viruses of other chicken tumors, such as Rous sarcoma.

The difference in the average size of the virus particles examined with the electron microscope on ultrathin sections (80 mμ) as compared with that on dehydrated virus shadowed with metal, that is 102 to 120 mμ for the virus of erythroblastosis and myeloblastosis respectively (Beard, 1957), may be due to the different techniques employed. Sizes determined on dehydrated and shadowed virus, may be relatively large because of flattening of the particles, and the thickness of the metal layer covering the individual particles. It is unlikely, however, that the diameter of particles examined on ultrathin sections indicates exactly the size of the virus particles *in vivo*. The dehydration and embedding in preparation for thin sections produce shrinkage which may influence to a considerable degree the size of the particles revealed on electron microscopy of ultrathin sections.

Further electron microscopic studies of avian myeloblastosis were made in 1958 by Parsons and his colleagues in Beard's laboratory. Examination of ultrathin sections of circulating myeloblasts, and of such cells grown in tissue culture, revealed only rarely the presence of virus particles. This was a rather unexpected finding, since myeloblasts were known to liberate the virus at a high rate in tissue culture; large amounts of extracellular virus could be detected in tissue culture fluid, as well as in blood plasma. In contrast, when ultrathin sections were prepared from cells other than myeloblasts, in the spleen, bone marrow, and liver of leukemic donors, intracytoplasmic virus particles could be detected in high concentrations, mostly in groups, in inclusion-like bodies.

More recently, Bonar and his associates (1960) in Beard's laboratory observed that under proper experimental conditions, virus particles could be observed consistently with the electron microscope in avian myeloblasts grown in tissue culture. In this study, the cells were examined at first immediately after they had been removed from diseased birds. Ultrathin sections were prepared from such cells and examined in the electron microscope. As in previous work (Parsons *et al.*, 1958), there was little evidence of the presence of virus particles in such cells. When, however, the myeloblasts, recovered from the circulating blood of the diseased birds, were placed in tissue culture under proper experimental conditions, i.e. in a medium consisting of 50 per cent chicken serum, supplemented by

---

FIG. 16. CHICKEN MYELOBLASTOSIS VIRUS PARTICLES IN PLASMA PELLET.

Ultrathin section of a high speed centrifugal pellet of plasma from a chicken with myeloblastosis. Innumerable spherical particles of uniform size and morphology, about 80 mμ in diameter, with distinct, centrally located, electron-dense nucleoids. Magnification 35,000 ×. Electron micrograph prepared by L. Dmochowski, P. L. Langford, and J. Furth, Department of Virology, University of Texas, M. D. Anderson Hospital and Tumor Institute, Houston.

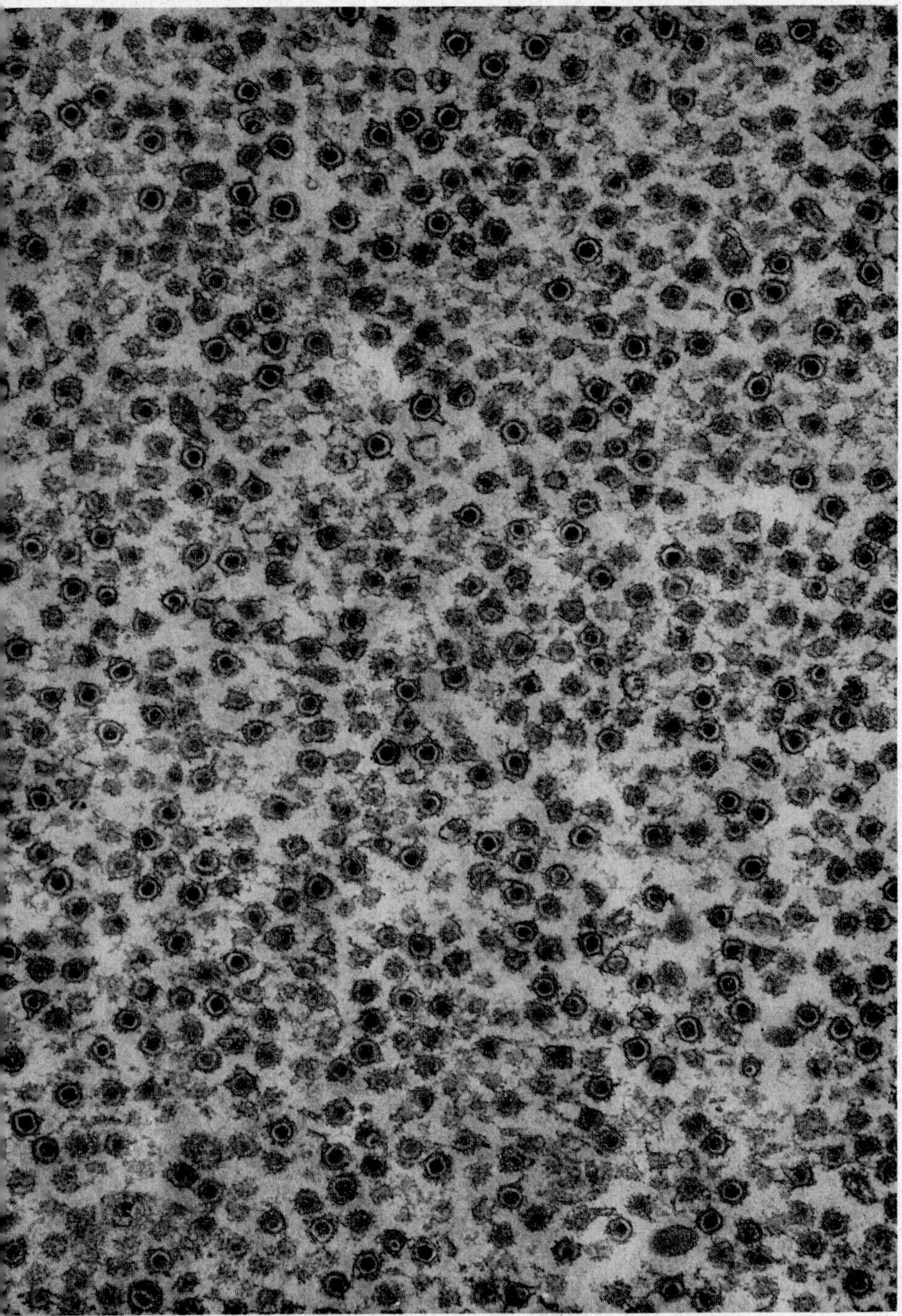

FIG 16. CHICKEN MYELOBLASTOSIS VIRUS PARTICLES IN PLASMA PELLET

vitamins B and folic acid in high concentration (Beaudreau *et al.*, 1960), within a few days only, large numbers of virus particles, either scattered or grouped in vacuoles, appeared in the cytoplasm of the tissue-culture-grown myeloblasts.

That same year (1958), L. Dmochowski of the M.D. Anderson Hospital in Houston, Texas, in collaboration with B. R. Burmester from the U.S. Dept. of Agriculture's Regional Poultry Research Laboratory of East Lansing, Mich., and their coworkers, carried out a cooperative study dealing with electron microscopy of ultrathin sections of avian erythroblastosis and myeloblastosis. In tumorous spleens and livers from chickens with either form of leukemia, particles were found, essentially similar to those reported previously, but slightly smaller in size. The particles were spherical, varying in diameter from 57 to 77 mμ, with an average of about 67 mμ. They had an inner dense core having a diameter averaging 26 mμ. Inclusion-like bodies filled with very large numbers of particles were found in the cytoplasm of the cells. Some of the particles were found outside of cells, in intercellular spaces. The size of the particles was slightly larger (average 73 mμ) in a subsequent study of erythroblastosis carried out by Dmochowski and his associates (1959).

There was essentially no difference, either in morphology or in size, between the particles observed on ultrathin sections of organs from chickens with myeloblastosis, as compared with those from chickens with erythroblastosis. The slight differences between the size of particles observed by Bernhard and his coworkers, and those reported by Dmochowski and his colleagues, may be due to differences in the technique of preparing sections and possibly also in the calibration of the electron microscopes.

Iwakata and Amano, at the Institute for Virus Research, Kyoto University in Japan (1958), also carried out electron microscopic studies of ultrathin sections of bone marrow from chickens infected with erythroblastosis (the virus was originally obtained from Dr. J. W. Beard, Duke University). The Japanese investigators observed spherical particles distributed in groups in the cytoplasm and also outside of cells. The particles were oval in shape and varied in diameter from 65 to 102 mμ. They had an electron-dense centrally located nucleoid about 27 to 30 mμ in diameter.

AVIAN LYMPHOMATOSIS

Visceral Lymphomatosis, Neural Lymphomatosis, Ocular Lymphomatosis, and Osteopetrosis

The outstanding characteristic of this group of the chicken leukosis complex is the fact that in most instances the leukemic cells do not penetrate into the peripheral blood circulation, but remain in tissues, infiltrating internal organs in a diffuse manner, or forming tumors.

Are the different forms of avian lymphomatosis caused by different viruses? What is the true nature of neurolymphomatosis, ocular lymphomatosis, or osteopetrosis? What is the etiological relationship of the disease entities, as well as that of the various sarcomas and related tumors, to avian lymphomatosis or to the leukemias? What is the etiological relation of visceral lymphomatosis or osteopetrosis to erythroblastosis or myeloblastosis? Are they all caused by the same virus, or by a family of related oncogenic agents?

We have no answers to these fundamental questions, but shall discuss this problem again at the end of this chapter.

Studies on Avian Lymphomatosis

Incidence and Epidemiology. Visceral and neural lymphomatosis are among the most destructive diseases of the fowl. It is estimated that over 50 million mature chickens, with a total value exceeding 60 million dollars, die each year from lymphomatosis in the United States alone. From 1949 to 1952, a sample test was conducted in which 26 poultrymen from different sections of the country entered their stock for 3 years. The yearly average total mortality of the hens hatched as chicks was approximately 35 per cent. Lymphomatosis was responsible for 14.5 per cent of this loss, two-thirds of which was caused by the visceral form of the disease.

The causative agent, which has many properties of a common virus, spreads by direct contact, by aerogenous route, and is also found in many apparently healthy carriers; it is present in washings from oral and nasal passages of chicks with visceral lymphomatosis, and also in feces from certain chickens. Furthermore, the virus of visceral lymphomatosis is transmitted from parents to offspring through hatching eggs. All these features suggest that avian lymphomatosis, and presumably also neural lymphomatosis, are communicable diseases spread by a naturally transmissible virus.

Actually some forty years ago, visceral lymphomatosis occurred only sporadically in the United States. More recently, however, this disease has become widely spread and destructive to the poultry stocks. About 1920, the poultry industry of the United States began to use mass production methods: enormous incubators and rearing stations containing large numbers of chickens of relatively pure breed, mass brooding, and widespread interstate shipments of day-old chicks. The mass production methods applied in chicken hatcheries, and the breeding of many thousands of birds of susceptible strains, facilitated to a considerable extent the spread of this disease, and supplied favorable conditions for the propagation of the virus. Gradually, visceral lymphomatosis assumed epidemic proportions.

At about that time, neural lymphomatosis also became a serious problem and appeared to spread across the country from east to west like an infectious disease. At the same time ocular lymphomatosis began to appear more frequently. Similar observations on the spread of the disease were noted in England, Australia, and Japan, beginning about 1930, when those countries modernized their poultry industries.

Because of the staggering loss to the poultry industry, the U.S. Department of Agriculture established in 1937 a Regional Poultry Laboratory in East Lansing, Michigan, to conduct research, with the main purpose of determining the cause of avian lymphomatosis and developing measures for its prevention and control.

The Different Manifestations of Avian Lymphomatosis and Related Forms of the Avian Leukosis Complex

As we have already stressed before, our current information is insufficient to warrant a clear and documented classification of the various forms of the chicken leukosis complex on the basis of their etiology. With these reservations in mind, we are going to review on the following pages the forms of the avian leukosis complex in which the principal pathologic manifestation consists of the formation of lymphoid tumors.

There are three principal pathologic forms of avian lymphomatosis, namely: visceral, neural, and ocular; these designations indicate the primary location of the lesions whose common characteristic is the infiltration and proliferation of cells of the lymphoid series. In spite of this similarity, there are differences in the character of the lesions, and in epizootiology, which have led some investigators to separate visceral lymphomatosis from neural and ocular lymphomatosis. In addition, we will also discuss in this group osteopetrosis, a curious disease manifested principally by the enlargement of leg bones.

A separate group, also included in this discussion, consists of soft tissue tumors, the various fibrosarcomas, myxosarcomas, and also renal carcinomas or nephroblastomas.

Visceral Lymphomatosis (*"Lymphoid Leukosis"* or *"Big Liver Disease"*)

This is the most common and destructive form of the chicken leukosis complex. It occurs frequently, particularly in commercial flocks.

There exist several forms of chicken lymphomatosis. The principal form, called "visceral lymphomatosis," is that in which multiple tumors form in internal organs, particularly in spleen and liver. The liver, spleen, ovaries, and other organs become infiltrated with leukemic cells and increase considerably in size; the chickens invariably die.

Lymphomatosis may be either acute or chronic. Pullets will become droopy and succumb eventually. Laying hens may cease laying eggs abruptly and die within one month. Other birds may be droopy in appearance for a relatively long time, gradually lose weight, become emaciated, and die after a long illness. The principal manifestation is that of a very large liver; accordingly, the term "big liver disease" has been used by the poultrymen to describe this form of lymphomatosis.

A more detailed description of experimental studies on visceral lymphomatosis will follow on subsequent pages.

Neural Lymphomatosis
(*"Range Paralysis" or "Marek's Disease"*)

This very common form of avian lymphomatosis, first described by Marek in 1907, affects the nerves and often results in paralysis. More recently neurolymphomatosis was also described by Pappenheimer and his colleagues (1926, 1929). As a main manifestation of this disease the nerve trunks become thick and swollen as a result of infiltration with lymphoid cells. In advanced stages, the nerve trunks leading from the spinal column to one or both legs, or one or both wings, or to the neck, may show irregular enlargements. Clinical manifestations are a drooping of one or both wings, and weakness and lack of coordination of the legs. This usually leads to inability to stand or walk; the chicken may lie on its side with one leg extended forward and the other backward. Eventually, most of the paralyzed chickens die.

Neural paralysis is generally considered to be a form of the chicken leukosis complex, and hence its designation "neural lymphomatosis" or "neurolymphomatosis." The true nature of this disease, however, has not yet been clarified; its etiological relationship to other forms of the chicken leukosis complex has not been established. The apparent relationship of neural and visceral lymphomatosis is often evident on pathologic examination, which reveals presence of lymphoid tumors not only infiltrating brain and peripheral nerves, but in some instances also visceral organs, particularly the ovaries.

Neural lymphomatosis (range paralysis, or "Marek's disease," as it is also called) is endemic in certain poultry areas, and may from time to time assume epidemic proportions, affecting mostly younger birds, and causing considerable loss to the poultry industry. The causative virus is probably transmitted among very young chicks directly by contact, and by contaminated environment, possibly also through the eggs.

When grown in tissue culture in chick embryo fibroblasts, the virus of neurolymphomatosis does not induce resistance to Rous sarcoma virus ("RIF-negative"). In this respect it is different from the virus of lymphoid leukosis or visceral lymphomatosis.

Transmission Experiments. It has been observed previously that when the virus of lymphoid leukosis was propagated by serial cell-free passages in chickens, most of the inoculated animals developed visceral lymphomatosis and osteopetrosis; among the inoculated birds, some developed neural lymphomatosis (Burmester and Cottral, 1947); the same filtrates induced also erythroblastosis (Burmester *et al.*, 1959). Neural lymphomatosis could be considered, therefore, to be a form of the chicken leukosis spectrum, and transmitted by inoculation of tumor extracts as a part of the chicken leukosis complex. However, on the basis of an assumption that neurolymphomatosis may be caused by an agent distinct from visceral lymphomatosis, or from other forms of the avian leukosis complex, attempts have been made recently to isolate an infective agent which would induce predominantly neural lesions.

Biggs and Payne (1963, 1964) isolated an infective agent from ovarian lymphoid tumors of a typical field case of neurolymphomatosis; this virus strain, designated B14, has been serially passed 15 times and consistently produced typical neurolymphomatosis following intraperitoneal inoculation into 1- or 2-day-old chickens. Paresis or spastic paralysis of the legs, wings, and sometimes neck and eyelids developed as a result of inoculation. Many different nerves were affected: the vagus, coeliac plexus, brachial and sciatic plexuses were most commonly involved; in addition, lymphoid tumors, primarily involving the ovaries, developed in some of the inoculated chickens.

Ocular Lymphomatosis ("Gray Eye Disease")

In this disease, which is also considered to be a form of the chicken leukosis complex, lymphoid cells infiltrate the iris, resulting in an impairment of the vision, leading eventually to complete blindness in one or both eyes. The size and shape of the pupil of the eye change, and the iris becomes gray. Ocular lymphomatosis appears to be in some manner related to lymphomatosis; the etiology of ocular lymphomatosis is obscure, however, and its neoplastic nature is still questionable.

Osteopetrosis ("Big Bone Disease")

This condition often occurs in birds with visceral lymphomatosis, but may also develop separately. The main manifestation is an enlargement of the leg bones; other bones of the body, however, may also become involved. The principal lesion is excessive formation of hard bone caused by a hypertrophic activity of the periosteum and endosteum. Again, the true nature of this disease and its etiological relationship to avian lymphomatosis remain to be determined.

Osteopetrosis is a curious form of the avian leukosis complex. The principal manifestations concern bone lesions characterized by abnormal, symmetrical, or irregular enlargement of long bones. The initial observation was made by Jungherr and Landauer (1938) who found that the disease could be transmitted with whole blood, bone marrow, or with cellular suspensions prepared from lymphomatous tumors often observed in such birds. Brandley and his colleagues (1942) observed osteopetrosis following inoculation of chicks with whole blood from donors with no evidence of bone disease, but suffering from neural lymphomatosis. Burmester and his colleagues (1946, 1947) noted the appearance of osteopetrosis and lymphomatosis following inoculation of filtrates prepared from donors with osteopetrosis alone, or following injection of the virus of visceral lymphomatosis.

Holmes (1958, 1959, 1964) carried out extensive studies on experimental osteopetrosis. It was difficult to induce only osteopetrosis in the inoculated birds. Most of the inoculated birds developed both osteopetrosis and visceral tumors, although some developed only osteopetrosis. Among the 400 birds in which osteopetrosis was induced, 63 birds had soft tissue tumors. Among 491 control birds, only 9 had soft tissue tumors. Accordingly, the incidence of chickens having soft tissue tumors and osteopetrosis was 15.8 per cent, as compared with only 1.8 per cent incidence of tumors in the controls. Visceral lymphomatosis predominated among the neoplasms observed.

The best results in transmission experiments were obtained following inoculation of whole blood into either one-day-old chicks, or into the amnion of chick embryos. The overall incidence of induced osteopetrosis was 39 per cent. The disease could also be transmitted by filtrates; however, the incidence of induced disease was lower under such conditions.

Whether osteopetrosis is caused by a distinct osteopetrosis virus, or

---

FIG. 17. CHICKEN MYELOBLASTOSIS VIRUS PARTICLES IN PLASMA PELLET.

Ultrathin section of a pellet that resulted from ultracentrifugation of plasma from a chicken with myeloblastosis. Innumerable spherical particles having a diameter of approximately 75 to 80 mμ and a distinct external membrane; this membrane is often double when observed in pictures of high resolution. The particles also have a centrally located electron-dense nucleoid approximately 35 to 40 mμ in diameter. Magnification 130,000 ×. Electron micrograph from a study by W. Bernhard, R. A. Bonar, D. Beard and J. W. Beard. (From: *Proc. Soc. Exp. Biol. & Med.*, **97**: 48, 1958.)

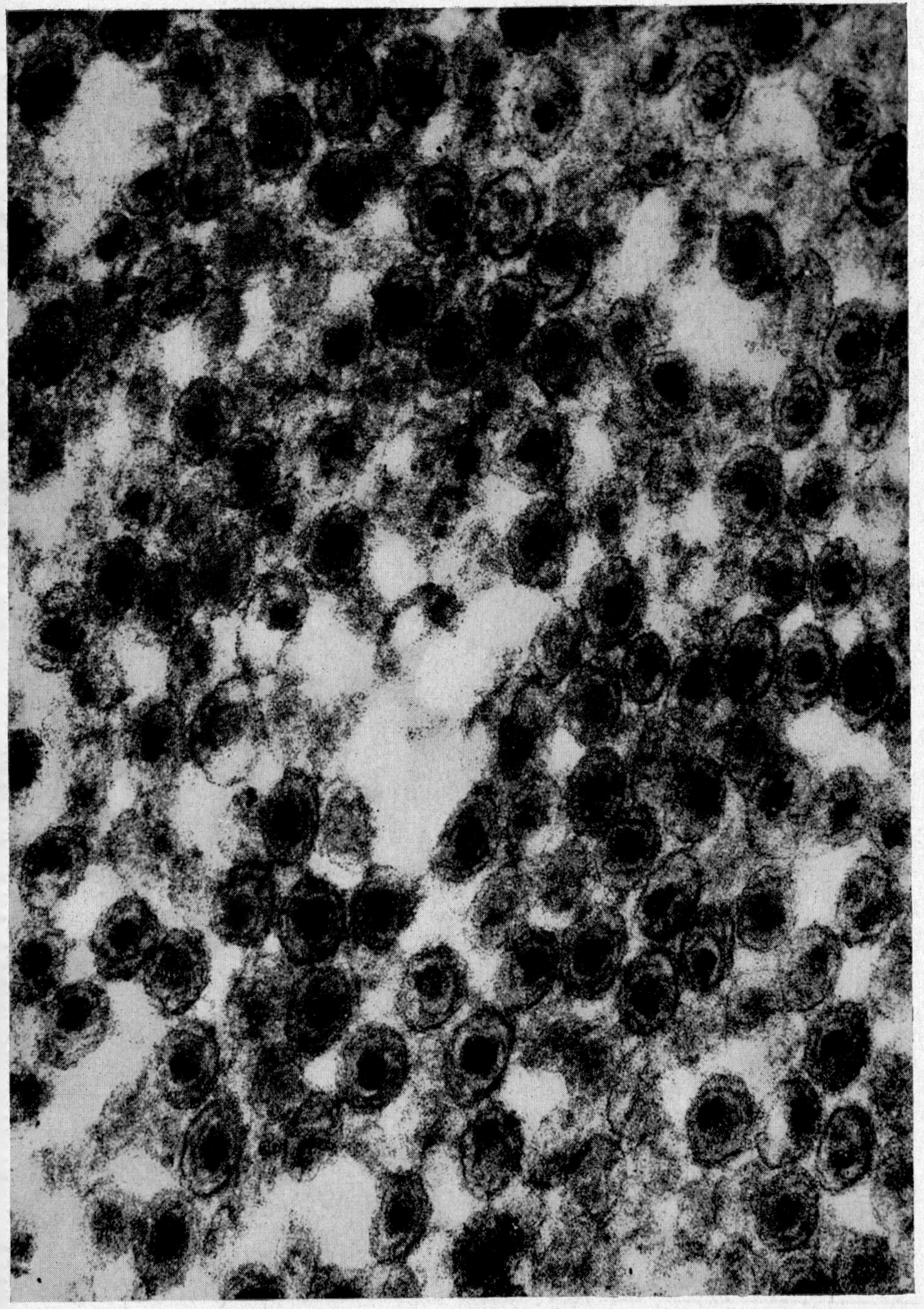

Fig. 17. Chicken Myeloblastosis Virus Particles in Plasma Pellet.

whether it is caused by a virus which may cause other forms of avian leukosis, has not yet been determined.

Under natural life conditions, the disease is probably spread by mouth in the first few days of life, possibly also through the egg.

Transmission of Osteopetrosis to Turkeys. In the field, osteopetrosis appears to be confined to the domestic fowl, but it has been experimentally reproduced in the turkey (Holmes, 1963) by use of fresh blood taken initially from an active case in a fowl, and subsequently passed through an infected turkey. Of 42 turkey poults inoculated when one day old, 19 subsequently developed bone lesions resembling those seen in the fowl. In general, they took about twice as long to develop as in chickens, which may account in part for the disease not having been reported in the field.

Fibrosarcomas, Myxosarcomas, and Other Tumors

The often concurrent development of various types of sarcomas, such as fibrosarcomas, myxosarcomas, osteochondrosarcomas, endotheliomas, hemangiomas, and also of renal tumors (nephroblastomas), in chickens with induced or naturally occurring leukemias, has long been observed. In certain instances such tumors could be induced with filtrates prepared from some of the forms of the chicken leukosis complex, without a concurrent development of leukemia. Many of these tumors could be transmitted by inoculation of tumor filtrates, or of plasma of donor animals; such inoculation induced similar tumors, with or without a concurrent development of leukemia, or produced leukemia alone in the inoculated birds.

The Renal tumors (nephroblastomas), similar to Wilms' tumors in man, form a separate interesting group related to the avian leukosis complex.

Experimental Studies on Avian Lymphomatosis

Transmission of Avian Lymphomatosis by Cell Transplantation. Successful transmission of lymphoid tumors in chickens by cell transplantation was reported by several investigators, among others by Furth, Pentimalli, Olson, Burmester and his associates. Extracts containing viable cells, prepared from organs of birds with naturally occurring lymphomatosis, were inoculated into susceptible chickens. Tumors developed usually within days or weeks at the site of inoculation, spreading later and killing the hosts. Some tumors were readily transplanted; others could be transplanted only with difficulty, or could not be transplanted at all.

It is quite apparent that many factors, such as genetic susceptibility of the recipient host, age at time of inoculation, route of inoculation, and malignancy of the transplanted tumor cells may influence the success of transplantation of avian lymphoid tumors. In this respect, conditions determining the success of transplantation of chicken lymphomatosis do not differ fundamentally from those encountered in the transplantation of other tumors.

Several strains of transplantable avian lymphoid tumors derived from spontaneously occurring visceral lymphomatosis have been established. At the Regional Poultry Research Laboratory in East Lansing, such tumor strains were designated by the symbol RPL (abbreviation of Regional Poultry Laboratory) with added numbers, such as RPL 14 or RPL 15, each number indicating a different passage strain. Many of these tumors grew rapidly, producing growth within 7 to 10 days after intramuscular implantation. Some of the transplanted tumors persisted only temporarily, then regressed completely. Most of the tumors, however, grew progressively and eventually caused secondary, metastatic tumors in internal organs, frequently involving the liver.

Experimental Transmission of Visceral Lymphomatosis by Filtrates

It has been known since the original observations of Ellermann and Bang (1908) that erythro-myeloblastic chicken leukemia could be transmitted by filtrates. Evidence, however, that avian lymphomatosis could also be transmitted by filtrates has been obtained only more recently. Furth reported, in 1933, the transmission by filtrates of a rather unusual form of lymphomatosis characterized by the appearance in peripheral blood and in internal organs of large lymphocytes, with occasional formation of lymphoid tumor-like nodules in the liver; furthermore, endotheliomas and myelomas were reported to have appeared occasionally in the inoculated birds.

It was not until 1946 that a thorough and systematic study dealing with cell-free transmission of naturally occurring lymphomatosis was carried out by Burmester, Prickett and Belding. A transplantable strain of chicken lymphomatosis, designated by the symbol RPL 12, was used for these fundamental experiments. This strain originated as a field case of visceral lymphomatosis in Massachusetts, in 1941. Initially transplanted by Olson, it was carried later by successive cell-passages at the Regional Poultry Research Laboratory in East Lansing, Michigan. After some 200 additional cell transfers, tumors, and in some instances blood, from tumor-bearing donors were used for the preparation of cell-free filtrates.

Three experiments were performed. In the first experiment, an extract was prepared from lymphoid tumors removed from the pectoral muscle and liver; the extract was centrifuged at 3000 r.p.m. for 20 minutes; the supernate was removed, and again centrifuged at 3000 r.p.m. for 20 minutes; the second supernate was then used for inoculation. In the second experiment, the tumor extract was centrifuged for 20 minutes at 19,000 r.p.m., and the supernate was used for inoculation. Finally, in the third experiment, blood from birds bearing 7-day-old tumors of the pectoral muscle was obtained by cardiac puncture. After centrifugation, the plasma was passed through Seitz filter pads and used for inoculation.

The centrifuged extracts and the filtrate were inoculated into 2 to 3-day-old chicks of a pedigreed White Leghorn line, known to be susceptible to lymphomatosis, yet free from spontaneous disease when maintained under quarantine conditions.

The chicks inoculated with the cell-free preparations did not show any evidence of tumor formation until they were at least 10 weeks old. Clinical symptoms resembling osteopetrosis then began to make appearance; later visceral tumors also began to appear. Out of a total of 80 inoculated birds, 84 per cent developed tumors of the bone, viscera, or nerves, within 6 months. Of the 67 birds that were positive, 20 had osteopetrosis, 29 had visceral tumors, and 16 had a combination of osteopetrosis and visceral tumors; the remaining two had neurolymphomatosis. Of the 29 birds with visceral lymphomatosis, one had also neurolymphomatosis. Out of 29 non-inoculated controls, two chickens developed neural, and one visceral lymphomatosis. There was essentially no difference between the centrifuged extracts and the filtrates in their potency to induce tumors.

These experiments demonstrated conclusively that chicken lymphomatosis could be transmitted by filtrates and that the causative agent of this disease is presumably a filterable virus. Whether a single virus was responsible for the induction of the different forms of lymphomatosis, or whether the filtrates contained a mixture of viruses, remained to be determined.

Serial, Cell-free Passage of the Virus of Visceral Lymphomatosis

In the initial experiment performed by Burmester and his coworkers (1946), the lymphomatosis virus was obtained from a transplantable strain (RPL 12). This strain had been propagated through a considerable number of serial passages by transplants of tumor cells; thus the agent was propagated in the tumor cells and passed along in each graft. Relatively large amounts of the virus must soon have appeared in the blood stream of tumor-bearing birds, since filtered plasma from a bird only one week after intramuscular implantation was as potent in inducing lymphomatosis on inoculation tests as were centrifuged cell-free extracts prepared from the primary tumors.

In subsequent experiments carried out by Burmester and Cottral (1947), the filterable agent or agents inducing osteopetrosis and visceral lymphomatosis were propagated through 6 cell-free serial passages in 1 to 3-day-old chicks. The potency of the extracts was increased after passage. Of 189 inoculated chicks, 81 per cent developed tumors within 6 months. Among the positive cases, 88 per cent had visceral tumors, 55 per cent had osteopetrosis, and 6 per cent had neural lymphomatosis. Filtered plasma obtained from tumor-bearing birds induced about as high an incidence of tumors as did the filtrates prepared from lymphomatous livers.

Filtrates prepared from donors showing only osteopetrosis induced about the same incidence of visceral tumors and osteopetrosis as did filtrates prepared from donors with only visceral tumors.

No tumors developed in any of the 31 non-inoculated controls.

Active and Inactive Filtrates

Some of the tumors yielded very active extracts, whereas filtrates prepared from other tumors were only slightly active, or, in some experiments, inactive on inoculation tests. Some tumors were highly active at first, but inactive in subsequent transfers. This variation in potency of tumors could be explained by assuming that the infective virus particles may be present in tumors in different quantities, that they may be in some tumors neutralized by antibodies or inhibitors, or that the particles may be present in some tumors in a latent, non-infective form. A similar phenomenon has been observed in experiments dealing with many other tumors, such as Rous sarcoma or mouse leukemia.

Some Properties of the Virus

The agent of avian visceral lymphomatosis could be stored for at least one year, and possibly longer, without loss of infectivity, at −70°C, in carbon dioxide dry ice.

The virus was found to be relatively sensitive to heating; it could be completely inactivated by heating in a waterbath for 30 minutes at 55°C.

Dosage and Route of Inoculation. A series of experiments was performed by Burmester and Gentry (1956), dealing with the dosage of filtrates prepared from strain RPL 12. The filtrates, in serial dilutions, were inoculated into 1-day-old chicks of the susceptible Single Comb White Leghorn line 15. In experiments involving 1458 chickens, filtered plasma and lymphomatous liver filtrates from strain RPL 12 were inoculated. The incidence of induced lymphomatosis ranged from 55 to 90 per cent. Dilutions up to 1 : 10,000,000 still induced a significant incidence of lymphoid tumors. Osteopetrosis occurred to a variable extent in all groups of inoculated chickens. Females were slightly more susceptible to visceral lymphomatosis, whereas males were slightly more susceptible to osteopetrosis. Some cases of erythroblastosis developed among the chicks as early as 22 days after inoculation of high doses of the RPL 12 virus. Most of the tumors developed, however, in from 2 to 4 months, visceral lymphomatosis developing seldom earlier than 100 days after inoculation.

The virus of avian lymphomatosis could be inoculated with about equal effect by either intramedullary, intracranial, intraperitoneal or intravenous routes. Somewhat less effective were the intramuscular and subcutaneous routes. Still less effective, though infectious, were the nasal, ocular, tracheal, and oral routes.

Difference in Susceptibility of Different Strains of Chickens. The various strains of chickens were found to differ widely in their susceptibility to the virus of lymphomatosis. At the Regional Poultry Research Laboratory in East Lansing, Michigan, several lines of White Leghorn chickens were inbred and tested for their resistance or susceptibility to the virus of lymphomatosis. The isolated subline (15-I) of the Single Comb White Leghorn line 15 was found to be most suitable for these tests. For over 12 years the birds making up this subline have been maintained in strict isolation to reduce the extent of natural infection with lymphomatosis. The incidence of spontaneous disease was less than 3 per cent when the birds were maintained for periods of about one year of age. Chickens of this particular subline were used for routine experiments dealing with the inoculation of the virus of lymphomatosis.

The same line 15 was also found to be suitable for experiments dealing with the inoculation of the virus of erythroblastosis and myeloblastosis.

Influence of Age on Susceptibility to Inoculation with the Virus. There was a marked influence of age of the chickens on susceptibility to the inoculation with the virus. Newly hatched, 1- to 2-day-old chicks were found most susceptible. There was a gradual decrease of susceptibility with increasing age: 3-week-old birds were substantially less susceptible than 1-day-old chicks. The susceptibility further decreased in older birds. In some of the representative experiments, the incidence of lymphomatosis induced by inoculation of 1- to 2-day-old chicks was as high as 95 per cent; on the other hand, this incidence was reduced to only 50 per cent when the same virus was inoculated into 30-day-old chicks; the incidence dropped further to only 31 per cent when 114-day-old chickens were inoculated.

Because of the marked influence of age on susceptibility to the virus, 1- or 2-day-old chicks were used routinely for the inoculation tests.

Natural Transmission of the Virus of Visceral Lymphomatosis. The Role of the Infected Egg

It has long been suspected that the virus of avian visceral lymphomatosis is transmitted from parents to offspring through the embryonated eggs (Cottral, 1950, 1952). Experimental evidence, however, has been furnished only more recently by Cottral, Burmester, Waters, and Gentry, at the Regional Poultry Research Laboratory in East Lansing, Michigan. In a series of experiments reported in 1954 by Cottral and his coworkers, either cell suspensions or filtrates were prepared from livers of chicken embryos from eggs laid by normal appearing hens. All the dams used to supply eggs in these experiments were clinically healthy at the time they were used, and very few of them developed lymphomatosis later on. The extracts were inoculated into 1-day-old chicks of the susceptible Single Comb White Leghorn line 15. Of 1135 chicks inoculated with the extracts, 29.6 per cent developed visceral lymphomatosis. The incidence varied among the different groups; in some of the inoculated groups the incidence of induced lymphomatosis was as high as 88 per cent. Among the 137 non-injected controls, which remained in contact with the inoculated birds ("contact controls"), 11 per cent developed visceral lymphomatosis. Among 141 isolated controls, only 4 per cent developed lymphomatosis. Neural lymphomatosis, although present in the parent flock, was not transmitted to any significant degree.

These results furnished the first direct evidence that the causative agent of visceral lymphomatosis could be transmitted from hens to their progeny through the eggs, and that normal appearing chickens may carry the virus.

In a subsequent report published in 1955 by Burmester and his colleagues, a study was made of the shedding of the virus of lymphomatosis in eggs laid over a 2-year period by 22 normal, apparently healthy, White Leghorn hens from an infected stock, and also in the eggs of their progeny. Seventeen hens were of susceptible inbred lines, and 5 were of a line relatively free from lymphomatosis. The eggs were incubated for 15 days; on the fifteenth day the eggs were washed in a detergent, rinsed in water, then immersed in a 0.1 per cent solution of mercury bichloride for half a minute. The embryos were then removed from the eggs, and the livers excised aseptically. The livers from 4 embryos of each dam were pooled and ground. The extracts so prepared were then injected intraperitoneally into 1-day-old chicks of the susceptible line 15. Each group injected with a pool of livers from 4 embryos consisted of about 50 susceptible chicks.

FIG. 18. CHICKEN ERYTHROBLASTOSIS VIRUS.

Ultrathin section of bone marrow from a young chick infected with the virus of erythroblastosis. Intercellular space showing a large number of spherical virus particles approximately 75 to 80 mμ in diameter. The particles have an external membrane which appears double at high magnification; they also have a centrally located nucleoid about 35 to 40 mμ in diameter. These particles are indistinguishable from those found in chickens infected with the myeloblastosis virus. Magnification 240,000×. Electron micrograph prepared by E. L. Benedetti and W. Bernhard, Institut de Recherches Scientifiques sur le Cancer, Villejuif (Seine), France. (From: *J. Ultrastructure Research*, **1**: 309, 1958.)

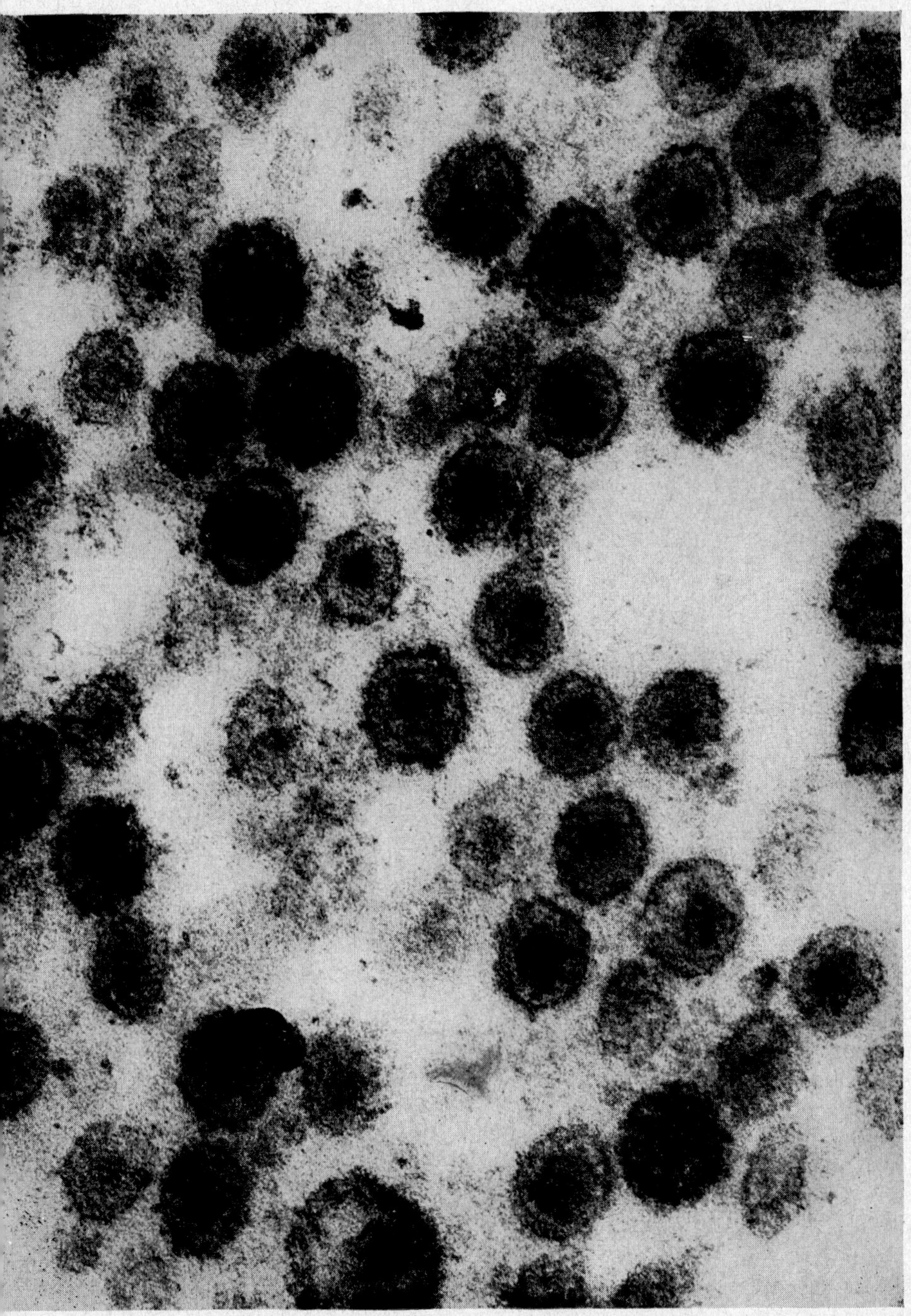

FIG. 18. CHICKEN ERYTHROBLASTOSIS VIRUS.

Sixteen of the 17 hens of susceptible lines contained enough virus to produce a significant incidence of visceral lymphomatosis in the inoculated chicks. On the other hand, only one out of the 5 hens from the resistant line shed the virus into her eggs.

The incidence varied according to the source of the eggs serving for the preparation of extracts; the highest incidence of induced lymphomatosis was 63.5 per cent in chickens observed during an experimental period of 270 days.

The hens carrying the virus shed a significant amount of virus when tested 3 and 6 months later. The level of the transmitted virus was much lower, however, when the same hens were tested when 2 and 3 years old. It was apparent, therefore, that young hens of a susceptible line were more apt to shed the virus of lymphomatosis into their eggs than older birds. The eggs laid by the progeny of the virus-carrying hens were also tested for the presence of virus. Out of 14 virus-carrying hens, 9 were found to shed significant levels of virus in their eggs.

The eggs carrying the virus hatched well, and the chicks appeared perfectly healthy. Thus, the virus of lymphomatosis may be present in eggs, in newly hatched chicks, or in adult hens, and yet the embryos, the chicks, and the mature hens may appear perfectly normal.

Although both the neural and visceral forms of lymphomatosis occurred in the flock that supplied the eggs for infectivity tests, visceral lymphomatosis alone was observed in the inoculated chicks.

The curious fact was observed that although the carrier hens transmitted the virus to their own progeny, very few of them developed lymphomatosis, even though they carried and shed the virus. Only 3 out of 22 hens died of lymphomatosis; one died a week after the eggs for the test were laid, and the other 2 died almost a year later. Similarly, chicks hatched from the infected eggs, i.e. the progeny of heavy shedders of the virus, if left alone, remained in good health.

These observations suggested that the presence or absence of the virus of lymphomatosis in the embryo is not the only important factor determining whether or not chickens hatched from such embryos will develop the disease.

It is conceivable that embryos which carry the virus also carry antibodies; they may also have a certain degree of natural resistance to the virus. Further experiments suggested that a high incidence of lymphomatosis may occur when a susceptible flock of chicks is exposed to the virus at brooding time, without the benefit of protection by either antibodies or natural resistance. Thus, if chicks carrying the virus are reared together with susceptible, relatively virus-free chicks, the latter will suffer heavy losses from visceral lymphomatosis, whereas the actual carriers may remain free from disease. It is quite probable, therefore, that families, or strains of chickens suffering heavy losses from visceral lymphomatosis, acquired the virus from another flock of chickens. The virus-carrying stock, coming from dams having a latent infection (which may be manifested only by a low incidence of this disease) is the likely source of infection. The progeny of the virus-carriers also contain and spread the virus, but will suffer only nominal losses. Thus, despite conclusive evidence that significant amounts of the virus of lymphomatosis may be found in embryonated eggs, laid by many normal appearing hens of an infected population, it is apparent that such an infection does not necessarily result in a significant incidence of disease in the virus-carrying progeny. It is important to realize this aspect of egg-borne infection. Such infection may not cause losses in the progeny of infected hens. The infected eggs and chicks, however, appear to be an important source of the infection for chicks of dams having no significant latent infection. The brooding period was found to be far more important than the hatching period in the transmission of the virus of visceral lymphomatosis.

Transmission of the Virus of Visceral Lymphomatosis by Contact

Many investigators have noticed that chicks of a flock relatively free from lymphomatosis developed a high incidence of this disease when they were reared in the same brooder units with chicks from infected flocks. Actually, such chicks developed a higher incidence of lymphomatosis than that occurring spontaneously in the infected flock. The age of the chicks at the time of exposure appeared to be of great importance, since it was found that the younger the birds at the time of exposure, the greater was the incidence of disease.

In a series of experiments carried out by Burmester and Gentry (1954) at the Regional Poultry Research Laboratory, it was demonstrated that the virus of lymphomatosis was present in the debris of an incubator that had been used to hatch chicks of an infected flock. Furthermore, the virus is apparently eliminated in the saliva of carrier-birds. Studies showed that oral washings from naturally and experimentally infected birds were highly infectious. When chicks were inoculated with the virus of lymphomatosis at one day of age, highly infectious oral washings were obtained as early as 10 days later; the saliva remained infectious for as long as 180 days. Further experiments suggested that chickens exposed to infected birds acquired the virus and soon began to shed the virus in their own saliva.

The oral washings of normal birds of an infected flock and also of the progeny were infectious, as were oral washings from chickens which actually had visceral lymphomatosis. Thus, the virus was shed not only by diseased chickens, but also by normal carriers.

Oral washings were not the only samples containing the virus. The agent was also found in the feces or droppings, and was also disseminated by the dried extra-embryonic fluids and other hatching debris. In addition, the infected chicks shed the virus in their saliva and feces during the brooding period and contaminated the feed, water, and other material and equipment of the brooder unit, providing a source of infection for susceptible penmates.

Further experiments have indicated that chickens may be infected through many of the natural body openings in the following descending order of effectiveness: tracheal, nasal, cloacal, conjunctival, and oral.

Antigenic Properties of the Virus of Visceral Lymphomatosis

Antisera for the neutralization tests were obtained from hens that had received a series of injections of filtrates containing live virus of strain RPL 12 of visceral lymphomatosis. Serum collected from such immunized hens was inactivated at 56°C for 30 minutes and then used for the neutralization tests. Live virus of strain RPL 12 lymphomatosis in serial dilutions was mixed with the immune serum and left at 0°C for 2 to 3 hours. The mixtures were then inoculated intraperitoneally into 1-day-old chicks. The immune serum neutralized the virus, though not completely, and only when mixed with higher dilutions of the virus. Normal chicken serum did not have a neutralizing effect.

In further experiments, mature hens received several successive inoculations of live virus of strain RPL 12 lymphomatosis. Chicks hatched from eggs laid by such hens proved to have a higher resistance to a challenging inoculation with the same virus than chicks hatched from eggs laid by untreated dams.

Attempt to Propagate the Virus of Visceral Lymphomatosis in Embryonated Eggs

Gentry and Burmester (1955) at the Regional Poultry Research Laboratory propagated the virus of visceral lymphomatosis in embryonated chicken eggs. Filtrates containing live virus of lymphomatosis were inoculated into the yolk of embryonated chicken eggs. The presence of the virus in subsequent serial passages was determined by the inoculation of susceptible chicks with the harvested embryonic material. The embryos used for the passage of the virus were obtained from hens which had been hatched and reared in complete isolation and had no evidence of natural infection with the virus. The material was harvested after a period of incubation of 7 days for each egg passage. A total of 5 passages was made in the embryos. The harvested extracts were injected into 1-day-old chicks. Of the chicks inoculated with the material from the 1st, 3rd, and 5th embryo passage, 65, 75, and 80 per cent, respectively, developed visceral lymphomatosis. Uninoculated chicks, and chicks receiving material from untreated embryos, remained free from tumors.

These experiments suggested that the virus of avian lymphomatosis could be propagated serially in embryonated chicken eggs, although no gross microscopic lesions could be detected in such embryos.

Attempts to grow the virus of visceral lymphomatosis in normal chick-embryo-liver cells, in tissue culture, have been reported. Filtrates prepared from leukemic livers from donors with RPL 12 virus-induced lymphomatosis were used by Fontes, Sharpless and their associates (1958) for the inoculation of tissue culture tubes seeded with chick embryo liver cells. A cytopathogenic effect was observed at the third serial passage, but was later found to be unrelated to the lymphomatosis virus (Burmester *et al.*, 1960).

Only fluids from the first few serial passages of the virus induced visceral lymphomatosis or erythroblastosis in some of the inoculated chickens. Of 25 chicks inoculated with fluids from the 3rd passage, 13 died from visceral lymphomatosis, and 2 of erythroblastosis. Attempts to induce visceral lymphomatosis or other forms of the chicken leukosis complex with tissue culture fluid from subsequent serial passages have not been successful. Results thus far obtained were not entirely satisfactory. They did not prove that the agent was actually propagated under such conditions. Sufficient quantity of the virus could have been used for the initial inoculation of the tissue culture cells to induce, in higher dilutions, some of the tumors resulting from inoculation of the subsequent early passage fluids.

Electron Microscopic Studies of Avian Lymphomatosis. In a cooperative study carried out by L. Dmochowski of the M. D. Anderson Hospital in Houston, and B. R. Burmester of the Regional Poultry Research Laboratory in East Lansing, and their associates (1957, 1959), ultrathin sections prepared from spleens of chicken donors with either virus-induced or naturally occurring visceral lymphomatosis were examined in the electron microscope. Spherical particles were observed in the cytoplasm of the cells; the particles were present frequently in agglomerations in cytoplasmic vacuoles, or in inclusion-like bodies. Similar particles could also be found in intercellular spaces. The particles were spherical, about 64 to 82 mμ in diameter, with an average diameter of 72 mμ. The external membrane surrounded a less dense zone. There was a dense internal center, about 30 mμ in diameter.

The particles detected in tumorous spleens from chickens with induced or naturally occurring visceral lymphomatosis resembled in morphology particles described in erythroblastosis and myeloblastosis, and were of about similar size (Dmochowski *et al.*, 1958. Benedetti *et al.*, 1958).

Distribution of Virus Particles in Different Organs and Different Cells. The distribution of virus in organs of chickens and chick embryos congenitally infected with avian leukosis virus was studied by Dougherty and Di Stefano (1967) at the State University of New York in Syracuse. The sites of virus multiplication in cells of various tissues were determined by electron microscopy. The presence of infectious virus, determined by bio-assay, was detected in all organs examined, and the highest titers were found in liver and kidney. The adult female reproductive system also contained large amounts of virus, while lesser amounts were found in spleen, intestine, muscle, brain, and blood.

The presence of virus budding revealed on electron microscopic studies was used as evidence of virus multiplication in specific cells of various tissues and organs. Virus multiplication was found to take place in cells derived from all 3 embryonic germ layers, and virus budding was seen in cells of every type of tissues examined except nervous tissue.

Cells in which the avian leukosis virus multiplied included all 3 types of muscle, chondroblasts, fibroblasts, epidermal cells, lining epithelial cells of digestive organs, glandular epithelium of digestive organs and salivary glands, epithelial cells of kidney, reticular epithelium of thymus and bursa of Fabricius, endothelium, mesothelium, and primitive reticular cells of the spleen.

Studies on Virus-induced Renal Carcinomas, i.e. Nephroblastomas

Carr reported (1956) that renal adenocarcinomas, as well as erythroblastic leukemia, were induced in chickens inoculated with the ES-4 tumor strain of Engelbreth-Holm. He later reported (1960) that the MH-2 reticuloendothelioma also caused renal adenocarcinomas. Transmission of virus-induced avian kidney tumors was reported by Thorell (1958, 1959), who referred to these tumors as adenosarcomas. Both leukemia and renal tumors could be induced following inoculation of cell-free extracts prepared from tumors, or following inoculation of plasma from the leukemic birds.

In more recent experiments, Walter, Burmester, and Cunningham (1962) observed that inoculation of White Leghorn chickens of the inbred line 15-I with a well-known strain of avian leukosis, BAI strain A, more generally known as the myeloblastosis strain of Beard, resulted in the development of osteopetrosis and also of tumors of the renal parenchyma. The renal tumors were at first identified as renal adenocarcinomas; further histopathologic studies showed, however, that these tumors were of a complex morphology. The Armed Forces Institute of Pathology in Washington, D.C., confirmed the observations concerning the complex nature of the renal neoplasms, and considered these tumors to be nephroblastomas, histologically comparable to Wilms' tumors of man.

The nephroblastoma was readily transplantable by inoculation of cell suspensions. After nine transplant passages, the tumor apparently lost its ability to cause myeloblastosis. Although the twelth-passage tumor filtrate no longer induced the leukemic lesions, it did cause a high incidence of renal tumors and a moderate incidence of visceral lymphomatosis, and of osteopetrosis.

How Many Oncogenic Viruses?

It would be of great interest to determine whether the different forms of the chicken leukosis complex are caused by a single virus or whether they are induced by distinct, although possibly related, oncogenic agents. Experimental data thus far available are insufficient to provide an answer to this fundamental question.

It is quite possible that several related oncogenic viruses are involved. It would be rather surprising to find that osteopetrosis and the various solid tumors, such as fibromyxosarcomas, osteochondrosarcomas and renal tumors (nephroblastomas), are caused by the same virus, which may also be able to induce visceral lymphomatosis, neural lymphomatosis, myeloblastosis, and erythroblastosis.

Induction of Visceral Lymphomatosis, Erythroblastosis, Osteopetrosis, and a Spectrum of Tumors (Fibrosarcomas, Myxosarcomas, Hemangiomas) with Visceral Lymphomatosis RPL 12 Virus

It has long been observed that experimental transmission of avian leukosis could result in the induction of one or more different forms of this disease complex. Ellermann (1922) concluded in his early studies that myeloblastosis, erythroblastosis, and lymphomatosis were produced by a single virus.

The etiological relationship between the principal forms of the chicken leukosis complex became apparent in experiments carried out by B. R. Burmester and his colleagues (1959). A strain of visceral lymphomatosis, designated by the symbol RPL 12, and carried in East Lansing, consistently induced visceral lymphomatosis, and only occasionally related neoplasms, when inoculated routinely in cell-free passages into susceptible chicks. When, however, after several passages, RPL 12 filtrates were inoculated into 1 to 2-week-old chicks of the White Leghorn strain 15, some of the birds developed typical erythroblastosis, and others developed visceral lymphomatosis. Osteopetrosis, and now and then fibrosarcomas, myxosarcomas, and hemangiomas also were induced. Heavy doses, as a rule, induced erythroblastosis, killing the birds within 100 days after inoculation, the peak of mortality occurring at 40 to 50 days after inoculation. Higher dilutions induced visceral lymphomatosis, but not until some 100 to 120 days after inoculation.

Several other strains of visceral lymphomatosis, including naturally occurring field cases, were also tested, and it was found that all sources of virus that caused visceral lymphomatosis also caused erythroblastosis.

Filtrates of some of the lymphoid tumor strains also caused osteopetrosis, in addition to erythroblastosis and visceral lymphomatosis.

Induction of Erythroblastosis, Visceral Lymphomatosis, Osteopetrosis, or Renal Carcinomas (Nephroblastomas), with Virus of Erythroblastosis. When, in a series of similar experiments, Burmester and his colleagues (1959) inoculated various dilutions of cell-free preparations of a presumably pure strain R (Beard) of erythroblastosis into young chicks, most chickens developed and died from erythroblastosis in 12 to 100 days, usually in less than 33 days. Among those which survived that critical period, a large number of chickens developed visceral lymphomatosis. Thus, in a sample of 26 birds that had been inoculated with the erythroblastosis virus and survived 100 days, 11 developed visceral lymphomatosis. Moreover, a few chickens developed osteopetrosis or renal carcinomas.

Induction of Myeloblastosis, Visceral Lymphomatosis, Osteopetrosis, and Renal Carcinomas (Nephroblastomas) with Virus of Myeloblastosis. In another series of experiments, Burmester and his colleagues (1959) used for inoculation filtrates prepared from a presumably pure strain A of myeloblastosis (granuloblastosis) that had been carried by Dr. J. W. Beard and his group at Duke University. This particular strain was considered to be a relatively pure strain of myeloblastosis. In Dr. Beard's laboratories this virus had been passed routinely by plasma filtrates, inducing consistently typical myeloblastosis, and killing the chicks within 2 to 3 weeks.

In a series of experiments carried out by Burmester and his associates (1959), high dilutions of this particular virus strain were inoculated into 1 to 2-week-old White Leghorn line 15 chicks. Some of the chicks died after only a short period of time from typical myeloblastosis. Among those that survived, however, and were kept for observation for about one year, a considerable number developed visceral lymphomatosis and/or osteopetrosis; some of the birds, quite unexpectedly, developed multiple or single adenocarcinomas of the kidneys. All combinations were observed, except a concurrent development of myeloblastosis and visceral lymphomatosis.

Visceral lymphomatosis, osteopetrosis, and kidney carcinomas developed usually in older birds, some 6 or 7 months after the inoculation of the filtrates. This could explain why most of these different forms of tumors had not been observed in previous experiments dealing with cell-free passage of myeloblastosis; such passage involved as a rule only short range experiments, and usually required rather large doses of the virus. In Burmester's experiments, high dilutions of the myeloblastosis virus strains were injected, and the inoculated birds were observed for long periods of time.

The development of kidney carcinomas in some of the chickens following inoculation of myeloblastosis filtrates was a striking phenomenon. It was similar to the earlier report of Carr, from Edinburgh, who also observed (1956) the development of multiple renal carcinomas following inoculation of filtrates from a strain of avian erythroblastosis into young chicks.

More recently, Fredrickson and his coworkers (1964) studied the oncogenic spectrum of virus strains isolated from lymphomatous chickens of 5 different farm flocks. Four strains of visceral lymphomatosis were isolated from farm flocks, and one from a spontaneous nephroblastoma. These virus strains had been studied in chickens of the inbred line 15-I, and each had been characterized as a strain of avian tumor virus. Serial tenfold dilutions of virus were inoculated into line 15-I chickens 1 to 14 days of age and into 11-day-old embryos. Intravenous, intraabdominal, and intramuscular routes of inoculation were employed.

Neoplasms induced included visceral lymphomatosis, erythroblastosis, osteopetrosis, fibrosarcomas, endotheliomas, and nephroblastomas. In addition, hemorrhages, with or without any concomitant neoplastic condition, were observed in many birds.

The response of the host was influenced by factors connected with administration of the virus. Incidence of hemorrhages and endotheliomas was greatest among chickens inoculated with large amounts of virus given intravenously or intraperitoneally. Increase in dose, decrease in age, and inoculation by the intravenous route tended to increase the incidence of erythroblastosis.

Dose of virus and route of inoculation, but not age at inoculation, had a similar significant effect on the incidence of fibrosarcomas. The route of inoculation appeared to influence the incidence of fibrosarcomas. Visceral lymphomatosis was induced only in chickens given low doses of virus, and among these there was low mortality from other neoplasms. All strains of virus investigated induced a multiple pathologic response. Each virus strain induced its own oncogenic spectrum. There were variations in the incidence of different forms of the chicken leukosis complex induced with the individual virus strains following inoculation into susceptible chickens.

Induction of Visceral Lymphomatosis and Erythroblastosis with the Bryan Strain of Rous Sarcoma Virus

It has been shown recently (Burmester and Walter, 1961) that under certain experimental conditions inoculation of the Bryan strain of Rous sarcoma virus induced in susceptible chickens not only typical Rous sarcomas, but also visceral lymphomatosis and less frequently erythroblastosis. The virus was inoculated intravenously into 9-day-old chicks of the White Leghorn line 15-I. In this experiment doses of the Rous virus

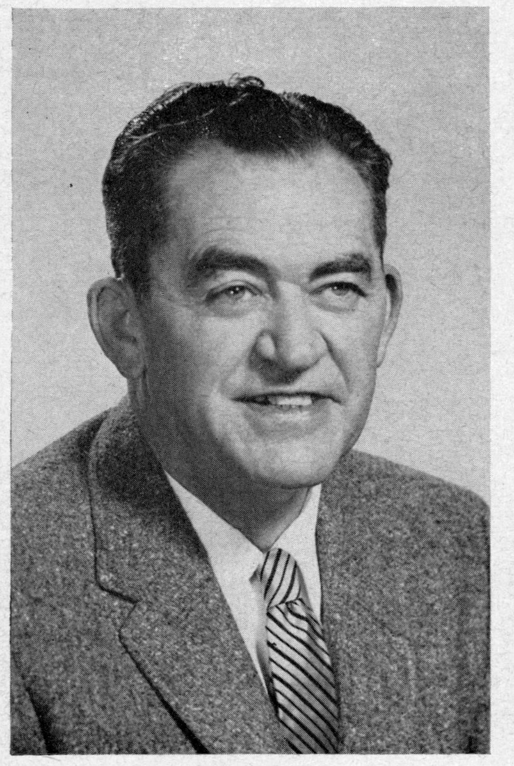

Joseph W. Beard

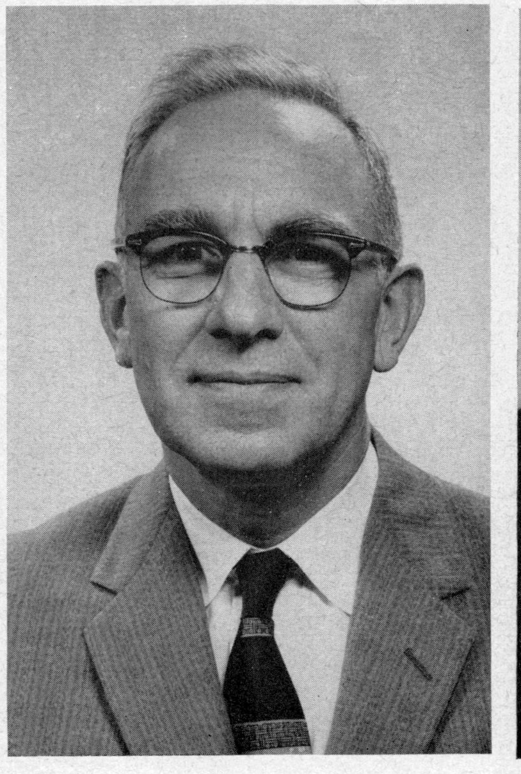

Ben R. Burmester

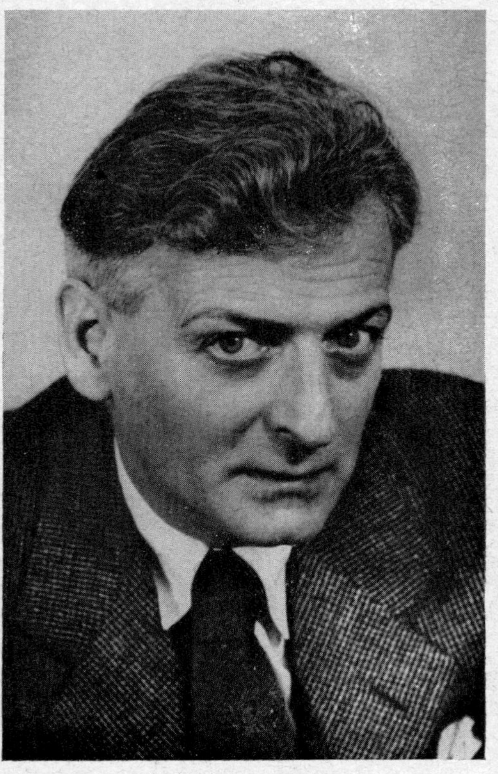

F. Duran-Reynals

FIG. 19

had to be sufficiently low so that an appreciable number of birds survived the period during which sarcomas would have been induced. When a dilution was injected which did not induce Rous sarcoma because of low content of virus inoculated, some of the chickens still developed visceral lymphomatosis. Most of the chickens inoculated with relatively large doses of the virus developed and died from sarcomas; however, among 262 birds inoculated with higher dilutions of the virus, and surviving the time period of mortality resulting from the development of solid tumors, 53 chickens developed visceral lymphomatosis, and 6 developed erythroblastosis. None of the 99 control birds developed any neoplasms during the same 270-day experimental period.

* * *

Interference between the Virus of Avian Leukosis, and the Rous Sarcoma Virus

The Transmissible "Resistance Inducing Factor" (RIF). It was pointed out in the preceding chapter that the presence of avian leukosis virus in chick embryo fibroblasts grown in tissue culture inhibits their susceptibility to infection with the Rous sarcoma virus (Rubin, 1960).

Inoculation of Rous sarcoma virus on chick embryo fibroblasts in tissue culture produces discrete foci of transformed cells with a characteristic rounded appearance. Some of the chick embryo cell pools showed relative resistance to the inoculation of Rous sarcoma virus. This resistance was found to be due to the presence of a congenitally transmitted "resistance inducing factor" (RIF), which was subsequently identified as a virus of the avian leukosis group (Rubin and Vogt, 1962. Hanafusa *et al.*, 1963).

The reports of Rubin and his coworkers prompted the introduction of a new and rather confusing terminology, which seems to have gained acceptance among the students of avian tumor viruses. The term "RIF-positive" has been applied to chickens infected congenitally with the avian leukosis virus. The term "RIF-positive" implies that chickens so designated carry a "resistance inducing factor," i.e. a factor which induces in such birds resistance to inoculation with the Rous sarcoma virus. Since this transmissible factor actually represents the virus of avian lymphomatosis, it would appear more simple, and it would add clarity, if such chickens were designated as natural carriers of a latent leukosis virus.

The Concept of a "Defective Virus" and of a "Helper Virus" or "Rous Associated Virus" (RAV)

Some of the recently developed concepts referring to a "defective virus," and to a "helper virus," are here briefly summarized. They were also discussed in the preceding chapter.

According to this concept, the Bryan high-titer strain of Rous sarcoma contains a "defective virus," unable in higher dilutions to produce infective virus particles. Tumors induced with such a virus do not yield infective virus particles on extraction procedures.

The avian leukosis virus is frequently present in filtrates containing certain strains of Rous sarcoma virus, such as the Bryan strain.

Called also a "Rous associated virus" (RAV), or a "helper virus," the avian leukosis virus was found to be necessary for the maturation of the "defective" Rous sarcoma virus, providing the necessary protein coat and thereby assisting in the formation of infective Rous sarcoma virus particles (Rubin, 1960. Rubin and Vogt, 1962. Vogt and Rubin, 1962. Hanafusa *et al.*, 1963, 1964. Hanafusa, 1964). However, according to a recent study by Vogt (1967), the Bryan high-titer strain of Rous sarcoma virus could be regarded as being defective only in a quantitative sense.

All viruses of the avian leukosis complex thus far tested, including the visceral lymphomatosis virus and avian myeloblastosis virus, serve as "helpers" for the activation of Rous sarcoma virus. Viruses which are structurally similar to Rous sarcoma virus but biologically distinct from it, such as Newcastle disease virus, are ineffective as helpers.

Paradoxically, the helper viruses can also induce resistance to infection by Rous sarcoma virus if they infect the cells before, or at the same time as, Rous sarcoma virus. Once the Rous sarcoma infection is established, the helper virus can no longer prevent multiplication of virus or its action on the cells; the helper viruses then serve in activating the formation of infective Rous sarcoma virus particles (Hanafusa, 1964).

The resistance induced by infection with the avian leukosis viruses is apparently specific for Rous sarcoma virus, since such cells are fully susceptible to infection with unrelated viruses, such as Newcastle disease, western equine encephalomyelitis, and vaccinia viruses (Rubin, 1960. Hanafusa, 1964).

This subject is also discussed in the chapter on Rous sarcoma, and the interested reader is referred for further information to the preceding pages of this monograph and to the references quoted.

The Complement Fixation Test for Avian Leukosis Virus (COFAL)

Inoculation of the Schmidt-Ruppin strain of Rous sarcoma virus into newborn hamsters or guinea pigs results in the development of tumors at the site of inoculation. Such tumors, particularly those induced in hamsters, grow progressively, and may attain large size; they can be transplanted by cell-graft within the same species. This is discussed in more detail in the preceding chapter of this monograph.

Huebner and his coworkers recently observed (1963) that sera of hamsters and guinea pigs carrying large primary or transplanted tumors induced with the Schmidt-Ruppin strain contain specific complement-fixing antibodies. These antibodies were found to react specifically not only with the Schmidt-Ruppin, and also with the Bryan strain of the Rous sarcoma virus, but also with a field strain of the avian leukosis virus. Subsequent studies (Sarma *et al.*, 1964. Huebner *et al.*, 1964) showed that these complement-fixing antibodies are also specific for several avian leukosis virus strains, such as RPL 12, or field isolates of avian leukosis virus, and erythroblastosis or myeloblastosis viruses. This group-specific complement-fixation reaction occurred despite antigenic differences demonstrated in the neutralization tests between the Schmidt-Ruppin strain of Rous sarcoma, and the avian leukosis viruses (Sarma *et al.*, 1963).

In subsequent experiments this group-specific complement-fixation reaction was applied for quantitative assays of avian leukosis viruses grown in tissue cultures of chicken embryo fibroblasts (Sarma *et al.*, 1964); it appeared well suited for the detection of latent avian leukosis viruses which produce little or no visible effect in tissue culture.

This test proved to be useful for the detection and assay of naturally occurring virus of chicken leukosis in viremic sera, chicken embryos, tissues, and secretions of chickens carrying the avian leukosis virus. In preliminary experiments, it also appeared useful for direct demonstration of viral antigens in tissues of naturally infected chickens and chicken embryos.

In the hands of the investigators who developed this method, the complement-fixation test for avian leukosis (COFAL) proved to be as useful and sensitive *in vitro* assay system for avian leukosis viruses, as the "resistance inducing factor" (RIF), i.e. interference between the avian leukosis virus and the Rous sarcoma virus, described by Rubin (1960).

* * *

Relationship of Thymus and Bursa of Fabricius to Virus-induced Visceral Lymphomatosis. Inhibiting Effect of Bursectomy

The thymus plays a crucial role in the development of leukemia, particularly of its lymphatic form, in mice and rats. It has been known for some time that removal of thymus by surgical procedure may inhibit, or at least considerably delay, the development of either spontaneous (McEndy *et al.*, 1944. Furth, 1946), or radiation-induced (Kaplan, 1950. Gross, 1958) leukemia in mice. More recently, following the isolation of the mouse leukemia virus, it was determined that the development of virus-induced leukemia in mice could also be inhibited or considerably delayed by thymectomy performed preferably during the first 3 weeks of life (Gross, 1959. Levinthal *et al.*, 1959. Miller,

1959). The incidence of virus-induced leukemia could also be reduced following thymectomy in rats (Gross, 1963. Kunii and Furth, 1964). Furthermore, the incidence of myeloid leukemia was higher in virus-injected thymectomized mice (Gross, 1960) and rats (Gross, 1963. Kunii and Furth, 1964) than in non-thymectomized controls.

It was of interest, therefore, to determine a possibly similar effect of thymectomy on virus-induced leukosis in chickens. In the fowl, however, this problem is more complex, since there is another lymphoid organ of apparently similar function, namely the bursa of Fabricius. The thymus is located on each side of the neck as a string-like structure along the carotid arteries.

The bursa of Fabricius is a small lymphoid organ adherent to the dorsal surface of the distal cloaca; it can readily be freed from its fascial attachment and cut free from the cloaca by a surgical procedure. The removal of thymus, particularly of its lower lobes, is more difficult, because of its location along the carotid arteries.

In a series of experiments performed by Peterson, Burmester, Fredrickson, Purchase, and Good (1964), it was determined that surgical removal of the bursa of Fabricius in White Leghorn line 15-I chickens during the first month of life prevented the development of visceral lymphomatosis ordinarily induced by virus RPL 12. Such an effect was noted whether the bursectomy was performed at one day or at 29 days of age, or whether the infectious virus was administered at one day or at 28 days of age.

Surgical removal of the thymus performed at hatching, or when the bird was 29 days old, had no effect on the incidence of visceral lymphomatosis. The incidence of erythroblastosis, which also developed in some of the inoculated chickens, was unaffected by any of the surgical procedures.

In a continuation of these studies, Peterson and his colleagues (1966) defined more precisely the relationship of the bursa of Fabricius, and also of thymus, to virus-induced visceral lymphomatosis. Removal of the bursa of Fabricius performed at any time during the first 3 months of life prevented almost completely the development of visceral lymphomatosis. Bursectomy performed even as late as at 5 months of age significantly reduced the incidence of this disease. In some animals, both the bursa of Fabricius and the thymus were removed; however, the effect of such a dual operation was not superior to the result of the removal of the bursa alone.

Complete surgical removal of the bursa of Fabricius was not entirely innocuous for the birds. There was a considerably higher non-neoplastic mortality rate in the bursectomized chickens, as compared with the non-bursectomized controls. The cause of this non-neoplastic mortality was not fully determined.

It was of considerable interest that the incidence of osteopetrosis, the curious form of chicken leukosis complex manifested by periosteal proliferation and formation of new bone, was higher in bursectomized birds than in the controls. However, bursectomy increased the frequency of osteopetrosis only if bursectomy was performed in newly hatched chicks. Both groups of chickens, the bursectomized group and the control group, were inoculated with the visceral lymphomatosis virus filtrate intra-abdominally at one day of age.

The observation that osteopetrosis occurred more frequently in bursectomized chickens than in the control animals was rather unexpected. This observation was perhaps comparable to the higher incidence of myeloid leukemia developing in thymectomized mice following inoculation of the passage A virus (Gross, 1960). The mouse leukemia virus usually induces lymphatic leukemia; in thymectomized mice the total incidence of induced leukemia is reduced; among the thymectomized mice which eventually develop leukemia, there is a higher incidence of the myelogenous form. If one virus is capable of inducing either lymphatic or myelogenous leukemia, one could speculate that lack of susceptible target cells necessary for development of lymphatic leukemia may lead to the induction by the same virus of another form of this disease. Could a similar concept be employed to explain the higher incidence of osteopetrosis in bursectomized chickens? However, other explanations of this interesting observation are also possible.

In any event, it was of considerable interest that surgical removal of the bursa of Fabricius in young chickens prevented the development of visceral lymphomatosis in such animals suggesting that at least this form of the avian leukosis complex is a malignancy depending on the presence of lymphoid tissue derived from the bursa of Fabricius, which presumably serves as a target organ for the virus.

* * *

Epidemiology of Chicken Leukosis Under Natural Life Conditions

Under natural conditions the virus of visceral lymphomatosis is transmitted from parents to offspring via the egg, and from bird to bird within hatching and rearing units. Chickens heavily infected as embryos, or shortly after hatching, develop a low grade infection which persists for long periods without the development of detectable antibodies. Such chickens produce infected eggs, and shed virus in their body excretions and secretions. Most chickens exposed when several weeks old, experience a transient infection followed by the development of antibodies. Most infections of either type do not result in the development of lymphomatosis or other tumors.

Very little is known concerning the natural transmission of some of the other forms of avian leukosis. Neural paralysis, also called Marek's disease, is endemic in many commercial flocks, and may often assume epidemic proportions, resulting in very high mortality among the infected birds, particularly those in the younger age group. Although no precise experimental data are available concerning natural transmission of the causative agent of this disease, it is quite apparent from field observations that it may spread by contact, possibly by air, among chicks housed in close quarters, and also through contaminated environment. The possibility of transmission through carriers must also be considered.

Transmission of myeloblastosis and erythroblastosis under natural life conditions has not been determined experimentally; the virus is possibly transmitted through the eggs from one generation to another, and also directly by contact. The same is presumably true also for the natural transmission of fibrosarcomas, nephroblastomas, and osteopetrosis.

REFERENCES

BALUDA, M. A., Properties of cells infected with avian myeloblastosis virus. Basic mechanisms in animal virus biology. *Cold Spring Harbor Symposia on Quantitative Biology*, **27**: 415–425, 1962.

BALUDA, M. A., and GOETZ, I. E., Morphological conversion of cell cultures by avian myeloblastosis virus. *Virology*, **15**: 185–199, 1961.

BALUDA, M. A., GOETZ, I. E., and OHNE, S., Induction of differentiation in certain target cells by avian myeloblastosis virus: An *in vitro* study. pp. 387–400 in: Viruses, Nucleic Acids, and Cancer. *17th Ann. Symp. on Fundamental Cancer Research, Univ. of Texas*, M. D. Anderson Hospital and Tumor Institute, Williams & Wilkins, Baltimore, Md., 1963.

BALUDA, M. A., MOSCOVICI, C., and GOETZ, I. E., Specificity of the *in vitro* inductive effect of avian myeloblastosis virus. pp. 449–458 in: *Internat. Conference on Avian Tumor Viruses, Nat. Cancer Inst. Monograph No. 17*, U.S. Publ. Health Service, Bethesda, Md., 1964.

BEARD, D., and BEARD, J. W., Virus of avian erythroblastosis. VI. Further studies on neutralization by antiserum to normal chicken protein. *J. Nat. Cancer Inst.*, **19**: 923–939, 1957.

BEARD, D., BEAUDREAU, G. S., BONAR, R. A., SHARP, D., and BEARD, J. W., Virus of avian erythroblastosis. III. Antigenic constitution and relation to the agent of avian myeloblastosis. *J. Nat. Cancer Inst.*, **18**: 231–259, 1957.

BEARD, J. W., The fallacy of the concept of virus "masking": A review. *Cancer Research*, **16**: 279–291, 1956.

BEARD, J. W., Virus of avian myeloblastic leukosis. *Poultry Sci.*, **35**: 203–223, 1956.

BEARD, J. W., Nature of the viruses of avian myeloblastosis and erythroblastosis. pp. 336–344 in: *Proc. Third Nat. Cancer Conference (1956)*, J. B. Lippincott, Philadelphia, 1957.

BEARD, J. W., Etiology of avian leukosis. *Ann. N.Y. Acad. Sci.*, **68**: 473–486, 1957.

BEARD, J. W., Isolation and identification of tumor viruses. *Texas Rep. Biol. & Med.*, **15**: 627–658, 1957.

BEARD, J. W., Etiologic aspects of the avian leukemias. *Progress in Hematol.*, **3**: 105–135, 1962.

Beard, J. W., Viral tumors of chickens with particular reference to the leukosis complex. *Ann. N.Y. Acad. Sci.*, **108**: 1057–1085, 1963.

Beard, J. W., Bonar, R. A., Heine, U., de Thé, G., and Beard, D., Studies on the biological, biochemical, and biophysical properties of avian tumor viruses. pp. 345–373 in: Viruses, Nucleic Acids, and Cancer. *17th Ann. Symp. on Fundamental Cancer Research, Univ. of Texas,* M. D. Anderson Hospital and Tumor Institute, Williams & Wilkins, Baltimore, Md., 1963.

Beard, J. W., Sharp, D. G., Eckert, E. A., Beard, D., and Mommaerts, E. B., Properties of the virus of the fowl erythromyeloblastic disease. *Proc. Second Nat. Cancer Conference,* **2**: 1396–1411, 1952.

Beaudreau, G. S., and Becker, C., Virus of avian myeloblastosis. X. Photometric microdetermination of adenosinetriphosphatase activity. *J. Nat. Cancer Inst.*, **20**: 339–349, 1958.

Beaudreau, G. S., Becker, C., Sharp, D. G., Painter, J. C., and Beard, J. W., Virus of avian myeloblastosis. XI. Release of the virus by myeloblasts in tissue culture. *J. Nat. Cancer Inst.*, **20**: 351–382, 1958.

Beaudreau, G. S., Becker, C., Bonar, R. A., Wallbank, A. M., Beard, D., and Beard, J. W., Virus of avian myeloblastosis. XIV. Neoplastic response of normal chicken bone marrow treated with the virus in tissue culture. *J. Nat. Cancer Inst.*, **24**: 395–415, 1960a.

Beaudreau, G. S., Becker, C., Stim, T., Wallbank, A. M., and Beard, J. W., Virus of avian myeloblastosis. XVI. Kinetics of cell growth and liberation of virus in cultures of myeloblasts. pp. 167–187 in: *Symposium, Phenomena of the Tumor Viruses, Nat. Cancer Inst. Monograph No. 4,* U.S. Publ. Health Service, Bethesda, Md., 1960b.

Beaudreau, G. S., Bonar, R. A., Beard, D., and Beard, J. W., Virus of avian erythroblastosis. II. Influence of host age and route of inoculation on dose-response. *J. Nat. Cancer Inst.*, **17**: 91–100, 1956.

Benedetti, E. L., Présence de corpuscules identiques à ceux du virus de l'érythroblastose aviaire chez l'embryon du poulet et les poussins normaux. *Bull. du Cancer,* **44**: 473–482, 1957.

Benedetti, E. L., and Bernhard, W., Recherches ultrastructurales sur le virus de la leucémie érythroblastique du poulet. *J. Ultrastructure Research,* **1**: 309–336, 1958.

Benedetti, E. L., Bernhard, W., and Oberling, C., Présence de corpuscules d'aspect virusal dans des cellules spléniques et médullaires de poussins leucémiques et normaux. *Compt. Rend. Acad. Sci. (Paris),* **242**: 2891–2894, 1956.

Bernhard, W., Electron microscopy of tumor cells and tumor viruses. A review. *Cancer Research,* **18**: 491–509, 1958.

Bernhard, W., and Guérin, M., Présence de particules d'aspect virusal dans les tissus tumoraux de souris atteintes de leucémie spontanée. *Compt. Rend. Acad. Sci. (Paris),* **247**: 1802–1805, 1958.

Bernhard, W., Bonar, R. A., Beard, D., and Beard, J. W., Ultrastructure of viruses of myeloblastosis and erythroblastosis isolated from plasma of leukemic chickens. *Proc. Soc. Exp. Biol. & Med.*, **97**: 48–52, 1958.

Biggs, P. M., and Payne, L. N., Transmission experiments with Marek's disease (fowl paralysis). *Vet. Rec.*, **75**: 177–179, 1963.

Biggs, P. M., and Payne, L. N., Relationship of Marek's disease (neural lymphomatosis) to lymphoid leukosis. pp. 83–98 in: *Internat. Conference on Avian Tumor Viruses, Nat. Cancer Inst. Monograph No. 17,* U.S. Publ. Health Service, Bethesda, Md., 1964.

BONAR, R. A., BEARD, D., BEAUDREAU, G. S., SHARP, D. G., and BEARD, J. W., Virus of avian erythroblastosis. IV. pH and thermal stability. *J. Nat. Cancer Inst.*, **18**: 831–842, 1957.

BONAR, R. A., BEAUDREAU, G. S., SHARP, D. G., BEARD, D., and BEARD, J. W., Virus of avian erythroblastosis. V. Adenosinetriphosphatase activity of blood plasma from chickens with the disease. *J. Nat. Cancer Inst.*, **19**: 909–922, 1957.

BONAR, R. A., PARSONS, D. F., BEAUDREAU, G. S., BECKER, C., and BEARD, J. W., Ultrastructure of avian myeloblasts in tissue culture. *J. Nat. Cancer Inst.*, **23**: 199–225, 1959.

BONAR, R. A., SHARP, D. G., BEARD, D., and BEARD, J. W., Identification of avian erythroblastosis virus by precipitation with chicken immune serum. *Proc. Soc. Exp. Biol. & Med.*, **92**: 774–778, 1956.

BONAR, R. A., WEINSTEIN, D., SOMMER, J. R., BEARD, D., and BEARD, J. W., Virus of avian myeloblastosis. XVII. Morphology of progressive virus-myeloblast interactions *in vitro*. pp. 251–290 in: *Symposium, Phenomena of the Tumor Viruses, Nat. Cancer Inst. Monograph No. 4*, U.S. Publ. Health Service, Bethesda, Md., 1960.

BRANDLEY, C. A., NELSON, N. M., and COTTRAL, G. E., Serial passage of lymphomatosis-osteopetrosis in chickens. *Am. J. Vet. Research*, **3**: 289–295, 1942.

BRYAN, W. R., CALNAN, D., and MOLONEY, J. B., Biological studies on the Rous sarcoma virus. III. The recovery of virus from experimental tumors in relation to initiating dose. *J. Nat. Cancer Inst.*, **16**: 317–335, 1955.

BURMESTER, B. R., The cytotoxic effect of avian lymphoid tumor antiserum. *Cancer Research*, **7**: 459–467, 1947.

BURMESTER, B. R., Studies on the transmission of avian visceral lymphomatosis. II. Propagation of lymphomatosis with cellular and cell-free preparations. *Cancer Research*, **7**: 786–797, 1947.

BURMESTER, B. R., The propagation of lymphoid tumors in the anterior chamber of the chicken eye. *Am. J. Vet. Research*, **13**: 246–251, 1952.

BURMESTER, B. R., Studies on fowl lymphomatosis. *Ann. N.Y. Acad. Sci.*, **54**: 992–1003, 1952.

BURMESTER, B. R., *In vitro* and *in vivo* neutralization of the virus of visceral lymphomatosis. *Proc. Soc. Exp. Biol. & Med.*, **50**: 284–286, 1955.

BURMESTER, B. R., Immunity to visceral lymphomatosis in chicks following injection of virus into dams. *Proc. Soc. Exp. Biol. & Med.*, **88**: 153–155, 1955.

BURMESTER, B. R., Bioassay of the virus of visceral lymphomatosis. I. Use of short experimental period. *J. Nat. Cancer Inst.*, **16**: 1121-1127, 1956.

BURMESTER, B. R., The shedding of the virus of visceral lymphomatosis in the saliva and feces of individual normal and lymphomatous chickens. *Poultry Sci.*, **35**: 1089–1099, 1956.

BURMESTER, B. R., Recent studies on the natural transmission of visceral lymphomatosis in chickens. *J. Am. Vet. Med. Assoc.*, :**131** 496–499, 1957.

BURMESTER, B. R., The vertical and horizontal transmission of avian visceral lymphomatosis. *Cold Spring Harbor Symposia on Quantitative Biology*, **27**: 471–477, 1962.

BURMESTER, B. R., and BELDING, T. C., Immunity and cross immunity reactions obtained with several avian lymphoid tumor strains. *Am. J. Vet. Research*, **8**: 128–133, 1947.

BURMESTER, B. R., and COTTRAL, G. E., The propagation of filtrable agents producing lymphoid tumors and osteopetrosis by serial passage in chickens. *Cancer Research*, **7**: 669–675, 1947.

BURMESTER, B. R., and DENINGTON, E. M., Studies on the transmission of avian visceral lymphomatosis. I. Variation in transmissibility of naturally occurring cases. *Cancer Research*, **7**: 779–785, 1947.

BURMESTER, B. R., and FREDRICKSON, T. N., Experimental transmission of avian visceral lymphomatosis and related neoplasms. pp. 101–122 in vol. 13, *Proc. Thirteenth Symp. Colston Research Soc., Univ. Bristol*, Butterworths Scientific Publ., London, 1961.

BURMESTER, B. R., and FREDRICKSON, T. N., Transmission of virus from field cases of avian lymphomatosis. I. Isolation of virus in line 15 I chickens. *J. Nat. Cancer Inst.*, **32**: 37–63, 1964.

BURMESTER, B. R., and GENTRY, R. F., The presence of the virus causing visceral lymphomatosis in the secretions and excretions of chickens. *Poultry Sci.*, **33**: 836–842, 1954.

BURMESTER, B. R., and GENTRY, R. F., A study of possible avenues of infection with the virus of avian visceral lymphomatosis. *Proc. 91st Ann. Meeting Am. Vet. Med. Assoc.*, pp. 311–316, 1954.

BURMESTER, B. R., and GENTRY, R. F., The transmission of avian visceral lymphomatosis by contact. *Cancer Research*, **14**: 34–42, 1954.

BURMESTER, B. R., and GENTRY, R. F., The response of susceptible chickens to graded doses of the virus of visceral lymphomatosis. *Poultry Sci.*, **35**: 17–26, 1956.

BURMESTER, B. R., and PRICKETT, C. O., The development of highly malignant tumor strains from naturally occurring avian lymphomatosis. *Cancer Research*, **5**: 652–660, 1945.

BURMESTER, B. R., and WALTER, W. G., Occurrence of visceral lymphomatosis in chickens inoculated with Rous sarcoma virus. *J. Nat. Cancer Inst.*, **26**: 511–518, 1961.

BURMESTER, B. R., and WATERS, N. F., The role of the infected egg in the transmission of visceral lymphomatosis. *Poultry Sci.*, **34**: 1415–1429, 1955.

BURMESTER, B. R., and WATERS, N. F., Variation in the presence of the virus of visceral lymphomatosis in the eggs of the same hens. *Poultry Sci.*, **35**: 939–944, 1956.

BURMESTER, B. R., and WITTER, R. L., An outline of the diseases of the avian leukosis complex. *Production Research Report No. 94*, p. 8, Agricultural Research Service, U.S. Dept. of Agriculture, Washington, D.C., 1966.

BURMESTER, B. R., BRANDLEY, C. A., and PRICKETT, C. O., Viability of a transmissible fowl tumor (Olson) upon storage at low temperature. *Proc. Soc. Exp. Biol. & Med.*, **55**: 203–204, 1944.

BURMESTER, B. R., CUNNINGHAM, C. H., COTTRAL, G. E., BELDING, R. C., and GENTRY, R. F., The transmission of visceral lymphomatosis with live virus Newcastle disease vaccines. *Am. J. Vet. Research*, **17**: 283–289, 1956.

BURMESTER, B. R., FONTES, A. K., and WALTER, W. G., Pathogenicity of a viral strain (RPL12) causing avian visceral lymphomatosis and related neoplasms. III. Influence of host age and route of inoculation. *J. Nat. Cancer Inst.*, **24**: 1423–1442, 1960.

BURMESTER, B. R., FONTES, A. K., WATERS, N. F., BRYAN, W. R., and GROUPÉ, V., The response of several inbred lines of White Leghorns to inoculation with the viruses of strain RPL 12 visceral lymphomatosis-erythroblastosis and of Rous sarcoma. *Poultry Sci.*, **39**: 199–215, 1960.

BURMESTER, B. R., GENTRY, R. F., and WATERS, N. F., The presence of the virus of visceral lymphomatosis in embryonated eggs of normal appearing hens. *Science*, **34**: 609–617, 1955.

Burmester, B. R., Gross, M. A., Walter, W. G., and Fontes, A. K., Pathogenicity of a viral strain (RPL12) causing avian visceral lymphomatosis and related neoplasms. II. Host-virus interrelations affecting response. *J. Nat. Cancer Inst.*, **22**: 103–127, 1959.

Burmester, B. R., Prickett, C. O., and Belding, T. C., A filtrable agent producing lymphoid tumors and osteopetrosis in chickens. *Cancer Research*, **6**: 189–196, 1946.

Burmester, B. R., Sharpless, G. R., and Fontes, A. K., Virus isolated from avian lymphomas unrelated to lymphomatosis virus. *J. Nat. Cancer Inst.*, **24**: 1443–1447, 1960.

Burmester, B. R., Walter, W. G., and Fontes, A. K., The immunological response of chickens after treatment with several vaccines of visceral lymphomatosis. *Poultry Sci.*, **36**: 79–87, 1957.

Burmester, B. R., Walter, W. G., Gross, M. A., and Fontes, A. K., The oncogenic spectrum of two "pure" strains of avian leukosis. *J. Nat. Cancer Inst.*, **23**: 277–291, 1959.

Carr, J. G., Renal adenocarcinoma induced by fowl leukemia virus. *Brit. J. Cancer*, **10**: 379–383, 1956.

Carr, J. G., Kidney carcinomas of the fowl induced by the MH2 reticuloendothelioma virus. *Brit. J. Cancer*, **14**: 77–82, 1960.

Cottral, G. E., Avian lymphomatosis, another egg-borne disease. *Proc. 53rd Ann. Meeting of the U.S. Livestock Sanitary Assoc.*, pp. 183–192, 1950.

Cottral, G. E., The enigma of avian leukosis. *Proc. 89th Ann. Meeting Am. Vet. Med. Assoc.*, pp. 285–293, 1952.

Cottral, G. E., Burmester, B. R., and Waters, N. F., Egg transmission of avian lymphomatosis. *Poultry Sci.*, **33**: 1174–1184, 1954.

Di Stefano, H. S., and Dougherty, R. M., Virus multiplication in the oviduct of hens infected with an avian leukosis virus. *Virology*, **26**: 156–159, 1965.

Di Stefano, H. S., and Dougherty, R. M., Mechanisms for congenital transmission of avian leukosis virus. *J. Nat. Cancer Inst.*, **37**: 869–883, 1966.

Dmochowski, L., and Grey, C. E., Electron microscopy of tumors of known and suspected viral etiology. *Texas Rep. Biol. & Med.*, **15**: 704–756, 1957.

Dmochowski, L., Grey, C. E., and Burmester, B. R., Studies on submicroscopic structure of chicken lymphomatosis tumors. (Abstract.) *Proc. Am. Assoc. Cancer Research*, **2**: 196, 1957.

Dmochowski, L., Grey, C. E., Burmester, B. R., and Fontes, A. K., Submicroscopic morphology of avian neoplasms. I. Studies on erythroblastosis. *Proc. Soc. Exp. Biol. & Med.*, **98**: 662–665, 1958a.

Dmochowski, L., Grey, C. E., Burmester, B. R., and Walter, W. G., Submicroscopic morphology of avian neoplasms. II. Studies on granuloblastosis (myeloblastosis). *Proc. Soc. Exp. Biol. & Med.*, **98**: 666–669, 1958b.

Dmochowski, L., Grey, C. E., Burmester, B. R., and Gross, M.A., Submicroscopic morphology of avian neoplasms. III. Studies on visceral lymphomatosis. *Proc. Soc. Exp. Biol. & Med.*, **100**: 514–516, 1959.

Dmochowski, L., Grey, C. E., and Burmester, B. R., Submicroscopic morphology of avian neoplasms. IV. Studies on erythroblastosis of strain RPL 12. *Proc. Soc. Exp. Biol. & Med.*, **100**: 517–519, 1959.

Doljanski, L., and Pikovski, M., Agent of fowl leukosis in tissue cultures. *Cancer Research*, **2**: 626–631, 1942.

Dougherty, R. M., and Di Stefano, H. S., Sites of avian leukosis virus multiplication in congenitally infected chickens. *Cancer Research*, **27**: 322–332, 1967.

DURAN-REYNALS, F., The reciprocal infection of ducks and chickens with tumor-inducing viruses. *Cancer Research*, **2**: 343–369, 1942.

ECKERT, E. A., BEARD, D., and BEARD, J. W., Dose-response relations in experimental transmission of avian erythro-myeloblastic leukosis. II. Host response to whole blood and to washed primitive cells. *J. Nat. Cancer Inst.*, **13**: 1167–1184, 1953.

ECKERT, E. A., BEARD, D., and BEARD, J. W., Dose-response relations in experimental transmission of avian erythro-myeloblastic leukosis. III. Titration of the virus. *J. Nat. Cancer Inst.*, **14**: 1055–1066, 1954.

ECKERT, E. A., BEARD, D., and BEARD, J. W., Dose-response relations in experimental transmission of avian erythro-myeloblastic leukosis. V. Influence of host age and route of virus inoculation. *J. Nat. Cancer Inst.*, **15**: 1195–1207, 1955.

ECKERT, E. A., BEARD, D., and BEARD, J. W., Virus of avian erythroblastosis. I. Titration of infectivity. *J. Nat. Cancer Inst.*, **16**: 1099–1120, 1956.

ECKERT, E. A., GREEN, I., SHARP, D. G., BEARD, D., and BEARD, J. W., Virus of avian erythromyeloblastic leukosis. V. pH stability of the virus particles, the infectivity and the enzyme dephosphorylating adenosine triphosphate. *J. Nat. Cancer Inst.*, **15**: 1209–1215, 1955.

ECKERT, E. A., GREEN, I., SHARP, D. G., BEARD, D., and BEARD, J. W., Virus of avian erythromyeloblastic leukosis. VII. Thermal stability of virus infectivity; of the virus particle and of the enzyme dephosphorylating adenosinetriphosphate. *J. Nat. Cancer Inst.*, **16**: 153–161, 1955.

ECKERT, E. A., NELSON, F. W., BURMESTER, B. R., BEARD, D., and BEARD, J. W., Dose-response relations in experimental transmission of avian erythromyeloblastic leukosis. IV. Strain differences in host-response to the virus. *J. Nat. Cancer Inst.*, **14**: 1067–1080, 1954.

ECKERT, E. A., SHARP, D. G., BEARD, D., and BEARD, J. W., Variation in infectivity and virus-particle content of individual plasmas from birds with erythromyeloblastic leukosis. *J. Nat. Cancer Inst.*, **13**: 533–542, 1952.

ECKERT, E. A., SHARP, D. G., MOMMAERTS, E. B., REEVE, R. H., BEARD, D., and BEARD, J. W., Virus of avian erythromyeloblastic leukosis. III. Interrelations of plasma particles, infectivity, and the enzyme dephosphorylating adenosinetriphosphate. *J. Nat. Cancer Inst.*, **14**: 1039–1053, 1954.

ECKERT, E. A., SHARP, D. G., BEARD, D., GREEN, I., and BEARD, J. W., Virus of avian erythromyeloblastic leukosis. IX. Antigenic constitution and immunologic characterization. *J. Nat. Cancer Inst.*, **16**: 593–643, 1955.

ECKERT, E. A., SHARP, D. G., BEARD, D., GREEN, I., and BEARD, J. W., Neutralization and precipitation of the virus of avian erythromyeloblastosis with serum of hyperimmunized chickens. *Proc. Soc. Exp. Biol. & Med.*, **88**: 181–187, 1955.

ECKERT, E. A., WATERS, N. F., BURMESTER, B. R., BEARD, D., and BEARD, J. W., Dose-response relations in experimental transmission of avian erythromyeloblastic leukosis. IV. Strain differences in host-response to the virus. *J. Nat. Cancer Inst.*, **14**: 1067–1080, 1954.

ELLERMANN, V., The leucosis of fowls and leucemia problems. 105 pp., Gyldendal, London, 1922.

ELLERMANN, V., and BANG, O., Experimentelle Leukämie bei Hühnern. *Centralbl. f. Bakt.*, Abt. I (Orig.), **46**: 595–609, 1908.

ELLERMANN, V., and BANG, O., Experimentelle Leukämie bei Hühnern. *Zeitschr. f. Hyg. & Infektionskr.*, **63**: 231–272, 1909.

ENGELBRETH-HOLM, J., Spontaneous and experimental leukaemia in animals. 245 pp., Oliver and Boyd, Publ., Edinburgh and London, 1942.

Engelbreth-Holm, J., and Rothe Meyer, A., Bericht über neue Erfahrungen mit einem Stamm Hühner-Erythroleukose. *Acta Path. & Microbiol. Scand.*, **9**: 293–332, 1932.

Febvre, H., Rothschild, L., Arnoult, J., and Haguenau, F., *In vitro* malignant conversion of rat embryonic cell lines with the Bryan strain of Rous sarcoma virus. pp. 459–477 in: *Internat. Conference on Avian Tumor Viruses, Nat. Cancer Inst. Monograph No. 17*, U.S. Publ. Health Service, Bethesda, Md., 1964.

Feldman, W. H., and Olson, C., Jr., The pathology of spontaneous leukosis of chickens. *J. Am. Vet. Med. Assoc.*, **82**: 875–900, 1933.

Feldman, W. H., and Olson, C., Jr., Leukosis of the common chicken. *J. Am. Vet. Med. Assoc.*, **84**: 488–498, 1934.

Fontes, A. K., Burmester, B. R., Walter, W. G., and Iseler, P. E., Growth in tissue culture of cytopathogenic agent from strain of virus which produces avian lymphomatosis. *Proc. Soc. Exp. Biol. & Med.*, **97**: 854–857, 1958.

Fredrickson, T. N., Purchase, H. G., and Burmester, B. R., Transmission of virus from field cases of avian lymphomatosis. III. Variation in the oncogenic spectra of passaged virus isolates. pp. 1–29 in: *Internat. Conference on Avian Tumor Viruses, Nat. Cancer Inst. Monograph No. 17*, U.S. Publ. Health Service, Bethesda, Md., 1964.

Friedmann, J.-C., Lévy, J.-P., Lasneret, J., Thomas, M., Boiron, M., and Bernard, J., Induction de fibromes sous-cutanés chez le hamster doré par inoculation d'extraits acellulaires de papillomes bovins. *Compt. Rend. Acad. Sci. (Paris)*, **257**: 2328–2331, 1963.

Fujinami, A., and Inamoto, K., Ueber Geschwülste bei japanischen Haushühnern insbesondere über einen transplantablen Tumor. *Zeitschr. f. Krebsforsch.*, **14**: 94–119, 1914.

Fujinami, A., and Suzue, K., Contribution of pathology of tumours growth. Experiments on transplantable chicken sarcoma. *Trans. Japan. Path. Soc.*, **15**: 281–293, 1925.

Furth, J., Erythroleukosis and the anemias of the fowl. *Arch. Path.*, **12**: 1–30, 1931.

Furth, J., Studies on the nature of the agent transmitting leukosis of fowls. I. Its concentration in blood cells and plasma and relation to the incubation period. *J. Exp. Med.*, **55**: 465–478, 1932.

Furth, J., Studies on the nature of the agent transmitting leukosis of fowls. III. Resistance to desiccation, to glycerin, to freezing and thawing; survival at ice box and incubator temperatures. *J. Exp. Med.*, **55**: 495–504, 1932.

Furth, J., Lymphomatosis, myelomatosis, and endothelioma of chickens caused by a filterable agent. I. Transmission experiments. *J. Exp. Med.*, **58**: 253–275, 1933.

Furth, J., Lymphomatosis in relation to fowl paralysis. *Arch. Path.*, **20**: 379–428, 1935.

Furth, J., The relation of leukosis to sarcoma of chickens. II. Mixed osteochondrosarcoma and lymphomatosis (strain 12). III. Sarcomata of strains 11 and 15 and their relation to leukosis. *J. Exp. Med.*, **63**: 127–155, 1936.

Furth, J., Prolongation of life with prevention of leukemia by thymectomy in mice. *J. Gerontology*, **1**: 46–52, 1946.

Furth, J., and Breedis, C., Attempts at cultivation of viruses producing leukosis in fowls. *Arch. Path.*, **24**: 281–302, 1937.

Furth, J., and Miller, H. K., Studies on the nature of the agent transmitting leukosis of fowls. II. Filtration of leucemic plasma. *J. Exp. Med.*, **55**: 479–493, 1932.

FURTH, J., and STUBBS, E. L., Tissue culture studies on relation of sarcoma to leukosis of chickens. *Proc. Soc. Exp. Biol. & Med.*, **32**: 381–383, 1934.

GENTRY, R. F., and BURMESTER, B. R., Tumor incidence in the progeny of hens repeatedly injected as adults with visceral lymphomatosis virus. *Poultry Sci.*, **34**: 44–47, 1955.

GENTRY, R. F., and BURMESTER, B. R., The propagation of the virus of visceral lymphomatosis in embryonated eggs. *Science*, **34**: 669–672, 1955.

GREEN, I., The ATPase activity of avian erythromyeloblastic leukosis virus. Competitive inhibition by ADP. *Acta Biochim. and Biophys.*, **18**: 43–48, 1955.

GREEN, I., and BEARD, J. W., Virus of avian erythromyeloblastic leukosis. VI. Properties of the enzyme associated with the virus in dephosphorylating adenosine triphosphate. *J. Nat. Cancer Inst.*, **15**: 1217–1229, 1955.

GREEN, I., and BEARD, J. W., Virus of avian erythromyeloblastic leukosis. VIII. Dephosphorylation of inosinetriphosphate. *J. Nat. Cancer Inst.*, **16**: 163–172, 1955.

GREEN, I., and SHARP, D. G., The ATPase activity of avian erythromyeloblastic leukosis virus. Introductory kinetics. *Acta Biochim. and Biophys.*, **18**: 36–42, 1955.

GREEN, I., BEARD, D., ECKERT, E. A., and BEARD, J. W., Quantitative aspects of micro ATPase measurements on plasma from chicks with erythromyeloblastic leukosis. *Proc. Soc. Exp. Biol. & Med.*, **85**: 406–409, 1954.

GREEN, I., BEARD, D., and BEARD, J. W., Elevation of blood magnesium and potassium in avian erythromyeloblastic leukosis. *Proc. Soc. Exp. Biol. & Med.*, **87**: 189–191, 1954.

GROSS, L., Attempt to recover filterable agent from X-ray induced leukemia. *Acta Haemat.*, **19**: 353–361, 1958.

GROSS, L., Effect of thymectomy on development of leukemia in C3H mice inoculated with leukemic "passage" virus. *Proc. Soc. Exp. Biol. & Med.*, **100**: 325–328, 1959.

GROSS, L., Development of myeloid (chloro-) leukemia in thymectomized C3H mice following inoculation of lymphatic leukemia virus. *Proc. Soc. Exp. Biol. & Med.*, **103**: 509–514, 1960.

GROSS, L., Serial cell-free passage in rats of the mouse leukemia virus. *Proc. Soc. Exp. Biol. & Med.*, **112**: 939–945, 1963.

GROSS, M. A., BURMESTER, B. R., and WALTER, W. G., Pathogenicity of a viral strain (RPL12) causing avian visceral lymphomatosis and related neoplasms. I. Nature of the lesions. *J. Nat. Cancer Inst.*, **22**: 83–101, 1959.

GROUPÉ, V., DUNKEL, V. C., and MANAKER, R. A., Improved pock counting method for the titration of Rous sarcoma virus in embryonated eggs. *J. Bact.*, **74**: 409–410, 1957.

HAGUENAU, F., ROUILLER, C., and LACOUR, F., Corpuscules d'aspect virusal dans l'endothéliome de Murray-Begg. Étude au microscope électronique. (Note préliminaire.) *Bull. du Cancer*, **42**: 350–357, 1955.

HALBERSTAEDTER, J., DOLJANSKI, L., and TENENBAUM, E., Experiments on the cancerization of cells *in vitro* by means of Rous sarcoma agent. *Brit. J. Exp. Path.*, **22**: 179–187, 1941.

HANAFUSA, H., Nature of the defectiveness of Rous sarcoma virus. pp. 543–556 in: *Internat. Conference on Avian Tumor Viruses, Nat. Cancer Inst. Monograph No. 17*, U.S. Publ. Health Service, Bethesda, Md., 1964.

HANAFUSA, H., HANAFUSA, T., and RUBIN, H., The defectiveness of Rous sarcoma virus, *Proc. Nat. Acad. Sci., USA*, **49**: 572–580, 1963.

HANAFUSA, H., HANAFUSA, T., and RUBIN, H., Analysis of the defectiveness of Rous sarcoma virus. I. Characterization of the helper virus. *Virology*, **22**: 591–601, 1964.

HANAFUSA, H., HANAFUSA, T., and RUBIN, H., Analysis of the defectiveness of Rous sarcoma virus. II. Specification of RSV antigenicity by helper virus. *Proc. Nat. Acad. Sci., USA*, **51**: 41–48, 1964.

HANAFUSA, T., HANAFUSA, H., and RUBIN, H., Differential responsiveness of Rous sarcoma virus stocks to specific cellular resistance induced by avian leukosis viruses. *Virology*, **22**: 643–645, 1964.

HAYASHI, N., Experimenteller Beitrag zu Myxosarkoma von Hühnern. *Verh. jap. path. Ges.*, **3**: 123, 1913.

HAYASHI, N., Einige experimentelle Untersuchungen von Hühnergeschwülsten. *Verh. jap. path. Ges.*, **5**: 130, 1915.

HLOŽÁNEK, I., DONNER, L., and SVOBODA, J., Malignant transformation *in vitro* of Chinese hamster embryonic fibroblasts with the Schmidt-Ruppin strain of Rous sarcoma virus and karyological analysis of this process. *J. Cell. Physiol.*, **68**: 221–235, 1966.

HOLMES, J. R., Experimental transmission of avian osteopetrosis. *J. Comp. Path.*, **68**: 439–448, 1958.

HOLMES, J. R., Further studies on the experimental transmission of avian osteopetrosis. *J. Comp. Path.*, **69**: 385–389, 1959.

HOLMES, J. R., Experimental osteopetrosis in the turkey. *J. Comp. Path.*, **73**: 136–145, 1963.

HOLMES, J. R., Avian osteopetrosis. pp. 63–79 in: *Internat. Conference on Avian Tumor Viruses, Nat. Cancer Inst. Monograph No. 17*, U.S. Publ. Health Service, Bethesda, Md., 1964.

HUEBNER, R. J., ARMSTRONG, D., OKUYAN, M., SARMA, P. S., and TURNER, H. C., Specific complement-fixing viral antigens in hamster and guinea pig tumors induced by the Schmidt-Ruppin strain of avian sarcoma. *Proc. Nat. Acad. Sci., USA*, **51**: 742–750, 1964.

HUEBNER, R. J., ROWE, W. P., TURNER, H. C., and LANE, W. T., Specific adenovirus complement-fixing antigens in virus-free hamster and rat tumors. *Proc. Nat. Acad. Sci., USA*, **50**: 379–389, 1963.

Internat. Conference on Avian Tumor Viruses. JOSEPH W. BEARD, Edit. p. 803, *Nat. Cancer Inst. Monograph No. 17*, U.S. Publ. Health Service, Bethesda, Md., 1964.

IWAKATA, S., and AMANO, S., Causative virus of chicken erythroblastosis observed in ultrathin sections under the electron microscope and the modus of intracellular proliferation of this virus. *Acta Haemat., Japan*, **21**: 60–75, 1958.

JARMAI, K., Infektionsversuche bebrüteter Eier mit dem "Virus" der Hühner-Erythroleukose. *Deutsche tierärztl. Wochenschr.*, **41**: 418–420, 1933.

JARMAI, K., Zur Produktion und Artspezifität des Agens der Hühnerleukose. *Arch. f. Wissenschaft. und Praktische Tierheilk.*, **70**: 62–70, 1935.

JUNGHERR, E., and LANDAUER, W., Studies on fowl paralysis. 3. A condition resembling osteopetrosis (marble bone) in the common fowl. Storrs Agric. Exp. Station Bull. 222, pp. 1–34, 1938.

KAPLAN, H. S., Influence of thymectomy, splenectomy, and gonadectomy on incidence of radiation-induced lymphoid tumors in strain C57 Black mice. *J. Nat. Cancer Inst.*, **11**: 83–90, 1950.

KREBS, C., RASK-NIELSEN, H. C., and WAGNER, A., The origin of lymphosarcomatosis and its relation to other forms of leucosis in white mice—Lymphomatosis infiltrans leucemica et aleucemia. *Acta Radiol., Suppl. X*, pp. 1–53, 1930.

KUNII, A., and FURTH, J., Inhibition of lymphoma induction in virus-infected rats by thymectomy. An affinity of the lymphoma virus for myeloid cells. *Cancer Research*, **24**: 493–497, 1964.

LAGERLÖF, B., *In vitro* and *in vivo* investigations of fowl erythroleukemia. *Acta Path. & Microbiol. Scand., Suppl. 138*, **49**: 1–19, 1960.

LANGLOIS, A. J., and BEARD, J. W., Converted-cell focus formation in culture by strain MC29 avian leukosis virus. *Proc. Exp. Biol. & Med.*, **126**: 718–722, 1967.

LEVINTHAL, J. D., BUFFETT, R. F., and FURTH, J., Prevention of viral lymphoid leukemia of mice by thymectomy. *Proc. Soc. Exp. Biol. & Med.*, **100**: 610–614, 1959.

MCENDY, D. P., BOON, M. C., and FURTH, J., On the role of thymus, spleen and gonads in the development of leukemia in a high-leukemia stock of mice. *Cancer Research*, **4**: 377–383, 1944.

MANAKER, R. A., and GROUPÉ, V., Discrete foci of altered chicken embryo cells associated with Rous sarcoma virus in tissue culture. *Virology*, **2**: 838–840, 1956.

MAREK, J., Multiple Nervenentzündung (Polyneuritis) bei Hühnern. *Deutsche tierärztl. Wochenschr.*, **15**: 417–421, 1907.

MILLER, J. F. A. P., Role of the thymus in murine leukaemia. *Nature*, **183**: 1069, 1959.

MLADENOV, Z., HEINE, U., BEARD, D., and BEARD, J. W., Strain MC29 avian leukosis virus. Myelocytoma, endothelioma, and renal growths: Pathomorphological and ultrastructural aspects. *J. Nat. Cancer Inst.*, **38**: 251–285, 1967.

MOMMAERTS, E. B., BEARD, D., and BEARD, J. W., Screening of chicks with erythromyeloblastic leukosis for plasma activity in dephosphorylation of adenosine triphosphate. *Proc. Soc. Exp. Biol. & Med.*, **83**: 479–483, 1953.

MOMMAERTS, E. B., ECKERT, E. A., BEARD, D., SHARP, D. G., and BEARD, J. W., Dephosphorylation of adenosine triphosphate by concentrates of the virus of avian erythromyeloblastic leucosis. *Proc. Soc. Exp. Biol. & Med.*, **79**: 450–455, 1952.

MOMMAERTS, E. B., SHARP, D. G., ECKERT, E. A., BEARD, D., and BEARD, J. W., Virus of avian erythromyeloblastic leukosis. I. Relation of specific plasma particles to the dephosphorylation of adenosine triphosphate. *J. Nat. Cancer Inst.*, **14**: 1011–1025, 1954.

OBERLING, C., and GUÉRIN, M., Nouvelles recherches sur la production de tumeurs malignes avec le virus de la leucémie transmissible des poules. *Bull. du Cancer*, **22**: 326–360, 1933.

OBERLING, C., and GUÉRIN, M., La leucémie érythroblastique ou érythroblastose transmissible des poules. *Bull. du Cancer*, **23**: 38–81, 1934.

OLSON, C., Jr., A study of transmissible fowl leukosis. *J. Am. Vet. Med. Assoc.*, **89**: 681–705, 1936.

OLSON, C., Jr., A transmissible lymphoid tumor of the chicken. *Cancer Research*, **1**: 384–392, 1941.

PALADE, G. E. A study of fixation for electron microscopy. *J. Exp. Med.*, **95**: 285–298, 1952.

PAPPENHEIMER, A. M., DUNN, L. C., and CONE, V., A study of fowl paralysis (neuro-lymphomatosis gallinarum). Storrs Agric. Exp. Station Bull. 143, pp. 185–290, 1926.

PAPPENHEIMER, A. M., DUNN, L. C., and CONE, V., Studies on fowl paralysis (neurolymphomatosis gallinarum); Clinical features and pathology. *J. Exp. Med.*, **49**: 63–86, 1929.

Pappenheimer, A. M., Dunn, L. C., and Sedlin, S. M., Studies on fowl paralysis (neurolymphomatosis gallinarum); Transmission experiments. *J. Exp. Med.*, **49**: 87–102, 1929.

Parsons, D. F., Painter, J. C., Beaudreau, G. S., Becker, C., and Beard, J. W., Tissue culture and circulating myeloblasts of avian leukemia studied in electron micrographs of ultrathin sections. *Proc. Soc. Exp. Biol. & Med.*, **97**: 839–844, 1958.

Pentimalli, F., Transplantable lymphosarcoma of the chicken. *Cancer Research*, **1**: 69–70, 1941.

Peterson, R. D. A., Burmester, B. R., Fredrickson, T. N., and Good, R. A., Prevention of lymphatic leukemia in the chicken by the surgical removal of the bursa of Fabricius. *Proc. 36th Ann. Meeting. J. Lab. & Clin. Med.*, **62**: 1000, 1963.

Peterson, R. D. A., Burmester, B. R., Fredrickson, T. N., Purchase, H. G., and Good, R. A., Effect of bursectomy and thymectomy on the development of visceral lymphomatosis in the chicken. *J. Nat. Cancer Inst.*, **32**: 1343–1354, 1964.

Peterson, R. D. A., Purchase, H. G., Burmester, B. R., Cooper, M. D., and Good, R. A., Relationships among visceral lymphomatosis, bursa of Fabricius, and bursa-dependent lymphoid tissue of the chicken. *J. Nat. Cancer Inst.*, **36**: 585–598, 1966.

Porter, K. R., and Blum, J. A., A study in microtomy for electron microscopy. *Anat. Record*, **117**: 685–710, 1953.

Prince, A. M., Quantitative studies on Rous sarcoma virus. V. An analysis of the mechanism of virulence of the Bryan "high titer" strain of RSV. *Virology*, **11**: 371–399, 1960.

Rothe Meyer, A., and Engelbreth-Holm, J., Experimentelle Studien über die Beziehungen zwischen Hühnerleukose und Sarkom an der Hand eines Stammes von übertragbarer Leukose-Sarkom-Kombination. *Acta Path. & Microbiol. Scand.*, **10**: 380–428, 1933.

Rubin, H., A virus in chick embryos which induces resistance *in vitro* to infection with Rous sarcoma virus. *Proc. Nat. Acad. Sci., USA*, **46**: 1105–1119, 1960.

Rubin, H., Response of cell and organism to infection with avian tumor viruses. *Bact. Rev.*, **26**: 1–13, 1962.

Rubin, H., The immunological basis for non-infective Rous sarcomas. *Cold Spring Harbor Symposia on Quantitative Biology*, **27**: 441–452, 1962.

Rubin, H., Carcinogenic interactions between virus, cell, and organism. *J. Am. Med. Assoc.*, **190**: 727–731, 1964.

Rubin, H., and Hanafusa, H., Significance of the absence of infectious virus in virus-induced tumors. pp. 508–525 in: Viruses, Nucleic Acids, and Cancer. *17th Ann. Symp. on Fundamental Cancer Research, Univ. of Texas*, M.D. Anderson Hospital and Tumor Institute, Williams & Wilkins, Baltimore, Md., 1963.

Rubin, H., and Temin, H. M., Infection with the Rous sarcoma virus *in vitro*. *Fed. Proc.*, **17**: 994–1003, 1958.

Rubin, H., and Vogt, P. K., An avian leukosis virus associated with stocks of Rous sarcoma virus. *Virology*, **17**: 184–194, 1962.

Rubin, H., Cornelius, A., and Fanshier, L., The pattern of congenital transmission of an avian leukosis virus. *Proc. Nat. Acad. Sci., USA*, **47**: 1058–1069, 1961.

Ruffilli, D., Infezioni in vitro di esplanti di cuore embrionale con cellule del sangue di polio eritroleucemico. *Boll. Soc. Italiana di Biologia Sperimentale*, **13**: 146–148, 1938.

SARMA, P. S., HUEBNER, R. J., and ARMSTRONG, D., A simplified tissue culture tube neutralization test for Rous sarcoma virus antibodies. *Proc. Soc. Exp. Biol. & Med.*, **115**: 481–486, 1963.

SARMA, P. S., TURNER, H. C., and HUEBNER, R. J., Complement fixation test for the detection and assay of avian leukosis viruses. pp. 481–493 in: *Internat. Conference on Avian Tumor Viruses, Nat. Cancer Inst. Monograph No. 17*, U.S. Publ. Health Service, Bethesda, Md., 1964.

SARMA, P. S., TURNER, H. C., and HUEBNER, R. J., An avian leukosis group-specific complement fixation reaction. Application for the detection and assay of non-cytopathogenic leukosis viruses. *Virology*, **23**: 313-321, 1964.

SHARP, D. G., and BEARD, J. W., Counts of virus particles by sedimentation on agar and electron micrography. *Proc. Soc. Exp. Biol. & Med.*, **81**: 75–79, 1952.

SHARP, D. G., and BEARD, J. W., Virus of avian erythromyeloblastic leukosis. IV. Sedimentation, density and hydration. *Acta Biochim. and Biophys.*, **14**: 12–17, 1954.

SHARP, D. G., BEARD, D., and BEARD, J. W., Morphology of characteristic particles associated with avian erythroblastosis. *Proc. Soc. Exp. Biol. & Med.*, **90**: 168–173, 1955.

SHARP, D. G., ECKERT, E. A., BEARD, D., and BEARD, J. W., Morphology of the virus of avian erythromyeloblastic leucosis and a comparison with the agents of Newcastle disease. *J. Bact.*, **63**: 151–161, 1952.

SHARP, D. G., ECKERT, E. A., BURMESTER, B. R., and BEARD, J. W., Particulate component of plasma of fowls with avian lymphomatosis. *Proc. Soc. Exp. Biol. & Med.*, **79**: 204–208, 1952.

SHARP, D. G., MOMMAERTS, E. B., ECKERT, E. A., BEARD, D., and BEARD, J. W., Virus of avian erythromyeloblastic leukosis. II. Electrophoresis and sedimentation of the plasma particles and the enzyme dephosphorylating adenosine triphosphate. *J. Nat. Cancer Inst.*, **14**: 1027–1037, 1954.

SHARPLESS, G. R., DEFENDI, V., and COX, H. R., Cultivation in tissue culture of the virus of avian lymphomatosis. *Proc. Soc. Exp. Biol. & Med.*, **97**: 755–757, 1958.

STECK, F. T., and RUBIN, H., The mechanism of interference between an avian leukosis virus and Rous sarcoma virus. I. Establishment of interference. *Virology*, **29**: 628–641, 1966.

STUBBS, E. L., and FURTH, J., The relation of leukosis to sarcoma of chickens. I. Sarcoma and erythroleukosis (strain 13). *J. Exp. Med.*, **61**: 593–615, 1935.

SVOBODA, J., and CHÝLE, P., Malignization of rat embryonic cells by Rous sarcoma virus *in vitro*. *Folia Biol.* (*Praha*), **9**: 329–342, 1963.

THORELL, B., Modification of the host reaction towards leukemia virus. *Proc. VII Internat. Congress Internat. Soc. Hematology, Rome*, pp. 582–592, Sept. 7–13, 1958.

THORELL, B., Induction av Njurtumör med Leukämivirus. *Nord Med.*, **59**: 762–764, 1958.

THORELL, B., Virusinducerad njurtumör hos Höns. *Nord Med.*, **62**: 1687–1688, 1959.

U.S. Dept. Agriculture. Lymphomatosis in chickens. Circular No. 970, p. 17, U.S. Government Printing Office, Washington, D.C., 1955.

VAN DEN BERGHE, L., and D'URSEL, F., Culture en tissus du virus de l'érythroblastose de la poule (souche O.G.). *Compt. Rend. Soc. Biol.*, **131**: 1301–1302, 1939.

VERNE, J., OBERLING, C., and GUÉRIN, M., Tentatives de culture *in vitro* de l'agent de la leucémie transmissible des poules. *Compt. Rend. Soc. Biol.*, **121**: 403–405, 1936.

Vogt, P. K., Avian tumor viruses. *Advances in Virus Research*, **11**: 293–385, Academic Press, New York and London, 1965.

Vogt, P. K., A virus released by "nonproducing" Rous sarcoma cells. *Proc. Nat. Acad. Sci., USA*, **58**: 801–808, 1967.

Vogt, P. K., and Rubin, H., The cytology of Rous sarcoma virus infection. Basic mechanisms in animal virus biology. *Cold Spring Harbor Symposia on Quantitative Biology*, **27**: 395–405, 1962.

Wallbank, A. M., Sperling, F. G., Stubbs, E. L., and Hubben, K., Studies of avian sarcoma and erythroblastosis (strain 13). II. Virus susceptibility to ether and chloroform. *Proc. Soc. Exp. Biol. & Med.*, **110**: 809–811, 1962.

Walter, W. G., Burmester, B. R., and Cunningham, C. H., Studies on the transmission and pathology of a virus-induced avian nephroblastoma (embryonal nephroma). *Avian Dis.*, **6**: 455–477, 1962.

Waters, N. F., Etiological relationship of visceral and neural lymphomatosis. *Poultry Sci.*, **33**: 365–373, 1954.

Waters, N. F., and Burmester, B. R., Mode of inheritance of resistance to induced erythroblastosis in chickens. *Poultry Sci.*, **42**: 97–102, 1963.

Waters, N. F., and Bywaters, J. H., Influence of age of chickens at contact exposure on incidence of lymphomatosis. *Poultry Sci.*, **28**: 254–261, 1949.

Waters, N. F., Burmester, B. R., and Walter, W. G., Genetics of experimentally induced erythroblastosis in chickens. *J. Nat. Cancer Inst.*, **20**: 1245–1256, 1958.

Young, D., Some characteristics of the virus responsible for osteopetrosis in chickens. *J. Comp. Path.*, **76**: 45–48, 1966.

CHAPTER 8

The Development of Inbred Strains of Mice, and its Impact on Experimental Cancer Research

Some forty years ago, shortly after World War I, it became apparent to a small group of geneticists in the United States that it would be most desirable to develop uniformly susceptible strains of mice for certain biological studies, and principally for experimental cancer research. Studies dealing with implantations of tumors or the tumor-inducing action of certain carcinogenic chemicals were handicapped by the lack of uniformly susceptible animals. A group of mice bought from a dealer and used for an experiment would show great differences in individual response under apparently identical conditions, even though all animals used might have been of the same sex and of similar age.

It is now common knowledge that among mice of unknown ancestry and different genetic make-up, treated with the same dose of carcinogenic chemicals, some may develop tumors, while others may show partial or complete resistance. Implantation of fragments of a transplantable tumor under otherwise apparently similar experimental conditions may give different results; in some animals the implanted tumors may grow progressively, in others they may "take," then grow temporarily and eventually regress, or they may not grow at all. On the other hand, when carcinogenic chemicals are applied to a group of homozygous mice of an inbred line, or if bits of transplantable tumors are implanted into such animals, the results are far more uniform: the chemicals may or may not induce tumors; the implanted tumors may either grow, or the animals may remain in good health. This is only an example, but it illustrates the importance of using groups of pedigreed mice of similar genetic constitution in experimental cancer research, as well as in other biological studies which require animals for inoculation, in order to assure uniform susceptibility under otherwise similar experimental conditions.

The development of inbred strains of mice in which the degree of biological variability could be carefully controlled was initiated by C. C. Little and a few other pioneer geneticists, in an attempt to obtain animals of similar susceptibility, and thus enable the investigator, using mice as a biological tool, to conduct his studies on a "quantitative" basis, similar to experiments carried out by a chemist using pure chemicals. A system of pedigreed mating was introduced; all animals were given individual identifying numbers early in life, and complete vital records of each animal were individually entered in permanent form. As a rule, in each successive generation, a brother was mated to his own sister. Occasionally, an offspring was mated to his or her parent, the younger of the two parents being used for such a purpose.

Dr. C. C. Little was first, in 1909, at Harvard University in Boston, to develop, by recombination of coat-color genes, the dilute-brown (DBA) strain of mice. Several lines were continued by brother-to-sister mating. Later on, after Little moved to the Carnegie Institution, Cold Spring Harbor, Long Island, N.Y., a severe epidemic of mouse paratyphoid completely wiped out his colony of DBA mice during the summer of 1919. Fortunately, he had left a part of his DBA colony of mice with E. E. Tyzzer, at Harvard University. This precaution saved the DBA strain. At the end of the summer, in 1919, three dilute-brown mice were received at Cold Spring Harbor from Dr. Tyzzer. These mice, almost one year of age, formed a new nucleus, from which, by pedigreed inbreeding, the DBA strain has been developed.

Another partially inbred colony of mice at Cold Spring Harbor was the so-called Bagg-albino. This stock was imported in 1906 from a dealer in Ohio by Dr. Halsey J. Bagg (1920, 1925) who was then associated with the old Memorial Hospital in New York City. Some brother-to-sister mating had been employed in that stock, but most of the stock had been carried by pen mating, which meant that several females and males were kept together in one cage. Gradually, by pedigreed inbreeding, the well known strain BALB/c was developed from this initial nucleus.

In 1920, L. C. Strong obtained two mice from the laboratory of the Department of Genetics, Carnegie Institution, in Cold Spring Harbor. One of these mice was a male from the above mentioned dilute-brown strain of Dr. Little, and the other was a Bagg-albino female. This female was mated first to the dilute-brown male, and later on to one of her sons obtained from the above cross. Eventually, this female mouse developed a spontaneous mammary carcinoma, as did many of her female descendants. From this initial nucleus, by pedigreed inbreeding over a period of 15 years, the well known high-mammary-tumor strain C3H was developed by L. C. Strong (1935). After a fair degree of inbreeding had been initially established, the various resulting substrains were designated by letters of the alphabet; later on, it also became necessary to add numbers for classification. Thus, the now well known symbol C3H was eventually given by Strong to a selected substrain gradually developed by selective inbreeding for its high-breast-tumor incidence. The black agouti pattern in mice of

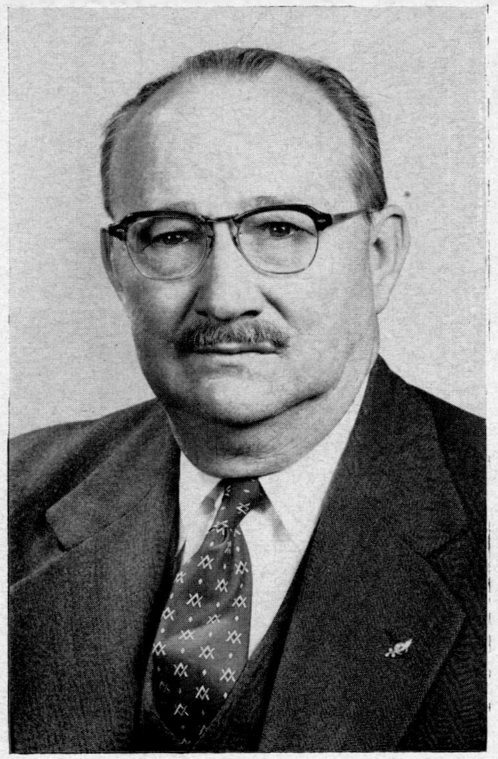

L. C. Strong

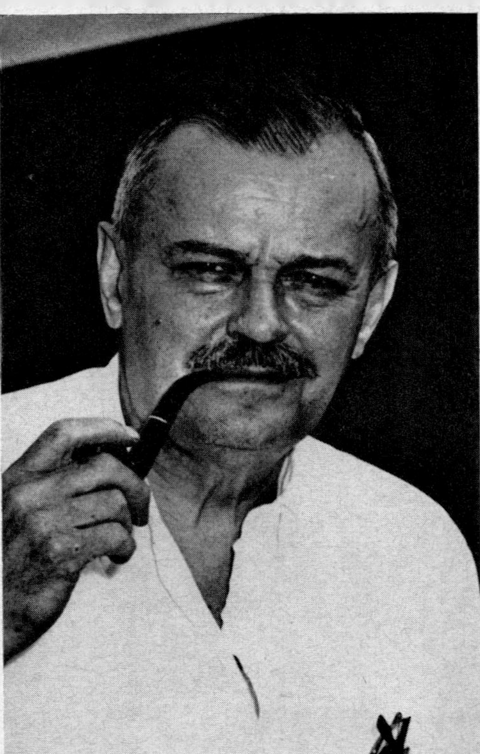

C. C. Little

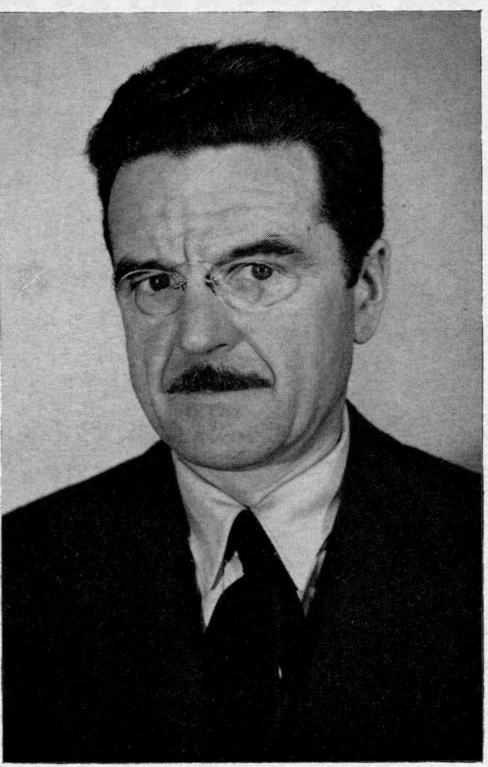
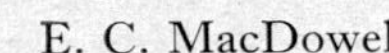

E. C. MacDowell

FIG. 20

this strain was derived from the unpedigreed albino mouse used in its origin.

Strain C3H was not the only one developed by Strong. Between 1920 and 1925, four unpedigreed pairs of mice from various sources were selected and pedigreed inbreeding was started (Strong, 1942). Later on several other pairs of mice were added to the breeding colonies. Continuous selection was applied in each generation, the breeding being continued primarily by brother-to-sister mating. From this initial nucleus, a series of sublines was established according to color combinations or other characteristics. These lines have been separated and continued by pedigreed inbreeding as separate sublines. They are the well-known strains A, C3H, CBA, etc., all related to each other to some extent, but differing among themselves in the incidence of spontaneous mammary tumors, and also in certain other respects, such as color, etc.

These were not the only strains of mice developed by pedigreed inbreeding. Many others, such as C57 Black, C57 Brown, C58, etc., were developed by C. C. Little, E. C. MacDowell, and other geneticists (Table 2).

After fifteen to twenty successive generations, the process of brother-to-sister, or parent-to-offspring, mating resulted eventually in a high degree of genetic uniformity in all animals of a particular inbred line. For practical purposes, these animals were now as alike as identical twins, and they also proved equally susceptible, or equally resistant, to the implantation of certain tumors. Thus, a tumor that developed spontaneously, or was induced, in an animal of one of these inbred lines, would grow without difficulty when implanted into any animal of the same line. Similarly, such animals would be uniformly susceptible, or resistant, to the tumor-inducing action of certain carcinogenic chemicals. They also proved of great value in studies dealing with nutritional requirements, sensitivity to hormones, or to certain pharmacological compounds, etc.

* * *

At about the same time, Maud Slye (1914, 1931) reported in a series of publications, that among mice bred in her laboratory, tumors occurred much more frequently in successive generations of certain families of mice than in others.

Actually, it has long been observed that families of mice having a markedly higher incidence of tumors or leukemia than the average population could be segregated. The influence of some hereditary factors predisposing to cancer has been suspected by numerous observers. Many geneticists have shown that by proper manipulation of the process of heredity, i.e. by selective inbreeding, it was possible to control, at least to some degree, the incidence of spontaneous tumors developing in certain families of mice.

Table 2. Some of the Inbred Lines of Mice More Frequently Used in Cancer Research

Symbol	Color	Mammary tumor incidence* per cent	Leukemia incidence* per cent	Strain initially developed by
A	albino	90†	1	Strong
Ak	albino	1	85	Furth
BALB	albino	2	15	Bagg
CBA	black agouti	3	1	Strong
C3H	black agouti	90	<1‡	Strong
C57 Brown	non-agouti brown	4	5	Little
C57 Black	black	1	5	Little
C58	black	1	85	MacDowell
DBA/2	non-agouti dilute-brown	60	30	Little
I	dilute-brown, piebald pink-eyed	1	5	Strong
R III	albino	75	3	Dobrovolskaia-Zavadskaia
Swiss**	albino	15–20	5–11	Lynch

* Approximate only; the figures indicated may vary in different laboratories and particularly in certain substrains by as much as 25 per cent, or even more. For example, in some laboratories BALB/c mice have a low incidence of spontaneous leukemia (<5 per cent), whereas in other laboratories incidence up to 35 per cent has been recorded, particularly in mice 15 to 24 months old. Incidence of spontaneous pulmonary tumors, hepatomas, etc., is not included in this table.

** Only some of the substrains employed are inbred, or partially inbred. For that reason, the characteristics may vary among the different sublines.

† In breeding females only. The incidence in virgin females is 5 per cent.

‡ In the Bittner substrain of the C3H line, bred in our laboratory, we have observed an incidence of spontaneous leukemia approximately 0.5 to 1 per cent. In another substrain (maintained at the National Cancer Inst., and also at the Jackson Lab.) a 5 per cent incidence of spontaneous leukemia has been reported.

One of the greatest contributions made by the development of inbred strains of mice was the introduction of families of mice with either a high, or a low, incidence of spontaneous tumors, such as mammary carcinomas or leukemia. It was soon realized, however, that the development of these various neoplasms in certain families of mice could not be explained consistently by the established laws of inheritance. Nevertheless, strains of mice have been developed, such as lines C3H, A (Strong, 1935, 1936), and R III (Dobrovolskaia-Zavadskaia, 1933), in which the great majority of females developed spontaneously mammary carcinomas upon reaching approximately one year of age, whereas other strains of mice were found to be essentially free from these tumors. Pulmonary adenomas or hepatomas were observed to occur in middle-aged mice of certain strains. A particularly high incidence of pulmonary tumors, exceeding 55 per cent in animals that lived 10 months or longer, was observed in strain A mice. MacDowell developed at Cold Spring Harbor a strain of black mice, designated by the symbol C58; he observed with Richter (1935) that most of these mice died with large spleens, and realized that they had been breeding a strain of mice showing a high incidence of leukemia. Later on, Furth and his associates (1933) developed by design a high leukemic inbred line of mice, designated by the symbol Ak, by breeding selectively relatives of leukemic mice, and continuing such selective inbreeding through a number of successive generations.

The development of selected pure strains of mice* was a tedious process, requiring years of pedigreed inbreeding; it was necessary to restrict descendants by discarding mice in collateral lines, even though they descended from the same original stock. Now and then, the breeding was interrupted by intercurrent and unexpected diseases, which at times decimated valuable stocks of mice. The Roscoe B. Jackson Memorial Laboratory in Bar Harbor, Maine, has maintained and made available to other investigators mice of various inbred strains. Unfortunately, the forest fire that swept through the Jackson Laboratory in 1947 destroyed many priceless inbred lines of mice. Considerable efforts were required to replace most of the destroyed strains, fortunately preserved in other laboratories, and gradually to rebuild the priceless collection of inbred lines of mice at the Jackson Memorial Laboratory.

The development of inbred strains of mice has made possible observations of a fundamental nature, such as the discovery of the mouse mammary carcinoma virus transmitted through the milk of nursing females, and that of the mouse leukemia virus transmitted directly through the embryos from one generation to another. These observations might not have been made otherwise. Furthermore, mice of the various strains proved their value in many other fields of experimental cancer research, as well as in general biological studies requiring uniformly susceptible mice for inoculations.

Mice of the Swiss stock should also be mentioned here, since they are frequently employed in experimental cancer research. The Swiss mice were introduced to the United States by Clara Lynch of the Rockefeller Institute in New York. Dr. Lynch† brought 2 male mice and 7 females of this particular stock from the laboratory of Dr. A. de Coulon in Lausanne, Switzerland, in

* The interested reader is referred to the list of inbred strains of mice prepared by the Committee on Standardized Genetic Nomenclature for Mice (1952, 1960, 1964, 1968).

† Personal communication to the author from Dr. Clara Lynch (1960).

1926. Some of the Swiss mice were maintained, for a certain period of time at least, as a pedigreed colony in the laboratory of Dr. Lynch. During the intervening years, however, mice of this stock were given to other laboratories, and also to commercial dealers. Several substrains of mice of the Swiss stock are now available; most of them are non-inbred stocks, although some are inbred, or partially inbred. Mice of the Swiss stock are characterized by a high incidence of pulmonary tumors (about 44 per cent) and a relatively high incidence of spontaneous mammary carcinomas appearing in breeding females (approximately 15 to 20 per cent). The incidence of spontaneous leukemia varies from 5 to 11 per cent, approximately.

A strain of mice with a high incidence of spontaneous bone tumors was developed by Pybus and Miller (1938a). Among mice of the Simpson strain (Pybus and Miller, 1934), which they maintained in their laboratory since 1929, they noted that a few animals developed bone tumors. An inbreeding by brother-to-sister mating of the progeny of these mice was initiated, and as a result the incidence of bone tumors increased considerably in several substrains which were thus developed. In one "Special Strain" the incidence of bone tumors exceeded 50 per cent; the tumors developed much more frequently in females than in males (Pybus and Miller, 1938b). The interested reader is referred for further details to the chapter on Mouse Osteosarcoma in this monograph.

REFERENCES

BAGG, H. J., Individual differences and family resemblances in animal behavior. A study of habit formation in various strains of mice. *Arch. Psychol.*, **6**: 1–58, 1920.

BAGG, H. J., The functional activity of the breast in relation to mammary carcinoma in mice. *Proc. Soc. Exp. Biol. & Med.*, **22**: 419–421, 1925.

Committee on Standardized Nomenclature for Inbred Strains of Mice. Standardized nomenclature for inbred strains of mice. *Cancer Research*, **12**: 602–613, 1952.

Committee on Standardized Genetic Nomenclature for Mice. Standardized nomenclature for inbred strains of mice. Second listing. *Cancer Research*, **20**: 145–169, 1960.

Committee on Standardized Genetic Nomenclature for Mice. Prepared by Joan Staats. Standardized nomenclature for inbred strains of mice. Third listing. *Cancer Research*, **24**: 147–168, 1964. Fourth listing. *Cancer Research*, **28**: 391–420, 1968.

DOBROVOLSKAIA-ZAVADSKAIA, N., La fréquence des cancers chez les souris procrées par des mères cancereuses. *Compt. Rend. Soc. Biol.*, **107**: 466–469, 1931.

DOBROVOLSKAIA-ZAVADSKAIA, N., Heredity of cancer. *Radiology*, **18**: 805–808, 1932.

DOBROVOLSKAIA-ZAVADSKAIA, N., Heredity of cancer susceptibility in mice. *J. Genetics*, **27**: 181–198, 1933.

FURTH, J., SEIBOLD, H. R., and RATHBONE, R. R., Experimental studies on lymphomatosis of mice. *Am. J. Cancer*, **19**: 521–604, 1933.

LITTLE, C. C., The genetics of cancer in mice. *Biol. Reviews*, **22**: 315–343, 1947.

LITTLE, C. C., Biological aspects of cancer research. *J. Nat. Cancer Inst.*, **20**: 441–464, 1958.

MACDOWELL, E. C., and RICHTER, M. N., Mouse leukemia. IX. The role of heredity in spontaneous cases. *Arch. Path.*, **20**: 709–724, 1935.

PYBUS, F. C., and MILLER, E. W., Hereditary mammary carcinoma of mice. (A description of 100 consecutive tumors.) *Newcastle Med. J.*, **14**: 151–169, 1934.

PYBUS, F. C., and MILLER, E. W., Spontaneous bone tumors of mice. *Am. J. Cancer*, **33**: 98–111, 1938a.

PYBUS, F. C., and MILLER, E. W., A sex-difference in the incidence of bone tumors in mice. *Am. J. Cancer*, **34**: 248–251, 1938b.

SLYE, M., The incidence and inheritability of spontaneous tumors in mice. *J. Med. Research*, **30**: 281–298, 1914.

SLYE, M., The relation of heredity to the occurrence of spontaneous leukemia, pseudo-leukemia, lymphosarcoma and allied diseases in mice. Preliminary report. *Am. J. Cancer*, **15**: 1361–1368, 1931.

SLYE, M., The relation of heredity to cancer occurrence as shown in strain 621. Studies in the incidence and inheritability of spontaneous tumors in mice: 31st report. *Am. J. Cancer*, **15**: 2675–2726, 1931.

STRONG, L. C., The establishment of the C3H inbred strain of mice for the study of spontaneous carcinoma of the mammary gland. *Genetics*, **20**: 586–591, 1935.

STRONG, L. C., The establishment of the "A" strain of inbred mice. *J. Heredity*, **27**: 21–24, 1936.

STRONG, L. C., The origin of some inbred mice. *Cancer Research*, **2**: 531–539, 1942.

STRONG, L. C., The origin of some inbred mice. II. Old techniques and new. *J. Nat. Cancer Inst.*, **15**: 1417–1426, 1955.

CHAPTER 9

Mouse Mammary Carcinoma

FILTERABLE VIRUS (BITTNER) CAUSING MOUSE MAMMARY CARCINOMA, AND ITS NATURAL TRANSMISSION THROUGH MILK OF NURSING FEMALE MICE

It has long been observed that cancer of the mammary gland developed spontaneously more frequently in certain families of mice than in others. By a tedious process of selective inbreeding, strains of mice having a very high incidence of mammary tumors have been developed; these strains have remained in marked contrast to other inbred strains of mice in which spontaneous breast cancer has been seen only occasionally.

Two outstanding inbred strains of mice developed by L. C. Strong in the United States, and designated by the symbols C3H and A respectively, have been characterized by a very high incidence of mammary tumors developing spontaneously in middle-aged females. In mice of the C3H strain, the mammary tumors appear in over 90 per cent of both virgin and breeding females; in mice of the A strain, on the other hand, the breeding females have a very high incidence of mammary tumors (over 90 per cent), whereas the incidence is relatively low (5 per cent) in virgin females. Microscopically, these tumors have a typical morphology of adenocarcinomas of the mammary glands. They usually begin to appear in females about 5 to 6 months old; the incidence rises rapidly, reaching a peak at about 8 to 12 months of age, then gradually decreases. Other strains of mice such as CBA, BALB/c, C57 Black, etc., developed at the same time by L. C. Strong, H. J. Bagg, C. C. Little, and other geneticists in the United States, have a low or negligible incidence of spontaneous mammary carcinoma.

The objection could have been raised that pure inbred lines of mice represented the outcome of artificial laboratory conditions of pedigreed inbreeding not occurring under natural conditions of life. In an attempt to answer the question whether mammary tumors would also be "inherited" under conditions of breeding more similar to those occurring in nature, N. Dobrovolskaia-Zavadskaia, at the Radium Institute in Paris, carried out (1930–1931) the following experiment: five middle-aged female mice bearing spontaneous breast carcinomas were mated to 5 healthy males. All these mice were plain market mice, with no family records available, but apparently unrelated genetically, and purchased from different commercial dealers. These 5 cancerous mothers initiated 5 typical cancer families; all female offspring of the F_1 generation that lived more than 6 months, and 67 per cent of those of the F_2 generation, developed mammary carcinomas.

It was quite apparent that the development of breast cancer in mice depended, to some extent at least, on inherited susceptibility and hormonal stimulation; the tumors obviously favored certain families, and, among untreated animals, developed exclusively in females. Interesting as these factors were, however, they could not fully explain the development of breast cancer in mice. Thus, for many years, the etiology of mouse mammary carcinoma remained obscure.

The Extra-chromosomal, Maternal "Influence"

Lathrop and Loeb noticed as early as 1918 that the incidence of mammary tumors in hybrid mice of certain crosses more often depended on the tumor incidence of the ancestry of the mothers than on that of the fathers; this phenomenon was explained, however, by the assumption of the existence of a partial linkage of a hypothetical determiner of the tumor rate with the sex determinant. At that time pure inbred strains of mice were not yet generally available.

The clarification of this problem became possible only some 15 or 18 years later, after the high-breast-cancer and low-tumor strains of mice had been developed. In a series of fundamental experiments* performed at the Roscoe B. Jackson Memorial Laboratory in Bar Harbor, Maine, and published by the Staff† of the laboratory in 1933, female mice of strains having a high incidence of breast cancer were mated to males of low-

* According to information obtained by the author from Dr. John J. Bittner, the following investigators of the staff of the laboratory carried out experiments which contributed to the results published: C. C. Little, W. S. Murray, John J. Bittner, and Charles V. Green.

† The following is an excerpt from a letter received by the author (1959) from Dr. Clarence C. Little, referring to the discovery of the "extra-chromosomal influence":

> " ... Murray and I had made reciprocal crosses between DBA and C57 black and had raised thousands of animals. When we tabulated our F_1 and F_2 results, the presence of maternal influence was strikingly shown. We then went to Bittner and Green who had made reciprocal crosses between 'high' and 'low' tumor strains, and got them to tabulate their data in the way that *we* had. Their figures supported ours.
>
> I then published the communication as a 'Staff' contribution, for I felt, and still feel, that we were all on the same general track and were a 'team' which I wanted to recognize and encourage ... "

tumor strains. The female offspring resulting from this cross had a high incidence of mammary tumors. When, in another experiment, the parental partners were reversed, and fathers of high-mammary-tumor strains were mated to females of low-tumor strains, their offspring remained relatively free from breast tumors. Four reciprocal crosses were made between three strains of mice having a high incidence of spontaneous mammary carcinomas, and four strains with a low incidence of these tumors. In every cross, the females of the first hybrid generation which had mothers from the strain with a high tumor incidence also developed breast carcinomas. On the other hand, those hybrid mice which had mothers from the low-tumor strains developed few tumors only. Had the genetic principles of inheritance alone been responsible for the transmission of a factor determining the incidence of breast cancer in hybrid mice, either parent should have had an equal influence. Since this was not the case, it appeared necessary to assume the existence and the transmission from parents to offspring, of an extra-chromosomal, i.e. non-genetic, factor, inducing mammary tumors in mice, and transmitted from parents to offspring through the mother. Similar conclusions were reached at about the same time (1934) by Korteweg, in Holland, who, using strains of mice obtained from the R. B. Jackson Memorial Laboratory, also noticed in his cross-mating experiments the existence of an extra-chromosomal maternal influence.

The Discovery of the "Milk Influence"

An extra-chromosomal factor, responsible for the transmission of breast tumors in mice, could have been passed from mothers to their offspring (a) by way of the cytoplasm of the ovum, (b) during intra-uterine life, or (c) by way of mothers' milk. While other investigators at the Jackson Laboratory explored the first two possibilities, John J. Bittner, then a member of the staff, suspected that the extra-chromosomal factor responsible for the development of breast cancer in mice is transmitted in mothers' milk to suckling mice. In an experiment which was initiated in January, 1934, and published as a brief preliminary report in the August 14, 1936 issue of *Science*, three litters of mice of strain A, which has a breast cancer incidence of 88 per cent, were removed from their mothers when less than 24 hours old and were transferred for nursing to females of the low-tumor strain X (Strong's CBA). There were 9 females in the 3 foster-nursed litters, and of these only 3 developed mammary tumors, whereas the expected incidence would have been 7 or 8. A similarly reduced incidence was observed among the 40 descendants of these mice. Bittner concluded that "while the number of animals used in this preliminary work has been small, a larger group of females fostered by C57 Black stock mice are giving observations which are indicative of similar results. Should further study demonstrate that the incidence of mammary gland tumors in mice may be affected by nursing, an explanation may be offered for the so-called extra-chromosomal influence as a cause in the development of this type of neoplasm."

Bittner now extended his experiments, using larger numbers of mice of several strains. Suckling mice, born to high-cancer strain A females, were removed, when less than 24 hours old, from their potentially cancerous mothers, and were transferred for foster-nursing to females of the low-breast-cancer CBA(X), or C57 Black, lines. Of 127 foster-nursed females, only 10 (8 per cent) developed breast tumors; the remaining 117 females died at an average age of 18 months without tumors. Of 376 female relatives of the same A line that had been left undisturbed with their own strain A mothers, serving as controls, 92 per cent developed breast tumors at an average age of 10 months.

These fundamental observations have been confirmed and extended by other investigators using several high-breast-cancer and low-breast-tumor lines of mice. It was soon realized that even a very small quantity of milk containing the tumor agent was sufficient to transmit the potentially pathogenic agent. For that reason, in order to prevent the transmission of the tumor agent, newborn mice had to be removed from their mothers immediately after birth, before they had a chance to ingest even a few drops of milk. H. B. Andervont (1941) at the National Cancer Institute in Bethesda, Md., observed that the development of mammary tumors in female descendants of high-tumor lines could be almost entirely prevented by removing these animals, shortly before birth, at full term, by Caesarean section, from their mothers' womb, and transferring them for nursing to foster-mothers of low-tumor lines.

Since the offspring of the foster-nursed mice also remained essentially free from breast tumors, it became clear that a high-breast-cancer inbred line could now be changed, by foster-nursing of one generation, into a low-tumor line. When Bittner removed newborn mice of the high-tumor C3H line from their potentially cancerous mothers and transferred them for the purpose of nursing to foster-mothers of the low-tumor C57 Black line, only two mice out of 165, through five successive generations, developed breast tumors. Among 214 C3H mice left with their own mothers as controls, 97 per cent developed breast tumors at an average age of 9 months. It soon became apparent that breast cancer in mice could not only be prevented by foster-nursing, but that it could also be acquired by the ingestion, in early infancy, of milk containing the tumor agent. In a series of experiments performed by Bittner (1939–1940), Andervont (1940–1945), and followed by other investigators,* newborn mice of low-

* The interested reader is referred to reviews by Andervont (1945), Bittner (1946–1947, 1948, 1958), Dmochowski (1953) and others.

tumor lines were transferred for nursing to foster-mothers of high-breast-cancer strains. The incidence of spontaneous mammary tumors resulting in the foster-nursed females varied, but was high when a susceptible stock was used. Offspring of such foster-nursed mice of susceptible stocks also developed breast tumors. Thus, a low-tumor line could be changed into a high-breast-cancer line, following foster-nursing of only one generation of mice.

Actually, therefore, mammary cancer in mice was found to be a "communicable" disease, the causative agent being transmitted from mothers to their offspring by way of milk. The nursing mothers were in perfect health at the time they transmitted the virus to their offspring. Mammary tumors developed in some of the mothers later, after they had reached middle age; other mothers remained for the balance of their lives in good health, even though they carried the tumor agent and transmitted it to their offspring (see also Gross, 1944, 1949).

It was soon determined that the agent responsible for the induction of mammary carcinomas, and transmitted through the milk, is so small that it could pass Seitz filter pads (Bittner, 1942) or Berkefeld filter candles (Andervont and Bryan, 1944) which retained all visible microbes. It became apparent that the mammary tumor agent (called also "milk influence" or "milk factor") actually belongs to the broad group of filterable viruses, although it was realized that mouse mammary carcinoma is in certain respects different from the common virus-caused diseases.

The Role of Hormones

The role of hormones has been apparent since the earliest observations on spontaneous mammary cancer; these tumors developed spontaneously in females of susceptible families, but not in untreated males. It was quite apparent therefore that hormonal influence was essential in the development of these tumors.

Lathrop and Loeb attempted in 1916 to prevent the development of spontaneous mammary carcinomas by removing ovaries, early in life, in female mice of families having a relatively high incidence of these tumors; these early experiments met with only relative success. Twelve years later, in 1928, using a different approach to test the effect of hormones, W. S. Murray established the role of ovarian hormones by inducing mammary carcinomas in 15 out of 210 males of a high-tumor line, in which, after castration, ovaries had been implanted. In 1932, Lacassagne, at the Radium Institute in Paris, reported the development of breast cancer in male mice following prolonged treatment with estrogenic hormones: three male mice of the high-breast-cancer R III strain received, when 2 weeks old, folliculine injections; this hormonal treatment was repeated every week. After 5 to 6 months, all 3 males developed breast carcinomas.

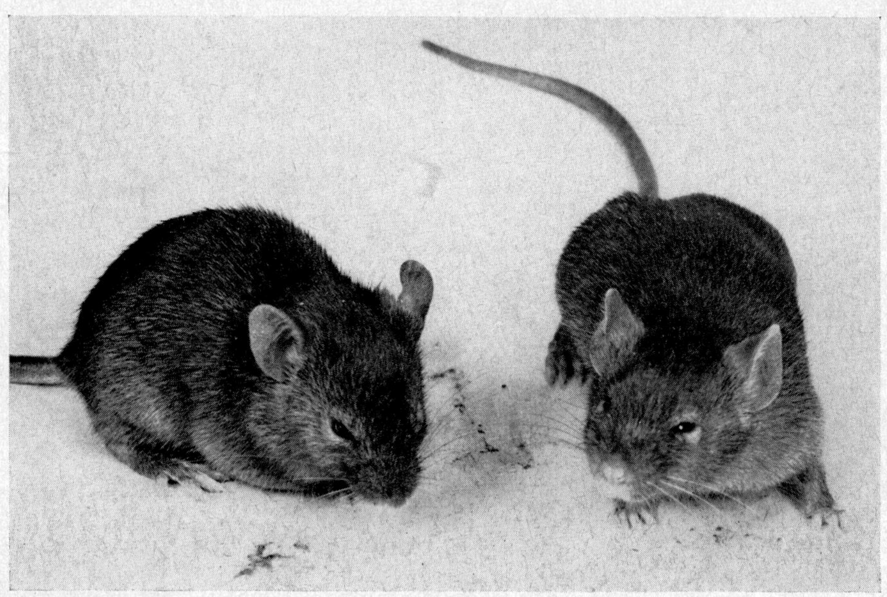

FIG. 21a. C3H MICE.

Young male and female of the C3H inbred line. These mice remain in perfect health when they are young. Most of the females of this strain, however, develop spontaneously mammary carcinoma after they reach 5 to 12 months of age. The incidence varies, but may exceed 90 per cent. The mouse mammary carcinoma virus is transmitted at the time of nursing from mothers to offspring through the milk.

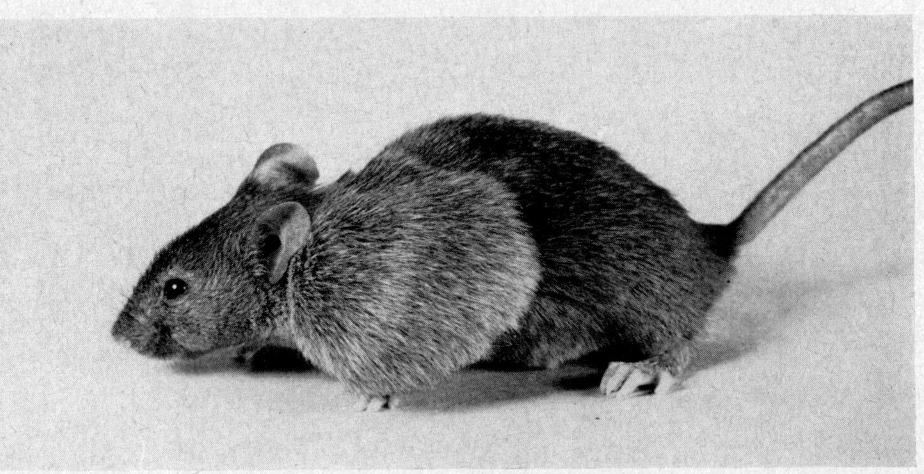

FIG. 21b. MOUSE MAMMARY CARCINOMA.

Spontaneous mouse mammary carcinoma in a 7½-month-old C3H female.

This fundamental observation was soon repeated and confirmed in other laboratories; it became clear, however, that estrogenic hormones will induce mammary tumors only in males of inbred strains having a high incidence of spontaneous mammary carcinomas in females; if males of low-breast-cancer strains were treated with estrogenic hormones, no mammary tumors resulted. These differences were at first interpreted as being genetic. After the discovery of the mammary tumor "milk-agent," however, the role of estrogenic hormones was re-evaluated in its relation to the induction of mammary tumors in the male. It was then realized that breast cancer could be induced with estrogenic hormones in the male mouse, provided that the milk agent was also present. If the males carried the tumor agent, which they had received from their mothers or foster-mothers of high-tumor lines, then mammary tumors could be subsequently induced in such male mice by treatment with estrogenic hormones. On the other hand, estrogenic hormones did not induce mammary tumors in male mice of low-tumor lines, or those born to high-tumor line mothers, but nursed by low-tumor line foster-mothers. The role of estrogenic hormones in the induction of mammary tumors could thus be explained in an indirect manner. Apparently, properly developed and stimulated mammary glands, which are principally under hormonal control, represent an essential condition allowing the agent to induce tumors.

Under certain not yet fully clarified conditions, castration of agent-carrying male mice, without any injection of estrogenic hormones, may sufficiently disturb the hormonal balance to induce the development of mammary tumors. Bittner and Huseby observed that castration alone of certain hybrid mice carrying the mammary tumor agent was sufficient to induce spontaneous mammary carcinomas in up to 80 per cent of the castrated males at an average age of 15 months, as compared with no mammary tumors at all in the intact male controls.*

Higher Incidence of Mammary Carcinomas in Breeding Female Mice as Compared with Virgin Females of Certain Inbred Lines

Breeding females often had a higher incidence of mammary tumors than non-breeding females of the same stock. This observation was made by Lathrop and Loeb in 1913. Later on, studies on mice of pure inbred strains fully substantiated these early observations. Breeding females of strain A have an incidence of spontaneous mammary tumors of over 90 per cent, whereas virgin females of the same stock have a mammary tumor incidence of only 5 per cent. The difference between breeding and non-breeding

* Bittner, J. J., and Huseby, R. A. Unpublished experiments. (Communicated to the author by Dr. J. J. Bittner.)

females is less striking in other high-tumor lines and almost non-existent in females of the C3H line in which over 90 per cent of either breeding or virgin females develop spontaneous mammary carcinomas, although in virgin females these tumors tend to appear a month or so later than in breeders. The hormonal pattern determining the incidence, and to some extent also the time of appearance, of spontaneous mammary tumors in mice carrying the agent is different in different inbred strains and is apparently inherited.

Difference in Monthly Hormonal Pattern between Human Females and Female Mice

The fact that virgin female mice have, in general, and particularly in certain inbred strains, such as strain A, a lower incidence of mammary tumors than breeding females, cannot be compared directly with human data. There is a difference in the hormonal monthly pattern between human females and female mice. Women that have never been pregnant cannot be compared with virgin female mice, but possibly only with those female mice that have had spurious pregnancies. In women, the ovaries complete each month a full hormonal cycle, the secretion of estrogenic hormones being followed by that of progesterone. In virgin female mice, the hormonal cycle is not completed unless the animals are either pregnant, or the pregnancy conditions are simulated by a spurious pregnancy. It was not surprising, therefore, that the incidence of mammary tumors in virgin female mice of the A strain was raised from 5 per cent to 26 per cent in Law's experiments when such virgin females were mated to vasectomized strain A males, and thus hormonal conditions of pseudopregnancy were simulated (1941).

Adair (1925), Bagg (1925), Fekete (1936) and their colleagues reported that non-suckling, resulting in stagnation of milk in the breast, predisposed toward the appearance of mammary tumors in mice. This work attracted attention since the relationship between stagnation of milk in the breast and mammary carcinoma was supported by statistical data in humans. Experimental results in mice were not conclusive, however, and could not be supported in other laboratories.

Bittner (1948) studied several groups of high-breast-cancer strain C3H females: in the first group, the females were not permitted to nurse their progeny, but were immediately returned to the breeding pen ("forced breeding"). In the second group, the females were permitted to nurse their progeny for only 12 days. Finally, in the third group, the females were permitted to nurse their progeny normally until weaning time (21 days). The lowest incidence (74 per cent) of breast cancer was observed in those females that were permitted to nurse their progeny for 12 days. And yet, their mammary glands were found engorged with an accumulation of stagnated milk, following removal of their offspring on the 12th day of nursing; the engorgement of glands persisted for several days. The females subjected to "forced breeding" had no evidence whatever of engorgement of mammary glands with milk, after removal of their progeny immediately after birth; yet, this group showed an incidence of 81 per cent of spontaneous mammary carcinomas. The highest incidence (93 per cent) was observed in those females that were allowed to nurse their progeny normally. Bittner concluded that if rapid breeding and the prevention of nursing exert any influence on the development of mammary cancer in mice, it could be explained by the increased hormonal stimulation due to the additional number of litters, and not necessarily by the retention and stagnation of milk in the mammary ducts.

Bio-Assay for Presence of the Virus. Susceptibility of Various Strains. Importance of Age of Host at Time of Inoculation

The presence of the virus could only be determined by a bio-assay consisting of introducing the virus, by feeding or injection of extracts tested, into susceptible mice. If the inoculated mice developed mammary tumors, it was possible to assume that the sample tested contained the virus. Mice used for bio-assay had to be susceptible to, but at the same time free from, the mammary tumor virus. In the initial experiments, suckling mice ingested the virus with the milk of their mothers. Later on, the extracts tested for the presence of the virus were introduced orally, by means of a blunt needle; however, this route of administration was found to be cumbersome. It was soon determined that inoculation of extracts containing the virus by intraperitoneal route was a more sensitive and satisfactory method of administration. Not only newborn, suckling mice, but 3-week-old weanlings as well, and even young mice up to 6 weeks old, were found to be susceptible. Adult mice were thought at first to be resistant. It was demonstrated, however, independently by Dmochowski, Bittner, Andervont, and Mühlbock, that inoculation of large doses of the mouse mammary carcinoma virus into adult females of a susceptible strain also induced mammary tumors.

For routine inoculation of the virus, some investigators now use suckling mice, 1 to 2 weeks old; others use 3-week-old weanlings.

Many of the strains tested were found to be relatively susceptible, but wide differences in the degree of susceptibility were observed, even among sublines of certain strains. Some strains, such as certain sublines of C57 Black, were found to be relatively resistant, whereas other strains, such as BALB/c, were found highly susceptible. Susceptibility depended also on the virus strain employed. The various mammary tumor viruses carried by different high-breast-cancer strains, such as C3H, A, R III, etc., are most probably closely related; it has not yet been determined whether they represent the same virus prototype, or its substrains.

Induction of Mammary Carcinoma in Wild Mice. Andervont and Dunn (1956) carried out a series of experiments on wild house mice. When kept under observation, 3 out of 73 breeding wild female mice, that had lived to be over one year of age, developed mammary tumors spontaneously; this suggested that wild house mice carry a mammary tumor virus of low activity. The wild house mouse virus also induced mammary tumors following administration either by nursing, or by injection, into mice of low-tumor strain BALB/c or agent-free, foster-nursed mice of strains C3H or R III. That the wild mice are also relatively susceptible to the mammary tumor virus carried by C3H mice, was evident from an experiment in which 11 per cent of wild mice developed breast carcinomas, following foster-nursing by female mice of the high-mammary-tumor strain C3H.

Distribution and Properties of the Mouse Mammary Carcinoma Virus

It is now quite clear that mouse mammary carcinoma is caused by a filterable and transmissible oncogenic virus. The term "mammary carcinoma virus" would therefore be the most logical and appropriate. However, other related terms have been employed for many years as substitute designations of this virus. The term "mammary tumor agent," or its abbreviation "M.T.A.," has been widely employed. Also the term "milk agent" has gained wide acceptance, since the virus has been known to be transmitted principally through the milk of nursing female mice. In recent years the term "Bittner virus" has been gradually accepted, but has not yet replaced the more frequently employed term "Mammary Tumor Agent."

In this chapter the terms referred to above have been used interchangeably. They are all synonymous, and designate the same mouse mammary carcinoma virus.

The mammary tumor agent was first discovered in the milk of nursing female mice; it was soon realized, however, that the virus is widely distributed in the body of the mouse.

On bio-assay tests it was found that normal organs of mice of high-breast-cancer strains contain the agent; thus, the virus was found in the spleen, thymus, blood, and particularly in normal lactating mammary glands. Furthermore, the agent was also found in spontaneous and transplanted mammary tumors. There was some indication that the agent was present in higher concentration in spontaneous than in transplanted tumors, and that the activity of the extracts decreased when such extracts were made from tumors that had been transplanted for a large number of passages.

Properties of the Mouse Mammary Carcinoma Virus. The virus could be filtered through Seitz filter pads (Bittner, 1942), or through Berkefeld N filter candles (Andervont and Bryan, 1944). It could be stored for a few days in 50 per cent glycerin, and for up to 6 months when desiccated by lyophilization. Heating to 56°C or 61°C for 30 minutes inactivated the agent (Bittner, 1942. Andervont *et al.*, 1944. Barnum *et al.*, 1944). The mammary tumor virus could be sedimented after centrifugation in an ultracentrifuge at 60,000 × g, or at 110,000 × g, for one hour, or at 23,000 × g, for 90 minutes (Bryan *et al.*, 1942. Barnum *et al.*, 1946, 1950).

The concentration of the agent in the milk in the lactating mammary glands, or in spontaneous mammary tumor extracts, was tested by Bittner (1945), and by Barnum and Huseby (1950). Dilutions representing up to 10^{-6} gram equivalents, injected intraperitoneally into susceptible agent-free mice, still gave rise to tumors. Dilutions, however, comparable to LD 50, i.e. inducing tumors in about 50 per cent of animals, were those corresponding to somewhere between 10^{-4} and 10^{-5} gram equivalents. Extracts prepared from lactating mammary glands had a higher concentration of the agent than those prepared from mammary tumors (Bittner, 1945. Barnum *et al.*, 1946, 1950).

Antigenic Properties of the Mouse Mammary Carcinoma Virus. When injected into rabbits, guinea pigs, or rats, the virus stimulated the development of specific antibodies (Andervont and Bryan, 1944. Green *et al.*, 1946). The serum from such immunized animals neutralized the virus *in vitro*. Furthermore, such serum injected into one-week-old mice, prior to the inoculation of the virus, prevented the development of breast tumors. However, treatment with the immune serum of mice that had received the agent by nursing from their high-breast-cancer line mothers did not prevent the development of mammary tumors.

Attempt to Propagate the Mouse Mammary Carcinoma Virus in Tissue Culture. Several attempts have been made to propagate the mouse mammary tumor virus in tissue culture (Lasfargues *et al.*, 1958, 1959, 1960. Lasfargues, 1964). The virus was introduced into tissue culture containing fragments of normal mammary glands, and could be passed in such cultures from one tube to another, demonstrating a moderate multiplication in the presence of normal mouse mammary gland tissue fragments. However, no evidence of any prolonged virus multiplication could be obtained in attempts in which the virus was introduced into tissue cultures containing monolayers of mouse mammary gland epithelium. Under these experimental conditions, presence of virus in tissue culture could be determined on the basis of bio-assay studies only during the first 3 months of culture passage. Apparently the virus requires for multiplication the presence of cells of the glandular stroma (Lasfargues, 1964).

Hemolytic Action of Mouse Mammary Carcinoma Extracts on Red Blood Cells In Vitro. Filtered extracts prepared from spontaneous mouse mammary carcinomas, a transplantable mouse sarcoma, rat carcinoma and spontaneous or transplanted mouse leukemia, hemolyzed mouse red blood cells *in vitro* after incubation at 37°C for 2½ hours (Gross, 1947, 1948). Similar results were observed with extracts prepared from human tumors (Gross, 1949).

Although the association of cancer with anemia has long been observed, no satisfactory explanation of the mechanism of this relationship has yet been furnished. Experiments reported in these studies appear to suggest that at least in the case of certain mouse and rat tumors a direct destructive action of a filterable substance contained in the tumor cells on the erythrocytes of the host should be taken into consideration. This is discussed again in more detail in the chapter on Mouse Leukemia.

Transmission of the Mammary Tumor Virus by the Male. Development of Mammary Carcinomas in Mice Presumably Free from the Milk Agent

The initial observation which led to the discovery of the mouse mammary tumor agent was based on the fact that the agent was transmitted through the mother. Hence, the observation of the existence of an "extra-chromosomal maternal factor" and, later on, of the "milk influence."

In 1945 Andervont reported that when females of the low-tumor strain BALB/c were mated to males of the high-breast-cancer strain C3H, 60 per cent of their female offspring developed mammary carcinomas. In only a few of these tumors, however, could the presence of the mammary tumor agent be demonstrated. These observations were considerably extended by studies of Andervont and Dunn, Foulds, Bittner, Mühlbock, Dmochowski and others. It became well established that males of cancerous strains may transfer the tumor agent and infect agent-free females at coitus. The infected females at times did, and sometimes did not, develop mammary tumors; they transmitted the agent, nevertheless, to their offspring; as a result, mammary tumors developed in F_1 hybrid progeny. When Bittner mated BALB/c females with strain C3H males (carrying the agent), 56 per cent of the BALB/c females developed tumors, and up to 96 per cent of their hybrid-offspring also developed mammary carcinomas. Considerable differences were noticed in the ability of agent-carrying males of different strains to transmit the agent during coitus. When hybrid progeny was observed after mating low-tumor strain BALB/c females to agent-carrying males of strains C3H, DBA/2, or R III, female offspring born to C3H fathers showed a higher incidence of mammary tumors.

The situation became more complicated, however, when it was found

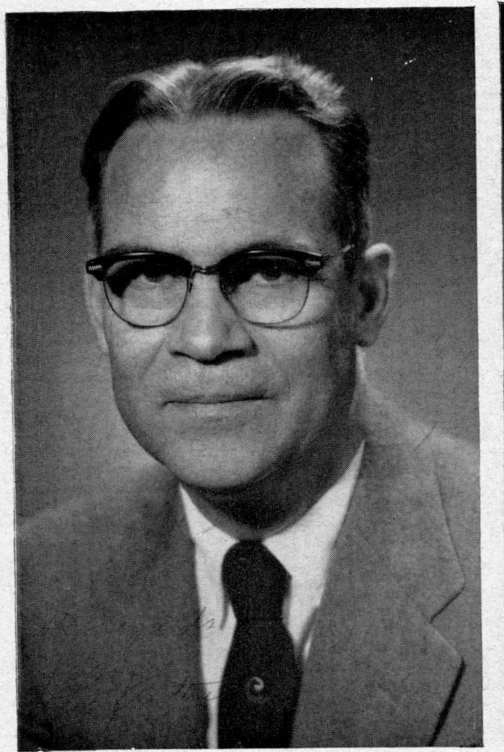

John J. Bittner

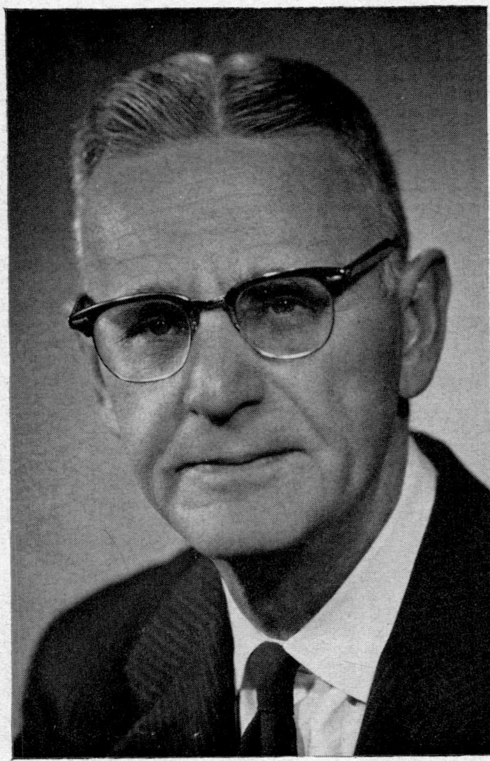

H. B. Andervont

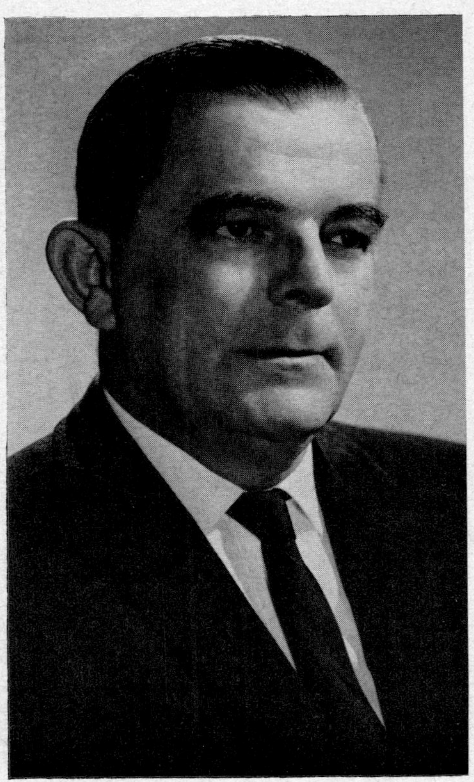

Leon Dmochowski

FIG. 22

by Andervont and Dunn, Bittner, Mühlbock, Dmochowski and others, that mammary tumors may develop also in hybrid progeny, following mating of low-tumor line females with agent-free males. Andervont and Dunn determined that when low-tumor strain BALB/c females were mated to agent-free (foster-nursed) C3H males, the incidence of mammary tumors in their hybrid progeny was as high as 60 per cent, i.e. as high as in a similar progeny from agent-carrying fathers. The tumors appeared at an average age in excess of 20 months. These observations were confirmed by Bittner.

The difficulty was increased by the fact that attempts to demonstrate the presence of a filterable tumor agent in most of these tumors failed.

The Induction of Mammary Tumors in "Agent-free" Females with Carcinogenic Chemicals and Hormones

Foster-nursing of mice of a high-breast-cancer strain by low-cancer strain females eliminates to a large extent the milk-transmitted agent, i.e. the Bittner virus. Under normal life conditions, the foster-nursed females will then remain relatively free from mammary carcinoma. Yet, under certain experimental conditions, namely after application of carcinogenic chemicals, or following intense hormonal stimulation, mammary tumors can be induced in such presumably agent-free females. Dmochowski and Orr (1949) induced mammary tumors in agent-free mice following application of a carcinogenic chemical, i.e. methylcholanthrene. Biological tests failed to reveal the presence of a cell-free agent in such tumors.

Heston and his associates (1950), at the National Cancer Institute, observed that mammary tumors could also be induced in up to 40 per cent of foster-nursed, and presumably agent-free, C3H females, provided that such females had been bred in rapid succession, and were permitted to have as many litters as possible. The average cancer age in the agent-free females was in excess of 20 months; again, the presence of a cell-free agent could not be demonstrated when extracts from 24 tumors were assayed.

By weekly subcutaneous grafting of several hypophyses, Mühlbock demonstrated (1956) that mammary cancer could be induced in a high percentage of agent-free females of certain inbred strains and their hybrids; no agent could be detected in the induced tumors by biological tests.

The Limitations of the Bio-Assay Test for the Presence of Mammary Tumor Agent

It should be emphasized, however, that our present means of determining the presence of a cell-free tumor agent are not conclusive. The test consists of preparing a cell-free extract from the tumor and inoculating such an extract, intraperitoneally or subcutaneously, into very young (usually 1 to 2 weeks old, or slightly older) mice of a presumably susceptible, but agent-free, strain. The methods of preparing the extracts vary in different laboratories. Most extracts are prepared in physiological saline solution, but some are made in sterile water. In one of the leading laboratories in routine testing of mammary tumors for the presence of a cell-free agent, a tumor extract of 10 per cent concentration is prepared in distilled water, and centrifuged, in an ordinary centrifuge, at room temperature, at 2000 to 3000 r.p.m. for 20 to 30 minutes; the supernate is then diluted with distilled water to obtain 1 : 50 and 1 : 1000 concentrations. These two concentrations are inoculated into 3-week-old, presumably susceptible and agent-free, mice. The inoculated mice are then observed for the development of mammary tumors. Their progeny is not always observed. In other laboratories, extracts are prepared in physiological saline solution and higher concentrations (such as 1 : 10) are injected. In most instances, only the inoculated mice are observed, not their progeny.

If the inoculated animals later develop mammary tumors, it is concluded that the sample tested contained the agent. If no tumors develop, it is usually concluded that the sample tested did not contain the agent, and that, under the circumstances, the tumors tested were "agent-free." Usually, such tumors cannot be transmitted through the milk.

It is apparent, however, that the extracts tested might have contained very small quantities of the agent. The methods of preparing extracts for testing may not always be those actually required for optimal conditions of bio-assay. There may exist several types of mammary tumor agents, and not all of them may tolerate suspension in distilled water, or centrifugation at room temperature. The agent may be present in such small quantities, that dilutions of 1 : 1000, or even only 1 : 50, may prevent the induction of tumors requiring a minimum quantity of infective particles. The presumably susceptible animals used for inoculation may be relatively resistant to the particular agent tested. Furthermore, it is being more and more realized that small quantities of agent may not induce tumors in the inoculated animals (or in those that acquired the agent by nursing), but tumors may, nevertheless, develop later on in their progeny. It is quite apparent, therefore, that in order to be relatively dependable, bio-assay of tumors for the presence of a cell-free agent would require careful technique, since it could be assumed that the agent may be present in low concentrations in the samples tested; should some of the extracts contain only very small quantities of infective virus particles, concentration of the extract by ultracentrifugation may be needed, rather than dilution. A sufficient number of mice of different strains would have to be inoculated and then observed through at least two successive generations. Such tests would be tedious and time consuming. Small amounts of agent would still frequently escape detection. Furthermore, the possibility is at hand that in some tumors the agent may be present in a non-infective form.

And yet, on the basis of negative inoculation tests carried out under routine conditions, many leading investigators in the field of mouse mammary carcinoma are now of the opinion that there exist "agent-free" mammary tumors. Accordingly, there would exist two groups of mouse mammary tumors: (a) one group of mammary tumors containing a filterable agent, usually transmitted by mothers' milk, but under certain conditions also transmitted by males, and (b) another group of presumably "agent-free" mammary tumors in which no filterable agent could be detected on biological tests.

A Working Hypothesis

Let us assume, on the other hand—as a working hypothesis at least—that *all* mouse mammary carcinomas contain a tumor agent, which we may or may not be able to detect with our present biological tests. In certain mammary tumors, the agent may be present in very small quantities, or in a non-infective form. There may be other reasons for the failure to detect the agent with our present, rather crude methods of bio-assay, in certain, presumably "agent-free," tumors.

There may exist several distinct types of mammary tumors which may be caused by different, although possibly related, agents. Some of the agents may be transmitted mainly by way of mothers' milk. The Bittner mammary tumor virus would represent such a type of a mammary tumor agent. Even among those transmitted mainly through the milk of nursing mothers, there may exist differences among the various high-mammary-cancer strains tested.

It has been suggested, as a working hypothesis (Gross, 1944), that at least certain human mammary tumors may be similar in their origin to those observed in mice. On the basis of such a concept it was suggested that women of families with any malignant tumors in their ancestry refrain from nursing their children. Since no more than a few hours of breast feeding, or even less, may suffice to transmit the hypothetical tumor-agent, breast feeding should be abandoned in such families *from birth* and artificial feeding substituted (Gross, 1946, 1949. Gross *et al.*, 1950). Feeding of pasteurized human milk should also be considered; a brief boiling of human milk, such as is routinely done in certain human milk banks, would serve the same purpose. Artificial feeding of a single human generation would interrupt the chain of vertical transmission of the hypothetical oncogenic agent. Breast feeding could then be again resumed.

It is realized, however, that no experimental, clinical, or statistical evidence is yet available to suggest that human breast cancer is actually caused by a milk-transmitted oncogenic virus. Statistical data do not support such a possibility (Macklin, 1959).

It is also realized that there exist certain mammary tumors in mice which are not transmitted through the milk, and in which the detection of an oncogenic virus by electron microscopy or bio-assay is most difficult, or has failed under the experimental conditions employed. Furthermore, even the Bittner mouse mammary carcinoma virus, although transmitted mainly through the milk of nursing females, is also disseminated through other routes, and also by the male.

There seems to exist a difference between mammary carcinoma occurring in female mice of certain high-mammary-carcinoma inbred lines, such as C3H, A, or R III, and human breast cancer. Electron microscopic studies of mouse mammary carcinoma reveal consistently the presence of characteristic virus particles. In contrast, electron microscopic studies of human breast cancer thus far performed, failed to detect the presence of virus-like particles in spite of careful and systematic search for such structures (Haguenau, 1959). (For review of more recent electron microscopic studies of human breast cancer, see pp. 875 and 876).

In addition, however, there may also exist other oncogenic agents, capable of inducing mammary carcinomas, which may follow a different route of transmission. As in the case of mouse leukemia, such agents may be transmitted from one generation to another directly through the germinal cells (Gross, 1949), and possibly also by other routes. Many of them would remain latent, causing no tumors, unless prompted by carcinogenic chemicals, hormones, or other inducing factors. Relatively small quantities of an agent, or the presence of the agent in a non-infective form, may cause great difficulties in experimental attempts to detect its existence on routine biological tests.

These different oncogenic agents may cause carcinomas of the mammary glands or other tumors.* There may exist morphological and other differences among the various types of mammary tumors induced by different agents. In most instances, these differences may be too subtle to be detected with our present methods.

It is realized, however, that most of the milk-agent-carrying mammary tumors develop much earlier than those presumably free from the agent. Morphologically, mammary tumors containing the milk agent are more frequently typical adeno-carcinomas with acinar structure, hemorrhagic cyst formation, alveolar, or atypical glandular form. On the other hand, among the "agent-free" mammary tumors, induced with carcinogenic chemicals, some, at least, have the morphology of squamous cell carcinomas, even with epithelial pearl formation. However, considerable variations of forms can be found among both the milk-factor-induced, and the presumably agent-free tumors.

Environmental Factors. Effect of Caloric Food Restriction

It became quite clear that mice may carry the tumor agent, transmit it to their offspring, and never themselves develop mammary carcinomas.

* Mammary carcinoma could also be induced in mice with the parotid tumor (polyoma) virus (see chapter 18).

The most obvious example would be that of a young high-breast-cancer strain C3H female. Such a mouse ingests the agent early in life with the milk of her mother, but remains in perfect health until she reaches 7 to 9 months of age. This mouse could have died, however, at the age of 4 or 5 months, before she ever had a chance to reach the tumor age; and yet, she not only carried the agent, but transmitted it to her offspring as well. In another example, a female of the high-cancer-strain A, which also carries a highly potent tumor agent, most frequently remains free from mammary cancer, even if she lives to be more than one year old, unless she was mated and became pregnant.

The development of breast cancer in females carrying the tumor agent depends not only on such obvious factors as inherited susceptibility, hormonal stimulation, and age of the carrier at the time of observation, but also on other experimental conditions, not all of them fully understood.

One of the most interesting observations dealing with the influence of environmental factors, was that dealing with the influence of restriction of the food intake on the incidence of mammary tumors developing in mice of high-breast-cancer strains.

Many investigators have studied the influence of food restriction on the development and growth of tumors (Sivertsen and Hastings, 1938). The most comprehensive studies were carried out by A. Tannenbaum in Chicago. In 1940 and in subsequent publications, Tannenbaum reported that the incidence of spontaneous tumors in mice of high-breast-cancer lines could be considerably reduced by caloric restriction of the food intake. It did not actually matter what type of food was restricted, provided that the overall total of caloric intake was reduced. The mice did not have to be starved. In order to cut down the incidence of spontaneous mammary tumors to a considerable extent, it was sufficient to reduce the food intake by 30 per cent; in some experiments, significant inhibition occurred with even smaller reduction in food intake.

The inhibition of formation of spontaneous breast tumors could be effected if caloric restriction was instituted at any time before the tumors began to appear. Definite inhibition occurred whether the mice were 2 or 5 months old at the time the caloric restricted diet was initiated. Mice on the restricted diet appeared healthy, and in general outlived the control mice, which received food without limitation.

Visscher and his associates reported (1942) that a reduction (by restriction of fat and carbohydrate intake) of approximately one-third of the total calories ingested resulted in a decrease of spontaneous mammary carcinoma incidence in virgin C3H females from 67 per cent in the controls, to zero in the caloric restricted group. The life span of the mice subsisting on the restricted diet was considerably increased over that of fully fed controls.

These studies were also confirmed and extended by White and his colleagues (1944) at the National Cancer Institute. A 50 per cent reduction in calories, without alteration in the amount of dietary essentials, reduced the incidence of mammary tumors in females of the high-cancer-strain C3H from 97 per cent to 12.5 and 18 per cent in virgin and breeding females respectively.

The most probable mechanism of the reduction of the incidence of mammary tumors by caloric restriction was through the reduction or abolishment of estrus activity mediated probably through the thyroid gland. Many physiological functions, particularly those concerned with reproduction, are depressed in such animals. However, caloric food restriction not only reduced the incidence of spontaneous mammary carcinomas, but also that of either spontaneous or carcinogen-induced leukemias, and, moreover, that of sarcomas induced with carcinogenic hydrocarbons. It would be rather difficult to explain fully this inhibitory effect of caloric restriction on the development of these different neoplasms by a hormonal mechanism.

Caloric restriction inhibited the development of either spontaneous tumors or those induced by carcinogens. It had only a limited influence, however, on the growth of tumors already established.

The influence of restricted food intake on the survival of mice with spontaneous mammary carcinomas was investigated by Tannenbaum and Silverstone (1953). Strain C3H mice with small single tumors were paired according to age and body weight, as well as size and location of the neoplasms. A total of 163 pairs of mice was used. One of each pair was fully fed (13 calories daily), the other restricted (7.4 calories). Limitation of food intake was achieved by either proportionate reduction of all dietary components (underfeeding), or by decrease of carbohydrates only (caloric restriction).

The average survival time of the tumor-bearing mice on the low-caloric rations was about 20 per cent longer than that of the fully fed controls. Furthermore, in two-thirds of the pairs, the restricted mouse outlived its respective mate. The limitation of food intake also resulted in a decreased rate of growth of the tumors, and lower frequency of metastases to the lungs (Tannenbaum and Silverstone, 1953).

Fig. 23. Mouse Mammary Carcinoma Virus.
Mature Type B Virus Particles.

Section of a spontaneous mouse mammary carcinoma from a C3H female mouse. Characteristic type B mature virus particles in intercellular spaces. The particles are spherical and have an average diameter of about 100 to 105 mμ. Most of the virus particles contain eccentrically located electron-dense nucleoids surrounded by a membrane. Magnification 90,000 $\times$. Electron micrograph prepared by W. Bernhard, Institut de Recherches Scientifiques sur le Cancer, Villejuif (Seine), France.

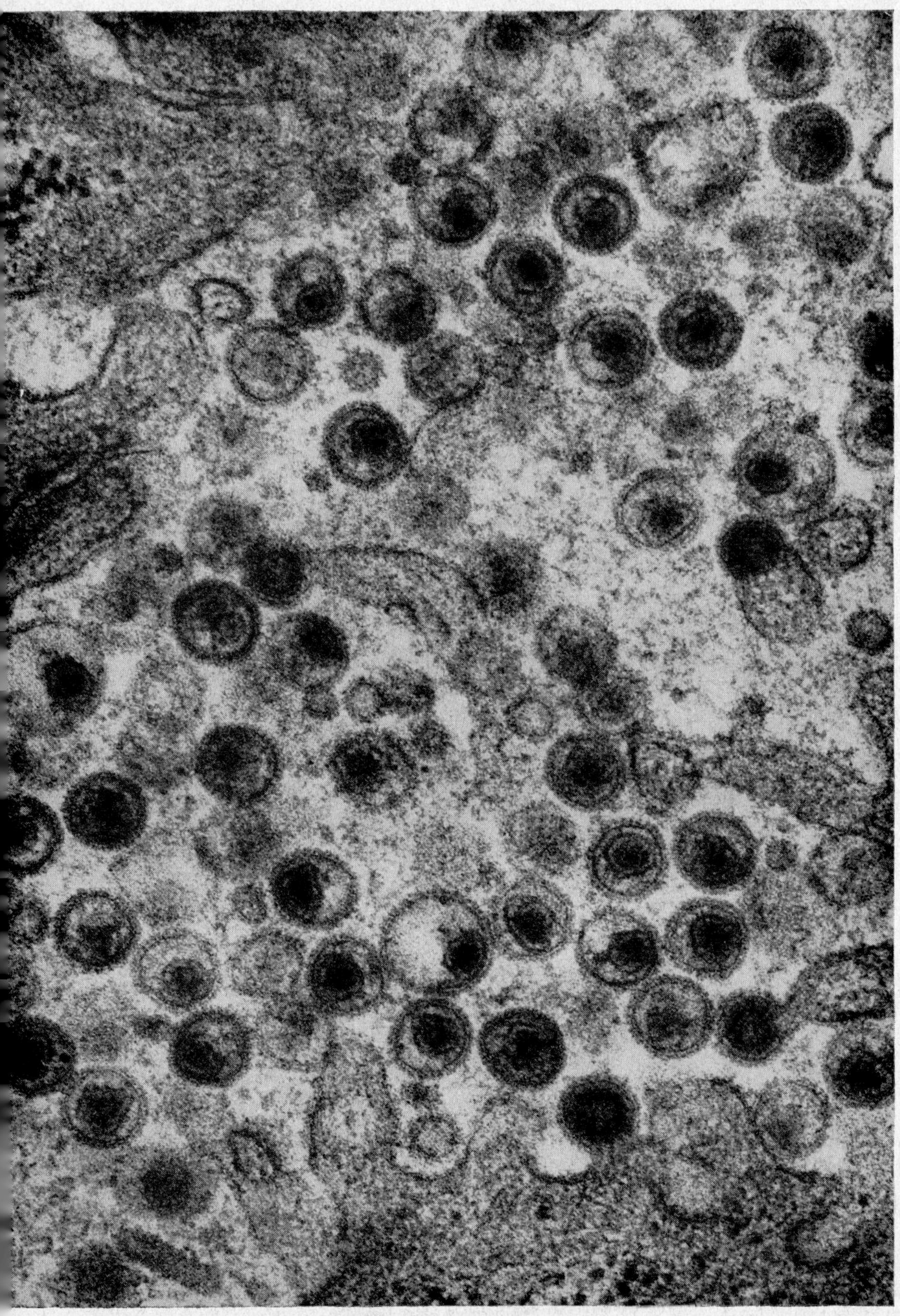

Fig. 23. Mouse Mammary Carcinoma Virus.
Mature Type B Virus Particles.

Inclusion Bodies

M. Guérin (1955, 1956) at the Institut de Recherches sur le Cancer, in Villejuif, Seine, in France, studied the occurrence of inclusion bodies in mouse mammary carcinoma. The first group of tumors studied consisted of mice of a low-breast-cancer strain I.C., developed in his laboratories by pedigreed inbreeding. Thirty adult females of this strain received a single total-body irradiation of 300 R, and 10 of them developed mammary tumors. Of these, 5 tumors showed typical cytoplasmic inclusion bodies. In addition, 52 mammary tumors of different origin, some of them transplanted, were also examined, and 6 of them had inclusion bodies. Finally, 26 spontaneous mammary tumors that developed in high-breast-cancer strain XXXIX (Dobrovolskaia-Zavadskaia) were also examined, and 4 of them had inclusion bodies.

The inclusion bodies observed by Guérin were cytoplasmic, round or oval, about 2 to 8μ in diameter, and appeared brick-red when stained routinely with hematoxylin-eosin, or with the trichrome stain of Masson. They were located in the epithelial cells of mammary adenocarcinomas, but could also be found occasionally in normal epithelial cells of the mammary gland, in the immediate vicinity of the tumor cells.

Examination of normal mammary gland cells from healthy mice, free from tumors, failed to reveal the presence of similar inclusion bodies. Whether the presence of inclusion bodies was a peculiarity of the mammary tumors examined by Guérin in his laboratory, or whether such inclusion bodies also exist in mammary tumors developing in mice of other high-mammary-tumor strains, remains to be determined. Inclusion bodies are not always readily detected; careful re-examination of microscopic slides of many mammary tumors may be needed. Special staining may be required. It is possible that inclusion bodies will be found at least in some of the mouse mammary tumors developing in strains used in other laboratories. Guérin also noticed typical inclusion bodies in some of the spontaneous mammary carcinomas developing in milk-agent-carrying C3H mice.*

Hyperplastic Alveolar Nodules in Mammary Glands of Old Female Mice. In mice carrying the mammary tumor agent the formation of hyperplastic alveolar nodules in mammary glands is common; these nodules are now considered to represent early preneoplastic lesions. The nodules appear in adult female mice of susceptible strains carrying the mammary tumor virus; they develop usually after one or several pregnancies. The initial lesions appear in some of the alveolar cells which differentiate from the duct system.

Not all nodules which develop in the mammary glands eventually change into mammary tumors. The number of nodules developing in susceptible

* Guérin, M., Personal communication to the author (1959).

mice carrying the mammary tumor virus is far greater than the number of mammary carcinomas that eventually develop in such mice. Furthermore, hyperplastic alveolar nodules can be induced in mice not only following infection with the mammary carcinoma virus; they can also develop in mice, and in rats, after application of certain carcinogenic chemicals. Such nodules do not necessarily become neoplastic. In fact, most of the nodules do not lead to the development of tumors.

DeOme and his coworkers (1959) provided experimental evidence suggesting that these hyperplastic alveolar nodules represent precancerous lesions. In their experimental studies, portions of the subcutaneous tissue and fat in the inguinal area, containing growing mammary glands, were removed in 3-week-old C3H female mice. The cleared "fat pad" sites were then employed for implantation of fragments of mouse mammary glands containing hyperplastic alveolar nodules from old C3H females. The implanted alveolar nodules gave rise to mammary tumors more frequently, and in a shorter time, than did, in control experiments, fragments of normal resting mammary glands removed from the same donor mice, and implanted under similar experimental conditions.

During the first 29 weeks after transplantation into the cleared inguinal fat pads of 3-week-old female C3H mice, 9 out of 19 nodule transplants produced mammary tumors within 21 weeks, whereas in a control experiment only 2 out of 19 normal mammary gland transplants produced tumors after 24 weeks. The transplantation of samples of normal mammary tissues resulted in outgrowths of normal mammary glands which resembled the hosts' own glands.

Electron microscopic examination of the hyperplastic alveolar nodules, which developed in mammary glands of mice carrying the mammary tumor virus, revealed presence of type B virus particles indistinguishable in morphology and abundance from those seen in mammary carcinomas in mice (Pitelka *et al.*, 1960, 1964).

Development of Alveolar Foci in Organ Cultures. When mammary tumor fragments from virus-carrying pregnant R III female mice were explanted as organ cultures on a nutrient medium, and when such explants were stimulated *in vitro* by ovarian and hypophyseal hormones, foci of epithelial alveolar hyperplasia eventually developed (Lasfargues and Murray, 1964). On electron microscopic examination, these foci were also found to be a site of viral, type B, particle production (Lasfargues and Feldman, 1963).

Induction of Hyperplastic Alveolar Nodules in Mammary Glands as a Bioassay Test for Mammary Carcinoma Agent. A high incidence of hyperplastic alveolar nodules could be induced in female mice and in castrated males of a substrain of BALB/c line (BALB/cCrgl) infected naturally, or by experimental inoculation, with the mouse mammary carcinoma virus, and following prolonged hormonal treatment; such nodules developed only occasionally in mice of the same strain observed under similar experimental conditions, but not infected with the mammary tumor virus. On this basis a bio-assay test was proposed (Nandi, 1963) for relatively early detection of mouse mammary carcinoma. This test consists of inoculating biological samples tested into newborn BALB/c mice, which are subjected subsequently to prolonged hormonal stimulation. Development of hyperplastic alveolar nodules in mammary glands of such mice after 3 to 4 months is considered a positive test result for the presence of mammary tumor agent in the samples tested.

However, there is not sufficient evidence to suggest that this test is specific. Hyperplastic alveolar nodules are frequently observed in mammary glands of female mice of certain strains, such as C3H(f) and others, which develop only a very low incidence of mammary carcinomas, or do not develop mammary tumors at all. Furthermore, similar nodules can also be induced in mammary glands of mice and rats following treatment with chemical carcinogens.

Presence of Mouse Mammary Carcinoma Virus in Blood of Virus-carrying Mice. The demonstration of the presence of mouse mammary carcinoma virus in the blood of virus-carrying mice was demonstrated by Woolley and his coworkers (1941), Bittner (1945), Hummel and Little (1949). The presence of viral activity was found to be present not only in the blood plasma, but also in the cellular fractions. In these early studies induction of mammary carcinomas was considered as the end-point of bio-assay tests determining the presence or absence of the virus in the blood of the animal donors.

More recently, Nandi and his coworkers (1966), employing the alveolar hyperplastic mammary nodule induction bio-assay test, reported that the mouse mammary carcinoma virus was associated with the red blood cell fraction in the blood of virus-carrying mice. However, the interpretation of these experiments would be more convincing if actual induction of mammary carcinomas would be the end-point of the bio-assay tests.

Electron Microscopic Studies of Mouse Mammary Carcinoma

Porter and Thompson were first, in 1948, to describe virus-like particles in mammary tumor cells grown *in vitro*. They suspected that these particles may represent a virus. At that time, however, morphological identification of such particles was not yet possible.

Examination, in the electron microscope, of shadow-cast preparations of mouse milk known, on the basis of biological tests, to contain the mammary tumor agent, was also suggestive in some experiments, and revealed the presence of spherical particles (Graff *et al.*, 1949. Passey *et al.*, 1950). Similar particles were also observed on electron microscopic examination of milk samples obtained from nursing women having a family record of cancer (Gross *et al.*, 1950, 1952. Dmochowski *et al.*, 1952). Women having a family record apparently free from cancer had fewer particles. No definite conclusions could be reached, however, in experiments dealing either with mouse or human milk, since it was, for all practical purposes, impossible to differentiate such particles from casein and lipoprotein particles also present in the milk preparations.

A new era began when the technique of ultrathin sections was developed following introduction of the ultramicrotome by Porter and Blum (1953). The method of preparation of the specimens for sectioning, including fixation procedure (Palade, 1952), was also improved. The newly developed microtome made it possible to cut not only through the cells, but also through individual virus particles. The ultrathin sections were only 20 to 40 mμ in thickness. The structure of the particles could thus be revealed, differentiating virus particles, presumably representing the tumor agent, from certain other cell components. Similarly, on ultrathin sections, the virus particles could now be readily differentiated, on the basis of their inner structure, from amorphous spherical droplets of lipoproteins or casein, in milk ducts and in milk pellet preparations.

> Kinosita and his coworkers reported (1953) the presence of particles revealed on electron microscopic examination of ultrathin sections of mouse mammary carcinomas. The particles, 140 to 180 mμ in diameter, were found in the cytoplasm and in the nucleus. The particles showed a dense region surrounded by a pale zone with a well defined boundary. This observation, made at an early stage of electron microscopy of tissue sections, was only in part correct, however, since it now has been well established that mouse mammary carcinoma particles could not be found in the cell nucleus; moreover, they are of a smaller diameter.

In a preliminary study, Dmochowski (December, 1954) reported the presence in mouse mammary carcinoma of typical particles most probably representing the causative agent. These particles were found in the cytoplasm and in intercellular spaces, and they had a characteristic internal structure, showing an electron-dense nucleoid. Only a few months later (March, 1955), in an independent study, Bernhard and Bauer reported very similar electron micrographs of spherical particles found in the cytoplasm and in the intercellular spaces of mouse mammary carcinomas. Bernhard and his colleagues (1955, 1956) gave a thorough description, differentiating between particles found in the cytoplasm and those observed outside the cellular membranes, in intercellular spaces, and inside milk ducts. All these particles were spherical, but their diameters and details of inner structure varied. In some tumors, the particles were found in large numbers; in other tumors, only very few particles could be found.

Bernhard observed (1960) that essentially two distinct types of particles could be found in mouse mammary tumors: one, designated "type A," predominantly cytoplasmic, and another, predominantly extracellular, and designated "type B." The extracellular type was characterized by an eccentric electron-dense nucleoid. This classification proved very useful in electron microscopy of tumor viruses. Even though it later became necessary to make modifications and adjustments based on more recent data and information, the currently accepted classification (*J. Nat. Cancer*

Inst., **37**: 395–397, 1966), which includes "immature" and "mature" B particles, is still based on the initial suggestions made by Bernhard, and has retained some of his original recommendations.

Classification of Virus Particles Observed in Mouse Mammary Carcinoma. The virus particles observed on electron microscopic examination of ultra-thin sections of mouse mammary carcinoma can be divided into the following three principal groups:

The A Particles. These are doughnut-shape particles with double membranes, approximately 75 mμ in diameter, with an electron-translucent center; they can be found located freely in the cytoplasmic matrix, frequently agglomerated in substantial clusters. They are often located in the area of the Golgi apparatus. They may also be found in considerable numbers surrounding the cytoplasmic vacuoles.

The vesicular-like type A particles were described by Bernhard and his coworkers (1955, 1956) in mammary tumors of mice of strains CI and C3H. The same particles were described in mammary tumors of mice of the R III and C3H strains by Dmochowski and his colleagues (Dmochowski *et al.*, 1955. Dmochowski, 1956. Dmochowski and Grey, 1957a), and more recently also in normal mammary glands of high-mammary-cancer strain DBA females (Feldman, 1963).

The Immature B Particles. The immature B particles are essentially similar to the A particles, except that they are located in the extracellular spaces and are slightly larger. These are again doughnut-shape particles, about 105 mμ in diameter, with four layers or shells of concentric membranes, and with an electron-translucent center. The four layers can be seen distinctly on electron microscopic examination of particles which are in the process of their formation by budding, or shortly after their separation from the cells. These particles are found singly, or in groups, most often in intercellular spaces, but occasionally also in cytoplasmic vacuoles.

The Mature B Particles. These particles are most characteristic for the mouse mammary carcinoma. As a rule, they can be found either singly, or more often in groups, in extracellular spaces; occasionally, however, they can be found also in cytoplasmic vacuoles. These particles are spherical, about 105 mμ in diameter; their appearance is striking, and they can be usually recognized at once, because they contain an eccentrically located electron-dense nucleoid, about 35 mμ in diameter, surrounded by a thin membrane. Occasionally, two nucleoids can be found in one particle. The particles are surrounded by two distinct layers, or shells, of outer membranes.

The B particles are so characteristic for mouse mammary carcinoma that their recognition on electron microscopic examination justifies the conclusion that the donor host, whose tissues were examined, carries the mouse mammary carcinoma virus. Usually these particles can be found in intercellular spaces, in groups consisting of both mature (with electron-dense nucleoids) and immature (with translucent centers) virus particles.

Formation of Virus Particles by Budding. Although reliable information on the sequence of virus formation is not yet available, it is possible to reconstruct tentatively the presumable manner of virus formation on the basis of serial electron micrographs thus far obtained.

The extracellular particles appear to be formed gradually by a process of budding from the cell membranes of mammary epithelium in which the virus particles are replicated. At first, a thickened crescent-shaped protrusion forms along the edge of the cell membrane. This protrusion consists of four distinct layers: two outer layers derived from the cell membrane, and two additional inner layers. Occasionally, the two inner shells are made up of intracytoplasmic type A particles previously described.

The protrusions grow, and gradually change into villiform protuberances extending finger-like from the edge of cell membranes. Eventually these protuberances become detached from the cell; the particles break off, taking with them fragments of the protuberances, which now may form circular, closed membranes around the separated particles. After the particles form, and become separated from the cells, they make their way into the intercellular spaces, then into the acini, and later into the lumen of the mammary ducts; if the mouse is lactating, the particles are then excreted with the milk.

It is possible to speculate that in some instances the cytoplasmic type A particles may represent an earlier phase of virus formation, and that they are later transformed into the extracellular types. Although details of such a transformation—if it occurs at all—have not yet been clarified, it is conceivable that the cytoplasmic type A particles gradually make their way out of the cell; after they reach the cell membrane, they leave the cell through one of the finger-like membrane protuberances resulting from the budding process. In the extracellular space, the newly formed particles are now larger than the cytoplasmic type A particles, since they acquired during the process of budding new external double membranes from the cell cytoplasm. The mechanism of the formation of the eccentric electron-dense nucleoid, seen in the mature B particles, is unknown.

In some instances, type B particles may bud from vacuolar membranes in the cytoplasm into the vacuolar spaces of the cell. As a rule, however, they

---

FIG. 24. MOUSE MAMMARY CARCINOMA VIRUS.
INTRACYTOPLASMIC TYPE A VIRUS PARTICLES.

Section of spontaneous mammary carcinoma from a $7\frac{1}{2}$-month-old C3H female mouse. Numerous type A virus particles are present in the cytoplasmic matrix. The particles are spherical, about 65 to 75 mμ in diameter; they have two concentric membranes and no internal nucleoid. Magnification 54,000 $\times$. (D. G. Feldman and L. Gross, unpublished.)

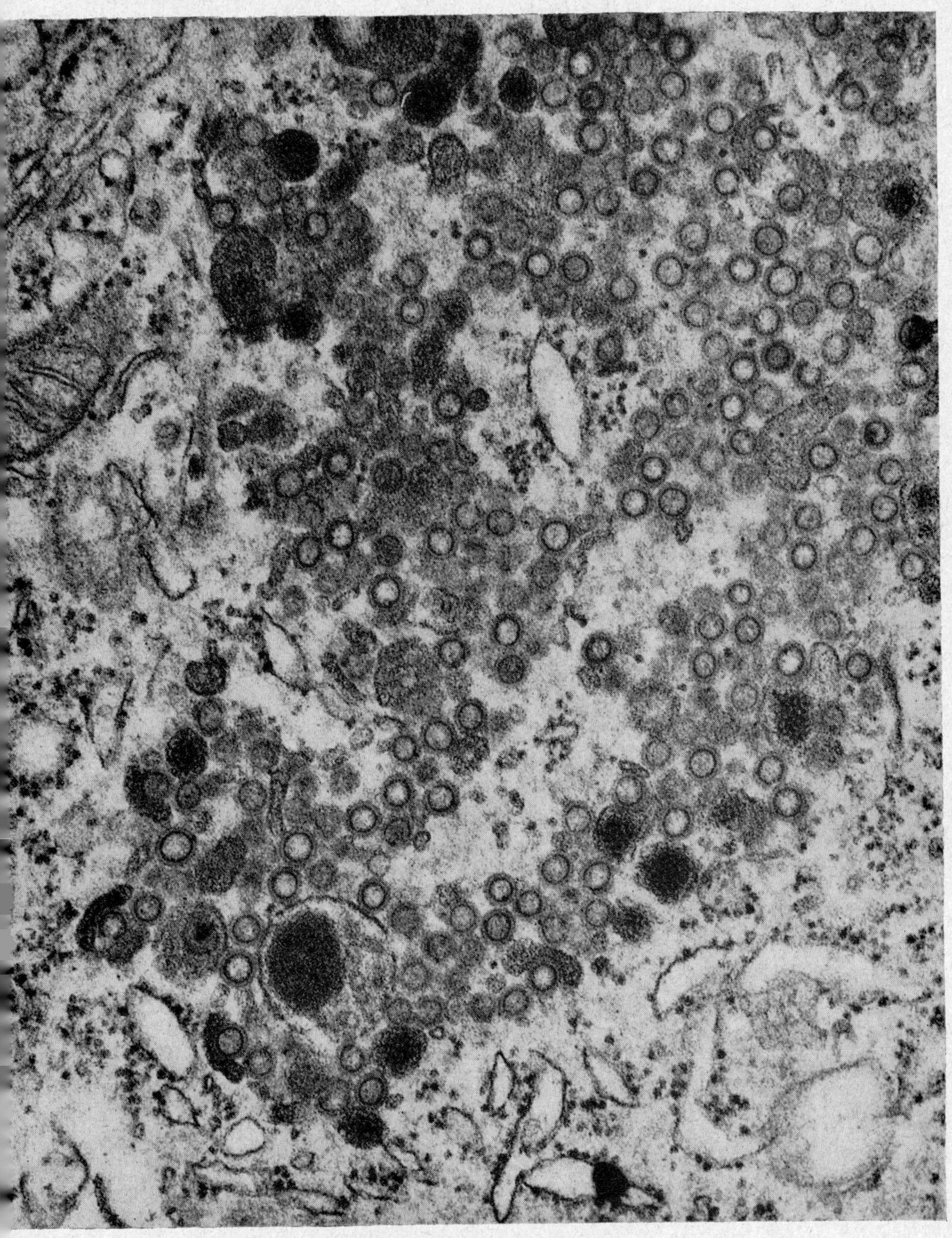

Fig. 24. Mouse Mammary Carcinoma Virus. Intracytoplasmic Type A Virus Particles.

form at the edge of the cell membranes, are then separated, and make their way into the extracellular spaces.

Most virus particles are found in spontaneous mammary carcinomas, and also in hyperplastic alveolar nodules which precede the formation of mammary tumors. Large numbers of particles can also be found in normal mammary glands during pregnancy and during lactation in mice carrying the mammary carcinoma virus.

The Presumptive Relation of the Particles Observed in the Electron Microscope to the Etiology of Mouse Mammary Carcinoma. Although the relation of the particles found on electron microscopic examination of mouse mammary tumors to the etiology of this neoplasm in mice has not been conclusively established, experimental evidence thus far accumulated is rather convincing, particularly for the B particles. In the course of years, the relation of the B particles to the causation of mouse mammary carcinoma has become more and more apparent. These particles, always of the same size and similar morphology, have now been found in mammary tumors of different strains of mice known to carry the Bittner tumor agent. Type B virus particles have been found in most of the mammary cancers of mice examined; some observers found them in every single mouse mammary carcinoma examined. In addition to their rather consistent presence in mouse mammary carcinoma cells, the type B particles can also be found in presumably normal mammary glands of pregnant or lactating female mice, and in middle-aged virgin female mice, of high-mammary-carcinoma strains, carrying the mammary carcinoma virus. There now seems to be little doubt that the type B particles are intimately connected with the mammary carcinoma in mice, and that they most probably represent the mouse mammary carcinoma virus.

The nature of the intracytoplasmic type A particles has not yet been clarified. However, they have been found consistently in mouse mammary carcinoma cells, and it is reasonable to assume that they represent a form of the mammary carcinoma virus.

Innumerable type A particles were found by Bernhard and his coworkers in the inclusion bodies described by Guérin in some of the mammary tumors examined. The inclusion bodies, filled with particles, appear in close contact with the Golgi apparatus in the cytoplasm. The development of inclusion bodies in mammary carcinomas, however, has not been generally observed.

Presence of Virus Particles in Genital Organs of Male Mice. Electron microscopic examination revealed the presence of type B virus particles in genital organs of R III and DBA male mice carrying the agent (Moore *et al.*, 1963). Similar observations were also reported by Smith (1965) who examined ultrathin sections of cauda epididymis and seminal vesicles of C3H/AnWi males carrying the mammary tumor agent.

Significantly, particles of the same size and morphology, but relatively fewer in numbers, have been found also in presumably "agent-free" mammary tumors by both Dmochowski and Bernhard. In some of the "agent-free" mammary tumors, Bernhard had to examine up to 100 cells in order to detect the presence of particles. Even though such an examination was not complete, and a few particles might have been missed in some of the cells, it illustrates the difficulties encountered. Theoretically, four hundred to six hundred ultrathin serial sections would be needed to cut through one single cell. In most of the tumors examined, however, particles could be found without too much difficulty, although they were relatively less frequent in "agent-free" mammary tumors than in mammary carcinomas known to be caused by the Bittner virus.

The presence of particles in presumably "agent-free" tumors could be explained by assuming that such tumors may appear free from an agent only on bio-assay, because the agent may be present in too small a quantity, or in a non-infective form. Actually, however, these tumors may also carry a tumor agent.

Examination of normal, healthy tissues, particularly mammary glands of young healthy mice of low-mammary-carcinoma strains presumably free from the agent, did not reveal the presence of particles. Here again, however, it would be difficult to state categorically that a prolonged search would not eventually detect the presence of a few particles. Healthy mice may carry the agent in small quantities, or in a non-infective form, even though they may remain free from tumors.

We are faced with similar problems in electron microscopic studies of mouse leukemia. Virus particles, presumably representing the mouse leukemia virus, can be found frequently in normal healthy mice of strains relatively free from spontaneous leukemia. This will be discussed in more detail in the chapter on Mouse Leukemia.

Interference between the Mouse Mammary Carcinoma Virus and the Mouse Leukemia Virus

There appears to exist a competitive interference between the mouse mammary carcinoma virus and the mouse leukemia virus. This was observed in the early studies dealing with the induction of leukemia in mice with cell-free mouse leukemia extracts. Following inoculation of the mouse leukemia virus into newborn mice of strains C3H(f) and C3H, a substantially higher incidence of leukemia developed in C3H(f) mice free from the mammary carcinoma agent, as compared with the incidence of leukemia induced under otherwise similar experimental conditions in mice of the C3H strain carrying the mammary carcinoma virus (Gross, 1957).

Recent studies by J. and C. Mouriquand (1960, 1965) in Grenoble, France, on the incidence of mammary carcinoma and leukemia developing spontaneously in a strain of mice are also suggestive of a possible interference between the viruses causing mammary tumors and leukemia. These investigators raised by brother-to-sister mating a colony of albino mice which they designated by the symbol PS. Mice of this strain apparently carry both viruses, one causing mammary carcinoma and the other leukemia. In the 13th generation of inbreeding, in a group of 212 females which reached the average tumor age (10 to 13 months), the incidence of spontaneous mammary carcinomas was 38.5 per cent, and the incidence of spontaneous leukemia was 31.5 per cent. Only 8 per cent of mice in this group developed concurrently both mammary carcinomas and leukemia.

These interesting observations, and related studies, will be discussed in more detail in the chapter on Mouse Leukemia on subsequent pages of this monograph.

REFERENCES

ADAIR, F. E., and BAGG, H. J., Breast stasis as the cause of mammary cancer. *International Clinics*, **4** (S.35): 19–26, 1925.

ANDERVONT, H. B., Susceptibility of mice to spontaneous, induced, and transplantable tumors. A comparative study of eight strains. *Public Health Reports*, **53**: 1647–1665, 1938.

ANDERVONT, H. B., The influence of foster nursing upon the incidence of spontaneous mammary cancer in resistant and susceptible mice. *J. Nat. Cancer Inst.*, **1**: 147–153, 1940.

ANDERVONT, H. B., Spontaneous tumors in a subline of strain C3H mice. *J. Nat. Cancer Inst.*, **1**: 737–744, 1941.

ANDERVONT, H. B., Effect of ingestion of strain C3H milk in the production of mammary tumors in strain C3H mice of different ages. *J. Nat. Cancer Inst.*, **2**: 13–16, 1941.

ANDERVONT, H. B., Note on the transfer of the strain C3H milk influence through successive generations of strain C mice. *J. Nat. Cancer Inst.*, **2**: 307–308, 1941.

ANDERVONT, H. B., Influence of hybridization upon the occurrence of mammary tumors in mice. *J. Nat. Cancer Inst.*, **3**: 359–365, 1943.

ANDERVONT, H. B., Fate of the C3H milk influence in mice of strains C and C57 Black. *J. Nat. Cancer Inst.*, **5**: 383–390, 1945.

ANDERVONT, H. B., Susceptibility of young and of adult mice to the mammary tumor agent. *J. Nat. Cancer Inst.*, **5**: 397–401, 1945.

ANDERVONT, H. B., The milk influence in the genesis of mammary tumors. pp. 123–139 in *Symp. on Mammary Tumors in Mice. Publ. Am. Assoc. Adv. Sci.*, No. 22, 1945.

ANDERVONT, H. B., Biological studies on the mammary tumor inciter in mice. *Ann. N.Y. Acad. Sci.*, **54**: 1004–1011, 1952.

ANDERVONT, H. B., Genetic, hormonal and age factors in susceptibility and resistance to tumor-inducing viruses. *Tex. Rep. Biol. & Med.*, **15**: 462–476, 1957.

ANDERVONT, H. B., and BRYAN, W. R., Properties of the mouse mammary-tumor agent. *J. Nat. Cancer Inst.*, **5**: 143–149, 1944.

ANDERVONT, H. B., and DUNN, T. B., Mammary tumors in mice presumably free of the mammary tumor agent. *J. Nat. Cancer Inst.*, **8**: 227–233, 1948.

Andervont, H. B., and Dunn, T. B., Influences of heredity and the mammary tumor agent on the occurrence of mammary tumors in hybrid mice. *J. Nat. Cancer Inst.*, **14**: 317–327, 1953.

Andervont, H. B., and Dunn, T. B., Studies of the mammary tumor agent carried by wild house mice. *Acta Internat. Union Against Cancer*, **12**: 530–543, 1956.

Andervont, H. B., Dunn, T. B., and Canter, H. Y., Susceptibility of agent-free inbred mice and their F_1 hybrids to estrogen-induced mammary tumors. *J. Nat. Cancer Inst.*, **21**: 783–811, 1958.

Andervont, H. B., and McEleney, W. J., Incidence of spontaneous tumors in a colony of strain C3H mice. *Public Health Reports*, **52**: 772–780, 1937.

Andervont, H. B., and McEleney, W. J., The influence of non-breeding and foster nursing upon the occurrence of spontaneous breast tumors in strain C3H mice. *Public Health Reports*, **53**: 777–783, 1938.

Bagg, H. J., The functional activity of the breast in relation to mammary carcinoma in mice. *Proc. Soc. Exp. Biol. & Med.*, **22**: 419–421, 1925.

Barnum, C. P., Ball, Z. B., Bittner, J. J., and Visscher, M. B., The milk agent in spontaneous mammary carcinoma. *Science*, **100**: 575–576, 1944.

Barnum, C. P., Ball, Z. B., and Bittner, J. J., Some properties of the mammary tumor milk agent. *Cancer Research*, **6**: 499, 1946.

Barnum, C. P., and Huseby, R. A., The chemical and physical characteristics of preparations containing the milk agent virus: A review. *Cancer Research*, **10**: 523–529, 1950.

Bernhard, W., Electron microscopy of tumor cells and tumor viruses. A review. *Cancer Research*, **18**: 491–509, 1958.

Bernhard, W., The detection and study of tumor viruses with the electron microscope. *Cancer Research*, **20**: 712–727, 1960.

Bernhard, W., and Bauer, A., Mise en évidence de corpuscules d'aspect virusal dans des tumeurs mammaires de la souris. Étude au microscope électronique. *Compt. Rend. Acad. Sci. (Paris)*, **240**: 1380–1382, 1955.

Bernhard, W., and Guérin, M., Évaluation quantitative du virus dans les tumeurs mammaires spontanées ou greffées de différentes souches de souris et étude de ses rapports avec l'appareil de Golgi. *Proc. Second Internat. Symp. on Mammary Cancer, Perugia*, pp. 627–639, 1957.

Bernhard, W., and Guérin, M., Présence de particules d'aspect virusal dans les tissue tumoraux de souris atteintes de leucémie spontanée. *Compt. Rend. Acad. Sci. (Paris)*, **247**: 1802–1805, 1958.

Bernhard, W., Bauer, A., Guérin, M., and Oberling, C., Étude au microscope électronique de corpuscules d'aspect virusal dans des épithéliomas mammaires de la souris. *Bull. du Cancer*, **42**: 163–178, 1955.

Bernhard, W., Guérin, M., and Oberling, C., Mise en évidence de corpuscules d'aspect virusal dans différentes souches de cancers mammaires de la souris. Étude au microscope électronique. *Acta Internat. Union Against Cancer*, **12**: 544–557, 1956.

Bittner, J. J., The breeding behavior and tumor incidence of an inbred albino strain of mice. *Am. J. Cancer*, **25**: 113–121, 1935.

Bittner, J. J., Some possible effects of nursing on the mammary gland tumor incidence in mice. *Science*, **84**: 162, 1936.

Bittner, J. J., Relation of nursing to the extra-chromosomal theory of breast cancer in mice. *Am. J. Cancer*, **35**: 90–97, 1939.

Bittner, J. J., Breast cancer in mice as influenced by nursing. *J. Nat. Cancer Inst.*, **1**: 155–168, 1940.

BITTNER, J. J., Further studies on active milk influence in breast cancer production in mice. *Proc. Soc. Exp. Biol. & Med.*, **45**: 805–810, 1940.

BITTNER, J. J., Changes in the incidence of mammary carcinoma in mice of the A stock. *Cancer Research*, **1**: 113–114, 1941.

BITTNER, J. J., The influence of estrogens on the incidence of tumors in foster nursed mice. *Cancer Research*, **1**: 290–292, 1941.

BITTNER, J. J., The preservation by freezing and drying in vacuo of the milk-influence for the development of breast cancer in mice. *Science*, **93**: 527–528, 1941.

BITTNER, J. J., The influence of foster nursing on experimental breast cancer. *Tr. & Stud. Coll. Physicians, Phila.*, **9**: 129–143, 1941.

BITTNER, J. J., Milk-influence of breast tumors in mice. *Science*, **95**: 462–463, 1942.

BITTNER, J. J., Observations on the genetics of susceptibility for the development of mammary cancer in mice. *Cancer Research*, **2**: 540–545, 1942.

BITTNER, J. J., Possible relationship of the estrogenic hormones, genetic susceptibility, and milk influence in the production of mammary cancer in mice. *Cancer Research*, **2**: 710–721, 1942.

BITTNER, J. J., Mammary cancer in fostered and unfostered C3H breeding females and their hybrids. *Cancer Research*, **3**: 441–447, 1943.

BITTNER, J. J., Observations on the inherited susceptibility to spontaneous mammary cancer in mice. *Cancer Research*, **4**: 159–167, 1944.

BITTNER, J. J., The genetics and linkage relationship of the inherited susceptibility to mammary cancer in mice. *Cancer Research*, **4**: 779–784, 1944.

BITTNER, J. J., Inciting influences in the etiology of mammary cancer in mice. *Research Conference on Cancer. Am. Assoc. Adv. Sci.*, pp. 63–96, 1945.

BITTNER, J. J., Characteristics of the mammary tumor milk agent in serial dilution and blood studies. *Proc. Soc. Exp. Biol. & Med.*, **59**: 43–44, 1945.

BITTNER, J. J., The causes and control of mammary cancer in mice. Harvey Lectures, **42**: 221–246, 1946–1947.

BITTNER, J. J., Some enigmas associated with the genesis of mammary cancer in mice. *Cancer Research*, **8**: 625–639, 1948.

BITTNER, J. J., The genesis of breast cancer in mice. *Tex. Rep. Biol. & Med.*, **10**: 160–166, 1952.

BITTNER, J. J., Transfer of the agent for mammary cancer in mice by the male. *Cancer Research*, **12**: 387–398, 1952.

BITTNER, J. J., Tumor-inducing properties of the mammary tumor agent in young and adult mice. *Cancer Research*, **12**: 510–515, 1952.

BITTNER, J. J., Studies on the inherited susceptibility and inherited hormonal influence in the genesis of mammary cancer in mice. *Cancer Research*, **12**: 594–601, 1952.

BITTNER, J. J., Assay of spontaneous and transplanted mammary tumors for the mammary tumor agent. *Cancer Research*, **13**: 361–366, 1953.

BITTNER, J. J., Mammary cancer in mice observed in different laboratories and during the war period. *J. Nat. Cancer Inst.*, **15**: 359–366, 1954.

BITTNER, J. J., Mammary cancer in mice of different ages and stocks following the administration of the mammary tumor agent. *Cancer Research*, **16**: 1038–1042, 1956.

BITTNER, J. J., Activity of the mammary tumor agent in mice of different ages and their progeny. *J. Nat. Cancer Inst.*, **18**: 65–76, 1957.

BITTNER, J. J., Recent studies on the mouse mammary tumor agent. *Ann. N.Y. Acad. Sci.*, **68**: 636–648, 1957.

BITTNER, J. J., Survival of the mouse mammary tumor agent (MTA) in frozen tissue. *Cancer Research*, **18**: 706–707, 1958.

BITTNER, J. J., Genetic concepts in mammary cancer in mice. *Ann. N.Y. Acad. Sci.*, **71**: 943–975, 1958.

BITTNER, J. J., Mammary-cancer-inducing and inhibitory inherited hormonal patterns in mice. *J. Nat. Cancer Inst.*, **21**: 631–640, 1958.

BITTNER, J. J., Influence of the mammary-tumor agent on the genesis of mammary cancer in agent-free mice after male transmission. *J. Nat. Cancer Inst.*, **25**: 177–199, 1960.

BITTNER, J. J., and FRANTZ, M. J., Sensitivity of females of the C stock to male infection with the mammary tumor agent. *Proc. Soc. Exp. Biol. & Med.*, **86**: 698–701, 1954.

BITTNER, J. J., and HUSEBY, R. A., Relationship of the inherited susceptibility and the inherited hormonal influence in the development of mammary cancer in mice. *Cancer Research*, **6**: 235–239, 1946.

BITTNER, J. J., and IMAGAWA, D. T., Assay of frozen mouse mammary carcinoma for the mammary tumor milk agent. *Cancer Research*, **10**: 739–750, 1950.

BITTNER, J. J., and IMAGAWA, D. T., The mammary tumor agent in extracts of frozen and unfrozen mammary cancers. *Cancer Research*, **13**: 525–528, 1953.

BITTNER, J. J., and IMAGAWA, D. T., Effect of the source of the mouse mammary tumor agent (MTA) upon neutralization of the agent with antisera. *Cancer Research*, **15**: 464–468, 1955.

BITTNER, J. J., EVANS, C. A., and GREEN, R. G., Survival of the mammary tumor milk agent of mice. *Science*, **101**: 95–97, 1945.

BITTNER, J. J., HUSEBY, R. A., VISSCHER, M. B., BALL, Z. B., and SMITH, F., Mammary cancer and mammary structure in inbred stocks of mice and their hybrids. *Science*, **99**: 83–85, 1944.

BOOT, L. M., and MÜHLBOCK, O., The mammary tumor incidence in the C3H mouse strain with and without the agent (C3H; C3Hf; C3He). *Acta Internat. Union Against Cancer*, **12**: 569–581, 1956.

BRYAN, W. R., KAHLER, H., SHIMKIN, M. B., and ANDERVONT, H. B., Extraction and ultracentrifugation of mammary tumor inciter of mice. *J. Nat. Cancer Inst.*, **2**: 451–455, 1942.

DEOME, K. B., The role of the mammary tumor virus in mouse mammary noduligenesis and tumorigenesis. pp. 498–507 in: Viruses, Nucleic Acids, and Cancer, *17th Annual Symp. on Fundamental Cancer Research, Univ. of Texas.* M. D. Anderson Hospital and Tumor Inst., Williams and Wilkins, Baltimore, Md., 1963.

DEOME, K. B., and NANDI, S., The mammary-tumor system in mice, a brief review. pp. 127–137 in: *Viruses Inducing Cancer.* Univ. of Utah Press, Salt Lake City, Utah, 1966.

DEOME, K. B., FAULKIN, L. J., JR., BERN, H. A., and BLAIR, P. B., Development of mammary tumors from hyperplastic alveolar nodules transplanted into gland-free mammary fat pads of female C3H mice. *Cancer Research*, **19**: 515–520, 1959.

DMOCHOWSKI, L., Age and dosage in the induction of breast cancer in mice by the mouse mammary tumour agent. *Brit. J. Exp. Path.*, **26**: 192–197, 1945.

DMOCHOWSKI, L., Mammary tumour inducing factor and genetic constitution. *Brit. J. Cancer*, **2**: 94–102, 1948.

DMOCHOWSKI, L., Some data on the distribution of the milk factor. *Brit. J. Cancer*, **3**: 525–533, 1949.

DMOCHOWSKI, L., Behaviour of the mammary tumour inducing agent in a transplantable mammary tumour in mice. *Brit. J. Cancer*, **6**: 249–253, 1952.

DMOCHOWSKI, L., The milk agent in the origin of mammary tumors in mice. *Advances in Cancer Research*, **1**: 103–172, Academic Press, New York, 1953.

DMOCHOWSKI, L., Discussion in: Proceedings, Symposium on 25 years of progress in mammalian genetics and cancer. *J. Nat. Cancer Inst.*, **15**: 785–787, 1954.

DMOCHOWSKI, L., A biological and biophysical approach to the study of the development of mammary cancer in mice. *Acta Internat. Union Against Cancer*, **12**: 582–618, 1956.

DMOCHOWSKI, L., and GREY, C. E., Subcellular structures of possible viral origin in some mammalian tumors. *Ann. N.Y. Acad. Sci.*, **68**: 559–615, 1957.

DMOCHOWSKI, L., and GREY, C. E., Electron microscopy of tumors of known and suspected viral etiology. *Tex. Rep. Biol. & Med.*, **15**: 704–756, 1957.

DMOCHOWSKI, L., and ORR, J. W., Chemically induced breast tumours and the mammary tumour agent. *Brit. J. Cancer*, **3**: 520–525, 1949.

DMOCHOWSKI, L., and PASSEY, R. D., Attempts at tumor virus isolation. *Ann. N.Y. Acad. Sci.*, **54**: 1035–1066, 1952.

DMOCHOWSKI, L., GREY, C. E., PADGETT, F., and SYKES, J. A., Studies on the structure of the mammary tumor-inducing virus (Bittner) and of leukemia virus (Gross). pp. 85–121 in: Viruses, Nucleic Acids, and Cancer, *17th Annual Symp. on Fundamental Cancer Research, Univ. of Texas*, M. D. Anderson Hospital and Tumor Inst., Williams and Wilkins, Baltimore, Md., 1963.

DMOCHOWSKI, L., GREY, C. E., LANGFORD, P. L., MIGLIORI, P. J., SYKES, J. A., WILLIAMS, W. C., and YOUNG, E. L., Viral factors in mammary tumorigenesis. pp. 211–256, in: Carcinogenesis: A Broad Critique. *20th Annual Symp. on Fundamental Cancer Research, Univ. of Texas*, M. D. Anderson Hospital and Tumor Inst., Williams and Wilkins, Baltimore, Md., 1967.

DMOCHOWSKI, L., HAAGENSEN, C. D., and MOORE, D. H., Studies of sections of normal and malignant cells of high- and low-cancer-strain mice by means of electron microscope. *Acta Internat. Union Against Cancer*, **11**: 640–645, 1955.

DOBROVOLSKAIA-ZAVADSKAIA, N., Sur une tumeur de souris à évolution lente et discontinue et son comportement héréditaire. *Compt. Rend. Soc. Biol.*, **103**: 994–996, 1930.

DOBROVOLSKAIA-ZAVADSKAIA, N., La fréquence des cancers chez les souris procrées par des mères cancereuses. *Compt. Rend. Soc. Biol.*, **107**: 466–469, 1931.

DOBROVOLSKAIA-ZAVADSKAIA, N., Heredity of cancer. *Radiology*, **18**: 805–808, 1932.

DOBROVOLSKAIA-ZAVADSKAIA, N., Heredity of cancer susceptibility in mice. *J. Genetics*, **27**: 181–198, 1933.

DOBROVOLSKAIA-ZAVADSKAIA, N., and ROUYER, M., Réaction à certain agents cancerigènes d'une lignée de souris exempte du cancer spontané de la mamelle (lignée XXX). *Compt. Rend. Soc. Biol.*, **127**: 383–386, 1938.

FEKETE, E., and GREEN, C. V., The influence of complete blockage of the nipples on the incidence and location of spontaneous mammary tumors in mice. *Am. J. Cancer*, **27**: 513–515, 1936.

FEKETE, E., and LITTLE, C. C., Observations on the mammary tumor incidence of mice born from transferred ova. *Cancer Research*, **2**: 525–530, 1942.

FEKETE, E., LITTLE, C. C., and RICHARDSON, F. L., The influence of blockage of the nipples on the occurrence of hyperplastic nodules in the mammary glands of C3H mice. *Cancer Research*, **12**: 219–221, 1952.

FELDMAN, D. G., Origin and distribution of virus-like particles associated with mammary tumors in DBA strain mice. I. Virus-like particles in mammary gland tissues. *J. Nat. Cancer Inst.*, **30**: 477–501, 1963.

Feldman, D. G., Origin and distribution of virus-like particles associated with mammary tumors in DBA strain mice. II. Virus-like particles in the blood and organs. *J. Nat. Cancer Inst.*, **30**: 503–515, 1963.

Feldman, D. G., Origin and distribution of virus-like particles associated with mammary tumors in DBA strain mice. III. Virus-like particles in transplanted tumors. *J. Nat. Cancer Inst.*, **30**: 517–531, 1963.

Foulds, L., Mammary tumours in hybrid mice: the presence and transmission of the mammary tumour agent. *Brit. J. Cancer*, **3**: 230–239, 1949.

Graff, S., Moore, D. H., Stanley, W. M., Randall, H. T., and Haagensen, C. D., Isolation of mouse mammary carcinoma virus. *Cancer*, **2**: 755–762, 1949.

Green, R. G., and Bittner, J. J., Neutralization of the mouse mammary cancer virus with antiserum. *Cancer Research*, **6**: 499, 1946.

Green, R. G., Moosey, M. M., and Bittner, J. J., Antigenic character of the cancer milk agent in mice. *Proc. Soc. Exp. Biol. & Med.*, **61**: 115–117, 1946.

Gross, L., Is cancer a communicable disease? *Cancer Research*, **4**: 293–303, 1944.

Gross, L., The possibility of exterminating mammary carcinoma in mice by a simple preventive measure. Its practical implication for human pathology. *New York State J. Med.*, **46**: 172–176, 1946.

Gross, L., The possibility of preventing breast cancer in women. Is artificial feeding of infants justified? *New York State J. Med.*, **47**: 866–867, 1947.

Gross, L., Hemolytic action of mouse mammary carcinoma filtrate on mouse erythrocytes *in vitro*. *Proc. Soc. Exp. Biol. & Med.*, **65**: 292–293, 1947.

Gross, L., Destructive action of mouse and rat tumor extracts on red blood cells *in vitro*. *J. Immunol.*, **59**: 173–188, 1948.

Gross, L., Destructive action of human cancer extracts on red blood cells *in vitro*. *Proc. Soc. Exp. Biol. & Med.*, **70**: 656–662, 1949.

Gross, L., The "vertical epidemic" of mammary carcinoma in mice. Its possible implications for the problem of cancer in general. *Surgery, Gynecology and Obstetrics*, **88**: 295–308, 1949.

Gross, L., Studies on the nature and biological properties of a transmissible agent causing leukemia following inoculation into newborn mice. *Ann. N.Y. Acad. Sci.*, **68**: 501–521, 1957.

Gross, L., Gessler, A. E., and McCarty, K. S., Electron-microscopic examination of human milk particularly from women having family record of breast cancer. *Proc. Soc. Exp. Biol. & Med.*, **75**: 270–276, 1950.

Gross, L., McCarty, K. S., and Gessler, A. E., The significance of particles in human milk. *Ann. N.Y. Acad. Sci.*, **54**: 1018–1034, 1952.

Guérin, M., Corps d'inclusion dans les adénocarcinomes mammaires de la souris. *Bull. du Cancer*, **42**: 14–28, 1955.

Guérin, M., Influence des rayons X sur l'apparition d'adénocarcinomes mammaires chez des souris inoculées avec de telles tumeurs contenant des corps d'inclusion. *Bull. du Cancer*, **43**: 23–36, 1956.

Guérin, M., and Vigier, P., Adéno-carcinome mammaire transmissible chez la souris adulte par un agent filtrable, cultivable dans l'oeuf et assimilable au facteur lacté de Bittner. *Bull. du Cancer*, **42**: 145–162, 1955.

Haguenau, F., Le cancer mammaire de la souris et de la femme. Étude comparative au microscope électronique. *Path. Biol.* (Paris), **7**: 989–1015, 1959.

Hairstone, M. A., Sheffield, J. B., and Moore, D. H., Study of B particles in the mammary tumors of different mouse strains. *J. Nat. Cancer Inst.*, **33**: 825–836, 1964.

HESTON, W. E., DERINGER, M. K., DUNN, T. B., and LEVILLAIN, W. D., Factors in the development of spontaneous mammary gland tumors in agent-free strain C3Hb mice. *J. Nat. Cancer Inst.*, **10**: 1139–1155, 1950.

HUMMEL, K. P., and LITTLE, C. C., Studies on the mouse mammary tumor agent. I. The agent in blood and other tissues in relation to the physiologic or endocrine state of the donor. *Cancer Research*, **9**: 129–134, 1949.

HUMMEL, K. P., and LITTLE, C. C., Studies on the mouse mammary tumor agent. III. Survival and propagation of the agent in transplanted tumors and in hosts that grew these tumors in their tissues. *Cancer Research*, **9**: 137–138, 1949.

ICHIKAWA, Y., and AMANO, S., A new type of virus found in a spontaneous mammary tumor of SL mice and its proliferating modus observed in ultrathin sections under the electron microscope. *Gann*, **49**: 57–64, 1958.

KILHAM, L., Isolation in suckling mice of a virus from C3H mice harboring Bittner milk agent. *Science*, **116**: 391–392, 1952.

KILHAM, L., and MURPHY, H. W., A pneumotropic virus isolated from C3H mice carrying the Bittner milk agent. *Proc. Soc. Exp. Biol. & Med.*, **82**: 133–137, 1953.

KINOSITA, R. ERICKSON, J. O., ARMEN, D. M., DOLCH, M. E., and WARD, J. P., Electron microscope study of mouse mammary carcinoma tissue. *Exp. Cell. Research*, **4**: 353–361, 1953.

KORTEWEG, R., Proefondervindelijke onderzoekingen aangaande erfelijkheid van kanker. *Nederland. Tijdschr. v. Geneesk.*, **78**: 240–245, 1934.

KORTEWEG, R., On the manner in which the disposition to carcinoma of the mammary gland is inherited in mice. *Genetics*, **18**: 350–371, 1936.

LACASSAGNE, A., Apparition de cancers de la mammelle chez la souris mâle, soumise à des injections de folliculine. *Compt. Rend. Acad. Sci.* (*Paris*), **195**: 630–632, 1932.

LACASSAGNE, A., Relationship of hormones and mammary adenocarcinoma in the mouse. *Am. J. Cancer*, **37**: 414–424, 1939.

LASFARGUES, E. Y., Étiologie virale des tumeurs mammaires de la souris. *Laval Médical*, **35**: 901–908, 1964.

LASFARGUES, E. Y., and FELDMAN, D. G., Hormonal and physiological background in the production of B particles by the mouse mammary epithelium in organ cultures. *Cancer Research*, **23**: 191–196, 1963.

LASFARGUES, E. Y., and MURRAY, M. R., Cell differentiation and the primary lesion in mouse mammary carcinogenesis. *Nature*, **204**: 593–594, 1964.

LASFARGUES, E. Y., and MURRAY, M. R., Comparative hormonal responses in vitro of mouse mammary glands from agent-carrying and agent-free strains. Formation of hyperplastic nodules. *Acta Internat. Union Against Cancer*, **20**: 1458–1462, 1964.

LASFARGUES, E. Y., MOORE, D. H., and MURRAY, M. R., Maintenance of the milk factor in cultures of mouse mammary epithelium. *Cancer Research*, **18**: 1281–1285, 1958.

LASFARGUES, E. Y., MOORE, D. H., MURRAY, M. R., HAAGENSEN, C. D., and POLLARD, E. C., Production of the milk agent in cultures of mouse mammary carcinoma. *J. Biophys. and Biochem. Cytol.*, **5**: 93–96, 1959.

LASFARGUES, E. Y., MURRAY, M. R., and MOORE, D. H., Cultivation of the mouse mammary carcinoma virus. pp. 167–187 in: *Symposium, Phenomena of the Tumor Viruses, Nat. Cancer Inst. Monograph No.* 4, U.S. Publ. Health Service, Bethesda, Md., 1960.

LASFARGUES, E. Y., MURRAY, M. R., and MOORE, D. H., Induced epithelial hyperplasia in organ cultures of mouse mammary tissues. Effects of the milk agent. *J. Nat. Cancer Inst.*, **34**: 141–152, 1965.

LATHROP, A. E. C., and LOEB, L., The influence of pregnancies on the incidence of cancer in mice. *Proc. Soc. Exp. Biol. & Med.*, **11**: 38–40, 1913.

LATHROP, A. E. C., and LOEB, L., Further investigations on the origin of tumors in mice. III. On the part played by internal secretion in the spontaneous development of tumors. *J. Cancer Research*, **1**: 1–19, 1916.

LATHROP, A. E. C., and LOEB, L., Further investigation on the origin of tumors in mice. V. The tumor rate in hybrid strain. *J. Exp. Med.*, **28**: 475–500, 1918.

LAW, L. W., Effect of pseudopregnancy on mammary carcinoma incidence in mice of the A stock. *Proc. Soc. Exp. Biol. & Med.*, **48**: 486–487, 1941.

LITTLE, C. C., The genetics of cancer in mice. *Biol. Reviews*, **22**: 315–343, 1947.

LITTLE, C. C., Biological aspects of cancer research. *J. Nat. Cancer Inst.*, **20**: 441–464, 1959.

MACKLIN, M. T., Comparison of the number of breast-cancer deaths observed in relatives of breast-cancer patients, and the number expected on the basis of mortality rates. *J. Nat. Cancer Inst.*, **22**: 927–951, 1959.

MARTINEZ, C., and BITTNER, J. J., Effect of ovariectomy, adrenalectomy and hypophysectomy on growth of spontaneous mammary tumors in mice. *Proc. Soc. Exp. Biol. & Med.*, **86**: 92–95, 1954.

MOORE, D. H., Mouse mammary tumour agent and mouse mammary tumours. *Nature*, **198**: 429–433, 1963.

MOORE, D. H., CHOPRA, H. C., LUNGER, P. D., and LYONS, M. J., Unpublished data. See Moore, 1963.

MOURIQUAND, J., and MOURIQUAND, C., Tumeurs mammaires et leucémies de la souche PS. Considérations étiologiques. *Path. Biol.*, **13**: 630–642, 1965.

MOURIQUAND, J., MOURIQUAND, C., and PETAT, J., Premières observations à propos d'une nouvelle souche de souris hautement cancérigène. *Compt. Rend. Soc. Biol.*, **154**: 632–633, 1960.

MÜHLBOCK, O., Mammary tumor agent in the sperm of high-cancer-strain male mice. *J. Nat. Cancer Inst.*, **10**: 861–864, 1950.

MÜHLBOCK, O., Studies on the transmission of the mouse mammary tumor agent by the male parent. *J. Nat. Cancer Inst.*, **12**: 819–837, 1952.

MÜHLBOCK, O., The hormonal genesis of mammary cancer. *Advances in Cancer Research*, **4**: 371–391, Academic Press, New York, 1956.

MÜHLBOCK, O., Biological studies on the mammary tumor agent in different strains of mice. *Acta Internat. Union Against Cancer*, **12**: 665–681, 1956.

MURRAY, W. S., Ovarian secretion and tumor incidence. *Science*, **66**: 600–601, 1927.

MURRAY, W. S., Ovarian secretion and tumor incidence. *J. Cancer Research*, **12**: 18–25, 1928.

NANDI, S., New method for detection of mouse mammary tumor virus. I. Influence of foster nursing on incidence of hyperplastic mammary nodules in BALB/cCrgl mice. *J. Nat. Cancer Inst.*, **31**: 57–73, 1963.

NANDI, S., New method for detection of mouse mammary tumor virus. II. Effect of administration of lactating mammary tissue extracts on incidence of hyperplastic mammary nodules in BALB/cCrgl mice. *J. Nat. Cancer Inst.*, **31**: 75–89, 1963.

NANDI, S., HANDIN, M., and YOUNG, L., Strain-specific mammary tumor virus activity in blood of C3H and BALB/c f. C3H mice. *J. Nat. Cancer Inst.*, **36**: 803–808, 1966.

NANDI, S., KNOX, D., DEOME, K. B., HANDIN, M., FINSTER, V. V., and PICKETT, P. B., Mammary tumor virus activity in red blood cells of BALB/c f. C3H mice. *J. Nat. Cancer Inst.*, **36**: 809–815, 1966.

OBERLING, C., Progrès récents dans l'étude des virus cancérigènes. *Presse Méd.*, **64**: 525–529, 1956.

PALADE, G. E., A study of fixation for electron microscopy. *J. Exp. Med.*, **95**: 285–298, 1952.

PASSEY, R. D., DMOCHOWSKI, L., ASTBURY, W. T., REED, R., and JOHNSON, P., Electron microscope studies of normal and malignant tissues of high- and low-breast-cancer strains of mice. *Nature*, **165**: 107, 1950.

PASSEY, R. D., DMOCHOWSKI, L., REED, R., and ASTBURY, W. T., Biophysical studies of extracts of tissues of high- and low-breast-cancer-strain mice. *Acta Biochim. and Biophys.*, **4**: 391–409, 1950.

PITELKA, D. R., BERN, H. A., NANDI, S., and DEOME, K. B., On the significance of virus-like particles in mammary tissues of C3Hf mice. *J. Nat. Cancer Inst.*, **33**: 867–885, 1964.

PITELKA, D. R., DEOME, K. B., and BERN, H. A., Virus-like particles in precancerous hyperplastic mammary tissues of C3H and C3Hf mice. *J. Nat. Cancer Inst.*, **25**: 753–777, 1960.

PORTER, K. E., and BLUM, J., Study in microtomy for electron microscopy. *Anat. Record*, **117**: 685–710, 1953.

PORTER, K. R., and THOMPSON, H. P., A particulate body associated with epithelial cells cultured from mammary carcinoma of mice of a milk factor strain. *J. Exp. Med.*, **88**: 15–24, 1948.

RUDALI, G., and YOURKOVSKI, N., L'élevage des souris de lignée pure à la Fondation Curie. *Presse Méd.*, **64**: 2045–2047, 1956.

SIVERTSEN, I., and HASTINGS, W. H., A preliminary report on the influence of food and function on the incidence of mammary gland tumor in "A" stock of albino mice. *Minnesota Med.*, **21**: 873–875, 1938.

SLYE, M., The incidence and inheritability of spontaneous tumors in mice. *J. Med. Research*, **30**: 281–298, 1914.

SMITH, G. H., The role of the milk agent in the disappearance of mammary tumors in inbred C3H/SiWi mice. (Abstract). *Proc. Am. Assoc. Cancer Research*, **6**: 60, 1965.

STAFF OF ROSCOE B. JACKSON MEMORIAL LABORATORY, *per* C. C. Little, *Director*, The existence of non-chromosomal influence in the incidence of mammary tumors in mice. *Science*, **78**: 465–466, 1933.

STRONG, L. C., The establishment of the C3H inbred strain of mice for the study of spontaneous carcinoma of the mammary gland. *Genetics*, **20**: 586–591, 1935.

STRONG, L. C., The establishment of the "A" strain of inbred mice. *J. Heredity*, **27**: 21–24, 1936.

STRONG, L. C., The origin of some inbred mice. *Cancer Research*, **2**: 531–539, 1942.

Suggestions for the classification of oncogenic RNA viruses. *J. Nat. Cancer Inst.*, **37**: 395–397, 1966.

TANNENBAUM, A., The initiation and growth of tumors. Introduction. I. Effects of underfeeding. *Am. J. Cancer*, **38**: 335–350, 1940.

TANNENBAUM, A., The genesis and growth of tumors. II. Effects of caloric restriction per se. *Cancer Research*, **2**: 460–467, 1942.

TANNENBAUM, A., The genesis and growth of tumors. III. Effects of a high-fat diet. *Cancer Research*, **2**: 468–475, 1942.

TANNENBAUM, A., and SILVERSTONE, H., The influence of the degree of caloric restriction on the formation of skin tumors and hepatomas in mice. *Cancer Research*, **9**: 724–727, 1949.

TANNENBAUM, A., and SILVERSTONE, H., Nutrition in relation to cancer. *Advances in Cancer Research*, **1**: 451–501, Academic Press, New York, 1953.

TANNENBAUM, A., and SILVERSTONE, H., Effect of limited food intake on survival of mice bearing spontaneous mammary carcinoma and on the incidence of lung metastases. *Cancer Research*, **13**: 532–536, 1953.

TAYLOR, A., CARMICHAEL, N., and NORRIS, T., A further report on yolk sac cultivation of tumor tissue. *Cancer Research*, **8**: 264–269, 1948.

VISSCHER, M. B., BALL, Z. B., BARNES, R. H., and SIVERTSEN, I., The influence of caloric restriction upon the incidence of spontaneous mammary carcinoma in mice. *Surgery*, **11**: 48–55, 1942.

VISSCHER, M. B., GREEN, R. G., and BITTNER, J. J., Characterization of milk influence in spontaneous mammary carcinoma. *Proc. Soc. Exp. Biol. & Med.*, **49**: 94–96, 1942.

WEIL, R., The hemolytic reactions in cases of human cancer. *J. Med. Research*, **19**: 281–293, 1908.

WHITE, F. R., WHITE, J., MIDER, G. B., KELLY, M. G., and HESTON, W. E., Effect of caloric restriction on mammary-tumor-formation in strain C3H mice and on the response of strain DBA to painting with methylcholanthrene. *J. Nat. Cancer Inst.*, **5**: 43–48, 1944.

WOOLLEY, G. W., Increase in mammary carcinoma incidence following inoculations of whole blood. *Proc. Nat. Acad. Sci., USA*, **29**: 22–24, 1943.

WOOLLEY, G. W., LAW, L. W., and LITTLE, C. C., The occurrence in whole blood of material influencing the incidence of mammary carcinoma in mice. *Cancer Research*, **1**: 955–956, 1941.

CHAPTER 10

Mouse Osteosarcoma

Malignant tumors of the bone develop only occasionally in mice and other animal species, but can be induced readily following administration of radium or radioactive material, particularly following oral or parenteral administration of certain radioactive isotopes, such as strontium-90, which localize in the bones.

Spontaneous Development of Bone Sarcomas in Mice. A low incidence of spontaneous bone tumors has been occasionally observed in certain strains of mice. This incidence was considerably increased by selective inbreeding of descendants of tumor-bearing mice.

This was illustrated in the following study: Pybus and Miller (1934) maintained since 1929 in their laboratory mice of the Simpson strain (Marsh, 1929). They observed in these mice in addition to a relatively high incidence of mammary carcinomas also pulmonary and liver tumors, and occasionally subcutaneous sarcomas. In 1933 it was noted that among the descendants of the original pair of mice bred in their laboratory, three animals developed bone tumors, and two developed subcutaneous sarcomas. An inbreeding by brother-to-sister mating of the progeny of the tumor-bearing mice was initiated (Pybus and Miller, 1938a); as a result of the inbreeding, the incidence of bone tumors in certain sublines increased considerably. Several substrains were developed and among them a "Special Strain" producing a very high proportion of bone tumors (Pybus and Miller, 1938a). This strain, originally developed from 3 females and 1 male, which all had developed bone tumors, had been carried through 8 generations of brother-to-sister inbreeding (Pybus and Miller, 1938b) and at that time the incidence of spontaneous bone tumors reached 53 per cent. Of 195 mice, which died after they reached the tumor age, 104 had bone tumors. The tumors were much more common in females than in males. The average age at which the tumors developed was about 15 months for females and slightly over 17 months for males. The tumors, which were frequently multiple, included osteomas, osteosarcomas with or without giant cells, chondro-osteosarcomas, and spindle-cell sarcomas (Pybus and Miller, 1938c, 1940).

At the time these experiments were carried out, the general approach to the study of the development of spontaneous tumors in mice was based on genetic considerations. However, there have been considerable changes in this approach during the last two decades, and it is now realized that many, perhaps most, of the tumors in mice are caused by oncogenic viruses. The development of spontaneous tumors in successive generations of mice may be due to the presence of an oncogenic virus transmitted from one generation to another in such animals. This is true for the mouse mammary carcinoma and for mouse leukemia, and it may also be true for mice which develop bone tumors. It is therefore possible to speculate that the development of bone tumors in mice of the Simpson strain could have been caused by the presence of an oncogenic virus transmitted in these animals from one generation to another.

Induction of Bone Tumors Following Inoculation of Oncogenic Viruses. Not many experiments have been reported on the induction of bone tumors following inoculation of oncogenic viruses. Occasionally, however, bone tumors have been induced; this was observed, for instance, in mice following inoculation of the polyoma virus. However, the development of bone tumors in such animals was unpredictable and rather rare; most of the inoculated animals developed other tumors, such as salivary gland tumors or soft tissue sarcomas. Bone tumors have been occasionally also observed following inoculation of other oncogenic viruses, including the virus of the chicken leukosis complex (osteopetrosis).

Recently, however, an oncogenic virus was isolated from a mouse osteosarcoma, which could be passed serially, and which consistently induces osteosarcomas following inoculation into newborn mice.

Isolation of a Transmissible, Filterable Agent Causing Osteosarcoma in Mice

In experiments carried out recently at Argonne National Laboratory, near Chicago, Illinois, an attempt was made by M. P. Finkel and her co-workers, Biskis and Jinkins (1966), to isolate a transmissible virus from bone sarcomas in mice. This study was prompted by evidence accumulated in recent years that most of the malignant tumors in mice, such as mammary carcinoma, salivary gland tumors, soft tissue sarcomas, as well as leukemia and lymphosarcomas, are caused by oncogenic viruses. Accordingly, a search was made for the presence of a viral agent in mouse osteogenic sarcoma. In this study, partially inbred, commercially available mice of strain CF1 (Carworth Farms line ♯ 1) were employed. Mice of this strain occasionally develop bone sarcomas; however, the incidence of osteosarcomas developing spontaneously in mice of this strain usually does not exceed 1 to 2 per cent. Similar bone tumors could be induced in mice of this strain following administration of certain radioactive isotopes, such as strontium-90 (Finkel *et al.*, 1961, 1968).

In the initial study, an attempt was made to recover a transmissible virus from 7 radiation-induced, and from 4 spontaneous mouse osteosarcomas. Centrifuged cell-free extracts prepared from the bone tumors were inoculated into newborn CF1 mice. Among the extracts tested, only one, prepared from a spontaneous bone tumor, proved to be oncogenic on inoculation tests.

Filtration of the Extracts, and Serial Virus Passage. The osteosarcoma from which the extract was prepared appeared spontaneously in a 260-day-old male mouse of the CF1 strain. The tumor, which involved the 10th, 11th, and 12th thoracic vertebrae, and the 12th rib, was removed under sterile conditions, ground in a mortar with physiological saline solution; the cell suspension thus obtained was centrifuged at 2,500 r.p.m. for 20 minutes at 0°C; the supernate was removed and again centrifuged for additional 20 minutes at 3,500 r.p.m. The second supernate was then injected subcutaneously into a newborn CF1 litter consisting of 5 mice. One of the mice that had received the extract died with an osteosarcoma of the cervical spine after 9 months. Another mouse developed a large tumor mass extending from the lower thoracic to mid-lumbar spine 11 months after inoculation. A new centrifuged extract was prepared from this tumor and injected subcutaneously into 4 newborn CF1 litters. In 9 months 12 of 24 mice developed bone tumors. Among mice in this group, 5 mice had palpable bone tumors after only $2\frac{1}{2}$ months. Four mice of this group were sacrificed, and each was found to have 2 osteosarcomas; 5 of the 8 tumors were in the spine, 2 were in the ribs, and one was in the humerus.

The tumors were removed, pooled, and again an extract was prepared; this time the extract was filtered through a 0.45 mμ HA type millipore filter. Both the centrifuged and the filtered extracts were inoculated into newborn CF1 mice; after less than 2 months tumors began to develop in both groups, i.e. in mice that received either the centrifuged extracts or the filtrate.

A third passage was made; this time only filtrates were prepared and inoculated into newborn mice of the CF1 strain. The latency elapsing between the inoculation of the extracts and the development of tumors decreased in the third passage, and in some animals tumors began to appear after only 35 days.

During a two year experimental period, 22 consecutive passages were made from the original sarcoma, and bone tumors only were induced in each passage. Some litters were resistant, whereas other litters were uniformly susceptible. In one litter 10 mice were inoculated, and within 3 months all developed osteosarcomas; most of these mice developed multiple bone tumors in the ribs, femur, tibia, pelvis, scapula, or in other bones.

Most of the tumors grew progressively and eventually invaded also the adjacent tissues; some resulted in fracture of the bone. In a few instances a small bone tumor which started to develop, later on regressed. The latent period, which frequently did not exceed 3 weeks following inoculation of the virus, was considerably shorter than that observed for radioisotope-induced bone tumors in mice. The radiographic identification of such neoplasms was made 98 days after the optimum carcinogenic amount of strontium-90 had been injected (Finkel *et al.*, 1961).

Microscopic Morphology of the Induced Bone Tumors. The virus-induced osteosarcomas appeared anywhere along the bones, first as cortical thickening and as small areas of increased density in the soft tissues adjacent to bone. Proliferative activity seemed to begin at the periosteum, and growth proceeded at first peripherally with deep cortical bone becoming involved relatively late. Microscopic examination of the induced bone tumors revealed presence of cell types ranging from fibroblasts to giant cells and osteocytes.

Electron Microscopic Studies. Electron microscopic examination of ultra-thin sections of the tumors revealed presence of virus-like particles, essentially similar in their morphology to the mouse leukemia virus. The particles were present in the intercellular spaces; some were also found budding at the edge of cell membranes; however, no adequate electron microscopic studies have yet been made which would allow a more precise description of the morphology, formation, and location of these particles in relation to cell structure. A study of the possible presence of such particles in different organs of the tumor-bearing animals would also be of interest.

Only Osteogenic Sarcomas Developed in the Inoculated Mice. The newly isolated virus appears to induce only osteosarcomas following inoculation into newborn mice. This is of particular interest since other oncogenic viruses, which may very occasionally induce bone tumors, more often cause the development of other tumors. This is true for the polyoma virus in mice, for the leukosis virus in chickens, etc.

It is therefore of considerable interest that the newly isolated virus has induced thus far, on inoculation, bone tumors only, and no other neoplasms; the relatively short latency period elapsing between the time of inoculation and the development of the tumors is also interesting.

However, it must be stressed that the information thus far available is only preliminary. The physical, biological, and pathogenic properties of this virus have not yet been adequately studied. It is possible that this virus may be capable of inducing not only osteosarcomas, but other tumors also.

The host range of the newly isolated virus will also have to be determined, as well as its possible relation to other known oncogenic viruses in mice and in related species.

Attempt to transmit human osteosarcomas to hamsters. In recent studies, Finkel and her coworkers (1968) inoculated centrifuged extracts, prepared from 38 human osteosarcomas, into newborn Syrian hamsters. Among 461 animals inoculated with extracts from the first 7 patients, 6 hamsters

(1.3 per cent) developed osteosarcomas. Electron microscopic examination of ultrathin sections revealed the presence of virus-like particles in 5 out of 6 hamster osteosarcomas examined.

REFERENCES

FINKEL, M. P., BERGSTRAND, P. J., and BISKIS, B. O., The latent period, incidence, and growth of Sr^{90}-induced osteosarcomas in CF1 and CBA mice. *Radiology*, **77**: 269–281, 1961.

FINKEL, M. P., BISKIS, B. O., and JINKINS, P. B., Virus induction of osteosarcomas in mice. *Science*, **151**: 698–700, 1966.

FINKEL, M. P., and BISKIS, B. O., Experimental induction of osteosarcomas. *Prog. Exp. Tumor Res.*, **10**: 72–111, 1968.

FINKEL, M. P., BISKIS, B. O., and FARRELL, C., Osteosarcomas appearing in Syrian hamsters after treatment with extracts of human osteosarcomas. *Proc. Nat. Acad. Sci.*, USA, **60**: 1223–1230, 1968.

FINKEL, M. P., JINKINS, P. B., TOLLE, J., and BISKIS, B. O., Serial radiography of virus-induced osteosarcomas in mice. *Radiology*, **87**: 333–339, 1966.

MARSH, M. C., Spontaneous mammary cancer in mice. *J. Cancer Research*, **13**: 313–339, 1929.

PYBUS, F. C., and MILLER, E. W., Hereditary mammary carcinoma of mice. (A description of 100 consecutive tumours.) *Newcastle Med. J.*, **14**: 151–169 1934.

PYBUS, F. C., and MILLER, E. W., Spontaneous bone tumours of mice. *Am. J. Cancer*, **33**: 98–111, 1938a.

PYBUS, F. C., and MILLER, E. W., A sex-difference in the incidence of bone tumours in mice. *Am. J. Cancer*, **34**: 248–251, 1938b.

PYBUS, F. C., and MILLER, E. W., Multiple neoplasms in a sarcoma strain of mice. *Am. J. Cancer*, **34**: 252–254, 1938c.

PYBUS, F. C., and MILLER, E. W., The gross pathology of spontaneous bone tumours in mice. *Am. J. Cancer*, **40**: 47–53, 1940.

PYBUS, F. C., and MILLER, E. W., The histology of spontaneous bone tumours in mice. *Am. J. Cancer*, **40**: 54–61, 1940.

CHAPTER 11

Mouse Leukemia

BIOLOGICAL PROPERTIES OF THE MOUSE LEUKEMIA VIRUS AND ITS PATHOGENIC POTENCY FOR MICE AND RATS

The interest in experimental mouse leukemia has been more general than that referring to leukemia in chickens. There are several reasons which account for this attitude. The anatomy, physiology, and pathology of man appear more closely related to mice than to chickens. To take an example, the chicken has no peripheral lymph nodes; even in advanced lymphatic leukemia there is, therefore, no peripheral lymph node enlargement in the chicken, whereas the lymph node enlargement is characteristic in mouse and human lymphatic leukemia. The thymus, apparently of fundamental importance in the development of certain forms of lymphatic leukemia, is located in the mediastinum in mice as well as in humans. In certain forms of leukemia, thymic tumors are common in mice and in humans. In the chicken, on the other hand, the elongated, string-like thymus is located along the deep veins of the neck and does not appear to play a particularly dominant role in the common forms of avian leukemia.

The morphology of the normal chicken blood is different from that in mice or humans, since normal red blood cells circulating in the peripheral blood of the chicken contain nuclei; on the other hand, mouse and human erythrocytes circulating in the peripheral blood do not contain nuclei. This difference may, or may not, be related to the development of certain forms of leukemia such as erythroblastosis in the chicken, very rare in man or mice. These few examples are quoted to illustrate some of the differences between the leukemias in the chicken and in man, and to stress the possibly closer relationship between normal and pathological conditions encountered in mice and humans.

Furth and his coworkers (1935) published photomicrographs in which, side by side, the morphology of human and mouse leukemic tissues and leukemic blood smears were compared; they concluded that leukemia in man is essentially the same disease as leukemia in mice. This referred to both the acute and chronic forms of lymphatic, as well as myeloid, leukemias. In mice, however, lymphoid leukemia is far more frequent than myeloid, whereas these two forms of leukemia occur with approximately equal frequency in humans.

The interest in mouse leukemia had an additional stimulus. Since 1908 (Ellermann and Bang) it has been known that chicken leukemia is caused by a transmissible virus. Obviously, it was of great interest to determine whether mouse leukemia is also of similar etiology, and whether it could be transmitted by filtrates.

It was understandable, therefore, that the study of leukemia in mice attracted the attention of many investigators. The great difficulty, however, was the lack of a sufficient number of leukemic mice for experimental investigation. The study of mouse leukemia became possible only after inbred strains of mice with a high incidence of spontaneous leukemia had been developed.

Incidence of Spontaneous Disease. The natural incidence of spontaneous leukemia developing in a large segment of a mixed population of mice is probably very low, although exact data are not available. Figures are available only on the incidence of leukemia and allied diseases in mice of certain inbred strains.

It can be safely stated that it would be difficult to find a strain of mice entirely free from leukemia or allied diseases. Now and then, particularly in older mice, leukemia or lymphosarcomas develop in most of the strains known, although the incidence is generally quite low. In some strains, such as C3H or C57 Brown, leukemia develops only occasionally. In other strains, the development of this disease is more frequent.

Even in mice of strains having a very low incidence of spontaneous leukemia, thymic lymphosarcomas or generalized leukemia can be frequently induced by total body X-ray irradiation, by application of estrogenic hormones, or by certain chemical carcinogens, such as methylcholanthrene or dibenzanthracene.

THE LEUKEMIC STRAINS OF MICE

Development of Spontaneous Leukemia in Certain Families of Mice. Maude Slye reported in 1931 the development of spontaneous leukemia and lymphosarcomas in mice of certain "tumor strains." It was apparent even at that time that leukemia may develop more frequently in certain families of mice than in others. This was attributed to genetic factors.

Later on, several inbred strains of mice having an incidence of spontaneous leukemia varying from 25 to 75 per cent were gradually developed by the untiring efforts of Little, MacDowell, Strong, Furth, and others.*

* See also "The Development of Inbred Strains of Mice ... etc." on page 229 of this monograph.

Two outstanding high-leukemic inbred lines are now available, namely strain C58 Black and the albino strain Ak. Up to 90 per cent of mice of either of these inbred lines develop leukemia spontaneously. In several other strains, a relatively high incidence of leukemia has also been observed. In DBA/2 (subline 2 of strain DBA), one of the oldest strains developed initially by Little, an incidence of spontaneous leukemia ranging from 30 to 40 per cent has been observed. In strain F, developed by Strong, an incidence of up to 40 per cent of spontaneous leukemia, mostly lymphatic, some myelogenous, has been observed by Kirschbaum and Strong (1939). In a strain of mice reported by Mercier (1937, 1940), over 30 per cent of mice developed lymphosarcomas in successive generations.

Leukemic Strain C58

The ancestors of strain C58 were brought to the Department of Genetics, Carnegie Institution of Washington, at Cold Spring Harbor, in Long Island, N.Y., in 1920 by Dr. C. C. Little.* At that time pedigreed inbreeding was initiated in several strains of mice at Cold Spring Harbor. Some of these strains were related to each other to some extent, but differed among themselves in the incidence of spontaneous tumors and in some other respects, such as color. The mice were bred by brother-to-sister mating, and several strains were developed.

Dr. E. C. MacDowell developed strain C58 Black from mating of littermates, female 58 and male 5, of Miss Lathrop's stock. This strain was then further studied by MacDowell and M. N. Richter (1935).

Before the eighteenth generation, several animals with greatly enlarged spleens were casually noted. Their occurrence in this strain was recognized as characteristic, but no particular attention was paid to them; most

* The following excerpts from a letter written to the author by Dr. C. C. Little on August 19, 1959, refer to the origin of strain C58:

> " ... When I was at Cold Spring Harbor 1919–22, I obtained, among the mice purchased from Miss A. E. C. Lathrop of Granby, Mass., two black females, C57 and C58.
>
> "I gave the latter and her descendants derived from mating her with her brother (also from Miss Lathrop) to Dr. E. C. MacDowell, my associate, in 1921.
>
> " ... The purpose of developing both C58 and C57 strains was to provide non-irradiated control lines for strains 85 and 86 (also of Lathrop origin) which Dr. Halsey Bagg and I exposed to X-rays at the old Memorial Hospital in New York City and from which we obtained genetic abnormalities.
>
> " ... The appearance of leukemia in mice of strain C58 was not premeditated or expected. MacDowell, however, was keen enough to perpetuate it by continued genetically controlled inbreeding."

animals were killed early, as soon as breeding became reduced. A few animals with large spleens were preserved, however, and later on, from microscopic sections, their condition was diagnosed as lymphatic leukemia.

In 1928 a study was made on a group of 637 mice of the C58 strain that lived at least 6 months. This was a purely random sample of mice born from generations 18 to 23. Over 85 per cent of these mice developed leukemia spontaneously. Most of these leukemias were lymphatic. Only 6 out of a total of 543 leukemias were diagnosed as myeloid, and 3 additional as "probably myeloid." Strain C58 continued to display a high incidence of spontaneous leukemia in further breeding and became a very useful tool in experimental leukemia research.

Actually, therefore, strain C58 was developed in a genetic study not related to leukemia. Later on, it was casually observed that mice of that particular strain developed spontaneously large livers and spleens; this was diagnosed as leukemia. Thus, accidentally, a leukemic strain was developed.

Strain C58 represents an excellent experimental tool providing mice which develop spontaneously lymphatic leukemia at an average age ranging from 9 to 11 months. This is the oldest inbred line outstanding for its remarkably high incidence of spontaneous leukemia.

Our own experience (Gross, 1956) with the C58 strain of mice has been as follows:

In April 1952 a litter of C58 mice was obtained from Dr. George W. Woolley of the Sloan-Kettering Institute in New York. A colony of these mice has been raised in our laboratory by brother-to-sister mating from this nucleus.

It would be difficult to estimate accurately the incidence of spontaneous leukemia among the C58 mice of our colony, because many mice were removed from records and sacrificed before they had an opportunity to reach the age at which leukemia might have developed. Some of the males and females were removed when young and healthy for either transplantation of leukemic cells or for other experiments requiring adult animals for inoculation. Among those used for breeding, many animals, particularly males, were removed from the colony and sacrificed when in good health, after they had passed their optimal age for breeding.

The earliest age at which spontaneous leukemia occurred in our colony of C58 mice was 5½ months in females, and 6½ months in males. If animals that died, or were sacrificed prior to that age, were excluded from tabulation, and if, among the surviving animals, only those were included that were allowed to die a natural death, the incidence of spontaneous leukemia in our C58 mice would be as follows:

In a sample of 132 females, 108 (82 per cent) developed leukemia at ages varying from 5½ to 18½ months (average age 9 months). In a sample of 61 males, 52 (85 per cent) developed leukemia at ages varying from 6½ to 17 months (average age 10.8 months).

Thus, the incidence of spontaneous leukemia in our colony of C58 mice was approximately 85 per cent, essentially similar to that described some twenty-five years earlier by MacDowell and Richter.

Forms of Leukemia Developing Spontaneously in C58 Mice. In a sample of 44 mice (32 females and 12 males) of the C58 strain, which developed leukemia spontaneously at ages varying from 5.5 to 17 months (average age 9.8 months), 38 mice (86 per cent) developed lymphoid tumors in the thymus, spleen, peripheral and visceral lymph nodes, and frequently also in the liver; the remaining 6 mice (14 per cent) developed no thymic tumors, but had enlarged spleens and livers, and also enlarged peripheral and visceral lymph nodes. All 44 mice in the sample studied had multiple lymphosarcomas; three mice in this group developed also reticulum-cell sarcomas in the liver and in cervical lymph nodes.

In the total group studied, 23 mice (52 per cent) with multiple lymphosarcomas had essentially no pathologic changes in peripheral blood. These 23 mice were considered to have "lymphatic leukemia," even though their peripheral blood reflected no definite basis for the diagnosis of this disease (aleukemic form). In the remaining 21 mice (48 per cent), leukemia could be recognized on the basis of examination of peripheral blood smears, which showed elevation in white blood cell counts and presence of abnormal cells. The peripheral white blood cell counts in these mice ranged from 29,000 to 163,000 (average 76,000) per mm^3. A moderate anemia was present in most of the leukemic mice examined; in a few mice anemia was pronounced; the lowest hemoglobin level was 5.9 grams per 100 ml of blood. Among 21 mice with leukemic blood changes, 13 developed lymphatic leukemia, one developed stem-cell leukemia, and 7 developed well differentiated myelogenous leukemia.

Microscopic examination of tissues of 31 leukemic mice of this group showed, in all animals, diffuse infiltration with leukemic cells not only of organs of the hematopoietic system, but also of liver, kidney, salivary glands, etc.

To summarize, in a sample of 44 spontaneous C58 mouse leukemias, the form of leukemia could be classified as lymphatic (including the aleukemic group) in 36 mice (82 per cent), myeloid in 7 mice (16 per cent), and stem-cell in one mouse (2 per cent).

As discussed in more detail elsewhere in this chapter, the term "lymphatic leukemia" is here employed in its broad meaning; it also includes aleukemic forms representing essentially localized or generalized lymphosarcomas, without significant changes in peripheral blood morphology.

Leukemic Strain Ak

Dr. Jacob Furth became interested in experimental leukemia when working about 1930 in the laboratories of Dr. Eugene L. Opie at the Department of Pathology, Cornell University Medical College, in New York City.

Dr. Furth felt that mice would be most suitable for experimental leukemia research, since from a clinical and morphological point of view mouse leukemia bears many similarities to leukemia in humans. Yet, leukemic mice could not readily be acquired for investigation. Under the circumstances, Furth decided to develop his own leukemic strain of mice.

Mice of an albino stock designated arbitrarily by the symbol A were purchased from a commercial dealer.* This stock was unrelated to Strong's stock A, or, in fact, to any other inbred strains then available. It was a non-inbred, commercial stock, claimed by the dealer to yield many cancers, including leukemias.

This stock was inbred in Furth's laboratories; it was split up into a number of families. The inbreeding proceeded by brother-to-sister mating, selection being made to breed close relatives of leukemic mice, and eliminating from breeding descendants of those mice that remained free from the disease. The inbred families were designated by a second small letter added to the capital A. In this manner, individual families designated by the symbols Aa, Ab, Ac, Ad, Ae, Af, etc., were developed. The inbreeding of several individual families was continued, and the incidence of spontaneous leukemia was recorded in each group. After some 25 generations of brother-to-sister mating, the inbred family Ak proved to have a relatively high incidence of spontaneous leukemia, about 70 per cent of mice developing lymphatic leukemia upon reaching approximately one year of age.

With great generosity, Dr. Jacob Furth offered his precious stock of mice to all interested in experimental leukemia research. The Ak leukemic stock of mice became one of the most valuable and readily obtainable tools in experimental mouse leukemia research (Furth *et al.*, 1933).

The Various Sublines of the Ak Strain. The Ak strain has been maintained in several laboratories. The stock maintained in the laboratories of the Rockefeller Institute, in New York, (Lynch, 1954) was designated AKR, or RIL (Rockefeller Institute Leukemic strain).

We obtained a litter of Ak mice in November 1945, directly from Dr. Furth, then at Cornell University. A colony of Ak mice, designated Ak-n, has been raised by brother-to-sister mating from this litter in our laboratory (Gross, 1950).

> The symbols AkR and AKR are synonymous and are both used in this chapter interchangeably. The Committee on Standardized Genetic Nomenclature for Mice (1960) recommended the symbol AKR. Some investigators, however, use the symbol AkR (see references at the end of this chapter). Actually the strain Ak was developed, and so designated, by Furth and his associates (1933). The additional letter R was added later to the Ak symbol to designate that particular subline of the Ak strain, which was maintained at the Rockefeller Institute in New York.

Actually, both the AKR and the Ak-n stocks are sublines of the same Ak inbred line. Although these sublines have now been separated for some

* The dealer's name was Detwiler, in Norristown, Pa. (Personal communication from Dr. J. Furth to the author).

20 years, each maintained by brother-to-sister mating, the incidence of spontaneous leukemia has been essentially the same in both of them. This refers also to other sublines of the Ak strain maintained in different laboratories. From time to time, however, slight variations have been recorded in the incidence of spontaneous leukemia developing in different Ak sublines. For that reason, when an experiment is carried out, each group of experimental animals should be matched with controls consisting of related mice of the same subline, and if possible also of the same generation.

The incidence of spontaneous leukemia in Ak mice varies slightly in different laboratories, but is generally higher in females than in males. In females, the incidence varies from 71 to 85 per cent, occasionally reaching 90 per cent, or even more. In males, the incidence is lower, varying from 52 to 77 per cent.

Our experience referring to spontaneous Ak leukemia (Ak-n) has been, with only few exceptions, limited to female micc. In some instances we have observed leukemia also developing in Ak males kept for a sufficiently long period of time in the breeding colony of this strain in our laboratory. We have not kept large numbers of Ak males for prolonged periods of time, however, because Ak males, when kept in cages together, fight ferociously.*

The incidence of spontaneous leukemia in a sample of 500 Ak females was, in our laboratory, 94 per cent at 8.6 months average age (Gross, 1958). Spontaneous leukemia, usually of the lymphatic type, begins to develop in Ak females approximately at 4 months of age; this incidence rises rapidly, reaching its peak at 7 to 9 months, then declines gradually.

Forms of Leukemia Developing Spontaneously in Ak Mice. In a sample of 97 mice (79 females and 18 males) of the Ak strain, which developed leukemia spontaneously at ages varying from 5.5 to 18 months (average age 8.8 months), 93 mice (96 per cent) developed lymphoid tumors in the thymus and spleen, in peripheral and visceral lymph nodes, and frequently also in the liver; four mice had thymic tumors only.

In the total sample studied, 60 mice (62 per cent) were "aleukemic," i.e. had essentially no pathologic changes in peripheral blood. All these 60 mice were considered to have developed "lymphatic leukemia," even though their peripheral blood reflected no definite basis for the diagnosis of this disease (aleukemic form). The 4 mice with thymic tumors only were in the aleukemic group.

* The hostility of Ak males could be inhibited by daily treatment with one of the tranquilizers added to the drinking water supply. Several Ak males treated in such a manner could be raised without difficulty in the same cage. This treatment did not affect the incidence of spontaneous leukemia (Dr. J. D. Levinthal, Boston. Personal communication to the author, 1959).

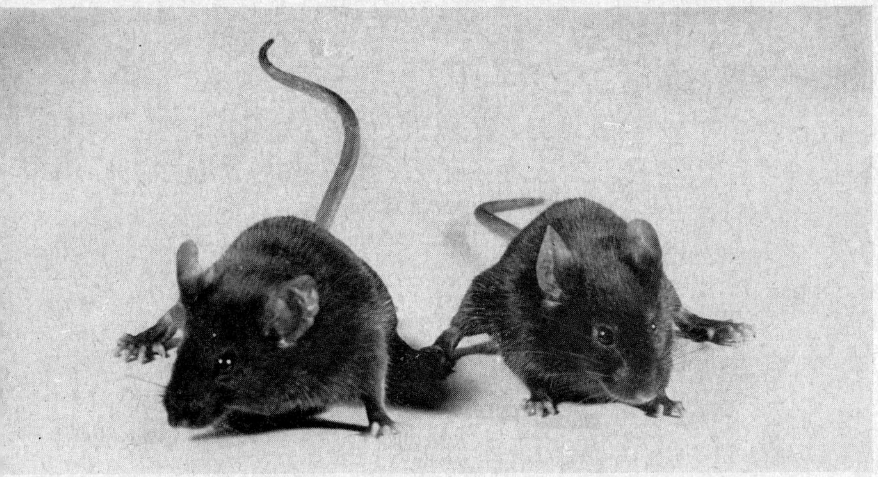

FIG. 25a. C58 MICE.

Mice of the C58 line are perfectly healthy when young. However, approximately 85 per cent of these mice develop spontaneously disseminated lymphosarcomas, or leukemia, usually of the lymphatic form, after they reach 6 months of age. (From: L. Gross, *Cancer*, **9**: 778, 1956.)

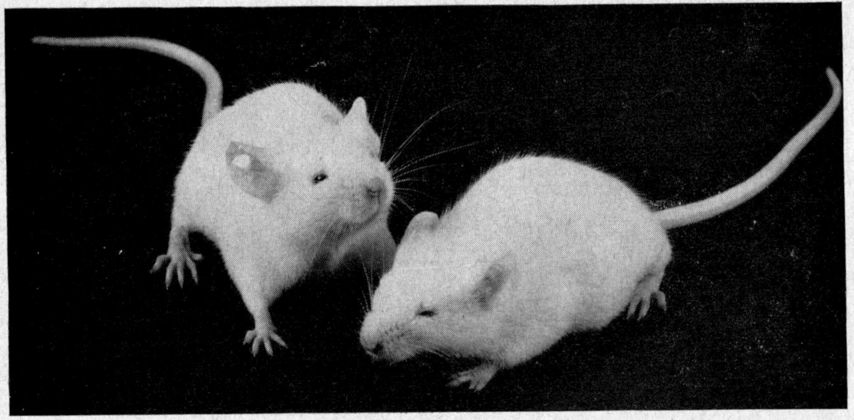

FIG. 25b. AK MICE.

Young adult male and female of the Ak inbred line. These mice remain in perfect health through early adult age. However, at the age of 6 to 9 months approximately 70 to 90 per cent of these animals develop spontaneously thymic or disseminated lymphosarcomas, or generalized leukemia, usually of the lymphatic form.

In the remaining 37 mice (38 per cent) of this total sample studied, leukemia could be recognized on the basis of examination of peripheral blood smears, which showed elevation in white blood cell counts and presence of abnormal blast cells. The peripheral white blood cell counts in these mice ranged from 23,000 to 125,000 (average 55,000) per mm^3. A moderate anemia was present in most of the leukemic mice examined. In a few mice anemia was pronounced; the lowest hemoglobin level was 2 grams per 100 ml of blood. Among the 37 mice with leukemic blood changes, 28 developed lymphatic leukemia, 5 developed stem-cell leukemia, and 4 had well differentiated myeloid leukemia.

Microscopic examination of tissues of all 97 leukemic mice in the sample studied showed in 91 mice (94 per cent) diffuse infiltration with leukemic cells not only of organs of the hematopoietic system, but also of liver, kidneys, lungs, salivary glands, etc.; in some of these mice, the infiltration was general and involved most of the internal organs; in other animals, only a few of the internal organs were infiltrated. One mouse, with multiple lymphosarcomas, developed also a Hodgkin-like lesion in one of the cervical lymph nodes. Only 6 mice (6 per cent) with lymphosarcomas in thymus only, or in thymus, spleen, and peripheral lymph nodes, had no generalized infiltration of internal organs with leukemic cells; these 6 mice were in the "aleukemic" group, i.e. they had no pathologic changes in their peripheral blood morphology.

To summarize, in a sample of 97 spontaneous Ak mouse leukemias, the form of leukemia could be classified as lymphatic (including the aleukemic group) in 88 mice (91 per cent), stem-cell in 5 mice (5 per cent), and myeloid in 4 mice (4 per cent).

It should be emphasized, as discussed in more detail elsewhere in this chapter, that the term "lymphatic leukemia" is here employed in its broad meaning, and that it also includes aleukemic forms representing essentially localized (thymic) or generalized lymphosarcomas without significant changes in peripheral blood morphology.

Host Factors Influencing Development of Spontaneous Leukemia in Mice of Leukemic Strains

Influence of Sex on the Development of Spontaneous Leukemia. Mercier was probably the first, in 1937, to notice a higher incidence of lymphosarcomas developing spontaneously in females (60 per cent) as compared with males (38 per cent) of a susceptible stock.

Cole and Furth reported in 1941 that in their colony of Ak mice the incidence of spontaneous leukemia in a sample of 118 Ak females was 71 per cent as compared with 67 per cent in a sample of 94 males. In some of the sublines of their Ak stock, this difference between the two sexes was more pronounced. In line f of the Ak stock, for example, the incidence of leukemia was 64 per cent in a sample of 161 females, as compared with only 42 per cent in a sample of 126 males. Furthermore, females developed leukemia earlier than males. Cole and Furth also reviewed the data reported by MacDowell and Richter (1935) on spontaneous leukemia developing in C58 mice; there was an incidence of 90.2 per cent in 336 females, as compared with 88.9 per cent in 270 males. The C58 strain has apparently such a high general incidence of spontaneous leukemia, that the difference between the two sexes is only very slight. When, however, in a subline of the C58 stock, the general incidence of spontaneous leukemia was lower, a difference between the two sexes could also be noticed. Law (1947) observed a higher incidence of spontaneous leukemia in C58 females as compared with males among mice of the C58 stock raised in his laboratory.

The Influence of Gonadectomy on the Incidence of Spontaneous Leukemia in Ak Mice. Ovariectomy performed by McEndy, Boon and Furth (1944) on Ak female mice, 1 to 2 months old, reduced the incidence of leukemia from 74 per cent among the controls, to 45 per cent among the ovariectomized females. When the testicles were removed from Ak males, 1 to 2 months old, the incidence of leukemia was increased from 52 per cent among the controls, to 60 per cent among the operated males. It was evident from this series of experiments that removal of ovaries inhibited, whereas the removal of testicles increased, the incidence of spontaneous leukemia in Ak mice.

Rudali and his colleagues (1956) at the Radium Institute in Paris recorded an incidence of 83 per cent of spontaneous leukemia developing at an average age of 227 days among females, as compared with 65 per cent developing at an average age of 297 days in males of their AkR stock of mice. Following ovariectomy, the incidence was reduced to 67 per cent. In males, on the other hand, orchidectomy increased the incidence of leukemia from 65 to 84 per cent. These results were essentially similar to those previously reported by McEndy and his colleagues.

Murphy reported in 1944 the results of similar experiments carried out on a Rockefeller Institute subline of the Ak strain of mice (designated RIL). The incidence of spontaneous leukemia in intact males was 53 per cent; castrated males, on the other hand, had an incidence of 97 per cent. The effect of gonadectomy was not significant in females, however. Ovariectomized females had an incidence of leukemia of 90 per cent, as compared with 88 per cent in intact control females. Treatment with testosterone proprionate of ovariectomized females decreased the incidence of spontaneous leukemia to 53 per cent.

Law (1947) carried out similar experiments on mice of the leukemic C58 strain. Orchidectomy of immature C58 males increased significantly the incidence of leukemia from 44 per cent in the controls to 76 per cent in the gonadectomized males. Ovariectomy, on the other hand, had no significant effect (60 per cent in the controls as compared with 65 per cent in the ovariectomized females).

Treatment with cortisone reported by Upton and Furth (1954), and also by Woolley and Peters (1953), decreased the incidence and delayed the development of spontaneous leukemia in mice of the Ak strain.

Effect of Splenectomy. Studies reported in 1944 by McEndy and his colleagues, and in 1950 by Law and Miller, indicated that splenectomy had no significant effect on the incidence of spontaneous leukemia in mice of either the Ak or C58 strain.

The Role of the Thymus in the Development of Spontaneous Leukemia in Ak Mice. Effect of Thymectomy

A remarkable observation referring to the effect of the removal of the thymus on the development of spontaneous leukemia in mice of the high leukemic strain Ak was reported by McEndy, Boon and Furth in 1944.

McEndy and his colleagues noticed that the thymus is almost always involved in leukemia affecting the high leukemic stock Ak. It was sometimes the only organ involved, whereas the degree of leukemic infiltration in spleen, other organs, and in lymph nodes was variable. Thus, the thymus seemed to be the most common site of the neoplastic process, and consequently it appeared advisable to determine what effect the removal of thymus, performed at an early age, would have on the incidence of spontaneous leukemia.

An experiment was therefore carried out in which young, healthy mice, 1 to 2 months old, of the leukemic Ak line, were operated on; the thymus was removed, and the mice were then kept under observation in order to determine whether the removal of the thymus would have any effect on the subsequent development of spontaneous leukemia in such animals.

The influence of thymectomy on the incidence of spontaneous leukemia was striking. Surgical removal of thymus in young, normal Ak mice, performed at 1 to 2 months of age, inhibited the development of spontaneous leukemia to a considerable degree; only 11 per cent of the 46 thymectomized males and 8 per cent of 40 thymectomized females developed spontaneous leukemia, as compared with 61 per cent and 77 per cent in males and females of the control groups.

Thymectomy did not cause a reduction of weight in the animals, neither did it inhibit their fertility.

Law and Miller (1950) at the National Cancer Institute confirmed these findings in a series of experiments carried out on mice of the leukemic strains Ak and C58. Using a substrain of the Ak stock, designated by the symbol RIL, they observed that total thymectomy, performed at 4 weeks of age, reduced the incidence of spontaneous leukemia from 83 per cent to 15 per cent. In mice of the strain C58, thymectomy reduced the incidence of leukemia from 91 per cent to 35 per cent.

It was difficult to explain the fundamental role of the thymus in the development of spontaneous leukemia in either strain Ak or C58, unless the assumption was made that the leukemic process actually originated in the thymus itself. Among mice of the leukemic strains, particularly of the strain C58, those developing spontaneous leukemia do not always show predominant involvement of the thymus. It would be possible to assume, however, that even though the process originates in the thymus, it may rapidly spread to other organs and areas of lymphoid tissues.

In a limited series of experiments Furth also investigated the incidence of leukemia in offspring of thymectomized animals (1946), and did not notice any reduction in such an incidence, as compared with that in normal, non-thymectomized, Ak mice.

More recently, an attempt was made (Gross, 1960) to determine whether removal of thymus, prior to breeding age, in males and females of several successive generations of the Ak strain, would not eventually reduce the incidence of spontaneous leukemia in descendants of thymectomized mice. Accordingly, young Ak males and females were thymectomized when approximately 3 weeks old. They were then mated. Their offspring were again thymectomized when about 3 weeks old. This procedure was repeated in the third and fourth generations. *Untreated* offspring of thymectomized mice were then observed in each generation. The incidence of spontaneous leukemia in descendants of thymectomized mice was essentially similar to that observed in offspring of normal, non-thymectomized Ak mice; neither was there a difference in the average age at which the disease appeared in both groups.

In a similar study carried out independently, Miller (1962) also observed offspring of Ak mice through 8 successive generations of thymectomized parents, and did not notice any significant difference in the incidence or time of appearance of spontaneous leukemia in descendants of thymectomized mice, as compared with controls.

*The Inhibition of the Development of Spontaneous Leukemia by Underfeeding**

Statistical data have long established a relation between body weight and the development of tumors. Experimental studies which have been discussed in the chapter on Mouse Mammary Carcinoma of this monograph have indicated that caloric restriction alone may reduce the incidence of such tumors as breast cancer in mice.

* A moderate inhibiting effect of caloric food restriction on virus-induced leukemia in mice is discussed on p. 419 of this chapter.

Saxton, Boon, and Furth (1944), at the Department of Pathology, Cornell University Medical College, in New York City, carried out a series of experiments in which a group of 47 Ak males and 47 Ak females received an amount of food permitting only the minimum of growth and gain in weight compatible with life. A mouse could be maintained on about 2 gm. of bread and milk and 1.5 gm. of dog food pellets, given on alternate days. The amount of food was determined according to the daily and weekly weight of mice, and was adjusted from time to time.

Another group of Ak males and females consisting of 52 Ak males and 59 Ak females served as controls. These mice were given the same diet, but in unlimited amounts.

At 400 days of age the underfed mice weighed about two-thirds as much as the controls. The caloric restriction inhibited fertility; during the first 6 months of the experiment, the underfed mice were grouped in cages without regard to sex, but none of the females became pregnant. At autopsy the uterus was invariably thin and the ovaries appeared inactive. In males, the seminal vesicles remained small.

The underfed mice appeared physiologically younger than the controls of corresponding age. Not only were they small, but their fur remained thick and fine in texture at an age when that of normal mice appeared more sparse and coarse. The underfed mice lived longer than the controls. The underfeeding prolonged both the average and the maximum life span. The development of leukemia in the group receiving a limited amount of food was substantially inhibited.

Mice which died when less than 6 months old were omitted from tabulation; after this adjustment, the results were as follows:

The incidence of spontaneous leukemia in the control group of Ak mice was 65 per cent in 100 normally fed control mice. In 79 related mice which received a limited amount of an otherwise adequate diet, the incidence of leukemia was only 10 per cent.

The mechanism of the retardation or prevention of leukemia by underfeeding was not quite clear. The fact that hormonal balance of the underfed mice was disturbed, as evidenced by the inhibition of the development of female and male sexual organs, was probably significant, but was hardly sufficient to explain fully the striking decrease in the incidence of spontaneous leukemia in such mice.

General Considerations Concerning the Development of Spontaneous Leukemia in Leukemic Strains

The development of inbred strains of mice having a high incidence of spontaneous leukemia was of the greatest importance in experimental leukemia research. It provoked, nevertheless, a number of questions which could not be answered at that time. The fundamental problem concerned the actual cause of the development of spontaneous leukemia. It was obvious that one of the principal responsible factors was genetic, and therefore inherited from one generation to another. It was clear, however, that genetic factors alone could not be fully responsible for the development of spontaneous leukemia in mice of a high-leukemic inbred line. Even in strain C58 having an incidence of up to 90 per cent of spontaneous leukemia, or in those sublines of the Ak strain which had a similarly high leukemic incidence, there remained always at least some 10 per cent of mice that lived their normal life span and somehow escaped the development of either leukemia or allied diseases, such as lymphosarcomas. These mice were genetically not different from their brothers and sisters which, under apparently similar conditions, developed leukemia. And yet, they remained free from this disease. Furthermore, the offspring of such non-leukemic mice developed leukemia as frequently as did the offspring of leukemic mice. Already in the early studies it became quite apparent, therefore, that genetic factors alone were not sufficient to determine the development of leukemia in mice.

Non-genetic factors also influenced the development of leukemia in mice of the leukemic strains. Among the non-genetic factors already discussed were the hormonal influence and the effect of nutrition. Females developed leukemia earlier and more frequently than males; ovariectomy or treatment with cortisone decreased, and orchidectomy increased, the incidence of spontaneous leukemia in mice of the high-leukemic stocks. Caloric restriction inhibited the development of leukemia in both sexes.

In an experiment carried out by Mori-Chavez (1958) in Lima, Peru, the incidence of spontaneous leukemia in a group of mice of the C58 strain placed in a laboratory located at the top of a high mountain, at Morococha, at an altitude of 14,900 feet, was compared with the incidence recorded in a control group consisting of mice of the same strain, sex, and age, placed in a laboratory at sea level in Lima. The same temperature, humidity, and nutritional conditions were maintained for both groups. The total number of mice tabulated for the high altitude group was 329, and 448 for the sea level group. The incidence of spontaneous leukemia among males was 45 per cent at high altitude, as compared with 66.4 per cent at sea level. Among females, 68 per cent of those kept at high altitude developed leukemia, as compared with 77.8 per cent at sea level.

It would be only logical to assume that there may exist other non-specific factors influencing the actual development of leukemia in mice of the high-leukemic strains. Such factors may include the possible influence of light, environmental temperature,* crowding, and many other obscure and difficult to evaluate conditions.

*See also p. 420 in this chapter.

It is apparent, therefore, that there may exist many non-genetic factors influencing the incidence of spontaneous leukemia in mice of leukemic strains. Only very few of these factors are known or understood.

EXPERIMENTAL INDUCTION OF LEUKEMIA BY IONIZING RADIATION, CARCINOGENIC CHEMICALS, OR HORMONES

Even in strains having a very low incidence of spontaneous leukemia, thymic lymphosarcomas or generalized leukemia could be induced in a relatively high number of animals by total-body X-ray irradiation, by application of certain carcinogenic hydrocarbons, such as methylcholanthrene, or by estrogenic hormones.

One of the most convenient and dependable methods of inducing leukemia in mice of a low-leukemic strain is fractionated total-body X-ray irradiation. This will be discussed in a more detailed manner in chapter 13 of this monograph.

Leukemia could also be induced with *chemicals.* It would be beyond the scope of this monograph to present a complete review of the literature dealing with the induction of leukemia with the various carcinogenic chemicals and hormones. In the earlier attempts, leukemia could be induced at least in some mice with benzol (Lignac, 1933), indol (Büngeler, 1932), or tar (Brues and Marble, 1939). The induction of leukemia was more readily accomplished by treatment with one of the many carcinogenic hydrocarbons, such as by repeated injections of 1,2,5,6-dibenzanthracene (Burrows and Cook, 1936), or 1,2-benzpyrene (Furth and Furth, 1938). Morton (1941), Law (1940), Kirschbaum (1940), Engelbreth-Holm (1941) and their coworkers found that cutaneous painting with, or injections of, carcinogenic hydrocarbons in mice susceptible to the development of leukemia, increased the incidence and hastened the appearance of the disease. Furth and Barnes (1941) found that even mice of a low-leukemic stock could readily be rendered leukemic by painting with methylcholanthrene.

Lacassagne reported in 1937 that prolonged treatment with *estrogenic hormones* may induce the development of leukemia in mice of a low-leukemic strain. In extensive experiments, Gardner and his colleagues (Gardner, 1937. Gardner *et al.*, 1940, 1944) induced leukemia in up to 12 per cent of mice of different low-leukemic strains by prolonged treatment with estrogenic hormones; the incidence of spontaneous leukemia in untreated controls ranged from 0 to 5 per cent.

Synergistic action of the various inducing factors, such as carcinogenic chemicals and either radiation or hormones, has also been investigated. In certain instances, a combination of inducing factors resulted in a substantially higher incidence of leukemia than the application of one inducing factor alone. Kirschbaum and his coworkers reported (Kirschbaum *et al.*, 1953) a considerably increased incidence of leukemia induced in mice of low-leukemic strains by the combined action of estrogenic hormones and either radiation or carcinogenic hydrocarbons. Kawamoto, Kirschbaum and Taylor (1958) reported that urethan was not leukemogenic for low-leukemic strains of mice when administered alone, but remarkably increased the incidence of induced leukemia when applied together with either X-rays or estrogenic hormones.

Attempt at Classification of Leukemia-inducing Factors. Fundamental Differences Between Radiation, Carcinogenic Chemicals, or Hormones, and Leukemogenic Viruses

It is quite evident from the foregoing that leukemia could be induced in mice of otherwise low-leukemic strains by a number of non-specific factors, which could be classified into three main groups: (a) ionizing radiation, (b) carcinogenic chemicals, and (c) estrogenic hormones. It should be stressed, however, that these factors are essentially not specific, and that they can exert their oncogenic potential on different species of hosts. As a rule, these inducing factors cannot be recovered from tumors they induced. Chemical carcinogens or hormones are metabolized, decomposed, and/or excreted. And yet, they induce a progressive disease.

On the other hand, there exist biological agents which are leukemogenic, but have a relatively narrow and specific host range. They can induce leukemia usually in one or two host species. These leukemogenic agents actually multiply in the inoculated hosts, and for that reason they can be recovered from the diseased tissues and passed on by inoculation indefinitely from one host to another. They are submicroscopic particles, which are thermolabile, and belong to the broad group of viruses. This method of inducing leukemia differs therefore fundamentally from the non-specific induction by carcinogenic factors previously described. It is possible to speculate that the causative agent responsible for the development of leukemia is a specific and transmissible virus, which may be carried in a non-pathogenic form by many healthy hosts. The non-specific leukemogenic factors, such as ionizing radiation, or carcinogenic chemicals, may act only in an indirect manner, activating a hitherto latent virus, and thereby causing the development of disease.

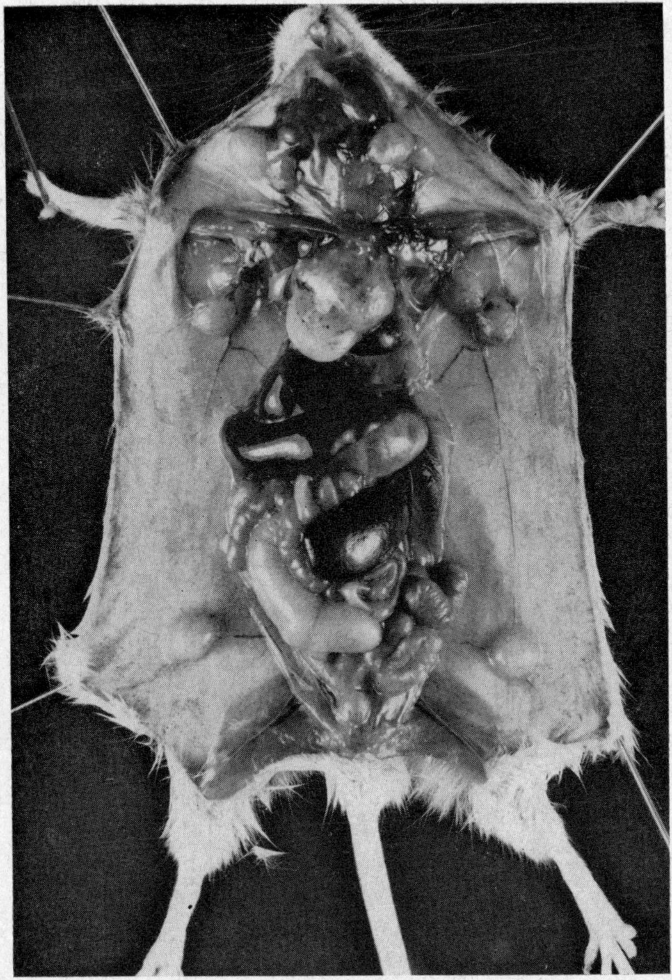

Fig. 26. Spontaneous Ak Leukemia.

Spontaneous lymphatic leukemia in an 8-month-old female mouse of the Ak-n strain. Large thymic tumor, large spleen and liver, large tumorous lymph nodes in the mesentery, in the groins, in axillary pits, and in the submaxillary area.

MORPHOLOGY OF THE MOST FREQUENTLY OBSERVED FORMS OF SPONTANEOUS OR INDUCED LEUKEMIA AND LYMPHOMAS IN MICE

The term "mouse leukemia" refers to a limited variety of forms of this disease which in mice develop either spontaneously or can be induced by X-ray irradiation, by carcinogenic chemicals, or by hormones. The most frequently observed form is lymphatic.

This is true for the great majority of strains of mice as well as for the general mouse population. The usual prominent feature of this form of leukemia is a large thymic lymphosarcoma; there is often, but not always, a concomitant enlargement of spleen, and less frequently also that of the liver. In the fully developed disease there may also be present a prominent enlargement of axillary and inguinal, as well as mesenteric, lymph nodes. Microscopic sections of internal organs, such as spleen, liver, lungs, or kidneys, show infiltration with leukemic cells, particularly in animals with generalized leukemia; this is not always the case, however, since in some mice in early phases, when the disease is limited to a thymic lymphosarcoma, there may not be any apparent infiltration of internal organs. The degree of maturation of the leukemic cells, of invasion of peripheral blood, and of infiltration of internal organs may vary; in certain instances, acute lymphoblastic or stem-cell leukemia can be observed. It is quite probable that all these pathological manifestations represent different phases of the same progressive disease rather than distinct disease entities.

Generalized Lymphosarcoma the Most Frequent Form of "Leukemia" in Mice

In the majority of mice that develop leukemia spontaneously, the peripheral blood morphology does not reflect the presence of this disease. In such animals the disease can actually be designated as a localized or, more frequently, disseminated lymphosarcoma. Many animals develop only thymic lymphosarcomas. In other animals multiple lymphosarcomas can be observed, involving thymus, spleen, liver, and peripheral lymph nodes. Less frequently, particularly in old mice, lymphosarcomas involving only the spleen or the mesenteric lymph node can be found.

The most common form, particularly in mice of the Ak inbred line, is thymic lymphosarcoma, with or without concomitant development of disseminated lymphoid infiltration of other organs. The very important, and not yet fully understood, role of the thymus in the development of spontaneous and virus-induced mouse leukemia will be discussed in more detail on subsequent pages of this chapter.

It is of interest that, according to recent studies (Siegler and Rich, 1963), the initial development of lymphosarcoma in the thymus involves at first only one of the thymic lobes. According to this study, the left and right thymus lobes of Ak mice are separate and distinct. Morphologic changes are different in these two lobes in the preleukemic period. When lymphoma develops, it usually does so only in the altered thymus lobe, and involves the opposite lobe only at a later time.

The most common form of "mouse leukemia" is therefore a localized or generalized lymphosarcoma. It is obvious that the term "leukemia" can be applied to this form of disease only in its broad and general meaning; it does not necessarily imply changes in peripheral blood morphology. Actually, the most commonly occurring form of leukemia in mice does not show leukemic manifestations in peripheral blood, and could be designated as a generalized lymphosarcoma. This form of lymphoid leukemia in mice is essentially similar to visceral lymphomatosis in the fowl, the most common form of the chicken leukosis complex.*

Myeloid leukemia also occurs spontaneously or can be induced in certain strains of mice, but is considerably less frequent than the lymphatic form. In some instances it may be difficult to recognize the myeloid form on the basis of the macroscopic picture alone. In certain instances, we have seen moderately large thymic tumors, even though such animals had myeloid leukemia. More often, however, in myeloid leukemia the thymic tumor is small, or the thymus may not be enlarged at all; on the other hand, the spleen is usually considerably enlarged. The examination of the peripheral blood and of sections of the internal organs reveals the presence of white blood cells of the myeloid series, in different degrees of maturation.

TRANSPLANTATION OF MOUSE LEUKEMIA BY CELL-GRAFT

Since we have reviewed the various methods of inducing leukemia, it should be recalled at this point that leukemia, like other malignant neoplasms, can be transmitted to normal hosts by the implantation of live leukemic cells from a genetically related donor. The transmission of leukemia from one host to another by transplantation of leukemic cells differs, however, fundamentally from the previously discussed methods of inducing leukemia by non-specific, or specific and submicroscopic, leukemogenic factors.

The biological, transmissible entities capable of inducing leukemia by

* For more detailed information on the chicken leukosis complex, the reader is referred to Chapter 7 of this monograph.

experimental inoculation can be essentially divided into two principal groups: (a) leukemic cells, and (b) filterable oncogenic viruses. Thus, leukemia, in mice, as well as in chickens, can be transmitted either by cell-graft or by inoculation of a filterable virus. Fundamentally, these two methods are also applicable to many other experimental animal tumors.

Experimental Transmission of Mouse Leukemia by Cell-Graft. Leukemia which developed spontaneously, or was induced with a carcinogenic chemical or by irradiation, can be transplanted by inoculating whole blood, or a cell suspension prepared from the leukemic organs, into another host of the same species, and preferably also of the same, or a genetically related, inbred line. In some instances, transplantation may also succeed if genetically unrelated hosts are used; this is particularly true when newborn mice are used for inoculation, and will be discussed later in a more detailed manner.

Richter and MacDowell, in the United States, first reported, in 1929, the transmission of lymphoid leukemia by cell-graft in *mice of an inbred strain* in which this leukemia originated. Mice of the leukemic strain C58, that developed spontaneously lymphoid leukemia, were used as donors. Either blood or lymphoid tumor emulsions were used for intraperitoneal or subcutaneous inoculation of young C58 mice. Leukemia resulted in from 2 to 4 weeks, and could be carried through more than 30 successive generations. Inoculation of mice of other strains did not result in the development of leukemia (Richter and MacDowell, 1929, 1930).

That same year, in 1929, Korteweg, in Amsterdam, also reported successful transmission of mouse leukemia by cell-graft. His leukemic material originated in a single mouse in which leukemia was induced by intratracheal application of tar. Transmission of this leukemia by inoculation of whole blood, or leukemic tumor emulsions, into *mice of a non-inbred stock* resulted in the development of leukemia in some of the inoculated mice. Korteweg carried his leukemic strains by successive cell-grafts through 20 generations.

In 1931, Furth and Strumia, in New York, also reported successful transmission of spontaneous lymphoid mouse leukemia. Mice with spontaneous leukemia of Furth's stock A (which served as a basis for the subsequent development of the leukemic strain Ak) were used as donors. Either whole blood or lymphoid tumor cell suspensions prepared from such donors were inoculated into young adult mice of either stock A or of the unrelated stock R. Transplantation succeeded in both stocks, though the incidence varied. Leukemia developed within 2 to 4 weeks, in some animals in less than 2 weeks, after inoculation of the leukemic cells.

In 1930 Krebs and his associates, in Denmark, successfully transmitted mouse leukemia by transplanting leukemic cells into mice of a non-inbred stock whose resistance had been lowered by preceding exposure to X-rays, but failed to transplant leukemia to non-irradiated mice of the same stock.

* * *

These were the early attempts dealing with transmission of mammalian leukemias. Transplantation of mouse leukemia became a routine procedure in many laboratories, serving as a dependable tool in experimental cancer research. This became possible after the inbred strains of mice became available for such studies.

Transplanted leukemias, i.e. leukemias carried by cell-grafts in certain strains of mice, can be essentially divided into the following three main groups: (a) those which originated as a spontaneous leukemia in a host of a high-leukemic line, such as C58 or Ak, and have been subsequently carried by cell transplantation in susceptible mice, usually of the same or a related strain; (b) those which originated as a spontaneous leukemia in a host of a low-leukemic strain, and have then been carried by cell-graft in susceptible mice, usually of the same or a related line; and, finally, (c) those which originated as a leukemia resulting from application of either ionizing radiation, or a chemical carcinogen, or hormones, in an animal, usually of a low-leukemic line, and have been carried by cell transplantation in susceptible mice of the same or a related strain.

As a rule, leukemia that developed spontaneously, or was induced by radiation, carcinogenic chemicals or hormones, in a mouse of a particular inbred line, can be transplanted by cell-graft into mice of the same, or a closely related, inbred strain. This specificity becomes less narrow after a large number of successive transplantations. In this respect, mouse leukemia does not essentially differ from other mouse tumors. After a large number of successive cell transfers, such tumors grow faster and may be transplanted, in certain instances at least, to strains other than those in which they originated. The growth of such transplanted tumors or leukemias in unrelated strains may be only temporary, and the incidence of "takes" variable, whereas transplantation in inbred strains of origin succeeds as a rule in all instances and is uniformly fatal.

The strain specificity of the transplanted leukemias is evident when adult mice are used for inoculations. The conditions are fundamentally different, however, when newborn mice are inoculated with the leukemic cell suspensions.

The Use of Newborn Mice for the Inoculation of Leukemic Cells

It has long been observed that very young animals frequently show less resistance to the implantation of tumor cells than older hosts.

Actually, the developing embryo is relatively most susceptible. Rous and

Murphy were first, in 1911, to utilize the chick embryo for the propagation of tumors. They showed that the Rous sarcoma could be grown in various parts of the embryo and its membranes. Later on, in 1912, Murphy showed that tumors of foreign species would also grow in the chicken embryo.

Immediately after birth, the newly born infant is still very susceptible. Tumors from donors of the same, or genetically related, inbred strains can be transplanted readily to newborn hosts. In certain instances, tumors from mice of genetically unrelated stocks also can be implanted successfully into newborn mice.

In certain instances, tumors that grew only with great difficulty in adult hosts could be propagated readily in newborn animals. Bunting reported in 1941 that a transplantable mammary carcinoma, which originated in a female mouse of the A strain, could be transplanted with great difficulty into adult Bagg albino mice: of 47 inoculated mice only 20 per cent developed tumors; 36 per cent of these regressed spontaneously. The same tumor, however, grew progressively and without difficulty in suckling mice of the same strain: 49 suckling mice, 1 to 2 days old, were inoculated, and 78 per cent of them developed tumors; none regressed.

Rogers, Kidd, and Rous reported in 1950 that it was most difficult to transplant into adult animals cancers arising from virus-induced papillomas in domestic rabbits. They had no difficulty, however, in growing such tumors in newborn mongrel rabbits.

Under certain conditions, tumors of foreign species could also be grown in newborn hosts. Purdy (1932) and later, in more extensive studies, Duran-Reynals (1942) used newly hatched, less than 24-hour-old, ducklings for the propagation of chicken sarcoma; within 30 days after tumor cell inoculation, solitary spindle-cell sarcomas, very similar to the original tumor, appeared at the site of implantation.

Certain mouse tumors could be grown in newborn rats, and, conversely, rat tumors could be grown in suckling mice. The growth of such transplanted tumors was usually only temporary; the tumors had to be removed and transplanted into new hosts before they regressed in the foreign soil.* In some instances, however, heterologous tumors may grow progressively in the suckling animals of the foreign species; such was the case, for example, with mouse Sarcoma 180 transplanted by Patti and Moore (1950) into suckling rats.

In 1949, it was observed in our laboratory that newborn mice of the C3H strain are highly susceptible to the implantation of Ak leukemic cells (Gross, 1950). The origin of this observation will be discussed in a more detailed manner on the subsequent pages of this chapter.

It was found that the susceptibility of the newborn C3H mouse to the

* The reader will find in the review of Woglom (1929) some of the early references dealing with the use of very young animals for the transplantation of tumors.

implantation of Ak leukemic cells decreases rapidly with increasing age. Newborn, less than 16-hour-old, C3H mice are practically 100 per cent susceptible. This susceptibility decreases gradually during the first week, and much more rapidly during the second week of life. At weaning age, i.e. when the mice are about 21 days old, they are, with only rare exceptions, resistant to the implantation of Ak leukemic cells. This resistance is substantial, and the young mouse will tolerate perhaps 1000 or 10,000 tumor-inducing doses. However, an overwhelming quantity of tumor cells, such as, for example, 2 cc. of a 20 per cent tumor cell suspension, inoculated intraperitoneally, may still induce leukemia in some of the inoculated mice.

When other strains are used for the inoculation of Ak leukemic cells, the decline in susceptibility of the newborn may be even more rapid. Newborn mice of the C57 Black strain, for example, are fully susceptible; very rapidly, however, with increasing age, their susceptibility diminishes. Suckling mice, only a few days old, are already resistant. Adult C57 Black mice are completely resistant to the inoculation of Ak leukemic cells.

These observations refer to the inoculation of cell suspensions prepared from spontaneous Ak leukemia. Such leukemia retains its strain specificity. Cell suspensions prepared from spontaneous Ak leukemia will consistently reproduce leukemia when inoculated into mice of the Ak strain, but will not induce leukemia when injected into adult mice of foreign strains, such as C3H or C57 Black. When, however, spontaneous Ak leukemia is successively transplanted in Ak mice, it may gradually lose its strain specificity. After some one or two hundred consecutive passages, such leukemia may be successfully transplanted to adult mice of certain genetically related strains.

This is true for other transplantable tumors also. Certain tumors, such as Sarcoma 180, or Sarcoma 37, or certain Ehrlich carcinomas, have been transplanted for many years through hundreds of successive hosts; as a result they eventually lost their strain specificity, and now grow in adult mice of several strains, including non-inbred stocks.

The Nature of Leukemia Resulting from Implantation of Ak Leukemic Cells into Newborn C3H Mice

When leukemic cells from Ak spontaneous leukemia are inoculated subcutaneously into a newborn mouse of the C3H strain, the implanted cells multiply rapidly, forming, at first, a local tumor at the site of implantation. This tumor appears within about 7 to 12 days. A few days later generalized leukemia follows, and all such mice die within the next few days. Leukemia thus developing in the newborn C3H mouse retains its original Ak strain specificity. The lymphoid tumors can be removed from the young C3H mouse and transplanted without difficulty back to adult

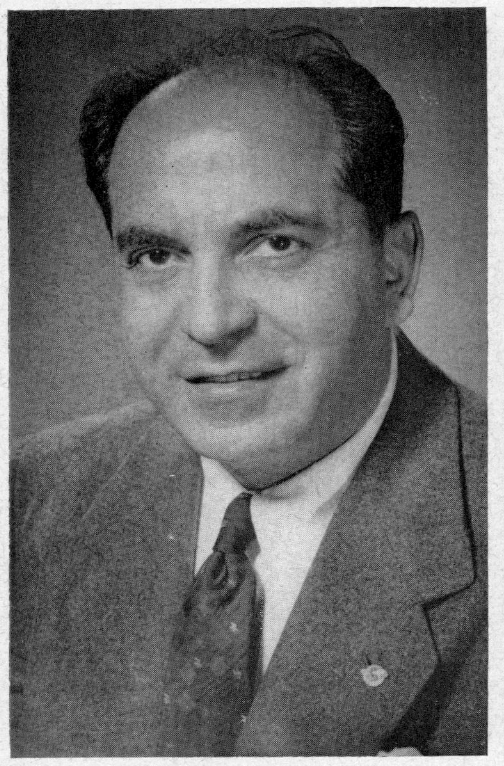

Ludwik Gross

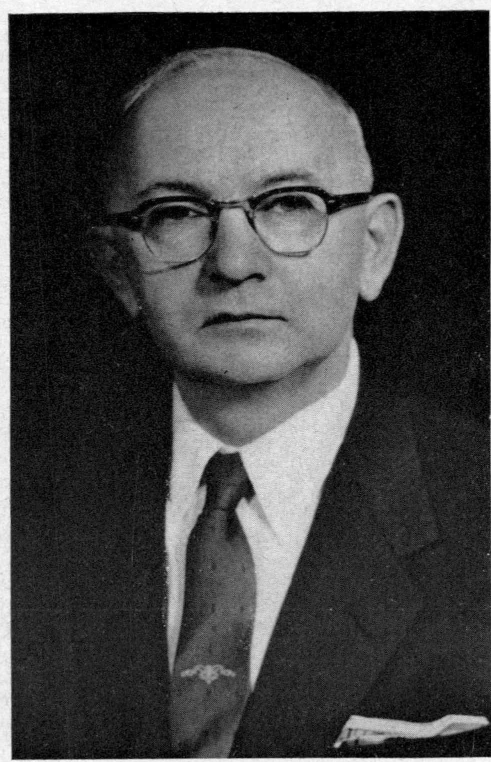

Jacob Furth

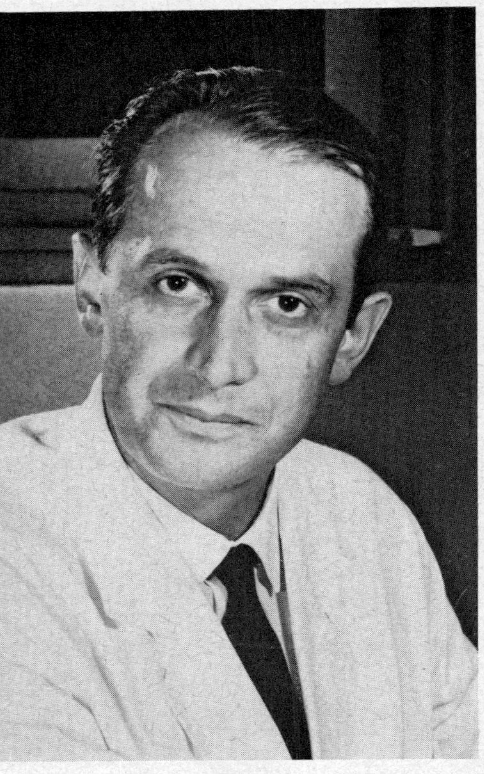

Wilhelm Bernhard

Fig. 27

Ak mice, inducing promptly leukemia in the inoculated Ak mice. In most instances these lymphoid tumors cannot be transplanted to adult C3H mice.

Such transplantation tests provide an excellent illustration demonstrating that the transplanted Ak cells retain their genetic (Ak) specificity even though they are grown in the C3H host. The latter serves only as a suitable medium providing food and shelter for the multiplying Ak cells.

Adaptation of the implanted Ak cells to the new environment may occasionally occur, however. Now and then, the Ak leukemic tumors growing in newborn C3H hosts may gradually acquire the ability to grow, on subsequent transplantation, in adult hosts of both the Ak and C3H strains.

* * *

The observation that newborn mice of an otherwise resistant strain were susceptible to the inoculation of leukemic cells prepared from a donor of an alien strain was interesting not only from a theoretical, but also from a practical point of view. Mouse leukemia could now be transplanted from one strain to another, provided that newborn hosts were used for inoculation; not all strain barriers, however, could be bridged.

The method of using newborn hosts for the propagation of leukemia, first devised on mice, was soon applied to rats. Shay and his coworkers, at Temple University in Philadelphia, had difficulty in transplanting a methylcholanthrene-induced lymphatic leukemia in adult rats of a random-bred Wistar colony. After the successful use of newborn C3H mice for transplantation of Ak leukemia was reported, however, Shay and his colleagues employed suckling rats, 1 to 7 days old, instead of adult animals, for the transplantation of their methylcholanthrene-induced leukemia. All suckling rats in this age group developed leukemia following inoculation of the leukemic cells. Transfer of leukemia succeeded uniformly also to suckling rats, 1 to 7 days old, of the random-bred Sherman and Long-Evans strains (Shay *et al.*, 1950).

"*Acquired Tolerance*"

The fact that newborn C3H mice were susceptible to the implantation of leukemic cells prepared from a donor of Ak strain could be considered essentially similar to the phenomenon of "acquired tolerance" to grafts of normal tissues, induced experimentally in very young hosts by Billingham, Brent and Medawar, at the University College, in London. The English authors reported in 1953 an ingenious method consisting of inoculating embryos of one mouse strain with blood, or suspensions of other types of living tissue cells, from another, unrelated strain. After birth, such pre-treated hosts could then be grafted with fragments of normal tissues, such as skin, from the original foreign donor strain; these animals were incapable of reacting immunologically against the foreign implants. This "tolerance" was specific and extended only to grafts from the foreign strain used to provide cells for the intra-embryonic inoculation (Billingham *et al.*, 1953, 1956).

For example, mouse embryos of the A strain were injected, usually on the 16th or 17th day of fetal life, while they were carried in the wombs of their mothers, with suspensions of living cells prepared from normal adult donors of a different inbred line, such as CBA. After birth, when several weeks old, such pre-treated hosts could then be grafted with CBA skin. These skin homografts became incorporated, and grew a batch of dark hair surrounded by the white color of the strain A host's normal hair. Tolerance could also be induced by inoculating intravenously foreign cells into newborn hosts within a few hours after birth.

The acquired tolerance induced in a given host did not always last for a prolonged period of time, i.e. it was not necessarily complete. Furthermore, it could be summarily abolished by inoculating the tolerant animal with a cell suspension prepared from the regional lymph nodes of other members of its own strain. If, for example, an A strain mouse carried a homograft from a donor of CBA strain, then tolerance could be abolished, and the tolerated homograft could be caused to slough away, by either of the following methods: (a) injecting the tolerant A mouse with cells from lymph nodes of normal A mice which had been previously sensitized ("immunized") by homografts of CBA strain skin; or, (b) by injecting the tolerant mouse with cells from lymph nodes of normal, non-sensitized A mice. The former method was rapid: the involution of the, until then, tolerated homografts began within a few days and was completed within 2 weeks. The injection of normal lymph node cells from non-sensitized animals was a slower method, but also resulted in the abolition of tolerance.

There is, on the surface at least, a striking similarity between the "acquired tolerance" to foreign cells, described by Billingham and his colleagues in 1953, and the susceptibility of newborn C3H or C57 Black mice to the implantation of Ak, leukemic cells (Gross, 1950).

Actually, however, there are certain differences between these two phenomena.

"Acquired tolerance" is not a natural, physiological state of the host, but is induced experimentally by inoculating foreign cells either during the host's fetal life or immediately after birth. The state of tolerance thus acquired as a consequence of this early exposure to the foreign cells is revealed experimentally on the basis of the subject's inability to reject a subsequent test graft from the original donor strain.

In contrast, the newborn C3H or C57 Black mouse is naturally susceptible (or "tolerant") to the implantation of Ak leukemic cells. No preparatory treatment is necessary. The implanted leukemic cells multiply in the host, which is naturally susceptible at that early age to the graft of leukemic cells originating from a foreign strain.

Once the Ak leukemic cells have been successfully grafted in the newborn C3H or C57 Black mice, they multiply rapidly; the resulting tumors grow progressively and almost invariably kill their hosts. No immunological procedure is yet known that is capable of abolishing the susceptibility of the inoculated newborn C3H or C57 Black mice to the growing tumors, transplanted from the foreign strain.

This is in striking contrast to the phenomenon of "acquired tolerance," which can be abolished, at will, by the injection of a cell suspension prepared from either sensitized or normal animals of the host's strain.

This interpretation, however, was not shared by Dr. R. E. Billingham, then at the Wistar Institute in Philadelphia, who felt that the two phenomena were, in fact, identical. Excerpts from Dr. Billingham's letter to the author, written on October 21, 1959, and referring to this matter, follow:

"The inoculation of newborn C3H or C57 Black mice with Ak leukemic cells is, in effect, a treatment or exposure of these mice to the Ak tissue cells, just as in our own experiments inoculation of newborn A strain mice with CBA cells was. In both of our studies there is every reason for believing, or in fact knowing, that some of the inoculated cells survived indefinitely and continued to proliferate in the foreign host. You inferred this from the appearance of tumors; we have been able to establish this by doing appropriate chimera tests. In our own experiments the grafting of skin to neonatally inoculated animals was a simple test to find out whether or not they were tolerant and, by implication, whether the inoculated cells still survived within them. It is therefore questionable whether your own hosts are *naturally* susceptible to the grafted leukemic cells of foreign origin.

It does not surprise me that you cannot abolish the once established susceptibility of your inoculated mice to the growing tumors. We found this in our own work when we used tumor test grafts instead of those of skin. This is simply a function of the ability of tumors to over-ride even high degrees of immunological opposition. So here again, I think, the evidence available does not separate the two phenomena under discussion."

"Acquired tolerance" could also be applied, in a more direct manner, to experimental cancer research. Koprowski, in 1955, induced in Swiss mice "tolerance" to normal C3H cells by injecting whole blood from C3H mice into Swiss strain embryos, between their 16th and 17th day of fetal life. Trypan blue dye was injected simultaneously, in order to identify, after birth, those mice that actually received the injection at the time they were carried in their mothers' wombs. When the pre-treated mice were 6 to 8 weeks of age, they were inoculated with a cell suspension of a transplantable ascites tumor known to grow progressively only in mice of the C3H strain. The pre-treated Swiss mice developed tumors, demonstrating thereby that following treatment with C3H blood during fetal life they had acquired "tolerance" for C3H cells.

Technique of Transmitting Mouse Leukemia by Cell-Graft

There are several methods of transplanting mouse leukemia by cell-graft from one host to another. Essentially, these methods consist of inoculating leukemic cells, such as whole blood, or preferably a lymphoid tumor cell suspension, into a susceptible host. The inoculation should be performed under aseptic conditions. Intraperitoneal route is probably most suitable and sufficiently sensitive. The intravenous route is probably somewhat more sensitive, but also more difficult in the mouse, and has more strict limitations as to the volume that can be inoculated. The subcutaneous route is less sensitive and, furthermore, often leads to the development, at first, of a lymphoid tumor at the site of inoculation of the leukemic cells; generalized leukemia follows only later.

Some investigators use small fragments of lymphoid tumors, or leukemic spleen, for subcutaneous, intramuscular, or intraperitoneal implantations performed by means of a trocar. A similar method has long been used for the routine transplantation of solid tumors, such as sarcomas or carcinomas, in mice and rats.

We prefer to use leukemic cell suspensions sufficiently homogenized to allow inoculation by means of a syringe and a very small, 26 gauge, needle. Such a method is very convenient and dependable; it allows proper dosage, and the entire procedure can be carried out under aseptic conditions. This is in marked contrast to transplantation by a trocar of a fragment of tumor. Actually, it is most difficult, if at all possible, to perform a trocar transplantation under conditions of complete sterility.

* * *

The following technique of transplanting mouse leukemia by cell-graft has been employed in our laboratory:

> The leukemic donor, such as an Ak female with spontaneous leukemia, is sacrificed by ether inhalation, placed on a cork plate, and immobilized in supine position, with glass-headed pins piercing each of the paws. The skin of the abdomen and chest is then sponged with 95 per cent ethyl alcohol. A longitudinal incision, through the skin only, running in the middle line, from tail to the lower jaw, is made with sterile scissors; the skin is gently separated, retracted, and pinned down to the cork plate, exposing abdomen and chest. With another sterile forceps and scissors, the peritoneum is opened, and the sternum also removed. The instruments are again changed, and a sterile forceps and scissors are used to remove fragments of liver (care being taken not to disturb the gallbladder), spleen, mesenteric and mediastinal tumors, possibly also a peripheral lymph node, and a fragment of neck tissue. Before the mouse is discarded, fragments of tissue from neck, and fragments of liver and spleen, etc., are separately removed for routine microscopical sections, and the findings are dictated to an assistant.

The aseptically removed tissue fragments are weighed on a small sterile gauze, then transferred into a sterile mortar, cut with small, sterile scissors, then ground with a pestel, 0.85 per cent sterile chilled sodium chloride solution being added in sufficient quantity to obtain a cell suspension of 20 per cent concentration. After grinding for about 3 minutes, the cell homogenate is passed through a sterile voile, or organdy, cloth filter, which retains the larger tissue fragments. The resulting fine, homogenous cell emulsion is then placed in a sterile test tube which is immersed in a container filled with ice cubes (0°C).

A routine inoculation of tryptose phosphate broth is then made with a drop of the leukemic cell suspension, to check for bacterial sterility. The inoculated broth is incubated for 24 hours at 37°C and is expected to remain sterile. (Should bacterial contamination become evident, it is preferable to destroy those animals that might have been in the meantime inoculated with the contaminated cell extract, and prepare a new one under aseptic conditions.)

Once removed from the leukemic donor, the leukemic cells should be inoculated into a new host with a minimum of delay, either immediately or within an hour or two, the leukemic cell extract remaining in the meantime at 0°C in a sterile glass tube immersed in a glass container filled with ice cubes. At that temperature, suspended in physiological saline solution, mouse leukemic cells can be kept for at least 3 or 4 days without losing their ability to reproduce leukemia on transplantation. At 37°C, on the other hand, the leukemic cells become inactivated within approximately 6 to 8 hours (Gross, unpublished).

The leukemic cell suspension is inoculated intraperitoneally (0.10 to 0.25 cc. of a 20 per cent cell suspension), using a tuberculin syringe and a 26 gauge needle. The skin of the recipient mouse is moistened with a drop of 95 per cent ethyl alcohol prior to inoculation, at the point where the needle will pierce the abdomen.

Routinely, if the leukemic cell suspension is prepared from an Ak leukemic donor, young adult Ak mice (about 4 to 6 weeks old) are used for inoculation. It is preferable to inoculate Ak females, since Ak males fight ferociously when kept together in a cage. As discussed on preceding pages, however, the Ak leukemic cells can be also inoculated into newborn or suckling mice of other strains, such as C3H, C57 Black, etc. Leukemia develops usually in the inoculated mice within 10 to 15 days.

The leukemic cell suspensions can be diluted considerably, such as to 10^{-4} dilution and may still retain their ability to reproduce leukemia when inoculated into mice of the same strain; when small doses are injected, however, the latency period is usually prolonged.

THE SEARCH FOR A LEUKEMIC VIRUS IN MICE

Early Attempts to Transmit Mouse Leukemia by Cell-free Extracts. It has long been suspected that mouse leukemia is caused by a transmissible virus. Ellermann and Bang demonstrated as early as 1908 that erythromyeloblastic chicken leukemia could be transmitted by filtrates. It was only logical to assume that under proper experimental conditions it would be possible to transmit mouse leukemia also by cell-free extracts.

All attempts, however, to transmit leukemia in mice by filtrates failed prior to 1951. Transmission of leukemia appeared possible only when live, undamaged leukemic cells were transplanted. Whenever cell-free extracts prepared from leukemic donors were employed for inoculation, no leukemia resulted.

Richter and MacDowell reported in 1933 a series of experiments carried out on mice of the C58 strain, and demonstrated that no successful transmission of leukemia could be accomplished under conditions employed in their studies, unless intact, living cells were inoculated. MacDowell and his colleagues again reviewed in 1939 their attempts to transmit C58 leukemia by filtrates, or by dried, or otherwise treated, material in which the cells had been killed. All these attempts failed to transmit leukemia.

Furth and his coworkers carried out their experiments on mice of the Ak line, and also failed to transmit leukemia by cell-free extracts. They reported in 1933 that procedures which destroy leukemic cells, but fail to affect viruses, such as addition of glycerin to the leukemic tissue fragments, or drying of leukemic cells, inactivate the leukemogenic potential of the inoculated material. Later on, in 1937, Barnes and Furth again reported experiments dealing with attempts to transmit mouse leukemia by cell-free extracts in mice of strain A. Leukemia was induced in a mouse of this strain by the intrasplenic injection of benzpyrene. The disease could be readily transmitted to mice of the stock in which this leukemia originated. Transmission was accomplished, however, only with material containing living cells, but failed with cell-free material. Transmission did not succeed with Berkefeld filtrates, or with either dried or glycerinated leukemic tissues.

Attempts to transmit leukemia in mice by inoculation of cells that had been irradiated with a dose expected to destroy the cells, but not to affect the more resistant virus, also failed (Rask-Nielsen, 1938. Furth *et al.*, 1938).

In 1938 Engelbreth-Holm and Fredericksen, in Copenhagen, believed that they had transmitted mouse leukemia to young adult Ak mice by means of presumably cell-free, centrifuged extracts of leukemic organs from donors of the same strain. The extracts, prepared under anaerobic conditions, were centrifuged at 3600 r.p.m. for 15 minutes. The supernate was again centrifuged at 3600 r.p.m. for another 15 minutes. The resulting supernate was then injected into normal, healthy Ak mice. Nine experiments were performed, and a total of 179 mice was inoculated. Of these, 36 developed leukemia, 1 to 3 months after inoculation. Some of the positive mice approached an age at which spontaneous leukemia already might have appeared; other mice, however, were much younger, some only 2 or 3 months old, i.e. they were of an age at which spontaneous leukemia did not yet appear. Furthermore, no spontaneous leukemia appeared among control Ak mice injected with similar extracts, prepared under aerobic conditions.

Attempts to repeat these observations, reported by MacDowell and his coworkers in 1939, and also by Engelbreth-Holm in 1948, failed, however. Engelbreth-Holm expressed in 1942 the view that the findings in his initial experiment might have been the result of an acceleration of spontaneous leukemia rather than that of a transmission of the disease. The picture was more confused when MacDowell and his associates reported in 1939 that acceleration of the development of spontaneous leukemia in mice of the C58 strain could be accomplished by the injection of the medium alone (a cobalt-sulfate-cysteine solution) which was used in Englebreth-Holm's experiments for the preparation of the extracts; repetition of that experiment, however, gave negative results. Engelbreth-Holm concluded in 1948 that the most natural way to explain his initial positive results was to assume that, despite the precautions taken, the centrifuged extracts used in his 1938 experiments did contain a number of intact leukemic cells, floating in the injected supernate, sufficient to induce the development of leukemia in some of the inoculated mice. None of his extracts was filtered.

A similar reservation should probably be applied to the experiments of Stasney and his associates, who reported in 1950 transmission of a rat lymphosarcoma by inoculation of presumably cell-free, isolated cytoplasmic or nuclear components of tumor cells. Lymphosarcoma extracts, fractionated by the differential centrifugation technique of Claude, and containing the mitochondria or chromatin fractions, were inoculated. Tumors developed in from 3 to 18 days at the site of inoculation and were followed by generalized leukemia. Klein (1952) repeated these experiments, using two transplantable mouse lymphosarcomas that originated and grew in genetically controlled strains of mice. The tumors induced by inoculation of chromatin fractions, however, did not possess the genetic constitution of the host in which they arose; genetically, they were not different from the original tumor. Klein suggested that the most probable explanation of these findings was a contamination of the chromatin fractions with surviving cells. The same explanation probably also applied to the findings of Stasney and his associates. Such a possibility should always be considered when centrifuged extracts are used for inoculation.

Transmission of Mouse Leukemia by a Single Cell

Furth and Kahn demonstrated in 1937 that, under favorable experimental conditions, a single leukemic cell may be sufficient to reproduce the disease following intravenous inoculation into a susceptile mouse of the same strain in which the leukemia originated. Three out of 65 mice of strain S2, and two out of 32 mice of strain Ak developed leukemia following intravenous inoculation of a single leukemic cell isolated by means of a micromanipulator and inoculated intravenously. The latency was short, varying from 15 to 50 days. When mice received a dose larger than 20 cells, all developed leukemia.

All of 52 mice inoculated under similar conditions with cell-free material remained in good health.

This finding was a warning, suggesting the necessity of a careful assessment of any reported transmission by means of a presumably cell-free material.

* * *

It was thus apparent that only transmission of mouse leukemia by a filtrate, under strictly controlled experimental conditions, could demonstrate in a convincing manner the existence of a transmissible, cell-free agent.

The existence of such a filterable agent, though long suspected, was not established, however, until 1951, when experimental conditions under which mouse leukemia could be transmitted by filtrates were recognized.

Preliminary Attempts to Transmit Mouse Leukemia by Filtrates into Suckling Mice

Early in 1945, the author, still on duty with the U.S. Army Medical Corps, was assigned to the Veterans Administration Hospital in Bronx, New York City, and there had an opportunity to carry on, in spare time, experimental cancer research. This was done in a former oxygen-tank room, in the basement of Building F of the hospital, with a minimum of equipment and a staff consisting of one technical assistant. A small colony of mice of the leukemic strain Ak was raised by brother-to-sister mating from a nucleus of these mice generously supplied by Dr. Jacob Furth, then at Cornell University Medical College. At the same time, a colony of C3H mice was also raised from a litter initially obtained from Dr. J. J. Bittner, University of Minnesota.

At that time the idea that mouse leukemia might be caused by a virus had been virtually abandoned, since all previous attempts to transmit this disease by filtrates had failed.

We felt, however, that additional experiments should be carried out along this line. In previous studies only adult mice were used for the inoculation of the leukemic filtrates. Yet, during the preceding decade it had gradually become clear that certain oncogenic viruses had to be injected into very young animals in order to induce the disease. Were not suckling, less than 2 or 3-week-old, mice particularly susceptible to the inoculation of the mouse mammary carcinoma virus?

It appeared reasonable to speculate in 1945 that the susceptibility of mice to inoculation with the hypothetical leukemic agent might also be limited to the first three, or perhaps even to the initial two weeks of life.

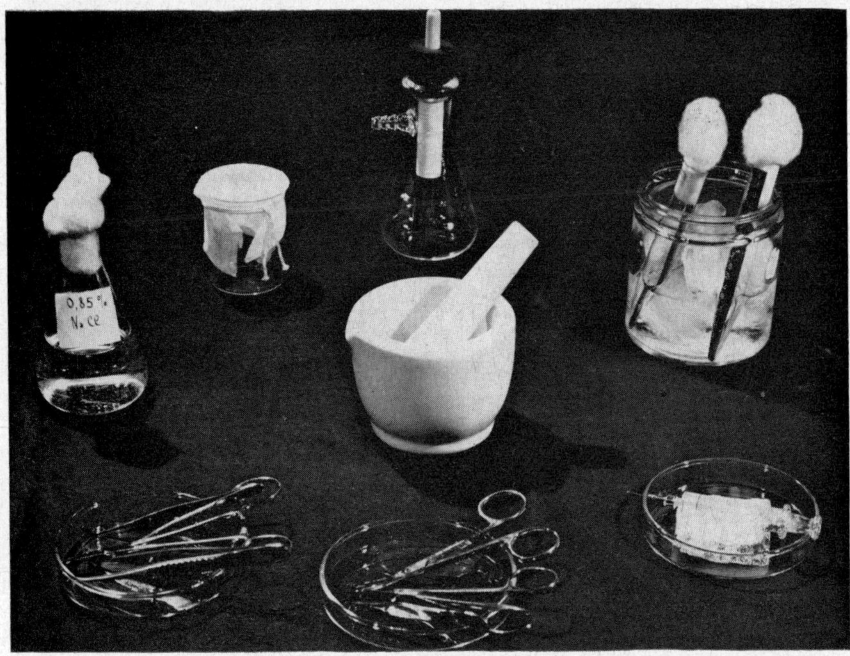

FIG. 28a. PREPARATION OF FILTRATE.

Set of instruments for the preparation of a leukemic filtrate, including a Selas porcelain filter candle.

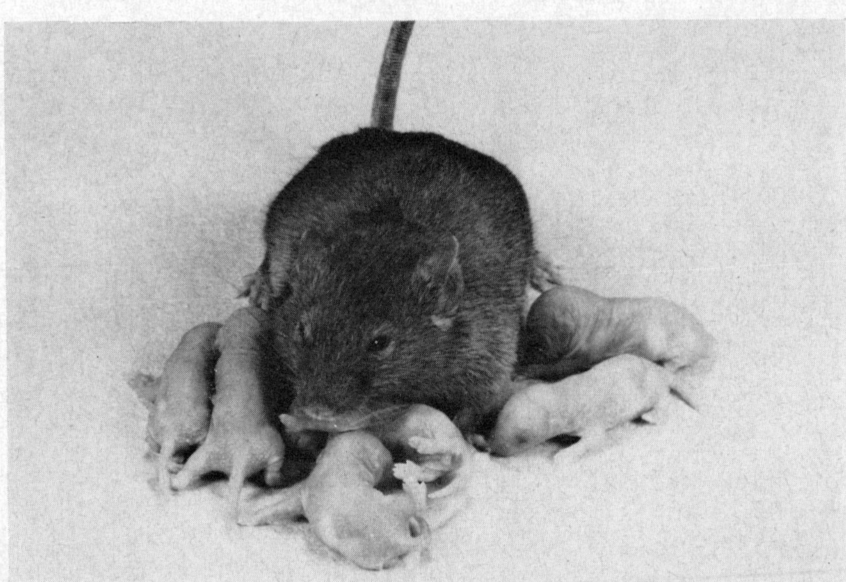

FIG. 28b. NEWBORN C3H LITTER.

Young healthy C3H female with a newly born litter. Newborn C3H mice are employed for the inoculation of leukemic filtrates. Newborn mice of several other inbred strains, such as C57 Brown or BALB/c, are also susceptible to the induction of lymphosarcomas and leukemia with the mouse leukemia virus.

The Disappointing and Time-consuming Project Ready to be Abandoned

The preliminary plan was as follows: extracts were to be prepared from organs of Ak donors with spontaneous or transplanted leukemia; these extracts were to be centrifuged, then passed through Seitz filters; the resulting filtrates were then to be inoculated into suckling C3H mice about 7 to 10 days old. That particular age was selected tentatively, since mouse mammary carcinoma virus was known to induce tumors readily when injected into susceptible mice 7 to 14 days old (Andervont and Bryan, 1944), and even into weanlings 21 days of age (Bittner, 1944).

At that time it was not realized that still younger mice should have been inoculated with the leukemic filtrates.

Since inoculation of the mammary carcinoma virus into suckling mice was followed by the development of tumors only after a latency of some 7 to 12 months, it was anticipated that inoculation of suckling mice with the leukemic filtrates might also be followed by an equally long latency period preceding the eventual development of leukemia. It was obvious, therefore, that mice of a leukemic strain, such as C58 or Ak, could not be used for the bio-assay, since spontaneous leukemia develops in a great majority of these mice before they reach one year of age.

It appeared necessary to use for inoculation only mice of a low-leukemic strain, i.e. animals that would not develop leukemia spontaneously.

Since C3H mice were available in the same laboratory, and since these mice have long been known to have a very low incidence of spontaneous leukemia, it was decided to use mice of this particular strain for the inoculation of the Ak leukemic filtrates.

These early experiments were continued for the next five years with very little success. Only an insignificant number of the injected C3H mice developed leukemia. The incidence was too low to justify any conclusions. The latency was prohibitive, since the few cases of leukemia developed in mice 18 to 27 months of age; most of the inoculated mice died before they reached such an advanced age.

In 1949, the disappointing and time-consuming project was ready to be abandoned.

* * *

In retrospect, the principal reasons for the failure of these early attempts were probably as follows:

(a) Mice used for inoculation were too old.

(b) Most of the C3H mice used were of the less susceptible An subline. This will be discussed later in a more detailed manner.

(c) Seitz filter pads, used for the filtration of leukemic extracts, were not particularly suitable, since they retained most of the virus. Diatomaceous earth (Berkefeld) or unglazed procelain (Selas) filter candles would have been more suitable.

(d) Extracts prepared from single leukemic Ak donors may often be inactive on inoculation tests. Pooled extracts from several donors would have been preferable.

THE USE OF NEWBORN MICE FOR INOCULATION OF LEUKEMIC EXTRACTS

In 1948 and 1949, G. Dalldorf and his coworkers at the New York State Department of Health, in Albany, reported that suckling mice 4 to 5 days old, and in certain experiments newborn mice less than 48 hours old, had to be used for inoculation of an agent recovered from feces of children having symptoms similar to poliomyelitis. This agent, designated "Coxsackie virus" (since the first recognized human cases were residents of that New York State village) proved to be pathogenic for suckling mice and hamsters, inducing severe destructive lesions in striated muscles. Newborn mice were found to be susceptible, but the resistance of these animals rapidly increased with age. Dalldorf had the idea of employing such very young mice for the bio-assay leading to the discovery of the new agent, because previous studies in his laboratory suggested that newborn mice were unusually susceptible to certain neurotropic viruses.

The experiments with chicken tumors and lymphomatosis were then recalled. In 1942, Duran-Reynals demonstrated that the chicken tumor virus could be successfully transmitted to ducks, provided that newly hatched, less than 24-hour-old, ducklings were inoculated. Burmester and his associates reported in 1946 that chicken lymphomatosis could be transmitted by filtrates into newly hatched, 1 or 2-day-old, chicks.

It gradually became apparent that the 7 to 10-day-old C3H mice used in the preliminary experiments for the inoculation of Ak leukemic filtrates might have been too old for such a purpose.

* * *

It was decided, therefore, to repeat the experiments dealing with the cell-free transmission of mouse leukemia. Newborn C3H mice, only a few hours old, were to be used. Furthermore, before injecting filtered extracts, it was thought advisable to inject in a preliminary experiment unfiltered leukemic cell homogenate, so as to administer an extract possibly richer in the content of the virus. Mice of the C3H strain were considered refractory to the grafting of Ak leukemic cells, but it was hoped that they might be susceptible to the leukemic virus.

For a preliminary experiment carried out in 1949, a newly born, less than 24-hour-old, C3H litter was located in the laboratory. A leukemic cell suspension was prepared from an Ak donor with transplanted leukemia. The uncentrifuged and unfiltered cell homogenate was then inoculated into both parents, and also into all 5 newborn infants. The parents remained in good health, as was expected, since adult C3H mice were known to be resistant to the implantation of Ak leukemic cells. Surprisingly, however, all 5 inoculated infant mice developed acute leukemia within 12 days after inoculation.

It was soon realized that leukemia developing in the suckling C3H mice within only 2 weeks after inoculation of Ak leukemic homogenate was not induced by a virus, but was the result of multiplication of the implanted Ak leukemic cells. The lymphoid tumors that developed in the inoculated suckling C3H mice could be readily transplanted, by cell-graft, back to adult Ak mice, but not to those of the C3H line.

In view of the susceptibility of the newborn C3H mouse to the inoculation of Ak leukemic cells, it was decided to re-evaluate previous experiments. A comprehensive series of experiments was carried out to determine the influence of age of the suckling C3H mice on susceptibility to implanted Ak leukemic cells. The susceptibility was found to be highest immediately after birth, and then to decline quite rapidly with each passing day (Gross, 1950).

Since newborn C3H mice, only a few hours old, were found to be substantially more susceptible to the implantation of Ak leukemic cells than suckling mice, 7 to 10 days old, it was felt that susceptibility to the inoculation of the hypothetical leukemic virus could also be linked to the early age of the mouse used for inoculation. For that reason, experiments dealing with inoculation of leukemic filtrates were repeated, using newborn C3H mice, instead of employing test animals 7 to 10 days old. Most of the mice now used were less than 16 hours old at the time of inoculation; some were less than 24 hours old; in addition, the susceptibility of suckling mice, 1 to 7 days old, was also tested.

Transmission of Mouse Leukemia by Centrifuged Cell-free Extracts Inoculated into Newborn and Suckling Mice

The first series of experiments in which newborn mice were used for inoculation of cell-free leukemic extracts was initiated in January, 1950, and reported in 1951 (Gross).

The extracts were prepared from Ak mice with either spontaneous or transplanted leukemia. Fragments of livers, spleens, mediastinal and mesenteric tumors were removed aseptically, weighed, cut with small scissors, then

> ground by hand in a mortar for about 5 minutes, sterile chilled physiological saline solution being added to obtain cell suspensions of approximately 20 per cent concentrations. After passing through a sterile voile cloth filter, which retained larger tissue pieces, the resulting homogeneous extracts were centrifuged at 3000 r.p.m. for 15 minutes in a refrigerated PR-1 centrifuge at 0°C. The supernate was removed, placed in a new tube, and again centrifuged at 3000 r.p.m. for additional 15 minutes. The final supernate was then removed carefully with a syringe, and used immediately for inoculation.

A group of 14 newborn, less than 12-hour-old, C3H mice was inoculated subcutaneously and/or intraperitoneally, and 7 of them developed generalized leukemia at 8 to 11 months of age; later on, 5 additional mice developed leukemia in this group, making it a total of 12 out of 14 inoculated mice.

Another group of newborn and suckling C3H mice was inoculated with centrifuged extracts, and the results were reported later that same year (Gross, 1951). Of 44 C3H mice inoculated in the second group, 29 (66 per cent) developed leukemia at ages varying from 4 to 20 months.

There was a rather striking difference in latency time elapsing between the inoculation of the extracts and the development of disease, depending on the age at the time of inoculation. Most of those mice that were inoculated when less than 24 hours old developed leukemia 7 to 9 months later, whereas those inoculated when 3 to 6 days old developed leukemia only after 18 to 20 months.

In a third series of experiments (Gross, 1953), 41 newborn C3H mice were inoculated when less than 24 hours old with centrifuged Ak leukemic extracts, and 19 of them (46 per cent) developed leukemia at ages varying from $3\frac{1}{2}$ to $11\frac{1}{2}$ months.

Cell Transplantation of Leukemia that Developed in the Inoculated C3H Mice

The development of leukemia in C3H mice following inoculation of centrifuged Ak leukemic extracts was most probably the result of the leukemogenic action of a transmissible cell-free agent present in the injected extracts. Theoretically, however, it was possible to assume that a few leukemic cells could have been injected with the supernate. Only injection of filtrates would have precluded such a possibility.

An indication suggesting that the induced leukemia was not the result of an accidental transplantation of leukemic cells was obtained in a series of experiments in which leukemia resulting in C3H mice inoculated with the centrifuged extracts was transplanted to adult C3H and Ak mice.

There exist certain experimental procedures dealing with transplantation of tumors, which may be of assistance in determining whether leukemic tumors induced in animals of a certain inbred line were the result of an accidental implantation of neoplastic cells from a different strain's donor, or whether such tumors were induced by an oncogenic action of a cell-free agent on the cells of the recipient host.

Ak leukemic cells can be readily transplanted to mice of the same inbred strain, but usually will not grow when implanted into adult C3H mice.

Let us assume that leukemia which developed in C3H mice inoculated with the centrifuged Ak extracts was the result of an accidental transplantation of Ak leukemic cells introduced with the supernate. It would then follow that such a leukemia was the result of multiplication of the implanted Ak cells, and that the resulting lymphoid tumors consisted of Ak leukemic cells growing in a genetically foreign host. Such Ak cells could be readily transplanted back to adult mice of the strain of origin, i.e. Ak, but not to adult mice of the C3H strain. Similar experimental conditions exist when newborn C3H mice are inoculated with Ak leukemic cell suspensions. The resulting lymphoid tumors, even though developing in suckling C3H mice, can be transplanted to adult Ak mice (strain of origin of the implanted leukemic cells), but usually not to adult C3H mice (recipient strain).

As another theoretical possibility, let us now assume that leukemia which developed in C3H mice inoculated with the centrifuged Ak extracts was the result of a leukemogenic action of a cell-free agent (inoculated with the Ak extracts) on the hitherto normal cells of the injected host, i.e. on C3H cells. The resulting leukemia would thus consist of cells having the genetic constitution of the inoculated host. It would be a C3H leukemia, consisting of C3H leukemic cells, and should prove to be readily transplantable to other C3H mice, but not to adult mice of the Ak strain.

Accordingly, leukemic cell suspensions were prepared in the usual manner, from livers, spleens, and mesenteric tumors of those C3H mice that developed leukemia as a result of inoculation, in their infancy, with the centrifuged Ak leukemic extracts.

In eight separate experiments, 33 adult C3H mice were inoculated with the leukemic cell suspensions thus prepared, and 29 developed transplanted leukemia within 2 weeks; the remaining 4 mice also developed leukemia within 2 months.

Under apparently identical experimental conditions, 34 adult Ak mice were inoculated with the same C3H leukemic cell suspensions, and only 2 of them developed transplanted leukemia after 60 and 72 days respectively. Of the 34 Ak mice, 32 proved resistant to the implantation of the C3H leukemic cells.

The results of these transplantation experiments were consistent with the assumption that in the initial experiment the C3H mice inoculated with the centrifuged Ak leukemic extracts developed leukemia as a result of inoculation of a cell-free leukemic agent, rather than because of an accidental implantation of a few Ak leukemic cells inadvertently floating in the injected supernate.

The final proof, however, of cell-free transmission of mouse leukemia was furnished only when it was demonstrated that this disease could be reproduced by inoculation of leukemic filtrates.

TRANSMISSION OF MOUSE LEUKEMIA BY FILTRATES

A turning point in the study of experimental mouse leukemia was marked in 1951,* when transmission of leukemia in mice was accomplished by inoculation of filtrates prepared from leukemic mouse tissues and inoculated into newborn mice of a susceptible, but relatively free from spontaneous leukemia, inbred line. This observation changed the concept of genetic origin of mouse leukemia, and suggested that not only in chickens, as had been known previously, but also in mice, leukemia is of viral origin.

In our experiments, centrifuged (3000 r.p.m. for 15 minutes) leukemic extracts, prepared from Ak donors with either spontaneous or transplanted leukemia, were passed through Seitz (S-1) filter pads. The filters were impervious to *E. coli*, as determined by tests carried out immediately after the filtration of each leukemic extract.

> In 5 experiments, 25 newborn, less than 12-hour-old, mice of the C3H strain, were inoculated with the leukemic filtrates, and 7 of them (28 per cent) developed generalized lymphatic leukemia at 6½ to 9 months of age. When an older group consisting of 7 suckling, 8-day-old, C3H mice was inoculated with the filtrates, only 2 developed leukemia, at 23 and 27 months of age.

The incidence of leukemia induced with the filtrates (28 per cent) was significant, since mice of the C3H strain used for the inoculation of the leukemic filtrates had a very low incidence of spontaneous leukemia, usually not exceeding 0.5 per cent.

Leukemia developing in C3H mice following inoculation of the leukemic filtrates was usually of the lymphatic type and resembled that which develops spontaneously in mice of the Ak strain.

* Successful transmission of mouse leukemia by filtrates (Gross, L., *Proc. Soc. Exp. Biol. & Med.*, **78**: 342, 1951) was first reported by the author on November 17, 1951, at a Conference on "Viruses as Causative Agents in Cancer" held by the New York Academy of Sciences at the Barbizon Plaza Hotel in New York City.

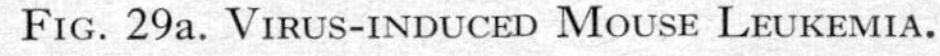

Fig. 29a. Virus-induced Mouse Leukemia.

This C3H(f) female mouse was inoculated, when less than 8 hours old, with a centrifuged, cell-free extract prepared from organs of a leukemic Ak mouse, and developed lymphatic leukemia at the age of $7\frac{1}{2}$ months. Note the very large spleen and liver, large lymphoid mediastinal tumor, and large tumorous lymph nodes in the groin, in the axillary pits, and in the submaxillary area. (From: L. Gross, in CIBA Symposium on Leukemia Research, J. & A. Churchill, Publ., London, 1954.)

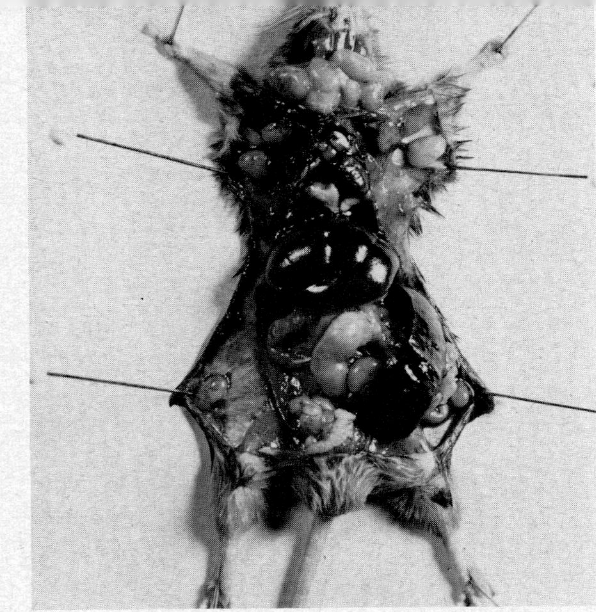

Fig. 29b. Virus-induced Mouse Leukemia.

This C57 Brown male mouse was inoculated, when less than 3 hours old, with a filtrate prepared from organs of a leukemic C58 mouse and developed generalized lymphatic leukemia at the age of 10 months. Note the very large ruptured spleen, large liver, and large tumorous lymph nodes in the mesentery, in the groins, in axillary pits, and in the submaxillary area. (From: L. Gross, *Cancer*, **9**: 778, 1956.)

In subsequent experiments dealing with the inoculation of Ak leukemic extracts into newborn C3H mice, the technique of preparing filtrates was modified. The use of Seitz filters was discontinued; Berkefeld filters, and later on Selas filter candles, were routinely employed.

*Technique of Preparation of Leukemic Filtrates.** The leukemic cell suspensions of 20 per cent concentration were prepared in the usual manner (described in detail on pages 316–317) from Ak leukemic donors with spontaneous or transplanted leukemia. As a rule, fragments of leukemic tissues from 2 or 3 leukemic donors were pooled.

After the initial centrifugation at 3000 r.p.m. (1400×g), at 0°C, for 15 minutes, the supernate was removed, placed in another tube and centrifuged at 9500 r.p.m. (7000×g) at 0°C, for 5 minutes. The second supernate was then passed through either Berkefeld (porosity N) or Selas (porosity 02 or 03) filter candles under a vacuum pressure of 20 to 25 mm of mercury. Each filter was tested, before and after filtration, and found to be impervious to *E. coli*. In most experiments the centrifuged leukemic extracts (10 to 15 cc.) were mixed, prior to filtration, with 0.5 to 1 cc. of a 1 : 2000 dilution of a fresh broth culture of *E. coli*, and then passed through the filter candles. The filters retained the *E. coli*, since the filtrates were found to be sterile, as evidenced by the inoculation of tryptose phosphate broth, incubated at 37°C for 48 hours and then inspected for *E. coli* growth. (After it was determined that the mouse leukemia virus is filterable, and that it passes through bacterial filters which retain *E. coli*, the routine addition of the *E. coli* to the extracts in the course of the preparation of the leukemic extracts was discontinued.)

The leukemic filtrates were immediately placed in sterile glass tubes immersed in larger glass containers filled with ice cubes. The filtrates were inoculated in most instances promptly after preparation. In some instances, when no newborn litters were available for immediate inoculation, the filtrates were inoculated within 24 hours (occasionally also within 48 hours) after their preparation, having been kept in the meantime at 0°C, in tubes immersed in containers filled with ice cubes, and placed in an electric refrigerator.

More recently it was realized that the leukemic filtrates could be frozen at −70°C and kept in sealed ampoules at carbon dioxide dry ice temperature for prolonged periods of time exceeding 2 years, without apparent loss of infectivity.

Additional Experiments Dealing with Inoculation of Ak Leukemic Filtrates into Newborn C3H Mice. The Unexpected Development of Parotid Gland Carcinomas

In an attempt to extend and confirm our own findings, additional filtration experiments were carried out (Gross, 1953).

* The technique here described refers to the initial experiments in which the original studies on cell-free transmission of mouse leukemia were carried out in the author's laboratory. For the description of a more recent technique of preparation of leukemic filtrates, now routinely employed for passage A and other similar virus strains, the reader is referred to page 350.

TABLE 3*. RESULTS OF INOCULATION OF FILTERED† AK LEUKEMIC EXTRACTS INTO NEWBORN C3H OR C3H(f) MICE‡

Strain	Sex	Fresh filtrate											Heated (65° to 68°C for ½ hour) filtrate									
		No. of mice inoc.	No. dev. leuk.	Leuk. inc. (%)	Avg. age (mos.)	No. dev. parotid tumors	Parotid tumors inc. (%)	Avg. age (mos.)	No. dev. subcut. sarcomas	Subcu. sarcomas inc. (%)	Avg. age (mos.)	Total leuk. and tumors inc. (%)	No. of mice inoc.	No. dev. leuk.	Leuk. inc. (%)	Avg. age (mos.)	No. dev. parotid tumors	Parotid tumors inc. (%)	Avg. age (mos.)	No. dev. subcut. sarcomas	No. died free from leuk. or tumors	Avg. age died free from leuk. or tumors (mos.)
C3H	F	90	22	24	9	13	14	4	0	0	—	39										
C3H	M	53	10	19	12	15	28	5	2	4	12	51										
Total C3H		143	32	22	10	28	20	6	2	1	12	43	71	0	0	—	1	1	8	0	70	16
C3H(f)	F	111	39	35	11	6	5	3	1	1	16	41										
C3H (f)	M	74	21	28	9	2	3	5	0	—	—	31										
Total C3H(f)		185	60	32	10	8	4	4	1	—	16	37	95	2	2	17	4	4	4	0	89	15
Total	F	201	61	30	10	19	10	4	1	—	—	40										
Total	M	127	31	24	10	17	13	7	2	—	—	39										
Grand total		328	92	28	10	36**	11	5	3	1	13	40	166	2	1	17	5	3	5	0	159	16

Those mice that died when less than 2 months old were not included in the tabulation. This refers particularly to the mortality, usually not exceeding 20 to 25 per cent, occurring among the infant mice within hours or days after inoculation.

† Seventy extracts were prepared, each from a different donor (44 from Ak donors with spontaneous leukemia and 26 from Ak donors with transplanted Ak leukemia). The extracts (20 per cent conc.), prepared from leukemic organs, were centrifuged ($7000 \times g$), and then filtered. Either Berkefeld N or Selas (porosity 02 or 03) filter candles were used. Of the total of 70 filtrates prepared (30 Berkefeld, and 40 Selas), only 52 proved to be active on inoculation.

‡ All mice used for inoculation in this series were of the Bittner substrain of the C3H line. Those designated by the symbol C3H(f) were of the same substrain, but free from the mammary tumor agent by foster nursing. Most mice were less than 12 hours old, many less than 6 hours old, and none more than 16 hours old, at the time of inoculation. The average age at inoculation was 10 hours. All inoculations were subcutaneous (0.1 cm^3 each). The extracts were used for inoculation within 48 hours, having been kept in the meantime in sterile tubes immersed in ice water, at 0°C. The heated (65° to 68°C., ½ hour) extracts were inoculated simultaneously into litter-mate control mice.

** Among the mice that developed parotid gland tumors, several also developed subcutaneous fibrosarcomas, usually near the groin, axilla, or within the abdominal wall, In one mouse a medullary adrenal tumor was also observed. Two mice developed, in addition to parotid gland tumors, carcinomas of the submaxillary gland, arising in small multiple foci. In one instance bilateral parotid gland carcinomas developed simultaneously with leukemia.

* From GROSS, L., *Ann. N.Y. Acad. Sci.*, **68**: 501–521, 1957.

In a first series, consisting of 16 individual experiments, 45 newborn C3H mice, less than 20 hours old (average age at inoculation 8 hours), were inoculated with leukemic filtrates passed through Berkefeld filter candles. Ten of the 45 inoculated mice (22 per cent) developed leukemia at 3 to 6 months of age. Two additional mice among those inoculated with the leukemic filtrates developed, surprisingly, carcinomas of the parotid glands.*

Thirty-nine litter-mate controls were injected simultaneously with heated (68°C for $\frac{1}{2}$ hour) leukemic filtrates, and none developed leukemia or salivary gland tumors.

In another series of 33 experiments, in which Selas filter candles were used for the filtration of Ak leukemic extracts, 84 newborn C3H mice, less than 16 hours old (average age at inoculation 12 hours), were inoculated with the leukemic filtrates, and 9 of them (11 per cent) developed leukemia at an average age of 4 months; however, 15 additional mice among those inoculated with the filtrates developed parotid gland carcinomas.

Fifty-seven litter-mate controls were inoculated simultaneously with heated (68°C for $\frac{1}{2}$ hour) filtrates, and none developed leukemia, but one developed parotid gland tumors.

The experiments dealing with the inoculation of leukemic filtrates into newborn C3H mice were continued, and additional data were accumulated. The completed results were later reviewed (Gross, 1957). They are presented in a separate table, summarizing the results of inoculation of either Berkefeld or Selas filtrates prepared from spontaneous or transplanted Ak leukemia into newborn C3H mice (Table 3).

Of a total of 328 newborn C3H mice inoculated with filtrates, 28 per cent developed leukemia at an average age of 10 months. This compared with an incidence of less than one per cent among 166 litter-mate controls, either non-treated or inoculated simultaneously with heated (65°–85°C for $\frac{1}{2}$ hour) leukemic extracts, and surviving to an average age of 16 months.

Again, some of the mice inoculated with the leukemic filtrates developed, instead of leukemia, parotid gland tumors or other related neoplasms.

* * *

* The unexpected development of parotid and submaxillary gland tumors, subcutaneous fibrosarcomas, occasionally mammary carcinomas, or medullary adrenal tumors, among those mice that had been inoculated with the leukemic filtrates, was caused by the presence of the parotid tumor, i.e. polyoma virus, in the extracts used for inoculation. This will be discussed in a more detailed manner in chapter 18 of this monograph.

Initial Difficulties. Low Potency of Extracts, and Variations in Susceptibility Among Strains of Mice Employed for Inoculation of the Filtrates

In our initial experiments the filtrates were prepared from leukemic mice of the Ak strain. Newborn mice of the Bittner subline of strain C3H were used as test animals for inoculation of the leukemic filtrates. Only some of the extracts proved to be potent and induced leukemia in the inoculated animals. The principal reason responsible for this difficulty was the fact, recognized only later, that in the great majority of leukemias developing in mice spontaneously, the lymphoid tumors and other tissues of such animals, which served for the preparation of our extracts, contained only small quantities of infective virus particles.

Since we were dealing with filtrates of relatively low potency, there were difficulties in reproducing consistently the initial transmission experiments. Cell-free extracts prepared from leukemic mouse tissues, but containing only small quantities of infective virus particles, induced a relatively low incidence of leukemia and had a narrow host range; newborn mice of only some of the inbred lines were found to be susceptible; differences in susceptibility were observed even among sublines of an inbred line.

In experiments described below, cell-free extracts were prepared from Ak mice with spontaneous leukemia. These extracts usually had a relatively low infective potency. Following inoculation into newborn mice of several strains tested, such extracts induced only a relatively low incidence of leukemia; furthermore, because of the low potency of these extracts, there was an apparent lack of susceptibility among mice of some of the inbred lines.

These initial difficulties disappeared as soon as a more potent mouse leukemia virus strain was developed by serial cell-free passage. The passaged virus was found to be infective for most of the strains tested, and consistently induced leukemia or lymphosarcomas in most of the inoculated animals. This will be discussed in more detail on subsequent pages of this chapter.

Difference in Susceptibility Among Sublines of Strain C3H to Inoculation with the Leukemic Agent. Following the initial report of successful transmission of mouse leukemia by filtrates, L. W. Law and his colleagues (1955) attempted to reproduce this observation. Cell-free leukemic extracts were inoculated into newborn mice of a C3H subline maintained at the National Cancer Institute. Of the 283 mice inoculated when less than 24 hours old, 22 (8 per cent) developed parotid gland tumors, and only 14 (5 per cent) developed leukemia. Of 161 controls, none developed parotid tumors, but 6 (4 per cent) developed leukemia at 21 months average age.

Since in our initial experiments a substantially higher incidence of leukemia could be induced in mice inoculated with the cell-free extracts, it appeared of interest to determine whether a difference in susceptibility between sublines of mice used for inoculation might not have been responsible for the discrepancy in the results obtained.

Two sublines of the C3H strain have been used in our laboratory. One subline consisted of descendants of C3H mice originally obtained from Dr. J. J. Bittner, University of Minnesota, in 1944. These mice, carrying the milk-transmitted mammary carcinoma agent, were designated in our laboratory by the symbol C3H. A separate colony has been simultaneously raised from a foster-nursed litter of the same substrain, and designated by the symbol C3H(f), or F. These mice were of the same subline, but free from the mammary carcinoma agent.

Another substrain of the C3H mice, also free from the milk agent by foster-nursing, was obtained in 1945 from Dr. H. B. Andervont, National Cancer Institute. These C3H mice have also been bred in our laboratory, and the colony raised from that particular substrain was designated by the symbol An, or C3H/An.

In our initial experiments we did not suspect any difference between these two sublines of the C3H strain to the inoculation of the cell-free leukemic extracts. The centrifuged or filtered leukemic extracts were inoculated in our laboratory into either C3H, C3H(f), or An litters, whichever were available. Proper identification of each injected litter was recorded in our protocols. No distinction, however, was made between the two different sublines when the total results were tabulated. All inoculated mice were recorded as those of the C3H strain.

When the difficulty in transmitting mouse leukemia by cell-free extracts at the National Cancer Institute became apparent, however, our experimental records were re-examined in order to determine whether any difference existed in susceptibility between the two different substrains of the C3H line. Our experiments were reviewed, and tabulated separately for each of the two sublines of the C3H line. The results were as follows (Gross, 1955a):

Of 320 C3H and C3H(f) mice of the Bittner substrain, inoculated with the Ak leukemic filtrates, 28 per cent developed leukemia.

Of 162 mice of the National Cancer Institute substrain (An), inoculated with the same leukemic filtrates, only 4 per cent developed leukemia.

Of 211 litter-mate control mice inoculated simultaneously with heated (65° to 68° C. for $\frac{1}{2}$ hour) leukemic filtrates, only 2 developed leukemia (1 per cent), but 5 developed parotid tumors.

It thus became apparent that C3H mice of the Bittner substrain are more susceptible to the leukemogenic action of filtered Ak leukemic extracts, than mice of the National Cancer Institute subline.

Actually, these two substrains of the C3H strain are quite distinct genetically, having been separated from the initial C3H parent stock for many years. Spontaneous mammary carcinomas that developed in mice of one substrain could be transplanted without difficulty into mice of the same, but not into those of the other subline of the C3H strain (Andervont, 1941). Later on we also found that leukemia induced by cell-free extracts in mice of one of these two sublines could be transplanted by cell-graft into adult mice of the same, but not to those of the other substrain (Gross, unpublished).

Susceptibility of Mice of the C57 Brown/cd strain to Inoculation with Ak Leukemic Extracts

It now appeared of interest to determine whether mice of other inbred strains are susceptible to inoculation with the cell-free leukemic extracts. Many viruses are known to have a narrow range of host specificity. Would a similar limitation apply also to the mouse leukemia agent?

Mice of the low-mammary-tumor inbred strain C57 Brown, subline cd, (C57BR/cd) were selected as test animals, because mice of this inbred line are essentially free from spontaneous leukemia.

According to information obtained from the Jackson Memorial Laboratory, Bar Harbor, Maine, only about 4 per cent of very old animals of this line have been observed to develop spontaneously neoplasms of reticular tissue, usually lymphosarcomas. From a litter obtained from the Jackson Laboratory in 1952, a small colony of C57 Brown mice was raised in our laboratory by brother-to-sister mating.

In a sample consisting of about 100 untreated mice of this strain observed in our laboratory, and surviving for 6 to 27 months (average 11 months), we have seen only one spontaneous leukemia in a female 6½ months old. However, most of our untreated C57 Brown mice were not observed for more than 15 months, and it is possible that a few more spontaneous leukemias might have been observed among older animals.

In a preliminary experiment, Ak leukemic cell suspensions were inoculated into suckling and adult C57 Brown mice. Suckling mice were found susceptible, whereas adult animals were resistant. Of 33 suckling, less than 2-day-old, C57 Brown mice inoculated with the Ak leukemic cell suspensions, 29 developed leukemia within 2 to 4 weeks. When, however, 53 young adult C57 Brown mice (2 months old) were inoculated, all remained in good health.

Leukemia developing in suckling C57 Brown mice as a result of implantation of Ak leukemic cells could readily be grafted to adult mice of the donor Ak strain, but not to mice of the recipient C57 Brown line.

In the second part of our study, the susceptibility of C57 Brown mice to the inoculation with the cell-free leukemic agent was tested.

Accordingly, centrifuged Ak leukemic extracts were prepared in the usual manner, and inoculated into 71 newborn C57 Brown mice (average age at inoculation 6 hours). As a result, 31 (44 per cent) of the inoculated mice developed leukemia at an average age of 10 months.

In another experiment, the leukemic extracts were filtered through Selas porcelain filter candles and inoculated into 42 newborn C57 Brown mice (average age at inoculation 7 hours). Fourteen (33 per cent) of the inoculated mice developed leukemia at an average age of 12 months (Gross, 1954).

Serving as controls, 43 litter-mates were inoculated simultaneously with heated (67° to 80°C for ½ to 1 hour) leukemic extracts, and 3 were untreated, but none developed leukemia.

Cell suspensions, prepared from those C57 Brown mice that developed leukemia as a result of inoculation of either centrifuged or filtered Ak leukemic extracts, reproduced, in most instances within a few weeks, acute leukemia, when transplanted into adult mice of the C57 Brown (recipient) line, but could not be grafted, with rare exceptions, to adult mice of the Ak (donor) strain.

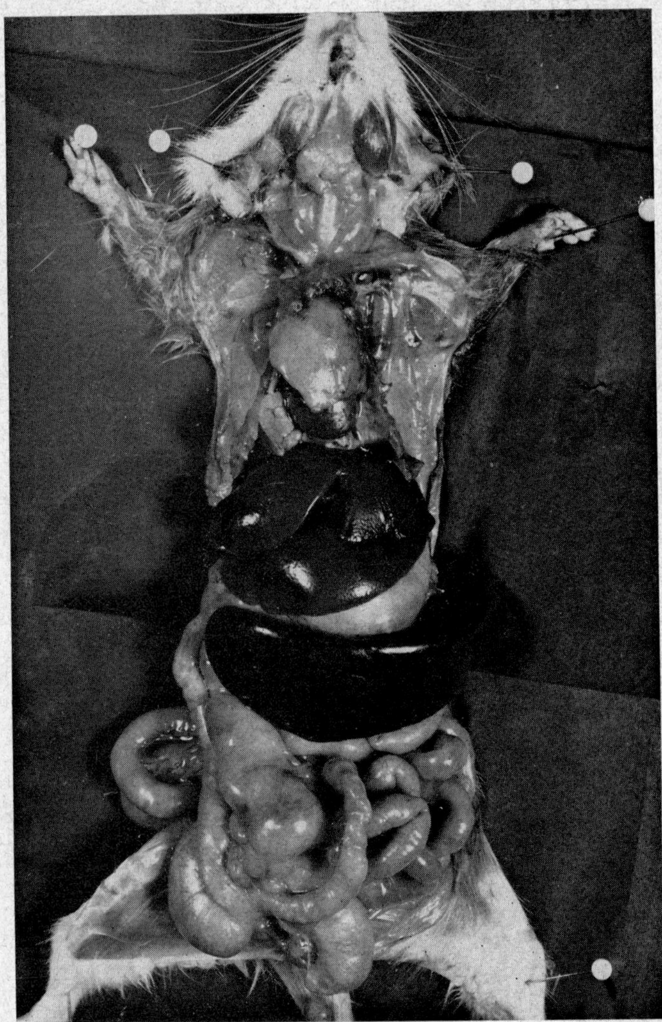

FIG. 30. STEM-CELL LEUKEMIA INDUCED IN A RAT WITH MOUSE LEUKEMIA VIRUS.

This Sprague-Dawley female rat was inoculated when one day old with passage A mouse leukemia virus (harvested from organs of a mouse donor with virus-induced leukemia). At the age of 4 months this rat developed an acute stem-cell leukemia (WBC 403,000/per mm^3 with 95% blast cells). Note a large thymic tumor and a considerably enlarged spleen. (From: L. Gross, *Proc. Soc. Exp. Biol. & Med.*, **106**: 890, 1961.)

When, in previous experiments, filtered Ak leukemic extracts were inoculated into newborn C3H mice, some of the inoculated animals developed leukemia, and others developed parotid gland carcinomas. When, however, filtered Ak leukemic extracts were inoculated into newborn C57 Brown mice, typical leukemia developed in some of them, but none developed salivary gland carcinomas.

This series of experiments suggested that mice of the C57 Brown strain, subline cd, are suitable for bio-assay of the Ak mouse leukemia agent. They have a relatively high susceptibility to the agent, and at the same time a low incidence of spontaneous leukemia.

Susceptibility of Mice of Strains A, BALB/c, and C57 Black to the Ak Leukemic Agent. A limited number of experiments was carried out in order to determine whether newborn mice of strains BALB/c, A, or C57 Black, are susceptible to inoculation with the cell-free mouse leukemia agent.

A small colony of BALB/c mice was raised in our laboratory by brother-to-sister mating from a nucleus obtained in 1954 from Jackson Memorial Laboratory, Bar Harbor, Maine. In a sample consisting of 33 untreated BALB/c mice that lived to an average age of 16 months (age range 9.5 to 22.5 months), only one mouse developed spontaneously leukemia at an age of 17 months.

Newborn BALB/c mice were inoculated at an average age of 8 hours with either centrifuged or filtered extracts prepared from Ak leukemic donors. Of 98 BALB/c mice inoculated with the cell-free extracts, 16 (18 per cent) developed leukemia at an average age of 16 months. Of 57 control BALB/c mice, 4 (7 per cent) developed leukemia at an average age of 22 months; the remaining 53 control mice died without signs of leukemia or tumors at an average age of 18 months (Gross, 1960).

A small colony of strain A mice was raised in our laboratory by brother-to-sister mating from a nucleus obtained from Dr. G. W. Woolley, Sloan Kettering Institute, in 1953. Newborn strain A mice were inoculated at an average age of 11 hours, with cell-free, either centrifuged or filtered, Ak leukemic extracts. Of 28 inoculated mice, only 3 (11 per cent) developed leukemia at an average age of 15 months. None of 14 control mice developed leukemia, and all lived to an average age of 17 months.* (Gross, 1960.)

In another small series of experiments, 44 newborn, less than 12-hour-old, C57 Black mice (C57 Bl) were inoculated with centrifuged Ak leukemic extracts, and 17 of them (39 per cent) developed leukemia at an average age of 17 months (Gross, 1954). No simultaneous controls were observed in this experiment, but the incidence of spontaneous leukemia in untreated mice of this strain was reported to be less than 10 per cent.

* Since none of the females of strain A used for the inoculation of the leukemic filtrates was allowed to breed, the sexes having been separated at weaning age, only 3 out of 25 strain A females used in this series of experiments developed spontaneous mammary carcinomas.

The results of experiments dealing with the susceptibility of newborn mice of several inbred strains to the inoculation of cell-free Ak leukemic extracts suggested that mice of the Bittner subline of the C3H strain or those of the C57 Brown/cd line were most suitable. Mice of both these strains proved to have a relatively high susceptibility to the leukemic agent, and a very low incidence of spontaneous leukemia.

Influence of Sex on the Incidence of Filtrate-induced Leukemia. Among a large group of C3H mice, inoculated when less than 16 hours old with filtered Ak leukemic extracts, females appeared to be more susceptible than males (Gross, 1957b).

Of 201 female mice inoculated with the filtrates, 30 per cent developed leukemia. Of 127 males inoculated simultaneously with the same filtrates, only 24 per cent developed leukemia (Table 3, page 332).

A similar influence of sex on the incidence of spontaneous leukemia developing in mice of high leukemic strains, such as Ak, had been previously recorded, and has already been discussed.

Higher Susceptibility of Foster-nursed C3H Mice, as Compared with those Carrying the Mouse Mammary Carcinoma Agent, to Filtrate-induced Leukemia

Two groups of C3H mice were inoculated when less than 16 hours old with filtered Ak leukemic extracts, under otherwise identical experimental conditions. One group consisted of males and females carrying the mammary carcinoma virus. Another group consisted of C3H mice of both sexes, free from the mammary tumor agent, since these mice were descendants of a C3H litter that had been foster-nursed by a C57 Black female free from the mammary carcinoma agent (Gross, 1951).

Surprisingly, the incidence of leukemia induced by the inoculation of newborn mice of both groups with the Ak leukemic filtrates was higher in the group free from the mammary carcinoma agent than in that carrying the mammary tumor virus (Table 3, p. 332).

Of 90 C3H females carrying the mammary carcinoma virus and inoculated with Ak leukemic filtrates, 24 per cent developed leukemia. Of 111 C3H(f) females free from the mammary carcinoma virus, and inoculated with the same filtrates, 35 per cent developed leukemia.

Of 53 C3H males carrying the mammary carcinoma agent, and inoculated with the leukemic filtrates, 19 per cent developed leukemia. On the other hand, of 74 C3H(f) males free from the mammary carcinoma virus, and inoculated with the same filtrates, 28 per cent developed leukemia.

It thus appeared that C3H mice carrying the mammary carcinoma agent were more resistant to the induction of leukemia following inoculation of the Ak leukemic filtrates than C3H mice free from the mammary carcinoma agent (Gross, 1957). A possible interference between the mammary carcinoma agent and the mouse leukemia virus had to be considered.

Transmission of C58 Leukemia by Filtrates into Newborn Mice of either C3H or C57 Brown/cd Inbred Lines

After it was demonstrated that leukemia developing spontaneously in mice of the high-leukemic Ak strain could be transmitted by filtrates into newborn mice of either strain C3H or C57 Brown, an attempt was made to determine whether leukemia developing spontaneously in another inbred strain, such as C58, could also be transmitted by cell-free extracts.

Leukemic extracts were prepared in the usual manner from C58 leukemic donors, then centrifuged and filtered through either Berkefeld (porosity N) or Selas (porosity 02 or 03) filter candles.

Newborn mice of the C57 Brown/cd strain were inoculated at an average age of 8 hours with the leukemic filtrates. Of 128 mice inoculated, 47 (37 per cent) developed leukemia at an average age of 10 months. Of 20 litter-mate controls inoculated with heated (70°C for ½ hour) extracts, or non-treated, only one mouse developed leukemia.

In a similar experiment, the leukemic filtrates were inoculated into 168 newborn (average 9 hours after birth) C3H mice (Bittner substrain); as a result, 38 (23 per cent) developed leukemia at an average age of 11 months. Of 46 litter-mate controls, either inoculated simultaneously with heated (70°C for ½ hour) leukemic extracts, or non-treated, only one mouse developed parotid tumors, none leukemia.

Leukemia induced in either C57 Brown or C3H mice as a result of inoculation of filtered C58 leukemic extracts could be transmitted by cell-graft to adult mice of the recipient line (C57 Brown or C3H, respectively), but not to mice of the donor (C58) strain.

The results of these experiments (Gross, 1956) suggested that leukemia developing spontaneously in mice of the C58 strain could also be transmitted by filtrates to newborn mice of the low-leukemic strains C3H or C57 Brown/cd.

Variations in Potency of Extracts Prepared from Ak Donors with Spontaneous Leukemia

Both the Ak and C58 leukemias were thus found to be readily transmissible by filtrates, provided that newborn mice of a susceptible strain were used for inoculation of the leukemic extracts. It soon became apparent, however, that the results of individual experiments may vary to a considerable degree, depending on the extract used. In our initial experiments, most of the cell-free extracts used for inoculation were prepared from Ak donors with spontaneous leukemia. Such extracts varied considerably in their leukemogenic potency. Some were completely inactive on inoculation tests. Thus, in a series of 70 leukemic filtrates tested in our laboratory, each prepared from a different Ak donor, 18 were found to be completely inactive on inoculation tests (Gross, 1957).

Other extracts were moderately active, and induced leukemia when inoculated into newborn, less than 16-hour-old mice of a susceptible strain, such as C3H or C57 Brown. When such filtrates were inoculated into suckling C3H mice, 2 to 12 days old, leukemia resulted in some of the inoculated animals, but only after a latency exceeding 14 months. Occasionally, leukemic filtrates prepared from Ak donors with spontaneous leukemia had a sufficiently high leukemogenic potential to induce leukemia after only 3 to 6 months when inoculated into suckling C3H mice, 1 to 7 days old (Gross, unpublished experiments). This was unpredictable, however. It was never possible to foresee whether a cell-free extract prepared from an Ak donor with spontaneous (or transplanted) leukemia would reproduce this disease following inoculation into newborn mice of a susceptible strain.

Initial Difficulties Followed by Confirmation of Cell-free Transmission of Mouse Leukemia

Transmission of mouse leukemia by filtrates marked a turning point and demonstrated conclusively the viral etiology of this disease. However, the original reports claiming cell-free transmission of mouse leukemia (Gross, 1951a,b) were received at first with doubt (Furth, 1951, 1952), and more often with considerable reservations (Kaplan, 1954. Kirschbaum, 1957a,b). Negative results of experiments carried out in order to verify the validity of this observation were reported from several leading laboratories. Law (1954) expressed criticism concerning the "design and interpretation" of the early reports (Gross, 1951a,b) of cell-free transmission of mouse leukemia. In an attempt to repeat these experiments, Law and his associates (1955), at the National Cancer Institute, inoculated 283 mice of the C3H strain, within 24 hours after birth, with cell-free, either centrifuged or filtered, extracts prepared from tissues of Ak, C58, or C3H/Fg mice with either spontaneous or transplanted leukemia, but did not observe any significant increase in the incidence of induced leukemia. Only 4.9 per cent of the inoculated mice developed leukemia, as compared with 3.7 per cent among the non-injected controls. Stewart (1955a), at the National Cancer Institute, inoculated 42 newborn C3H mice with cell-free Ak extracts, but none of them developed leukemia.* In a subsequent study, however, Stewart (1955b), employing newborn (C3Hf × AKR) F_1 hybrids as test animals, observed an increase in the incidence of leukemia following inoculation of cell-free extracts prepared from leukemic Ak mice.

Noriaki Ida (1957) in Dr. Kirschbaum's laboratory, in the Department of Anatomy at Baylor University in Houston, also attempted to reproduce, without success, our earlier experiments dealing with cell-free transmission of mouse leukemia (Gross, 1951, 1952, 1953). He employed filtered extracts prepared from C58 mice with spontaneous leukemia. The filtrates were injected into newborn C3H mice. Among 61 inoculated mice, 5 developed leukemia (8 per cent). This incidence was actually lower than that observed in the control group; the latter consisted of 164 untreated C3H mice, 22 of which (13.4 per cent) developed spontaneous leukemia. In another series, Ida inoculated centrifuged, cell-free extracts into newborn C3H mice. In this series again the incidence of induced leukemia was lower in the inoculated group (7 per cent among 106 injected mice) than that in untreated controls (approximately 20 per cent). He noticed, however, that leukemia appeared in the injected mice earlier than in the controls, even though the incidence was not increased. Ida, and also Kirschbaum (1957) concluded that there may possibly be some "acceleration" of spontaneous development of leukemia in mice inoculated at birth with leukemic extracts, but not an increase in the observed incidence. Reviewing the experiments of Ida (1957) and the studies of Gross (1951–1957), Kirschbaum (1957) stressed the multiplicity of factors presumably responsible for the development of leukemia, and questioned the necessity of a virus as an essential causative agent responsible for the development of this disease.

* * *

In analyzing the probable reasons for the initial difficulties, it is necessary to recall that transmission of mouse leukemia by filtrates was a new and rather striking development, contrasting sharply with previously reported negative results, and essentially inconsistent with the generally accepted genetic concept of the etiology of this disease. Furthermore, there were technical difficulties in reproducing transmission by cell-free filtrates of leukemia in mice. Preparation of active leukemogenic filtrates from organs of mouse donors with spontaneous leukemia was not readily accomplished, since most of them yielded filtrates of low infectivity. Considerable patience and repeated isolations were needed in order to obtain a relatively potent

* Some of the mice in both Law's and Stewart's experiments developed parotid gland tumors, instead of leukemia, an observation which had been reported previously (Gross, 1953. Stewart, 1953), and which will be discussed separately in more detail in the chapter on parotid tumor (polyoma) virus.

filtrate. Furthermore, in the early studies, the leukemogenic virus of relatively low potency recovered from mouse donors with spontaneous leukemia had a rather narrow host range; newborn mice of particular inbred strains were needed for bio-assay. Finally, because of the low content of infective virus present in filtrates employed for bio-assay, long latency periods, frequently exceeding one year, elapsed between inoculation of the filtrate and subsequent development of induced disease.

Gradually, however, the technique of transmission of mouse leukemia by filtrates became a routine procedure; with patience, and repeated efforts, more potent filtrates could be obtained from leukemic mouse donors. Eventually, several investigators working in different laboratories reported confirmatory experiments, and were able to transmit mouse leukemia by cell-free extracts.

Initial confirmation of cell-free transmission of mouse leukemia, accomplished by the use of newborn C3H mice for the inoculation of the leukemic filtrates, derived either from spontaneous Ak leukemias, or from C3H donors with Ak-agent-induced leukemias, was first reported by Woolley and Small in New York (1956). Confirmatory findings were subsequently also reported by Furth (1956), Dulaney (1957), Hays (1958), and their associates. Stewart (1955a) was at first unable to transmit Ak leukemia by cell-free extracts using newborn C3H mice for bio-assay, but succeeded in another series of experiments in which newborn (C3Hf × AKR) F_1 hybrids were employed for inoculation of the extracts (Stewart, 1955b).

"Acceleration" of Development of Spontaneous Leukemia Following Inoculation of Cell-free Leukemic Extracts into Newborn Mice

In an indirect manner confirmatory results were also obtained by Rudali, Duplan, and Latarjet at the Fondation Curie in Paris (1956b, 1957). The French authors used a modified method of bio-assay; instead of inoculating newborn C3H mice with cell-free leukemic Ak extracts, they employed newborn mice of the Ak strain as test animals. The inoculation of leukemic Ak extracts into newborn Ak mice resulted in the development of leukemia in 90 per cent of such animals after a relatively short latency of only 4½ months. Since mice of the Ak strain employed for inoculation are susceptible to the development of spontaneous leukemia, which is indistinguishable from that induced by inoculation of the virus, but which develops in such animals at a later age, the authors concluded (Rudali *et al.*, 1956b, 1957) that the injection of virus extracts "accelerated" the development of spontaneous leukemia in these mice. Among the non-injected controls, 84 per cent of mice developed spontaneous leukemia at an average

age of 9 months. In another control experiment, extracts prepared in a similar manner from mice of a non-leukemic line, and injected into newborn Ak mice, did not "accelerate" the development of leukemia.

"Acceleration" of Development of Spontaneous Leukemia, or Direct Induction of an Early Disease by the Inoculated Virus? It may be of interest to comment briefly on the results obtained by Rudali and his associates. The impression could have been gained (Rudali *et al.*, 1956b, 1957) that inoculation of the virus filtrate into newborn mice of the high-leukemic Ak strain resulted in an "acceleration" of the development of spontaneous leukemia in such animals, the disease appearing at $4\frac{1}{2}$ months of age, instead of developing at the usual age of $8\frac{1}{2}$ to 9 months. Another interpretation of these results is also possible. The early development of leukemia in the inoculated Ak mice could have been interpreted as an end-result of a direct, leukemogenic action of the injected virus, without affecting the potential susceptibility of such mice to a subsequent and unrelated development of spontaneous leukemia. Newborn mice of the Ak strain could therefore be compared with newborn mice of strain C3H or C57 Brown, all three strains being sensitive to the virus and susceptible to experimental induction of leukemia following inoculation of virus filtrate. The fact that Ak mice also carry, as a natural infection, a certain quantity of the same virus or of one of its close variants, transmitted in these mice naturally from one generation to another, may be unrelated to the susceptibility of such animals to an independent induction of this disease by inoculation of virus filtrate. Apparently, the presence of a small quantity of a latent mouse leukemia virus carried by such animals does not necessarily confer immunity to experimental inoculation of the same, or of a closely related, virus.

In subsequent experiments Jullien and Rudali (1960), at the Radium Institute in Paris, developed by serial cell-free passage a highly potent mouse leukemia strain originally isolated from one of the Ak leukemic donors. A cell-free leukemic extract prepared from organs of a mouse donor with spontaneous Ak leukemia was passed serially through newborn Ak mice, or through (AkR $\times$ RIIIf) F_1 hybrids. This method was based on experiments previously reported (Gross, 1957), dealing with passage A virus, and outlined in more detail on the following pages of this chapter, except that the passage A virus, also derived from Ak leukemic donors, was passed through suckling C3H mice. The highly active leukemogenic virus strain developed by the French investigators was designated "passage G." When inoculated into suckling Ak mice, this virus strain induced leukemia in practically 100 per cent of the injected animals after a brief latency of only 2 to 3 months.

THE DEVELOPMENT OF A HIGHLY POTENT MOUSE LEUKEMIA VIRUS STRAIN ("PASSAGE A")

It was of considerable practical importance that a consistently potent, leukemogenic virus strain could be isolated from spontaneous Ak leukemia.

The leukemogenic potency of cell-free extracts prepared from spontaneous mouse leukemia varied to a considerable extent. A particularly potent cell-free extract prepared from spontaneous Ak mouse leukemia was selected, and then passed serially, by successive cell-free passages, through several generations of newborn C3H mice. This procedure resulted eventually in the development of a highly potent strain of a filterable mouse leukemia virus, which was designated "passage A" (Gross, 1957a). After some 15 serial cell-free passages, this virus, when inoculated in the form of a filtrate into suckling, less than 7-day-old, C3H mice, induced lymphatic leukemia after only $2\frac{1}{2}$ to $3\frac{1}{2}$ months in over 95 per cent of the inoculated animals (Gross, 1960b).

Failure to obtain active filtrates from certain leukemic donors in mice, and the development of a consistently potent passage virus, recalled similar difficulties encountered in the early studies on cell-free transmission of the Rous chicken sarcoma. At first, when the filterable chicken tumor was discovered by Rous (1911), it was not always possible to reproduce cell-free transmission of the sarcoma, employing any tumor-carrying chicken as a donor for the preparation of the filtrate. In these early experiments it was observed that extracts prepared from certain chicken tumors yielded active tumor-inducing filtrates, whereas cell-free extracts prepared under apparently similar conditions from other chicken tumors proved to be inactive on inoculation tests. Gradually, it became apparent that different tumors contain different amounts of infective virus. Cell-free passage of the Rous sarcoma virus from one host to another—selecting as donors for successive passages always those animals that developed tumors after shortest latency—gradually increased the infective potency of such extracts (Bryan *et al.*, 1955). Employing for inoculation one of the highly potent passage strains of the Rous sarcoma virus, it is now possible to induce sarcomas in chicks with cell-free extracts in practically all animals after a short latency of less than 2 weeks.

"Passage A" Leukemic Virus in Mice Compared with "Fixed Virus" of Rabies of Pasteur

The initial method of transmitting mouse leukemia by filtrates prepared from Ak donors with spontaneous leukemia was frequently disappointing and always time consuming; persistence and many individual experiments, each dealing with a different extract, were needed in order to obtain positive results.

This situation changed fundamentally as soon as a highly active leukemic virus was isolated from one of the extracts tested, and then passed serially through newborn mice.

The leukemic "passage A" virus in mice is perhaps comparable to the

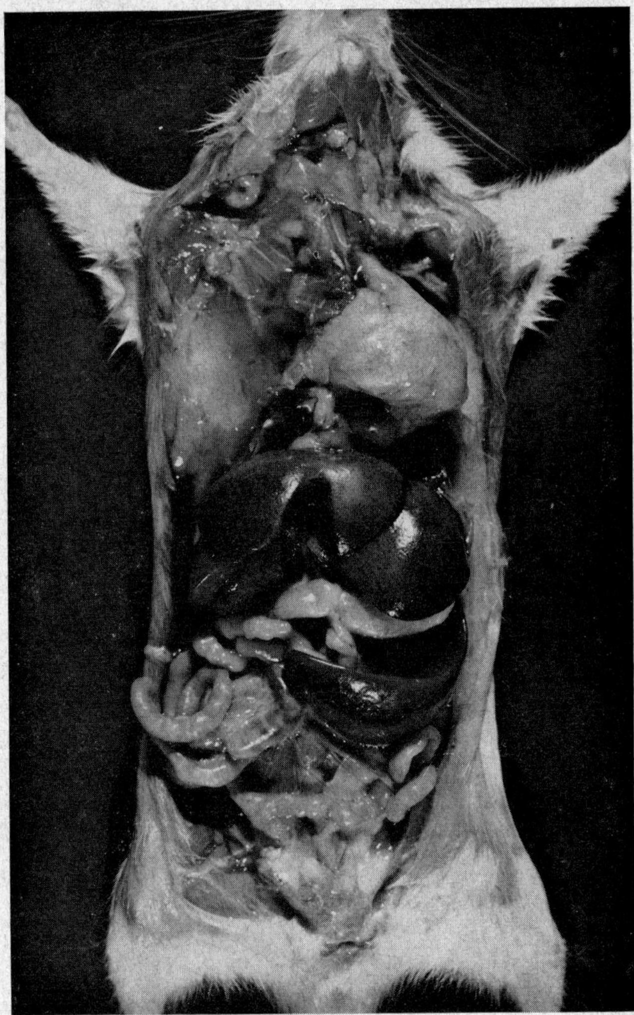

Fig. 31. Lymphatic Leukemia Induced in a Rat With Rat-adapted Mouse Leukemia Virus.

This Osborne-Mendel female rat was inoculated when 9 days old with rat-adapted mouse leukemia virus harvested from organs of a rat donor with virus-induced leukemia. At the age of 3 months this rat developed generalized lymphatic leukemia (WBC 72,000 per mm^3 with 51% blast cells and 40% lymphocytes; Hb 3 gm per 100 ml of blood). Note very large thymic tumor, spleen and liver; there was also a generalized infiltration of liver, kidneys and other organs with leukemic cells. (From: L. Gross, pp. 403–426 in: Viruses, Nucleic Acids, and Cancer, Williams & Wilkins Co., 1963.)

"fixed virus" of rabies of Pasteur, as contrasted with the "wild virus" encountered in animals developing disease spontaneously. After a considerable number of successive host-to-host passages, the pathogenic potency of the passage A virus gradually increased and became stabilized. When inoculated into susceptible hosts, this virus now regularly induces leukemia after a relatively short latency. Both the incidence of the induced leukemia and the latency are now consistent and predictable. By contrast, the virus recovered directly from spontaneous mouse leukemia is only occasionally potent; more often, such a "wild virus," as in the case of the "street virus" in rabies, is of an unpredictable, relatively low potency, and may induce disease in only some of the inoculated animals, and after a prolonged latency. Exceptions, however, exist and, in some instances, a relatively potent leukemic virus may be recovered directly from naturally occurring disease, i.e., from spontaneous leukemia.

Reproduction of Cell-free Transmission of Mouse Leukemia with Passage A Filtrates in Other Laboratories

As soon as passage A leukemic virus became available, the induction of mouse leukemia by inoculation of filtrates into newborn or suckling C3H mice could be reproduced without difficulty in other laboratories. Kassel and Rottino (1959), using the intravenous route for the inoculation of passage A filtrates into newborn C3H mice, observed the development of leukemia in 13 out of 13 injected mice in one group, and in 29 out of 36 injected mice (81 per cent) in another series, at an average age of 5 months. Of 28 alternate controls, observed up to 10 months of age, none developed leukemia. Levinthal, Buffet and Furth (1959), also using passage A filtrates for inoculation of suckling C3H mice, induced leukemia in 34 out of 58 inoculated animals (59 per cent), after an average latency of about 5 months. No leukemia was observed in 41 non-injected controls. Tennant and Syverton inoculated 38 C3H mice, 1 to 5 days old, with passage A filtrates; as a result, 31 of them (81.6 per cent) developed leukemia at an average age of 4.1 months. Miller (1959), at the Pollards Wood Research Station of the Chester Beatty Research Institute in England, inoculated passage A filtrates in four successive experiments into a total of 80 newborn or suckling C3H mice, inducing leukemia in all of them (100 per cent) after a latency varying from 2 to 4 months. W. P. Rowe and his associates at the National Institute of Health in Bethesda, Md., employing a more recent (20th and 21st) serial passage of this virus obtained from our laboratory, observed an incidence of leukemia of over 90 per cent, developing after a latency varying from $2\frac{1}{2}$ to $4\frac{1}{2}$ months, following inoculation of suckling, 3 to 7-day-old, C3H mice of the Bittner substrain, with passage A (Selas 02) leukemic filtrates. Similar reports have been received from several other laboratories.*

*Personal communications to the author (1959–1961) from J. R. Tennant, and J. T. Syverton, Dept. of Bacteriology, Univ. of Minnesota. W. P. Rowe, Nat. Inst. Health, Bethesda, Md. H. S. Kaplan, Stanford University, California. L. W. Law, Nat. Cancer Inst., Bethesda, Md. A. A. Axelrad, and H. C. Van der Gaag, Ontario Cancer Inst., Toronto.

Technique of Preparation of Passage A Leukemic Filtrate Employed in Our Laboratory

The extract is prepared from pooled tissues removed from 2 or 3 mice which developed leukemia as a result of inoculation with passage A virus. Preferably young mice which developed leukemia after a short latency of 2 to $2\frac{1}{2}$ months are used.

The instruments employed for removal of tissues are sterilized by boiling. Fragments of spleens, thymic and mesenteric tumors, peripheral lymph nodes, and livers (care being taken not to disturb the gallbladder) from all donor mice are removed aseptically, placed on a sterile gauze pad, and weighed. The tissue fragments are then placed in a sterile porcelain mortar, cut with small scissors and ground with a pestel by hand for about 3 minutes, sterile chilled physiological saline solution being added to obtain a cell suspension of approximately 20 per cent concentration.

The leukemic cell suspension is then centrifuged in a refrigerated International PR-2 centrifuge, at 3000 r.p.m. ($1400 \times g$), at 0°C, for 15 minutes. The supernate is removed, placed in another tube and again centrifuged in the PR-2 centrifuge at 0°C, this time at 9500 r.p.m. ($7000 \times g$) for 5 minutes. The second supernate is then passed through a Selas (porosity 0.2) porcelain filter candle under vacuum pressure of approximately 20 to 25 mm of mercury.

The leukemic filtrate thus obtained is immediately poured into a sterile glass tube, which is immersed in a larger glass container filled with ice cubes, and placed in an electric refrigerator (+4°C). The glass container should contain ice cubes at all times, assuring thereby that the filtrate's surrounding temperature is about 0°C.

The filtrate kept at 0°C can be used within a few hours after its preparation, but under these conditions the titer of the virus gradually decreases. It is preferable to inject the filtrate immediately after preparation. If a delay is necessary, the filtrate should be placed in glass ampoules, sealed, and quickly frozen at −70°C in carbon dioxide dry ice. Under such conditions the filtrate can be kept at least for 12 months, and according to our recent studies for up to 2 years, without appreciable loss of infective potency.

The passage A filtrate is inoculated in our laboratory intraperitoneally (approximately 0.3 to 0.4 cc. each) into suckling mice, 3 to 5 days old. Mice of a variety of strains are susceptible to the passage A virus; however, in order to obtain a uniformly consistent and high incidence of induced leukemia after a relatively short latency, it is suggested that mice of either strain C3H (Bittner subline), preferably free from the mammary carcinoma virus by foster-nursing, or mice of strain C57 Brown/cd, be used for inoculation of the filtrate. Generalized lymphatic leukemia will develop in over 95 per cent of the inoculated mice in about $2\frac{1}{2}$ to 3 months.

Influence of Age of the Host on Susceptibility to Inoculation of the Mouse Leukemia Virus

The introduction of newborn mice as test animals for inoculation of leukemic filtrates marked a turning point in the cell-free transmission of mouse leukemia. In subsequent experiments, when more knowledge was gained concerning the infectivity of leukemic extracts, and when more potent extracts were employed, it was realized that under certain experimental conditions young adult mice could also be used for inoculation. For all practical purposes, however, and under the usual experimental conditions, either newborn or suckling mice proved to be by far the most susceptible hosts.

In our initial experiments, newborn, less than 16-hour-old, mice were employed routinely for inoculation of the passage A filtrates. However, the immediate mortality following inoculation of newborn mice was relatively high. An attempt was made therefore to use, as test animals, suckling mice, 2 to 6 days old. We found, with some surprise, that such animals were at least as susceptible to the leukemogenic action of the passage A filtrates as were newborn mice (Gross, 1958a). The use of suckling, few-day-old, mice proved to be advantageous; larger doses of the filtrate could be inoculated; furthermore, the mortality was less pronounced than that following inoculation of newborn animals.

There was no particular advantage in inoculating embryos instead of newborn mice. In several experiments we have inoculated the passage A filtrate directly into C3H embryos exposed by laparotomy (Gross, unpublished studies, 1963). There was considerable mortality among the embryos thus inoculated, and several experiments performed in this manner were unsuccessful. In two experiments, however, in which the inoculated embryos survived, and were subsequently born at term, all developed later the usual forms of leukemia at ages varying from 2 to $3\frac{1}{2}$ months, i.e. not unlike those inoculated with the filtrate routinely after birth.

Suckling, 1 to 2-week-old, mice were also found to be highly susceptible to the inoculation of the leukemic virus. When inoculated into suckling, 1 to 14-day-old, but preferably less than 10-day-old, C3H or C57 Brown mice, the passage A filtrate induced leukemia in over 90 per cent of the inoculated mice after a latency of only 3 to $4\frac{1}{2}$ months (Gross, 1958). Gradually, however, the susceptibility of mice to the leukemogenic potency of the passage A virus decreased with increasing age.

The interesting observation was also made that following inoculation of leukemic filtrates containing a mixture of both the leukemic and the parotid tumor (polyoma) viruses, only leukemia resulted when suckling C3H mice, 2 to 14 days old, were inoculated. The same filtrates, however, induced either leukemia or parotid tumors, when newborn, less than 16-hour-old, mice of the same strain were inoculated (Gross, 1958a).

This striking difference in susceptibility, depending on the age of the host at the time of inoculation, afforded an opportunity to eliminate at will the induction of parotid tumors, by selecting recipient hosts of a proper age, even though extracts containing a mixture of both viruses were used for inoculation.

Susceptibility of Young Adult Mice to Inoculation of Passage A Filtrate

Previous attempts to transmit Ak leukemia by inoculation of filtrates into young adult C3H mice had not been successful. After the potency of the leukemic virus was increased through serial cell-free passage, however, it also became possible to induce leukemia by inoculating passage A leukemic filtrates into young adult mice of either the C3H or C57 Brown inbred lines.

In one of the experiments, 125 mice of the C3H strain were inoculated at the age of 1 to 2 months with the passage A filtrate (0.5 to 0.75 cc., i.p., each), and 98 of them (78 per cent) developed leukemia at $7\frac{1}{2}$ months of age. In another experiment, 12 mice of the C57 Brown strain were inoculated at the age of about 3 months with a similar dose of the virus, and 10 of them (83 per cent) developed leukemia at 11 months of age.

These and other similar experiments demonstrated that it was possible to induce leukemia by inoculating the potent passage A filtrate into adult mice of several different inbred lines; however, the incidence of leukemia was relatively lower, and the latency prolonged, as compared with results obtained following inoculation of newborn or suckling animals.

TABLE 4. SUSCEPTIBILITY OF MICE OF DIFFERENT STRAINS TO LEUKEMOGENIC ACTION OF PASSAGE A FILTRATES

Strain of mice	Serial pass. No.	No. of mice inoc.*	No. dev. leuk.	Leuk. inc. %	Avg. age leuk. dev. mos.
C3H/Bi†	27–28	189	187	99	2.7
C3H/An‡	21	37	26	70	3.9
C57 BR/cd	25–28	40	38	95	2.8
BALB/c	26–28	41	36	88	4.3
Swiss	30–31	53	42	79	3.5
I	29–30	17	11	65	5.2

*All mice inoculated i.p. when 1 to 5 days old, with 10 per cent to 20 per cent virus filtrate (0.2 to 0.3 cc. each).

†C3H/Bi, mice of Bittner subline of strain C3H, free from mouse mammary carcinoma virus by foster-nursing.

‡C3H/An, mice of Andervont subline of strain C3H, free from mouse mammary carcinoma virus by foster-nursing.

(From Gross, L., *Acta Haemat.*, **29**: 1, 1963.)

Susceptibility of Mice of Different Strains to the Leukemogenic Action of Passage A Virus

In the initial experiments, when filtrates prepared from spontaneous mouse leukemia of relatively low potency were employed, the virus was found to have a rather limited range of host specificity. The virus was leukemogenic for newborn or suckling mice of strains C3H/Bi and C57 Brown/cd (Gross, 1954 a, b, 1955 a, b, 1957b, 1960b), but was substantially less leukemogenic for mice of several other strains tested, such as inbred lines A, BALB/c, or Swiss (Gross, 1960b). When in more recent experiments substantially more potent passage A filtrates were employed for bioassay, the virus has shown a much broader host range (Gross, 1963b). Mice of several strains were tested, and all were found susceptible to the leukemogenic action of the passage A virus.

Suckling, 1 to 5-day-old, mice of several inbred lines, such as C3H/Bi, C3H/An, C57 Brown/cd, BALB/c, Swiss, and I, were inoculated intraperitoneally with passage A leukemic filtrates. The incidence of leukemia developing in the inoculated mice varied from 65 to 99 per cent, and the latency, i.e. the time elapsing between inoculation and development of disease, varied from 2.7 to 5.2 months. Mice of all strains tested were found to be susceptible to the leukemogenic action of the virus, though there were differences in the degree of susceptibility among the strains employed. Mice of the Bittner subline of the C3H strain were found to be most susceptible, 99 per cent of the inoculated animals developing leukemia, an observation consistent with results previously reported (Gross, 1955, 1957, 1960). The passage A virus appears to have a particular affinity for this substrain of mice. The Andervont subline of C3H strain showed a somewhat lower susceptibility. Mice of the C57 Brown/cd strain were almost as susceptible as those of the Bittner subline of the C3H strain. Mice of the BALB/c, and to a lesser extent those of the Swiss strain, were found to be also susceptible to the leukemogenic action of the passage A virus, 88 per cent and 79 per cent, respectively, developing leukemia following inoculation of the filtrates. Mice of the I line were also susceptible.

Symptoms and Course of Disease Developing in Mice Following Inoculation of the Passage A Virus

Leukemia developing in mice following inoculation of the passage A virus was essentially similar to the same disease developing spontaneously in mice of certain high-leukemic inbred lines, such as strain Ak. In most instances mice of the C3H strain inoculated with the passage A virus developed large thymic tumors, large spleens and livers, and also large tumorous lymph nodes in inguinal and axillary pits, and in the mesentery. All these tumors consisted of solid masses of lymphoid cells and could be classified as lymphosarcomas. In most animals the disease was generalized; in some, the disease was limited to only one or a few organs. The thymus appeared to be the principal target organ, since lymphoid tumors of varying size, replacing the thymic lobes, were found in practically all leukemic animals. In about 10 per cent of all leukemic mice, the disease was limited to a large mediastinal lymphosarcoma which originated in the thymus. In some instances, the thymic tumors filled out most of the chest cavity, without affecting appreciably other organs of the animals; for a few days before such mice died, their breathing was laborious; some of them died before the disease had an opportunity to become generalized.

It was, however, rather unusual to find the lymphoid neoplasm limited to the thymus. In the great majority of leukemic mice the spleens were also enlarged. The size of the spleens varied; quite frequently the spleen was of considerable volume. In many animals the liver was also enlarged. In those mice that had a fully developed and generalized disease, there were prominently enlarged peripheral lymph nodes, particularly noticeable in the axillary and inguinal pits, and also a characteristic reddish-white mesenteric tumor. In more advanced phases of the disease, the enlargement of the peripheral lymph nodes was readily recognized by inspection and gentle palpation of the inguinal and axillary pits. The enlargement of spleen could be also readily detected by palpation.

It is possible to speculate that even in such cases, the disease might have originated either in a single focus, or, what seems more probable, in a few isolated foci, located presumably within the thymus; generalization occurred, however, very early, and involved all the principal organs of the hematopoietic system, including spleen, liver, peripheral and visceral lymph nodes.

In all instances the disease was progressive. From the time leukemia was recognized in mice, they all died within 1 to 3 weeks. There was no case of spontaneous recovery.

FIG. 32. LEUKEMIC VIRUS PARTICLES IN ORGANS OF AK MOUSE WITH SPONTANEOUS LEUKEMIA AND C3H(F) MOUSE WITH VIRUS-INDUCED LEUKEMIA.

(A). Part of a phagocytic reticular cell from the thymus of an Ak mouse with spontaneous lymphatic leukemia. Several virus particles (c) in an intercellular space appear partially surrounded by cytoplasmic extensions (ce) of the cell. Magnification 33,600×. (D. G. Feldman and L. Gross, unpublished.) (B). A portion of a macrophage from lymph node of a C3H(f) mouse with lymphatic leukemia induced with passage A virus. Numerous vacuoles filled with large numbers of virus particles (c) are present in the partially disintegrated cell cytoplasm. Magnification 23,600×. (From: D. G. Feldman and L. Gross, *Cancer Research*, **24**: 1760, 1964.) Electron micrographs reproduced in Figs. 32 to 42 were prepared by Dr. D. G. Feldman in cooperation with the author.

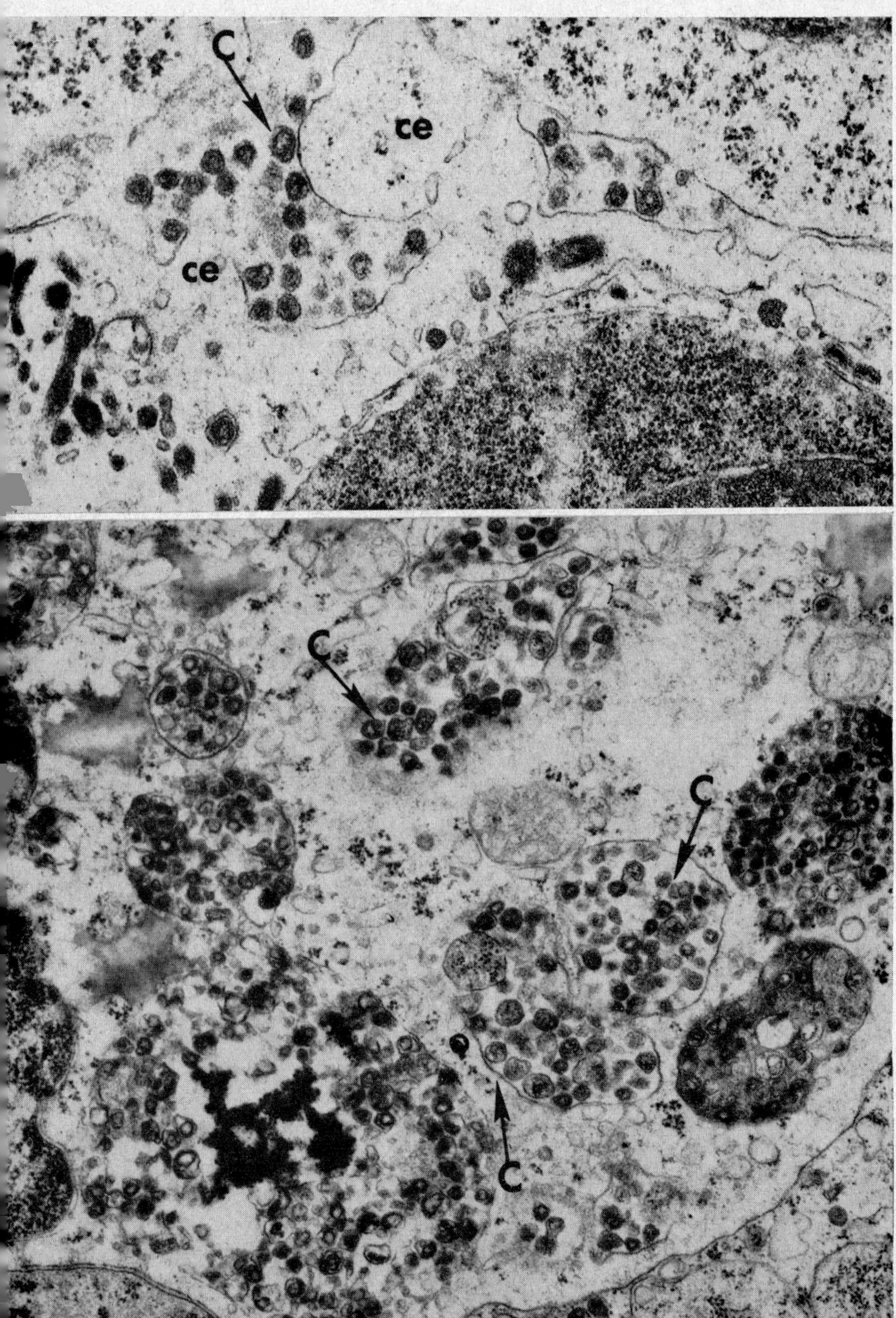

Fig. 32. Leukemic Virus Particles in Organs of Ak Mouse With Spontaneous Leukemia and C3H(f) Mouse With Virus-induced Leukemia.

In over 50 per cent of all C3H(f) mice with virus-induced leukemia, the peripheral blood picture did not reflect significant changes in the number and morphology of white blood cells. This form of "aleukemic" leukemia, quite similar to the most frequently occurring form of spontaneous mouse leukemia, could be considered to be essentially a generalized (in some instances a localized) lymphosarcoma. In most animals of this "aleukemic" group, the blood morphology remained essentially "normal" until the terminal phase of the disease, except for a frequently present and gradually progressing anemia. In some of the "aleukemic" mice, however, particularly in those with a more generalized form, as the disease progressed, the number of white cells in peripheral blood gradually increased, and later on abnormal cells, most frequently of the lymphatic series, could be seen; lymphoblasts eventually appeared. There were frequently also "smudge cells" present, which had no distinct morphology and were difficult to classify.

In less than 50 per cent of C3H mice with passage A virus-induced leukemia, the blood was leukemic from the early phases of the disease. Leukemia was in such animals either of the lymphatic or stem-cell form, and only very rarely myeloid.

Some animals had, apparently from the onset, a very high peripheral white blood count with large numbers of lymphoblasts. In such animals the disease was acute and generalized, and progressed rapidly from the beginning.

The femoral bone marrow of the leukemic mice was usually infiltrated with leukemic cells; however, in some of the leukemic mice in which the early disease was limited to a thymic lymphosarcoma, the bone marrow was found apparently normal, and was not infiltrated with leukemic cells at the time these mice were examined. It is possible that the leukemic process may initially develop in the thymus, or in another susceptible organ, such as spleen, then spread rapidly to other organs of the host, including the bone marrow. Accordingly, leukemic infiltration of the bone marrow may, in some instances at least, represent a secondary, and not necessarily a primary site in the progressive course of the disease.

On microscopic examination of different organs of leukemic mice, such as that of livers, kidneys, lungs, or salivary glands, there was noticeable in the majority of the animals a diffuse infiltration of parenchymal tissues with leukemic cells. This infiltration was more prominent around some of the larger vessels; this was particularly striking on examination of sections of livers.

All animals that had leukemic changes in their peripheral blood morphology, also had diffuse infiltration with leukemic cells of their internal organs. Among the animals with "aleukemic" leukemia, i.e. with either localized (thymic) or generalized lymphosarcomas, but with no leukemic changes in peripheral blood morphology, about 50 per cent had infiltration of internal organs with leukemic cells. It was of interest, therefore, that infiltration of internal organs with leukemic cells occurred quite frequently also in animals showing no leukemic changes in peripheral blood morphology.

The Various Forms of Leukemia and Lymphomas, Induced in Mice with Passage A Virus

At first, it was thought that the leukemic virus originally isolated from spontaneous Ak mouse leukemia could induce only the lymphatic form of this disease. More recently, however, it became clear that the passage A virus is capable of inducing a variety of different forms of leukemia and lymphomas in mice. The most frequently observed form was a generalized lymphosarcoma, involving predominantly the thymus, but usually also spleen, liver, and peripheral lymph nodes. This form, essentially similar to spontaneous leukemia observed in mice of high-leukemic strains, such as Ak or C58, was readily induced with the passage A virus in mice of strains C3H/Bi or C57 Brown/cd which we employed routinely in our laboratory for inoculation of the virus.

Acute lymphatic leukemia, and also stem-cell leukemia, sometimes involving in a striking manner the peripheral blood morphology, developed also quite frequently in C3H(f) or in C57 Brown mice, following inoculation of the passage A virus. Myelogenous leukemia, on the other hand, developed only exceptionally in mice of these inbred lines, following inoculation of the virus, unless they were thymectomized (Gross, 1960a). This will be discussed in more detail on subsequent pages of this chapter.

Influence of Genetic Susceptibility of the Host on the Forms of Virus-induced Leukemia and Lymphomas. Genetic susceptibility influenced to a considerable extent the form of leukemia developing in mice following inoculation of the passage A virus. Although this virus usually induced lymphatic or stem-cell leukemia, as well as lymphosarcomas in mice of strains C3H and C57 Brown, the same virus frequently induced myeloid leukemia following inoculations into mice of strain BALB/c (Gross, 1963b). Furthermore, not only lymphosarcomas, but also reticulum-cell sarcomas developed in spleens and lymph nodes of some of the BALB/c mice that had been inoculated with the passage A virus. Of particular interest were Hodgkin's-like lesions found in the lymph nodes and spleens, and occasionally also in livers of some of the leukemic mice. These lesions, similar to those described in mice by Dunn (1954), consisted of foci of pleomorphic infiltrates containing lymphocytes, histiocytes, plasma cells, eosinophils, and occasionally also multinucleated giant cells; these large multinucleated cells were, however, not typical Reed-Sternberg cells.

It should be stressed that microscopic examination of tissues, and study of peripheral blood morphology and bone marrow, were essential to determine the form of the induced disease. Only in some instances, and even then with considerable reservations, was it possible to suspect the probable form of leukemia on the basis of macroscopic examination alone. The presence of a very large thymic tumor, with the apparent absence of any other significant pathological changes, was suggestive of an aleukemic lymphatic disease. Generalized lymphatic and stem-cell leukemia frequently presented a similar macroscopic picture, i.e., a large or a moderately large thymic tumor, large spleen and liver, a large oblong mesenteric tumor, and considerably enlarged peripheral lymph nodes. Some cases of myelogenous leukemia could be suspected on the basis of a relatively small thymic tumor (or absence of a thymic tumor) and the presence of a very large spleen; in some of these animals the liver had a characteristic brownish color; occasionally there was also a slight amount of fluid present in the peritoneal cavity; these signs were far from consistent, however. In most instances, on macroscopic examination alone, myelogenous leukemia could not be distinguished from either lymphatic or stem-cell leukemia.

Forms of Leukemia Developing in C3H(f) Mice as a Result of Inoculation of Passage A Virus. A sample of 100 mice (53 females and 47 males) of the C3H(f) strain which developed leukemia at an average age of 2.7 months as a result of inoculation, within a few days after birth, with passage A virus filtrate was studied. In this sample, 96 mice (96 per cent) developed lymphoid tumors in the thymus, spleen, peripheral and visceral lymph nodes and frequently also in the liver; four mice (4 per cent) had thymic tumors only.

In the total sample studied, 64 mice (64 per cent) were "aleukemic," i.e. they had essentially no pathologic changes in their peripheral blood. The form of leukemia in these 64 mice was classified as "lymphatic," even though the peripheral blood in these animals reflected no definite basis for the diagnosis of this disease (aleukemic form). The four mice with thymic tumors only were in the aleukemic group.

In the remaining 36 mice (36 per cent) of this total sample studied, leukemia could be recognized on the basis of examination of peripheral blood smears, which showed an elevation in white blood cell counts and the presence of abnormal cells. The peripheral white blood cell counts in these mice ranged from 20,000 to 176,000 (average 49,000) per mm^3. A moderate anemia was present in most of the leukemic mice examined. In a few mice, anemia was pronounced; the lowest hemoglobin level was less than 2.0 grams per 100 cc. of blood. Among the 36 mice with leukemic blood changes, 23 developed lymphatic leukemia, 12 developed stem-cell leukemia, and one had myeloid leukemia.

To summarize, in a sample of 100 mice of the C3H(f) strain that developed leukemia as a result of inoculation with passage A virus filtrate, the form of leukemia could be classified as lymphatic (including the "aleukemic" group) in 87 mice (87 per cent), stem-cell in 12 mice (12 per cent), and myeloid in one mouse (1 per cent).

It should be emphasized, as discussed in more detail elsewhere in this chapter, that the term "lymphatic leukemia" is here employed in its broad meaning, and that it also includes localized (thymic) or generalized lymphosarcomas without significant changes in peripheral blood morphology.

Forms of Leukemia Developing in C57 Brown/cd Mice as a Result of Inoculation of Passage A Virus. A sample of 29 mice (18 females and 11 males) of the C57 Brown/cd strain which developed leukemia at an average age of 2.8 months as a result of inoculation, within a few days after birth, with passage A virus filtrate was studied. All 29 mice developed lymphoid tumors in the thymus, spleen, liver, visceral and peripheral lymph nodes.

In the total sample studied, 10 mice (34 per cent) were "aleukemic," i.e. they had no pathological changes in their peripheral blood morphology. In the remaining 19 mice leukemia could be recognized on the basis of examination of the peripheral blood; among the 19 mice with leukemic blood changes, 8 mice developed lymphatic leukemia, 10 mice developed stem-cell leukemia, and one mouse had myeloid leukemia.

Microscopic sections of tissues of 24 mice in this sample were studied, and all showed diffuse infiltration of internal organs with leukemic cells.

To summarize, in a sample of 29 mice of the C57 Brown/cd strain that developed leukemia as a result of inoculation with passage A virus filtrate, the form of leukemia could be classified as lymphatic (including the "aleukemic" group) in 18 mice (52 per cent), stem-cell in 10 mice (34 per cent), and myeloid in one mouse (4 per cent).

Forms of Leukemia Developing in BALB/c Mice as a Result of Inoculation of Passage A Virus. In a sample consisting of 53 mice of the BALB/c strain in which leukemia was induced with the passage A virus, 17 mice (32 per cent) developed lymphosarcomas, but had no significant changes in peripheral blood morphology (aleukemic form); in only two out of these 17 mice the lymphosarcomas were limited to the thymus; in the remaining 15 mice, either lymphosarcomas or reticulum-cell sarcomas developed in several organs, including thymus, spleen, and liver. In the remaining 36 mice of this group, leukemia could be recognized on the basis of examination of peripheral blood; among the 36 mice with leukemic blood changes, 2 mice developed lymphatic leukemia, 14 mice developed stem-cell leukemia, and 20 had myeloid leukemia. Lymphosarcomas or reticulum-cell sarcomas developed also in most of these animals.

To summarize, in a sample of 53 mice of the BALB/c strain that developed

> leukemia as a result of inoculation of passage A virus, the form of leukemia could be classified as lymphatic (including the "aleukemic" mice with lymphosarcomas) in 19 mice (36 per cent), stem-cell in 14 mice (26 per cent), and myeloid in 20 mice (38 per cent).

It is quite apparent, therefore, that the passage A mouse leukemia virus has a considerable oncogenic potential, and that it is capable of inducing in mice a variety of forms of leukemia and lymphomas, the form of the induced disease depending to a considerable extent on the individual response of the inoculated hosts.

TABLE 5. FORMS OF LEUKEMIA AND LYMPHOMAS INDUCED IN MICE AND RATS WITH MOUSE LEUKEMIA VIRUS

LEUKEMIAS

Lymphatic Leukemia
- (a) aleukemic
- (b) leukemic

Stem-cell Leukemia

Myelogenous Leukemia
- (a) undifferentiated
- (b) well differentiated

Chloro-Leukemia*

Erythroblastic Leukemia (atypical)*

Monocytic-like Leukemia

LYMPHOMAS

Lymphosarcomas
- (a) generalized
- (b) local lesions

Reticulum-cell Sarcomas

Hodgkin's-like Lesions

* In thymectomized mice only.

SUSCEPTIBILITY OF RATS TO THE MOUSE LEUKEMIA VIRUS

Rather unexpectedly newborn rats were found to be highly susceptible to the mouse leukemia virus.

Graffi and Gimmy (1957) were the first to observe that the mouse leukemia virus was also pathogenic for newborn rats; however, the incidence of leukemia induced with the Graffi strain of the mouse leukemia virus in rats was low and averaged only 10 per cent (Graffi, 1960). Moloney, employing for inoculation another mouse leukemia virus strain isolated from transplanted mouse sarcoma 37, was able to induce in rats an incidence of leukemia exceeding 70 per cent (Moloney, 1960).

When the passage A mouse leukemia virus was inoculated in the form of filtrates into newborn or suckling, less than 5-day-old, rats of either Sprague-Dawley or Osborne-Mendel strains, up to 70 per cent of the inoculated rats developed leukemia after a latency varying from $2\frac{1}{2}$ to $4\frac{1}{2}$ months (Gross, 1961). The virus could be readily recovered from the leukemic rats and passed serially by filtrate inoculation from rat to rat.

In order to harvest the virus, the extracts were prepared in the usual manner (described in more detail on page 350 of this chapter) from leukemic organs, mainly from thymic tumors and spleens of the leukemic rat donors. Briefly, the leukemic cell suspensions of either 10 per cent or 20 per cent concentration were first centrifuged at 3000 r.p.m. for 15 minutes, followed by a second centrifugation at 9500 r.p.m. for 5 minutes, and were then filtered through Selas (0.2) filter candles. Immediately after preparation, the filtrates were inoculated intraperitoneally (0.5 cc. each) into 1 to 7-day-old suckling rats.

For preservation and future use, the filtrates were sealed in glass ampoules, frozen in carbon dioxide dry ice, and kept at −70°C for several weeks or a few months, as needed, without any apparent loss of infectivity.

After only one or two successive serial rat-to-rat passages, the virus became adapted to the new species and induced leukemia in practically all inoculated rats; the incidence of induced leukemia exceeded 95 per cent, and the average latency decreased to less than 3 months (Gross, 1963).

The rat-adapted virus was at the time of this writing in its 27th serial rat-to-rat passage; following inoculation into less than 7-day-old suckling rats of the Sprague-Dawley strain, this virus induces leukemia and lymphomas in practically all instances.

We have been using most frequently 2 to 4-day-old rats for inoculation. In some instances we used newborn, less than 16-hour-old rats. When animals of the desired age group were not immediately available, we used 6 or 7-day-old rats, and occasionally we inoculated suckling rats 8 or 9 days old. Within this age range, we have found all animals fully susceptible to the leukemogenic action of the passage A virus.

Host Range in Rats. Strains of Rats Employed. The passage A virus was found to be leukemogenic for suckling rats of several strains. In our experiments we employed suckling rats of either the Sprague-Dawley, or Osborne-Mendel, and more recently also of Long-Evans strain. We found rats of all three strains about equally susceptible to the leukemogenic action of the passage A virus (Gross, 1961, 1963d). Newborn, non-inbred rats of the Wistar strain were also found to be highly susceptible to the induction of leukemia with the passage A virus (Kirsten *et al.*, 1962. Okano *et al.*, 1963). Other strains, such as Fischer rats, were also found susceptible.

From a nucleus of random-bred Sprague-Dawley rats received in June, 1960, from the Animal Production Unit, National Institute of Health, Bethesda, Maryland, a colony of rats has been raised in our laboratory by brother-to-sister mating.

In addition, from 2 litters of rats of the Osborne-Mendel strain, which we received from the same source in February, 1961, a separate colony of rats of that strain has been also raised for a limited study.

More recently, in April, 1966, we received from Dr. Charles Huggins, University of Chicago, a litter of Long-Evans rats. A small colony of these animals has been raised in our laboratory from this initial litter by brother-to-sister mating.

These three colonies have provided the only source of all rats employed for inoculation of the leukemic filtrates in our laboratory.

In our initial experiments we were using rats of both Sprague-Dawley and Osborne-Mendel strains, and we found them about equally susceptible to the leukemogenic action of the mouse leukemia virus. We then discontinued using rats of the Osborne-Mendel strain, and we have been using almost exclusively Sprague-Dawley rats.

Recently we have also been employing the Long-Evans rats for inoculation of the leukemic filtrates. We found these animals highly susceptible to the mouse leukemia virus; however, we found the Long-Evans rats slightly more difficult to handle, since they appear to be more excitable and less gentle than the Sprague-Dawley rats.

It is therefore apparent that suckling rats of several strains routinely employed in the laboratory are susceptible to the leukemogenic action of the mouse leukemia virus.

The use of suckling rats as experimental animals for studies of virus-induced leukemia presents certain advantages over the use of mice. The rat is highly susceptible to the virus, and develops a variety of forms of leukemia and lymphomas after a relatively short latency. Following inoculation of the virus, we have seen more often typical myeloid and acute stem-cell leukemia in rats than in mice. As a practical advantage, it should be noted that litters of rats are relatively large; it is not unusual to find 10 or 12 newborn rats in a single litter. Moreover, the infant mortality is generally low, and most of the injected animals can be raised in good health, and observed for subsequent development of leukemia. This contrasts with the frequent and relatively high infant mortality among the virus-injected mice. Furthermore, the virus can be readily recovered from leukemic rats. Because of its size, the rat donor offers a generous source for the harvesting of the leukemic virus. When working with mice, thymic tumors and spleens from several leukemic mouse donors have to be pooled to obtain source material for the preparation of relatively small quantities of the filtrate; on the other hand, similar organs from only one or two leukemic rat donors yield large quantities of potent virus filtrates. Moreover, because of its larger size, the rat is a better source of blood than the mouse; this is of importance in hematological and serological studies.

The incidence of spontaneous leukemia or lymphomas in rats of either strain employed in our laboratory appears to be extremely low. We have observed, however, mammary carcinomas developing quite frequently in middle-aged female rats, particularly those of the Sprague-Dawley strain.

We have observed thus far only a limited number of untreated rats of both strains. We have noticed an occasional development of spontaneous mammary carcinomas in old female rats, but not spontaneous development of either leukemia or lymphosarcomas. Two out of 27 breeding Sprague-Dawley female rats, observed for periods of time exceeding 7 months, developed spontaneous mammary carcinomas; none developed leukemia. In another group of rats consisting of 28 virgin females and 8 males of the Sprague-Dawley strain otherwise not treated, but born to virus-injected parents, 4 female rats developed mammary carcinomas at ages varying from 13 to 16 months; none developed leukemia; they were observed until they reached 16 months of age (Gross, 1963d).

Our experience with non-treated rats of the Osborne-Mendel strain has been limited to a small group of animals observed for periods of time varying from 5 to 10 months. Out of 13 breeding females and 13 males of that strain,

---

FIG. 33. THE FORMATION OF MOUSE LEUKEMIA VIRUS PARTICLES BY BUDDING FROM CELL MEMBRANES IN VIRUS-INJECTED RATS AND MICE.

(A). An area from bone marrow of a Sprague-Dawley rat with passage A virus-induced myeloid leukemia. Leukemia virus particles are shown in various stages of development. A virus particle (a) appears to be budding from the cell membrane (cm). Attached to the budding particle are 2 doughnut-like immature type C particles (b and c). A spherical mature type C particle (d) with a dense inner nucleoid and an irregularly shaped particle (e) with a less distinct nucleoid are shown. The probable sequence of development of the particles is from a to e. Magnification 122,000 ×. (From: D. G. Feldman and L. Gross, *Cancer Research*, **26**: 412, 1966.) (B). Portion of a macrophage from loose connective tissue from a C3H(f) mouse with passage A virus-induced lymphatic leukemia. Illustrated are budding virus particles in various stages of development (a to c), immature type C particles (d), and a mature type C particle (e) with a nucleoid. The probable sequence of development of the virus particles is from a to e. Magnification 54,250 ×. (D. G. Feldman and L. Gross, unpublished.)

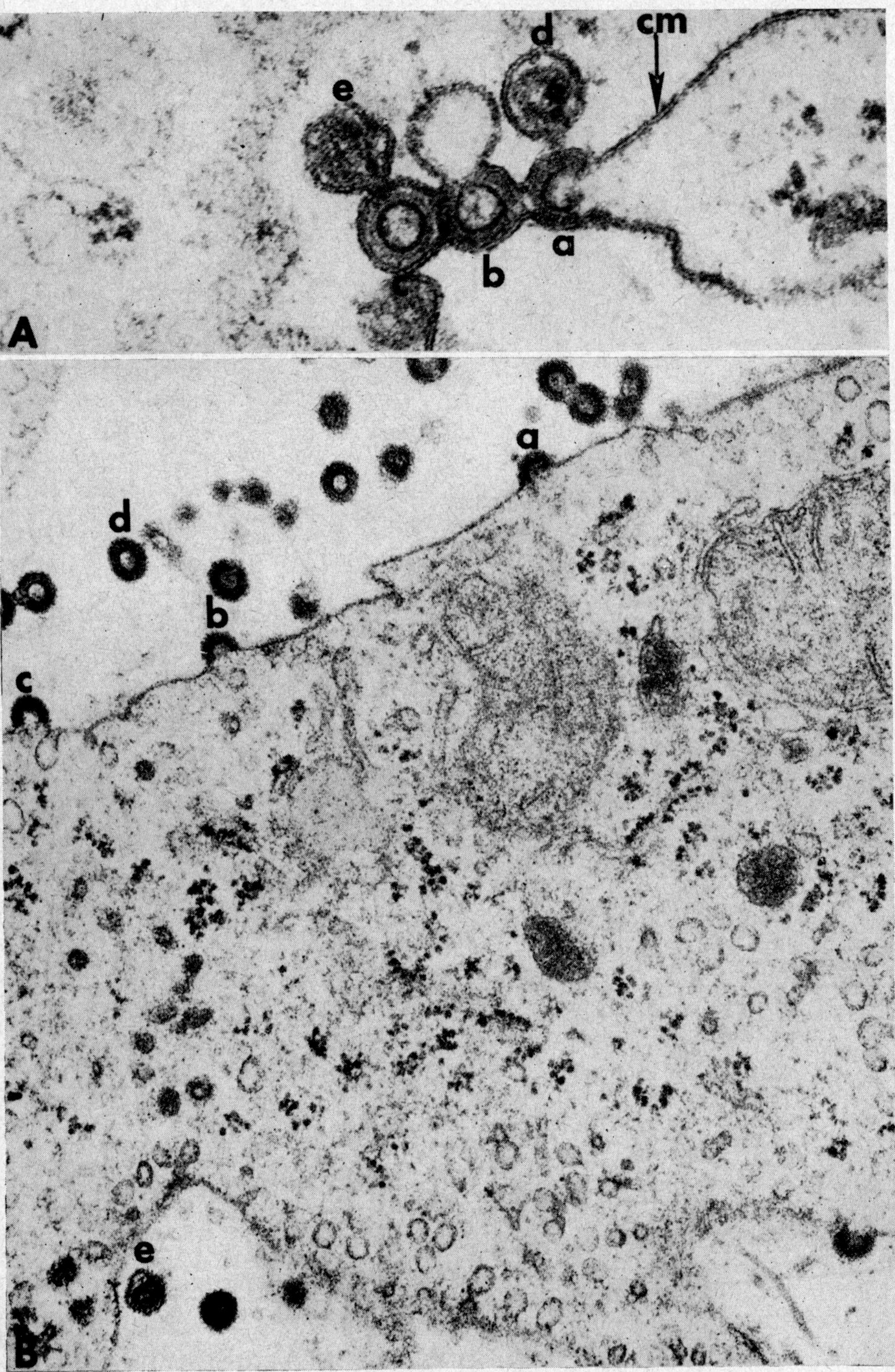

FIG. 33. THE FORMATION OF MOUSE LEUKEMIA VIRUS PARTICLES BY BUDDING FROM CELL MEMBRANES IN VIRUS-INJECTED RATS AND MICE.

one female developed mammary carcinoma at the age of $3\frac{1}{2}$ months. None developed leukemia (Gross, 1963d).

Rats have not been used as extensively in cancer research as have been the various strains of mice. However, there have been many reports in the literature on the incidence of spontaneous tumors in different strains of rats (Bullock and Curtis, 1930; Curtis, *et al.*, 1931; Ratcliffe, 1940; Saxton, *et al.*, 1948; Davis, *et al.*, 1956; Crain, 1958; Noble and Cutts, 1959; Kim, *et al.*, 1960).

Dr. Jacob Furth, who previously developed the Ak strain of mice known for their very high incidence of spontaneous leukemia, made an attempt to develop a similar inbred strain of rats. This opportunity seemed to be on hand when, about 15 years ago, numerous malignant lymphomas had been observed to develop spontaneously in rats of a partly inbred line of the Wistar strain in his laboratory. Dr. Furth began inbreeding rats of this strain by brother-to-sister mating, trying to develop eventually a strain of rats having a high incidence of spontaneous leukemia. This aim has not been achieved, however; in spite of continued inbreeding, leukemias and lymphomas developed in animals of this strain only in relatively small numbers (Kim, *et al.*, 1960).

TABLE 6. INCIDENCE OF LEUKEMIA INDUCED IN SPRAGUE-DAWLEY RATS WITH THE RAT-ADAPTED MOUSE LEUKEMIA (PASSAGE A) VIRUS

Serial rat-to-rat passage	No. of rats inoc.*	No. dev. leuk.†	Leuk. incid. %	Avg. latency mos.
1 to 5	204	158	77	3.4
6 to 10	208	189	91	3.0
11 to 15	113	108	96	3.1
16 to 20	98	95	97	3.6
21 to 25	107	101	94	4.4

* Suckling rats, 1 to 5 days old, were inoculated. Each rat received approx. 0.5 cc., i.p., of a 10 to 20 per cent filtrate.

† Most of the inoculated rats developed thymic and generalized lymphosarcomas.

Symptoms and Signs of Leukemia Developing in Rats Following Inoculation of the Passage A Virus

Examination of blood of rats which developed leukemia as a result of inoculation of the passage A virus revealed the presence of leukemia only in some animals. Over 30 per cent of leukemic rats had no significant changes in their peripheral (tail) blood morphology. These rats had only large lymphoid thymic tumors, and in addition frequently also lymphosarcomas in spleens, livers, and lymph nodes. As was the case in mice, in rats also this form of "aleukemic" lymphatic leukemia could be designated as a generalized (or in some instances localized) lymphosarcoma.

Gradually we have learned to suspect the development of leukemia in rats, and in more advanced cases to recognize the disease, on the basis of certain clinical features. Among the more characteristic signs, labored breathing was indicative of a mediastinal, i.e., thymic tumor. Enlargement of spleen could be detected by gentle palpation. In certain advanced cases, characteristic pin-point hemorrhages around the eyelids were also present. Gradually, leukemic rats developed muscular weakness, and in some instances paralysis of one or two limbs; the hind limbs appeared more frequently involved. In more advanced phases, there was a marked loss of weight. Ruffled fur in the leukemic rats was also quite characteristic and contrasted sharply with the smooth, shiny fur of healthy animals.

There was as a rule no difficulty in recognizing leukemia when the rat died or was sacrificed. Most of the leukemic rats had large thymic tumors; in about 10 to 15 per cent of all leukemic rats, the disease was limited to that organ. Most of the leukemic rats, however, had also large spleens and livers, and large mesenteric tumors. In a few animals the spleens, in some instances also the livers, were unusually large, occupying a considerable part of the abdominal cavity. Enlarged lymph nodes were often found in the submaxillary region. It is of interest, however, that in contrast to mice, with only rare exceptions, we have not observed in leukemic rats significantly enlarged inguinal or axillary lymph nodes.

In some leukemic rats we observed in the subcutaneous tissue, particularly in sternal, axillary, abdominal or dorsal areas, gelatinous-like soft swellings, which on microscopic examination had the structure of a myxoma.

All forms of leukemia observed were progressive. From the time leukemia was recognized in such animals, without exception they died within about 2 or 3 weeks; we have never observed spontaneous recovery.

Forms of Leukemia Induced in Rats with Passage A Virus

Most of the inoculated rats developed lymphatic leukemia; this designation included also those animals which developed the "aleukemic" form of the disease, i.e., had either thymic tumors only, or generalized lymphosarcomas, with no significant changes in peripheral blood morphology. Stem-cell leukemia developed also quite frequently in some of the inoculated rats; this form of disease was frequently associated with the presence of very high numbers of lymphoblasts in peripheral blood. Finally, about 5 to 8 per cent of the inoculated rats developed myelogenous leukemia; in these animals the number of white blood cells in peripheral blood circulation was considerably increased, and included primitive cells of the myeloid series in various phases of maturation, including myelocytes and myeloblasts.

The majority of leukemic rats had a rapidly progressing anemia; the hemoglobin level was in some animals exceedingly low, in a few instances below 3 grams per 100 cc. of blood. It was our impression that the number of platelets was not appreciably diminished. Microscopic examination revealed in spleens, livers, and kidneys of some of the leukemic animals a marked extramedullary hematopoiesis. In the majority of leukemic rats, particularly in those with generalized disease, microscopic examination revealed diffuse infiltration of internal organs, such as liver, spleen, kidneys, lungs, salivary glands, etc. with leukemic cells. This infiltration was very similar to that observed in leukemic mice.

Lymphosarcomas were very common. They could be readily recognized on microscopic examination in the spleens, livers, kidneys, and other organs infiltrated with leukemic cells. Reticulum-cell sarcomas were also found, though less frequently, in lymph nodes and spleens, occasionally in livers. Furthermore, as was the case in mice, in some of the leukemic rats also, Hodgkin's-like lesions were found in thymic tumors, spleens, livers, and lymph nodes. These lesions consisted of foci of pleomorphic infiltrates containing lymphocytes, histiocytes, plasma cells, eosinophils, and occasionally also multinucleated giant cells; they did not contain, however, typical Reed-Sternberg cells.

In a group of Sprague-Dawley rats in which leukemia developed following inoculation of passage A virus *harvested from leukemic mice*, the incidence of the various forms of leukemia and lymphomas was as follows:

> Out of 44 leukemic rats examined, 20 (45 per cent) developed lymphatic leukemia; among rats in this group, 15 animals (34 per cent) had the aleukemic form, i.e. localized or generalized lymphosarcomas with no significant changes in peripheral blood morphology. Twenty-one rats (48 per cent) developed stem-cell leukemia, and 3 (7 per cent) developed myelogenous leukemia. Among the 29 rats with leukemic blood changes, the white blood cell counts ranged from 18,000 to 1,456,000 per mm^3, with an average of 194,000. Most leukemic rats had a rapidly progressing anemia; the lowest hemoglobin level was <2 grams per 100 cc. of blood.
>
> Eight rats (18 per cent) had lymphoid tumors limited to the thymus only; all other rats had, in addition to thymic tumors, also lymphosarcomas involving spleen, liver, lymph nodes, and frequently also other organs; one rat had a reticulum-cell sarcoma, and one had Hodgkin's-like lesions in the spleen, liver, and lymph nodes. The majority of leukemic rats had also diffuse infiltration of liver and other internal organs with leukemic cells. Two leukemic rats had extensive, gelatinous-like, subcutaneous swellings which had the microscopic morphology of myxomas.

In another group of Sprague-Dawley rats in which leukemia was induced with the passage A virus *harvested from leukemic rat donors*, the incidence of the various forms of leukemia and lymphomas was as follows:

> Out of 38 leukemic rats examined, 22 (58 per cent) developed lymphatic leukemia; among rats in this group, 15 animals (39 per cent) had the aleukemic

form, i.e. localized or generalized lymphosarcomas with no significant changes in their peripheral blood morphology. Fourteen rats (37 per cent) developed stem-cell leukemia, and 2 rats (5 per cent) developed myelogenous leukemia. Among the 23 rats with leukemic blood changes, the white blood cell counts ranged from 22,000 to 600,000 per mm^3, with an average of 81,400. Almost all leukemic rats examined had anemia. The lowest hemoglobin level was 2.4 grams per 100 cc. of blood.

Five rats (13 per cent) developed thymic tumors only. One rat had lymphosarcomas in spleen and liver but had no thymic tumor. All other rats had not only thymic tumors, but also lymphosarcomas in spleens, livers, lymph nodes, and other organs. Six rats developed Hodgkin's-like lesions in the thymic tumors, spleens, lymph nodes, and/or livers. All rats, except 10 animals in the aleukemic group, had diffuse infiltration of liver and other internal organs with leukemic cells.

In some instances only, and then with considerable reservation, was it possible to suspect the probable form of leukemia by macroscopic examination. Presence of a very large thymic tumor with concurrent absence of any other significant pathology was suggestive of aleukemic lymphatic disease; such rats usually had no enlargement of spleen or liver. Subcutaneous petechial hemorrhages accompanying generalized leukemia were frequently indicative of an acute stem-cell form of the disease. However, stem-cell leukemia was also observed without concurrent hemorrhagic manifestations. Generalized lymphatic and myelogenous leukemia frequently presented a similar picture to the naked eye; only microscopic examination of blood, bone marrow, and tissue sections revealed the specific form of the disease. Bone marrow was infiltrated with leukemic cells in many, but not in all, cases. Some rats in which the disease was limited to a large thymic tumor had apparently normal bone marrow; these, however, presented a relatively small minority.

In summary, the forms of leukemia and lymphomas induced in rats with the mouse leukemia virus were essentially similar to those induced with the same virus in mice. We had, however, the impression that myeloid leukemia and also acute stem-cell leukemia, both forms with high white cell counts in peripheral blood, were more frequently observed in rats than in mice.

* * *

We were therefore faced with the fact that a leukemogenic virus isolated from mice proved to be pathogenic not only for mice, but also for rats, inducing in both species the same disease, i.e. leukemia and/or lymphomas in their usual variety of morphological forms.

In certain instances, the mouse leukemia virus could be transmitted directly from spontaneous mouse leukemia to rats, without a preliminary serial passage of the virus in mice prior to its transfer into rats. Kirsten and his colleagues (1962) prepared filtered cell-free extracts from pooled organs of AkR mice that had developed spontaneous leukemia. The filtrates were inoculated into newborn rats of the Wistar strain. Thirty-four out of 79 inoculated rats (43 per cent) developed leukemia after a latency varying from $3\frac{1}{2}$ to 10 months. The virus could be readily recovered from the leukemic rats, and passed serially through newborn animals of that species. The incidence of leukemia in the second and third passage increased to over 90 per cent, and the average latency decreased to $3\frac{1}{2}$ months.

It was of considerable interest that the leukemic virus could be readily recovered from leukemic rats, and that it could be passed serially, from rat to rat, without any apparent loss of its pathogenic potency.

When, after 21 to 25 consecutive rat-to-rat passages, the virus filtrate was inoculated into a total of 107 suckling, less than 7-day-old Sprague-Dawley rats, 101 animals (94 per cent) developed leukemia after an average latency of 4.4 months (Gross, 1967–1968, unpublished data).

Furthermore, the passage of the virus in rats did not measurably decrease its pathogenic potency for mice; when, after several consecutive rat-to-rat passages, the virus was inoculated back into newborn mice, leukemia developed in over 95 per cent of the inoculated animals.

The mouse was, nevertheless, more susceptible to the passage A virus than the rat. This was evident from titration experiments which revealed that substantially higher dilutions of the virus filtrate induced leukemia in mice than in rats. Even after 7 to 12 successive rat-to-rat passages, the virus still retained a considerable higher potency for the mouse, i.e. its species of origin, than for the rat. This might not have been apparent when relatively high concentrations of the virus were inoculated, such as a 10 per cent or even a 10^{-2} dilution of the filtrate; such concentrations induced in either mice or rats an incidence of leukemia approaching 100 per cent. When, however, 10^{-4} or 10^{-5} dilutions of the filtrate, harvested from leukemic rat donors, were inoculated into suckling mice and rats in simultaneous titration experiments, an incidence of leukemia of 83 per cent or 73 per cent, respectively, was induced in mice, as compared with an incidence of leukemia of only 25 per cent, or 9 per cent, induced with the same dilutions in the inoculated rats (Gross, 1965).

Attempts to Transmit the Mouse Leukemia Virus to Hamsters

The passage A leukemia virus, harvested from leukemic mice after 37th to 39th serial passages in that species, was inoculated (0.5 to 0.75 cc. of a 10 per cent or 20 per cent filtrate i.p.) into newborn or suckling, less than 4-day-old, hamsters. Only those animals that survived at least 4 months were included in the tabulation. Forty-four hamsters were observed, and all died without evidence of either leukemia, lymphomas, or any other malignant neoplasms, 4 to 17 months following inoculation (average survival time, 10.5 months).

In a second group, the leukemic virus was first passed serially through 10 to 12 consecutive rat-to-rat passages, and then harvested from leukemic rats, and inoculated (0.5 to 0.75 cc. of 10 per cent or 20 per cent filtrate i.p.) into suckling, less than 5-day-old, hamsters. Only those animals that survived at least 4 months were included in the tabulation. Forty-one hamsters were observed, and all died without evidence of either leukemia, lymphomas, or any other malignant tumors, 4 to 17 months following inoculation (average survival time, 9 months).

Inoculation of the Mouse Leukemia Virus into Chickens

In a joint project (1964, unpublished) carried out by Dr. B. R. Burmester at the Regional Poultry Research Laboratory in East Lansing, Michigan, with the author, an attempt was made to determine whether the passage A leukemic virus would be pathogenic for chickens. In the first experiment, passage A filtrate of 20 per cent concentration, prepared in the usual manner from leukemic rats, was inoculated either undiluted, or in a 1 : 10 dilution. Among the 177 chickens of line 15 I that had been inoculated either as embryos (91 chickens) or as one-day-old chicks (86 chickens), and which survived an observation period of up to 310 days, there were 9 cases of visceral lymphomatosis, 2 erythroblastosis, 6 neurolymphomatosis, and 2 osteopetrosis, a total of 19 leukemias or related tumors (total 11 per cent). There was only one case of erythroblastosis among 83 control chickens that had been inoculated either as embryos (39 chickens) or as one-day-old chicks (44 chickens) with the diluent only, without the virus.

Although the incidence of visceral lymphomatosis and related tumors was higher in the virus-inoculated group than in the controls, the results did not appear sufficiently convincing to warrant a definite conclusion. For that reason this experiment was repeated. In the second experiment, the passage A virus, again harvested from leukemic rats, was inoculated into 100 one-day-old chicks of line 15 I. These chickens were observed for 310 days, and none developed either visceral lymphomatosis or any other form of a related neoplasm.

In a control experiment, 100 one-day-old chicks of line 15 I were inoculated with physiological saline solution, and none developed either visceral lymphomatosis or any other related tumors.

In conclusion, it appears that under experimental conditions employed, the mouse leukemia virus had no demonstrable oncogenic effect in chickens.

PROPERTIES AND PATHOGENIC POTENCY OF THE MOUSE LEUKEMIA VIRUS

Filterability and Size. The mouse leukemia virus is a spherical particle about 100 mμ in diameter, which readily passes through bacteria-tight filters, such as Seitz (S-1) filter pads, Berkefeld-N or Selas (porosity 02 or 03) filter candles (Gross, 1951a,b, 1953a, 1956). Gradocol filtration experiments, in which membranes of known porosity were employed, suggested that the diameter of the leukemic virus particles probably averages somewhere between 70 and 100 mμ (Gross, 1957b).

In electron microscopic studies, which will be discussed in more detail on subsequent pages of this chapter, the diameter of the virus particles varied from 75 to 125 mμ, and even within wider limits (Dmochowski and Grey, 1957. Bernhard and Gross, 1959). Recent electron microscopic studies of ultrathin sections of leukemic tissues from either mice (Feldman and Gross, 1964) or rats (Dmochowski *et al.*, 1962. Dmochowski, Padgett and Gross, 1964), with passage A virus-induced leukemia, suggested that the average diameter of the virus particles is about 100 mμ.

Sedimentation of the Mouse Leukemia Virus in an Ultracentrifuge. Ultracentrifugation studies suggested that the mouse leukemia virus could be sedimented in about 30 minutes at 40,000 r.p.m. in a Spinco Model L ultracentrifuge (Gross, 1957b).

Cell-free leukemic extracts prepared in the usual manner (described on page 350 of this chapter), and derived either from organs of Ak donors with spontaneous leukemia or from C3H donors with Ak leukemic filtrate-induced leukemia, were centrifuged in Spinco Model L ultracentrifuge, using Swinging Bucket Rotor SW 39 at maximum speed 40,000 r.p.m. (average 125,000 $\times$ g). After ultracentrifugation for 30 minutes the supernate was, with only some exceptions, inactive on inoculation tests, whereas the sediment consistently reproduced leukemia (Gross, 1957b,c).

Sensitivity of the Virus to Heating. The mouse leukemia virus was found to be relatively sensitive to moderate heating. In preliminary experiments, it could be destroyed after heating for 30 minutes at 68°C (Gross, 1953). More recent experiments have shown that heating in a water bath at 50°C for 30 minutes inactivated the leukemogenic potency of passage A filtrates (Gross, 1960b).

The virus, in the form of a filtrate, could be preserved without any apparent and substantial loss of infectivity in a bacteriological incubator at 37°C for at least 7 to 12 hours. However, no titration experiments have been carried out in these studies, and it is quite probable that partial loss of infectivity occurred under such conditions. After 24 hours at 37°C loss of potency was apparent since only 19 out of 27 suckling C3H(f) mice (70 per cent) inoculated with such extracts developed leukemia after an average latency of 4.8 months. In a simultaneous control experiment the same extracts kept at 0°C and inoculated into 36 suckling C3H(f) mice induced leukemia in all animals (100 per cent) after an average latency of only 2.8 months. The potency of the extracts was further decreased after an incubation at 37°C for 48 hours: out of 20 suckling mice inoculated with such extracts, only 8 (40 per cent) developed leukemia after an average latency of 6.4 months. The extract was completely inactivated after an incubation at 37°C exceeding 48 hours. Seventeen suckling mice were inoculated with extracts that had been incubated at 37°C for 72 hours, but none developed leukemia, although they reached an average age of 17 months.

The relative resistance of the virus to incubation at 37°C was in contrast to the considerable sensitivity of leukemic cells to *in vitro* incubation at 37°C. The leukemic cell suspensions, suspended in physiological saline solution, lost their ability to grow on implantation into susceptible mice, and to induce transplanted leukemia, after incubation *in vitro* at 37°C for only 8 hours.

Sensitivity of the Virus to Ether. When the leukemic filtrate was mixed *in vitro* with ethyl ether, its leukemogenic potency was promptly destroyed. This observation suggested that the mouse leukemia virus belongs to the group of ether-sensitive viruses.

Preliminary experiments were carried out with extracts prepared either from spontaneous Ak leukemia, or from C3H donor mice in which leukemia was induced by inoculation of cell-free Ak extracts. Leukemic cell suspensions of 20 per cent concentration prepared in physiological saline solution were mixed with equal amounts of ethyl ether (Gross, 1956a); the tubes were left overnight in a refrigerator. The next morning the extracts were centrifuged; the upper ether layer was then aspirated with a syringe and discarded; the remaining traces of ether were removed by evaporation; the extracts were then again centrifuged, and the supernate was inoculated into 105 newborn, C3H or C3H(f) mice. Out of 101 mice inoculated with the ether-treated extracts, 53 survived, and only one of them (2 per cent) developed leukemia. In a control series, out of 169 mice inoculated with non-treated extracts, 124 survived, and 44 of them (35 per cent) developed leukemia at an average age of 7 months (Gross, 1956a).

In more recent experiments (Gross, unpublished, 1964) passage A filtrates of either 10 or 20 per cent concentration harvested from leukemic C3H(f) donor mice were mixed with ethyl ether in 4 : 1 proportion; in each test tube, 1 cc. of ethyl ether was added to 4 cc. of the virus filtrate. The test tubes were then tightly plugged, vigorously shaken at frequent intervals, and then left overnight in a refrigerator. The next morning (after a total exposure to ether for 17 to 24 hours), the mixtures were poured into sterile 125 cc. volume vacuum flasks, and the ether was removed by evaporation under a light vacuum of approximately 20 to 25 mm of mercury. The filtrate was then inoculated into suckling C3H(f) mice. Out of a total of 24 mice inoculated

---

FIG. 34. LEUKEMIC VIRUS PARTICLES IN MOUSE THYMIC LYMPHOMA AND IN RAT MYELOID LEUKEMIA INDUCED WITH PASSAGE A VIRUS.

(A). Necrotic area from a thymic lymphoma induced in a C3H(f) mouse with passage A virus. Large numbers of virus particles are present among cellular debris in an intercellular space. Magnification 30,000×. (D. G. Feldman and L. Gross, unpublished.) (B). Section of a spleen from a Sprague-Dawley rat; this animal developed myeloid leukemia as a result of inoculation with rat-adapted passage A virus filtrate. Several mature type C virus particles (c) containing nucleoids are present in the intercellular space. Magnification 37,450×. (From: L. Gross, *Acta Haemat.*, **35**: 200, 1966.)

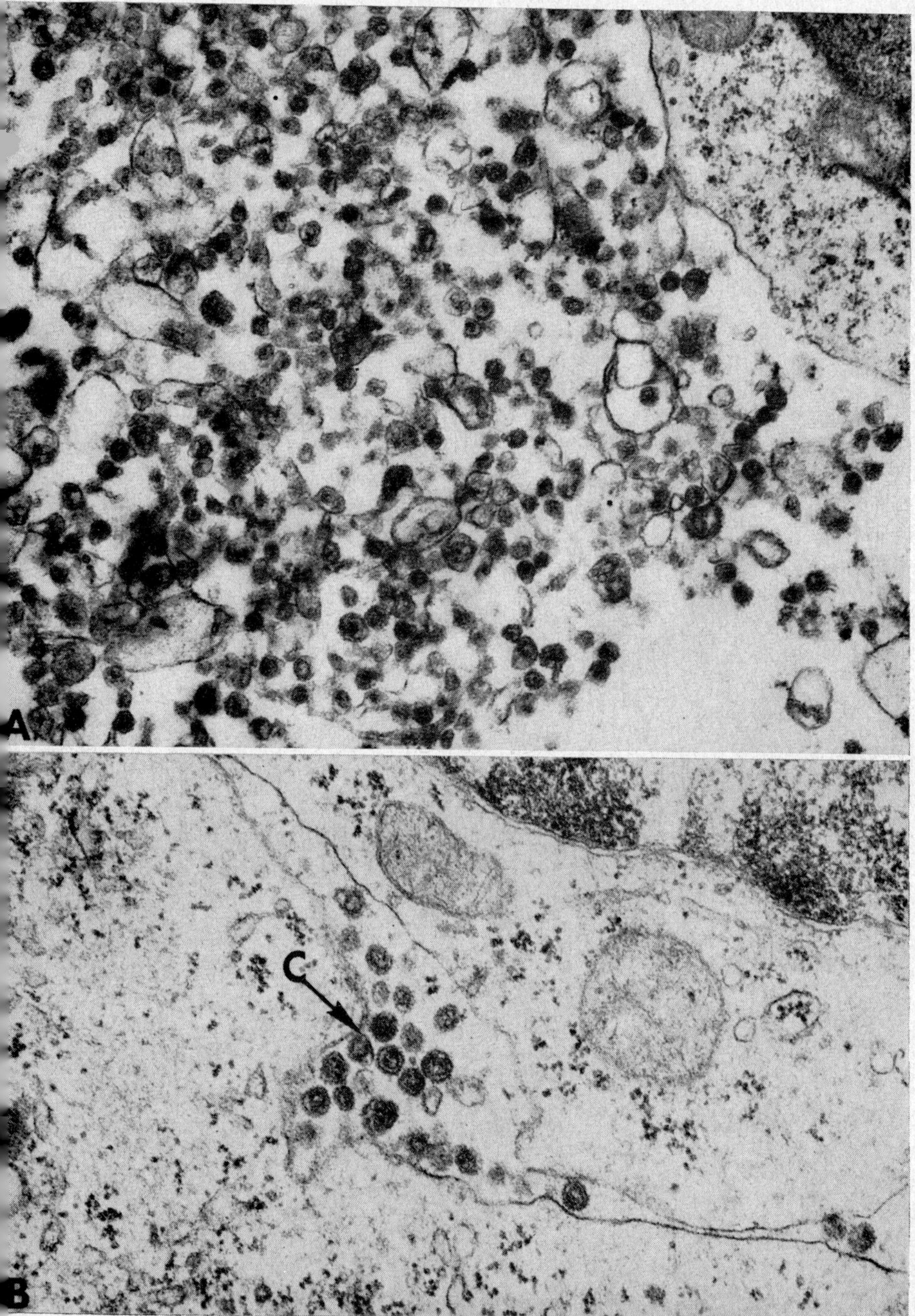

Fig. 34. Leukemic Virus Particles in Mouse Thymic Lymphoma and in Rat Myeloid Leukemia Induced With Passage A Virus.

with ether-treated extracts and observed for 10 months, none developed leukemia. In a simultaneous control experiment, physiological saline solution, instead of ether, was added to the leukemic filtrates; the extracts were then kept overnight in a refrigerator, and were submitted next morning to an evaporation procedure similar to that employed for the ether-treated extracts. Suckling C3H(f) mice, litter-mates of animals employed for bio-assay of the ether-treated extracts, were used as test animals in the control experiment. Out of 51 mice inoculated with the control extracts, 25 developed leukemia (49 per cent) at an average age of 3.8 months.

Preservation of the Virus at −70°C. The leukemic filtrates could be preserved without any apparent loss of infectivity for at least two years at −70°C in carbon dioxide dry ice (Gross, 1957a,b, also 1966 unpublished data), and for at least six months at −20°C in an electric freezer (Gross, 1963, also unpublished data). However, titration experiments have not yet been completed, and it is possible that partial loss of the titer of the frozen virus occurred gradually, particularly when the ampoules with frozen virus were kept at −20°C.

The leukemic virus could also be preserved in 50 per cent glycerin, or by lyophilization (Gross, 1956, 1957a,b); partial loss of infectivity occurred, however, under such conditions.

Titration Experiments. Potency of the Passage A Virus Carried in Mice. In order to determine the concentration of the virus in the filtrates employed for inoculation, serial dilutions of passage A filtrates (serial passage 33 to 42), harvested from leukemic mice, were prepared and inoculated (0.3 cc. i.p., each) into suckling C3H(f) mice).

An incidence of leukemia of approximately 100 per cent could be induced with either full strength filtrates of either 10 or 20 per cent concentration, or with 10^{-2} dilutions. The incidence of induced leukemia was reduced to over 95 per cent when a 10^{-3} dilution of the filtrate was employed. The incidence was further reduced to 91 or 56 per cent, respectively, when 10^{-4} or 10^{-5} dilutions were inoculated; a 14 per cent incidence of leukemia could still be induced with a 10^{-6} dilution of the filtrate.

The latency increased gradually from 2.8 months in the 10^{-2} group to 5 and 9 months in those mice which received the 10^{-5} and 10^{-6} dilutions of the filtrate (Gross, 1958, 1960, 1965). A more recent titration experiment, with slightly different figures, is summarized in Table 7.

The apparent relationship between the inoculated dose and the latency was similar to that observed previously in studies with the Rous sarcoma virus (Bryan *et al.*, 1955). The latency period elapsing between the time of inoculation and the development of leukemia in mice, or Rous sarcoma in chickens, was longer in animals receiving smaller quantities of virus.

Potency of Rat-adapted Virus. Since the mouse leukemia virus was also potent for newborn or suckling rats, serial passage through rats was carried for some 5 to 13 consecutive cell-free rat-to-rat transfers; the virus was then harvested from leukemic rats ("rat-adapted virus") and inoculated in serial dilutions into newborn rats. At the same time newborn mice were also inoculated with the rat-adapted virus.

When the rat-adapted virus was inoculated into newborn rats, 10^{-2} dilution induced a 100 per cent incidence of leukemia. An incidence exceeding 76 per cent could be induced with the 10^{-3} dilution. The

TABLE 7. TITRATION OF THE PASSAGE A MOUSE LEUKEMIA VIRUS* IN SUCKLING C3H(f) MICE

Virus filtrate dilution	No. of mice inoc.†	No. dev. leuk.	Leuk. incid. %	Avg. latency mos.
10^{-2}	8	8	100	3.8
10^{-3}	20	19	95	3.6
10^{-4}	12	12	100	3.9
10^{-5}	34	28	82	5.6
10^{-6}	11	3	27	11.5

* Serial 39 to 42 mouse-to-mouse filtrate passage. Virus harvested from leukemic C3H(f) mice.

† Suckling mice, 1 to 6 days old, were inoculated. Each mouse received approx. 0.3 cc. i.p. of the filtrate.

TABLE 8. TITRATION OF RAT-ADAPTED* PASSAGE A VIRUS IN SUCKLING RATS AND MICE

Titration in suckling rats†					Titration in suckling mice‡				
Virus fil. dil.	No. of rats inoc.	No. dev. leuk.	Leuk. incid. %	Avg. latency mos.	Virus fil. dil.	No. of mice inoc.	No. dev. leuk.	Leuk. incid. %	Avg. latency mos.
10^{-1}	6	6	100	2.8	10^{-1}	6	6	100	3.1
10^{-2}	13	13	100	4.3	10^{-2}	14	14	100	4.9
10^{-3}	25	19	76	4.2	10^{-3}	17	15	88	4.8
10^{-4}	20	5	25	6.1	10^{-4}	23	19	83	4.5
10^{-5}	23	2	9	3.0	10^{-5}	15	11	73	5.2

* 7th to 12th serial rat-to-rat passage. Virus harvested from leukemic rats.

† <7-day-old Sprague-Dawley rats, inoculated 0.4 cc. i.p. each.

‡ <6-day-old C3H(f) mice, inoculated 0.3 cc. i.p. each.

incidence dropped, however, to 25 per cent when a 10^{-4} dilution was inoculated, and to only 9 per cent when the 10^{-5} dilution was employed.

It was noted with interest that newborn mice were more susceptible than newborn rats to the inoculation of the rat-adapted virus. The incidence of leukemia following inoculation of serial dilutions of the rat-adapted virus into newborn mice was approximately 100 per cent when a 10^{-2} dilution was inoculated, and about 88 per cent when a 10^{-3} dilution was injected. The incidence dropped to 83 per cent and 73 per cent, respectively, when 10^{-4} and 10^{-5} dilutions were employed (Gross, 1965a).

Intraperitoneal, Intramuscular, and Subcutaneous Routes of Inoculation. We have employed in our studies routinely in both mice and rats the intraperitoneal route of inoculation of the virus filtrates. In some instances we employed also the subcutaneous and intramuscular routes, and we found them also suitable. No comparative titration experiments have been carried out thus far, and for that reason we have no exact way of comparing in a precise manner the possible differences in susceptibility between these three different routes of inoculation employed. However, on the basis of experiments thus far performed on a large number of animals, we have gained the impression that for all practical purposes all three routes of inoculation are equally suitable, and that there are no fundamental differences in host susceptibility among these three routes employed.

Infection by Oral Route. It may be of interest to mention at this point that the oral route is also suitable for inoculation of the mouse leukemia virus. This became apparent as soon as it was demonstrated that under certain experimental conditions leukemia could be transmitted to suckling mice through milk of virus-carrying mothers (Law and Moloney, 1961. Gross, 1962a). However, these foster-nursing experiments suggested that only newborn mice may be susceptible to infection by oral route. In our more recent experiments (Gross, 1968), we have also demonstrated that young adult mice may be susceptible to oral infection with the mouse leukemia virus.

In this study, which is still in progress, 12 C3H(f) mice, 3 to 4 weeks old, shortly after weaning, were kept without food or water for 16 hours, and were then given a meal consisting of bread soaked in milk and mixed with a finely ground cell suspension prepared from spleen, liver, and lymphoid tumors of mouse donors with passage A virus-induced leukemia. No forced feeding was employed. The food was placed in sterile, open Petri dishes at the bottom of the cage, and the mice were allowed to feed. A few hours later they received their regular Purina Laboratory Chow food pellets and water.

All 12 mice which received the leukemic cell suspension in their food developed generalized lymphatic leukemia at ages varying from 4 to 12 months (average age 7.6 months). In a control group consisting of 8 mice which received heated (56°C for ½ hour) leukemic cell extracts in their food, under otherwise similar experimental conditions, none developed leukemia up to the age of 16 months, when this part of the experiment was terminated. Another experiment dealing with an attempt to transmit mouse leukemia by feeding of virus filtrate, instead of leukemic cell suspension, is now in progress (Gross, 1968).

Resistance of the Mouse Leukemia Virus to In Vitro Gamma Rays Irradiation

The mouse leukemia passage A virus (Gross) harvested from leukemic rats was exposed, in the form of filtrates of 10 or 20 per cent concentration sealed in glass ampoules, to gamma irradiation. This was performed using fresh spent radioactive fuel elements from the nuclear reactor at Industrial Reactor Laboratories, AMF Atomics, Plainsboro, New Jersey. Following irradiation, the filtrates were inoculated into suckling, less than 7-day-old, Sprague-Dawley rats. Irradiation of up to 750,000 R had no apparent effect on the leukemogenic potency of the virus. Of 38 rats inoculated with filtrates that received up to 750,000 R *in vitro*, 37 animals developed generalized lymphosarcomas at an average age of 4.3 months (Gross *et al.*, 1965). Higher doses of irradiation, varying from 1,000,000 to 3,000,000 R, had at best only a partially inactivating effect. However, irradiation with 4,500,000 R gamma rays *in vitro* inactivated the virus completely (Gross, Roswit, Malsky, Dreyfuss and Amato, 1968). The same dose of 4,500,000 R also inactivated completely the Friend virus (Gross, *et al.*, to be published, 1968).

In contrast to the considerable resistance of the virus to *in vitro* gamma irradiation was the relative sensitivity of leukemic cells. Irradiation with less than 5,000 R (Cobalt-60) *in vitro* of 5 or 10 per cent leukemic cell suspensions, prepared from organs of C3H(f) mice with passage A virus-induced leukemia, inhibited their ability to induce transplanted leukemia following inoculation into young adult C3H(f) mice.

PROPAGATION OF THE MOUSE LEUKEMIA VIRUS IN TISSUE CULTURE

The mouse leukemia virus could be propagated *in vitro* either on normal mouse or rat cells, or in cultures of virus-induced mouse or rat lymphoma cells. The virus replicated in the infected cells and was continuously released in the tissue culture fluid under such experimental conditions. Electron microscopic studies revealed formation of virus by budding in the infected cells. Bio-assay performed on newborn mice or rats led to the development of typical leukemia or lymphosarcomas in the inoculated animals.

Propagation of the Mouse Leukemia Virus on Normal Mouse Cells. In the early studies (Gross, Dreyfuss and Moore, 1961), normal C3H/Bi mouse embryo cells were inoculated with passage A leukemic filtrate and placed at 37°C. The nutrient fluid (modified Eagle's medium with 10 per cent inactivated horse serum) was changed every 3 or 4 days. No cytopathogenic effect was observed, but fluids harvested on 16th and 24th days were leukemogenic when inoculated into suckling C3H(f) mice; 2 out of 5 in the first, and 3 out of 5 in the second bio-assay developed leukemia after 3 to 5 months.

On the 28th day, the culture fluid was transferred into tubes containing freshly prepared normal C3H(f) embryo cells. Fluid harvested from the second culture after 8 days was inoculated into 6 suckling C3H(f) mice and induced leukemia in all of them; one leukemia was of an unusually acute form (1,200,000 WBC, with 99 per cent primitive stem-cells per mm^3). Additional bio-assays performed with fluids harvested on 14th, 18th, 25th and 32nd days, were all positive; most of the inoculated mice in each respective group developed leukemia after 3 to 4½ months. The majority were stem-cell leukemias, a few were lymphatic, and 2 were myelogenous. The virus could also be grown on Swiss mouse embryo cells. Again, no cytopathic effect was observed, but fluids harvested through several successive subcultures induced leukemia on inoculation tests (Gross *et al.*, 1961, also unpublished data, 1962).

In a similar study, Manaker and his coworkers at the National Cancer Institute (1960) propagated the mouse leukemia virus (Moloney strain) on normal mouse spleen cells. Several passages at 2-week intervals were made, using the overlying culture fluid for inoculation of fresh normal mouse spleen cells. No evidence of cytopathic effect was detected. The presence of the virus, however, and its continuous multiplication, was determined on bio-assay. When newborn and suckling mice were inoculated with either unfiltered or filtered tissue culture fluids, leukemia resulted in the inoculated mice after a latency varying from 2½ to 4½ months.

The virus required at least 2 weeks for the initial growth. After this preliminary interval of time, the production of virus was continuous. The nutrient fluid was changed three times weekly, and in each sample of the collected and replaced fluid the presence of virus could be detected on bio-assay. Sixteen successive passages were made; some of the spleen cells that had been seeded with the virus could be maintained for at least 3 months, remaining viable and consistently reproducing the virus. The harvested tissue culture fluid was, however, less potent on bio-assay than were the usual cell-free extracts prepared from leukemic mouse tissues.

Ginsburg and Sachs (1962) propagated successfully the mouse leukemia virus (Moloney strain) on cultures of normal Swiss mouse embryo and kidney cells. No cytopathic effect was observed, but the virus replicated, as evidenced on bio-assay tests. Lemonde and Clode (1962) propagated mouse leukemia virus, isolated from spontaneous Ak leukemia, on normal C3H(f) spleen cells. Two passages were made at 14-day-intervals. The supernatant fluid from both passages inoculated into newborn C3H(f) mice induced leukemia in up to 25 per cent of the inoculated animals.

In more recent experiments, Manaker and his coworkers (1964) established long-term cell-culture lines from normal spleens of suckling BALB/c mice. The cultures were then infected with the mouse leukemia virus (Moloney strain). No clear cytopathic changes were noted, but the infected cells continuously released virus during the 4 years of observation. The fluids from the infected cultures proved leukemogenic for newborn mice and were pathogenic in 10^{-2} dilutions; however, only a very low incidence of leukemia could be induced with a 10^{-3} dilution of the fluid. The leukemogenic activity was therefore estimated to be about 100 times lower than that observed with virus extracted from leukemic mouse donors.

Graffi and his coworkers (1963) also propagated the mouse leukemia virus (Graffi strain) in tissue culture on normal mouse embryo cells. The virus multiplied in the infected cells for several weeks. Filtrates prepared from the tissue culture fluid induced leukemia on bio-assay in mice. Electron microscopic studies revealed presence and formation of virus particles predominantly on the outer membranes of the infected cells propagated in tissue culture.

Propagation of the Mouse Leukemia Virus on Normal Rat Embryo Thymus Cells. Malignant Transformation in Long-term Cultures. The passage A mouse leukemia virus was propagated successfully for a prolonged period of time in cultures of normal embryonal rat thymus cells (Ioachim, 1967). In this study thymuses of normal Wistar/Fu rat embryos were collected, minced

---

Fig. 35. Leukemic Virus Particles in Plasma Pellet, in a Peripheral White Blood Cell and in a Blood Platelet from a Rat with Virus-induced Leukemia.

(A). Section of a plasma pellet from blood of a Long-Evans rat with myelogenous leukemia induced by rat-adapted passage A virus. Both immature type C leukemia virus particles (ic) and mature type C particles (c) containing nucleoids are present in this preparation. Magnification 46,500 ×. (D. G. Feldman and L. Gross, unpublished.) (B). Part of a white blood cell from buffy coat from a Sprague-Dawley rat with stem-cell leukemia induced by rat-adapted passage A virus. A leukemic virus particle (b) is illustrated budding from the cell membrane. Magnification 46,500 ×. (D. G. Feldman and L. Gross, unpublished.) (C). An area of buffy coat from a Sprague-Dawley rat with stem-cell leukemia induced by rat-adapted passage A virus. Part of a platelet is shown. Within the vacuoles of the platelet appear immature (ic) and mature type C virus particles (c) containing nucleoids. Magnification 32,100 ×. (D. G. Feldman and L. Gross, unpublished.)

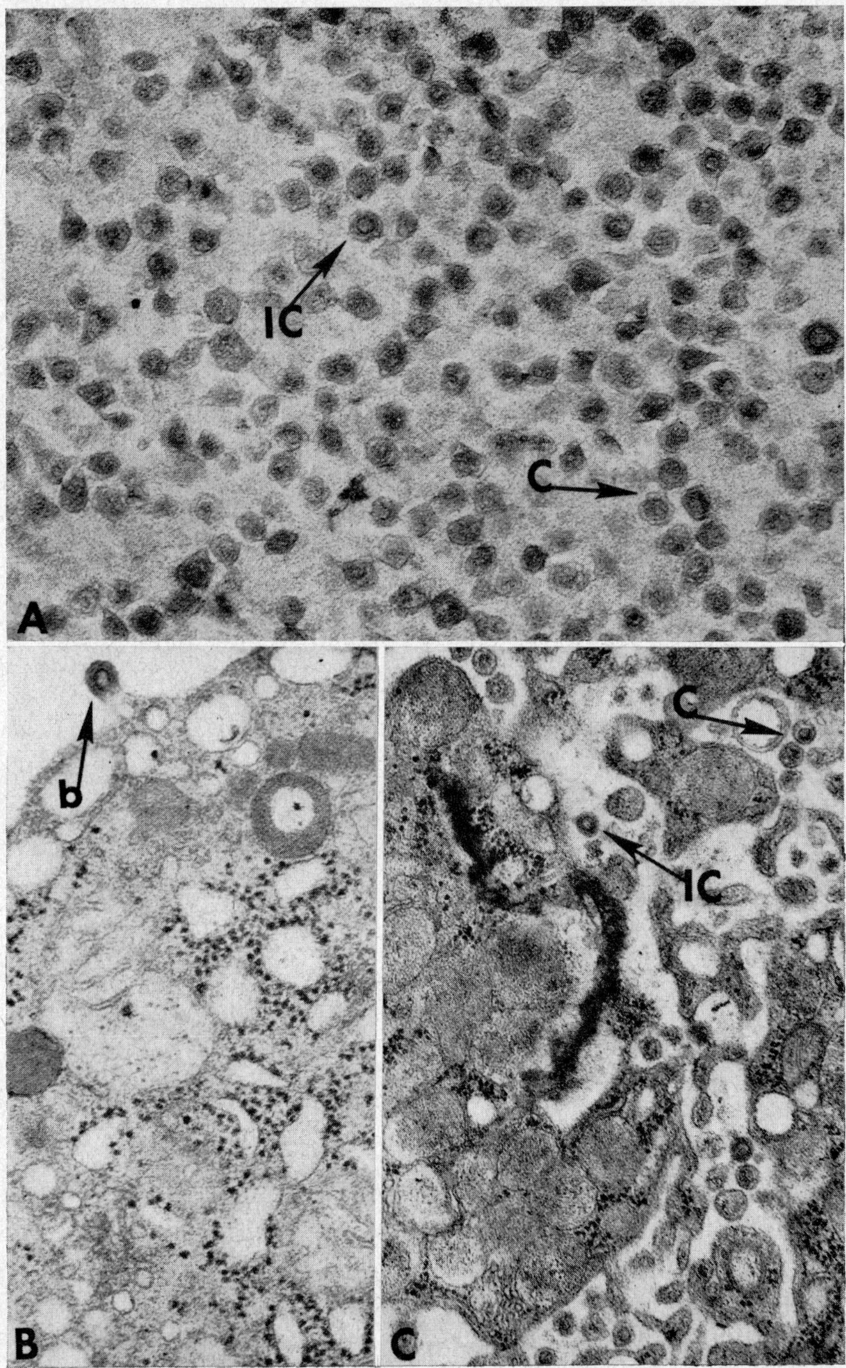

Fig. 35. Leukemic Virus Particles in Plasma Pellet, in a Peripheral White Blood Cell and in a Blood Platelet from a Rat with Virus-induced Leukemia.

and suspended in Puck's medium. The mouse leukemia virus (Gross) was then added. The thymic cells were deposited in plasma drops and placed in Petri dishes. Monolayer cultures were obtained at the end of one month, and were then subcultured.

After about 3 months morphologic changes were observed in the infected cells and also in control cultures. The infected cultures grew more abundantly and required shorter intervals between subculturing. Piling up and criss-cross growth of cells, although seen occasionally in normal cultures, appeared more frequently in the infected cells. The epithelioid pattern was more common in the infected cells and presence of large cells with atypical nuclei, sometimes with two or three nuclei, was also noted. Viral replication constantly took place in the virus-infected thymic cells during the 20 months of experimental observation; the infected cells continuously released the virus. Electron micrographs displayed large numbers of virus particles in the virus-infected cell cultures. On bio-assay, following inoculation into newborn mice or rats, the supernatant fluid, as well as cell-free filtrates prepared from the tissue culture fluid, induced leukemia in practically 100 per cent of inoculated animals of both species after an average latency of about 3 months.

The virus-infected thymic cells acquired a malignant potential during their culture *in vitro*. This was revealed upon their transplantation into newborn Wistar/Fu rats. Thymic and generalized lymphosarcomas were induced following intraperitoneal implantation of the tissue-culture-grown virus-infected cells. Many of the inoculated animals also developed local tumors at the site of inoculation as well as innumerable lymphoid tumors in the peritoneal cavity. Histologically the pattern of the tumors resembled that of a reticulum-cell sarcoma (Ioachim, 1967).

In a similar experiment, cultures of normal rat embryo spleen and kidney cells were also infected with the mouse leukemia virus (Ioachim, 1966). However, the virus did not replicate in the spleen and kidney cell cultures. Tissue culture fluids collected from such cultures failed to produce leukemia on bio-assay.

Accordingly, long-term thymus cultures proved to be most favorable for the replication of the mouse leukemia virus *in vitro*. The use of rat cells in the tissue culture study was important since it avoided interference with certain oncogenic viruses naturally carried by mice (Ioachim and Berwick, 1968).

Propagation of the Mouse Leukemia Virus in Leukemic Mouse Cells in Tissue Culture. Ginsburg and Sachs (1962) at the Weizmann Institute of Science in Rehovoth, Israel, studied the growth of the mouse leukemia virus (Moloney strain) in long and short-term tissue cultures of mouse cells. The virus was grown in five independently originating long-term cultures of virus-induced leukemic cells, which were maintained on feeder layers of spleen cells. Culture fluids were then inoculated into suckling Swiss mice, and the presence of virus was determined by the induction of leukemia in the inoculated animals. A high leukemogenic activity was recovered in all tests made from cultures that had been maintained for 9 to 290 days *in vitro*.

Propagation of the Mouse Leukemia Virus on Leukemic Rat Cells in Tissue Culture. In a study carried out by Ioachim and Furth (1964) thymic lymphomas were induced in Wistar/Fu rats with rat-adapted Gross passage A virus. Tissue cultures from the thymic lymphomas were studied for 300 days in parallel experiments with cultures of normal, embryonal and adult rat thymuses. Unlike normal lymphoid cells, the neoplastic cells apparently could be grown indefinitely. The tissue-culture-grown lymphoblasts caused lymphomas which grew progressively when inoculated into young Wistar/Fu rats and killed their hosts within 2 to 3 weeks.

In a more recent study (Ioachim *et al.*, 1965), leukemic lymphoblasts originating from a thymic lymphoma induced by the Gross passage A virus in Wistar/Fu rats were cultured *in vitro* for over 18 months. The presence of virus in these cultures was established by bio-assay in rats and mice. In continuation of these experiments, two cultures of leukemic cells were established from Gross virus-induced rat thymomas and grown *in vitro* for 29 and 36 months. A constant virus yield was obtained; when cell-free fluid from these cultures, collected at intervals varying from 8 to 30 months of growth *in vitro*, was inoculated into newborn Ak/C3H/F_1 hybrid mice, generalized lymphosarcomas developed in 97 per cent of the inoculated mice after an average latency of 3 months. Electron microscopic studies of these cultures confirmed the abundance of virus particles, and permitted observations on formation, release, and phagocytosis of virus particles by the leukemic cells (Ioachim *et al.*, 1966).

* * *

In summary, long-term propagation of the mouse leukemia virus *in vitro* has been achieved in cultures of both normal and leukemic mouse and rat cells, and particularly in rat thymus cells. Cell cultures of virus-induced rat thymic lymphomas were propagated *in vitro* for over 4 years, continuously releasing the virus. In another system, normal rat thymic cell cultures infected once with the mouse leukemia virus have been also replicating the virus for over 20 months. In both cases the production of infectious virus particles was demonstrated by electron microscopy, and also on bio-assay in susceptible animals.

The following is a personal communication from Dr. H. L. Ioachim referring to his recent studies with the mouse leukemia virus:

"In summarizing our work with the Gross mouse leukemia virus (*GLV*), I consider that the following are the most pertinent findings:

1. Long-term cultures were established, in which *GLV* replicates abundantly, constantly, and indefinitely. Permanent lines are available now in our laboratory in which *GLV* has been replicating for up to five years. The *GLV* is carried in both cultures of leukemic lymphoblasts (derived from rats with virus-induced thymomas) and in cultures of normal rat thymus cells, infected *in vitro*.

2. Neoplastic cellular transformation *in vitro* was obtained upon infection of embryonal rat thymus cells with *GLV*. The cultures display the features considered characteristic for cellular transformation and produce tumors upon isotransplantation."

ELECTRON MICROSCOPIC STUDIES OF THE MOUSE LEUKEMIA VIRUS

In the early studies, carried out prior to the development and refinement of precise technique of ultrathin sections, filtrates prepared from C3H donors with Ak virus-induced leukemia, were placed on collodium covered screens, fixed in osmic acid vapor, shadowed with chromium, and examined in an electron microscope. Spherical particles varying in diameters from 30 to 70 mμ could be seen in some of the leukemic filtrates examined (Gross, 1956). However, the method of examining drop preparations shadowed with metal vapor was not sufficiently precise to allow a distinction between viral particles and unrelated protein particles of similar shape and size.

More detailed studies leading to the identification of the virus particles became possible only after the development of the technique of ultrathin tissue sections in electron microscopy. Such sections, actually cutting through the virus particles, revealed not only their shape and size, but also their inner structure.

Initial Studies and Identification of the Mouse Leukemia Virus. In the initial studies, mice with spontaneous leukemia, as well as those with virus-induced leukemia, were used. Ultrathin sections were prepared from organs of mice of high-leukemic strains Ak and C58, which developed spontaneous leukemia; in addition, sections were also prepared from organs of mice of low-leukemic strains C3H and C57 Brown, in which leukemia had been induced by inoculation of virus filtrates. Electron microscopic examinations of these sections revealed the presence, in some of the tissues, of characteristic spherical particles, some with double membranes, with or without electron-dense centrally located nucleoids. Numerous particles were scattered in intercellular spaces, frequently along the edges of cell membranes, some also in the cytoplasm (Dmochowski and Grey, 1957. Bernhard and Guérin, 1958. Bernhard and Gross, 1959). These particles could be found in tissues of over 50 per cent of all leukemic animals examined, i.e. in mice with spontaneous leukemia, as well as in those with virus-induced leukemia.

Bernhard and Guérin (1958) examined ultrathin sections of 16 mice of strains AkR, I.P., and XVII, with spontaneous leukemia, and found virus particles in organs of 9 mice. In another study (Bernhard and Gross, 1959) 23 C3H and C57 Brown mice, in which leukemia had been induced by inoculation of passage A virus filtrates, were used as donors for the preparation of ultrathin sections from thymic tumors, peripheral lymph nodes, spleens, etc. In organs of 13 of these mice virus particles were found, identical in their morphology and location with those found in organs of mice with spontaneous leukemia.

Gradual Improvement in the Technique of Electron Microscopy. Considerable progress has been accomplished in recent years in electron microscopy, and this progress has been reflected also in the study of the mouse leukemia virus; as a result, in more recent studies described on the following pages, it became possible to reveal the presence of virus particles in practically all leukemic mice and rats examined.

The development of electron microscopes with higher resolution power, the improvements in the embedding of tissue specimens, and in the technique of cutting ultrathin sections, the introduction and improvement of staining methods, provided means of obtaining excellent high resolution electron micrographs of relatively undistorted cells and their components. More detailed studies of cell structure, of the morphology and location of cell components, and their relation to the virus particles, became possible. The electron microscopic study of the virus particles revealed with more precision not only the size and shape of the virus, but also the presence and number of outer membranes, their width and spacing, the presence, size and location of the electron-dense nucleoids within the virus particles, and other characteristics of virus morphology. Furthermore, actual formation of the virus and its emergence from cell surface, or into cytoplasmic vacuoles, could also be observed. All these observations, although still fragmentary, led gradually to the recognition and identification of the characteristic morphology of the mouse leukemia virus. The results of these studies could be summarized as follows:

Recent Electron Microscopic Studies of Tissues of Mice with Virus-induced Leukemia

Structural changes in cell morphology were essentially limited to cells of the hematopoietic system and particularly to leukemic cells forming lymphoid tumors, circulating in the blood, and infiltrating internal organs. When ultrathin sections of leukemic cells from thymic tumors, spleens, or other organs from leukemic mouse or rat donors were examined, destructive changes in cell structure could be observed in some of the cells, even at low magnification. These changes varied in degree, were in some instances only minimal, and in others considerably advanced to the point of total destruction of the cells. In general, they could be summarized as follows: the cell membranes were frequently ruptured; the intercellular spaces were frequently filled with cellular debris; some cells had a bizarre configuration; there was sometimes an overall increase, or a decrease, in the density of the cytoplasm; the mitochondria were swollen, and their normal structure partially destroyed, with disappearance, in part or total, of their cristae. Characteristic inclusion bodies, containing granular or opaque material, were frequently found in the cytoplasm. The nuclear chromatin appeared clumped or pyknotic. Under higher magnification small granules varying in size and shape could often be observed in the nucleus; numerous small granules could also be observed scattered in the cytoplasm.

In addition to the general structural changes in the morphology of certain cells, characteristic spherical virus particles could be found in the cytoplasm, usually in clusters located within vacuoles, and more frequently scattered in the intercellular spaces. Particles were also found in the course of their formation, budding either into cytoplasmic vacuoles, or from cell membranes into the intercellular spaces. Furthermore, curious cylindrical structures, apparently related to the formation of virus particles, which will be described later in this chapter, were observed within the cytoplasm of some of the cells, particularly in the megakaryocytes.

The destructive changes in cell morphology were not general, however, and varied considerably in their degree. Many immature or mature cells of the hematopoietic system, and most of the cells of other organs of the leukemic animals, had an apparently normal morphology.

It should be emphasized that not only cells unrelated to the hematopoietic system, such as connective tissue or epithelial cells, but also many cells directly related to the blood forming system, had an apparently normal and healthy morphology. Yet, some of them were infected and participated in the production of virus particles. In otherwise normal-appearing megakaryocytes, virus particles could be observed budding into the interior of cytoplasmic vacuoles. In other cells, virus particles were formed by budding from the cell membranes into the intercellular spaces; this was observed in many immature and mature cells of either the myeloid or lymphatic series, and also in erythroblasts; these cells had a perfectly normal morphology, except for the presence, in some instances, of isolated, partially formed and budding virus particles. Most striking, however, was the formation of virus particles by budding from the cell membranes of otherwise perfectly healthy appearing epithelial cells in mammary glands and also in salivary glands, pancreas, intestinal tract, and genital organs of leukemic, or non-leukemic but virus-injected, mice (Feldman and Gross, 1964, 1966, 1967. Feldman *et al.*, 1963, 1967. Gross, 1968).

Presence of Virus Particles in the Cytoplasm of Infected Cells, and in Intercellular Spaces

On electron microscopic examination of ultrathin sections of lymphoid cells, particularly those found in the thymus, bone marrow, spleen, or lymph nodes of leukemic mice and rats, characteristic spherical virus particles could be found in the cytoplasm and in intercellular spaces. In the cytoplasm of certain large cells, such as phagocytic reticular cells, or macrophages, either inclusion bodies or large vacuoles, surrounded by a thin membrane, were often found filled to capacity with clusters of virus particles. Occasionally, the virus particles could be detected scattered freely or in small clusters in disintegrated cytoplasm. Large numbers of particles could be found in intercellular spaces, between apparently normal cells, or scattered among debris of partially destroyed cells.

Examination of infected cells revealed isolated particles leaving the cell cytoplasm by budding, forming a villiform elongation of the protoplasmic cell membrane. Eventually the particles became separated from the cell, apparently carrying away, as their outer membranes, fragments of the cell cytoplasm.

It appears that budding from the cell membrane is one of the manners in which particles may originate, without any apparent damage to the cell. On the other hand, particularly in the megakaryocytes, the particles may be found in large numbers within the cytoplasmic vacuoles, presumably formed by budding from the cytoplasm into the lumen of vacuoles. One could speculate that at least some of the vacuoles may represent remnants of partially destroyed mitochondria; other vacuoles may represent true inclusion bodies, where virus particles are formed and agglomerate. The possibility should also be considered that in some of the cells, which appear to be phagocytic reticular cells or macrophages, the particles may be actually "ingested" by the cell and stored in cytoplasmic vacuoles by a process similar to phagocytosis.

Some of the cells, filled with virus particles, may eventually undergo total destruction and disintegration, liberating thereby large numbers of virus particles into the intercellular spaces.

Morphology and Classification of the Virus Particles

The mouse leukemia virus is a spherical particle about 100 mμ in diameter. The mature virus presumably consists of ribonucleic acid surrounded by a protein coat. The fully formed virus particles usually have two or three concentric membranes. Those with three membranes, but without nucleoids, have the appearance of doughnuts, and are assumed to be "immature" virus particles. Particles with electron-dense centers, i.e. nucleoids, considered to be "mature" virus particles, have usually two outer membranes. Both types can be found in vacuoles in cell cytoplasm, and also in intercellular spaces. Some particles, with or without nucleoids, have tail-like protuberances.

In previous studies, the mature and immature leukemic virus particles were considered to have one or two outer membranes, respectively. However, following the introduction of improved embedding and staining methods, and with better resolution of the more recent instruments, it is now generally accepted that the mouse leukemia virus particles are surrounded by either two or three outer membranes.*

Electron microscopic studies of the mouse leukemia virus were reported by Dmochowski and Grey (1957), Bernhard and Guérin (1958), Ichikawa (1958), Bernhard and Gross (1959), Amano and Ichikawa (1959), Heine *et al.* (1959), Dalton *et al.* (1961, 1962), Dalton (1962), Dmochowski *et al.* (1962, 1964), Granboulan and Rivière (1962), Feldman *et al.* (1963), Parsons (1963), Okano *et al.* (1963), Feldman and Gross (1964, 1966), Ioachim *et al.* (1966), and others.

According to the initial suggestions made by Bernhard (1960), and currently accepted with some modifications,* the virus particles observed in mouse leukemia can be classified as either immature or mature type C particles.

Doughnut-like or "Immature Type C" Particles. The doughnut-like particles usually have three concentric membranes; the center is electron-lucent. The measurement of over 100 doughnut-like particles indicated that the diameter of total particles varied from 80 to 110 mμ, the average being 96 mμ (Feldman and Gross, 1964). These particles are located in extracellular spaces, and in some instances also in the cytoplasm of the cells, i.e., in vacuoles, or in inclusion bodies. They occur singly, or in groups, or can be observed scattered among particles containing nucleoids.

Smaller doughnut-like particles can also be observed frequently in tissues of either leukemic or normal mice. These particles are different in size, structure, and location from the doughnut-like particles previously described. They are located in the cytoplasm in the endoplasmic reticulum. They are smaller, have an average diameter of 75 mμ, and have only two concentric membranes. According to current classification they are designated "intracisternal type A particles." Their significance is obscure, but they appear to have no relation to the mouse leukemia virus.

Particles with Nucleoids, or "Mature Type C" Particles. The particles with nucleoids have usually two concentric outer membranes; the nucleoids, usually located in the center of the particles, are either very opaque, or moderately electron-dense. Particles with nucleoids can be found usually in extracellular spaces. In the cytoplasm they can be found inside vacuoles and in inclusion bodies.

Measurement of at least 100 particles with nucleoids, studied on ultra-thin sections of organs of mice with virus-induced leukemia, indicated that their overall diameter ranged from 75 to 170 mμ, averaging about 105 mμ (Feldman and Gross, 1964). The average diameter of the nucleoid was

* The interested reader is referred to "Suggestions for the Classification of Oncogenic RNA Viruses," *J. Nat. Cancer Inst.*, **37**: 395–397, 1966.

about 68 mμ. The overall average diameter of all types of mature and immature particles, with or without nucleoids, studied in rats with virus-induced leukemia was approximately 99 mμ (Dmochowski, Gross, and Padgett, 1962).

Particles with Tail-like Structures. Mouse leukemia virus particles with tail-like protuberances were first reported in electron microscopic studies employing the negative staining technique (Dalton *et al.*, 1962. Dmochowski *et al.*, 1963), and subsequently also in studies of ultrathin sections of leukemic rat and mouse tissues (Okano *et al.*, 1963. Feldman *et al.*, 1963. Feldman and Gross, 1964. Dmochowski *et al.*, 1964). Whether these "tails" represent a real part of an undamaged leukemia virus particle, or whether they represent an artifact (de Harven and Friend, 1964) has not yet been determined. It is recalled that similar tail-like structures, believed to be an artifact, have been reported in previous electron microscopic studies of chicken erythro-myeloblastic leukosis (Sharp *et al.*, 1952) and of the Newcastle disease virus (Bang, 1949).

Cylindrical and Filamentous Structures. Cylindrical and filamentous structures of rather striking appearance were observed, particularly in megakaryocytes in spleen and bone marrow of mice and rats with virus-induced leukemia (Dalton *et al.*, 1961. Dmochowski *et al.*, 1962, 1964), apparently budding from vacuolar membranes of cytoplasmic channels, or from specific granules. Similar cylindrical structures were also found not only in the megakaryocytes, but also in cells of the lymphatic series, presumably in lymphocytes or lymphoblasts, in the thymus, spleen, and lymph nodes, budding from cytoplasmic membranes into the intercellular spaces (Feldman and Gross, 1964). The diameters of the outer and inner membranes of these cylinders corresponded to the diameters of the membranes forming the doughnut-like particles. Some of the cylinders appeared to be in the process of segmentation and budding, suggesting a phase leading to eventual formation of spherical virus particles.

Distribution of Virus Particles in Different Cells and Organs

Presence of Virus Particles in Leukemic Cells in Thymus, Bone Marrow, Lymph Nodes, Spleen, and in Blood Plasma. In our current studies carried out in our laboratory with D. G. Feldman, leukemic virus particles have been found in most of the organs of all leukemic mice and rats with passage A virus-induced leukemia thus far examined. This was consistent with results of experiments carried out on rats with virus-induced leukemia previously reported (Dmochowski, Padgett, and Gross, 1964). Considerable numbers of virus particles have been found in thymus, bone marrow, lymph nodes, and spleens of these animals. These organs represented the best source of finding, without too much effort, relatively large numbers of all forms of virus particles, including particles with nucleoids. Fully formed virus particles could also be found in pellets resulting from ultracentrifugation of blood plasma of leukemic mice and rats (Dalton *et al.*, 1963. Parsons, 1963. Okano *et al.*, 1963. Dmochowski, 1965). This observation was consistent with the results of bio-assay studies which demonstrated the presence of the leukemic virus in plasma of leukemic mice and rats.

Presence of Virus Particles in Mammary Glands, in Milk, and in Salivary Glands. It was of considerable interest that leukemic virus particles could be found not only in cells of the hematopoietic system, but also in organs apparently unrelated to the formation of blood cells. Thus, in virus-injected pregnant female mice, virus particles could be readily found in mammary glands; they were observed budding from the mammary epithelium into the intercellular spaces; fully formed, mature virus particles were also consistently found in the milk ducts of such mice (Feldman, Gross and Dreyfuss, 1963).

Under certain, rather limited, experimental conditions the mouse leukemia virus can also be transmitted through the milk (Law and Moloney, 1961. Gross, 1962), particularly when the nursing female is either suffering from leukemia, or is at the point of developing this disease (Gross, 1962). Recent electron microscopic studies of ultrathin pellet sections revealed the presence of large quantities of virus particles in the milk of C3H(f) female mice inoculated with the passage A virus, and also in the milk of female mice of the high-leukemic Ak strain (Dmochowski *et al.*, 1963).

Virus particles were also found in salivary glands, budding from epithelial cells into the acini (Feldman and Gross, 1964). Budding virus particles were also observed in the pancreas (Feldman and Gross, 1966) and in the epithelial cells of duodenum, jejunum, ileum, and colon (Feldman *et al.*, 1967. Gross, 1968).

Among other organs, virus particles were found in kidneys, livers, and lungs of leukemic animals, frequently in the vicinity of leukemic cells infiltrating such organs. In these organs, however, the virus particles were found as a rule fully formed.

Presence of Virus Particles in Genital Organs of Ak Mice and of Virus-injected C3H(f) Mice. An electron microscopic study of ultrathin sections of the genital organs of male and female mice carrying the mouse leukemia virus revealed the presence of virus particles in genital organs of Ak mice which naturally carry the virus, and also in organs of virus-injected C3H(f) mice. In this study, genital organs from 5 Ak males and 4 Ak females were examined, as well as those from virus-injected 7 males and 8 females of the C3H(f) strain. Three out of 9 animals in the first group, and 8 out of 15 mice in the second group had symptoms of leukemia at the time their organs were removed; the remaining animals were healthy and free from symptoms of leukemia at the time their organs were removed for electron microscopic studies. Virus particles were found in ovaries, oviducts, uteri, epididymis, vas deferens, seminal vesicles, and in the prostate of non-leukemic and leukemic Ak mice and of virus-injected non-leukemic and leukemic C3H(f) mice. In general, a larger number of particles appeared in the genital organs of leukemic than in non-leukemic virus-injected animals. There was no significant difference in the distribution and quantity of particles observed in the genitals of Ak and virus-injected C3H(f) mice. Budding of particles was observed from cells of the theca folliculi and corpus luteum of ovaries, and from epithelial cells and connective tissue fibroblasts of other genital organs. Occasionally, particles appeared to form from endothelial cells of capillaries and arterioles of ovaries or testes, from smooth muscle cells of arterioles of ovaries, and from smooth muscle cells of oviducts. Doughnut-like particles and also mature particles with nucleoids were usually present in intercellular spaces, or lying free within the tubular or glandular lumen of various organs. In a simultaneous control study, ultrathin sections of genital organs of normal non-injected 5 C3H(f) males and 5 C3H(f) females were also studied, but no virus particles were found in any of the genital organs examined (Feldman and Gross, 1967).

The implications of these observations will be discussed later in the final part of this chapter, dealing with the natural transmission of the mouse leukemia virus.

Presence of Virus Particles in a Variety of Cells. Considerable numbers of virus particles were observed in the megakaryocytes in bone marrow and spleen (Dalton *et al.*, 1961. Dmochowski *et al.*, 1962. Feldman and Gross, 1964), as was previously also observed in studies of the Friend virus (de Harven and Friend, 1958). Furthermore, virus particles were observed to bud off from a variety of cells of the hematopoietic system, such as lymphocytes, lymphoblasts, monocytes, monoblasts, eosinophils and neutrophils, plasma cells, erythroblasts, reticular cells, and megakaryocytes.

In the animals studied, production of particles by the above cells was not

---

FIG. 36. LEUKEMIC VIRUS PARTICLES IN SALIVARY GLANDS AND PANCREAS IN VIRUS-INJECTED C3H(F) MICE.

(A). Section of submaxillary salivary gland from a C3H(f) mouse with passage A virus-induced lymphatic leukemia. A virus particle (b) appears to be budding from the cell membrane into the intercellular space; many immature type C particles (IC) are present in the intercellular space. Magnification 33,200×. (From: L. Gross, *Acta Haemat.*, **29**: 1, 1963.) (B and C). Sections of pancreas from a C3H(f) mouse with passage A virus-induced leukemia. Illustrated are particles (b) budding from the cell membrane of pancreatic acinar cells, cylindrical particles (cl), and mature type C particles (C) containing nucleoids. Magnification 53,000×. (From: D. G. Feldman and L. Gross, *Cancer Research*, **26**: 412, 1966.)

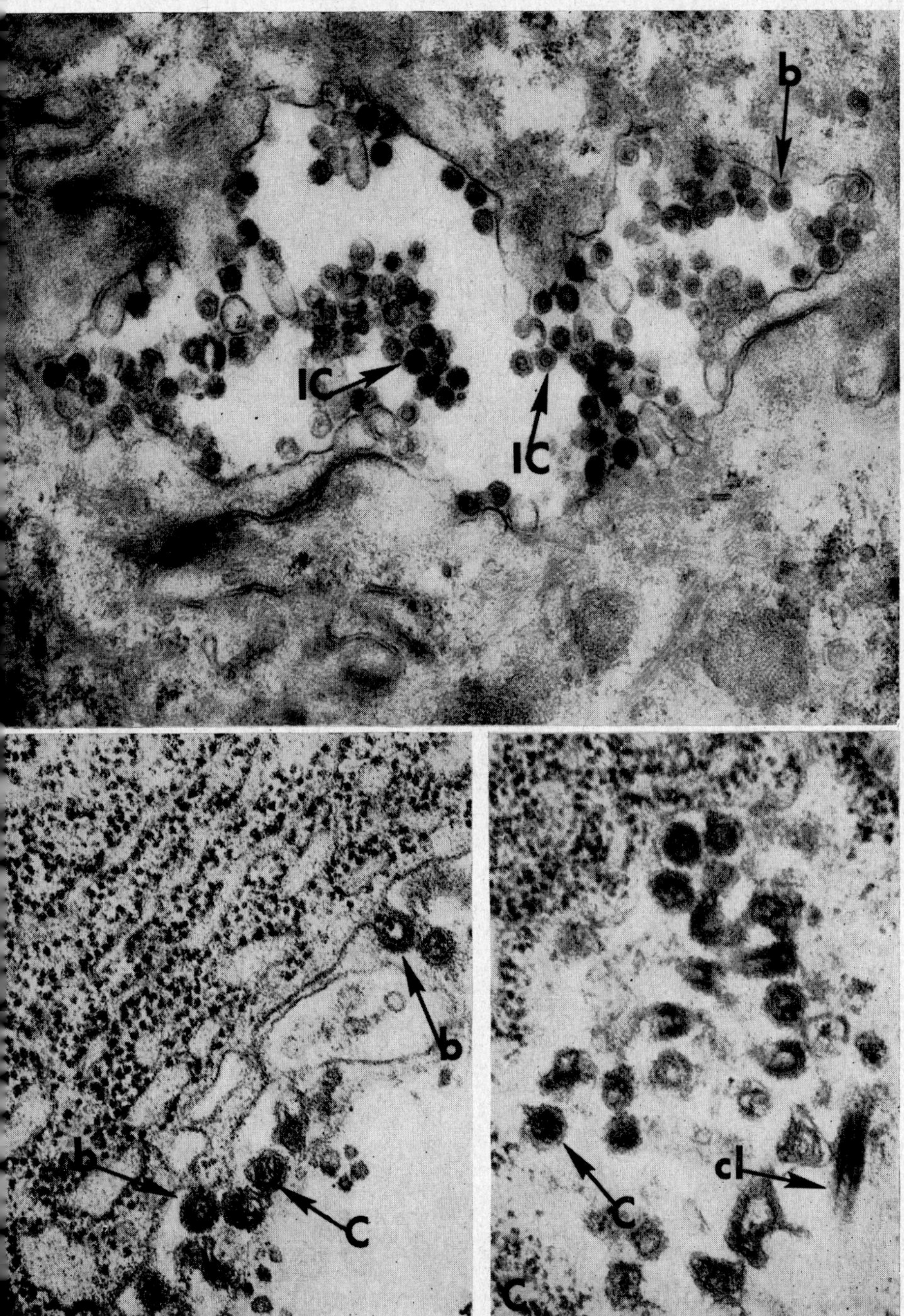

FIG. 36. LEUKEMIC VIRUS PARTICLES IN SALIVARY GLANDS AND PANCREAS IN VIRUS-INJECTED C3H(F) MICE.

always accompanied by an abnormal increase of the numbers of these cells in the blood or tissues, as revealed by light microscopy. It thus appears that the mouse leukemia virus can replicate in certain cell types, without inducing an abnormal multiplication of such cells.

How Often Could Virus Particles Be Found in the Organs of Leukemic Mice and Rats?

We have discussed on the preceding pages the fact that virus particles could be found frequently in organs of leukemic mice and rats. The distribution, forms, and numbers of virus particles varied considerably. Most frequently they were found in organs directly related to the hematopoietic system, such as thymus, bone marrow, spleen, lymph nodes, in blood plasma, etc.; virus particles were also found, however, in other cells, and in a variety of organs, including mammary and salivary glands. Particles, often in substantial numbers, could be found in most of these organs.

Although virus particles could be found in tissues of mice with either virus-induced or spontaneous leukemia, they were more numerous, and more readily found, in mice with virus-induced leukemia. This observation was consistent with the results of bio-assays previously performed (Gross, 1957) indicating higher potency of virus filtrates harvested from organs of mice in which leukemia was induced with the passage A virus, as compared with those prepared from Ak mouse donors with spontaneous leukemia.

In studies previously reported (Dmochowski, Padgett and Gross, 1964), virus particles were found in at least some of the organs of all 6 Osborne-Mendel and 12 Sprague-Dawley rats with passage A virus-induced leukemia examined. In our recent studies (1966) carried out with D. G. Feldman, electron microscopic examination of ultrathin sections of organs from 13 C3H(f) mice and 11 Sprague-Dawley rats, with passage A virus-induced leukemia, revealed the presence of virus particles in the thymus, bone marrow, and lymph nodes of all 24 animals examined. In another study (Okano *et al.*, 1963), ultrathin sections were examined of organs from 22 rats of W/Fu strain with passage A virus-induced leukemia; virus particles were found in the thymuses of all 22 rats examined, and in some of these animals also in other organs, such as bone marrow, lymph nodes, and blood plasma. Thus, in a total group of 64 mice and rats with passage A virus-induced leukemia, virus particles were found in at least some of the organs of all animals examined.

As referred to on preceding pages of this chapter, early electron microscopic studies of ultrathin sections of organs of AkR mice with spontaneous leukemia revealed the presence of virus particles in over 50 per cent of animals examined (Dmochowski and Grey, 1957. Bernhard and Guérin, 1958). In more recent studies, Granboulan and Rivière (1962), in Bernhard's laboratory, found mature virus particles, mostly in the thymus, in 21 out of 37 AkR mice with spontaneous leukemia.

Electron microscopic examination of ultrathin sections of organs of 10 Ak mice with spontaneous leukemia carried out recently with D. G. Feldman in our laboratory revealed the presence of both mature and immature virus particles in at least some of the organs of all 10 donors examined, but in lesser numbers than those observed in the study of mice or rats with passage A virus-induced leukemia.

Electron Microscopic Studies of Organs of Embryos from Virus-injected and from Healthy, Non-injected C3H(f) Mice

Presence of Virus Particles in Embryos of Virus-injected C3H(f) Parents. In a recent study carried out in our laboratory (Feldman, Dreyfuss and Gross, 1967), suckling, less than 5-day-old, mice of the C3H(f) strain were inoculated with passage A filtrate; shortly after weaning the injected males and females were mated. The embryos were removed by laparotomy from 10 female mice, after they became pregnant. At that time 5 of the pregnant females already had leukemia, and 5 were still in good health, although they also had received the virus.

In a simultaneous control study, ultrathin sections of embryos from normal, non-injected C3H(f) females were also examined. In this control experiment embryos were removed by laparotomy from 9 young, healthy, non-inoculated, pregnant, C3H(f) female mice taken from our pedigreed mouse colony.

Several organs, such as bone marrow, thymus, spleen, liver, and kidneys, were then removed aseptically from the embryos of both groups of animals, embedded, sectioned, and examined in the electron microscope. The examination consistently revealed the presence of very small numbers of characteristic, although usually isolated, virus particles in the bone marrow, in the thymus, spleen, and also in the liver of embryos from both virus-injected and normal control parents. The particles were, as a rule, of the immature doughnut-like form, without nucleoids. They appeared in approximately the same amounts and with similar frequency regardless of whether the embryos were removed from virus-injected or from normal female mice. Particles were observed budding from lymphocytes, lymphoblasts and epithelial cells in thymus, from erythroblasts and hemocytoblasts in liver and spleen, and from hemocytoblasts in bone marrow. The virus particles most frequently observed were either budding from the cell membranes into the intercellular spaces, or were doughnut-like; particles containing nucleoids appeared in only one specimen out of 8 of embryo thymuses from normal non-injected parents. Leukemic virus particles were not observed in kidney tissues from any of the embryos examined (Feldman, Dreyfuss and Gross, 1967).

Electron microscopic examination of ultrathin sections of organs from embryos of 3 virus-injected, and also of 3 normal, non-injected Sprague-Dawley rats did not reveal, in studies thus far performed, the presence of virus particles (Feldman, Dreyfuss and Gross, 1967).

Presence of Virus Particles in Embryos of Ak Females. Virus particles could also be found in organs of embryos removed from healthy mice of the high-leukemic AkR strain (Dmochowski *et al.*, 1963). These particles were either fully formed, of the immature type, or they were found budding from cell membranes into the intercellular spaces. More recently, mature virus particles, with nucleoids, were found in the bone marrow of AkR embryos (Dmochowski *et al.*, 1964).

In a similar study, carried out more recently in our laboratory (Feldman, Dreyfuss and Gross, 1967), examination of ultrathin sections of organs of mouse embryos removed from 4 young, healthy, pregnant, non-leukemic females revealed the presence of budding or doughnut-like virus particles in the thymus, spleen, and liver of the Ak embryos examined.

Presence of Virus Particles in Tissues of Normal, Adult, Healthy Mice of Low-leukemic Inbred Lines

On electron microscopic examination of organs of young adult healthy mice of low-leukemic strains, such as C3H or C3H(f), in most instances only isolated single particles could be found; with rare exceptions, these particles were found only in the thymus, and not in other organs. Furthermore, particles found in the normal control animals only very rarely had electron-dense nucleoids; with only few exceptions, the particles found in organs of healthy mice of low-leukemic strains were of the immature type. These particles were found budding from the cell membranes into the intercellular spaces, or from the cell cytoplasm into cytoplasmic vacuoles; others were found as fully formed doughnut-like particles in the cytoplasmic vacuoles, or in intercellular spaces. It should be stressed, however, that such particles could be found only after a prolonged search. This contrasted sharply with the relative ease with which similar particles could be found in organs of leukemic animals.

Among tissues of normal, healthy, young adult C3H(f) mice examined in our laboratory (Feldman and Gross, 1966), occasional, isolated particles could be found after a patient search in only 7 out of 10 mice examined. In one instance a single particle was found in the bone marrow and in another case in a lymph node. *All other particles were found in the thymus.* None was found in the spleen. Among the particles studied, only a few, appearing singly in the thymus, were of the mature form, i.e. had centrally located nucleoids; all other particles were of the immature form.

In general, one could summarize the overall impression that in normal, healthy mice of low-leukemic strains, such as C3H(f), virus particles could be found less frequently, were fewer in number, and were found in fewer areas; moreover, with rare exceptions, the virus particles were only of the immature form. On the other hand, in leukemic mice, in practically all animals examined, virus particles, either of the immature or of the mature form (with nucleoids), could be found readily, frequently in large numbers, and in a variety of organs.

It should be stressed that the presence of spherical particles, representing presumably the mouse leukemia virus, in tissues of normal, healthy mice of low-leukemic strains, and also in normal mouse embryos, should not be surprising. Mice of such low-leukemic strains as C3H or C57 Brown may be, under normal life conditions, essentially free from spontaneous leukemia; the same mice, however, develop a high incidence of leukemia following total body X-ray irradiation (Gross *et al.*, 1959). It is quite apparent therefore that these mice carry a latent leukemogenic virus which may not cause leukemia when undisturbed, but may be triggered into action by certain factors, such as radiation energy.

Smaller doughnut-like particles can also be found in normal mouse organs. They are different in location, size, and structure from the doughnut-like particles previously described. These particles, designated in current classification as "intracisternal type A" particles, are rather ubiquitous and can be found in many organs of normal mice examined, such as bone marrow, thymus, lymph nodes, spleen, liver, kidney, genital organs, mammary glands, connective tissue, etc. They have a characteristic location, since they can be found within the cell cytoplasm in the endoplasmic reticulum. They bud into the cisternae and can be frequently found lying free in the cisternal vacuoles. The morphology of these particles is different from that of the leukemic immature type C particles, since they have only two membranes, whereas the leukemic immature type C particles have three membranes. Furthermore, the intracisternal particles are smaller; the measurement of at least 50 particles of this type indicated that their overall diameter ranges from 65 to 85 mμ, with an average of 75 mμ (Feldman and Gross, 1964). The intracisternal type A particles can be found as frequently in normal as in leukemic mice. Their significance is obscure.

No Virus Particles in Organs of Normal Non-injected Rats. Finally, it was also of interest that no particles at all have been found thus far on electron microscopic examination of ultrathin sections of organs of healthy non-injected rats. This was demonstrated in earlier studies in which organs of non-injected 11 Sprague-Dawley and 4 Osborne-Mendel rats were examined (Dmochowski, Padgett and Gross, 1964), as well as in similar more recent electron microscopic studies of organs removed from 10 normal non-injected Sprague-Dawley rats (Feldman and Gross, 1966).

In contrast, as discussed on preceding pages, electron microscopic examination of ultrathin sections of organs of rats with virus-induced leukemia revealed in all animals examined the presence of characteristic virus particles. The virus particles could be found consistently in the thymus, in bone marrow, in the spleen and lymph nodes, and frequently also in other organs examined (Dmochowski, Gross, and Padgett, 1962. Okano, Kunii and Furth, 1963. Parsons, 1963. Dmochowski, Padgett and Gross, 1964. Feldman and Gross, 1966).

Do the Particles Found in Leukemic Mice and Rats Actually Represent the Mouse Leukemia Virus? We have been using rather confidently the term "mouse leukemia virus" when referring to the particles found, and described in some detail, in tissues of leukemic mice and rats.

It is necessary to stress that there is no conclusive evidence to prove that these particles actually represent the virus responsible for the development of leukemia in these species. It is true that the consistent presence of large numbers of characteristic particles in organs of all mice and rats with virus-induced leukemia is suggestive, and contrasts sharply with the only occasional presence of isolated particles in certain organs, particularly in the thymus of normal mice, and the apparent total absence of similar particles in tissues of normal rats, thus far examined. At the present time, nevertheless, there is only circumstantial evidence to suggest that the submicroscopic particles here described actually represent the mouse leukemia virus.

Antigenic Potency of the Leukemic Filtrate

In early, preliminary experiments (Gross, 1959), rabbits and guinea pigs were inoculated repeatedly with mouse leukemic organ filtrates; serum from such animals was collected and pooled. Normal serum was obtained from healthy rabbits and guinea pigs. All the sera were inactivated at 56°C for 30 minutes, because preliminary experiments indicated that fresh normal sera had a non-specific neutralizing effect on the mouse leukemia virus.

Undiluted serum from each group was then mixed with an equal volume of a freshly prepared passage A filtrate. This mixture was kept at room temperature (22°C) for 30 to 60 minutes, then for additional 2 to 20 hours in a refrigerator at +4°C, and was then inoculated into suckling C3H mice.

Results of these preliminary experiments indicated that the passage A immune serum had a moderate neutralizing effect on the mouse leukemia virus. The results were less distinct when guinea pig serum was used for neutralization tests. No neutralization occurred when normal rabbit or guinea pig serum was employed.

In more recent studies (Gross, 1965), the experimental conditions were modified and a more precise technique was employed. The virus filtrate was titrated prior to neutralization tests. Preliminary titration experiments suggested that a 10^{-3} dilution of the virus filtrate consistently induced leukemia in all inoculated animals; yet this quantity of virus was still suitable for neutralization tests. Higher concentrations of the virus filtrate could not be neutralized consistently with the immune serum prepared under the experimental conditions employed. Accordingly, 10^{-3} dilutions of the virus filtrate were employed routinely for the neutralization tests.

A more potent immune serum was obtained from rabbits that had received repeated injections of mouse leukemic organ filtrates mixed with Freund adjuvant. Control serum was obtained from rabbits which had received repeated injections of normal mouse organ filtrates mixed with Freund adjuvant. Sera obtained from several rabbits from each group were pooled, inactivated at 56°C for 30 minutes, and used for neutralization tests.

A 10^{-3} dilution of the virus filtrate was mixed with undiluted immune serum, incubated at room temperature for 30 minutes, then kept for additional 30 minutes at 37°C, and finally for 3 to 4 hours in a refrigerator at +4°C. The virus-serum mixtures were then inoculated into suckling C3H(f) mice. The inoculated mice were observed for the development of leukemia for about 10 to 12 months.

Results of these experiments suggested that under proper experimental conditions, the passage A mouse leukemia virus could be completely neutralized *in vitro* by an immune rabbit serum; this reaction was specific and quantitative. Neutralization occurred only when a 10^{-3} dilution of the virus filtrate was mixed with an equal amount of undiluted immune rabbit serum. When a higher concentration of virus filtrate, or either a less potent, or a more diluted, serum, was employed, neutralization was less pronounced, or did not occur at all.

In simultaneous control experiments, no neutralization of the passage A virus occurred when the virus filtrate was mixed with a serum obtained from rabbits that had received repeated injections of normal mouse organ filtrates.

FIG. 37. LEUKEMIC VIRUS PARTICLES IN THE INTESTINAL TRACT OF VIRUS-INJECTED C3H(F) MICE.

(A). Section of duodenum from a C3H(f) mouse with passage A virus-induced lymphatic leukemia. A virus particle (b) is budding from an epithelial cell; several mature type C particles (C) appear in an intercellular space. Magnification 42,800 ×. (From: L. Gross, *Acta Haemat.*, **40**: 1, 1968.) (B). An area of jejunum from a C3H(f) mouse with lymphatic leukemia induced by passage A virus. A virus particle (b) appears to be budding from an epithelial cell into an intercellular space. Magnification 62,000 ×. (D. G. Feldman and L. Gross, unpublished.) (C). Section of colon from a C3H(f) mouse with lymphatic leukemia induced with passage A virus. A group of mature type C leukemia virus particles (C) appear in an intercellular space. Magnification 33,600 ×. (D. G. Feldman and L. Gross, unpublished.)

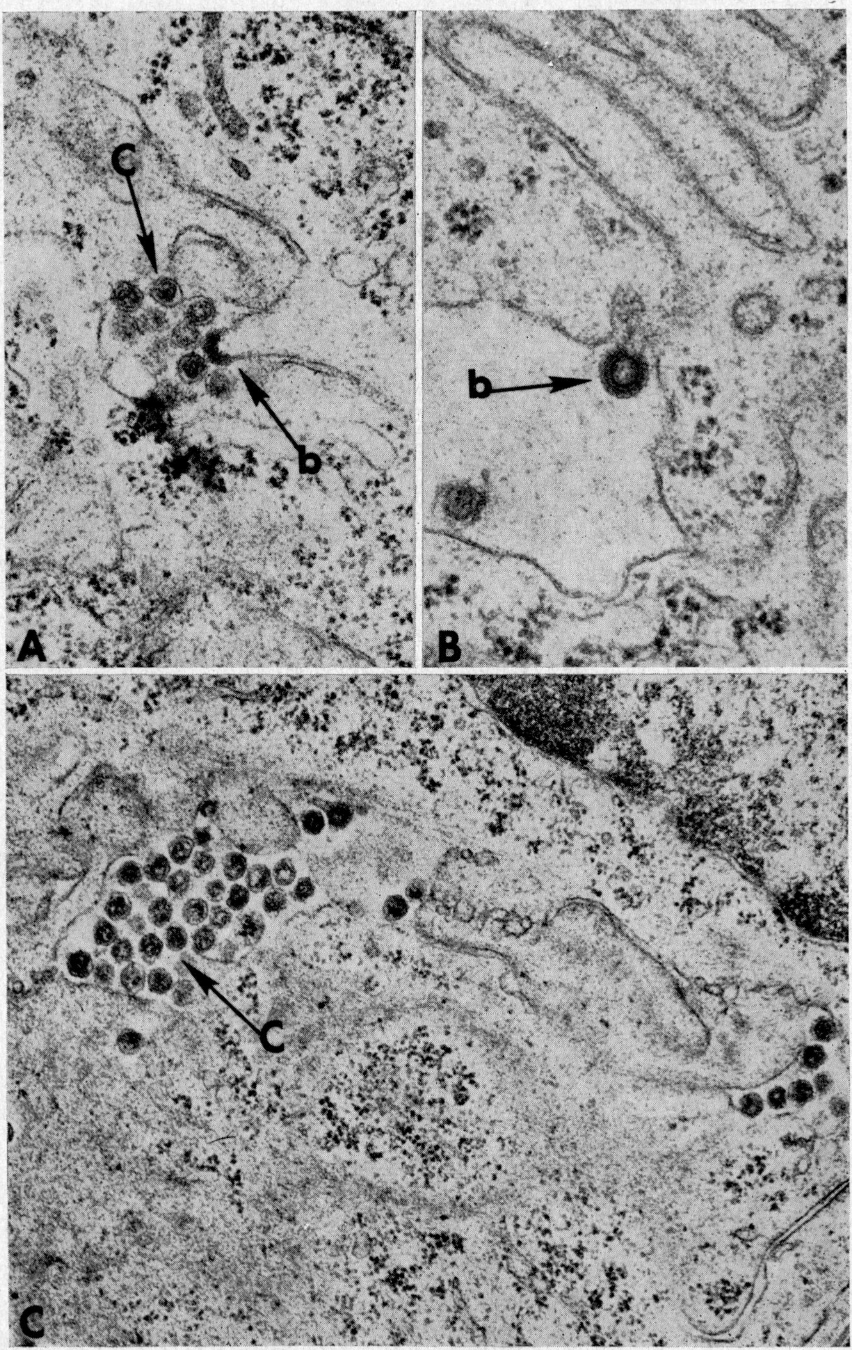

FIG. 37. LEUKEMIC VIRUS PARTICLES IN THE INTESTINAL TRACT OF VIRUS-INJECTED C3H(F) MICE.

These experiments suggested that neutralization of the mouse leukemia virus *in vitro* by an immune serum occurred only under carefully performed quantitative conditions. It also became quite apparent that results of serum neutralization tests of the mouse leukemia virus strains with immune sera could readily give results subject to erroneous interpretations. Thus, when a filtrate containing an unknown, and possibly highly potent, concentration of the mouse leukemia virus was mixed with a heterologous immune serum, neutralization did not always occur even though the serum contained specific antibodies. This difficulty was due to the usually low potency of the immune serum and the relatively high titer of virus present in routinely prepared filtrates.

Hemolytic Action of Tumor Extracts on Red Blood Cells In Vitro

It has long been observed that various forms of leukemia and lymphomas, as well as other malignant tumors in animals and in man, are frequently associated with a progressive anemia. It was of interest therefore that filtrates prepared from lymphoid mouse tumors were found to have a striking hemolytic effect on homologous red blood cells *in vitro* (Gross, 1947, 1948). A similar hemolytic effect was obtained when cell-free extracts prepared from several spontaneous or transplanted mouse tumors were mixed with mouse erythrocytes. A clumping of red blood cells was also observed, particularly when extracts from tumors were used (Gross, 1947, 1948. Salaman, 1948). The hemolytic action was more prominent than agglutination, however, and could be demonstrated by mixing a filtrate prepared from lymphoid mouse tumors, or from certain mouse carcinomas or sarcomas, with washed suspensions of mouse red blood cells. After such mixtures were placed in an incubator at 37°C, the red blood cells were hemolyzed after 2 or 3 hours. There was practically no hemolytic action observed when the mouse tumor extracts were mixed with red blood cells of other animal species. The hemolytic factor present in the tumor extracts was found to be very labile; the hemolytic potency of the tumor extracts promptly disappeared after the extracts were left at room temperature for only a few hours.

Experiments were also made with extracts made from human tumors; it was found that human tumor extracts also hemolyzed human red blood cells *in vitro* (Gross, 1949).

Although the association of malignant tumors, including lymphomas or leukemia, with anemia has long been observed, no satisfactory explanation of the mechanism of this relationship has yet been furnished. Experiments reported in the studies here described appear to suggest that, at least in the case of certain mouse and rat tumors and mouse leukemia, a direct destructive action of a filterable factor, contained in the tumor cells and in leukemic cells, on the circulating red blood cells of the host should be taken into consideration.

The agglutinating action of heated leukemic filtrates described more recently (Gross, 1959) differs fundamentally from that observed in our previous studies (Gross, 1947), or those carried out by Salaman (1948). The main difference is that the agglutinin described more recently (Gross, 1959) requires heating (55°C for ½ hour) prior to mixing with red blood cells, and that it is relatively stable; it is unaffected when standing for at least 5 hours at room temperature.

Attempt to Recover the Virus from Organs of Mice at Different Time Intervals, Following Virus Inoculation

The purpose of this series of experiments was to determine whether the leukemic virus could be recovered at various time intervals from newborn mice that had been inoculated with the passage A filtrate.

In the first group, the passage A leukemic filtrate was inoculated into newborn, less than 16-hour-old, C3H mice; after time intervals varying from 1 to 7 hours, the injected infant mice were sacrificed, cut with scissors, and ground in a mortar, physiological saline solution being added to make a cell suspension of 20 per cent concentration; the resulting extract was then centrifuged at 3000 r.p.m. for 15 minutes; the supernate was removed and again centrifuged at 9500 r.p.m. for 5 minutes; the final supernate was then inoculated into suckling, 1 to 5-day-old, C3H mice.

An incidence of leukemia exceeding 80 per cent could be induced with such extracts, indicating thereby that within the first few hours after inoculation the virus could still be recovered from the injected animals without loss of infectivity.

In a second group, 1 to 4-day-old newborn C3H mice were inoculated with passage A filtrates. After time intervals varying from 1 to 30 days, the injected mice were sacrificed; from pooled organs (thymus, spleen, and liver), removed from several donor mice, centrifuged extracts were prepared in the manner described above; the final supernate was then passed through Selas 02 filter candles and inoculated into suckling, less than 5-day-old, C3H mice.

Extracts prepared from mice that had been inoculated 1 to 4 days earlier with the leukemic filtrates had practically no leukemogenic effect on bio-assay. However, about one week after inoculation, the donor mice yielded infective virus; the presence of the leukemic virus could be detected on bio-assay in all experiments in which the virus was harvested at time intervals varying from 6 to 30 days after the inoculation of passage A filtrates. Filtered extracts prepared from pooled organs (spleen, liver, thymus) of such hosts induced an incidence of leukemia varying from 43 to 94 per cent following inoculation into suckling C3H mice (Gross, 1963).

Results of these experiments suggested, therefore, that the mouse leukemia virus could not be recovered from organs of inoculated mice during the time interval beginning about 24 hours after inoculation and lasting for about 3 to 4 days. After this initial transitory period of time, comparable to a phase of eclipse, the virus reappeared gradually in its infective form in organs of infected animals, and could then be detected consistently by means of bio-assay.

Accordingly, the leukemic virus could be recovered from tissues of the inoculated hosts a long time prior to the development of disease. This observation was consistent with results of our previous studies in which extracts prepared from normal embryos and from organs removed from healthy young mice of the high leukemic Ak and C58 inbred lines, naturally carrying the virus, induced leukemia on inoculation tests (Gross, 1951, 1955, 1956).

Presence of the Leukemic Agent in Blood Plasma and in Various Organs of the Leukemic Hosts

In this series of experiments, an attempt was made to determine whether blood plasma and different organs of leukemic mouse donors contained infective virus. In our routine procedure of preparing filtrates from leukemic mouse donors, fragments of thymic tumors and spleens were usually employed. Experiments here described were carried out in order to determine whether the virus could also be recovered in an appreciable and comparable quantity from blood plasma of leukemic donors as well as from several organs, such as peripheral and visceral lymph nodes, spleens, livers, thymic tumors, etc.

In order to determine whether the virus is present in plasma of leukemic donors, blood was removed directly from the heart of C3H mouse donors with passage A virus-induced leukemia. This was performed in ether anesthesia. A few drops of heparin solution were added to prevent clotting. The blood cells were removed by centrifugation, and the plasma, diluted with sterile physiological saline solution, was passed through Selas filter candles. The resulting plasma filtrate was then inoculated into suckling C3H mice. At the same time a cell suspension was prepared from pooled leukemic spleens, livers, thymic and mesenteric tumors of the same leukemic donors, then centrifuged, filtered, and inoculated into control groups of suckling C3H mice. Plasma filtrates were found to be almost as leukemogenic as organ filtrates on bio-assay. The incidence of leukemia induced in the inoculated mice with blood plasma filtrates was 84 per cent, as compared with an incidence of 98 per cent induced with pooled organs filtrates (Gross, 1960).

In another series of experiments, the presence of the leukemic virus in several individual organs of leukemic donors, such as thymic tumors, spleens, mesenteric tumors, peripheral lymph nodes, and livers, was determined by bio-assay. The results obtained suggested that the virus was approximately equally distributed in such organs of C3H mouse donors with passage A virus-induced generalized leukemia. Filtrates prepared either from thymic or lymphoid tumors, or from spleens or livers of leukemic mouse donors were equally active on inoculation tests (Gross, 1960). However, the brain of leukemic mice was relatively free from the leukemic virus, contrary to observations reported by Schwartz and his associates (1957).

These results were consistent with electron microscopic observations, discussed on preceding pages of this chapter, which revealed the presence of virus particles not only in thymic and lymphoid tumors, but also in a variety of organs, as well as in blood plasma, of mice and rats with virus-induced leukemia.

Leukemogenic Potency of Blood Plasma from Leukemic Rats. In more recent experiments, we have also tested rat plasma for its leukemogenic potency as compared with the potency of extracts prepared from leukemic organs of the same leukemic rat donors. In this study, the rat-adapted mouse leukemia virus (Gross) was inoculated into suckling Sprague-Dawley rats; after the inoculated rats developed leukemia, blood was drawn directly from their hearts in ether anesthesia. The blood plasma was then separated by centrifugation, diluted with physiological saline solution, and then passed through Selas 02 filter candles. At the same time, filtrates were also prepared from leukemic organs, such as thymus, spleen, and lymph nodes, of the same rat donors.

Suckling, less than 7-day-old rats were inoculated with serial dilutions of either plasma or organ filtrates. Ten rats were inoculated with the 10^{-2} dilution of the plasma filtrate, and all developed leukemia. Four rats were inoculated with 10^{-3}, and 5 additional rats with 10^{-4} plasma filtrate dilutions; all four rats in the first group, and 4 out of 5 in the second group, developed leukemia. In the same study, filtered extracts prepared from leukemic organs of the same rat donors induced leukemia in only 6 out of 10 rats inoculated with the 10^{-2} dilution, and in 3 out of 5 rats following inoculation of a 10^{-3} dilution. Only 1 out of 5 rats developed leukemia following inoculation of a 10^{-4} dilution of the organ filtrate. The average latency in both groups varied from $3\frac{1}{2}$ to 6 months.

It was apparent from this study that filtrates prepared from blood plasma of leukemic rats were more potent on bio-assay than those prepared from pooled organs of the same rat donors. However, it was noted in this particular experiment that the incidence of leukemia induced with filtrates prepared from leukemic rat organs was relatively lower than that usually observed in our routine rat-to-rat passage, in which such extracts are usually employed. For that reason the comparison between the leukemic potential of the blood plasma and pooled organs extracts will be again studied in a similar experiment. There seems to be little doubt, nevertheless, from results thus far obtained that blood plasma from leukemic rat donors represents an excellent source for harvesting of the leukemic virus. In this respect, plasma of leukemic rats is not different from blood plasma of mice with virus-induced leukemia.

HOST FACTORS DETERMINING THE DEVELOPMENT AND FORM OF INDUCED DISEASE

We have already discussed on the preceding pages of this chapter the differences among the various strains of mice in their response to the inoculation of the mouse leukemia virus, and we stressed the fact that the form of the induced disease may depend to a considerable extent on the genetic susceptibility of the host. The myeloid form of leukemia develops only rarely following inoculation of the virus into mice of such strains as C3H or C57 Brown, but develops quite frequently following inoculation of the same virus into mice of strain BALB/c, or into Sprague-Dawley rats. Many other factors may possibly influence the form of the induced leukemia and lymphomas; most of these factors have not yet been adequately studied and are actually unknown; such factors as age at inoculation, quantity and potency of the injected virus, age of the host in which the disease developed, etc., may be of some importance in determining the form of the induced disease, and may merit further investigation.

One of the most interesting factors determining the resistance of the animal to the inoculated virus, and to a considerable extent also the form of the induced leukemia, appears to be intimately related to the thymus.

Studies on the Role of Thymectomy on Virus-induced Leukemia in Mice

There exists a curious, and as yet not fully explained, relationship between the development of leukemia and the thymus, as determined by experimental removal of that organ in mice. The inhibiting effect of thymectomy on the development of spontaneous leukemia, first reported by McEndy, Boon and Furth (1944) in experiments dealing with mice of the high-leukemic Ak strain, has already been discussed. Thymectomy was also found to render mice of an otherwise susceptible strain resistant to radiation-induced leukemia (Kaplan, 1950). It appeared of interest, therefore, to determine whether leukemia induced by inoculation of a transmissible cell-free agent could also be inhibited by removal of the thymus, either preceding or following inoculation of the virus.

In experiments performed independently, and in rapid succession, in three different laboratories (Gross, 1959. Levinthal, Buffet and Furth, 1959. Miller, 1960), it was observed that when mice of a susceptible strain, such as C3H, were inoculated with passage A virus, and when their thymus lobes were removed by surgical procedure, many of them remained in good health, even though they received the virus. In our studies we examined the effect of thymectomy on mice either following or preceding the inoculation of the virus. It was observed in these studies that in mice of certain strains, such as C3H/Bi (Gross, 1959), or C57 Brown/cd (Gross, unpublished), the removal of thymus increased their resistance to the leukemogenic action of the virus. Furthermore, the interesting observation was also made in our laboratory that thymectomy increased considerably the incidence of myeloid leukemia in virus-injected mice (Gross, 1960).

Technique of Thymectomy. After some initial experiments with a variety of methods, we found the following technique most satisfactory, with a simplicity which allowed the acquisition of sufficient skill after a relatively short experience. This method represented our own modification of the technique which we observed a few years ago during our visit with Dr. R. H. Mole and Dr. J. F. Loutit at the Radiobiological Research Unit, in Harwell, England.

The procedure was performed under ether anesthesia. After skin incision, the upper part of sternum was bluntly exposed, and the manubrium sterni split longitudinally (about 3 to 4 mm) with fine scissors, exactly in the middle line. The fascia covering mediastinum was then exposed and gently lifted with an ophthalmic forceps; a small opening was made in the fascia to visualize the thymus. Both thymic lobes were then removed by suction, under vacuum pressure of about 20 to 25 mm of mercury, using a small glass tubing (eye-dropper-like) bent at right angle, and an electric suction pump. The wound was closed by 2 or 3 interrupted silk sutures involving only the skin. Immediate postoperative mortality did not exceed 10 per cent.

Influence of Thymectomy on Susceptibility to the Virus. In our initial studies, 39 young adult C3H mice about 4 to 6 weeks old were thymectomized; a few days later, they were inoculated with leukemic passage A filtrate. None developed leukemia although all these mice were observed until they reached an average age of 15 months. Of 41 control mice, not thymectomized and inoculated simultaneously with the same leukemic filtrate, 26 (63 per cent) developed leukemia at an average age of 8.7 months (Gross, 1959, 1960).

In a second and similar series carried out on a larger number of animals with an extended observation time, a few of the thymectomized mice that had been inoculated with passage A virus developed myelogenous leukemia after they reached 12 to 16 months of age (Gross, 1960).

The results were similar when thymectomy followed the inoculation of the virus. In this series the mice were inoculated within a few days after birth and were then thymectomized about one month later. Of 79 C3H mice inoculated with the passage A leukemic filtrate at an average age of 3.5 days, and thymectomized about one month later, at an average age of 33 days, only 34 (43 per cent) developed lymphatic leukemia at an average age of 8.8 months. In addition, however, among mice in this group, 11 (14 per cent) developed myelogenous leukemia, some of them chloroleukemia, noticeable because of the characteristic green lymphoid tumors, at an average age of 12.4 months (Gross, 1960, also 1961, unpublished). The remaining mice survived with no signs of leukemia to an average age of 14 months. Of 104 litter-mate controls, inoculated simultaneously with the same filtrates, but not thymectomized, 98, or 94 per cent, developed lymphatic leukemia, in most instances in its usual aleukemic form, after an average latency of only 3.4 months.

Accordingly, thymectomy inhibited the development of disease in some animals, or delayed it considerably in others. Furthermore, some of such animals developed unexpectedly myeloid leukemia, i.e. a form of leukemia observed in our laboratory only exceptionally in non-thymectomized, virus-injected mice of the C3H strain.

Anyone familiar with the technique of the removal of thymus in mice and rats will readily understand the difficulties in removing both thymic lobes without trace, in an operative technique requiring skill and speed to avoid hemorrhage and respiratory difficulties. It is possible to assume, therefore, that at least some of those mice that developed lymphatic leukemia in spite of thymectomy might have had parts of their thymic lobes left after the operation. In some of these mice, fragments of lymphoid tumors could be found in the mediastinum, at the site where the thymic lobes had been removed, suggesting thereby that thymectomy might not have been complete in such animals (Gross, 1960, unpublished).

Effect of Thymectomy on Susceptibility of Rats to Virus-induced Leukemia. Similar experiments were later performed on rats. In our initial studies 1 to 3-day-old Sprague-Dawley rats were inoculated with passage A virus harvested from leukemic rat donors. After inoculation, each litter was split; approximately half of the litter received no further treatment, serving as a control group. Rats of the other half of the litter were thymectomized when approximately 10 days old, employing exactly the same technique as that used in mice. Litter-mate animals injected simultaneously with the virus, but not thymectomized, served as controls. It was observed in these studies (Gross, 1963) that thymectomy delayed, and in some instances inhibited, the development of leukemia in the virus-injected rats. Furthermore, significantly, the incidence of myeloid leukemia was higher in the thymectomized animals (Gross, 1963, also unpublished data).

These results were confirmed and extended in a subsequent study carried out by Kunii and his colleagues (1965, 1966). In their studies, thymectomy performed on one-month-old rats reduced virus-induced leukemia from 97 to 59 per cent; furthermore, the incidence of myeloid leukemia among the thymectomized rats reached 12 per cent as compared with none in the control group. The inhibition of induction of leukemia was more marked following thymectomy performed on 1 to 3-day-old rats, the injection of the virus being performed on the same or next day (Kunii, Cali and Furth, 1965). Thymectomy performed at such early age reduced the induction of leukemia in virus-injected rats from 75 to 13 per cent in one experiment, and 93 to 19 per cent in another experiment carried out in these studies.

It must be stressed at this point that thymectomy carried out on newborn animals may not only present technical difficulties, particularly in newborn mice because of the small size of these animals, but may also disturb the immunological balance of the host, and result in the development of a wasting syndrome very similar to, if not identical with, the runt disease, causing high mortality in such animals.*

Restoration of Susceptibility to Virus-induced Leukemia in Thymectomized Mice by Implantation of Normal Thymus. Implantation of a normal mouse thymus into mice that had been thymectomized restored their susceptibility to inoculation of the mouse leukemia virus (Miller, 1959, 1960. Gross, 1960). In similar experiments performed previously by Law (1950), Kaplan (1956), Carnes (1956), and their associates, implantation of a normal thymus into thymectomized mice also restored their susceptibility to carcinogen- or radiation-induced leukemia, respectively. More recently Miller (1960) also observed that susceptibility of thymectomized C3H mice to inoculation of passage A mouse leukemia virus could be restored even several months after thymectomy, by implantation of a normal, homologous thymus. These experiments suggested that the thymus is not the only organ where the leukemic virus is stored. Animals that had been injected with the virus, and were later thymectomized, apparently still carried the virus.

The fact that removal of the thymus renders mice and rats of certain strains relatively resistant to the leukemogenic action of passage A virus

* Discussion of the role of the thymus in leukemogenesis in mice and rats as well as of the influence of this organ on immunological competency of the host would exceed the scope of this monograph. The interested reader is referred for further details to the volume on *The Thymus in Immunobiology* (R. A. Good, A. E. Gabrielsen, Edit., Hoeber Medical Division, Harper & Row, New York, p. 778, 1964).

FIG. 38. LEUKEMIC VIRUS PARTICLES IN MALE GENITAL ORGANS OF VIRUS-INJECTED C3H(F) MICE.

(A). Section through epididymis from a C3H(f) mouse with passage A virus-induced stem-cell leukemia. A virus particle (b) appears budding from an epithelial cell; several mature type C virus particles (C) with nucleoids are present in the intercellular space. Magnification 62,000×. (D. G. Feldman and L. Gross, unpublished.) (B). Portion of seminal vesicle from a C3H(f) mouse with passage A virus-induced lymphatic leukemia. A virus particle (b) is budding from the cell membrane into the lumen. Proximal to the virus particle within the lumen is a secretory droplet (s). Magnification 62,000×. (D. G. Feldman and L. Gross, unpublished.)

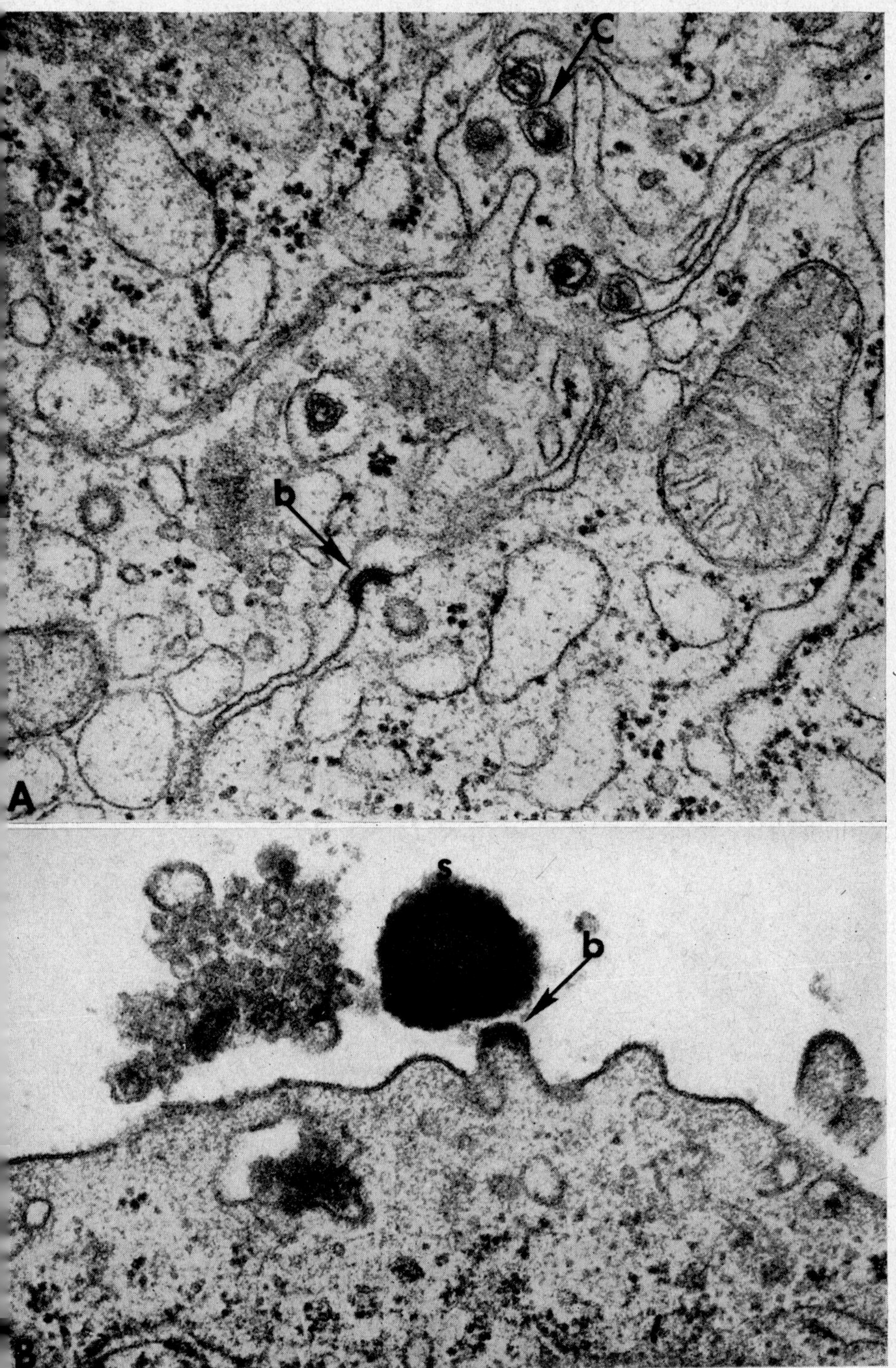

Fig. 38. Leukemic Virus Particles in Male Genital Organs of Virus-injected C3H(f) Mice.

filtrate is of considerable interest. As an explanation, it is possible to assume that the thymus represents the principal target organ where the injected leukemogenic agent may initiate its pathogenic potential. It is possible that in such animals the presence of the thymus is necessary for the leukemogenic action of the virus and the early development of disease. In the absence of thymus, the leukemic virus may select other organs, such as spleen or bone marrow, to initiate disease. A considerable delay, however, may occur in such instances; among such animals, many may live out their usual life span and may die from other causes before conditions favoring the development of leukemia may occur. Furthermore, if leukemia eventually develops in the absence of the thymus, it may be more frequently of the myeloid form than among non-thymectomized controls.

It appears therefore that a mouse in which the thymus was removed by a surgical procedure is relatively resistant to: (a) spontaneous leukemia, (b) radiation-induced leukemia, and (c) virus-induced leukemia. This observation would be consistent with the working hypothesis that at least in mice, a leukemogenic virus is the basic cause of spontaneous leukemia, as well as of leukemia induced by radiation or other carcinogenic factors, such as chemicals and hormones.

Thymectomy, and Susceptibility to Implantation of Leukemic Cells. It should be stressed at this point that although thymectomy may render the mouse relatively resistant to inoculation of the virus filtrate, i.e. to the induction of leukemia by a cell-free agent, it will not render such an animal resistant to the implantation of leukemic cells. As already discussed on the preceding pages of this chapter, mice of a given inbred line, such as Ak or C58, are susceptible to implantation of leukemic cell suspensions prepared from leukemic donors of the same respective inbred strain. The same is true for virus-induced leukemia in such strains as C3H or C57 Brown, for example; such leukemias are readily transplantable by cell-graft in mice of the same inbred lines.

It is of interest that removal of thymus will not alter the susceptibility of a mouse to implantation of leukemic cells. This observation was made in experiments dealing with cell transplantation of spontaneous mouse leukemia (Furth and Boon, 1944), as well as more recently on cell transplantation of leukemia induced in C3H mice with virus-filtrate (Gross, 1959). There appears to exist a fundamental difference in the mechanism of leukemogenesis between the induction of this disease by virus filtrate and by cell transplantation.

Finally, it should be also stressed that thymectomy had no therapeutic effect on the usual course of an established leukemia in the mouse (Gross, unpublished). After leukemia developed in the mouse, removal of the diseased thymic lobes was ineffective in controlling the course of this disease.

Increased Incidence of Myeloid Leukemia, Developing in Thymectomized Mice and Rats, Following Inoculation of the Passage A Virus

We have stressed on the preceding pages of this chapter that the passage A mouse leukemia virus, initially isolated from spontaneous Ak leukemia, induced in most instances the lymphatic form of this disease, usually thymic or generalized lymphosarcomas, following inoculation into suckling C3H or C57 Brown mice. The incidence of myeloid leukemia in untreated virus-injected mice of these inbred lines was very low; in a sample of 100 leukemic C3H mice examined it did not exceed 1 per cent. It was of considerable interest, therefore, to observe a relatively high incidence of myelogenous leukemia in C3H mice inoculated with the same virus, but thymectomized (Gross, 1960). A significant increase in the development of myelogenous leukemia was also observed following thymectomy of virus-injected mice of the C57 Brown/cd strain (Gross, unpublished), and more recently also in rats (Gross, 1963).

Myelogenous leukemia developing in thymectomized mice was characterized by the presence in peripheral blood of large numbers of white blood cells of the granulocytic series in all degrees of maturation. Undifferentiated stem-cell leukemias, and at least one or two cases of monocytic-like leukemia, were also observed among these mice. Most striking among the myelogenous leukemias observed were the chloroleukemias, noticeable because of the green tumorous lymph nodes. In two and possibly in three mice of this group, a form of leukemia was observed involving to a considerable extent the erythropoetic system; this form was manifested by the presence in the peripheral blood of very large numbers of nucleated red cells, and their precursors, with a hemoglobin level not exceeding 3 to 4 grams per 100 cc. of blood; this curious form of leukemia could be classified as a form of erythro-leukemia.

Transmission of the Virus-induced Myelogenous Leukemia in C3H Mice by Cell-Graft. The various forms of myelogenous leukemia, chloroleukemia, and also the erythroblastic form that developed in C3H mice, inoculated with passage A virus and subsequently thymectomized, could be transplanted by cell-graft to young adult mice of the same strain (Gross, 1960). We have carried a considerable number of such myeloid leukemias through consecutive cell transfers; the latency varied from less than 2 weeks to 6 or 8 weeks, or more. The myelogenous leukemias retained their original form on transplantation, at least through their first few consecutive cell transfers. This was also true for the chloroleukemic form, as well as for erythro-leukemia. In most of the myelogenous leukemias, nevertheless, with each successive cell transfer an increasing number of highly undifferentiated primitive cells, difficult to identify, appeared in the peripheral blood circulation. Gradually, following a number of additional cell transplantations, most of such leukemias lost their characteristic granulocytic character, and could only be designated as "stem-cell" leukemias. At this point the serial cell transfer of most of these leukemic cell lines was discontinued. In a few instances the cell passage was continued, however, and it was observed that with additional successive cell transplantations, the latency gradually increased and all the transplanted leukemias studied eventually reverted to the lymphatic form, manifested as a rule by the development of thymic or generalized lymphosarcomas, usually with no significant changes in peripheral blood morphology, i.e. a form similar to that initially induced with the original passage A virus filtrate.

Attempt to Transmit Myelogenous Leukemias by Filtrates. An attempt was made to transmit the myeloid leukemias in their particular forms by means of filtrates. The rather interesting observation was made that when filtrates prepared from mice with myeloid leukemia were inoculated into newborn C3H mice, lymphatic leukemia, usually in the characteristic form of thymic or generalized lymphosarcomas, developed in the great majority of the inoculated animals. Only exceptionally did myeloid leukemia develop following inoculation of such filtrates. Even then, however, an attempt to pass the myelogenous leukemia again by filtrates resulted eventually in the development of an aleukemic lymphatic form. The following is a summary of these experiments (Gross, 1960, 1962):

> Filtrates (Selas 02) were prepared from 45 individual leukemic mouse donors with 15 different forms of either primary or transplanted myeloid leukemia, including chloroleukemia, stem-cell leukemia, monocytic-like leukemia, and the erythroblastic form. Forty-five filtered extracts were prepared and inoculated into 354 suckling, less than 5-day-old, mice of the C3H strain. Among the inoculated mice, 247 developed lymphoid leukemia essentially similar to that which could be induced with the passage A virus, usually in the form of thymic or generalized lymphosarcomas, most frequently with no leukemic changes in peripheral blood morphology; only 12 mice, with 4 additional questionable classifications, i.e. at best 6 per cent of all forms of leukemia induced in this group, developed myeloid leukemia; none of the injected mice developed chloroleukemia (Gross, 1962). When the few myelogenous leukemias were again passed by filtrates, they induced usually on first, second, or third cell-free passage, the typical aleukemic lymphatic form of the disease, indistinguishable from that induced routinely with the passage A filtrates.

Accordingly, attempts to develop and maintain in mice a myelogenous form of leukemia which would preserve its myeloid character through serial cell-free passage have not succeeded. This was in contrast to the myeloid leukemia (myeloblastosis) in chickens which has been readily maintained by filtrate passage in the fowl (Beard, 1956).

It appears from the foregoing that, curiously, in mice of certain strains, such as C3H or C57 Brown, and also in rats, there may exist some regulatory mechanism which would favor the induction or spontaneous development of the lymphatic rather than the myeloid form of leukemia. It is of interest that under certain experimental conditions, such as removal of thymus in C3H mice inoculated with passage A virus, the myelogenous form of leukemia could be more readily induced. Even then, however, the myelogenous form could not be maintained serially by cell-free passage; in the course of such a passage, a gradual return to the lymphatic form was observed (Gross, 1960, 1962, also unpublished).

Effect of Splenectomy

Removal of spleen, either before or after the inoculation of the passage A virus, neither inhibited nor delayed the development of leukemia in C3H mice (Gross, 1962). Most of the virus-injected and splenectomized C3H mice developed the usual form of lymphatic leukemia, similar to that commonly induced with the passage A filtrate. Only one of these mice developed myelogenous leukemia; none developed chloroleukemia.

In the first group, 101 C3H mice were splenectomized when about 26 days old. One to three days later they were inoculated intraperitoneally (0.5 cc. each) with passage A filtrate. Eighty-one of them (80 per cent) developed leukemia at an average age of 6.4 months. Among the induced leukemias, 76 were of the usually observed lymphatic form, i.e. thymic or generalized lymphosarcomas, in most instances with no leukemic changes in peripheral blood morphology. Two mice developed stem-cell leukemia, one developed myeloid leukemia, and two mice developed a form of leukemia which was difficult to classify.

A control group consisting of 84 litter-mates was inoculated at the same time, and under otherwise similar experimental conditions, with passage A filtrate, except that none of these animals was splenectomized. Sixty-eight mice in this group (81 per cent) developed leukemia of the lymphatic form, i.e. mostly thymic or generalized lymphosarcomas, at an average age of 6.6 months.

In another experiment, 13 suckling C3H mice were inoculated at an average age of six days with passage A filtrate (0.3 to 0.4 cc. each, intraperitoneally); they were splenectomized when they were 30 to 32 days old. All developed leukemia of the lymphatic form at an average age of three months.

In a control group, 16 litter-mates were inoculated at the same time, and under similar experimental conditions, with the same leukemic filtrate, but were not splenectomized; all control mice developed lymphatic leukemia at an average age of three months.

It is apparent from results of these experiments that splenectomy performed on C3H mice did not alter the incidence or latency of the passage A virus-induced leukemia, and appeared to influence in isolated instances only, if at all, and only to a limited degree, the developing form of leukemia. This was in contrast to the removal of thymus previously described, which in most instances inhibited or considerably delayed the development of lymphatic leukemia, and frequently caused the myelogenous form to appear later in life.

Study of Other Host Factors. Inhibiting Effect of Food Restriction. There are several additional factors influencing the development of leukemia in the inoculated animals; only some of these factors are known. The influence of the hormonal factors was mentioned earlier in this chapter, and is reflected by the relatively higher incidence of induced leukemia and shorter latency period in virus-injected females, as compared with virus-injected males, in mice (Gross, 1957) and also in rats (Gross, unpublished data).

Among nonspecific factors influencing the induction of leukemia in mice, the inhibiting influence of caloric food restriction on development of spontaneous or virus-induced leukemia is of interest. Saxton, Boon, and Furth reported in 1944 that caloric food restriction inhibited the development of spontaneous mouse leukemia in mice of the Ak strain. A similar, although less striking influence could also be observed in experiments dealing with virus-induced leukemia in C3H mice.

In our recent studies (Gross, 1963, also unpublished data), passage A filtrates were inoculated into several litters of suckling C3H(f) mice. After weaning, at about three weeks of age, each litter was divided. One group, which served as controls, was raised under normal conditions, with an unlimited amount of Purina Laboratory Chow pellets and water available. Mice of the other group received daily only two grams, for each mouse, of the same food pellets, and once weekly some lettuce; the water intake was not limited.

All 24 control mice developed leukemia (100 per cent) at an average age of 2.6 months. In the experimental group, all 20 mice raised on the restricted diet also developed leukemia (100 per cent), but after a significant delay, at an average age of 4.5 months.

The effect of food restriction was evident therefore in delaying the appearance of leukemia in virus-injected mice; however, there was no complete inhibition of the development of the disease under the experimental conditions employed.*

These were only preliminary studies, however, and it is possible that under more precise experimental conditions, with proper dosage and quantity of the virus filtrate injected, and with more severe food restriction, better results could be obtained; it is possible to speculate that under such conditions the inhibiting effect of caloric food restriction could be perhaps more clearly determined; however, only additional experimental studies along this line could clarify this interesting possibility.

* It should be emphasized again at this point that the effect of food restriction influenced only, if at all, the actual induction of the disease, i.e. the presumable "activation" of the virus. Limitation of food intake did not in any way influence the growth rate of the tumors and the usual progress of the disease already established.

Study of the Possible Effect of Environmental Cold Temperature on Susceptibility to the Induction of Leukemia. An attempt was made to determine whether the resistance of adult C3H mice to intraperitoneal inoculation of passage A leukemic filtrates could be either increased or decreased by low environmental temperature (Gross, 1960). Accordingly, 24 C3H males, two months old, were inoculated with passage A leukemic filtrate (0.5 cc., i.p., each). They were divided into two groups, each consisting of 12 mice. One group was placed in a cold room in which the environmental temperature was constantly maintained at +4°C. The other group, serving as a control, was placed in the regular animal room, where the environmental temperature was maintained at approximately 20°C.

The results were as follows: Among the 12 C3H mice kept in the cold room, only 3 (25 per cent) developed leukemia at 6.8 months average age. The remaining 9 died, or were sacrificed, at an average age of 13.5 months. Among the 12 C3H control mice, kept at normal (20°C) room temperature, 8 developed leukemia (67 per cent) at 8.5 months average age; the remaining 3 died, or were sacrificed at 13.5 months average age.

The cold environmental temperature did not influence, however, the incidence of spontaneous leukemia in Ak mice, which are the natural hosts of the leukemic agent. In a series of experiments (Gross, 1960b), Ak females, approximately 2 months old, were divided, by splitting litters, into two groups: one group consisting of 33 females was placed in the cold room in which the temperature was maintained at 4°C; another group consisting of 23 littermates was kept, as a control, in the regular animal room in which the temperature was maintained at approximately 20°C.

Of the 33 females kept in the cold room, 31 (94 per cent) developed spontaneous leukemia at 8.9 months average age. Of 23 control Ak females, kept at the usual room (20°C) temperature, 20 (87 per cent) developed leukemia at 9.7 months average age.

Natural Transmission of the Mouse Leukemia Virus

We have reviewed on the preceding pages of this chapter the etiology and pathogenesis of mouse leukemia, and the experiments which led to the isolation of the mouse leukemia virus; we have also described some of the more important properties of the virus which causes this disease.

FIG. 39. LEUKEMIC VIRUS PARTICLES IN MALE GENITAL ORGANS OF VIRUS-INJECTED C3H(F) MICE.

(A). Section through the lumen of a prostate gland from a C3H(f) mouse with passage A virus-induced stem-cell leukemia. Within the lumen are mature type C virus particles (C) containing nucleoids. There is variation in the shape and size of type C particles as well as in the size and density of the inner nucleoids. Magnification 62,000×. (D. G. Feldman and L. Gross, unpublished.) (B). Intercellular space from seminal vesicle of a passage A virus-injected C3H(f) mouse sacrificed at the age of 5 weeks, prior to the development of leukemia. A particle (b) budding from an epithelial cell and mature type C virus particles (C) containing nucleoids are illustrated. Magnification 42,800×. (D. G. Feldman and L. Gross, unpublished.)

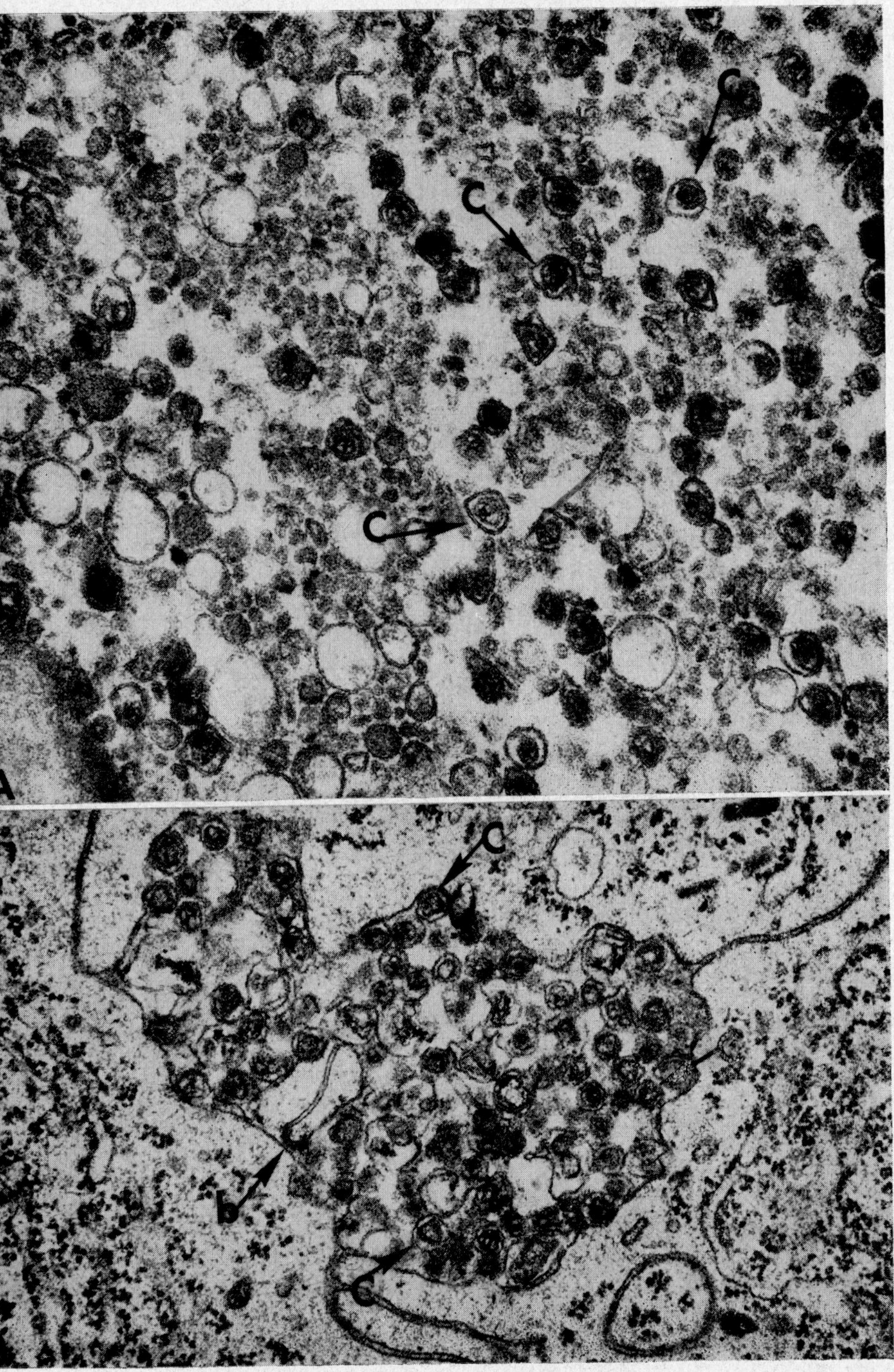

Fig. 39. Leukemic Virus Particles in Male Genital Organs of Virus-injected C3H(f) Mice.

It is now clear that leukemia in mice is caused by a virus which can be transmitted experimentally from one host to another by inoculation. It would be obviously of fundamental interest to determine as precisely as possible the manner in which this virus is transmitted from one host to another under natural life conditions. Unfortunately, the clarification of this problem presents considerable difficulties.

Leukemia is a relatively rare disease in a general mouse population, as it is rare also in most of the other animal species, including humans. In mice, leukemia and lymphomas develop here and there spontaneously, as a rule, in middle-aged animals; however, a more frequent development of this disease in several members of certain families of mice has been observed, as compared with the incidence in a general mouse population. Families of mice having a relatively high incidence of leukemia have been developed by selective inbreeding. In two most prominent leukemic families, designated by the symbols Ak and C58, most of the mice of both sexes develop "spontaneous" leukemia in each successive generation after they reach about 5 to 8 months of age. These families represent an interesting, although somewhat artificial model for the study of the actual host-to-host transmission of the virus causing this disease. The virus is obviously transmitted from one generation to another, since animals of each generation develop leukemia. However, how is this virus transmitted? Another point of considerable interest remains to be answered: why does the disease develop in mice of such families only after these animals reach, or pass, about 5 months of age?

Transmission of Virus Does Not Occur to any Significant Degree by Contact

It should be stressed at the onset of this discussion that leukemia, like other malignant tumors, is not transmitted by contact. When either Ak or C58 mice with spontaneous leukemia were placed in the same cages with young adult, normal, healthy mice of either the same or another inbred line, no transmission of the disease could be observed under such experimental conditions.

Experiments on Contact Transmission of Spontaneous Leukemia among Young Adult Mice. In a recent experiment carried out in our laboratory (Gross, 1964, unpublished), 20 Ak females and 20 C3H(f) females, about 3 to 4 weeks old, were placed together in 3 cages, each cage containing an equal number of mice of both strains. Mice of both strains were kept together for observation, to show the possible effect of contact transmission of the mouse leukemia virus. At the conclusion of this experiment, one Ak mouse and 3 C3H(f) females were not accounted for; they presumably died and were cannibalized, or they could have escaped from their cages in the course of the experiment; these 4 mice were not included in the tabulation of final results. Of the surviving animals, all 19 AK females developed spontaneous leukemia at ages varying from 5 to 14 months (average age 8.7 months). Of the 17 C3H(f) females, only one developed a reticulum-cell sarcoma in liver, spleen, and in the mesenteric lymph node, at 19 months of age. The remaining 16 C3H(f) females died without signs of leukemia or lymphomas at ages varying from 11 to 19 months (average age 16.7 months). The results of this experiment suggested that among young adult mice of strains Ak and C3H, transmission of the mouse leukemia virus does not occur to any significant degree.

Experiments on Contact Transmission of the Mouse Leukemia Virus Following Its Inoculation into Suckling Mice of Low-leukemic Strain C3H(f). The possibility of "horizontal," i.e. contact transmission of the mouse leukemia virus following its inoculation into newborn mice of a susceptible low-leukemic strain was also investigated in recent studies (Gross, 1962. Gross and Dreyfuss, 1967). Suckling, less than 6-day-old, C3H(f) mice were inoculated intraperitoneally with passage A virus filtrate. Each litter was divided; only about one half of each litter was inoculated with the virus. The injected mice had their tails tied and cut, as means of identification; immediately after inoculation they were returned to their cages and placed back in the nests with their non-injected litter-mates; these mice were then raised together.

Of the 130 mice injected with the virus, 128 (98 per cent) developed leukemia at 3 months of age.

The non-injected mice exposed to contact infection were divided into two groups; one group, consisting of 58 mice, was raised with the virus-injected mice through the period of nursing, but only until weaning age; these mice were weaned when about 3 to 4 weeks old, and were then separated from the virus-injected mice, and kept under observation; five of them (8.6 per cent) developed leukemia. Another group, consisting of 65 mice, was raised and remained with their virus-injected litter-mates, not only through their first few weeks of life, but also after weaning; in this group 4 mice (6.2 per cent) developed leukemia. It is apparent that there was very little, if any, difference between both groups of non-injected mice. Out of the total of 123 non-injected mice exposed to the possible contact infection in both groups, 9 mice (7.3 per cent) developed leukemia at an average age of 16 months. The incidence of leukemia developing among the non-injected mice which had been exposed to contact infection was relatively low, but nevertheless higher than the incidence of spontaneous leukemia observed in mice of our colony of the C3H(f) strain (less than 1 per cent).

It is possible to speculate on the basis of these experiments that "horizontal," i.e. contact, transmission of the leukemic virus may occur to some slight degree among newborn and suckling mice, although it may only very occasionally lead to the eventual development of the disease.

STUDIES ON THE EPIDEMIOLOGY OF MOUSE LEUKEMIA

Early Experiments on Spontaneous Mouse Leukemia Occurring in Families Naturally Infected with the Virus

Under experimental conditions thus far studied, there appears to exist a significant difference between the manner of transmission of "spontaneous" leukemia developing in mice of certain families naturally infected with an indigenous and potentially pathogenic mouse leukemia virus, and that of a passaged virus inoculated experimentally into mice of certain susceptible strains. This difference may be apparent only because of the experimental conditions employed. Mice of certain strains employed for inoculation of the virus may not be sufficiently susceptible to transmit the virus naturally. Other strains may have to be tested, or the experimental conditions thus far employed may have to be changed.

It seems appropriate, therefore, to discuss separately experiments on the epidemiology of spontaneous mouse leukemia developing in certain high-leukemic strains, such as Ak or C58.

Most of the experiments here discussed were carried out on mice of the high-leukemic strain Ak. The incidence of spontaneous leukemia in mice of this strain has varied somewhat in different laboratories, and at different times, and was about 60 per cent in Dr. Furth's laboratory at the time the early studies were carried out. At the present time, in our laboratory, the incidence of spontaneous leukemia in Ak mice has reached up to 77 per cent in males, and has exceeded 90 per cent in females.

The incidence of spontaneous leukemia in strain C58 was about 90 per cent (MacDowell and Richter, 1935) and in strain F about 55 per cent (Kirschbaum and Strong, 1939, 1942).

The incidence of spontaneous leukemia in mice of low-leukemic strains, such as C3H, NH, Af, Rf, etc., has varied from 0 to 4 per cent. In our laboratory, the incidence of spontaneous leukemia in mice of our colonies of strains C3H(f) and C57 Brown/cd has been less than 1 and 5 per cent, respectively.

The interested reader is referred for more details concerning the incidence of leukemia in high-leukemic inbred lines, particularly C58 and Ak, to preceding pages of this chapter, and also to the chapter on the Development of Inbred Strains of Mice in this monograph, as well as to the original publications of the authors quoted.

How Is the Virus Transmitted?
Possibility Studied of Transmission of the Virus in Mothers' Milk. Experiments on Spontaneous Mouse Leukemia

The possibility of the transmission of a causative agent responsible for the development of leukemia in certain leukemic inbred strains of mice in the milk of nursing mothers had been investigated experimentally in the early studies, even before it was realized that leukemia in mice is caused by a transmissible virus, and prior to the initial preliminary report by Bittner in 1936 of the transmission through the milk of the mouse mammary carcinoma virus.*

MacDowell and Richter reported in 1935 that in an experiment in which suckling mice of the high-leukemic C58 line were foster-nursed by females of

*The interested reader is referred to the chapter on Mouse Mammary Carcinoma in this monograph.

the low-leukemic strain StoLi, there was no reduction in the incidence of leukemia in the foster-nursed animals, and no induction of leukemia in reciprocal nursing experiments in which StoLi mice were nursed by C58 foster-mothers.

No further details or figures were given; it should be stressed, however, that at the time these early foster-nursing experiments were carried out, the existence of a subcellular, transmissible leukemic agent in mice could only be suspected; no experimental evidence of its actual existence was yet available.

Results of foster-nursing experiments carried out on mice of the high-leukemic strain Ak, and those of the low-leukemic strains Rf, Af, and C3H, were reported by Barnes and Cole in 1941, and by Furth and his colleagues in 1942; Kirschbaum and Strong (1942) also reported similar experiments carried out on mice of the high-leukemic strain F, foster-nursed by female mice of several low-leukemic strains, such as CBA, I, A, C3H, and NH.

In all these experiments, foster-nursing of mice of high-leukemic inbred strains by female mice of low-leukemic lines decreased significantly the incidence of leukemia in the foster-nursed animals. In the experiments of Barnes and Cole (1941), the incidence of leukemia in Ak mice, foster-nursed by females of the low-leukemic lines Rf or Af, was decreased from 60 to 32 per cent. In another series carried out by Furth, Cole and Boon (1942), the incidence of leukemia in Ak mice foster-nursed by C3H females was decreased from 58 to 27 per cent. However, they noted that if the foster-nursed Ak mice were again bred among themselves, the incidence of leukemia in the next generation was considerably increased, reaching about the same level (59 per cent) as that observed in the original Ak strain prior to the foster-nursing experiment.

It appeared from these early experiments that the incidence of spontaneous leukemia in mice of certain high-leukemic inbred lines could be significantly reduced, but could not be inhibited, by foster-nursing of such mice by females of low-leukemic inbred lines. It should be stressed, however, that at no time could a high-leukemic inbred line be changed by foster-nursing into a non-leukemic strain. This was in striking contrast to experiments on mouse mammary carcinoma in which, as discussed in more detail in a separate chapter of this monograph, the incidence of spontaneous mammary carcinomas in certain inbred lines, such as C3H or A, could be virtually eliminated by foster-nursing.

In all these experiments, suckling mice of the leukemic strains, such as Ak, were removed from their mothers, and were transferred for nursing to their foster-mothers when they were about 12 to 24 hours old. The possibility had to be considered that under such experimental conditions the newborn mice might have ingested the virus with small quantities of milk swallowed prior to removal of such animals from their own mothers. Accordingly, of considerable interest were several crucial experiments which demonstrated that the development of leukemia in mice of the high-leukemic strain Ak could not be prevented, even if such animals were removed prior to birth by laparotomy from the wombs of their mothers, and were transferred for foster-nursing to low-leukemic line females. Such animals did not ingest even the smallest amount of their mothers' milk. If they developed leukemia, as many of them did, the disease could not have been caused by a milk-transmitted virus.

Development of Spontaneous Leukemia in Ak Mice Raised from Full Term Infant Mice (or from Transferred Ova) Removed by Laparotomy from Pregnant Ak Females, and Nursed by Low-leukemic Strain Foster-Mothers

Furth (1945) removed by laparotomy at full term infant mice from pregnant healthy Ak females, and transferred them for foster-nursing to low-leukemic stock Rf females. Among the 30 Ak mice (17 females and 13 males) foster-nursed by Rf mice, 9 developed leukemia (30 per cent). The incidence of leukemia in the 112 offspring of these foster-nursed mice (68 females and 44 males) rose, however, to 79 per cent.

In a similar experiment carried out more recently in our laboratory (Gross, 1952), full-term infant mice were removed by laparotomy from the womb of a pregnant, healthy, 2½-month-old, Ak female, and were transferred to a foster-mother of the C57 Black strain, known to have been free from spontaneous leukemia for at least 15 preceding generations. From these transferred and foster-nursed Ak mice, three survived; two of them (females) developed spontaneous leukemia at the age of 6 and 10 months, respectively, and the third mouse, a male, was found dead at the age of 17 months, with enlarged peripheral lymph nodes, but no other conclusive evidence of leukemia. These three foster-nursed mice had 13 offspring; eleven of them (85 per cent) developed leukemia at an average age of 8 months.

In another similar experiment, Fekete and Otis (1954) removed Ak infant mice, at term, by laparotomy from the wombs of two Ak females, and transferred these mice to C3H foster-mothers. Of the original 10 animals in this group, 7 developed leukemia, and 3 died of other causes. Among the foster-nursed mice and their descendants, a total of 77 mice, 64 (83 per cent) developed leukemia.

In another ingenious experiment, Fekete and Otis (1954) removed fertilized ova from the oviducts of pregnant Ak female mice, and transplanted these ova into the uteri of pregnant C3H females. All 10 mice born from transplanted ova,* and nursed by their C3H foster-mothers, developed

* The albino Ak mice born among the dark brown (technically designated as "black agouti") C3H mice could be readily spotted and recognized as having been born from Ak ova.

leukemia. Among 97 offspring of these 10 mice, 75 (77 per cent) developed leukemia. This compared with an 84 per cent incidence of leukemia in the original Ak strain carried in their laboratory.

* * *

Accordingly, a relatively large number of mice of a leukemic strain developed spontaneous leukemia, even though they did not ingest a single drop of their mothers' milk. Another route of virus passage from parents to offspring had to be investigated. These mice had been apparently infected with the virus prior to birth. On the other hand, it should also be pointed out that although the results of these experiments demonstrated that in a leukemic inbred line of mice, mothers' milk is not the principal route of virus transmission, they did not preclude the possibility that a small quantity of the virus could be transmitted in the milk. Such an assumption would be consistent with the observation that foster-nursing of Ak mice by low-leukemic strain females reduced the incidence of leukemia in the foster-nursed animals. Although such mice had been infected with the virus prior to birth, they could have received, nevertheless, a lesser amount of virus than those which received an additional, even though relatively small, quantity of virus in the milk of their mothers.

In recent studies the presence of the mouse leukemia virus in milk of Ak females was demonstrated in electron microscopic studies by Dmochowski and his colleagues (1963). Virus particles were also found on electron microscopic examination of mammary glands of pregnant C3H(f) females that had been injected with the mouse leukemia virus (Feldman, Gross and Dreyfuss, 1963).

Attempts to Induce Leukemia in Mice of Low-leukemic Strains by Foster-Nursing. Even before the existence of the mouse leukemia virus was experimentally demonstrated, attempts had been made to induce leukemia in mice of low-leukemic strains by foster-nursing, employing Ak females as foster-

---

FIG. 40. LEUKEMIC VIRUS PARTICLES IN FEMALE GENITAL ORGANS OF VIRUS-INJECTED C3H(F) MICE.

(A). Section through ovary from a C3H(f) mouse with passage A virus-induced leukemia. Shown are follicular epithelium (fe) and theca folliculi (tf). A higher magnification of part of the theca folliculi (b) illustrates 2 virus particles (b inset) budding from the cell membrane of a thecal cell. Magnification Fig. A: 17,400 ×. Inset: 42,800 ×. (D. G. Feldman and L. Gross, unpublished.) (B). An area from uterus of a C3H(f) mouse with passage A virus-induced leukemia. Indicated are the epithelium (e), connective tissue fibroblasts (f), and collagen (c). Higher magnification of part of a fibroblast (b) illustrates a leukemia virus particle (b inset) budding from the cell membrane. Magnification Fig. B: 9,200 ×. Inset: 62,000 ×. (D. G. Feldman and L. Gross, unpublished.)

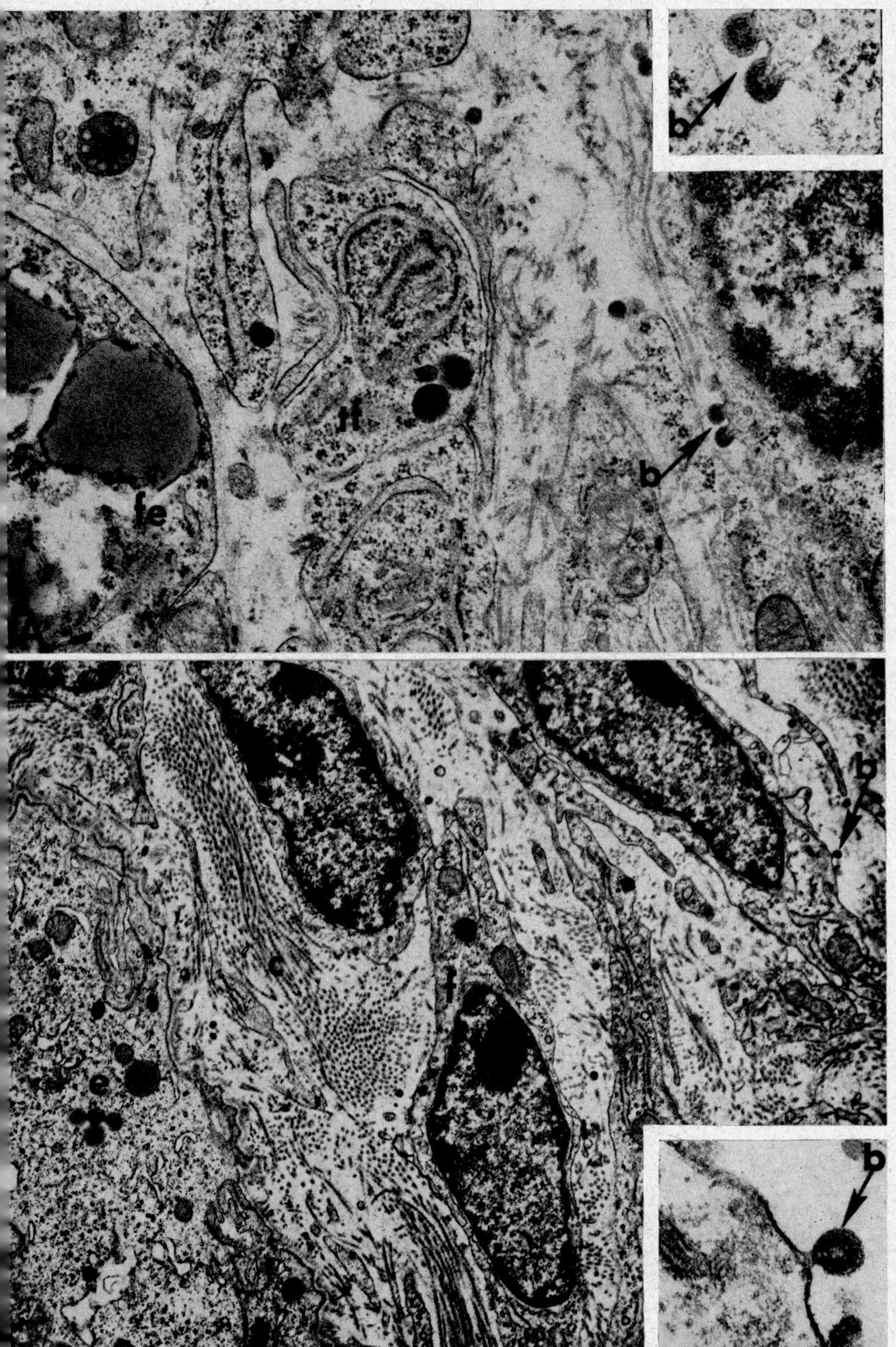

Fig. 40. Leukemic Virus Particles in Female Genital Organs of Virus-injected C3H(f) Mice.

mothers. Most of these experiments were inspired by the results of earlier studies on mouse mammary carcinoma, in which the development of these tumors could be induced in mice of low-mammary carcinoma strains by foster-nursing of such animals by high-mammary carcinoma strain females. However, it soon became apparent that leukemia could not be induced in mice of low-leukemic strains by foster-nursing.

Barnes and Cole (1941) transferred 181 mice of low-leukemic strains* Rf and Af to foster-mothers of the Ak strain. Only 4 of the foster-nursed Rf and Af mice (2 per cent) developed leukemia. In a similar study, Furth and his colleagues (1942) transferred 215 mice of the low-leukemic strain C3H to Ak females for foster-nursing; none of the foster-nursed C3H mice developed leukemia. Law also reported that in his studies (1954) none of the mice of the low-leukemic strain NH, that were foster-nursed by high-leukemic strain AKR females, developed leukemia.

Recent Experiments on Transmission of the Mouse Leukemia Virus Through Milk, Employing Healthy or Leukemic Ak Females as Foster-Mothers. In our recent studies (Gross and Dreyfuss, 1967) we have examined the effect of foster-nursing by Ak females on mice of our C3H(f) colony. The Ak female mice had their own litters one to two days old removed and sacrificed, and replaced by C3H(f) litters of about the same age. These C3H(f) mice were then nursed and raised by their Ak foster-mothers; at the age of 3 to 4 weeks they were weaned, separated by sexes, and then kept under observation for the possible development of leukemia. A total of 132 C3H(f) females and males, foster-nursed by Ak females, was observed until they reached an average age of 16.6 months; only 4 of them (3 per cent) developed leukemia at an average age of 14 months.

In this experiment the Ak females employed as foster-mothers were still in good health at the time of nursing, but developed leukemia later on. Since we have observed in our more recent studies, which will be reported on subsequent pages of this chapter, that C3H(f) females injected with the mouse leukemia passage A virus shed the virus in milk to a much higher degree when they are either leukemic or at the point of developing this disease at the time of nursing, an attempt was also made to determine whether Ak females would not transmit leukemia to foster-nursed C3H(f) mice if they had leukemia at the time they nursed these mice. Three such Ak females were employed as foster-mothers; they nursed 16 C3H(f) mice (6 females and 10 males), but none of them developed leukemia, although they lived to an average age of 16 months.

In another experiment, three Ak females, injected when newborn with passage A virus, were employed as foster-mothers; all three of them had

* For incidence of spontaneous leukemia in these and other strains of mice referred to in this discussion, see p. 425 and also Table 2 on p. 234.

leukemia at the time of nursing. They nursed 11 C3H(f) mice, but none of the foster-nursed mice developed leukemia during an observation time exceeding 16 months (Gross and Dreyfuss, 1967).

Results of these experiments indicated clearly that leukemia could not be induced in mice of low-leukemic strains by foster-nursing by females of the high-leukemic Ak inbred line. Even though milk of Ak female mice may contain the mouse leukemia virus, the quantity of virus present in such milk may not be sufficient to induce a significant incidence of leukemia in mice of low-leukemic strains, following foster-nursing.

Transmission of Virus to Offspring by Either Mother or Father of the High-leukemic Ak or C58 Strains. Reciprocal Mating Experiments

As soon as C58 and Ak strains of mice, having a very high incidence of spontaneous leukemia, were developed, it became of considerable interest to the geneticists, and also to investigators interested in cancer and leukemia research, in particular, to study the possible genetic inheritance in such families. The strikingly high incidence of an otherwise rare disease in successive generations of such families was puzzling; the presence of a virus, logically suspected as a causative agent, was thought to be excluded in view of the failure of all previous attempts to transmit this disease by filtrates. Thus, genetic inheritance was thought to be solely responsible, and an interpretation in genetic terms was thought to offer the most promising, if not the only avenue of approach to this difficult problem.

Among the first experiments carried out in these early studies were those in which reciprocal matings between mice of the high-leukemic inbred lines and those of families having a very low incidence of leukemia were initiated. Since these experiments were planned and were carried out before it was known that leukemia is caused by a virus, the results obtained were interpreted in terms of genetic inheritance. MacDowell and Richter (1935) were first to have at their disposal the C58 inbred line which had an incidence of spontaneous leukemia of approximately 85 per cent. Since there was also available at the same time another strain of mice, StoLi, having a negligible (not exceeding 1 per cent) incidence of spontaneous leukemia, it was a simple matter to carry out reciprocal mating experiments, in which only one parent, i.e. either the mother or the father, was of the leukemic strain C58. Results of these early experiments, interpreted in genetic terms, indicated clearly that either parent could transmit leukemia to the offspring. It was noted, however, that the incidence of leukemia was higher if the mothers were of the leukemic C58 strain, i.e. 62 per cent, as compared with 42 per cent in experiments in which the mating was reversed, i.e. low-leukemic StoLi strain mothers were mated to high-leukemic strain C58 fathers.

A few years later Cole and Furth (1941) carried out similar experiments using mice of the high-leukemic strain Ak and of the low-leukemic strains Rf and C3H. The incidence of spontaneous leukemia in mice of the Ak strain in their laboratory was 69 per cent, as contrasted with the low-leukemic strain Rf, which had an incidence of leukemia of about 2 per cent. The results were as follows: when Ak females were mated to Rf males, the incidence of leukemia in F_1 hybrids was 22 per cent; on the other hand, when Rf females were mated to Ak males the incidence of leukemia in F_1 hybrids was 12 per cent.

In another study, Furth and his coworkers (1942) mated mice of the high-leukemic Ak strain with those of the low-leukemic C3H inbred line. The results were as follows: when Ak females were mated to C3H males, the incidence of leukemia in 201 F_1 hybrids was 50 per cent; on the other hand, when C3H females were mated to Ak males, the incidence of leukemia in 205 F_1 hybrids was 34 per cent. Similar results were obtained by Law (1954) who mated mice of the high-leukemic C58 strain to those of the low-leukemic NH line.

Recent Reciprocal Mating Experiments Carried Out in Our Laboratory. The Unexpected Development of High Incidence of Myeloid Leukemia in F_1 Hybrids

In our more recent experiments (Gross and Dreyfuss, 1967) we have carried out reciprocal matings between mice of the high-leukemic strain Ak and those of the low-leukemic strains C3H(f) and C57 Brown, respectively.

The results were as follows: when Ak females were mated to C3H(f) males, the incidence of spontaneous leukemia, developing at an average age of 9.8 months in 160 F_1 hybrids, was 71 per cent. When C3H(f) females were mated to Ak males, the incidence of leukemia developing at an average age of 10.6 months in 122 F_1 hybrids was 57 per cent. Among the leukemic mice of both groups of F_1 hybrids the incidence of myelogenous leukemia was unexpectedly high, 14 and 11 per cent in each group, respectively.

Instead of assuming that virus transmission took place directly through the fertilized ova, the possibility had to be considered that a virus-carrying male, such as Ak, could infect, during mating, the female, which, in turn, might have subsequently transmitted the virus to its offspring.*

In order to clarify such a possibility, 8 young adult C3H(f) females, 4 to 6 weeks old, were mated to 8 young healthy Ak males of about the same age.

* See chapter on Mouse Mammary Carcinoma.

Each female had one or two litters from this mating; these hybrid F_1 litters were destroyed, and the Ak males were then removed.

The same C3H(f) females were then mated again, this time, however, to their C3H(f) brothers, and each female had two additional litters from this second mating. These C3H(f) F_1 offspring were then raised by their mothers, weaned, separated by sexes, and kept under observation. A total of 60 C3H(f) F_1 mice was observed (32 females and 28 males); only two mice in this group (3 per cent) developed lymphosarcomas at 16.5 months of age; the remaining 58 mice remained in good health until the experiment was terminated when they reached approximately 14 to 19 months of age (average age 17 months).

The incidence of leukemia in this group was therefore only slightly higher than that observed in mice of our untreated colony of this strain (less than 1 per cent); it is doubtful whether the difference observed was truly significant, and whether it was actually related to the mating of the C3H(f) females to Ak males.

In another reciprocal mating experiment, Ak females were mated to C57 Brown/cd males. The incidence of leukemia in 102 F_1 hybrids was 48 per cent (among the leukemic animals, 16 per cent developed myelogenous leukemia). On the other hand, when C57 Brown/cd females were mated to Ak males, the incidence of leukemia developing in 122 F_1 hybrids was 38 per cent (the incidence of myelogenous leukemia in this group was 32 per cent). In both groups, leukemia developed at an average age of 15 months.

The very high incidence of myelogenous leukemia observed in F_1 hybrids born in the course of this series of reciprocal mating was striking. These animals had very high numbers of primitive cells of the myeloid series in peripheral blood and in the bone marrow. In some of these leukemic mice, the peripheral white blood cell counts were strikingly high, exceeding in at least three animals 600,000 WBC per mm^3, i.e. figures which we have seen only on exceedingly rare occasions in our previous studies on mouse leukemia. On microscopic study the internal organs were also found to be infiltrated with myeloid cells.

The Role of the Male in Transmitting the Virus in Experiments Performed on Mice of High and Low-leukemic Strains. Results of experiments dealing with reciprocal mating of high and low-leukemic strain mice indicated clearly that although the incidence of leukemia in F_1 hybrids was relatively higher when the mother was of the leukemic strain, the father was also able to transmit the disease to the offspring. This point was of considerable interest. In the early experiments in which the reciprocal mating experiments were instituted, the results were interpreted by genetic factors; under such conditions either parent could have been considered responsible for the transmission of genetic inheritance. Since it is realized now that leukemia is caused by a transmissible virus, a new interpretation of the results of reciprocal mating experiments is needed. Even though a precise mechanism of the parent-offspring transmission has not yet been determined, the results of the reciprocal mating experiments thus far obtained point clearly to the fact that transmission of the virus from one generation to another occurs not only through the mother, but also through the father. Apparently, the virus can be transmitted either through the ovum or through the sperm; thus, prior to fertilization, either of the germinal cells can carry the infection. The fertilized ovum is infected, the embryo formed from such an ovum also carries the infection and so does the host developing from the embryo. The quantity of the virus may then be increased in the suckling mouse by the relatively small amount passed in the milk of the mother; however, even without this additional quantity of virus, the amount of virus acquired prior to birth may be sufficient to cause the subsequent development of disease at a later date in some of the virus-carrying animals.

Transmission of the Mouse Leukemia Virus in Mice of the High-leukemic Ak and C58 Strains Through the Embryos. Direct Bio-Assay Experiments. As soon as the existence of the mouse leukemia virus was demonstrated, experiments were carried out to determine whether extracts prepared from embryos removed from pregnant, young, healthy female mice of the leukemic inbred lines Ak and C58 had a leukemic potential on bio-assay, i.e. whether they contained the virus and whether such extracts would induce leukemia on inoculation into newborn mice of susceptible low-leukemic inbred lines.

In experiments carried out in our laboratory (Gross, 1951, 1954, 1956), normal healthy embryos were removed aseptically from young, pregnant Ak or C58 females. The female mice serving as donors were about 2 months old, and therefore of an age at which leukemia would not yet develop spontaneously.

The embryos were cut into small pieces with scissors, then ground in a mortar with physiological saline solution added. Either the cell suspension thus obtained, or the supernate resulting from centrifugation of such normal embryo cell suspension, was used for inoculation of newborn C3H or C57 Brown/cd mice. The results were as follows:

Of 57 newborn C3H(f) or C3H mice inoculated with the normal Ak embryo cell suspensions, 12 animals (21 per cent) developed leukemia at an average age of 14 months, and 2 mice developed salivary gland carcinomas. In another series of experiments, the supernate resulting from centrifugation of normal Ak embryo cell suspensions was inoculated into newborn C3H mice. Of 35 inoculated mice, 10 developed salivary gland carcinomas and 2 developed leukemia at 11 months of age.

That the leukemic agent is present in normal C58 embryos was evident from a series of experiments in which centrifuged extracts were prepared from normal, healthy C58 embryos and inoculated into newborn mice of either the C57 Brown or C3H lines. Of 21 C57 Brown mice, 6 developed leukemia (28 per cent) and 1 parotid tumors. Of 63 C3H mice, 6 developed leukemia (10 per cent) and 7 parotid tumors.

In a control series, centrifuged extracts were prepared from normal embryos removed from young, healthy mice of the low-leukemic C3H and C57 Brown/cd lines. These extracts were then injected into 62 newborn C3H mice. Four of the inoculated mice developed parotid gland carcinomas, but none developed leukemia.

The results of these experiments suggested that extracts prepared from normal Ak or C58 embryos had a leukemogenic potential. The incidence of leukemia induced by inoculating such extracts into susceptible mice was relatively lower than that which followed inoculation of extracts prepared from Ak or C58 leukemic donors. It was only logical to assume, however, that the content of infective virus particles was lower in extracts prepared from normal, healthy embryos of the Ak or C58 lines than in either Ak or C58 donors with fully developed leukemia.

The incidence of leukemia induced with such extracts was significant, however, when compared with results obtained with normal embryo extracts prepared from mice of low-leukemic lines, such as C3H or C57 Brown. Such extracts had no leukemogenic effect.

The fact that inoculation of extracts prepared from normal organs of mice of either high-leukemic or low-leukemic lines induced in some instances the development of parotid tumors was of considerable interest, and will be further discussed in a separate chapter on the parotid tumor (polyoma) virus in the latter part of this monograph. This phenomenon had no apparent relation, however, to the induction of leukemia with Ak or C58 embryo extracts.

The observation that Ak or C58 embryo extracts had a leukemogenic potential which could be revealed on bio-assay was of considerable importance and implied that such embryos actually contain the leukemic agent. This further implied that the agent of mouse leukemia is transmitted in certain families of mice, such as the Ak or C58 inbred lines, from one generation to another directly through the embryos. In this respect mouse

---

Fig. 41. Leukemic Virus Particles in Mammary Glands of Pregnant Virus-injected C3H(f) Mice.

(A). Section of mammary epithelium from a pregnant C3H(f) mouse with passage A virus-induced thymic lymphoma. Three virus particles (b) are shown budding from the cell membrane. Magnification 62,000×. (From: D. G. Feldman, L. Gross and Y. Dreyfuss, *Cancer Research*, **23**: 1604, 1963.) (B). Lumen of mammary gland from a pregnant C3H(f) mouse with passage A virus-induced thymic lymphoma. Within the lumen are protein droplets (p) and several mature type C leukemia virus particles (C). Magnification 34,900×. (From: D. G. Feldman, L. Gross and Y. Dreyfuss, *Cancer Research*, **23**: 1604, 1963.)

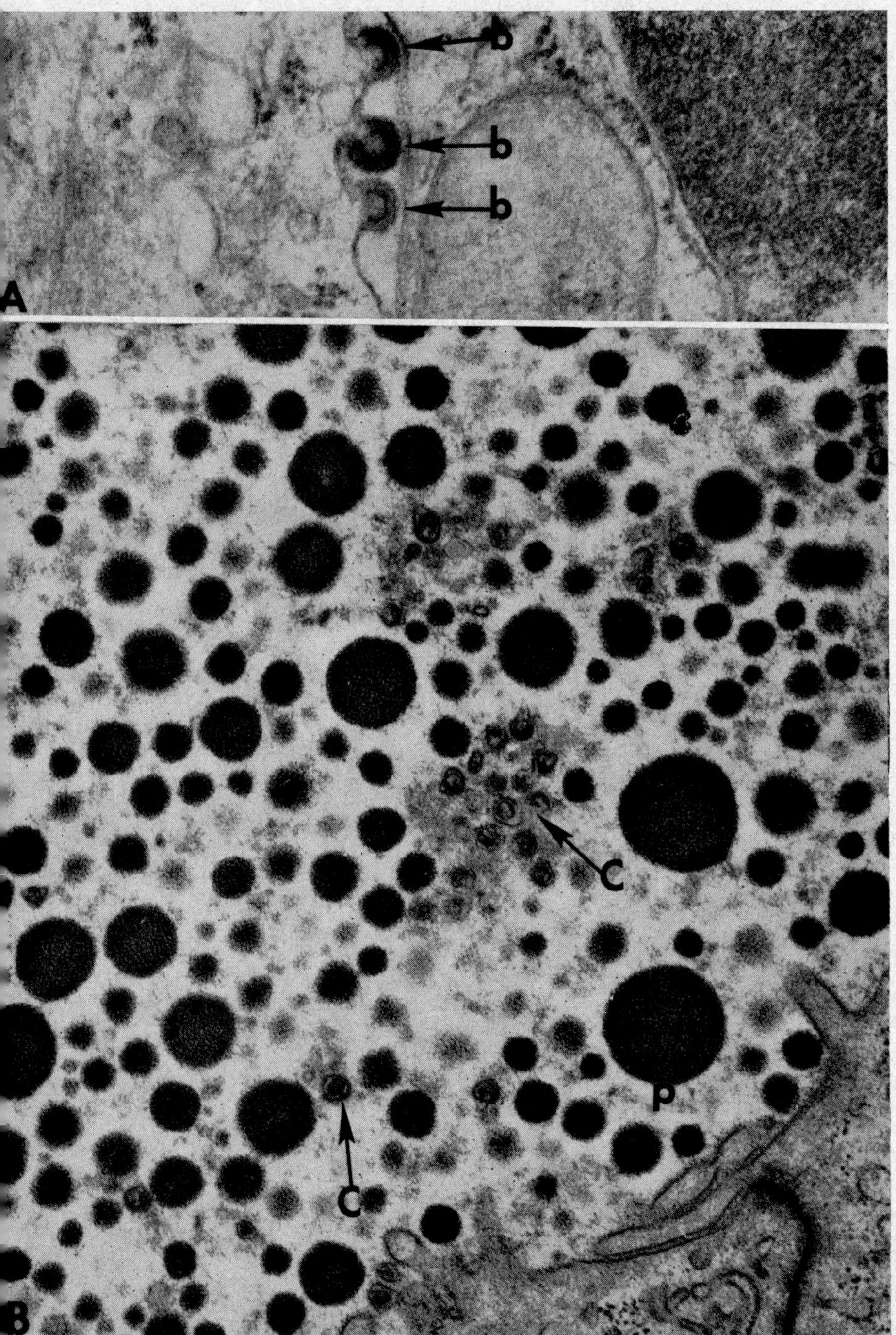

Fig. 41. Leukemic Virus Particles in Mammary Glands of Pregnant Virus-injected C3H(f) Mice.

leukemia was therefore found to be essentially similar to chicken lymphomatosis: apparently, both are egg-borne virus diseases.

In continuation of these studies, an attempt was made to determine whether extracts prepared from normal testes and ovaries of young, healthy Ak mice contain a virus. Accordingly, cell-suspensions were prepared from normal testes and ovaries removed aseptically from young, 6 to 12-week-old, healthy males and females of the Ak inbred line. The extracts were prepared by cutting and then grinding the testes or the ovaries with a hand pestle in a mortar, with a small quantity of physiological saline solution added; the extracts were then passed through a sterile voile cloth and inoculated into newborn, less than 15-hour-old, mice of the C3H(f) strain.

In a first series, 12 C3H(f) mice were inoculated with testicular extracts, and 8 of them developed leukemia at an average age of 12 months. In another series, out of 14 C3H(f) mice inoculated with ovarian extracts, 6 developed leukemia at an average age of 15 months (Gross, 1953).

Leukemia that developed in the C3H(f) mice as a result of inoculation of either the testicular or ovarian extracts could be transferred by cell-graft to C3H(f) mice, but not to mice of the Ak strain, suggesting thereby that this disease did not develop in the inoculated mice as a result of implantation of some dormant Ak cells, but that it was induced in the inoculated mice by a cell-free agent, introduced with the testicular or ovarian extracts, respectively.

Studies on Natural Transmission of the Mouse Leukemia Virus Following Experimental Inoculation into Mice of Low-leukemic Strains

On the preceding pages we have discussed the natural transmission of the mouse leukemia virus, as observed in experiments with spontaneous mouse leukemia; these studies concerned a virus carried naturally, and transmitted from one generation to another in certain inbred lines, such as Ak, or C58, which have a high incidence of this disease developing spontaneously.

The studies which will be discussed on the following pages refer to the same virus inoculated into mice of inbred lines essentially free from spontaneous leukemia, such as C3H or C57 Brown. These studies were carried out in order to determine whether a leukemic family of mice could be developed in the laboratory by introducing the mouse leukemia virus into a strain of mice hitherto relatively free from this disease.

Accordingly, several newborn males and females of the low-leukemic strain C3H were inoculated with cell-free extracts prepared from spontaneous Ak mouse leukemia. After the inoculated mice reached sexual maturity, they were mated, and their non-injected descendants were then observed, without any further treatment through several successive generations, for the development of leukemia. In some experiments only the F_1 generation was observed, and no attempt was made to extend observation beyond the untreated offspring of the inoculated mice. In other experiments, four successive generations of the injected mice were observed for the possible development of leukemia or lymphomas (Gross, 1951, 1955).

The results varied. In some experiments, the incidence of leukemia developing spontaneously in untreated F_1 offspring of the inoculated C3H mice was relatively high. An attempt to develop experimentally a "leukemic C3H strain" did not succeed, however. The incidence of this disease in the F_2, F_3, and F_4 generations was relatively low, leukemia developing in some of these animals, if at all, relatively late (Gross, 1955, also unpublished data). The disease appeared in a spotty manner, only in some of the descendants of the inoculated mice; even though the incidence of leukemia was not high, it was significant, however, since mice of the particular subline of the C3H strain raised in our laboratory, and employed in these experiments, only rarely develop spontaneous leukemia.

Inoculation of Passage A Virus (Gross) into Suckling Mice of a Low-leukemic Strain. Study of Its Natural Transmission

The early experiments on natural transmission of the leukemic virus were recently repeated and extended, employing a mouse leukemia virus of considerably increased potency (Gross, 1962, also unpublished data, 1966, 1967). Suckling, less than 6-day-old, mice of the C3H(f) strain were inoculated with the passage A virus; they were then mated, and their offspring were observed for the development of leukemia. In a similar parallel series, only part of the newborn C3H(f) litter was injected with the passage A virus; the injected mice were marked by having their tails tied and cut for identification. After these mice reached sexual maturity, they were selected for mating in such a manner that only one of the future parents, either the female or the male, had previously received inoculation of the virus.

Studies on the Transmission of Mouse Leukemia Through Virus-injected Females. Transmission of Mouse Leukemia Virus Through Milk

Results of initial experiments indicated that transmission of the virus from injected parents to non-injected offspring may occur readily, particularly if the mother received inoculation of the virus (Gross, 1962).

In recent experiments (Gross, 1966, 1967, unpublished data), 7 C3H(f) virus-injected females were mated to their virus-injected brothers. Among their 29 untreated offspring, 21 (72 per cent) developed leukemia at an average age of 6 months.

In another experiment 9 virus-injected C3H(f) females were mated to non-injected C3H(f) males. Among their 22 untreated offspring, 13 (59 per cent) developed leukemia at an average age of 6 months.

The mouse leukemia passage A virus was found to be readily transmitted in the milk of nursing female mice, provided that these animals had leukemia or were at the point of developing the disease at the time they were nursing (Gross, 1962).

C3H(f) females inoculated with the passage A mouse leukemia virus (Gross) were mated to their virus-injected brothers. Litters born to these females were removed promptly after birth, and were replaced by litters of similar age, born to non-injected healthy female mice from our C3H(f) colony. The virus-injected female mice served then as foster-mothers. In some experiments they were employed only for a few days as foster-mothers; the foster-nursed litters were then returned to their own mothers. Most of the foster-nursed mice developed leukemia (Gross, 1962, also unpublished experiments, 1966).

Similar observations were reported by Law and Moloney (1961) as well as Krischke and Graffi (1963). The mouse leukemia virus strains which they employed for their experiments, and which will be discussed in more detail in the next chapter of this monograph, could be readily transmitted through the milk of nursing female mice.

The results of these experiments demonstrated clearly that under certain experimental conditions, using a highly potent mouse leukemia virus, transmission of the virus from one generation to another could take place through the milk of nursing females. This was a striking observation, suggesting that not unlike mouse mammary carcinoma, the mouse leukemia virus could also be transmitted through the milk, and, furthermore, that the virus could enter and effectively infect new hosts through the digestive tract. However, mice that received the virus in the milk did not transmit the virus in any significant quantity to their own offspring (Gross, 1962, also unpublished). The incidence of leukemia in descendants of the foster-nursed mice, i.e. in F_2 and F_3 generations, was again very low. This contrasted sharply with the mouse mammary carcinoma. As discussed in more detail in a separate chapter dealing with that subject in this monograph, foster-nursing of mice of low-tumor lines by high mammary carcinoma line females caused not only the development of mammary carcinomas in the foster-nursed generation, but subsequently also a high incidence of mammary tumors in their descendants.

The fact that the mouse leukemia virus could be transmitted under certain experimental conditions through milk did not necessarily imply that this is the only manner of its transmission from mothers to their offspring; transmission through the placenta, or directly through the ova, had to be considered. Previous experiments dealing with reciprocal mating of high and low-leukemic line mice suggested clearly that the virus could be transmitted from parents to their offspring by means other than milk. Furthermore, experiments dealing with direct bio-assay studies suggested that extracts prepared from embryos of virus-injected parents contain the virus, since such extracts induced leukemia following inoculation into newborn mice of susceptible strains.

Studies on the Incidence of Leukemia Developing in Untreated Offspring of Virus-injected C3H(f) Males. In this series of experiments, suckling, less than 7-day-old, C3H(f) mice were inoculated with the passage A mouse leukemia virus. Only part of a litter was injected; the injected mice were marked by having their tails tied and cut for identification. After these mice reached sexual maturity, non-injected females were mated to virus-injected males. The untreated offspring born to such parents were then observed for the development of leukemia. In the initial experiments (Gross, 1962), among 31 offspring born to non-injected mothers and virus-injected fathers, 7 mice (23 per cent) developed leukemia; the disease appeared late, at 14 to 17 months of age.

In a recent and more extensive series (Gross, 1966, 1967, unpublished data) 43 non-injected C3H(f) females were mated to virus-injected males. Among a total of 266 of their untreated F_1 offspring, 21 mice (8 per cent) developed leukemia or lymphosarcomas at an average age of 16 months.

This incidence was not high, but significant, since the incidence of spontaneous leukemia and lymphomas observed in untreated mice of our colony of C3H(f) mice observed during the preceding years in our laboratory has not exceeded 1 per cent.

Studies on the Transmission of Mouse Leukemia Virus Through Embryos of Virus-injected C3H(f) Parents. Bio-Assay Experiments

In this series of experiments, suckling, less than 6-day-old, mice were inoculated with the passage A virus. After these mice reached sexual maturity, they were mated. In one group, both prospective parents were inoculated with the virus. In another series, either the mother or the father received the virus, and was later mated to a normal, untreated litter-mate. After the females became pregnant, their embryos were removed in ether anesthesia, by laparotomy; among the pregnant females that received inoculation of the virus, only those were employed as donors that had no symptoms of leukemia at the time their embryos were removed.

The embryos were removed aseptically, washed carefully with sterile physiological saline solution, then cut with small scissors and ground in a mortar, with physiological saline solution added to obtain a cell suspension of 10 to 20 per cent concentration. The extracts were then centrifuged at 3,000 r.p.m. for 15 minutes, followed by a second centrifugation at 9,500 r.p.m. The final supernate was inoculated into suckling, less than 6-day-old, C3H(f) mice.

In the first series both parents were injected with the passage A mouse leukemia virus. After 9 female mice became pregnant, their embryos were removed and used for the preparation of centrifuged extracts. Ninety suckling, less than 7-day-old, C3H(f) mice were inoculated with the extracts, and 36 of them (40 per cent) developed leukemia at an average age of 5 months.

In a second series, virus-injected C3H(f) females were mated to non-injected males of the same strain. Embryos removed later from 5 pregnant females were used for the preparation of extracts. Fifty-five suckling, less than 5-day-old, C3H(f) mice were inoculated with the embryo extracts, and 32 of them (58 per cent) developed leukemia at an average age of 5 months.

In a third series, non-injected C3H(f) female mice were mated to virus-injected C3H(f) males. Embryos removed later from 11 pregnant females were used for the preparation of extracts. One hundred and twenty-one suckling, less than 7-day-old, C3H(f) mice were inoculated with the extracts, and 11 of them (9 per cent) developed leukemia at an average age of 16 months.

In a simultaneous control experiment, healthy, non-injected C3H(f) females were mated to their non-injected brothers. Embryos were later removed from 9 pregnant females of this group, and were used for the preparation of extracts. The extracts were then inoculated into 119 suckling, less than 7-day-old, C3H(f) mice. Only 4 of the inoculated mice (3 per cent) developed leukemia at an average age of 16 months.

The experiment was terminated in all groups after the mice reached 17 months of age.

The results of these experiments were consistent with those dealing with the observation of untreated offspring of virus-injected parents and reviewed on the preceding pages. Natural transmission of the virus following its inoculation into mice of the C3H(f) strain occurred readily through the females; transmission through the male also occurred, but to a considerably lesser degree. This was in striking contrast to the transmission of the naturally carried virus through males of the high-leukemic Ak inbred line.

Summary and Recapitulation of Our Present Knowledge of the Transmission of the Mouse Leukemia Virus Under Natural Life Conditions

All experimental data are not yet on hand to form a clear and reasonably accurate picture of the manner of the natural transmission of the mouse leukemia virus. Although incomplete, however, our present information on this subject could be summarized as follows:

Contact, or "horizontal" transmission of the virus seems to occur only to a very limited degree, and presumably only among newborn mice; however, even under favorable conditions it may only rarely lead to the development of disease.

It appears that the principal route of transmission of the mouse leukemia virus follows a "vertical" pattern; the virus is transmitted in certain families of mice from one generation to another directly through the embryos. This is particularly clear in experiments carried out on mice of high-leukemic strains. Under certain conditions a small quantity of the virus may be also excreted in the milk*; the quantity of virus transmitted in milk may vary, however, and may be larger at the time when the nursing females develop symptoms of the disease; the main route of virus transmission is through the embryos, and possibly directly through the germinal cells. A small quantity of the virus transmitted in the milk may increase the total amount of virus transmitted to a given host. However, even in absence of milk-transmitted virus, sufficient quantity of the virus is passed directly through the embryos to cause development of disease in successive generations of mice in certain inbred lines, such as Ak or C58.

* * *

There seem to exist differences between the transmission of the mouse leukemia virus in mice of high-leukemic lines, such as Ak or C58, which are natural carriers of the virus, and the transmission of the virus in experimentally inoculated mice of low-leukemic lines, such as C3H(f).

In mice of high-leukemic lines Ak or C58, the naturally carried virus is readily transmitted from one generation to another not only through the mothers, but also through the fathers; furthermore, the virus is only exceptionally, if at all, transmitted in the milk of nursing females.

In mice of the low-leukemic C3H(f) strain, inoculated with a highly potent passaged mouse leukemia virus, natural transmission of the virus from the inoculated parents to their offspring occurs mainly through the mothers, and often in mothers' milk. Transmission through the male is

* Recent electron microscopic studies (Gross and Feldman, unpublished) suggest that the virus may also be present in saliva and in pancreatic juice; no direct bio-assay evidence to that effect, however, is yet available.

apparently less frequent, but may occur through the germinal cells. Recent electron microscopic studies demonstrated presence of large numbers of virus particles in male and female genital organs of C3H mice that had been inoculated with the passage A mouse leukemia virus (Feldman and Gross, 1967).

It has not been possible, thus far, to change a low-leukemic strain of mice, such as C3H, C57 Brown, or BALB/c, into a high-leukemic line by inoculation of the mouse leukemia virus into the parents, or by foster-nursing of mice of such strains by virus-carrying foster-mothers. Even though leukemia may develop in some of the untreated F_1 offspring, the development of leukemia in the F_2 or F_3 generation becomes more and more rare. Eventually no spontaneous development of leukemia is observed in the successive generations (Gross, 1955, also, 1966, unpublished data).

Attempts to develop new leukemic lines by inoculating mice of low-leukemic strains, such as C3H or C57 Brown, with a potent mouse leukemia virus were only partially successful. It is apparent that mice of C3H or C57 Brown inbred lines may not be sufficiently susceptible to favor a continuous, generation-to-generation transmission of the inoculated virus. The leukemic virus, which was originally isolated from a different strain of mice, has been found to be consistently pathogenic for mice of strain C3H or C57 Brown as well as for those of several other inbred lines, following parenteral inoculation. The same virus, however, may not be readily transmitted under natural life conditions in mice of these strains, at least not in a quantity sufficient to cause a high incidence of disease in successive generations of such hosts. Under such conditions the virus may lose, at least to some degree, its pathogenic potential, causing only now and then development of leukemia. Eventually, after transmission through several successive host generations, the virus may either completely disappear, or it may become so submerged and masked, as to lose, with only occasional exceptions, its ability to become pathogenic spontaneously.

Certain fundamental differences between the milk transmission of the mouse leukemia virus and that of the mouse mammary carcinoma should be re-emphasized. In the case of mouse leukemia, the virus may be transmitted through the milk, particularly if the nursing female has symptoms of disease. However, the incidence of leukemia in descendants of foster-nursed mice was found to be very low, at least in experiments carried out in our laboratory. We have not been able to change a low-leukemic family into a high-leukemic strain by foster-nursing of one generation of mice by virus-injected females.

In the case of the mouse mammary carcinoma, a low-tumor line could be changed into a high-tumor line by a single foster-nursing of one generation of mice. Mice that acquired the mouse mammary carcinoma virus in the milk of their foster-mothers transmitted the virus to their own offspring and from then on to successive generations.

On the other hand, a high-mammary tumor line can be changed into a low-mammary tumor line by foster-nursing of a single generation of mice, i.e. by interrupting the chain of virus transmission occurring through the milk. This is not possible in the case of mouse leukemia. A high-leukemic inbred line, such as Ak or C58, could not be changed into a low-leukemic line by foster-nursing, or by any other experimental method thus far employed.

*Vertical Transmission of the Mouse Leukemia Virus**

The natural transmission of the mouse leukemia virus from one generation to another through the embryos was demonstrated in experimental studies on mice of high-leukemic inbred lines, such as Ak or C58.

Apparently, the virus can infect the ovum and sperm prior to fertilization, or it can infect the fertilized ovum. The embryo formed from the infected ovum then carries the virus.

The mechanism of natural transmission of the mouse leukemia virus from parents to offspring through the embryo has not yet been fully clarified. The manner by which the germinal cells, and subsequently the embryo, become infected with the virus requires further studies; however, results of recent electron microscopic investigations (Feldman and Gross, 1967) provide at least a partial clarification. In this study organs of male and female genital systems of both Ak and virus-injected C3H(f) mice were examined in order to determine the possible presence and sites of replication of the mouse leukemia virus. The ova and spermatozoa are apparently exposed to virus infection by numerous means. The ova develop in the

* The term "vertical transmission" was coined by the author and suggested to designate transmission of a latent, but potentially oncogenic, virus from one generation to another directly through germinal cells, occasionally also through milk of nursing females (Gross, 1944, 1951b, 1954c, 1955b, 1956b).

FIG. 42. LEUKEMIC VIRUS PARTICLES IN ORGANS OF NORMAL C3H(F) MICE AND IN ORGANS OF MOUSE EMBRYOS.

(A). Section of thymus from a normal 3-month-old non-injected C3H(f) mouse. Virus particles (b) are shown budding from vacuolar membranes of an epithelial cell. Magnification 62,000×. (From: D. G. Feldman and L. Gross, *Cancer Research*, **26**: 412, 1966.) (B). Part of an epithelial cell from the thymus of an embryo from normal non-injected C3H(f) parents, illustrating virus particles (b) budding from a vacuolar membrane, doughnut-like immature type C particles (IC), and mature type C particles (C) containing nucleoids within a vacuole. Magnification 62,000×. (From: D. G. Feldman, Y. Dreyfuss and L. Gross, *Cancer Research*, **27**: 1792, 1967.) (C). Part of an erythroblast from liver of an embryo from passage A virus-injected C3H(f) parents (the pregnant female was in good health when the embryos were removed for electron microscopic studies). A virus particle (b) appears budding from the cell membrane. Magnification 42,800×. (From: D. G. Feldman, Y. Dreyfuss and L. Gross, *Cancer Research*, **27**: 1792, 1967.)

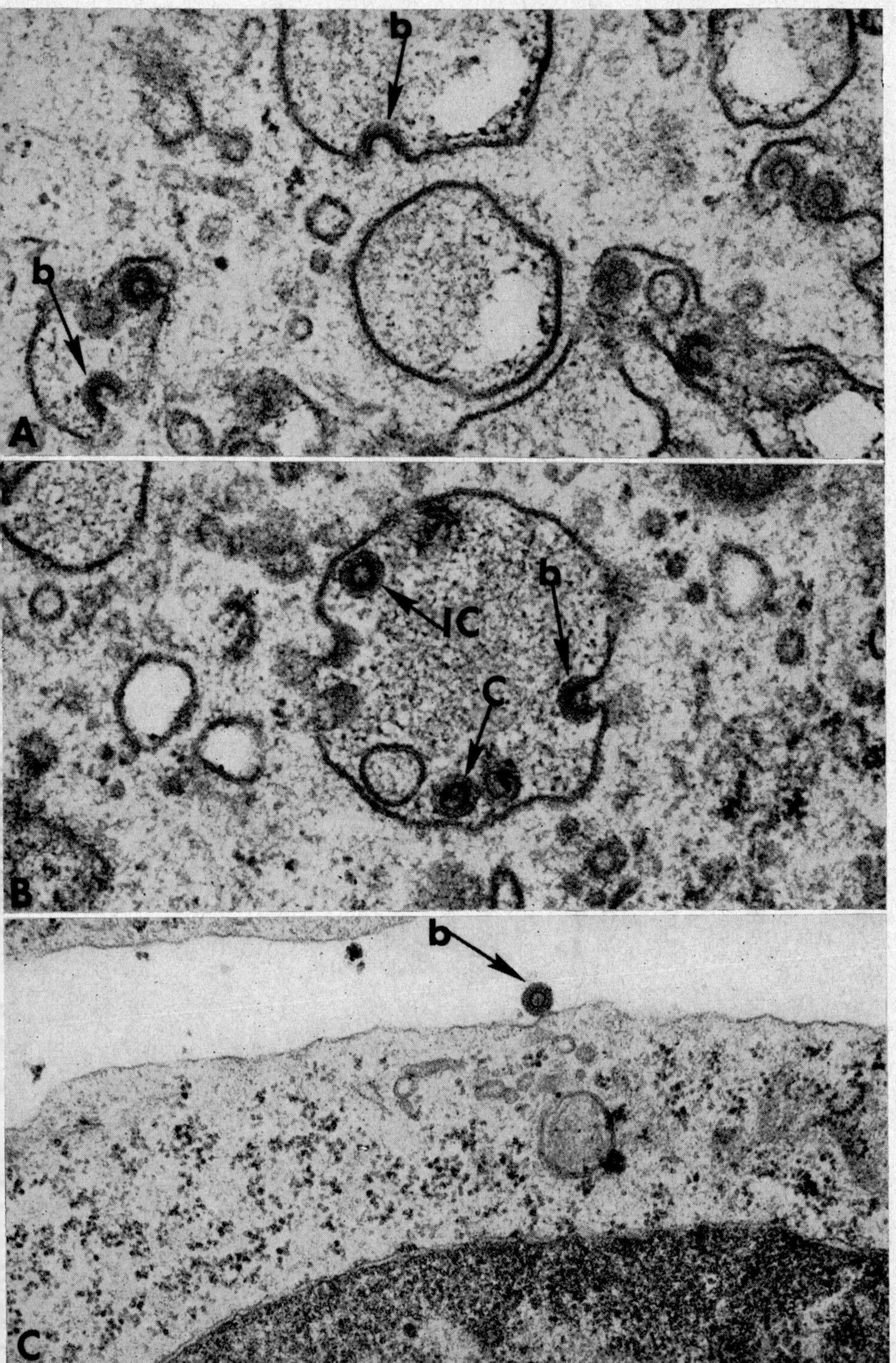

FIG. 42. LEUKEMIC VIRUS PARTICLES IN ORGANS OF NORMAL C3H(F) MICE AND IN ORGANS OF MOUSE EMBRYOS.

ovaries in which virus particles are formed in the theca folliculi and in the corpus luteum. The ova then pass through the oviduct, the mucosa and smooth muscle cells which also contain virus particles; here the ova are fertilized, thereby coming in contact with seminal fluid which contains virus particles formed from cells of the epididymis, vas deferens, seminal vesicle, and prostate. Finally, the ova are implanted in the uterus where virus particles are formed in the endometrium. Thus, the opportunity of the ovum to become infected is assured from its early development in the ovary, in its passage through the oviduct, until it reaches the uterus where it is finally embedded.

In the genital organs of males carrying the virus, the spermatozoa are also exposed to virus infection as they pass through the epididymis, vas deferens, and the seminal vesicle and prostate gland. Since virus particles are present in the genital tract of virus-infected females, the spermatozoa are also exposed to infection in their passage through the uterus and oviduct on their way to fertilize the ovum. There is ample opportunity, therefore, for the ova and spermatozoa to become infected, and eventually form an embryo also carrying the virus. Results of these studies are consistent with the concept of vertical transmission of the mouse leukemia virus, and explain the familial incidence of spontaneous leukemia in mice of certain high-leukemic inbred lines, such as Ak or C58.

The many similarities between the mouse leukemia and the chicken leukosis complex include the formation of virus particles in different organs of virus-carrying animals. It is of considerable interest that chicken lymphomatosis virus particles have been recently observed budding from epithelial cells of oviduct of infected hens (Di Stefano and Dougherty, 1965).

ISOLATION OF LEUKEMOGENIC VIRUSES FROM LEUKEMIAS AND LYMPHOSARCOMAS INDUCED WITH CARCINOGENIC CHEMICALS OR HORMONES

After the demonstration that spontaneous mouse leukemia is caused by a filterable and transmissible virus, it was only logical to look for the presence of a similar virus in leukemias and lymphosarcomas that had been induced in mice with carcinogenic chemicals or hormones.

In studies carried out by Toth (1963) in the laboratories of Dr. P. Shubik in the Division of Oncology at the Chicago Medical School, malignant lymphomas were induced in Swiss mice following injection at birth of dimethylbenzanthracene (DMBA). A filtered extract prepared from a thymic lymphoma from a 4-month-old male with DMBA-induced disease was inoculated into 8 newborn Swiss mice; 7 out of the 8 inoculated mice survived weaning. Of the surviving mice, 6 developed either thymic or generalized malignant lymphomas, at an average age of 13 months; the remaining mouse died at the age of 9 months with enlarged spleen, liver and lymph nodes. The incidence of spontaneous leukemia in untreated control mice varied from 3.5 to 17 per cent. However, several attempts to reproduce this experiment were not successful (Toth and Shubik, 1966).

In a similar study, Irino and his colleagues at the Department of Internal Medicine, Okayama University Medical School, in Japan (1963), induced leukemia by repeated (twice weekly for 4 months) painting of the dorsal skin of young adult Rf mice with a 5 per cent solution of methylcholanthrene in benzene. The incidence of carcinogen-induced leukemia in the treated mice was 8.8 per cent; among the induced leukemias, 48 per cent were lymphocytic and 40 per cent were myelogenous. The incidence of spontaneous leukemia in untreated mice was less than 1 per cent.

Inoculation of a cell-free filtrate prepared from the carcinogen-induced lymphocytic and myelogenous leukemias into newborn Rf mice induced lymphocytic leukemia in 4 out of 13 inoculated mice. Serial cell-free transmission of the induced leukemia was then accomplished through three successive passages.

In another study, Zilber and Postnikova, at the Gamaleya Institute in Moscow (1966), injected dimethylbenzanthracene into 2 to 6-day-old mice of 3 low-tumor strains carried in their laboratory.

Mice treated with the carcinogen developed sarcomas, papillomas, skin cancer, and leukemias. Newborn, less than 2-day-old, mice were inoculated with cell-free extracts prepared from either carcinogen-induced sarcomas, or from tissues of mice with carcinogen-induced leukemia. Eleven out of 175 mice (6 per cent) which received cell-free extracts prepared from carcinogen-induced sarcomas developed leukemia.

Similar results were obtained following inoculation of cell-free extracts prepared from carcinogen-induced leukemias. Eight out of a total of 46 mice inoculated with such extracts (17 per cent) developed leukemia. Some of the isolated viruses could be passed serially. Analysis of the experiments demonstrated that the leukemic agent could be detected in 3 out of the 22 sarcomas, and in 4 of the 7 leukemic extracts tested.

Ribacchi and Giraldo (1966) at the Division of Cancer Research, University of Perugia, in Italy, induced leukemia in BALB/c mice with either dimethylbenzanthracene (DMBA) or with urethan. The carcinogen treatment was initiated in newborn mice. Among the treated mice, 18 to 32 per cent of those that received DMBA and up to 19 per cent of those that received urethan developed lymphoid tumors.

Centrifuged cell-free extracts prepared from the carcinogen-induced lymphoid tumors were inoculated into newborn mice. The incidence of lymphoid tumors induced with such extracts varied from 30 to 55 per cent; the average latency was about 14 to 16 months.

Haran-Ghera at the Weizmann Institute of Science in Rehovoth, Israel (1967), induced thymic lymphomas in C57 Black mice with dimethylbenzanthracene (DMBA). The carcinogen dissolved in polyethylene glycol was applied to adult C57 Black mice by feeding through stomach tubes (10 times at weekly intervals). Thymic lymphomas developed in 60 per cent of the carcinogen-treated animals; the mean latent period from the beginning of the DMBA feeding was 6 months. Filtered extracts prepared from the carcinogen-induced thymic lymphomas were inoculated into 5 to 7-day-old thymus grafts under the kidney capsules of thymectomized, irradiated C57 Black mice, according to a bio-assay technique previously described (Haran-Ghera, 1966), and also discussed in the chapter on Radiation-induced Leukemia in this monograph.

Three series of filtrates prepared from the carcinogen-induced lymphomas were tested for their leukemogenic activity. The incidence of lymphomas induced in the inoculated mice varied from 15 to 27 per cent. Serial cell-free passage of the original filtrate-induced lymphomas revealed a similar leukemogenic activity.

Isolation of a Transmissible Leukemogenic Agent from Hormone-induced Leukemia in Mice. Kunii, Takemoto, and Furth (1965) isolated a transmissible leukemogenic agent from a lymphoma which had been induced with estrogenic hormones. Diethylstilbestrol pellets with cholesterol were implanted into adult Rf/Jax female mice.* The pellet implantations were repeated at 2 months intervals. As a result, thymic lymphomas developed in 63 per cent of the hormone-treated mice. A filtered extract prepared from one of the hormone-induced thymic lymphomas was found to be leukemogenic on inoculation tests: the filtrate injected into 2 to 4-day-old Rf/Jax mice induced lymphomas in 20 of the 48 inoculated mice (42 per cent) within 9 months after inoculation.

Filtrates prepared from other hormone-induced lymphomas were also tested, but were found essentially inactive on bio-assay; the incidence of lymphomas induced in 78 mice with filtrates prepared from the 2 other hormone-induced thymic lymphomas was only 2.6 per cent; this was about the same as spontaneous lymphoma incidence in Rf mice occurring within 9 months of age.

* * *

We have discussed on the preceding pages of this chapter the isolation of a leukemogenic virus from spontaneous mouse leukemia and lympho-

* The symbols Rf and RF are synonymous, and designate the same strain of mice. The term Rf/Jax refers to a subline of Rf mice.

sarcomas. The physical, biological, and pathogenic properties of the mouse leukemia virus have also been discussed.

The isolation of a transmissible virus from radiation-induced leukemia in mice is reviewed in a separate chapter of this monograph.

The isolation of transmissible, leukemogenic viruses from leukemias and lymphosarcomas induced in mice with carcinogenic chemicals, or with hormones, completes this chapter, and suggests that all leukemias and lymphosarcomas in mice, whether they develop spontaneously, or are induced by radiation, carcinogenic chemicals, or hormones, are actually caused by a transmissible, leukemogenic virus.

REFERENCES

AMANO, S., and ICHIKAWA, Y., Electron microscopical aspects of developing modes of the cancer virus and the problem of "pseudovirus particles." *Acta Path. Jap.*, **9**: 455–479, 1959.

ANDERVONT, H. B., Spontaneous tumors in a subline of strain C3H mice. *J. Nat. Cancer Inst.*, **1**: 737–744, 1941.

ANDERVONT, H. B., and BRYAN, W. R., Properties of the mouse mammary tumor agent. *J. Nat. Cancer Inst.*, **5**: 143–149, 1944.

BANG, F. B., Formation of filamentous forms of Newcastle disease virus in hypertonic concentration of sodium chloride. *Proc. Soc. Exp. Biol. & Med.*, **71**: 50–52, 1949.

BARNES, W. A., and COLE, R. K., The effect of nursing on the incidence of spontaneous leukemia and tumors in mice. *Cancer Research,* **1**: 99–101, 1941.

BARNES, W. A., and FURTH, J., A transmissible leukemia in mice with atypical cells. *Am. J. Cancer*, **30**: 75–94, 1937.

BARNES, W. A., and FURTH, J., A transmissible malignant neoplasm of mice originating in reticular or endothelial cells. *Am. J. Path.*, **16**: 457–465, 1940.

BARNES, W. A., and SISMAN, J. E., Myeloid leukemia and non-malignant extramedullary myelopoiesis in mice. *Am. J. Cancer*, **37**: 1–35, 1939.

BEARD, J. W., Virus of avian myeloblastic leukosis. *Poultry Sci.*, **35**: 203–223, 1956.

BERNHARD, W., The detection and study of tumor viruses with the electron microscope. *Cancer Research*, **20**: 712–727, 1960.

BERNHARD, W., and GROSS, L., Présence de particules d'aspect virusal dans les tissus tumoraux de souris atteintes de leucémies induites. *Compt. Rend. Acad. Sci. (Paris)*, **248**: 160–163, 1959.

BERNHARD, W., and GUÉRIN, M., Présence de particules d'aspect virusal dans les tissus tumoraux de souris atteintes de leucémie spontanée. *Compt. Rend. Acad. Sci. (Paris)*, **247**: 1802–1805, 1958.

BILLINGHAM, R. E., BRENT, L., and MEDAWAR, P. B., Actively acquired tolerance of foreign cells. *Nature,* **172**: 603–606, 1953.

BILLINGHAM, R. E., BRENT, L., and MEDAWAR, P. B., Quantitative studies on tissue transplantation immunity. III. Actively acquired tolerance. *Proc. Roy. Soc. B.*, **239**: 357–414, 1956.

BITTNER, J. J., Inciting influences in the etiology of mammary cancer in mice. *Research Conference on Cancer. Am. Assoc. Adv. Sci.*, pp. 63–96, 1944.

BREEDIS, C., and FURTH, J., The feasibility of preserving neoplastic cells in the frozen state. *Science*, **88**: 531–532, 1938.

BREEDIS, C., BARNES, W. A., and FURTH, J., Effect of rate of freezing on the transmitting agent of neoplasms of mice. *Proc. Soc. Exp. Biol. & Med.*, **36**: 220–224, 1937.

BRUES, A. M., and MARBLE, B. B., Lymphoblastoma in mice following administration of carcinogenic tar. *Am. J. Cancer*, **37**: 45–53, 1939.

BRYAN, R. W., CALNAN, D., and MOLONEY, J. B., Biological studies on the Rous sarcoma virus. III. The recovery of virus from experimental tumors in relation to initiating dose. *J. Nat. Cancer Inst.*, **16**: 317–335, 1955.

BUFFETT, R. F., COMMERFORD, S. L., FURTH, J., and HUNTER, M. J., Agent in Ak leukemic tissues, not sedimented at 105,000 g, causing neoplastic and non-neoplastic lesions. *Proc. Soc. Exp. Biol. & Med.*, **99**: 401–407, 1958.

BULLOCK, F. D., and CURTIS, M. R., Spontaneous tumors of the rats. *J. Cancer Research*, **14**: 1–115, 1930.

BÜNGELER, W., Die experimentelle Erzeugung von Leukämie und Lymphosarkom durch chronische Indolvergiftung der Maus. *Frankfurter Zeitschr. Path.*, **44**: 202–271, 1932.

BUNTING, H., Studies on regression in a transplantable tumor in mice. *Yale J. Biol. & Med.*, **13**: 513–522, 1941.

BURMESTER, B. R., PRICKETT, C. O., and BELDING, T. C., A filtrable agent producing lymphoid tumors and osteopetrosis in chickens. *Cancer Research*, **6**: 189–196, 1946.

BURMESTER, B. R., WALTER, W. G., GROSS, M. A., and FONTES, A. K., The oncogenic spectrum of two "pure" strains of avian leukosis. *J. Nat. Cancer Inst.*, **23**: 277–291, 1959.

BURROWS, H., and COOK, J. W., Spindle-cell tumours and leucaemia in mice after injection with a water soluble compound of 1 : 2 : 5 : 6-dibenzanthracene. *Am. J. Cancer*, **27**: 267–278, 1936.

CARNES, W. H., KAPLAN, H. S., BROWN, M. B., and HIRSCH, B., Indirect induction of lymphomas in irradiated mice. III. Role of the thymic graft. *Cancer Research*, **16**: 429–433, 1956.

CLAUDE, A., Fractionation of mammalian liver cells by differential centrifugation. I. Problems, methods, and preparation of extract. *J. Exp. Med.*, **84**: 51–59, 1946.

CLAUDE, A., Fractionation of mammalian liver cells by differential centrifugation. II. Experimental procedures and results. *J. Exp. Med.*, **84**: 61–89, 1946.

COLE, R. K., and FURTH, J., Experimental studies on the genetics of spontaneous leukemia in mice. *Cancer Research*, **1**: 957–965, 1941.

COMMITTEE on STANDARDIZED NOMENCLATURE for INBRED STRAINS of MICE. Standardized nomenclature for inbred strains of mice. *Cancer Research*, **12**: 602–613, 1952.

COMMITTEE on STANDARDIZED GENETIC NOMENCLATURE for MICE. Standardized nomenclature for inbred strains of mice. Second listing. *Cancer Research*, **20**: 145–169, 1960. Third listing. Prepared by Joan Staats. *Cancer Research*, **24**: 147–168, 1964. Fourth listing. Prepared by Joan Staats. *Cancer Research*, **28**: 391–420, 1968.

CONGDON, C. C., and LORENZ, E., Leukemia in guinea-pigs. *Am. J. Path.*, **30**: 337–359, 1954.

CRAIN, R. C., Spontaneous tumors in the Rochester strain of the Wistar rat. *Am. J. Path.*, **34**: 311–335, 1958.

CURTIS, M. R., BULLOCK, F. D., and DUNNING, W. F., A statistical study of the occurrence of spontaneous tumors in a large colony of rats. *Am. J. Cancer*, **15**: 67–121, 1931.

DALLDORF, G., The coxsackie group of viruses. *Science*, **110**: 594, 1949.

DALLDORF, G., and SICKLES, G., An unidentified, filtrable agent isolated from the feces of children with paralysis. *Science*, **108**: 61–62, 1948.

DALTON, A. J., Micromorphology of murine tumor viruses and of affected cells. *Fed. Proc.*, **21**: 936–941, 1962.

DALTON, A. J., HAGUENAU, F., and MOLONEY, J. B., Morphology of particles associated with murine leukemia as revealed by negative staining: Preliminary report. *J. Nat. Cancer Inst.*, **29**: 1177–1179, 1962.

DALTON, A. J., LAW, L. W., MOLONEY, J. B., and MANAKER, R. A., An electron microscopic study of a series of murine lymphoid neoplasms. *J. Nat. Cancer Inst.*, **27**: 747–791, 1961.

DAVIS, R. K., STEVENSON, G. T., and BUSCH, K. A., Tumor incidence in normal Sprague-Dawley female rats. *Cancer Research*, **16**: 194–197, 1956.

DE HARVEN, E., and FRIEND, C., Electron microscope study of a cell-free induced leukemia of the mouse: A preliminary report. *J. Biophys. and Biochem. Cytol.*, **4**: 151–156, 1958.

DE HARVEN, E., and FRIEND, C., Structure of virus particles partially purified from the blood of leukemic mice. *Virology*, **23**: 119–124, 1964.

DI STEFANO, H. S., and DOUGHERTY, R. M., Virus multiplication in the oviduct of hens infected with an avian leukosis virus. *Virology*, **26**: 156–159, 1965.

DMOCHOWSKI, L., Viruses and their relationship to animal and human tumors. *Texas Rep. Biol. & Med.*, **23**: 539–561, 1965.

DMOCHOWSKI, L., and GREY, C. E., Subcellular structures of possible viral origin in some mammalian tumors. *Ann. N.Y. Acad. Sci.*, **68**: 559–615, 1957.

DMOCHOWSKI, L., and GREY, C. E., Electron microscopy of tumors of known and suspected viral etiology. *Texas Rep. Biol. & Med.*, **15**: 704–756, 1957.

DMOCHOWSKI, L., GREY, C. E., PADGETT, F., and SYKES, J. A., Studies on the structure of the mammary tumor-inducing virus (Bittner) and of leukemia virus (Gross). pp. 85–121 in: Viruses, Nucleic Acids, and Cancer. *17th Ann. Symposium on Fundamental Cancer Research. Univ. of Texas*, M. D. Anderson Hospital and Tumor Inst. Williams & Wilkins, Baltimore, Md., 1963.

DMOCHOWSKI, L., GROSS, L., and PADGETT, F., Electron microscopic studies of rat leukemia induced with mouse leukemia virus. *Proc. Soc. Exp. Biol. & Med.*, **110**: 504-508, 1962.

DMOCHOWSKI, L., PADGETT, F., and GROSS, L., An electron microscope study of rat leukemia induced with mouse leukemia virus (Gross). *Cancer Research*, **24**: 869–899, 1964.

DMOCHOWSKI, L., RECHER, L., TANAKA, T., YUMOTO, T., SYKES, J. A., and YOUNG, L., Studies on the biologic relationship of some murine leukemia viruses. *Cancer Research*, **26**: 382–394, 1966.

DULANEY, A. D., Parotid gland tumors in AKR mice inoculated when newborn with cell-free Ak leukemic extracts. *Cancer Research*, **16**: 877–879, 1956.

DULANEY, A. D., GOSS, M. F., and MAXEY, M., Activity of cell-free extracts of Ak leukemic tissues for several strains of mice. (Abstract). *Proc. Am. Assoc. Cancer Research*, **2**: 197, 1957.

DULANEY, A. D., MAXEY, M., SCHILLIG, M. G., and GOSS, M. F., Neoplasms in C3H mice which received Ak-leukemic extracts when newborn. *Cancer Research*, **17**: 809–814, 1957.

DUNN, T. B., Normal and pathologic anatomy of the reticular tissue in laboratory mice, with a classification and discussion of neoplasms. *J. Nat. Cancer Inst.*, **14**: 1281–1433, 1954.

DUPLAN, J. F., La transmission de la leucémie lymphoide spontanée de la souris. *Revue d'Hématologie*, **11**: 190–215, 1956.

DURAN-REYNALS, F., The reciprocal infection of ducks and chickens with tumor-inducing viruses. *Cancer Research*, **2**: 343–369, 1942.

EDDY, B. E., ROWE, W. P., HARTLEY, J. W., STEWART, S. E., and HUEBNER, R. J., Hemagglutination with the SE polyoma virus. *Virology*, **6**: 290–291, 1958.

EDDY, B. E., STEWART, S. E., STANTON, M. F., and MARCOTTE, J. M., Induction of tumors in rats by tissue culture preparations of SE polyoma virus. *J. Nat. Cancer Inst.*, **22**: 161–172, 1959.

ELLERMANN, V., and BANG, O., Experimentelle Leukämie bei Hühnern. *Centralbl. f. Bakt., Abt. I* (Orig.), **46**: 595–609, 1908.

ELLERMANN, V., and BANG, O., Experimentelle Leukämie bei Hühnern, II. *Zeitschr. f. Hyg. & Infektionskr.*, **63**: 231–272, 1909.

ENGELBRETH-HOLM, J., *Spontaneous and experimental leukaemia in animals.* p. 245. Oliver and Boyd, London, 1942.

ENGELBRETH-HOLM, J., Is it possible to transmit or accelerate the development of mouse leukemia by tissue extracts? *Blood*, **3**: 862–866, 1948.

ENGELBRETH–HOLM, J., and FREDERIKSEN, O., The transmission of mouse leukemia to healthy animals by means of cell-free substance. *Acta Path. & Microbiol. Scand., Suppl.* **37**: 145–154, 1938.

ENGELBRETH-HOLM, J., and LEFEVRE, H., Acceleration of the development of leukemias and mammary carcinomas in mice by 9, 10-dimethyl-1, 2-benzanthracene. *Cancer Research*, **1**: 102–108, 1941.

FEKETE, E., and OTIS, H. K., Observations on leukemia in AKR mice born from transferred ova and nursed by low leukemic mothers. *Cancer Research*, **14**: 445–447, 1954.

FELDMAN, D. G., and GROSS, L., Electron-microscopic study of the mouse leukemia virus (Gross), and of tissues from mice with virus-induced leukemia. *Cancer Research*, **24**: 1760–1783, 1964.

FELDMAN, D. G., and GROSS, L., Electron microscopic study of the distribution of the mouse leukemia virus (Gross) in organs of mice and rats with virus-induced leukemia. *Cancer Research*, **26**: 412–426, 1966.

FELDMAN, D. G., and GROSS, L., Electron microscopic study of the distribution of the mouse leukemia virus (Gross) in genital organs of virus-injected C3Hf mice and of AK mice. *Cancer Research*, **27**: 1513–1527, 1967.

FELDMAN, D. G., DREYFUSS, Y., and GROSS, L., Electron microscopic study of the mouse leukemia virus (Gross) in organs of mouse embryos from virus-injected and normal C3Hf parents. *Cancer Research*, **27**: 1792–1804, 1967.

FELDMAN, D. G., GROSS, L., and DREYFUSS, Y., Electron microscopic study of the passage A mouse leukemia virus in mammary glands of pregnant, virus-injected, C3H(f) mice. *Cancer Research*, **23**: 1604–1607, 1963.

FLORY, C. M., FURTH, J., SAXTON, J. A., and REINER, L., Chemotherapeutic studies on transmitted mouse leukemia. *Cancer Research*, **3**: 729–743, 1943.

FRIEND, C., Cell-free transmission in adult Swiss mice of a disease having the character of a leukemia. *J. Exp. Med.*, **105**: 307–318, 1957.

FRIEND, C., Immunological relationships of a filterable agent causing a leukemia in adult mice. *J. Exp. Med.*, **109**: 217–228, 1959.

FURTH, J., Transmission of myeloid leukemia in mice. *Proc. Soc. Exp. Biol. & Med.*, **31**: 923–925, 1934.

FURTH, J., Transmission of myeloid leukemia of mice. Its relation to myeloma. *J. Exp. Med.*, **61**: 423–445, 1935.

FURTH, J., A neoplasm of monocytes of mice and its relation to similar neoplasms of man. *J. Exp. Med.*, **69**: 13–30, 1939.

FURTH, J., Nonhereditary nursing influence in leukemia. *Research Conference on Cancer (July 31–Aug. 4, 1944). Am. Assoc. Adv. Sci.*, pp. 106–107, Washington, D.C., 1945.

FURTH, J., Prolongation of life with prevention of leukemia by thymectomy in mice. *J. Gerontology*, **1**: 46–52, 1946.

FURTH, J., Recent studies on the etiology and nature of leukemia. *Blood*, **6**: 964–975, 1951.

FURTH, J., Recent experimental studies and current concepts on the etiology and nature of leukemia. *Proc. Inst. Med. Chicago*, **19**: 95–104, 1952.

FURTH, J., and BARNES, W. A., Differences between malignant blood cells from induced and spontaneous leukemias of mice. *Cancer Research*, **1**: 17–22, 1941.

FURTH, J., and BOON, M. C., The time and site of origin of the leukemic cell. *Research Conference on Cancer. Am. Assoc. Adv. Sci.*, pp. 129–138, Washington, D.C., 1944.

FURTH, J., and FURTH, O. B., Monocytic leukemia and other neoplastic diseases occurring in mice following intrasplenic injection of 1 : 2-benzpyrene. *Am. J. Cancer*, **34**: 169–183, 1938.

FURTH, J., and KAHN, M. C., The transmission of leukemia of mice with a single cell. *Am. J. Cancer*, **31**: 276–282, 1937.

FURTH, J., and KRUMDIECK, N., Splenic reticulum cell tumors in mice. *Am. J. Path.*, **16**: 449–456, 1940.

FURTH, J., and METCALF, D., An appraisal of tumor-virus problems. *J. Chronic Diseases*, **8**: 88–112, 1958.

FURTH, J., and STRUMIA, M., Studies on transmissible lymphoid leucemia of mice. *J. Exp. Med.*, **53**: 715–731, 1931.

FURTH, J., BOON, M. C., and KALISS, N., On the genetic character of neoplastic cells as determined in transplantation experiments. *Cancer Research*, **4**: 1–10, 1944.

FURTH, J., BUFFETT, R. F., BANASIEWICZ-RODRIGUEZ, M., and UPTON, A. C., Character of agent inducing leukemia in newborn mice. *Proc. Soc. Exp. Biol. & Med.*, **93**: 165–172, 1956.

FURTH, J., COLE, R. K., and BOON, M. C., The effect of maternal influence upon spontaneous leukemia of mice. *Cancer Research*, **2**: 280–283, 1942.

FURTH, J., FERRIS, H. W., and REZNIKOFF, P., Relation of leukemia of animals to leukemia of man. *J. Am. Med. Assoc.*, **105**: 1824–1830, 1935.

FURTH, J., SEIBOLD, H. R., and RATHBONE, R. R., Experimental studies on lymphomatosis of mice. *Am. J. Cancer*, **19**: 521–604, 1933.

FURTH, J., TUGGLE, A., and BREEDIS, C., Quantitative studies on the effect of X-rays on neoplastic cells. *Proc. Soc. Exp. Biol. & Med.*, **38**: 490–492, 1938.

FURTH, O. B., BARNES, W. A., and BROWER, A. B., Studies on resistance to transmissible leukemia in mice by means of parabiosis. *Arch. Path.*, **29**: 163–174, 1940.

GARDNER, W. U., Influence of estrogenic hormones on abnormal growths. Occas. Publ. Am. Assoc. Adv. Sci., Science Press, pp. 67–75, 1937.

GARDNER, W. U., and DOUGHERTY, T. F., The leukemogenic action of estrogens in hybrid mice. *Yale J. Biol. & Med.*, **17**: 75–90, 1944.

GARDNER, W. U., DOUGHERTY, T. F., and WILLIAMS, W. L., Lymphoid tumors in mice receiving steroid hormones. *Cancer Research*, **4**: 73–87, 1944.

GARDNER, W. U., KIRSCHBAUM, A., and STRONG, L. C., Lymphoid tumors in mice receiving estrogens. *Arch. Path.*, **29**: 1–7, 1940.

GINSBURG, H., and SACHS, L., Leukemia induction in mice by Moloney virus from long- and short-term tissue cultures, and attempts to detect a leukemogenic virus in cultures from X-ray-induced leukemia. *J. Nat. Cancer Inst.*, **28**: 1391–1410, 1962.

GOOD, R. A., and GABRIELSEN, A. E., Edit. *The thymus in immunobiology*. p. 778. Hoeber Med. Div., Harper & Row, New York, 1964.

GRAFFI, A., Chloroleukemia of mice. *Ann. N.Y. Acad. Sci.*, **68**: 540–558, 1957.

GRAFFI, A., Experimentelle Untersuchungen zur Ätiologie der Leukämien. *Zeitschr. Ges. Inn. Medizin & Grenzgebiete*, **23**: 961–971, 1958.

GRAFFI, A., Neuere Untersuchungen über das Virus der myeloischen Leukämie der Maus. pp. 112–161 in: *Progress in Experimental Tumor Research*. S. Karger, Basel, and J. B. Lippincott, Philadelphia, 1960.

GRAFFI, A., and GIMMY, J., Erzeugung von Leukosen bei der Ratte durch ein leukämogenes Agens der Maus. *Naturwissenschaften*, **44**: 518, 1957.

GRAFFI, A., and GIMMY, J., Rattenleukosen durch zellfreie Filtrate aus homologem leukämischem Gewebe. *Zeitschr. f. Naturforsch.*, **14**: 747–748, 1959.

GRAFFI, A., and KRISCHKE, W., Über Infektiosität und Übertragungsweise der virusbedingten myeloischen Leukämie der Maus. *Biolog. Zentralbl.*, **81**: 277–289, 1962.

GRAFFI, A., BAUMBACH, L., SCHRAMM, T., and BIERWOLF, D., Untersuchungen zur Frage der Züchtbarkeit des Virus der myeloischen Leukämie der Maus in der Gewebekultur. *Zeitschr. f. Krebsforsch.*, **65**: 385–395, 1963.

GRAFFI, A., BIELKA, H., and FEY, F., Leukämieerzeugung durch ein filtrierbares Agens aus malignen Tumoren. *Acta Haemat.*, **15**: 145–174, 1956.

GRANBOULAN, N., and RIVIÈRE, M. R., Étude au microscope électronique des particules virales présentes dans les lymphomatoses spontanées de la souris. *Journal de Microscopie*, **1**: 23–38, 1962.

GROSS, L., Is cancer a communicable disease? *Cancer Research*, **4**: 293–303, 1944.

GROSS, L., Hemolytic action of mouse mammary carcinoma filtrate on mouse erythrocytes *in vitro*. *Proc. Soc. Exp. Biol. & Med.*, **65**: 292–293, 1947.

GROSS, L., Increased hemolytic potency of mouse mammary carcinoma extracts following incubation with tumor cells. *Proc. Soc. Exp. Biol. & Med.* **67**: 341–343, 1948a.

GROSS, L., Destructive action of mouse and rat tumor extracts on red blood cells *in vitro*. *J. Immunol.*, **59**: 173–188, 1948b.

GROSS, L., Destructive action of human cancer extracts on red blood cells *in vitro*. *Proc. Soc. Exp. Biol. & Med.*, **70**: 656–662, 1949.

GROSS, L., Susceptibility of newborn mice of an otherwise apparently "resistant" strain to inoculation with leukemia. *Proc Soc. Exp. Biol. & Med.*, **73**: 246–248, 1950a.

GROSS, L., Susceptibility of suckling-infant and resistance of adult mice of the C3H and the C57 lines to inoculation with Ak leukemia. *Cancer*, **3**: 1073–1087, 1950b.

GROSS, L., "Spontaneous" leukemia developing in C3H mice following inoculation, in infancy, with Ak-leukemic extracts, or Ak-embryos. *Proc. Soc. Exp. Biol. & Med.*, **76**: 27–32, 1951a.

GROSS, L., Pathogenic properties, and "vertical" transmission of the mouse leukemia agent. *Proc. Soc. Exp. Biol. & Med.*, **78**: 342–348, 1951b.

Gross, L., Delayed effects of inoculation of Ak-leukemic cells in mice of the C3H line. A working hypothesis on the etiology of mouse leukemia. *Cancer*, **5**: 620–624, 1952a.

Gross, L., Mouse leukemia. *Ann. N.Y. Acad. Sci.*, **54**: 1184–1196, 1952b.

Gross, L., Biological properties of the mouse leukemia agent. *Cancer*, **6**: 153–158, 1953a.

Gross, L., A filterable agent, recovered from Ak leukemic extracts, causing salivary gland carcinomas in C3H mice. *Proc. Soc. Exp. Biol. & Med.*, **83**: 414–421, 1953b.

Gross, L., Presence of leukemic agent in normal testes and ovaries of young mice of Ak line. *Acta Haemat.*, **10**: 18–26, 1953c.

Gross, L., Neck tumors, or leukemia, developing in adult C3H mice following inoculation, in early infancy, with filtered (Berkefeld N) or centrifugated (144,000 × g) Ak-leukemic extracts. *Cancer*, **6**: 948–957, 1953d.

Gross, L., Transmissible mouse leukemia: Biological properties of the mouse leukemia agent. pp. 76–95 in: *CIBA Foundation Symposium on Leukaemia Research*. Little, Brown & Co., Boston, 1954a.

Gross, L., Transmission of Ak leukemic agent into newborn mice of the C57 Brown/cd inbred line. *Proc. Soc. Exp. Biol. & Med.*, **86**: 734–739, 1954b.

Gross, L., Is leukemia caused by a transmissible virus? A working hypothesis. *Blood*, **9**: 557–573, 1954c.

Gross, L., Difference in susceptibility to Ak leukemic agent between two substrains of mice of C3H line. *Proc. Soc. Exp. Biol. & Med.*, **88**: 64–66, 1955a.

Gross, L., Mouse leukemia: An egg-borne virus disease (with a note on mouse salivary gland carcinoma). *Acta Haemat.*, **13**: 13–29, 1955b.

Gross, L., Induction of parotid carcinomas and/or subcutaneous sarcomas in C3H mice with normal C3H organ extracts. *Proc. Soc. Exp. Biol. & Med.*, **88**: 362–368, 1955c.

Gross, L., Influence of ether, *in vitro*, on pathogenic properties of mouse leukemia extracts. *Acta Haemat.*, **15**: 273–277, 1956a.

Gross, L., Viral (egg-borne) etiology of mouse leukemia. Filtered extracts from leukemic C58 mice, causing leukemia (or parotid tumors) following inoculation into newborn C57 Brown, or C3H mice. *Cancer*, **9**: 778–791, 1956b.

Gross, L., Development and serial cell-free passage of a highly potent strain of mouse leukemia virus. *Proc. Soc. Exp. Biol. & Med.*, **94**: 767–771, 1957a.

Gross, L., Studies on the nature and biological properties of a transmissible agent causing leukemia following inoculation into newborn mice. *Ann. N.Y. Acad. Sci.*, **68**: 501–521, 1957b.

Gross, L., Filterable agent causing leukemia following inoculation into newborn mice. *Texas Rep. Biol. & Med.*, **15**: 603–626, 1957c.

Gross, L., High susceptibility of 1 to 14-day-old C3H mice to "passage A" leukemic filtrates. *Proc. Soc. Exp. Biol. & Med.*, **97**: 300–304, 1958a.

Gross, L., Viral etiology of "spontaneous" mouse leukemia: A review. *Cancer Research*, **18**: 371–381, 1958b.

Gross, L., Attempt to recover filterable agent from X-ray-induced leukemia. *Acta Haemat.*, **19**: 353–361, 1958c.

Gross, L., The aetiology of cancer and allied diseases. Development of a concept based on recent experiments dealing with a cell-free transmission of mouse leukaemia. *Brit. Med. J.*, **2**: 1–5, 1958d.

Gross, L., Serial cell-free passage of a radiation-activated mouse leukemia agent. *Proc. Soc. Exp. Biol. & Med.*, **100**: 102–105, 1959a.

GROSS, L., Effect of thymectomy on development of leukemia in C3H mice inoculated with "passage" virus. *Proc. Soc. Exp. Biol. & Med.*, **100**: 325–328, 1959b.

GROSS, L., Aetiology of leukaemia. Letter to the Editor. *Lancet*, **1**: 891, 1959c.

GROSS, L., Agglutinating action of heat-inactivated passage A mouse leukemia filtrates on mouse red blood cells. *Proc. Soc. Exp. Biol. & Med.*, **101**: 113–117, 1959d.

GROSS, L., Development of myeloid (chloro-) leukemia in thymectomized C3H mice following inoculation of lymphatic leukemia virus. *Proc. Soc. Exp. Biol. & Med.*, **103**: 509–514, 1960a.

GROSS, L., Biological and pathogenic properties of a mouse leukemia virus. *Acta Haemat.*, **23**: 259–275, 1960b.

GROSS, L., Viral aetiology of mouse leukaemia. Letter to the Editor. *Lancet*, **2**: 706–707, 1960c.

GROSS, L., Induction of leukemia in rats with mouse leukemia (passage A) virus. *Proc. Soc. Exp. Biol. & Med.*, **106**: 890–893, 1961a.

GROSS, L., Viral etiology of mouse leukemia. *Advances in Cancer Research*, **6**: 149–180. Academic Press, New York, 1961b.

GROSS, L., Transmission of mouse leukemia virus through milk of virus-injected C3H female mice. *Proc. Soc. Exp. Biol. & Med.*, **109**: 830–836, 1962a.

GROSS, L., Pathogenic properties of a filterable virus causing leukemia in rats. (Abstract). *Proc. Am. Assoc. Cancer Research*, **3**: 324, 1962b.

GROSS, L., Studies on pathogenic properties and natural transmission of a mouse leukemia virus. pp. 159–170 in: *CIBA Foundation Symposium on Tumour Viruses of Murine Origin.* J. & A. Churchill Ltd., London, 1962c.

GROSS, L., Properties of a virus isolated from leukemic mice, inducing various forms of leukemia and lymphomas in mice and rats. Bertner Foundation Lecture. pp. 403–426 in: Viruses, Nucleic Acids, and Cancer. 17*th Ann. Symposium on Fundamental Cancer Research. Univ. of Texas,* M. D. Anderson Hospital and Tumor Inst. Williams & Wilkins, Baltimore, Md., 1963a.

GROSS, L., Pathogenic potency and host range of the mouse leukemia virus. *Acta Haemat.*, **29**: 1–15, 1963b.

GROSS, L., Susceptibility of rats to leukemogenic action of passage A virus. Effect of thymectomy. (Abstract). *Proc. Am. Assoc. Cancer Research*, **4**: 25, 1963c.

GROSS, L., Serial cell-free passage in rats of the mouse leukemia virus. Effect of thymectomy. *Proc. Soc. Exp. Biol. & Med.*, **112**: 939-945, 1963d.

GROSS, L., How many different viruses causing leukemia in mice? *Acta Haemat.*, **32**: 44–62, 1964a.

GROSS, L., Attempt at classification of mouse leukemia viruses. *Acta Haemat.*, **32**: 81–88, 1964b.

GROSS, L., Neutralization *in vitro* of mouse leukemia virus by specific immune serum. Importance of virus titration. *Proc. Soc. Exp. Biol. & Med.*, **119**: 420–427, 1965a.

GROSS, L., Viral etiology of leukemia and lymphomas. Editorial. *Blood*, **25**: 377–381, 1965b.

GROSS, L., Are the common forms of spontaneous and induced leukemia and lymphomas in mice caused by a single virus? pp. 407–424 in: *Conference on Murine Leukemia. Nat. Cancer Inst. Monograph No.* 22, U.S. Publ. Health Service, Bethesda, Md., 1966a.

GROSS, L., Transmission of mouse leukemia virus (Gross) through embryos. (Abstract.). p. 259, *IXth Internat. Cancer Congress, Section I-11-g, Tokyo,* Japan, 1966b.

GROSS, L., Transmission of mouse leukemia by oral route. *Acta Haemat.*, **40**: 1–8, 1968.

GROSS, L., and DREYFUSS, Y., Studies on specificity and potency of passage A leukemic filtrates. (Abstract). *Proc. Am. Assoc. Cancer Research,* **3**: 24–25, 1959.

GROSS, L., and DREYFUSS, Y., How is the mouse leukemia virus transmitted from host to host under natural life conditions? pp. 9–21 in: Carcinogenesis: A Broad Critique. *20th Ann. Symposium on Fundamental Cancer Research. Univ. of Texas,* M. D. Anderson Hospital and Tumor Inst. Williams & Wilkins Co., Baltimore, Md., 1967.

GROSS, L., DREYFUSS, Y., and MOORE, L. A., Attempt to propagate "passage A" mouse leukemia virus on normal mouse embryo cells in tissue culture. (Abstract). *Proc. Am. Assoc. Cancer Research,* **3**: 231, 1961.

GROSS, L., EHRENREICH, T., DREYFUSS, Y., and MOORE, L. A., Development of high incidence of myeloid leukemia in F_1 hybrids born to C57 Brown × Ak parents. (Abstract). *Proc. Am. Assoc. Cancer Research,* **7**: 26, 1966.

GROSS, L., and FELDMAN, D. G. Electron microscopic studies of radiation-induced leukemia in mice: Virus release following total-body X-ray irradiation. *Cancer Research,* **28**: 1677–1685, 1968.

GROSS, L., ROSWIT, B., MADA, E. R., DREYFUSS, Y., and MOORE, L. A., Studies on radiation-induced leukemia in mice. *Cancer Research,* **19**: 316–320, 1959.

GROSS, L., ROSWIT, B., MALSKY, S. J., DREYFUSS, Y., and AMATO, C. G., Resistance of mouse leukemia virus to *in vitro* gamma rays irradiation. (Abstract). *Proc. Am. Assoc. Cancer Research,* **6**: 24, 1965.

GROSS, L., ROSWIT, B., MALSKY, S. J., DREYFUSS, Y., and AMATO, C. G., Inactivation of the mouse leukemia virus (Gross) with 4,500,000 r gamma irradiation. (Abstract). *Proc. Am. Assoc. Cancer Research,* **9**: 26, 1968.

GROUP of ELECTRON MICROSCOPISTS and VIROLOGISTS. Suggestions for the classification of oncogenic RNA viruses. *J. Nat. Cancer Inst.*, **37**: 395–397, 1966.

HAGUENAU, F., DALTON, A. J., and MOLONEY, J. B., A preliminary report of electron microscopic and bioassay studies on the Rous sarcoma I virus. *J. Nat. Cancer Inst.*, **20**: 633–649, 1958.

HALL, J. W., and KNOCKE, F. J., Transmission of chloroleukemia of mice. *Am. J. Path.*, **14**: 217–226, 1938.

HARAN-GHERA, N., Leukemogenic activity of centrifugates from irradiated mouse thymus and bone marrow. *Internat. J. Cancer,* **1**: 81–87, 1966.

HARAN-GHERA, N., Leukemogenic filtrable agent from chemically-induced lymphoid leukemia in C57BL mice. *Proc. Soc. Exp. Biol. & Med.*, **124**: 697–699, 1967.

HARAN-GHERA, N., LIEBERMAN, M., and KAPLAN, H. S., Direct action of a leukemogenic virus on the thymus. *Cancer Research,* **26**: 438–442, 1966.

HARTLEY, J. W., ROWE, W. P., CAPPS, W. I., and HUEBNER, R. J., Complement fixation and tissue culture assays for mouse leukemia viruses. *Proc. Nat. Acad. Sci., USA,* **53**: 931–938, 1965.

HAYS, E. F., and BECK, W. S., The development of leukemia and other neoplasms in mice receiving cell-free extracts from a high-leukemia (AKR) strain. *Cancer Research,* **18**: 676–681, 1958.

HAYS, E. F., SIMMONS, N. S., and BECK, W. S., Induction of mouse leukaemia with purified nucleic acid preparations. *Nature,* **180**: 1419–1420, 1957.

HEINE, U., GRAFFI, A., BIERWOLF, D., HELMCKE, J. G., and RANDT, A., Elektronenmikroskopische Untersuchungen an der zellfrei übertragbaren myeloischen Leukämie der Maus. *Acta Biol. Med. Germanica*, **3**: 608–623, 1959.

HENSHAW, P. S., Leukemia in mice following exposure to X-rays. *Radiology*, **43**: 279–285, 1944.

ICHIKAWA, Y., Electron microscopic observations on leukemia and lymphosarcomatosis in SL and Ak strain mice, with special reference to the distribution of viral particles as possible causative agents. Chapter 7, pp. 197–220 in: *Immunocytopathology, Virus Infection and Leukemia, Ann. Rep. Inst. for Virus Research,* Kyoto Univ., Publ., 1958.

IDA, N., Formal Discussion (following presentation of paper entitled "Filterable agent causing leukemia following inoculation into newborn mice," by L. Gross). *Texas Rep. Biol. & Med.*, **15**: 616–618, 1957.

IMAGAWA, D. T., and ISSA, H. A., Cultivation of Gross virus induced thymic lymphoma *in vitro*. (Abstract). *Fed. Proc.* **25**: 478, 1966.

IOACHIM, H. L., Long-term replication of Gross leukemia virus (GLV) in thymic cultures. (Abstract). *Proc. Am. Assoc. Cancer Research,* **7**: 33, 1966.

IOACHIM, H. L., Neoplastic transformation of rat thymic cells induced *in vitro* by Gross leukemia virus. *Science*, **155**: 585–587, 1967.

IOACHIM, H. L., and BERWICK, L., Continuous viral replication and cellular neoplastic transformation in cultures of normal rat thymus infected with Gross leukemia virus. *Internat. J. Cancer,* **3**: 61–73, 1968.

IOACHIM, H. L., BERWICK, L., and FURTH, J., Replication of Gross leukemia virus in long-term cultures of rat thymomas: Bioassays and electron microscopy. *Cancer Research*, **26**: 803–811, 1966.

IOACHIM, H. L., CALI, A., and SINHA, D., Age-dependent transplantability in rats of virus-induced thymic lymphoma cultured *in vitro*. *Cancer Research*, **25**: 132–139, 1965.

IOACHIM, H., and FURTH, J., Intrareticular cell multiplication of leukemic lymphoblasts in thymic tissue cultures. *J. Nat. Cancer Inst.*, **32**: 339–359, 1964.

IRINO, S., OTA, Z., SEZAKI, T., SUZAKI, M., and HIRAKI, K., Cell-free transmission of 20-methylcholanthrene-induced RF mouse leukemia and electron microscopic demonstration of virus particles in its leukemic tissue. *Gann*, **54**: 225–237, 1963.

JAKOBSSON, S. V., and WAHREN, B., Electron microscopy of Gross lymphoma cells treated with a tumor specific antiserum. *Exp. Cell Research*, **37**: 509–515, 1965.

JULLIEN, P., and RUDALI, G., Isolement et entretien par surinfections successives (passage G) d'un agent leucémigène de souris AkR régulièrement actif. *Compt. Rend. Acad. Sci.* (*Paris*), **250**: 1588–1589, 1960.

KAPLAN, H. S., Observations on radiation-induced lymphoid tumors of mice. *Cancer Research,* **7**: 141–147, 1947.

KAPLAN, H. S., Comparative susceptibility of the lymphoid tissues of strain C57 Black mice to the induction of lymphoid tumors by irradiation. *J. Nat. Cancer Inst.*, **8**: 191–197, 1948.

KAPLAN, H. S., Influence of age on susceptibility of mice to the development of lymphoid tumors after irradiation. *J. Nat. Cancer Inst.*: **9**, 55–56, 1948.

KAPLAN, H. S., Influence of thymectomy, splenectomy, and gonadectomy on incidence of radiation-induced lymphoid tumors in strain C57 Black mice. *J. Nat. Cancer Inst.*, **11**: 83–90, 1950.

KAPLAN, H. S., Radiation-induced lymphoid tumors of mice. *Acta Internat. Union Against Cancer*, **7**: 849–859, 1952.

KAPLAN, H. S., On the etiology and pathogenesis of the leukemias: A review. *Cancer Research*, **14**: 535–548, 1954.

KAPLAN, H. S., The pathogenesis of experimental lymphoid tumors in mice. pp. 127–143 in: *Proc. Second Canadian Cancer Conference*. Academic Press, New York, 1957.

KAPLAN, H. S., Radiation-induced leukemia in mice. A progress report. pp. 289–302 in: *Radiation Biology and Cancer*. Univ. of Texas, M. D. Anderson Hospital and Tumor Inst., Univ. of Texas Press, Austin, 1959.

KAPLAN, H. S., and BROWN, M. B., Further observations on inhibition of lymphoid tumor development by shielding and partial-body irradiation of mice. *J. Nat. Cancer Inst.*, **12**: 427–436, 1951.

KAPLAN, H. S., and BROWN, M. B., Mortality of mice after total-body irradiation as influenced by alterations in total dose fractionation, and periodicity of treatment. *J. Nat. Cancer Inst.*, **12**: 765–775, 1952.

KAPLAN, H. S., and BROWN, M. B., A quantitative dose-response study of lymphoid-tumor development in irradiated C57 Black mice. *J. Nat. Cancer Inst.*, **13**: 185–208, 1952.

KAPLAN, H. S., BROWN, M. B., and PAULL, J., Influence of bone-marrow injections on involution and neoplasia of mouse thymus after systemic irradiation. *J. Nat. Cancer Inst.*, **14**: 303–316, 1953.

KAPLAN, H. S., BROWN, M. B., HIRSCH, B. B., and CARNES, W. H., Indirect induction of lymphomas in irradiated mice. II. Factor of irradiation of the host. *Cancer Research*, **16**: 426–428, 1956.

KAPLAN, H. S., CARNES, W. H., BROWN, M. B., and HIRSCH, B. B., Indirect induction of lymphomas in irradiated mice. I. Tumor incidence and morphology in mice bearing nonirradiated thymic grafts. *Cancer Research*, **16**: 422–425, 1956.

KAPLAN, H. S., NAGAREDA, C. S., ROSSTON, B., and BROWN, M. B., Comparative activity of isologous versus homologous mouse bone marrow on lymphoid tumor production following irradiation. *Proc. Soc. Exp. Biol. & Med.*, **98**: 384–387, 1958.

KASSEL, R., BURTON, L., FRIEDMAN, F., and ROTTINO, A., Carcinogenic action of refined tumor factor isolated from mouse leukemia tissue. *Proc. Soc. Exp. Biol. & Med.*, **101**: 201–204, 1959.

KASSEL, R., and ROTTINO, A., Problems in the production of leukemia with cell-free extracts. *Cancer Research*, **19**: 155–158, 1959.

KAWAMOTO, S., IDA, N., KIRSCHBAUM, A., and TAYLOR, G., Urethan and leukemogenesis in mice. *Cancer Research*, **18**: 725–729, 1958.

KIM, U., CLIFTON, K. H., and FURTH, J., A highly inbred line of Wistar rats yielding spontaneous mammo-somatotropic pituitary and other tumors. *J. Nat. Cancer Inst.*, **24**: 1031–1055, 1960.

KIRSCHBAUM, A., Genetic and certain nongenetic factors with reference to leukemia in the F strain of mice. *Proc. Soc. Exp. Biol. & Med.*, **55**: 147–149, 1944.

KIRSCHBAUM, A., Rodent leukemia: Recent biological studies. A review. *Cancer Research*, **11**: 741–752, 1951.

KIRSCHBAUM, A., Genetic and nongenetic factors influencing the induction of mouse leukemia. Chapter 6, pp. 121–125 in: *The Leukemias. Etiology, Pathophysiology, and Treatment. H. Ford Hospital Internat. Symposium*. Academic Press, New York, 1957a.

KIRSCHBAUM, A., Formal Discussion (following presentation of paper entitled "Filterable agent causing leukemia following inoculation into newborn mice", by L. Gross). *Texas Rep. Biol. & Med.*, **15**: 618–620, 1957b.

KIRSCHBAUM, A., and KAPLAN, H. S., Induction of leukemia in mice. *Science*, **100**: 360–361, 1944.

KIRSCHBAUM, A., and MIXER, H. W., Induction of leukemia in eight inbred stocks of mice varying in susceptibility to the spontaneous disease. *J. Lab. & Clin. Med.*, **32**: 720–731, 1947.

KIRSCHBAUM, A., and STRONG, L. C., Leukemia in the F strain of mice: Observations on cytology, general morphology, and transmission. *Am. J. Cancer*, **37**: 400–413, 1939.

KIRSCHBAUM, A., and STRONG, L. C., Milk influence and leukemia in mice. *Proc. Soc. Exp. Biol. & Med.*, **51**: 404–406, 1942.

KIRSCHBAUM, A., SHAPIRO, J. R., and MIXER, H. W., Synergistic action of leukemogenic agents. *Cancer Research*, **13**: 262–268, 1953.

KIRSCHBAUM, A., STRONG, L. C., and GARDNER, W. U., Influence of methylcholanthrene on age incidence of leukemia in several strains of mice. *Proc. Soc. Exp. Biol. & Med.*, **45**: 287–289, 1940.

KIRSTEN, W. H., and MAYER, L. A., Morphologic responses to a murine erythroblastosis virus. *J. Nat. Cancer Inst.*, **39**: 311–335, 1967.

KIRSTEN, W. H., PLATZ, C. E., and FLOCKS, J. S., Lymphoid neoplasms in rats after inoculation with cell-free extracts of leukemic AKR mice. *J. Nat. Cancer Inst.*, **29**: 293–319, 1962.

KLEIN, G., The nature of mammalian lymphosarcoma transmission by isolated chromatin fractions. *Cancer Research*, **12**: 589–590, 1952.

KOPROWSKI, H., Actively acquired tolerance to a mouse tumour. *Nature*, **175**: 1087–1088, 1955.

KORTEWEG, R., Eine überimpfbare Leukosarkomatose bei der Maus. *Zeitschr. f. Krebsforsch.*, **29**: 455–476, 1929.

KREBS, C., RASK-NIELSEN, H. C., and WAGNER, A., The origin of lymphosarcomatosis and its relation to other forms of leucosis in white mice. Lymphomatosis infiltrans leucemica et aleucemica. *Acta Radiologica*, *Supplement* X, pp. 1–53, 1930.

KRISCHKE, W., and GRAFFI, A., The transmission of the virus of myeloid leukaemia of mice by the milk. *Acta Internat. Union Against Cancer*, **19**: 360–361, 1963.

KUNII, A., CALI, A., and FURTH, J., Effect of neonatal thymectomy on induction of leukemia by virus in rats. *Proc. Soc. Exp. Biol. & Med.*, **118**: 815–818, 1965.

KUNII, A., FURTH, J., and BERWICK, L., Studies on restoration of sensitivity of thymectomized rats to viral leukemia. *Cancer Research*, **26**: 48–59, 1966.

KUNII, A., TAKEMOTO, H., and FURTH, J., Leukemogenic filterable agent from estrogen-induced thymic lymphoma in RF mice. *Proc. Soc. Exp. Biol. & Med.*, **119**: 1211–1215, 1965.

LACASSAGNE, A., Sarcomes lymphoides apparus chez des souris longuement traitées par des hormones oestrogènes. *Compt. Rend. Soc. Biol.*, **126**: 193–195, 1937.

LACASSAGNE, A., Rôle du thymus dans la leucémie lymphoide chez la souris. *Le Sang*, **25**: 769–777, 1954.

LATARJET, R., La leucémie de la souris est-elle du à un virus? *Le Sang*, **25**: 777–787, 1954.

LATARJET, R., Leucémie de la souris et virus. La récolte de 1956. *Revue d'Hématologie*, **12**: 7–10, 1957.

LATARJET, R., REBEYROTTE, N., and MOUSTACCHI, E., Production de cancers multiplies chez des souris ayant reçu de l'acide nucleique extrait de tissus leucémiques isologues ou homologues. *Compt. Rend. Acad. Sci.* (*Paris*), **246**: 853–855, 1958.

LAW, L. W., Effect of gonadectomy and adrenalectomy on the appearance and incidence of spontaneous lymphoid leukemia in C58 mice. *J. Nat. Cancer Inst.*, **8**: 157–159, 1947.

LAW, L. W., Increase in incidence of leukemia in hybrid mice bearing thymic transplants from a high leukemic strain. *J. Nat. Cancer Inst.*, **12**: 789–805, 1952.

LAW, L. W., Recent advances in experimental leukemia research. *Cancer Research*, **14**: 695–709, 1954.

LAW, L. W., Genetic studies in experimental cancer. Advances in *Cancer Research*, **2**: 281–352, Academic Press, New York, 1954.

LAW, L. W., DUNN, T. B., and BOYLE, P. J., Neoplasms in the C3H strain and in F_1 hybrid mice of two crosses following introduction of extracts and filtrates of leukemic tissues. *J. Nat. Cancer Inst.*, **16**: 495–539, 1955.

LAW, L. W., and LEWISOHN, M., Induction of lymphomatosis in mice following painting with 9 : 10-dimethyl-1 : 2-benzanthracene. *Proc. Soc. Exp. Biol. & Med.*, **43**: 143–146, 1940.

LAW, L. W., and MILLER, J. H., The effect of thymectomy on the incidence, latent period, and type of leukemia in high leukemia strains of mice. (Abstract.) *Cancer Research*, **10**: 230, 1950.

LAW, L. W., and MILLER, J. H., Observations on the effect of thymectomy on spontaneous leukemias in mice of the high-leukemic strains, RIL and C58. *J. Nat. Cancer Inst.*, **11**: 253–262, 1950.

LAW, L. W., and MILLER, J. H., The influence of thymectomy on the incidence of carcinogen-induced leukemia in strain DBA mice. *J. Nat. Cancer Inst.*, **11**: 425–438, 1950.

LAW, L. W., and MOLONEY, J. B., Studies of congenital transmission of a leukemia virus in mice. *Proc. Soc. Exp. Biol. & Med.*, **108**: 715–723, 1961.

LEADING ARTICLE, The aetiology of leukaemia. *Lancet*, **2**: 30–31, 1958.

LEMONDE, P., and CLODE, M., *In vitro* culture of a leukaemic agent from spontaneous mouse leukaemia. *Nature*, **193**: 1191–1192, 1962.

LEVINTHAL, J. D., BUFFETT, R. F., and FURTH, J., Prevention of viral lymphoid leukemia of mice by thymectomy. *Proc. Soc. Exp. Biol. & Med.*, **100**: 610–614, 1959.

LIGNAC, G. O. E., Die Benzolleukämie bei Menschen und weissen Mäusen. *Klin. Wochenschr.*, **12**: 109–110, 1933.

LITTLE, C. C., Factors influencing the growth of a transplantable tumor in mice. *J. Exp. Zool.*, **31**: 307–326, 1920.

LYNCH, C. J., The R.I.L. strain of mice: Its relation to the leukemic Ak strain and AKR substrains. *J. Nat. Cancer Inst.*, **15**: 161–176, 1954.

MACDOWELL, E. C., POTTER, J. S., BOVARNICK, M., RICHTER, M. N., TAYLOR, M. J., WARD, E. N., LAANES, T., and WINTERSTEINER, M. P., Experimental Leukemia. *Year Book No. 38*, *Carnegie Inst. of Wash.*, pp. 191–195, 1939.

MACDOWELL, E. C., and RICHTER, M. N., Mouse leukemia. IX. The role of heredity in spontaneous cases. *Arch. Path.*, **20**: 709–724, 1935.

MACDOWELL, E. C., and TAYLOR, M. J., Mouse leukemia. XIII. A maternal influence that lowers the incidence of spontaneous cases. *Proc. Soc. Exp. Biol. & Med.*, **68**: 571–577, 1948.

MANAKER, R. A., JENSEN, E. M., and KOROL, W., Long-term propagation of a murine leukemia virus in an established cell line. *J. Nat. Cancer Inst.*, **33**: 363–371, 1964.

MANAKER, R. A., STROTHER, P. C., MILLER, A. A., and PICZAK, C. V., Behavior *in vitro* of a mouse lymphoid-leukemia virus. *J. Nat. Cancer Inst.*, **25**: 1411–1419, 1960.

MCENDY, D. P., BOON, M. C., and FURTH, J., Induction of leukemia in mice by methylcholanthrene and X-rays. *J. Nat. Cancer Inst.*, **3**: 227–247, 1942.

MCENDY, D. P., BOON, M. C., and FURTH, J., On the role of thymus, spleen and gonads in the development of leukemia in a high-leukemia stock of mice. *Cancer Research*, **4**: 377–383, 1944.

MERCIER, L., Hérédité du lymphosarcome de la souris dans les croisements d'hétérozygotes pour le couple de facteurs cancer-non cancer. *Compt. Rend. Soc. Biol.*, **124**: 403–405, 1937.

MERCIER, L., Hérédité du lymphosarcome de la souris. Résultats confirmatifs. *Compt. Rend. Soc. Biol.*, **133**: 29–31, 1940.

METCALF, D., The thymic lymphocytosis-stimulating factor. *Ann. N.Y. Acad. Sci.*, **73**: 113–119, 1958.

MIDER, G. B., and MORTON, J. J., The effect of methylcholanthrene on the latent period of lymphomatosis in dilute brown mice. *Am. J. Cancer*, **37**: 355–363, 1939.

MILLER, J. F. A. P., Role of the thymus in murine leukaemia. *Nature*, **183**: 1069, 1959.

MILLER, J. F. A. P., Fate of subcutaneous thymus grafts in thymectomized mice inoculated with leukaemic filtrate. *Nature*, **184**: 1809–1810, 1959.

MILLER, J. F. A. P., Studies on mouse leukaemia. Leukaemogenesis by cell-free filtrates inoculated in newborn and adult mice. *Brit. J. Cancer*, **14**: 83–92, 1960.

MILLER, J. F. A. P., Studies on mouse leukaemia. The role of the thymus in leukaemogenesis by cell-free leukaemic filtrates. *Brit. J. Cancer*, **14**: 93–98, 1960.

MILLER, J. F. A. P., Role of the thymus in virus-induced leukaemia. pp. 262–279 in: *CIBA Foundation Symposium on Tumour Viruses of Murine Origin*. J. & A. Churchill, London, 1962.

MILLER, J. F. A. P., TING, R. C., and LAW, L. W., Influence of thymectomy on tumor induction by polyoma virus in C57BL mice. *Proc. Soc. Exp. Biol. & Med.*, **116**: 323–327, 1964.

MILLS, K. C., and DOCHEZ, A. R., Specific agglutination of murine erythrocytes by a pneumonitis virus in mice. *Proc. Soc. Exp. Biol. & Med.*, **57**: 140–143, 1944.

MOLONEY, J. B., Biological studies on a lymphoid leukemia virus extracted from sarcoma S.37. I. Origin and introductory investigations. *J. Nat. Cancer Inst.*, **24**: 933–951, 1960.

MORI-CHAVEZ, P., Spontaneous leukemia at high altitude in C58 mice. *J. Nat. Cancer Inst.*, **21**: 985–997, 1958.

MORTON, J. J., and MIDER, G. B., Some effects of carcinogenic agents on mice subject to spontaneous leukoses. *Cancer Research*, **1**: 95–98, 1941.

MURPHY, J. B., Transplantability of malignant tumors to the embryos of a foreign species. *J. Am. Med. Assoc.*, **59**: 874, 1912.

MURPHY, J. B., The effect of castration, theelin, and testosterone on the incidence of leukemia in a Rockefeller Institute strain of mice. *Cancer Research*, **4**: 622–624, 1944.

MURPHY, J. B., and STURM, E., The transmission of an induced lymphatic leukemia and lymphosarcoma in the rat. *Cancer Research*, **1**: 379–383, 1941.

NETTLESHIP, A., Influence of age on the growth of lymphomas. *Am. J. Path.*, **21**: 147–165, 1945.

NOBLE, R. L., and CUTTS, J. H., Mammary tumors of the rat: A review. *Cancer Research*, **19**: 1125–1139, 1959.

OKANO, H., KUNII, A., and FURTH, J., An electron microscopic study of leukemia induced in rats with Gross virus. *Cancer Research*, **23**: 1169–1175, 1963.

OLD, L. J., BOYSE, E. A., and STOCKERT, E., Typing of mouse leukaemias by serological methods. *Nature*, **201**: 777–779, 1964.

PARSONS, D. F., Structure of the Gross leukemia virus. *J. Nat. Cancer Inst.*, **30**: 569–583, 1963.

PATTI, J., and BIESELE, J. J., Heterologous growth and passages of mouse sarcomas in hamsters (*Mesocricetus auratus*). *Cancer Research*, **11**: 540–542, 1951.

PATTI, J., and MOORE, A. E., Heterologous growth of sarcoma 180 with progression to death of hosts. *Cancer Research*, **10**: 674–678, 1950.

PURDY, W. J., The propagation of the Rous sarcoma No. I in ducklings. *Brit. J. Exp. Med.*, **13**: 473–479, 1932.

RASK-NIELSEN, H. C., and RASK-NIELSEN, R., Further studies on a transmissible myeloid leukosis in white mice. II. *Acta Path. & Microbiol. Scand.*, **15**: 169–175, 1938.

RATCLIFFE, H. L., Spontaneous tumors in two colonies of rats of the Wistar Institute of Anatomy and Biology. *Am. J. Path.*, **16**: 237–254, 1940.

REVERDY, J., RUDALI, G., DUPLAN, J.-F., and LATARJET, R., Leucémogenèse chez des souris AKR irradiées (rayons X) à la naissance. *Le Sang*, **29**: 796–804, 1958.

RIBACCHI, R., and GIRALDO, G., Leukemia virus release in chemically or physically induced lymphomas in BALB/c mice. pp. 701–711 in: *Conference on Murine Leukemia. Nat. Cancer Inst. Monograph No. 22*, U.S. Publ. Health Service, Bethesda, Md., 1966.

RICHTER, M. N., and MACDOWELL, E. C., The experimental transmission of leukemia in mice. *Proc. Soc. Exp. Biol. & Med.*, **26**: 362–364, 1929.

RICHTER, M. N., and MACDOWELL, E. C., Studies on leukemia in mice. I. The experimental transmission of leukemia. *J. Exp. Med.*, **51**: 659–673, 1930.

RICHTER, M. N., and MACDOWELL, E. C., Studies on mouse leukemia. VII. The relation of cell death to the potency of inoculated cell suspensions. *J. Exp. Med.*, **57**: 1–20, 1933.

RICHTER, M. N., and MACDOWELL, E. C., Experiments with mammalian leukemia. *Physiol. Reviews*, **15**: 509–524, 1935.

ROGEL, R., JULLIEN, P., RUDALI, G., and STERN, G., Étude de corpuscules contenant des acides nucléiques, dans les tissus leucosiques de souris AkR. *Le Sang*, **29**: 292–297, 1958.

ROGERS, S., KIDD, J. G., and ROUS, P., An etiological study of the cancers arising from the virus-induced papillomas of domestic rabbits. (Abstract). *Proc. Am. Assoc. Cancer Research*, **10**: 237, 1950.

ROUS, P., Transmission of a malignant new growth by means of a cell-free filtrate. *J. Am. Med. Assoc.*, **56**: 198, 1911.

ROUS, P., and MURPHY, J. B., Tumor implantations in the developing embryo. Experiments with a transmissible sarcoma of the fowl. *J. Am. Med. Assoc.*, **56**: 741–742, 1911.

RUBIN, H., The production of virus by Rous sarcoma cells. *Ann. N.Y. Acad. Sci.*, **68**: 449–472, 1957.

RUDALI, G., DESORMEAUX, B., and JULIARD, L., Action d'hormones mâles et femelles sur la leucémogenèse des souris AkR. *Bull. du Cancer*, **43**: 445–449, 1956a.

RUDALI, G., DUPLAN, J. F., and LATARJET, R., Latence des leucoses chez des souris Ak injectées avec un extrait leucémique a-cellulaire Ak. *Compt. Rend. Acad. Sci.* (*Paris*), **242**: 837–839, 1956b.

RUDALI, G., DUPLAN, J. F., and LATARJET, R., Leucémogenèse chez des souris AkR injectées à la naissance avec un extrait leucémique aqueux isologue. *Bull. du Cancer*, **44**: 440–443, 1957.

RUDALI, G., JULLIEN, P., and JULIARD, L., Action des hormones sur la leucémogenèse des souris. *Revue Française d'Études Cliniques et Biologiques*, **4**: 607–613, 1959.

RUDALI, G., and YOURKOVSKI, N., L'élevage des souris de lignée pure à la Fondation Curie. *Presse Med.*, **64**: 2045–2047, 1956.

SALAMAN, M. H., Haemagglutination by extracts of tumours and of some normal tissues. *Brit. J. Cancer*, **2**: 253–267, 1948.

SAXTON, J. A., JR., BOON, M. C., and FURTH, J., Observations on the inhibition of development of spontaneous leukemia in mice by underfeeding. *Cancer Research*, **4**: 401–409, 1944.

SAXTON, J. A., JR., SPERLING, G. A., BARNES, L. L., and MCCAY, C. M., The influence of nutrition upon the incidence of spontaneous tumors of the albino rat. *Acta Internat. Union Against Cancer*, **6**: 423–431, 1948.

SCHMIDT, F., Leukämie und Virus. Versuch einer Deutung experimenteller Ergebnisse bei Tier und Mensch. *Zeitschr. ges. Inn. Medizin & Grenzgebiete*, **12**: 337–348, 1957.

SCHOOLMAN, H. M., SPURRIER, W., SCHWARTZ, S. O., and SZANTO, P. B., Studies in leukemia. VII. The induction of leukemia in Swiss mice by means of cell-free filtrates of leukemic mouse brain. *Blood*, **12**: 694–700, 1957.

SCHRAMM, T., GRAFFI, A., and FÖRSTER, W., Weitere Versuche zum Nachweis einer infektiösen RNS aus virusinduzierten Mauseleukämien. *Arch. f. Geschwulstforsch.*, **25**: 212–214, 1965.

SCHWARTZ, S. O., and SCHOOLMAN, H. M., The etiology of leukemia: The status of the virus as causative agent—A review. *Blood*, **14**: 279–294, 1959.

SCHWARTZ, S. O., SCHOOLMAN, H. M., and SZANTO, P. B., Studies in leukemia. IV. The acceleration of the development of AKR lymphoma by means of cell-free filtrates. *Cancer Research*, **16**: 559–564, 1956.

SCHWARTZ, S. O., SCHOOLMAN, H. M., SZANTO, P. B., and SPURRIER, W., Studies in leukemia. IV. The induction of leukemia in AKR mice by means of cell-free brain filtrates of humans who died of leukemia. *Cancer Research*, **17**: 218–221, 1957.

SCHWARTZ, S. O., SCHOOLMAN, H. M., SZANTO, P. B., and SPURRIER, W., The induction of leukemia in AKR mice by cell-free filtrate of leukemic mouse and human brain. pp. 345–349 in: *Proc. Third Nat. Cancer Conference*. J. B. Lippincott Co., Philadelphia, 1957.

SCHWARTZ, S. O., SCHOOLMAN, H. M., SPURRIER, W., and YATES, L., Leukemia. VIII. Leukemogenic effect of brain filtrates after serial passage through mice. *Proc. Soc. Exp. Biol. & Med.*, **97**: 397–399, 1958.

SCHWARTZ, S. O., SPURRIER, W., YATES, L., and MADUROS, B. P., The induction of leukemia in Swiss mice with human leukemic brain extracts. (Abstract). *Proc. Am. Assoc. Cancer Research*, **3**: 149, 1960.

SEIBOLD, H. R., RATHBONE, R. R., and FURTH, J., Studies on transmissible lymphadenosis of mice. *Proc. Soc. Exp. Biol. & Med.*, **29**: 629–631, 1932.

SHARP, D. G., ECKERT, E. A., BEARD, D., and BEARD, J. W., Morphology of the virus of avian erythro-myeloblastic leucosis and a comparison with the agent of Newcastle disease. *J. Bact.*, **63**: 151–161, 1952.

SHAY, H., GRUENSTEIN, M., and GLAZER, L., Uniform transfer to random bred rats of lymphatic leukemia induced by gastric instillation of methylcholanthrene. *Proc. Soc. Exp. Biol. & Med.*, **75**: 753–754, 1950.

SHAY, H., GRUENSTEIN, M., MARX, H. E., and GLAZER, L., The development of lymphatic and myelogenous leukemia in Wistar rats following gastric instillation of methylcholanthrene. *Cancer Research*, **11**: 29–34, 1951.

SIEGLER, R., and RICH, M. A., Unilateral thymic lymphoma in AKR mice. *Trans. N.Y. Acad. Sci.*, **25**: 590–597, 1963.

SINKOVICS, J. G., SPURRIER, W. A., and SCHWARTZ, S. O., Studies in leukemia. XII. Interference and reactivation experiments with cell-free tissue extracts of leukemic Swiss mice. *Blood*, **15**: 95–102, 1960.

SLYE, M., The relation of heredity to the occurrence of spontaneous leukemia, pseudo-leukemia, lymphosarcoma and allied diseases in mice. Preliminary report. *Am. J. Cancer*, **15**: 1361–1368, 1931.

STASNEY, J., CANTAROW, A., and PASCHKIS, K. E., Production of neoplasms by injection of fractions of mammalian neoplasms. *Cancer Research*, **10**: 775–782, 1950.

STEWART, S. E., Leukemia in mice produced by a filterable agent present in AKR leukemic tissues with notes on a sarcoma produced by the same agent. (Abstract). *Anat. Record*, **117**: 532, 1953.

STEWART, S. E., Neoplasms in mice inoculated with cell-free extracts or filtrates of leukemic mouse tissues. I. Neoplasms of the parotid and adrenal glands. *J. Nat. Cancer Inst.*, **15**: 1391–1415, 1955a.

STEWART, S. E., Neoplasms in mice inoculated with cell-free extracts or filtrates of leukemic mouse tissues. II. Leukemia in hybrid mice produced by cell-free filtrates. *J. Nat. Cancer Inst.*, **16**: 41–53, 1955b.

STRONG, L. C., The establishment of the "A" strain of inbred mice. *J. Heredity*, **27**: 21–24, 1936.

STRONG, L. C., The origin of some inbred mice. *Cancer Research*, **2**: 531–539, 1942.

SYVERTON, J. T., and ROSS, J. D., The virus theory of leukemia. *Am. J. Med.*, **28**: 683–698, 1960.

THOMPSON, S. W., HUSEBY, R. A., FOX, M. A., DAVIS, C. L., and HUNT, R. D., Spontaneous tumors in the Sprague-Dawley rat. *J. Nat. Cancer Inst.*, **27**: 1037–1057, 1961.

TOCH, P., HIRSCH, B. B., BROWN, M. B., NAGAREDA, C. S., and KAPLAN, H. S., Lymphoid tumor incidence in mice treated with estrogen and X-radiation. *Cancer Research*, **16**: 890–893, 1956.

TOTH, B., Development of malignant lymphomas by cell-free filtrates prepared from a chemically induced mouse lymphoma. *Proc. Soc. Exp. Biol. & Med.*, **112**: 873–875, 1963.

TOTH, B., RAPPAPORT, H., and SHUBIK, P., Accelerated development of malignant lymphomas in AKR mice injected at birth with 7,12-dimethylbenz (a) anthracene. *Proc. Soc. Exp. Biol. & Med.*, **110**: 881–884, 1962.

TOTH, B., and SHUBIK, P., Studies with malignant lymphomas: possible interaction problems between chemical and viral-inducing agents. pp. 313–328 in: *Conference on Murine Leukemia. Nat. Cancer Inst. Monograph No. 22*, U.S. Publ. Health Service, Bethesda, Md., 1966.

UPTON, A. C., and FURTH, J., The effects of cortisone on the development of spontaneous leukemia in mice and on its induction by irradiation. *Blood*, **9**: 686–695, 1954.

WOGLOM, W. H., Immunity to transplantable tumours. *Cancer Review*, **4**: 129–214, 1929.

WOOLLEY, G. W., Occurrence of "neck tumors" in cortisone-treated leukemic-strain mice. (Abstract). *Proc. Am. Assoc. Cancer Research*, **1**: 53, 1954.

WOOLLEY, G. W., and PETERS, B. A., Prolongation of life in high-leukemia AKR mice by cortisone. *Proc. Soc. Exp. Biol. & Med.*, **82**: 286–287, 1953.

WOOLLEY, G. W., and SMALL, M. C., Experiments on cell-free transmission of mouse leukemia. *Cancer*, **9**: 1102–1106, 1956.

ZILBER, L. A., and POSTNIKOVA, Z. A., Induction of a leukemogenic agent by a chemical carcinogen in inbred mice. pp. 397–403 in: *Conference on Murine Leukemia. Nat. Cancer Inst. Monograph No. 22*, U.S. Publ. Health Service, Bethesda, Md., 1966.

CHAPTER 12

Isolation of the Mouse Leukemia Virus from Transplanted Mouse Tumors

In the preceding chapter we discussed the presence of the mouse leukemia virus in leukemic mice. The virus could be isolated not only from different organs, such as thymus, spleen, liver, lymphoid tumors, or blood, of leukemic mouse donors, but also from apparently normal and healthy tissues of mice that had been inoculated with the virus, but were used as donors prior to development of leukemia. Furthermore, the virus could be isolated also from normal embryos removed from Ak or C58 female mice, i.e. from animals of inbred lines known to have a high incidence of spontaneous leukemia.

After the viral etiology of mouse leukemia had been established, it was only logical to seek isolation of the causative agent either from organs of leukemic mouse donors, or from normal tissues of healthy mice known to carry the virus, and earmarked to develop disease later in life. Thus, isolation of the virus from such sources was to be expected, and has been accomplished repeatedly. However, it did not always succeed because of the relatively low potency of the virus carried in mice infected with the "wild" or naturally transmitted virus.

In continuation of the study of epidemiology of the mouse leukemia virus it gradually became apparent, however, that this virus is widely prevalent not only in virus-injected animals, or in mice of high-leukemic inbred lines, but also in mice of a variety of strains having a relatively low incidence of spontaneous leukemia. Furthermore, the rather surprising observation was made that the mouse leukemia virus could be recovered also from certain mouse tumors, such as induced or transplanted sarcomas or carcinomas, having no apparent relation to leukemia.

Studies dealing with the isolation of leukemogenic virus strains in mice from induced or transplanted tumors will be discussed in this chapter.

The Unexpected Development of Leukemia Following Inoculation of Filtrates from Parotid Carcinomas or Subcutaneous Sarcomas into Newborn Mice

When filtrates prepared from spontaneous Ak leukemias were inoculated into newborn C3H mice, some of the injected animals developed, instead of leukemia, carcinomas of the parotid glands, or subcutaneous fibromyxosarcomas (Gross, 1953).* An attempt was then made to transmit these tumors serially by filtrates. When, however, cell-free extracts, prepared from either parotid carcinomas or subcutaneous sarcomas, were inoculated into newborn C3H mice, only some of the injected animals developed carcinomas or sarcomas. Unexpectedly, 16 per cent of mice that had been inoculated with parotid tumor filtrates (Gross, 1955) and 7 per cent of those that had been inoculated with sarcoma filtrates (Gross, 1956, 1957) developed typical lymphatic leukemia. This incidence was considerably higher than that observed in untreated controls, or in those control groups that received injections of normal organ extracts.

This observation revealed the curious fact that filtrates prepared from non-leukemic mouse tumors, such as carcinomas or sarcomas, could induce leukemia following inoculation into newborn mice of a susceptible strain. It was possible to speculate that the tumors serving for the preparation of extracts contained a latent leukemic virus. Such an assumption appeared quite logical, at least in this limited series of experiments, since the tumors employed for preparation of the leukemogenic filtrates had been induced with extracts prepared from leukemic mouse tissues (Gross, 1955).

* * *

A similar observation was made independently, at about the same time and in considerably more extensive studies, by Graffi and his associates (1955, 1956) with filtrates prepared from transplanted mouse tumors. Before we describe in more detail this interesting observation, it is necessary to describe briefly the origin and nature of transplanted mouse tumors which have served for many years as a convenient experimental tool in leading cancer research laboratories.

Transplantation of Tumors by Cell-Graft, and the Establishment of Certain Transplantable Tumor Strains

During the past several decades, most of the routine experimental transmissions of tumors in various laboratories were accomplished by

* This interesting observation will be discussed in a more detailed manner in the chapter dealing with the Parotid Tumor (Polyoma) Virus.

cell-graft. The transplanted tumors, such as sarcomas or carcinomas, growing either in mice or rats, retained as a rule their morphology, with the exception of certain mouse carcinomas, which, in the course of transplantation, became more cellular and eventually changed into undifferentiated sarcomas (reviewed by H. L. Stewart *et al.*, 1959).

Many of the mouse tumors currently used for routine transplantation originated several decades ago as spontaneous mammary carcinomas in old female mice. Since no inbred strains of mice were available at that time, the transplantation of such tumors at first encountered considerable difficulties. Only a few of such tumors could be transplanted initially. On successive transplantations, however, some of these tumors grew more readily; a few eventually became adapted to the serial grafting.

At first, such tumors grew only in mice related to the hosts in which the initial tumors had developed. Gradually, however, the transplanted tumors became more independent and grew indiscriminately in hosts of different strains of the same species.

Paul Ehrlich collected in his laboratories in Frankfurt a large number of female mice with spontaneous mammary carcinomas. He attempted to transplant, by graft, over one hundred of them. Only 14 could be transplanted. The various Ehrlich tumors (Ehrlich and Apolant, 1905. Ehrlich, 1907), that have been carried since that time by successive cell-grafts in different laboratories, were derived from one or another of the original lines of Ehrlich's carcinomas. Changes in morphology occurred in some of the tumors in the course of successive transplantations. A few gradually became more cellular and eventually changed into sarcomas. Other tumors retained their essentially carcinomatous morphology.

Most of these tumors have been transplanted by the trocar method, by pushing small bits of tumor tissue under the skin or in the muscles of the animals. In some instances tumor cell suspensions were prepared and inoculated subcutaneously or intramuscularly. In other instances the tumor cell suspensions were inoculated intraperitoneally. In the course of successive serial intraperitoneal inoculations of tumor cell suspensions, some of the transplanted carcinomas gradually changed into ascites-forming tumors. A few retained such ascites-forming property through successive cell transfers.

Transplantable Tumors—A Convenient Tool in Experimental Cancer Research

Several types of transplantable tumors have thus been established in mice, and a few also in rats, during the past decades. Such tumor strains as the transplantable mouse carcinoma (Ehrlich), the transplantable mouse ascites carcinoma (Ehrlich), or the transplantable mouse sarcoma S.37, etc., have been carried through successive cell-grafts in many laboratories. Once established and stabilized, the transplanted tumors usually retained their morphology (see Stewart *et al.*, 1959).

The original tumor from which S.37 was derived was a spontaneous mammary adenocarcinoma, designated Carcinoma 37, that appeared in the thoracic region of an old female mouse of the Imperial Cancer Research Fund stock. The origin and early transplant generations of Carcinoma 37 and its gradual transformation to an anaplastic tumor were described by Haaland (1908) and Bashford (1911), and recently reviewed by H. L. Stewart *et al.* (1959).

On initial transplantation, only 8 out of 69 inoculated mice grew tumors. Gradually, the incidence of "takes" increased on successive transplantations. At the same time a sarcomatous transformation of the tumors occurred. Broad bands of atypical spindle-shaped cells appeared in the stroma, and these, in turn, were replaced by atypical polymorphous cells considered to be the sarcomatous components. Eventually the carcinomatous cell structure was entirely replaced by sarcoma. Once the sarcomatous pattern was firmly established, the tumors did not revert to a carcinoma. Coincidentally with these changes in morphology, the growth of the tumor was increased. A tumor of one of the sublines finally became stabilized as an atypical polymorphous-cell sarcoma and later became known as Sarcoma 37, or briefly S.37. This tumor, now widely used in many laboratories, grows in mice of many different strains. In some strains, such as C3H or C57 Black, S.37 grows only temporarily and frequently regresses. In other strains, such as BALB/c or DBA/2, Sarcoma 37 grows progressively, without regression, in more than 90 per cent of the inoculated mice. Actually, this tumor cannot be classified either as a sarcoma or as a carcinoma. It is an undifferentiated neoplasm. However, this tumor has been called Sarcoma 37 for over half a century, and it seems appropriate to retain its designation (see Stewart *et al.*, 1959).

A few of the transplantable tumor strains became useful tools in experimental cancer research and became widely used in many laboratories. The main advantage of using these tumors in cancer research was the fact that fast and progressively growing tumors could be obtained promptly, usually within two weeks, in large numbers of commercially available non-inbred mice. This was very convenient for such purposes as the investigation of the action of hormones on the growth of established tumors, etc., and particularly for chemotherapy studies.

INDUCTION OF MYELOID LEUKEMIA (CHLOROLEUKEMIA) WITH FILTRATES FROM TRANSPLANTED MOUSE TUMORS

The Experiments of Graffi

The successful cell-free transmission of spontaneous mouse leukemia, based on the use of newborn mice for the bio-assay of filtrates prepared from leukemic mouse tissues (Gross, 1951b), provided a renewed incentive for the search for filterable oncogenic agents in tumors hitherto thought to be of non-viral origin.

Arnold Graffi and his associates (1955, 1956), as well as Schmidt (1955, 1956, 1957) at the Institute for Medicine and Biology of the German Academy of Sciences in Berlin-Buch, carried out a series of experiments in an attempt to recover filterable oncogenic agents from a variety of transplanted mouse tumors. Newborn mice were employed for the inoculation of filtrates prepared from different tumors.

The curious and unexpected observation was made in these studies that such filtrates did not reproduce, as might have been anticipated, tumors similar to those that had served for the preparation of the extracts. Instead, a large number of the inoculated mice developed leukemia, usually of the myeloid form, with characteristic green discoloration of the lymph nodes (chloroleukemia).

Graffi realized at once the importance of this unexpected observation. During the succeeding years, in extensive studies, he and his coworkers carried out a large number of precise experiments which established the fundamental fact that certain transplanted mouse tumors can carry latent leukemic viruses, and that cell-free extracts, prepared from a variety of such tumors, could induce leukemia following inoculation into newborn mice of susceptible strains. Certain tumors yielded a considerable quantity of a potent leukemic virus; other tumors yielded only a relatively small quantity of the leukemogenic virus, or, in spite of repeated attempts, yielded no leukemic virus at all on bio-assay experiments.

Tumors Used for the Preparation of Filtrates in Graffi's Experiments

Several different transplanted mouse tumors were employed by Graffi and his associates for the preparation of filtrates. The tumor extracts of 20 or 10 per cent concentration were homogenized at 0°C, then centrifuged and filtered through Schott G 4 glass filters. The leukemogenic potency of the filtrates, as determined on bio-assay studies carried out on newborn mice, varied according to the tumors from which the filtrates had been prepared. Some of the tumors employed had a high leukemogenic potency. To this group belonged the Ehrlich ascites carcinoma which induced an incidence of over 50 per cent of leukemia, usually of the myeloid type, after an average latency of 8 months.

The best source of leukemogenic virus was found in two closely related reticulum-cell sarcomas, designated by Graffi by the symbols Sa I and Sa II. Both originated spontaneously in the same mouse and had been transplanted serially by cell-graft for 3 to 4 years prior to their use for the preparation of filtrates. It is conceivable that both were caused by the same virus.

Since reticulum-cell sarcomas represent a form of lymphoma, this particular virus strain isolated by Graffi was actually comparable to a mouse leukemia virus recovered directly from lymphoid tumors obtained from spontaneous or transplanted mouse leukemia. This was in contrast to the origin of other leukemogenic virus strains isolated by Graffi and his associates from mouse sarcomas and carcinomas unrelated to lymphomas, such as Ehrlich carcinoma, sarcoma S.37, etc.

Filtrates prepared from Sa I and Sa II and inoculated into newborn mice induced an incidence of up to 80 per cent of leukemia after an average latency of 8 months; again, most of the induced leukemias were of the myeloid form (chloroleukemia).

One of the leukemic tumors induced with Sa I filtrate, and designated by the symbol SOV 16, was again used for the preparation of filtrates. These filtrates were then inoculated into newborn mice, and induced an incidence of up to 85 per cent of leukemia after an average latency of only 4.2 months; approximately 37 per cent of these leukemias were of the myeloid form.

On the other hand, the leukemogenic potency of certain other tumors tested was low. "Carcinoma 450," originally induced with a carcinogenic hydrocarbon, yielded a filtrate which proved inactive on inoculation tests. Filtrates prepared from another carcinogen-induced tumor (DMBA sarcoma) induced an incidence of about 10 per cent of leukemia among the inoculated mice. Similarly, only 10 per cent of mice inoculated with filtrates prepared from the well-known transplantable mouse sarcoma S.37 developed leukemia (Graffi *et al.*, 1956).

The origin of the transplantable mouse sarcoma S.37 is discussed on page 473 of this chapter. It is of interest that this well-known transplantable mouse tumor did not yield a potent leukemogenic virus in Graffi's laboratory, whereas in experiments carried out by Moloney at the National Cancer Institute, which will be discussed on subsequent pages of this chapter, extracts prepared from sarcoma S.37 proved highly leukemogenic on bio-assay. It should be pointed out, however, that even though the individual strains of the S.37 sarcoma carried in different laboratories had the same initial origin, they could have picked up, nevertheless, different "passenger" viruses in the course of successive transplantations from host-to-host over periods of years. It is conceivable, therefore, that individual strains of S.37 tumor transplants, employed in different laboratories, could vary considerably in their capacity to serve as a source for the isolation of a virus inducing leukemia in mice.

Neither tumors nor leukemia could be induced when filtrates from heterologous rat tumors (Walker carcinoma or Jensen sarcoma) or when normal mouse tissue extracts were inoculated. Of a total of 332 newborn mice inoculated with such extracts in a control series, only one developed leukemia.

Svec and his coworkers in Bratislava, Czechoslovakia (1957), reported induction of myelogenous and/or erythroblastic leukemia in rats following inoculation of filtrates prepared directly from a transplantable rat sarcoma. In these experiments newborn rats of the Wistar strain were inoculated with the filtrates. Of 58 inoculated rats, 12 (20 per cent) developed myeloid leukemia after a latency varying from 6 to 9 months. Some of the leukemic rats also had a considerable involvement of the erythropoietic system, justifying a diagnosis of erythroblastic leukemia.

Mice Used for Inoculation. Influence of Age on Susceptibility to the Leukemic Agent. Several strains of mice were used for the bio-assay, namely the inbred strains Agnes-Bluhm (AB) (albino), as well as strains sg and db; in addition, non-inbred animals of the strains M and W were also used (Krischke *et al.*, 1956. Graffi, 1957). The incidence of spontaneous leukemia in mice of these strains was less than 1.3 per cent (Graffi, 1957, 1958. Graffi *et al.*, 1956).

All strains of mice employed for inoculation were susceptible to the leukemogenic potency of the filtrates. When filtrates from Sa I were inoculated into mice of strains AB, M, and W, the incidence of induced leukemia was 48 per cent in the AB strain, as compared with 61 and 63 per cent in strains M and W, respectively (Graffi *et al.*, 1956). In another series (Krischke *et al.*, 1956), filtrates prepared from Sa I were inoculated into newborn mice of strains AB, db and sg. The incidence of induced leukemia was 48 per cent in mice of strain AB, as compared with 30 and 36 per cent in strains db and sg, respectively.

Newborn and suckling mice up to 11 days of age were most susceptible, but adult animals could also be successfully inoculated. When newborn, less than one-day-old, mice were inoculated with the filtrates, 46 per cent developed leukemia. The incidence was about the same (42 per cent) following inoculation of suckling, 2 to 11-day-old, mice. Adult mice were relatively more resistant; following inoculation of the filtrates, up to 29 per cent of them developed leukemia after an average latency of 6.5 months (Gimmy *et al.*, 1956).

Transplantability of the Induced Leukemias. The leukemias induced by Graffi and his associates following inoculation of tumor filtrates into newborn mice proved only occasionally transplantable by cell-graft. Approximately 10 per cent of the induced leukemia could be transplanted to mice of the respective strains. Only a few leukemias could be carried serially by successive cell-transplantations (Graffi *et al.*, 1956).

Assuming that in Graffi's experiments homozygous mice of thoroughly inbred strains of mice were employed, this observation was difficult to explain, and was in marked contrast to that dealing with mouse leukemia induced in either C3H or C57 Brown mice with Ak or C58 leukemic filtrates. Such leukemias proved to be transplantable without difficulty by cell-graft (Gross, 1953, 1955, 1957). On the other hand, the parotid tumors, also induced with Ak leukemic filtrates in C3H mice, proved to be transplantable only with difficulty (Gross, 1957).

Serial Cell-free Passage of the Virus Isolated from Mouse Tumors. Induction of Different Forms of Leukemia with the Same Virus Strain

The leukemogenic virus isolated from transplanted mouse tumors could be readily passed serially, in the form of filtrates inoculated into newborn mice. The latency was shortened and the incidence of induced leukemia increased with successive passages. The forms of induced leukemia varied from one passage to another. In one of the experiments, in the first cell-free passage, the majority of induced leukemias was of the myeloid form (chloroleukemia); in the next passage, the majority of the induced leukemias was lymphatic, and only 25 per cent of the chloroleukemic form (Bielka *et al.*, 1955). Several leukemogenic virus strains, isolated from different tumors, but essentially similar in their biological and pathogenic properties, were studied and maintained in serial passages.

In more recent experiments, Graffi and his colleagues observed a variety of forms of leukemia developing in the course of serial passage of the virus in mice and in rats (Fey and Graffi, 1965. Graffi *et al.*, 1966). Although in some experiments the incidence of myeloid leukemia was higher following inoculation of extracts prepared from myeloid forms, attempts to develop and maintain a purely "myeloid" or a "lymphatic" virus strain, which would consistently induce only a single form of leukemia, did not succeed.

In this respect again the Graffi virus strain was essentially similar to the passage A virus, except that the incidence of myeloid leukemia was higher following inoculation of the Graffi virus. As reported in more detail in the preceding chapter, the passage A virus also induced a variety of forms of leukemia following inoculation into mice or rats; it was not possible, however, to develop and maintain a purely "lymphatic" or a "myeloid" variant of the mouse leukemia virus (Gross, 1962, 1963a,c).

Studies on Natural Transmission of the Virus. In studies on the natural transmission of the leukemogenic virus strain isolated from transplanted mouse tumors, Graffi and his coworkers made observations essentially similar to those recorded previously in our studies carried out with the passage A mouse leukemia virus, and discussed in more detail in the preceding chapter of this monograph.

Experiments on "Horizontal" Transmission of the Virus. In these studies, newborn mice of low-leukemic strains were inoculated with the virus. Only one half of each litter was injected; the inoculated mice were then placed in the same nests with their non-injected litter-mates, and were raised together. Among 97 mice exposed to contact infection, only 6 per cent developed leukemia. This compared with a less than 2 per cent incidence of spontaneous leukemia observed in control mice of the same inbred line. The incidence in mice exposed to contact infection was, therefore, only slighly higher than that expected to occur in normal controls, but was of interest, and probably significant, particularly in view of the fact that similar results were obtained in studies on contact transmission carried out independently in our laboratory with the passage A mouse leukemia virus (Gross, 1962).

Vertical Transmission of the Virus. Natural transmission of the virus from one generation to another was also investigated. Newborn mice of low-leukemic strains were inoculated with the virus; after they reached sexual maturity, they were mated. Non-treated offspring of virus-injected parents were then observed through several successive generations for development of leukemia. The incidence of leukemia developing in the F_1 generation was relatively high; in some of the individual experiments, 3 out of 5, or 3 out of 4, untreated offspring developed leukemia. This incidence diminished considerably in the second and third generation; leukemia was observed to develop only occasionally in some of these mice. The incidence of leukemia observed in the fourth generation of untreated offspring was negligible, and did not exceed that observed to develop spontaneously in mice of this strain (Krischke and Graffi, 1961. Graffi and Krischke, 1962). These results were essentially identical with results of similar studies carried out previously with the passage A virus (Gross, 1955).

Transmission of Virus Through the Milk. Graffi and his colleagues observed that under certain experimental conditions the mouse leukemia virus could be transmitted from virus-injected mothers to their offspring through the milk (Graffi and Krischke, 1962). A similar observation was made by Law and Moloney (1961), and also in our studies (Gross, 1962b), discussed in more detail in the preceding chapter.

*Induction of Leukemia in Rats with the Mouse Leukemia Virus.** Graffi and his associates (Graffi and Gimmy, 1957, 1959. Gimmy *et al.*, 1960) reported induction of leukemia in rats with the mouse leukemia virus which they had isolated from transplanted mouse tumors. This was the first time that a mouse leukemia virus was found to be leukemogenic for rats. Newborn or suckling rats of the Wistar strain were used for intracerebral or intraperitoneal inoculation of filtrates prepared from leukemic mouse donors. The latency period varied from about 3 to 8 months; either lymphatic or myelogenous leukemia developed in the inoculated rats. Thymic lymphomas were a common manifestation of the disease. Disseminated lymphosarcomas, and less frequently also reticulum-cell sarcomas, were found in a variety of organs, most frequently in lymph

* Induction of leukemia in rats with the mouse leukemia virus and passage of the virus from rats to rats are discussed in more detail in the preceding chapter of this monograph.

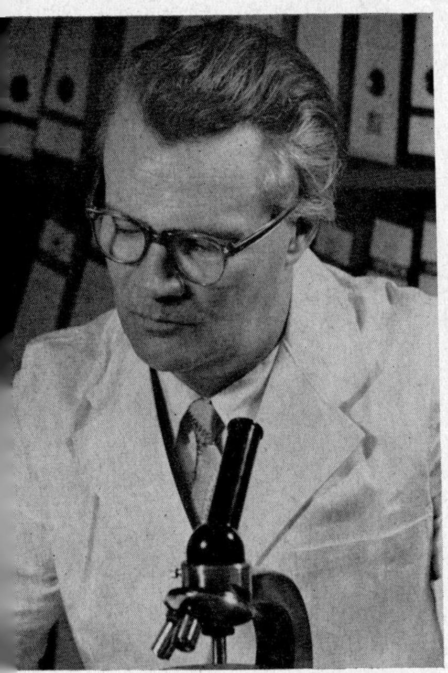

Arnold Graffi

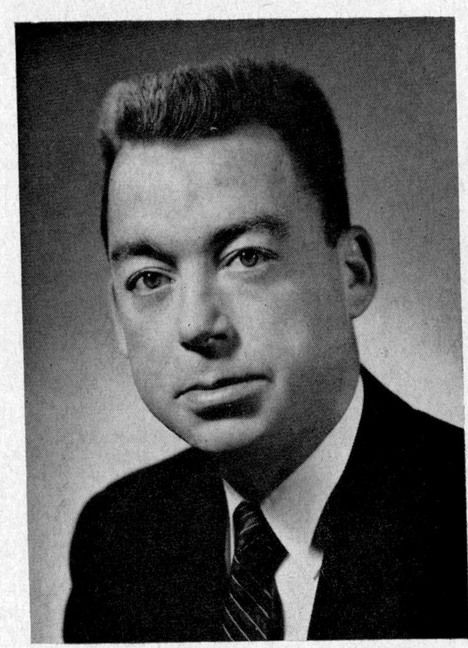

John B. Moloney

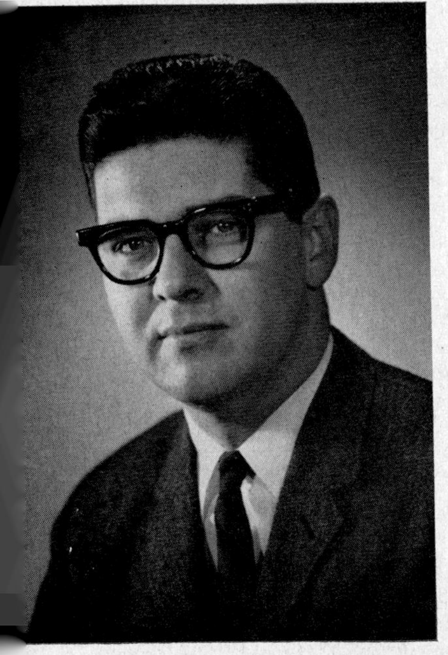

Frank J. Rauscher

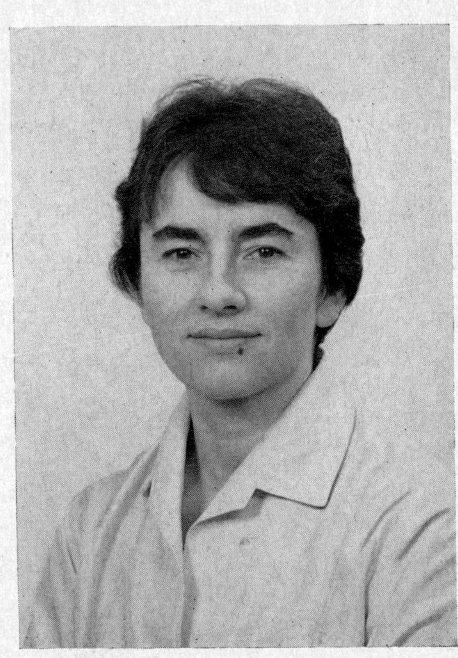

Jennifer J. Harvey

FIG. 43.

nodes, spleen, and liver. The incidence of induced leukemia varied, and was relatively high in some experiments, but averaged only about 10 per cent. Spontaneous leukemia was not observed in untreated animals. Graffi and Gimmy (1959) were able to pass, by filtrates, the leukemogenic virus not only from mice to rats, but also from rats to rats. The incidence of leukemia induced with the virus harvested from rats was about 30 per cent, and the latency varied from 3 to 13 months (Graffi, 1960).

Some Physical and Biological Properties of the Leukemogenic Virus Isolated by Graffi

Graffi and his colleagues studied the physical and biological properties of the leukemogenic virus strains recovered from transplanted mouse tumors. Essentially these properties were identical with those described in studies of the passage A mouse leukemia virus, described in the preceding chapter. The leukemogenic potency of the filtrates prepared from several different mouse tumors could be inactivated after heating to 65°C for 30 minutes (Graffi *et al.*, 1956).

In experiments reported by Lohmann and Schmidt (1957), and dealing with leukemogenic filtrates prepared from Ehrlich carcinoma, the leukemogenic potency of the filtrates was neutralized after heating to 56°C for 30 minutes. In our more recent experiments, in which we employed the Graffi virus strain, heating to only 50°C for 30 minutes inactivated completely the virus (Gross, 1964a). Thus, the Graffi virus strain was found to be inactivated by heating under the same experimental conditions as the passage A virus.

Exposure, *in vitro*, to ethyl ether inactivated completely the leukemogenic potency of the virus strain isolated by Graffi (Graffi and Bielka, 1959). The leukemogenic agent could be recovered from tumor tissues after storage in 50 per cent glycerin for one month; however, the potency of extracts prepared from such tissues was diminished (Graffi, 1958). The leukemogenic virus could be preserved at – 16°C for at least several weeks (Krischke *et al.*, 1956).

Graffi and his coworkers found that the leukemogenic virus present in tumor filtrates was antigenic. Sera prepared from rabbits immunized with the tumor filtrates neutralized *in vitro* the leukemogenic potency of the extracts (Graffi *et al.*, 1955, 1957). Normal rabbit serum, or serum from rabbits that had been immunized with normal mouse organs, had no neutralizing effect.

Electron Microscopic Studies. Ultrathin sections of leukemic tissues from mouse donors with virus-induced leukemia were studied in the electron microscope by Heine, Graffi and their coworkers (1959); these studies revealed presence in intercellular spaces, frequently adjacent to protoplasmic cell membranes, of spherical particles varying in diameter from 70 to over 100 mμ; many of the particles had electron-dense nucleoids.

In our laboratory, we have carried out, with Dr. Feldman, electron microscopic studies of the Graffi virus which we obtained recently from his laboratory (Gross, 1964a). In our studies we found that the virus particles present in the tissues of mice with Graffi virus strain-induced leukemia were in their size, morphology, and location, indistinguishable from those observed in our previous studies dealing with the passage A virus-induced leukemia, and described in more detail in the preceding chapter of this monograph.

A Review of Results of Graffi's Experiments, and Their Implications

After a review of the experiments of Graffi and his associates, it is apparent that these investigators isolated from transplanted mouse tumors leukemogenic virus strains pathogenic for mice and rats. Some of the virus strains isolated from a few transplanted tumors were very potent and induced a high incidence of leukemia in susceptible mice. Attempts to isolate leukemogenic viruses from certain other tumors, however, met with only partial success, or did not succeed at all.

The experiments of Graffi and his associates raised several fundamental questions. What was the nature of the causative factor responsible for the induction of leukemia resulting from inoculation of tumor extracts? Was the leukemogenic potency of such filtrates due to the presence of a distinct leukemia-inducing virus? If so, what was the relation, if any, of the leukemogenic virus, present in the tumor filtrates, to the tumor cells from which these extracts were prepared?

It was possible to speculate that the cell-free extracts prepared from transplanted mouse tumors contained a single multipotent oncogenic virus capable of inducing a variety of malignant tumors, as well as leukemia and lymphomas. It was difficult, however, to accept such an explanation. Filtrates prepared from transplanted tumors and inoculated into newborn mice consistently induced leukemia or lymphomas; they did not at any time induce solid tumors comparable in morphology to the sarcomas or carcinomas from which the extracts had been prepared. Furthermore, the leukemogenic virus isolated from tumors could be passed serially from mouse to mouse, invariably inducing leukemia and related lymphomas on subsequent bio-assays. The pathogenic potency of these filtrates increased with successive passages, but the induced disease remained the same.

It appeared, therefore, more reasonable to assume that the transplanted tumors carried a latent leukemogenic virus, only incidentally present in the tumor cells.

A Leukemogenic "Passenger" Virus?

It is conceivable that in the course of many successive transplantations through mice of different strains, the tumors, which had served as a source for the preparation of the extracts, might have picked up a leukemogenic "passenger virus," present in a latent form in some of the mice that carried the tumor implants. Such a latent, but potentially leukemogenic, virus might have then been carried along with the tumor-grafts from one transplantation to another. No leukemia appeared in the animals carrying the tumor-grafts as long as the transplantations were made by the usual cell-graft method, using adult mice for inoculation. Under favorable experimental conditions, however, i.e. following inoculation of filtrates prepared from such tumors into newborn mice of susceptible strains, the leukemogenic virus, hitherto latent, might have become pathogenic, causing then the development of leukemia in some of the inoculated mice.

This assumption was consistent with the results of studies of physical, biological, and pathogenic properties of the leukemic virus strains isolated by Graffi and his colleagues from transplanted mouse tumors. These properties were essentially identical with those observed in the study of the mouse leukemia virus isolated from spontaneous mouse leukemia, and described in the preceding chapter of this monograph.

A Comment on the Forms of Leukemia Induced with the Graffi Virus Strain. There appeared to exist only one significant difference between the leukemic virus strain isolated by Graffi and his colleagues and the passage A virus isolated from spontaneous mouse leukemia. The majority of leukemias induced in Graffi's laboratory with his virus strain were of the myeloid form, including chloroleukemia. This point was at first considered to be of considerable importance, possibly distinguishing the Graffi virus strains from the passage A virus, since the latter has been observed to induce usually the lymphoid form of leukemia on inoculation tests. However, more recently we have learned that the form of leukemia induced with virus filtrates in mice and rats depends to a considerable extent on the genetic susceptibility of the host; the passage A virus was found to be capable of inducing in mice of certain inbred lines, and also in rats, not only lymphatic leukemia, but also the myeloid form, particularly in thymectomized animals. It is, therefore, conceivable that in Graffi's experiments, in which mice of certain inbred lines not commonly used in our laboratories were employed, the relatively higher susceptibility of these mice to induction of myeloid leukemia could have been, at least to some extent, responsible for the high incidence of myeloid leukemia observed in these studies. This point requires further clarification. It should be emphasized, however, that such an explanation would be consistent with results of our recent studies (Gross, 1964) in which we inoculated the leukemogenic virus obtained from Graffi's laboratory into newborn mice of either C3H(f) or BALB/c inbred lines. In mice of strain C3H(f) the Graffi virus induced only either lymphatic or stem-cell leukemia, whereas in mice of strain BALB/c the same virus induced a 58 per cent incidence of lymphatic leukemia, a 15 per cent incidence of stem-cell leukemia, and a 27 per cent incidence of myeloid leukemia, figures essentially comparable to those obtained with the passage A virus (Gross, 1963a, 1964a). Similar results were obtained in experiments carried out by Fiore-Donati and Chieco-Bianchi (1964), in which mice of several inbred strains were inoculated with the Graffi virus. Although the Graffi virus has been described as myelogenous, different forms of leukemia, i.e. lymphatic, stem-cell, and myeloid, were induced with this virus in various strains of mice. In AKR mice inoculation of the virus caused almost exclusively lymphatic leukemia which developed after an average latency of 14 weeks. The results of their experiments indicated that the forms of leukemia developing after inoculation of the Graffi virus were similar to those resulting from inoculation of the Ak mouse leukemia virus.

* * *

After a review of experimental data thus far obtained, it appears that Graffi and his coworkers isolated from transplanted mouse tumors a mouse leukemia virus essentially similar to that isolated in our laboratory from spontaneous mouse leukemia. Quantitative titration and careful serological tests may be required for precise identification of the virus strain isolated by Graffi. In order to compare the Graffi virus strain with the passage A virus, the bio-assay studies should be performed on the same inbred lines of mice which served for the study of the passage A virus, such as mice of strains C3H(f), BALB/c, or C57 Brown/cd.

Presence of Latent Leukemogenic Viruses in Normal Mice

The fact that a leukemogenic virus could be recovered from transplanted mouse tumors appeared puzzling at first. After a review of experimental data accumulated during the preceding decade it is apparent, however, that latent leukemogenic viruses are rather ubiquitously present not only in leukemic mouse tissues, and in organs of mice of high-leukemic inbred families known to carry naturally transmitted virus, but also in normal, healthy mice of strains essentially free from spontaneous leukemia.

Since leukemogenic viruses can be carried in certain organs of normal, healthy hosts, it should not be surprising to observe their presence also in neoplastic cells, such as transplanted mouse tumors. Malignant, fast growing cells have long been known to represent an excellent medium for propagation of a variety of microorganisms, including certain viruses.

Many normal mice may carry potentially leukemogenic agents. This was evident from studies in which leukemia was induced in mice of low-leukemic strains, such as C3H or C57 Brown, by total-body X-ray irradiation; the radiation-induced leukemogenic agents could then be transmitted by filtrates to other mice (Gross, 1958, 1959a). These experiments will be discussed in more detail in the next chapter of this monograph.

ISOLATION OF A POTENT STRAIN OF MOUSE LEUKEMIA VIRUS FROM A TRANSPLANTED MOUSE SARCOMA

The Experiments of Moloney

After Graffi and his associates demonstrated that a leukemogenic virus could be isolated from certain transplanted mouse tumors, Dr. John B. Moloney (1959, 1960a) at the National Cancer Institute in Bethesda, Md., made an attempt to recover a similar leukemogenic virus from a mouse sarcoma that had been transplanted serially, by cell-graft, in one of the National Cancer Institute's laboratories. The tumor used for the preparation of the extracts was Sarcoma 37 (S.37).* This well-known transplantable mouse tumor had been carried for 195 successive transplantations in mice of the strain A/LN by Dr. M. K. Barrett in his laboratory at the National Cancer Institute, before it was used by Moloney for the preparation of the cell-free extracts. No leukemias had been observed by Dr. Barrett in mice of strain A/LN, carrying the Sarcoma 37 implants (Moloney, 1960a,b).

Preparation of Cell-Free Extracts. The method of preparation of cell-free extracts developed in the experimental studies on Rous chicken sarcoma (Bryan, 1955. Moloney, 1956. Bryan and Moloney, 1957) was applied by Dr. Moloney in the course of his experiments carried out on mouse sarcoma 37.

A tumor cell suspension of 10 per cent concentration was first prepared using approximately isotonic (0.153 M) solution of potassium citrate for homogenization of the tumor tissue. Two different extraction procedures carried out at 8°C were then applied. One method consisted essentially of a series of successive differential centrifugations; the cells were sedimented and discarded in three initial centrifugations (two successive centrifugations, 20 minutes each, at 2,300 $\times g$, followed by a brief (one minute) centrifugation at 10,000 $\times g$). The supernate from the third centrifugation was then used for the

* This tumor has been transplanted in mice of various strains for the past fifty years. It originated as a spontaneous carcinoma in an old female mouse (Haaland, 1908), and on successive transplantations changed gradually into an anaplastic sarcoma (reviewed by H. L. Stewart *et al.*, 1959). The tumor can now be transplanted in many different strains of mice.

preparation of the extract. The active sub-cellular particles were sedimented by ultracentrifugation ($30{,}000 \times g$ for one hour), and the resulting pellet was resuspended in a small volume of sodium citrate buffer, then cleared from aggregates by low speed centrifugation ($5{,}000 \times g$ for 8 minutes), and used for bio-assay.

The alternate procedure included, as a preliminary step, filtration of the tumor extract through either Selas (02), Berkefeld (N), or Mandler filter candles. The virus present in the filtrate was then sedimented by ultra-centrifugation at $30{,}000 \times g$ to $80{,}000 \times g$ for one hour. As a final step, the sedimented pellet was resuspended in a small volume of sodium citrate buffer solution,* and used for bio-assay.

In the initial series of experiments, filtrates were employed for the bio-assay. Once it was established that leukemia could be induced with filtrates, only differential centrifugation has been employed for routine preparation of cell-free extracts, since a certain amount of virus is lost when extracts are filtered.

Induction of Lymphatic Leukemia Following Inoculation of Sarcoma 37 Filtrates into Newborn or Suckling BALB/c Mice

In the initial experiment, filtered Sarcoma 37 extracts were inoculated into newborn, less than 16-hour-old, and also into suckling, 1 to 16-day-old, mice of the BALB/c strain.† There was no appreciable difference in susceptibility between the newborn and suckling mice of this age-range employed for inoculation. Of 32 newborn and suckling, less than 8-day-old, mice inoculated with the filtrates, all developed leukemia after an average latency of 8 months. Of 56 suckling mice, 9 to 16 days old, inoculated with the same filtrates, all developed leukemia after a latency of 8.7 months.

Susceptibility of Young Adult Mice to Inoculation of the Leukemic Agent· Not only newborn and suckling mice of the BALB/c strain, but young adult animals also, were found to be susceptible to the inoculation of the leukemic virus. When filtrates prepared from leukemic BALB/c mice were inoculated into 74 young adult, 1 to 2-month-old, mice of the same strain, 70 of the inoculated mice (95 per cent) developed leukemia after an average latency of 4.5 months.

* Previous studies on chicken tumors suggested that in such buffers the Rous sarcoma virus could be preserved for relatively long periods of time without loss of infectivity (Bryan, 1955).

† This is one of the oldest inbred lines, initially developed by Dr. Halsey J. Bagg some 50 years ago at the Memorial Hospital, New York City (see also the chapter on "The Development of Inbred Strains of Mice, etc.," in this monograph). There exist several different sublines of the BALB strain. The incidence of spontaneous tumors, including leukemia, in mice of this strain varies, depending on the subline. In certain sublines, the incidence of spontaneous leukemia and lymphomas, developing in old mice, reaches some 15 to 20 per cent.

Morphology of the Induced Leukemia and Lymphomas. The induced disease presented the usual picture of disseminated lymphosarcomas or generalized lymphatic leukemia with greatly enlarged spleens and livers, and massive involvement of the thymus, and of peripheral and mesenteric lymph nodes. Essentially the morphology of leukemia or lymphosarcomas induced with the virus strain isolated by Moloney was indistinguishable from that induced with the passage A virus (Gross) and described in the preceding chapter.

Recovery of Virus from Induced Leukemia. BALB/c mice in which leukemia was induced by inoculation of the S.37 extracts were then used as donors for the preparation of the extracts. Cell-free (centrifuged) extracts were prepared from spleens, lymph nodes, and livers of the leukemic donors, and inoculated into newborn or suckling, less than 36-hour-old, BALB/c mice. All inoculated mice developed leukemia after an average latency varying approximately from 3 to 4.5 months. Leukemia could be induced with 1: 1,000 dilution of the extract in all inoculated mice after an average latency of approximately 4 months. The incidence of induced leukemia was reduced to 82 per cent when a 1 : 10,000 dilution was used for inoculation.

Successive Transplantations of Sarcoma S.37, and Repeated Isolations of the Leukemogenic Virus. Sarcoma 37 was then transplanted in adult BALB/c mice, and from successive tumor generations new cell-free extracts were prepared and inoculated into newborn BALB/c mice; again leukemia could be induced with such extracts without difficulty. After 50 transplant generations, Sarcoma 37 still yielded the leukemogenic virus on bio-assay.

Susceptibility of Mice of Different Strains to Inoculations with the Virus. Newborn and suckling mice of eight different inbred strains, and also non-inbred Swiss mice, were inoculated with filtrates prepared from BALB/c leukemic donors.

In most of the inoculated mice leukemia was induced readily, the incidence varying from 67 per cent in mice of strain I, to 95 or 100 per cent in mice of strains A/LN, C3H, BALB/c, DBA/2, and R III. The average latency varied from 3.5 to 6.8 months. A relatively low incidence of only 29 per cent was obtained following inoculation of the filtrates into mice of the C57 Black strain.

Serial Cell-free Passage of the Leukemogenic Virus. An attempt was made to pass serially the leukemogenic virus recovered from S.37 tumors. The technique was similar to that which was found to increase the potency of the Rous sarcoma virus in chickens (Bryan *et al.*, 1955. Bryan and Moloney, 1957), and which was also applied more recently for the development of a highly potent passage A mouse leukemia virus (Gross, 1957). This technique consisted essentially of inoculating newborn mice with the extracts, and then using those mice that first developed leukemia as donors for the preparation of extracts serving for the next serial passage. With successive passages, the potency of the virus gradually increased, as evidenced by shortened latency time elapsing between the time of inoculation and the development of symptoms of disease.

Susceptibility of Suckling Rats to the Leukemogenic Potency of the Virus Isolated from Mouse Sarcoma. Graffi and his associates were first to observe (1957) that the leukemogenic virus isolated from transplanted mouse tumors was capable of inducing leukemia not only in mice but also in rats. Moloney (1960a,b) confirmed this observation, and reported that the virus, which he isolated from sarcoma S.37, was leukemogenic for mice as well as for rats. When centrifuged cell-free extracts prepared from leukemic mouse donors were inoculated into suckling, less than 2-day-old, rats of the Sprague-Dawley or Osborne-Mendel strain, about 80 per cent of the inoculated rats developed thymic lymphosarcomas after a latency varying from 3 to 4 months.

Propagation of the Mouse Leukemia Virus Strains Isolated by Graffi and Moloney in Tissue Culture. The virus strains of mouse leukemia isolated by Graffi and Moloney could be propagated in tissue culture on normal mouse embryo cells, or on other mouse cell lines. No cytopathic effect was induced, but the virus multiplied, as evidenced on bio-assay tests carried out on newborn mice (Manaker *et al.*, 1960. Ginsburg and Sachs, 1962. Graffi *et al.*, 1963). This is discussed in more detail in the preceding chapter, in which the propagation of the mouse leukemia virus in tissue culture is reviewed.

Sarcoma 37 Transplants May not Always Yield a Potent Leukemogenic Virus

Moloney isolated, as did Graffi and his colleagues, a mouse leukemia virus from Sarcoma 37 transplants. The rather interesting feature of Moloney's studies was the relatively high potency of the leukemogenic virus isolated from the mouse sarcoma cells.

It is of interest that in Graffi's experiments, Sarcoma 37 did not prove to be a good source of a leukemogenic virus (Graffi *et al.*, 1956). Following inoculation of S.37 filtrates into newborn mice in Graffi's laboratories, only 10 per cent of the inoculated mice developed leukemia. Furthermore, the morphology of the disease induced in Graffi's experiments was different from that observed by Moloney. However, the methods of preparing extracts were not the same in the two laboratories, and the inbred lines of mice employed for the bio-assay were different. Furthermore, the Sarcoma 37 strain used for the preparation of extracts in Graffi's experiments was different from that employed at the National Cancer Institute, even though both originated several decades ago from the same tumor (Haaland, 1908). In the course of successive transplantations through many different mice, these two Sarcoma 37 strains could have picked up, and might have then carried along, different latent leukemogenic virus strains.

The Moloney Virus Strain, and the Mouse Leukemia Passage A Virus (Gross). A Comparison of Physical, Biological and Pathogenic Properties.

The virus strain isolated by Moloney from Sarcoma 37 has been employed extensively in experimental mouse leukemia research. In many publications this virus strain has been referred to as "the Moloney virus," and the impression might have been gained that this is a distinct leukemogenic virus, different from the mouse leukemia virus originally isolated from spontaneous mouse leukemia (Gross, 1951, 1957), and carried under the term "passage A" in our, and other laboratories.

To clarify this problem, a series of experiments has been carried out in our laboratory with the Moloney strain, in order to compare this strain with the passage A mouse leukemia virus in some of their physical, biological, and pathogenic properties (Gross, 1964a, 1965b). Results of these experiments, outlined in more detail on the following pages of this chapter, suggested that there exist essentially no differences between these two virus strains.

In October, 1962, we received from Dr. Moloney several BALB/c mice inoculated with his virus strain. As soon as these mice developed leukemia, we prepared filtrates from their leukemic organs, using the method routinely employed in our laboratory for the preparation of passage A virus extracts (Gross, 1957), described in more detail on page 350 of this monograph. This simple method of preparation of filtrate was considerably less time consuming than the differential centrifugation method employed by Moloney (1960), outlined on page 485 of this chapter.

No Significant Difference in Virus Yield between Method of "Differential Centrifugation" and that of Simple Centrifugation of Extracts. Kirsten recently compared both methods of preparation of extracts, using Ak mice with spontaneous leukemia as donors of the leukemic tissues serving for preparation of extracts, and newborn rats as test animals. The difference between the method employed in our laboratory and the differential centrifugation method employed by Moloney was not significant, since the incidence of leukemia induced in rats with extracts prepared by the differential centrifugation method was 25 per cent, as compared with the 18 to 20 per cent incidence obtained by the method employed in our laboratory (W. H. Kirsten, personal communication to the author, 1965).

The filtrate was inoculated into suckling mice of strains C3H(f) and BALB/c. Of 74 mice of strain C3H(f), 72 developed leukemia at an average age of 4.2 months. Twenty-four BALB/c mice were inoculated, and all of them developed leukemia at an average age of 3.4 months. Leukemia induced in mice of both strains with the Moloney virus strain was indistinguishable from that induced in mice of either inbred line with the passage A virus. Most of the leukemic mice had large thymic tumors, considerably enlarged spleens and livers, large mesenteric tumors, and frequently also large peripheral lymph nodes. Microscopic examination of blood smears and tissues of 21 C3H(f) leukemic mice revealed that 14 had the lymphatic form (12 among these had generalized lymphosarcomas with no evidence of leukemia in peripheral blood morphology), and 7 had stem-cell leukemia. Among 14 leukemic BALB/c mice examined, 6 had lymphatic leukemia (5 of these had generalized lymphosarcomas), 2 had stem-cell leukemia, and 6 (43 per cent) had myeloid leukemia. Briefly, the forms of leukemia induced with the Moloney virus strain did not essentially differ from those induced with the passage A virus (Gross, 1960b, 1963a,c, 1964a).

Certain physical properties of the virus strain isolated by Moloney have been studied in our laboratory; again they were found indistinguishable from those found in our previous studies carried out with the passage A virus. In our experiments the Moloney virus strain was inactivated by heating to 50°C for 30 minutes; the same was true for the passage A virus.

Inactivation of the Moloney Strain of Mouse Leukemia Virus by Ether. We also found that the Moloney virus strain is sensitive to *in vitro* exposure to ethyl ether. Of 72 suckling mice inoculated with ether-treated Moloney strain filtrate, only 6 mice (8 per cent) developed leukemia, as compared with a 93 per cent incidence of leukemia induced in simultaneous control experiments, in which suckling mice were injected with untreated virus filtrate (Gross, 1964a).

These results were in contrast to a brief reference, which did not include more extensive experimental details, made by Moloney (1962) on the effect of ether on his virus strain. However, it is quite possible that in a single experiment reported by Moloney, particularly if the concentration of ether volume employed was not sufficient, some of the virus could have survived *in vitro* treatment with ether; in a more extensive study, such as that carried out in our laboratory, most of the Moloney virus strain was destroyed by ether, as was the case in a similar experiment carried out previously with the passage A virus (Gross, 1956).

Electron Microscopic Studies: No Difference in Morphology between the Virus Isolated by Moloney and the Passage A Mouse Leukemia Virus (Gross)

In the initial electron microscopic studies, the preliminary impression reported by Dalton and his associates (1961) was that the virus isolated by Moloney was larger in diameter than the passage A mouse leukemia virus and, furthermore, that certain characteristic cylindrical forms (Dalton, 1961), apparently related to the Moloney virus strains, as well as tail-like protuberances of virus particles (Dalton *et al.*, 1962), could be observed in studies of leukemic tissues from mouse donors with leukemia induced by the Moloney strain. No reference was made in these early studies to the presence of such characteristic features in tissues of leukemic mouse donors with passage A virus-induced leukemia. However, additional and more extensive electron microscopic studies of both virus strains revealed that there are essentially no differences between these two viruses either in size or morphology. On electron microscopic examination of ultrathin sections of leukemic tissues from mice and rats with virus-induced leukemia, the size of the virus isolated by Moloney, and that of the passage A mouse leukemia virus, were found to be the same, averaging about 100 mμ (Dmochowski *et al.*, 1962, 1964. Parsons, 1963. Feldman and Gross, 1964). Furthermore, the cylindrical structures and particles with "tails," previously described by Dalton and his colleagues (1961, 1962) in their studies of the Moloney virus strain, were found not to be limited to that particular virus. The same cylindrical structures apparently related to the formation of virus particles (Dmochowski *et al.*, 1962, 1964. Feldman and Gross, 1964), as well as characteristic particles with tail-like protuberances (Dmochowski *et al.*, 1963, 1964. Okano *et al.*, 1963. Feldman and Gross, 1964) could be found also in tissues of mice and rats with leukemia induced with the passage A virus. It became quite apparent, and generally agreed upon, that the virus isolated by Moloney and the passage A mouse leukemia virus (Gross) were indistinguishable on electron microscopic examination in their size, morphology and in their location in relation to cell forms and cell structures (Dmochowski *et al.*, 1962, 1964. Feldman and Gross, 1964. Gross, 1964. Dalton *et al.*, 1964).

Electron microscopic studies of the mouse leukemia virus are reviewed in detail in the preceding chapter of this monograph.

Neutralization of the Moloney Strain of the Mouse Leukemia Virus by Immune Passage A Rabbit Serum

Since the study of physical, biological, and pathogenic properties of the Moloney strain of the mouse leukemia virus did not suggest any significant differences between that virus isolate and the standard passage A mouse leukemia virus, an attempt was made to determine whether the Moloney virus filtrate could be neutralized with a specific immune serum prepared with the passage A virus. Results of these experiments demonstrated that both passage A virus and the Moloney virus strain could be neutralized *in vitro* by the same specific serum obtained from rabbits immunized by repeated injections of passage A virus filtrates with Freund adjuvant. The pooled serum was inactivated at 56°C for 30 minutes prior to its use for the neutralization test.

Virus filtrates containing either the passage A virus or the Moloney strain were mixed with equal amounts of undiluted serum, or with a 1 : 2 dilution of serum. The mixtures were thoroughly stirred, left at room temperature for 30 minutes, then for 3½ to 4 hours at +4°C. The virus-serum mixtures were then inoculated (0.3 cc., i.p., each) into suckling C3H(f) mice, less than 6 days old. The injected animals were then observed for development of leukemia. Four successive experiments were performed. Neutralization of both passage A virus and of the Moloney strain was obtained when 10^{-3} dilutions of the virus filtrates were mixed with equal amounts of undiluted serum obtained from rabbits that had received injections of passage A filtrates with adjuvant. When a higher concentration of virus filtrate, or a less potent serum, was employed, neutralization was less pronounced and affected only passage A virus, or did not occur at all. There was no neutralization of either virus when in control experiments serum was employed from rabbits that had received normal mouse organ filtrates with adjuvant (Gross, 1965) (Table 9, p. 495).

Results of experiments here reported suggest that neutralization of the virus *in vitro* by an immune serum will occur only under carefully performed quantitative conditions. When a filtrate containing an unknown, and possibly highly potent, concentration of the mouse leukemia virus is mixed with a heterologous immune serum, neutralization may not occur even though the serum contains specific antibodies. This difficulty is due to the low potency of the immune serum and the relatively high titer of virus present in routinely prepared filtrates.

FIG. 44. THE MOLONEY, GRAFFI, FRIEND, AND RAUSCHER VIRUS PARTICLES.

(A). Section of spleen from a C3H(f) mouse with stem-cell leukemia induced with the Moloney virus strain. The intercellular space is filled with mature type C virus particles (C) containing nucleoids. Magnification 33,600×. (B). Section of spleen from a BALB/c mouse with lymphatic leukemia induced with the Graffi virus strain. Several virus particles (b) appear budding from platelets; doughnut-like immature type C particles (IC) are present between the platelets. Magnification 43,800×. (C). Section of spleen from a C3H(f) mouse with erythroblastosis-like syndrome induced with the Friend virus. A group of mature type C particles (C) containing nucleoids are present in the intercellular space. Magnification 33,600×. (D). Part of a platelet from spleen of a C3H(f) mouse with erythroblastosis-like syndrome induced with the Rauscher virus strain. A particle (b) is shown budding from a vacuolar membrane and a group of mature type C particles (C) containing nucleoids appear within vacuoles. Magnification 38,750×. Electron micrographs prepared by Dr. D. G. Feldman in cooperation with the author. A, B, and D, unpublished; C, from L. Gross, *Acta Haemat.*, **35**: 200, 1966.

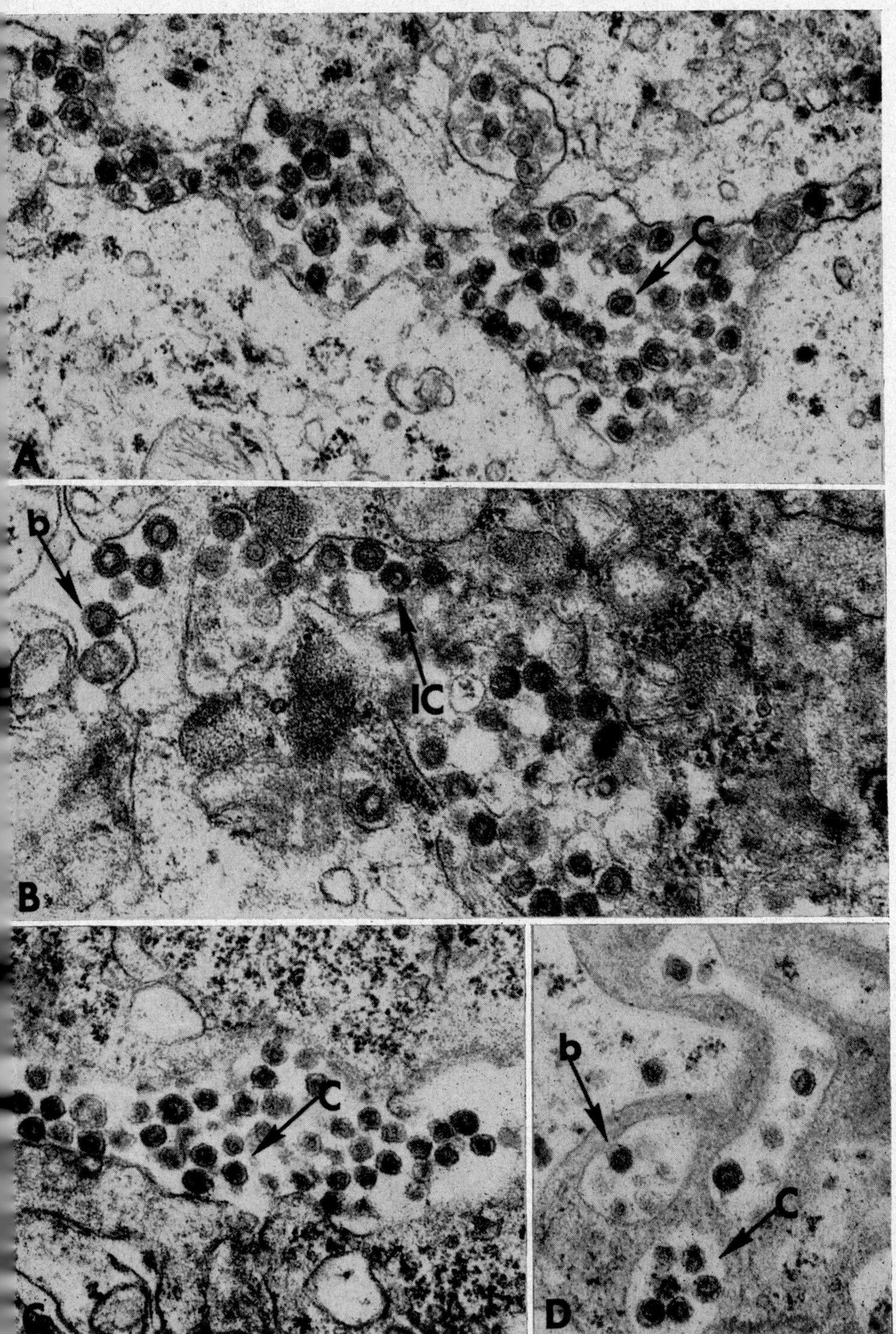

FIG. 44. THE MOLONEY, GRAFFI, FRIEND, AND RAUSCHER VIRUS PARTICLES.

To summarize, the passage A virus and the Moloney strain have identical physical properties; both can be inactivated by heating to 50°C for 30 minutes and are sensitive to ether; they are morphologically indistinguishable on electron microscopic examination; both have a similar

TABLE 9. NEUTRALIZATION OF PASSAGE A (GROSS) MOUSE LEUKEMIA VIRUS* AND OF MOLONEY VIRUS STRAIN BY IMMUNE PASSAGE A RABBIT SERUM†

Serum from rabbits immunized with	Serum dil.	Passage A virus			Moloney strain		
		Virus fil. dil.	No. of mice inoc.‡	No. dev. leuk.**	Virus fil. dil.	No. of mice inoc.‡	No. dev. leuk.**
Exp. 1							
Passage A virus (with adjuvant)	Undiluted	10^{-3}	8	0	10^{-3}	11	1
Normal mouse organs (with adjuvant)	Undiluted	10^{-3}	9	9	10^{-3}	13	13
Saline controls		10^{-3}	6	6	10^{-3}	3	2
Exp. 2							
Passage A virus (with adjuvant)	Undiluted	10^{-3}	8	0	10^{-3}	5	0
Passage A virus (with adjuvant)	1 : 2	10^{-3}	5	0	10^{-3}	5	1
Normal mouse organs (with adjuvant)	Undiluted	10^{-3}	4	4	10^{-3}	7	7
Normal mouse organs (with adjuvant)	1 : 2	10^{-3}	7	6	10^{-3}	11	11
Saline controls		10^{-3}	10	10	10^{-3}	8	8

* Virus filtrate mixed 1 : 1 with serum, incubated at room temperature for 30 minutes (in Exp. 1 also at 37°C for 25 minutes), and then at +4°C for 4 hours.

† Serum inactivated at 56°C for 30 minutes.

‡ Less than 6-day-old suckling C3H(f) mice inoculated intraperitoneally (0.3 cc. each).

** Leukemia developed at ages varying from 3 to 5 months. Surviving mice which did not develop leukemia were observed for periods of time varying from 9 to 13 months.

(From Gross, L., pp. 407–424, in: *Nat. Cancer Inst. Monograph No. 22*, 1966.)

host range, and both induce the same disease in mice and rats. Results of serum neutralization experiments suggesting that there are no fundamental antigenic differences between these two viruses, and that they both can be neutralized *in vitro* by the same immune serum, are consistent with the assumption that the passage A virus and the Moloney strain represent the same virus, or at best close variants of the same virus.

Under certain experimental conditions, a difference between the Moloney virus strain and the passage A virus filtrate could be detected when a special immunological procedure consisting of increasing host resistance against the implantation of leukemic cells was employed. As a preliminary step, the virus filtrate was inoculated into mice; this was followed by a subsequent implantation of leukemic cells derived from a host in which leukemia had been induced with the same, or with another, virus strain (Klein and Klein, 1962). This was a quantitative test procedure, and the number of leukemic cells implanted in order to determine the induced resistance of the host required careful dosage; immunity induced by the preliminary virus inoculation was limited and could be readily overwhelmed by a large challenging dose.

In another immunological procedure, cytotoxic neutralization tests based on the original studies of Gorer and O'Gorman (1946) were performed; in these tests the leukemic cells were examined for their sensitivity to *in vitro* incubation with a specific mouse serum. The sera were obtained from mice that had been rendered resistant to the implantation of virus-induced lymphomas either by implantation of genetically incompatible leukemic cells, or by treatment with subthreshold doses of leukemic cells of a genetically compatible lymphoma (Klein and Sjögren, 1960). Sera from such mice were found to be cytotoxic for leukemic cells, *in vitro*, in the presence of complement. The humoral antibodies appeared to be specific for a particular lymphoma of similar antigenic type (Slettenmark and Klein, 1962. Old *et al.*, 1964).

The Relatively High Titer of the Moloney Virus Strain. The only significant difference between the Moloney virus strain and the passage A mouse leukemia virus appears to be that of the titer. Prepared under similar experimental conditions, the Moloney strain filtrate has a higher titer than the passage A virus.

The Moloney strain was isolated from sarcoma S.37 which has been transplanted by cell-graft from mice to mice for over 50 years; it is possible to speculate that a leukemic virus picked up somewhere in the course of the Sarcoma 37 cell transplantations, and transmitted serially as a "passenger virus," increased considerably in potency after many years of consecutive mouse-to-mouse transfers, even though it remained latent in its carrier hosts.

Titration of Passage A Virus in Mice. Passage A mouse leukemia filtrate of 10 per cent concentration (10^{-2}) was prepared in the usual manner; this initial filtrate (10^{-2}) was serially diluted. Each dilution was then tested by inoculating suckling, less than 6-day-old, C3H(f) mice (0.3 cc., i.p., each).

The 10^{-2} through 10^{-4} dilutions induced an incidence of leukemia exceeding 91 per cent; this incidence dropped to 56 per cent when 10^{-5} dilution was inoculated, and to only 14 per cent when a 10^{-6} dilution was employed; the latency gradually increased from 2.8 months in the 10^{-2} group to 8.8 months in the 10^{-6} group.

Titration of the Moloney Strain. When, in a similar experiment, a filtrate prepared from the Moloney strain was inoculated in serial dilutions into suckling, less than 6-day-old, C3H(f) mice, the incidence of induced leukemia was 100 per cent when 10^{-2} and 10^{-3} dilutions were inoculated, exceeded 85 per cent when 10^{-4} and 10^{-5} dilutions were injected, and was still 77 per cent when 10^{-6} dilution was employed.

TABLE 10. NEUTRALIZATION OF THE GRAFFI VIRUS STRAIN* BY MOUSE LEUKEMIA VIRUS (GROSS) IMMUNE RABBIT SERUM†

Serum from rabbits immunized with	Virus fil. dil.	No. of mice inoc.‡	No. dev. leuk.**	Leuk. incid. per cent	Avg. age leuk. dev. mos.
Exp. 1					
Passage A virus (with adjuvant)	10^{-2}	11	1	9	7.0
Normal mouse organs (with adjuvant)	10^{-2}	9	9	100	3.0
Saline controls	10^{-2}	11	9	82	2.7
Exp. 2					
Passage A virus (with adjuvant)	10^{-3}	12	1	8	5.5
Normal mouse organs (with adjuvant)	10^{-3}	6	6	100	3.3
Saline controls	10^{-3}	6	6	100	3.2
Exp. 3					
Passage A virus (with adjuvant)	10^{-3}	10	0	—	—
Saline controls	10^{-3}	13	8	62	6.6

* Virus filtrate mixed 1 : 1 with undiluted serum, incubated at room temperature for 30 minutes, followed by incubation at 37°C for 30 minutes, and then at +4°C for 4 hours.

† Serum inactivated at 56°C for 30 minutes.

‡ Less than 6-day-old suckling C3H(f) mice inoculated intraperitoneally (0.3 cc. each).

** Surviving mice which did not develop leukemia were observed for periods of time varying from 9 to 13 months.

Neutralization of the Graffi Strain of Mouse Leukemia Virus with Immune Passage A Rabbit Serum

In a series of experiments similar to those performed with the Moloney virus strain, and described on the preceding pages of this chapter, an attempt was made to neutralize also the Graffi virus strain with immune rabbit serum directed against the Gross mouse leukemia virus. The serum was obtained from several rabbits immunized by repeated injections of passage A virus filtrates mixed with Freund adjuvant. The pooled serum was inactivated at 56°C for 30 minutes before being used for the neutralization test.

Graffi virus strain filtrates, in either 10^{-2} or 10^{-3} dilutions, were then mixed with equal amounts of undiluted immune rabbit serum. In a simultaneous control series, the Graffi virus strain filtrate was mixed with serum obtained from rabbits that had received normal mouse organ filtrates with adjuvant.

The virus-serum mixtures were thoroughly stirred, left at room temperature for 30 minutes, then incubated at 37°C for 30 minutes, and finally at +4°C for 4 hours. The virus-serum mixtures were then inoculated (0.3 cc., i.p., each) into suckling C3H(f) mice, less than 6 days old. Virus filtrate mixed with physiological saline solution was also inoculated into an additional control group of mice in each experiment.

Three successive experiments were performed. Neutralization of both 10^{-2} and 10^{-3} dilutions of the Graffi virus strain was obtained with the undiluted passage A immune serum. There was no neutralization of the virus when serum was employed from rabbits that had received normal mouse organ filtrates. The experiments are summarized in Table 10 on page 497 (Gross, L., unpublished data, 1967).

ADDITIONAL ISOLATIONS OF MOUSE LEUKEMIA VIRUS STRAINS FROM LEUKEMIC OR NON-LEUKEMIC MOUSE TISSUES AND FROM TRANSPLANTED MOUSE TUMORS

After the experimental conditions were determined under which a leukemogenic virus could be isolated in mice, it gradually became a routine procedure to follow the established technique, and to isolate leukemogenic viruses from spontaneous mouse leukemia; more recently it also became apparent that similar leukemogenic viruses could be isolated, often without difficulty, from certain other sources, such as transplanted mouse tumors. Accordingly, many individual isolations of leukemogenic viruses in mice have been reported during the preceding decade from several laboratories.

The work of Graffi and his associates, as well as the more recent experiments of Moloney, have been reviewed on the preceding pages of this chapter. Among other isolations of mouse leukemia virus strains from a variety of sources, were the following:

Tennant (1962, 1965) isolated a leukemogenic virus from leukemic tissues of mice of strain C58 with either spontaneous or transplanted C58 leukemia. Cell-free extracts, some of them filtered, prepared from such mice were inoculated into newborn mice of strain BALB/c, inducing an incidence of leukemia varying from 11 to 25 per cent. Following serial passage of the virus through suckling mice, the incidence of induced leukemia was considerably increased, and the latency reduced. In our previous studies (Gross, 1956) we also employed mice of strain C58 with spontaneous leukemia as donors for the preparation of filtrates. In our studies, the cell-free extracts prepared from C58 leukemic donors were inoculated into newborn mice of strains C3H and C57 Brown. Leukemia was induced in both strains, but mice of strain C57 Brown were found to be more susceptible to the leukemogenic action of the virus strain isolated from C58 leukemia.

Franks and his colleagues (1959) observed development of leukemia in Swiss mice following inoculation of filtrates prepared from sarcoma S.37; leukemia also developed in mice following implantation, temporary growth, then regression of sarcoma S.37 cells.

Bather (1961) carried out additional experiments in Swiss mice with the leukemogenic virus obtained from Franks. In some instances enlargement of spleen was noticed after a short latency of only 2 weeks following inoculation of this virus; peripheral lymph nodes and thymus became also involved, but at a later date. Bather designated the induced leukemia as "monocytic," but stressed the resemblance to the disease induced by Friend virus (the latter will be discussed in more detail in a subsequent chapter of this monograph).

Stansly and his coworkers (1961) recovered a leukemogenic virus from Ehrlich mouse ascites carcinoma, using for bio-assay newborn BALB/c mice; the relatively large number of reticulum-cell sarcomas induced with this particular virus strain was emphasized by the authors.

Buffett and her colleagues (1964) reported isolation of a lymphoid leukemia virus from organs (spleen, liver and kidney) of a female Swiss mouse of the Ha/ICR strain, with a spontaneous mammary carcinoma. This donor mouse had been injected with a bone marrow filtrate prepared from a young woman with myeloid leukemia. There was no evidence suggesting a relation between the injection of the human extract and the subsequent development of mammary carcinoma in that mouse. The incidence of spontaneous leukemia in Swiss mice is relatively high (see Table 2 on page 234 of this monograph), and it is quite possible that the leukemogenic virus isolated by Buffett and her associates was a latent mouse leukemia virus naturally carried in the donor mouse.

Rask-Nielsen (1963) induced leukemia in mice with an extract prepared from non-leukemic hypertrophic mouse mammary tissue. The donor mouse had been grafted earlier, without apparent success, with leukemic tissues from a transplantable plasma-cell leukemia (Rask-Nielsen *et al.*, 1961).

Precerutti and Law (1963) observed development of leukemia in a C3H mouse that had received injection of polyoma virus. The parotid tumor, i.e. polyoma virus filtrates may contain also the mouse leukemia virus; as a result, some of the mice, injected when newborn with such filtrates, may develop either parotid tumors or leukemia (Gross, 1955, 1957).

Rich and his colleagues (1963, 1965) reported isolation of a leukemogenic virus from Swiss mice which received Friend virus filtrate. In relation to this observation, the more recent experiments are of interest, which suggest that the Friend virus filtrate may contain the conventional, i.e. "passage A" mouse leukemia virus (Gross, 1964b, 1966); it is, therefore, not surprising that under certain experimental conditions, inoculation of the Friend virus filtrate may result in the development of lymphatic leukemia in susceptible mice (Gross, 1964b, 1966) or rats (Mirand *et al.*, 1962. Gross, 1964, 1965).

Rudali and Jullien (1963) reported isolation of a leukemogenic virus from transplanted pulmonary mouse tumors. The particular pulmonary tumor used as a source for preparation of extracts containing the leukemogenic virus had originally been induced in a female mouse of strain XVII/G with methylcholanthrene, and was maintained by transplantation through 30 successive cell-grafts in mice of the same inbred line.

Schoolman and his coworkers (1957) isolated a leukemogenic virus from an old Swiss mouse with spontaneous lymphosarcoma. This lymphosarcoma was first transplanted by cell-graft to adult DBA and Swiss mice. Subsequently, cell-free filtrates prepared from the brains of the leukemic mice were inoculated into adult Swiss mice and induced leukemia in about 45 per cent of the inoculated animals after a short latency of only one to three weeks.

* * *

This is only a partial list. Other isolations of leukemogenic viruses in mice have also been reported.

The virus strains isolated from leukemias that were induced in mice with carcinogenic chemicals or hormones have been reviewed in the preceding chapter.

The leukemogenic virus strains isolated from radiation-induced leukemia in mice will be discussed in the next chapter of this monograph.

The Friend virus and the Rauscher virus strain will be discussed in a separate chapter, following the discussion of the radiation-induced leukemia in mice.

How Many Different Viruses Causing Leukemia in Mice?

The question remains to be answered whether the many leukemogenic viruses isolated during the preceding decade from leukemic, or from non-leukemic, mouse organs, and from transplanted mouse tumors, represent individually distinct viruses, or whether they represent isolations from different sources of the same mouse leukemia virus, or of some of its close variants.

The fact that some of these virus strains may induce predominantly lymphatic leukemia, others a relatively high incidence of myelogenous leukemia, and still others reticulum-cell sarcomas, etc., does not necessarily imply that they represent different viral agents. The variety of forms of leukemia and lymphomas induced on bio-assay depends to a considerable extent on the individual susceptibility of the host. We are therefore faced with the fact that practically all the usual forms of leukemia and lymphomas can be induced in mice and rats with several filterable mouse virus strains isolated from a variety of sources. These different virus strains have very similar biological, physical, and pathogenic properties. To identify and classify such virus strains, serological tests may be necessary.

It should not be surprising to find minor immunological differences between such virus variants; in many other virus diseases, individual virus strains isolated from different sources have been found to be immunologically distinct. Such variants represent, nevertheless, the same virus. Among oncogenic viruses one could mention, as an example, the several variants of the Rous sarcoma virus (Simons and Dougherty, 1963), or the immunologically distinct variants of the polyoma virus recently described (Hare, 1964); such variants may be distinct antigenically; some of them may even show differences in their pathogenic potency, evidenced on inoculation tests, or in tissue culture. Viruses are prone to mutate, and to form variants.

On the basis of experimental data thus far available it appears reasonable to assume that most of the individual isolations of leukemogenic viruses in mice represent recoveries, from different sources, of the same mouse leukemia virus or, at best, closely related variant strains; any of them may induce in mice the same disease.* Even though some of these virus strains may show minor immunological differences, it is only reasonable to assume that they all represent basically the same virus.

* A different form of a disease of the hematopoietic system, which also belongs to the broad group of leukemias, is caused by a virus isolated by Dr. Charlotte Friend; the leukemic virus strain isolated more recently by Dr. Frank J. Rauscher appears to be very similar to, if not identical with, the Friend virus. The disease induced by either the Friend virus or the Rauscher virus strain and its relation to the conventional forms of mouse leukemia is discussed in a separate chapter of this monograph.

REFERENCES

BANG, F. B., Formation of filamentous forms of Newcastle disease virus in hypertonic concentration of sodium chloride. *Proc. Soc. Exp. Biol. & Med.*, **71**: 50–52, 1949.

BASHFORD, E. F., The behaviour of tumour-cells during propagation. pp. 131–214 in: *Fourth Sci. Rep. Imperial Cancer Fund.* Taylor and Francis, London, 1911.

BATHER, R., Observations on murine monocytic leukemia induced by a virus isolated from S37 sarcoma. *Brit. J. Cancer*, **15**: 114–119, 1961.

BIELKA, H., FEY, F., and GRAFFI, A., Über mögliche Eigenschaftsänderungen eines onkogenen Agens nach zellfreier Passage. *Naturwissenschaften*, **42**: 563–564, 1955.

BIELKA, H., FEY, F., KRISCHKE, W., and GRAFFI, A., Über die Abhängingkeit der Leukämiehäufigkeit vom Alter der Tiere zur Zeit der Injektion zellfreier Tumorfiltrate. *Naturwissenschaften*, **42**: 563, 1955.

BRYAN, W. R., Biological studies on the Rous sarcoma virus. I. General introduction. II. Review of sources of experimental variation and of methods for their control. *J. Nat. Cancer Inst.*, **16**: 285–315, 1955.

BRYAN, W. R., and MOLONEY, J. B., Rous sarcoma virus: The purification problem. *Ann. N.Y. Acad. Sci.*, **68**: 441–453, 1957.

BRYAN, W. R., CALNAN, D., and MOLONEY, J. B., Biological studies on the Rous sarcoma virus. III. The recovery of virus from experimental tumors in relation to initiating dose. *J. Nat. Cancer Inst.*, **16**: 317–335, 1955.

BUFFETT, R. F., and FURTH, J., A transplantable reticulum-cell sarcoma variant of Friend's viral leukemia. *Cancer Research*, **19**: 1063–1069, 1959.

BUFFETT, R. F., GRACE, J. T., Jr., and MIRAND, E. A., Properties of a lymphoid leukemia agent isolated from Ha/ICR Swiss mice. (Abstract.) *Proc. Am. Assoc. Cancer Research*, **4**: 8, 1963.

BUFFETT, R. F., GRACE, J. T., Jr., and MIRAND, E. A., Properties of a lymphocytic leukemia agent isolated from Ha/ICR Swiss mice. *Proc. Soc. Exp. Biol. & Med.*, **116**: 293–297, 1964.

DALTON, A. J., Micromorphology of murine tumor viruses and of affected cells. *Fed. Proc.*, **21**: 936–941, 1962.

DALTON, A. J., HAGUENAU, F., and MOLONEY, J. B., Morphology of particles associated with murine leukemia as revealed by negative staining: Preliminary report. *J. Nat. Cancer Inst.*, **29**: 1177–1179, 1962.

DALTON, A. J., HAGUENAU, F., and MOLONEY, J. B., Further electron microscopic studies on the morphology of the Moloney agent. *J. Nat. Cancer Inst.*, **33**: 255–275, 1964.

DALTON, A. J., LAW, L. W., MOLONEY, J. B., and MANAKER, R. A., An electron microscopic study of a series of murine lymphoid neoplasms. *J. Nat. Cancer Inst.*, **27**: 747–791, 1961.

DE HARVEN, E., and FRIEND, C., Electron microscope study of a cell-free induced leukemia of the mouse: A preliminary report. *J. Biophys. and Biochem. Cytol.*, **4**: 151–156, 1958.

DE HARVEN, E., and FRIEND, C., Further electron microscope studies of a mouse leukemia induced by cell-free filtrates. *J. Biophys. and Biochem. Cytol.*, **7**: 747–752, 1960.

DMOCHOWSKI, L., GREY, C. E., PADGETT, F., and SYKES, J. A., Studies on the structure of the mammary tumor-inducing virus (Bittner) and of leukemia virus (Gross). pp. 85–121 in: Viruses, Nucleic Acids, and Cancer. *17th Ann. Symposium on Fundamental Cancer Research.* M. D. Anderson Hospital and Tumor Inst., Williams & Wilkins Co., Baltimore, Md., 1963.

DMOCHOWSKI, L., GROSS, L., and PADGETT, F., Electron microscopic studies of rat leukemia induced with mouse leukemia virus. *Proc. Soc. Exp. Biol. & Med.*, **110**: 504–508, 1962.

DMOCHOWSKI, L., PADGETT, F., and GROSS, L., An electron microscopic study of rat leukemia induced with mouse leukemia virus (Gross). *Cancer Research*, **24**: 869–899, 1964.

DUNN, T. B., Normal and pathologic anatomy of the reticular tissue in laboratory mice. With a classification and discussion of neoplasms. *J. Nat. Cancer Inst.*, **14**: 1281–1433, 1954.

EHRLICH, P., Experimentelle Studien an Mäusentumoren. *Zeitschr. f. Krebsforsch.*, **5**: 59–81, 1907.

EHRLICH, P., and APOLANT, H., Beobachtungen über maligne Mäusetumoren. *Berliner klin. Wochenschr.*, **42**: 871–874, 1905.

FELDMAN, D. G., and GROSS, L., Electron-microscopic study of the mouse leukemia virus (Gross), and of tissues from mice with virus-induced leukemia. *Cancer Research*, **24**: 1760–1783, 1964.

FELDMAN, D. G., GROSS, L., and DREYFUSS, Y., Electron microscopic study of the passage A mouse leukemia virus in mammary glands of pregnant virus-injected, C3H(f) mice. *Cancer Research*, **23**: 1604–1607, 1963.

FEY, F., and GRAFFI, A., Beeinflussung der myeloischen Filtratleukämie der Maus durch Splenektomie. *Naturwissenschaften*, **45**: 471–472, 1958.

FEY, F., and GRAFFI, A., Untersuchungen zur hämatologischen Aufsplitterung der durch das Virus der myeloischen Leukämie der Maus induzierten Leukosen. *Acta Haemat.*, **33**: 139–158, 1965.

FEY, F., and GRAFFI, A., Erythroblasten Leukämie nach Injektion von Virus der myeloischen Leukämie der Maus. *Zeitschr. f. Krebsforsch.*, **67**: 145–151, 1965.

FIORE-DONATI, L., and CHIECO-BIANCHI, L., Influence of host factors on development and type of leukemia induced in mice by Graffi virus. *J. Nat. Cancer Inst.*, **32**: 1083–1107, 1964.

FRANKS, W. R., MCGREGOR, A., SHAW, M. M., and SKUBLICS, J., Development of leukosis by cell-free filtrates of solid tumors or in mice surviving immune to these tumors. (Abstract.) *Proc. Am. Assoc. Cancer Research*, **3**: 19–20, 1959.

FRIEND, C., The isolation of a virus causing a malignant disease of the hematopoietic system in adult Swiss mice. (Abstract.) *Proc. Am. Assoc. Cancer Research*, **2**: 106, 1956.

FRIEND, C., Cell-free transmission in adult Swiss mice of a disease having the character of a leukemia. *J. Exp. Med.*, **105**: 307–318, 1957.

FRIEND, C., Leukemia of adult mice caused by a transmissible agent. *Ann. N.Y. Acad. Sci.*, **68**: 522–532, 1957.

FRIEND, C., A virus-induced leukemia of adult mice. pp. 231–244 in: *Perspectives in Virology*. John Wiley & Sons, New York, 1959.

FRIEND, C., and HADDAD, J., Local tumor formation with transplants of spleen or liver of mice with a virus-induced leukemia. (Abstract.) *Proc. Am. Assoc. Cancer Research*, **3**: 21, 1959.

FRIEND, C., and HADDAD, J. R., Tumor formation with transplants of spleen or liver from mice with virus-induced leukemia. *J. Nat. Cancer Inst.*, **25**: 1279–1289, 1960.

GIMMY, J., FEY, F., and GRAFFI, A., Hämatologische und histologische Untersuchungen an Rattenleukosen, die durch zellfreie Filtrate von Mäuseleukämien erzeugt wurden. *Arch. f. Geschwulstforsch.*, **16**: 118–128, 1960.

GIMMY, J., KRISCHKE, W., and GRAFFI, A., Über die leukämieerzeugende Wirkung zellfreier Tumorfiltrate nach Injektion in erwachsene Mäuse. *Naturwissenschaften*, **43**: 305, 1956.

GINSBURG, H., and SACHS, L., Leukemia induction in mice by Moloney virus from long- and short-term tissue cultures, and attempts to detect a leukemogenic virus in cultures from X-ray-induced leukemia. *J. Nat. Cancer Inst.*, **28**: 1391–1410, 1962.

GORER, P. A., and O'GORMAN, P., The cytotoxic activity of isoantibodies in mice. *Transpl. Bull.*, **3**: 142–143, 1946.

GRAFFI, A., Chloroleukemia of mice. *Ann. N.Y. Acad. Sci.*, **68**: 540–558, 1957.

GRAFFI, A., Zur Virusätiologie verschiedener Mäuseleukämien. *Acta Haemat.*, **20**: 49–62, 1958.

GRAFFI, A., Über einige Eigenschaften des virusartigen Agens der myeloischen Leukämie der Maus. *Acta Internat. Union Against Cancer*, **15**: 737–747, 1959.

GRAFFI, A., Neuere Untersuchungen über das Virus der myeloischen Leukämie der Maus. pp. 112–161 in: *Progress in Experimental Tumor Research.* S. Karger, Basel, and J. B. Lippincott, Philadelphia, 1960.

GRAFFI, A., Wirkungsweise und Eigenschaften des bei Maus und Ratte wirksamen Virus der myeloischen Leukämie. *Acta Internat. Union Against Cancer*, **17**: 181–197, 1961.

GRAFFI, A., and BIELKA, H., Zum Verhalten des leukämogenen Agens aus filtrierbaren Mäusetumoren gegenüber Glycerin und Gefriertrocknung. *Naturwissenschaften*, **44**: 382, 1957.

GRAFFI, A., and BIELKA, H., Versuche zur Frage der Beteiligung von Lipoiden am Aufbau des Virus der myeloischen Leukämie der Maus. *Acta Biologica et Medica Germanica*, **3**: 511–512, 1959.

GRAFFI, A., and FEY, F., Untersuchungen über die Antigen-Eigenschaften des leukämieerzeugenden Faktors aus dem Mäusetumor Sa I. *Naturwissenschaften*, **42**: 652, 1955.

GRAFFI, A., and GIMMY, J., Erzeugung von Leukosen bei der Ratte durch ein leukämogenes Agens der Maus. *Naturwissenschaften*, **44**: 518, 1957.

GRAFFI, A., and GIMMY, J., Rattenleukosen durch zellfreie Filtrate aus homologem leukämischem Gewebe. *Zeitschr. f. Naturforsch.*, **14**b: 747–748, 1959.

GRAFFI, A., and KRISCHKE, W., Über Infektiosität und Übertragungsweise der virusbedingten myeloischen Leukämie der Maus. *Biolog. Zentralbl.*, **81**: 277–289, 1962.

GRAFFI, A., and SCHMIDT, F., Methodische Versuche zur Frage einer subzellulären Übertragung von Mäusetumoren. *Deutsche Gesundheitswesen*, **9**: 1309–1319, 1954.

GRAFFI, A., BAUMBACH, L., SCHRAMM, T., and BIERWOLF, D., Untersuchungen zur Frage der Züchtbarkeit des Virus der myeloischen Leukämie der Maus in der Gewebekultur. *Zeitschr. f. Krebsforsch.*, **65**: 385–395, 1963.

GRAFFI, A., BIELKA, H., FEY, F., SCHARSACH, F., and WEISS, R., Gehäuftes Auftreten von Leukämien nach Injektion von Sarkom-Filtraten. *Wiener med. Wochenschr.*, **105**: 61–64, 1955.

GRAFFI, A., BIELKA, H., and FEY, F., Leukämieerzeugung durch ein filtrierbares Agens aus malignen Tumoren. *Acta Haemat.*, **15**: 145–174, 1956.

GRAFFI, A., FEY, F., BIELKA, H., HEINE, U., and HOFFMANN, F., Weitere Untersuchungen zur Charakterisierung des leukämieerzeugenden Agens aus Mäusetumoren. *Naturwissenschaften*, **43**: 63, 1956.

GRAFFI, A., FEY, F., HOFFMANN, F., and KRISCHKE, W., Inaktivierung des Leukämie erzeugenden filtrierbaren Agens aus Mäusetumoren durch heterologe Immunseren. *Klin. Wochenschr.*, **35**: 465–468, 1957.

GRAFFI, A., FEY, F., and SCHRAMM, T., Experiments on the hematologic diversification of viral mouse leukemias. pp. 21–31 in: *Conference on Murine Leukemia Nat. Cancer Inst. Monograph No. 22*, U.S. Publ. Health Service, Bethesda, Md., 1966.

GRAFFI, A., HEINE, U., HELMCKE, J.-G., BIERWOLF, D., and RANDT, A., Über den elektronenmikroskopischen Nachweis von Viruspartikeln bei der myeloischen Leukämie der Maus nach Injektion zellfreier Tumorfiltrate. *Klin. Wochenschr.*, **38**: 254–262, 1960.

GROSS, L., Is cancer a communicable disease? *Cancer Research*, **4**: 293–303, 1944.

GROSS, L., "Spontaneous" leukemia developing in C3H mice following inoculation, in infancy, with Ak-leukemic extracts, or Ak-embryos. *Proc. Soc. Exp. Biol. & Med.*, **76**: 27–32, 1951a.

GROSS, L., Pathogenic properties, and "vertical" transmission of the mouse leukemia agent. *Proc. Soc. Exp. Biol. & Med.*, **78**: 342–348, 1951b.

GROSS, L., A filterable agent, recovered from Ak leukemic extracts, causing salivary gland carcinomas in C3H mice. *Proc. Soc. Exp. Biol. & Med.*, **83**: 414–421, 1953.

GROSS, L., Induction of parotid carcinomas and/or subcutaneous sarcomas in C3H mice with normal C3H organ extracts. *Proc. Soc. Exp. Biol. & Med.*, **88**: 362–368, 1955.

GROSS, L., Filterable agent causing subcutaneous sarcomas following inoculation into newborn C3H mice. (Abstract.) *Proc. Am. Assoc. Cancer Research*, **2**: 112, 1956.

GROSS, L., Studies on the nature and biological properties of a transmissible agent causing leukemia following inoculation into newborn mice. *Ann. N.Y. Acad. Sci.*, **68**: 501–521, 1957.

GROSS, L., Attempt to recover filterable agent from X-ray-induced leukemia. *Acta Haemat.*, **19**: 353–361, 1958.

GROSS, L., Serial cell-free passage of a radiation-activated mouse leukemia agent. *Proc. Soc. Exp. Biol. & Med.*, **100**: 102–105, 1959a.

GROSS, L., Effect of thymectomy on development of leukemia in C3H mice inoculated with "passage" virus. *Proc. Soc. Exp. Biol. & Med.*, **100**: 325–328, 1959b.

GROSS, L., Development of myeloid (chloro-) leukemia in thymectomized mice following inoculation of lymphatic leukemia virus. *Proc. Soc. Exp. Biol. & Med.*, **103**: 509–514, 1960a.

GROSS, L., Biological and pathogenic properties of a mouse leukemia virus. *Acta Haemat.*, **23**: 259–275, 1960b.

GROSS, L., Studies on pathogenic properties and natural transmission of a mouse leukaemia virus. pp. 159–170 in: *CIBA Foundation Symposium on Tumour Viruses of Murine Origin*. J. & A. Churchill Ltd., London, 1962a.

GROSS, L., Transmission of mouse leukemia virus through milk of virus-injected C3H female mice. *Proc. Soc. Exp. Biol. & Med.*, **109**: 830–836, 1962b.

GROSS, L., Pathogenic potency and host range of the mouse leukemia virus. *Acta Haemat.*, **29**: 1–15, 1963a.

GROSS, L., Susceptibility of rats to leukemogenic action of passage A virus. Effect of thymectomy. (Abstract.) *Proc. Am. Assoc. Cancer Research*, **4**: 25, 1963b.

GROSS, L., Properties of a virus isolated from leukemic mice, inducing various forms of leukemia and lymphomas in mice and rats. Bertner Foundation Lecture. pp. 403–426 in: Viruses, Nucleic Acids, and Cancer. *17th Ann. Symposium on Fundamental Cancer Research.* M. D. Anderson Hospital and Tumor Inst., Williams & Wilkins Co., Baltimore, Md., 1963c.

GROSS, L., How many different viruses causing leukemia in mice? *Acta Haemat.*, **32**: 44–62, 1964a.

GROSS, L., Attempt at classification of mouse leukemia viruses. *Acta Haemat.*, **32**: 81–88, 1964b.

GROSS, L., Viral etiology of leukemia and lymphomas. Editorial. *Blood*, **25**: 377–381, 1965a.

GROSS, L., Neutralization *in vitro* of mouse leukemia virus by specific immune serum. Importance of virus titration. *Proc. Soc. Exp. Biol. & Med.*, **119**: 420–427, 1965b.

GROSS, L., Are the common forms of spontaneous and induced leukemia and lymphomas in mice caused by a single virus? pp. 407–424 in: *Conference on Murine Leukemia. Nat. Cancer Inst. Monograph No. 22*, U.S. Publ. Health Service, Bethesda, Md., 1966.

GROSS, L., DREYFUSS, Y., and MOORE, L., Attempt to propagate "passage A" mouse leukemia virus on normal mouse embryo cells in tissue culture. (Abstract.) *Proc. Am. Assoc. Cancer Research*, **3**: 231, 1961.

GROSS, L., ROSWIT, B., MALSKY, S. J., DREYFUSS, Y., and AMATO, C. G., Resistance of mouse leukemia virus to *in vitro* gamma rays irradiation. (Abstract.) *Proc. Am. Assoc. Cancer Research*, **6**: 24, 1965.

HAALAND, M., Contributions to the study of the development of sarcoma under experimental conditions. pp. 175-621 in: *Third Sci. Rep. Imperial Cancer Research Fund.* Taylor and Francis, London, 1908.

HARE, J. D., Transplant immunity to polyoma virus induced tumors. I. Correlations with biological properties of virus strains. *Proc. Soc. Exp. Biol. & Med.*, **115**: 805–810, 1964.

HEINE, U., GRAFFI, A., BIERWOLF, D., HELMCKE, J. G., and RANDT, A., Elektronenmikroskopische Untersuchungen an der zellfrei-übertragbaren myeloischen Leukämie der Maus. *Acta Biologica et Medica Germanica*, **3**: 608–623, 1959.

KLEIN, E., and KLEIN, G., Antigenic properties of lymphomas induced by the Moloney agent. *J. Nat. Cancer Inst.*, **32**: 547–568, 1964.

KLEIN, E., and SJÖGREN, H. O., Humoral and cellular factors in homograft and isograft immunity against sarcoma cells. *Cancer Research*, **20**: 452–461, 1960.

KLEIN, G., SJÖGREN, H. O., and KLEIN, E., Demonstration of host resistance against isotransplantation of lymphomas induced by the Gross agent. *Cancer Research*, **22**: 955–961, 1962.

KRISCHKE, W., and GRAFFI, A., Zur Frage der vertikalen Übertragung des Virus der myeloischen Leukämie der Maus. *Arch. f. Geschwulstforsch.*, **17**: 217–221, 1961.

KRISCHKE, W., and GRAFFI, A., The transmission of the virus of myeloid leukaemia of mice by the milk. *Acta Internat. Union Against Cancer*, **19**: 360–361, 1963.

KRISCHKE, W., GRAFFI, A., and HEYER, E., Untersuchungen über die Ansprechbarkeit genetische verschiedener Mäusestämme auf zellfreie Filtrate maligner Tumoren. *Naturwissenschaften*, **43**: 332, 1956.

LAW, L. W., and MOLONEY, J. B., Studies of congenital transmission of a leukemic virus in mice. *Proc. Soc. Exp. Biol. & Med.*, **108**: 715–723, 1961.

LEVINTHAL, J. D., BUFFETT, R. F., and FURTH, J., Prevention of viral leukemia of mice by thymectomy. *Proc. Soc. Exp. Biol. & Med.*, **100**: 610–614, 1959.

LOHMANN, K., and SCHMIDT, F., Über einige Eigenschaften des leukämieerzeugenden Agens aus Ehrlich-Ca-Filtraten der Maus. *Zeitschr. f. Krebsforsch.*, **61**: 520–526, 1957.

MANAKER, R. A., JENSEN, E. M., and KOROL, W., Long-term propagation of a murine leukemia virus in an established cell line. *J. Nat. Cancer Inst.*, **33**: 363–371, 1964.

MANAKER, R. A., STROTHER, P. C., and PICZAK, C. V., *In vitro* maintenance of a mouse lymphoid leukemia virus. (Abstract.) *Proc. Am. Assoc. Cancer Research*, **3**: 131, 1960.

MANAKER, R. A., STROTHER, P. C., MILLER, A. A., and PICZAK, C. V., Behavior *in vitro* of a mouse lymphoid-leukemia virus. *J. Nat. Cancer Inst.*, **25**: 1411-1419, 1960.

METCALF, D., FURTH, J., and BUFFETT, R. F., Pathogenesis of mouse leukemia caused by Friend virus. *Cancer Research*, **19**: 52–58, 1959.

MIRAND, E. A., and GRACE, J. T., Jr., Induction of leukemia in rats with Friend virus. *Virology*, **17**: 364–366, 1962.

MOLONEY, J. B., Biological studies on the Rous sarcoma virus. V. Preparation of improved standard lots of the virus for use in quantitative investigations. *J. Nat. Cancer Inst.*, **16**: 877–888, 1956.

MOLONEY, J. B., Preliminary studies on a mouse lymphoid leukemia virus extracted from Sarcoma 37. (Abstract.) *Proc. Am. Assoc. Cancer Research*, **3**: 44, 1959.

MOLONEY, J. B., Biological studies on a lymphoid leukemia virus extracted from sarcoma S.37. I. Origin and introductory investigations. *J. Nat. Cancer Inst.*, **24**: 933–951, 1960a.

MOLONEY, J. B., Properties of a leukemia virus. pp. 7–33 in: *Symposium, Phenomena of the Tumor Viruses. Nat. Cancer Inst. Monograph No. 4*, U.S. Publ. Health Service, Bethesda, Md., 1960b.

MOLONEY, J. B., The murine leukemias. *Fed. Proc.*, **21**: 19–31, 1962.

OKANO, H., KUNII A., and FURTH, J., An electron microscopic study of leukemia induced in rats with Gross virus. *Cancer Research*, **23**: 1169-1175, 1963.

OLD, L. J., BOYSE, E. A., and STOCKERT, E., Typing of mouse leukaemias by serological methods. *Nature*, **201**: 777–779, 1964.

PARSONS, D. F., Structure of the Gross leukemia virus. *J. Nat. Cancer Inst.*, **30**: 569–583, 1963.

PRECERUTTI, A., and LAW, L. W., Isolation of a murine leukaemogenic virus P-LLV. *Nature*, **198**: 801–803, 1963.

RASK-NIELSEN, R., Evidence of murine, virus-induced paraprotein-producing leukaemia and its relation to other virus-induced leukaemias. *Nature*, **200**: 440 and 453, 1963.

RASK-NIELSEN, R., HEREMANS, J. F., CHRISTENSEN, H. E., and DJURTOFT, R., Beta-2A (=Beta-3-II=Gamma-1A) mouse leukemia with "flame cells" in leukemic infiltrations and degenerative lesions in muscles. *Proc. Soc. Exp. Biol. & Med.*, **107**: 632–636, 1961.

RICH, M. A., and JOHNS, L. W., Jr., Morphology of an agent associated with a murine leukemia. *Virology*, **20**: 373–376, 1963.

RICH, M. A., GELDNER, J., and MEYERS, P., Studies on murine leukemia. *J. Nat. Cancer Inst.*, **35**: 523–536, 1965.

RUDALI, G., and JULLIEN, P., Production de leucémies verticalement transmissibles à l'aide d'extraits d'un adénocarcinome pulmonaire. *Acta Internat. Union Against Cancer*, **19**: 381–384, 1963.

SCHMIDT, F., Über Filtraversuche mit Mäusetransplantationstumoren. *Zeitschr. f. Krebsforsch.*, **60**: 445–455, 1955.

SCHMIDT, F., Über den intrazellulären Sitz des leukämieerzeugenden Faktors (Induktors) aus Substraten des Ehrlich-Karzinoms. *Zentralbl. f. Allg. Path. u. Path. Anat.*, **95**: 36–40, 1956.

SCHMIDT, F., Über Filtratversuche von Mäusetumoren mittels bakteriendichter G 5-Glasfilternutschen. *Zentralbl. f. Allg. Path. u. Path. Anat.*, **96**: 211–220, 1957.

SCHOOLMAN, H. M., SPURRIER, W., SCHWARTZ, S. O., and SZANTO, P. B., Studies in leukemia. VII. The induction of leukemia in Swiss mice by means of cell-free filtrates of leukemic mouse brain. *Blood*, **12**: 694–700, 1957.

SELBY, C. C., GREY, C. E., LICHTENBERG, S., FRIEND, C., MOORE, A. E., and BIESELE, J. J., Submicroscopic cytoplasmic particles occasionally found in the Ehrlich mouse ascites tumor. *Cancer Research*, **14**: 790–794, 1954.

SIMONS, P. J., and DOUGHERTY, R. M., Antigenic characteristics of three variants of Rous sarcoma virus. *J. Nat. Cancer Inst.*, **31**: 1275–1283, 1963.

SLETTENMARK, B., and KLEIN, E., Cytotoxic and neutralization tests with serum and lymph node cells of isologous mice with induced resistance against Gross lymphomas. *Cancer Research*, **22**: 947–954, 1962.

STANSLY, P. G., RAMSEY, D. S., and SOULE, H. D., Experiments on the transplantation and cell-free transmission of a reticulum cell sarcoma in BALB/c mice. (Abstract.) *Proc. Am. Assoc. Cancer Research*, **3**: 270, 1961.

STEWART, H. L., SNELL, K. C., DUNHAM, L. J., and SCHLYEN, S. M., Transplantable and transmissible tumors of animals. *Atlas of Tumor Pathology*. Sect. 12. Fasc. 40, p. 378. Am. Reg. Path., Armed Forces Inst. of Path., Washington, D.C., 1959.

SVEC, F., HLAVAY, E., THURZO, V., and KOSSEY, P., Erythroleukämie der Ratte, hervorgerufen durch zellfreie Karzinom-Filtrate. *Acta Haemat.*, **17**: 34–41, 1957.

TENNANT, J. R., Derivation of a murine lymphoid leukemia virus. *J. Nat. Cancer Inst.*, **28**: 1291–1301, 1962.

TENNANT, J. R., Susceptibility and resistance to viral leukemogenesis in the mouse. I. Biologic definition of the virus. *J. Nat. Cancer Inst.*, **34**: 625–632, 1965.

TENNANT, J. R., Susceptibility and resistance to viral leukemogenesis in the mouse. II. Response to the virus relative to histocompatibility factors carried by the prospective host. *J. Nat. Cancer Inst.*, **34**: 633–641, 1965.

TOTH, B., and SHUBIK, P., Studies with malignant lymphomas: Possible interaction problems between chemical and viral-inducing agents. pp. 313–328 in: *Conference on Murine Leukemia. Nat. Cancer Inst. Monograph No. 22*, U.S. Publ. Health Service, Bethesda, Md., 1966.

CHAPTER 13

Radiation-induced Leukemia in Mice

Carcinogenic Effect of Ionizing Radiation

It has long been known that frequent and prolonged exposures to X-rays and other forms of ionizing radiation may lead to the development of tumors and leukemia. X-rays were discovered in 1895 by the German physician W. C. v. Röntgen, and only 7 years later the first case of radiation-induced cancer was reported by Frieben (1902). This cancer developed on the back of the right hand of a technician who had tested for several years the proper functioning of X-ray tubes by projecting the image of his own fingers on the fluorescent screen. Other reports followed, and it soon became apparent that frequent and prolonged exposures to X-rays may lead to chronic dermatitis, followed by the development of very painful skin ulcers, then warts, and finally multiple skin cancers. It was soon realized that a similar effect may result from exposure to radium.

It also gradually became apparent that tumors may develop in remote organs following a local or general exposure to ionizing radiation. The history of a strange disease called "Bergkrankheit" among the miners of Schneeberg and Jachymov (Joachimsthal) in Czechoslovakia goes back several centuries, although only after the turn of this century was it realized that the majority of miners employed in these uranium mines died from primary carcinomas of the lungs (reviewed by Peller, 1939. Rajewsky *et al.*, 1943).

Most internal tumors in man, however, that have developed following exposure to either X-rays or radioactive substances have occurred in bones.

In some instances, bone tumors have developed as a result of repeated therapeutic irradiations given for such conditions as chronic joint infections (Hatcher, 1945). The accidental induction of primary osteogenic sarcomas by radioactive substances in watch dial painters, which claimed over 40 victims, was reported by Martland (1931). Between 1916 and 1925, luminous watch dial painters in New Jersey moistened, by licking, brushes which had been dipped into a compound containing radium and mesothorium. Ingested over a period of years, this radioactive material lodged in bones. Severe anemia resulted and was followed later by the development of primary bone sarcomas, and, as was more recently observed (Hasterlik *et al.*, 1964), also by development of other malignant tumors of adjoining epithelial organs, such as epidermoid carcinomas of the mastoid and paranasal sinuses.

Leukemogenic and Oncogenic Effect of Ionizing Radiation

The possible leukemogenic effect of total-body exposures to ionizing radiation was recognized early. In 1911, v. Jagić described four cases of leukemia among radiologists, and one in a radium worker, and suspected that long-continued exposure to X-radiation may cause this disease. Gradually it became apparent that frequent exposures to even very small doses of X-rays may increase the incidence of leukemia. Ulrich (1946) and March (1944, 1950) estimated that the incidence of leukemia among American radiologists was 8 to 10 times higher than that among other physicians.

The radiation hazard was increased with the development of atomic weapons. The explosion of atomic bombs in Hiroshima and Nagasaki was followed by increased incidence of leukemia developing among subjects exposed to radiation at distances less than 2000 meters, and the magnitude of increase was inversely related to the distance from the hypocenter (Folley *et al.*, 1952). During 1960–1964, almost 20 years after the bombing, persons who had been within 1500 meters of the hypocenters of the explosions were still manifesting a leukemia rate 6 or 7 times higher than those exposed at greater distances. A peak incidence of leukemia, evident in acute and in chronic myelocytic forms, occurred 5 to 8 years after exposure, but a second peak, evident only for acute cases, appeared 13 to 14 years after exposure. In the first 10 years after exposure 54 per cent of the cases were acute; 10 to 19 years after exposure 84 per cent were acute. A high incidence and short latency period for chronic myelocytic leukemia was observed in persons under 30 years of age at the time of exposure (Bizzozero *et al.*, 1966).

Development of Tumors or Leukemia Following Therapeutic or Diagnostic X-Ray Irradiation, or Application of Radioisotopes. Generally speaking, exposure to X-rays or other forms of ionizing radiation may induce leukemia as a predominant and most frequent manifestation. In other instances, however, it may result in the development of local tumors, such as skin carcinomas or subcutaneous sarcomas, or it may result in the induction of thyroid carcinomas, or bone sarcomas, or carcinomas of the lungs, or ovaries, or mammary glands.

It is now realized that radiation, even in relatively moderate or small doses, may eventually result in the development of leukemia or tumors, not only in animals, but also in man.

It appears that prenatal exposure to diagnostic radiation may increase the incidence of leukemia or cancer in childhood. Stewart and her colleagues (1956, 1958) reported in Oxford that mothers of children who died from leukemia, or other malignant tumors, had abdominal or pelvic X-rays with a higher frequency than did mothers of a sample of normal, healthy children of similar age groups. The incidence of leukemia or malignant tumors was approximately doubled in children that received "total-body" X-ray irradiation as foetuses, while *in utero*. This observation was more recently confirmed and extended by MacMahon in the United States (1962).

Evidence that therapeutic, or even diagnostic, irradiation can be leukemogenic became apparent from a British study carried out on patients whose ankylosing spondylitis had been treated with X-rays as long as 21 years prior to the development of leukemia. Continued follow-up examination of such patients confirmed the high incidence of leukemia in this group (Court-Brown and Doll, 1957, 1965). Furthermore, higher than expected rates have been observed for cancer of the pharynx, stomach, pancreas, lung, and lymph nodes, when these organs have been exposed to irradiation in the course of the therapeutic schedule for spondylitis.

In a similar category belongs the study of Simpson and her associates (1955), at the University of Rochester, indicating increased development of leukemia and thyroid adenomas and carcinomas, and in a few instances also osteochondromas, in persons that had received therapeutic irradiation of the thymus in childhood as long as 27 years earlier. Irradiation of a presumably "enlarged" thymus in children was a rather common practice some 20 or 30 years ago as treatment of an obscure syndrome designated "status lymphaticus."

The possibility that multiple fluoroscopies may increase the incidence of breast cancer also became apparent from another more recent study (MacKenzie, 1965) in which a series of 50 cases of carcinoma of the breast was presented in women who had previously had sanatorium treatment for pulmonary tuberculosis. Forty of these patients had received repeated fluoroscopic examinations of the chest over a considerable period of time in the course of pneumothorax treatment of tuberculosis.

* * *

It would be beyond the scope of this monograph to review the available data on the oncogenic effects of ionizing radiation, including the *leukemogenic and carcinogenic effects of radioisotopes* employed therapeutically, such as I^{131} in thyrotoxicosis, and P^{32} in polycythemia, and the development of carcinomas and sarcomas following the injection of thorotrast which was commonly used in the years 1928 to 1945 in diagnostic radiology, etc. These and other similar observations, as well as the corresponding bibliography, are reviewed in the recent reports of the U.N. Scientific Committee on Effects of Atomic Radiation (1964) and the International Committee on Radiological Protection (1966). The interested reader is also referred to several comprehensive reviews (Brues, 1951. Aub *et al.*, 1952. Furth and Lorenz, 1954. Miller, 1964. Casarett, 1965), and to the many special publications dealing with this subject.

EXPERIMENTAL INDUCTION OF TUMORS OR LEUKEMIA WITH IONIZING RADIATION

The investigator dealing with irradiation of animals may, to some extent at least, manipulate experimental conditions in an attempt to induce a desired tumor. This is possible only to a very limited degree. As a general rule, local exposure of a relatively small area of the body to repeated irradiations may eventually result in the development of a local tumor, whereas general irradiation may rather induce the development of internal tumors or, more frequently, leukemia. The results depend on the total dose of ionizing radiation employed, and on a variety of other factors, such as host species, genetic susceptibility, and age of the host at the time of irradiation; furthermore, several unknown but possibly most important factors have to be considered, such as the presence or absence in the irradiated hosts of potentially oncogenic viruses susceptible to the trigger effect of radiation injury.

A great variety of tumors, such as sarcomas and carcinomas, can be induced in mice, rats, and other animals, with X-rays or other forms of ionizing radiation, including radium and other radioactive substances. It is of considerable interest that total-body X-ray irradiation of mice of several different inbred strains results in the development of a relatively high incidence of leukemia. On the other hand, a similar total-body irradiation of rats usually induces a variety of solid tumors, mostly subcutaneous sarcomas, mammary carcinomas, ovarian carcinomas, etc., instead of leukemia. This curious species difference in host response to ionizing radiation is discussed in more detail at the end of this chapter.

The effects of nuclear detonation on a large population of young adult (6 to 12-week-old) mice of strain LAF_1, placed at various distances from the hypocenter, was reported by Furth (1954), Upton (1960), and their associates. The lethal dose (LD50, in 30 days) was approximately 755 R in both sexes. The first late effects were cataracts in eye lenses, atrophy of the iris, and graying of hair, appearing within 3 months after irradiation. Later on, thymic lymphomas, including other forms of generalized leukemia, appeared in some of the irradiated mice. In addition there was a high incidence of ovarian neoplasms, and the frequent development, particularly in females, of pituitary tumors. Among other tumors developing in the irradiated mice, were adenocarcinomas of the Harderian glands of the orbit, adenomas or carcinomas of lungs, liver, adrenals, and kidneys. Among those animals that received a dose above the 500 R level, fatal degeneration of kidneys (nephrosclerosis) occurred frequently.

In this chapter we shall limit our review mostly to the induction, and subsequent transmission, of mouse leukemia. This monograph deals essentially with oncogenic viruses. Radiation-induced leukemia is included, because recent experiments suggest that the true nature of this form of mouse leukemia is fundamentally not different from that of other mouse leukemias, since it can be transmitted serially by filtrates. It is thus apparent that radiation-induced leukemia in mice is actually caused by an oncogenic virus, and that the radiation energy serves only as an inducing mechanism, activating, possibly in an indirect manner, a hitherto latent oncogenic virus already present in the mouse.*

It is possible, indeed quite probable, that other forms of radiation-induced tumors may also be caused by oncogenic viruses. Such an assumption still remains to be proven, however. For that reason, and also because of limitation of space, a more detailed discussion of the induction with ionizing radiation of other tumors, such as sarcomas and carcinomas, is not included in this monograph.

Osteosarcomas are common among malignant tumors induced by ionizing radiation. No experimental evidence is yet available to suggest that radiation-induced osteosarcomas are caused by a virus. It is of interest, however, that at least some osteosarcomas in mice may be caused by filterable viruses. Evidence to that effect was obtained when it became apparent that under certain conditions the tissue-culture-grown polyoma virus can induce, among other tumors, also osteogenic sarcomas following inoculation into newborn mice (Stewart *et al.*, 1958). In more recent experiments, Finkel, Biskis, and Jinkins, at Argonne National Laboratory (1966), isolated a filterable virus from a spontaneous mouse osteosarcoma. The isolated virus could be transmitted serially, inducing osteosarcomas after a relatively short incubation period following inoculation into newborn mice.

Induction of Leukemia in Mice by X-Rays

It has long been observed that mice of otherwise low-leukemic strains may develop a significant incidence of leukemia following irradiation with X-rays. Krebs and his associates (1930) were the first to demonstrate experimentally the leukemogenic potency of X-rays. Of 5,500 mice exposed to sublethal doses of X-rays, 19 developed lymphoid leukemia (0.36 per

* Total-body X-ray irradiation may also activate another latent oncogenic virus in mice, namely the polyoma virus, which causes the development of salivary gland tumors and related neoplasms (Gross, 1958a. Gross *et al.*, 1959). For more detailed information, the interested reader is referred to the chapter on the Polyoma Virus in this monograph.

cent), as compared with only 6 mice among 10,500 non-irradiated controls (0·06 per cent). Hueper (1934) exposed mice bearing spontaneous mammary tumors to repeated doses of 30 to 80 R once a week for a period of up to 6 weeks and noticed a greatly increased incidence of leukemia among the irradiated mice. Furth and Furth (1936) exposed large numbers of mice of three different strains to one or several doses of 300 to 400 R and found a considerable increase in the incidence of leukemia among the irradiated mice.

Radiation, however, did not become a useful and convenient tool for the experimental induction of mouse leukemia until conditions were determined which made it possible to induce this disease by X-rays, almost at will, in the laboratory. These conditions were determined with remarkable precision by Kaplan and his associates at the Department of Radiology, Stanford University, California.

Influence of Host's Genetic Susceptibility, Age at Irradiation, and Sex. Mice of several low-leukemic strains were irradiated with X-rays in an attempt to determine the susceptibility of different strains to leukemogenic potency of ionizing radiation. Actually, all strains tested thus far were found to be susceptible to the development of radiation-induced leukemia, although the incidence varied from some 25 to 90 per cent. This refers to strains which, under normal conditions of life, have a negligible incidence of spontaneous leukemia. Mice of strains A, I, C3H, C57 Brown, C57 Black, etc., develop spontaneously leukemia only exceptionally, if at all. Yet, following fractionated total-body X-ray irradiation, an incidence of leukemia could be induced which varied from 27 per cent in mice of strain I, to 60 per cent in C3H or C57 Brown mice (Gross *et al.*, 1959), and even up to 90 per cent in C57 Black mice (Kaplan and Brown, 1952).

The studies of Kaplan (1947, 1948b) demonstrated that the incidence of radiation-induced leukemia was highest when 2 to 4-week-old mice were irradiated. This incidence decreased rapidly when mice more than 2 months old were used. Female mice were slightly, but significantly, more susceptible to the induction of lymphomas by X-rays than males (Kaplan and Brown, 1952).

The lowest dose employed, about 300 R, approached the minimal effective level below which no leukemia could be induced.

Fractionated, Total-body Irradiation: the Method of Choice to Induce Leukemia. In a series of fundamental experiments, Kaplan and Brown (1952) determined the precise conditions under which a high incidence of leukemia could be induced consistently in the irradiated mice. Fractionated irradiation at intervals of 4 to 8 days proved to be most suitable and yielded a higher incidence of leukemia and a shorter latency period. Increasing the interval to 16 days resulted in a decreased response. In order to induce leukemia the irradiation had to affect the entire host. In contrast to whole-body exposure, local irradiation of mice failed to increase consistently the incidence of leukemia (Kaplan, 1949). When C57 Black mice received total-body irradiation, 64 per cent developed leukemia; irradiation of the upper half of the body, under otherwise similar conditions, yielded leukemia in only 4 per cent, and that of the lower part of the body, in 2 per cent. As Kaplan has shown, the lymphoid tumors in irradiated C57 Black mice originated in most instances in the thymus, disseminating secondarily to other lymphoid tissues, internal organs, and ultimately to the blood. Yet, local irradiation of the thymic area alone was ineffective in inducing leukemia. Total-body irradiation was essential.

Partial Shielding During Irradiation Prevented the Development of Leukemia

The development of leukemia in the irradiated mice could be largely inhibited by placing a lead shield over the thigh or other peripheral region during the irradiation, despite the fact that the thymus received the same X-ray dose (Jacobson *et al.*, 1949, 1951. Jacobson, 1952). Shielding of thymus during the irradiation was also effective in preventing the development of leukemia (Toch *et al.*, 1956). Lorenz and his associates (1953) obtained the same result by shielding the exteriorized spleen, which in the young mouse normally contains much active extramedullary hematopoietic tissue.

Although repeated irradiation of only one-half of the body alone was ineffective, alternate irradiation of the upper and lower halves of the body yielded about the same lymphoma incidence as whole-body irradiation, provided that the interval of time between exposure of the two halves of the body was 24 hours or less (Kaplan and Brown, 1951, 1952).

The results of these experiments excluded the hypothesis that lymphoid tumors resulted from a direct effect of X-rays upon susceptible tissue, such as thymus. It seemed rather that an indirect mechanism was responsible for the development of radiation-induced leukemia (Kaplan and Brown, 1951). It was possible to speculate that a humoral factor was released from the irradiated tissue, and that such a factor could be destroyed or inactivated by non-irradiated tissue.

Prevention of Leukemia by Intravenous Injection of Normal Mouse Bone Marrow into Irradiated Mice

Further experiments carried out by Kaplan and his associates (1953b) have shown that intravenous injection of normal bone marrow cells into irradiated C57 Black mice had a distinct inhibitory influence on the development of lymphoid tumors, although the effect was not as significant as that of partial shielding. The injection of the bone marrow cells had to be made soon after the irradiation. Injection of the marrow as late as 12 days after irradiation was already without effect. Furthermore, the material was effective when given intravenously, distinctly less so when given intraperitoneally.

Tolerance of a Lethal Dose of X-Rays by Mice Whose Spleen was Shielded During Irradiation

In 1949, Jacobson and his associates reported that lead-shielding of surgically exteriorized spleen of adult mice during a single exposure to a lethal dose of X-rays had a remarkably protective effect against otherwise fatal radiation injury.

In a series of fundamental experiments carried out at the Argonne National Laboratory in Chicago, Jacobson and his associates (1949, 1951, 1952) determined that the survival of mice following exposure to a single lethal dose of total-body X-ray irradiation could be significantly increased by spleen-shielding. In one of the most striking experiments, 77 per cent of adult mice with exteriorized spleen shielded by lead survived exposure to 1,025 R of total-body X-ray irradiation, as compared with only 1.1 per cent of non-shielded control mice exposed to the same dose of X-rays. In another similar experiment, 55 per cent of mice with shielded spleen survived exposure to 1,100 R, whereas none survived among the unshielded controls.

Reduction of Radiation Mortality Following Injection of Normal Spleen or Bone Marrow Extracts. Similar, though less striking protective effect could be obtained in the irradiated mice by intraperitoneal implantation of normal mouse splenic tissue, by intraperitoneal inoculation of normal mouse spleen or embryo cell suspensions, or by either intraperitoneal or intravenous injections of homologous bone marrow cell suspensions (Jacobson, 1952. Cole *et al.*, 1952. Lorenz *et al.*, 1951–1954). Under certain experimental conditions, cell-free extracts prepared from normal mouse spleens were also found to be effective (Ellinger, 1958). Heterologous material from rats and even guinea pigs introduced into irradiated mice was also effective, although to a lesser degree than homologous or isologous material (Lorenz *et al.*, 1952. Lorenz and Congdon, 1954. Congdon and Lorenz, 1954. Ellinger, 1958, 1962. Katz and Ellinger, 1963).

Although some investigators felt that the protective effect might be caused by a *cellular* factor, introduced into the irradiated animals with the normal bone marrow cell suspensions (Loutit, 1954), other observations appeared to suggest that a *humoral* factor, present in normal spleen or bone marrow, was responsible for the stimulation of the recovery of the irradiated animals, and for the protective effect which reduced radiation mortality.

Inhibiting Effect of Normal Sheep Spleen Extracts on Radiation-induced Leukemia in Mice. Berenblum and his coworkers (1964, 1965) at the Department of Experimental Biology, Weizmann Institute of Science, in Rehovoth, Israel, reported that extracts from normal sheep spleens exerted an inhibiting effect on radiation-induced leukemia in mice. The extracts were prepared from sheep spleens, collected in a slaughter house. Either crude, homogenized, or centrifuged, cell-free extracts were prepared. C57 Black mice, 5 to 7 weeks old, serving as test animals, received fractionated total-body X-ray irradiation, 150 R per exposure, once a week, for 4 consecutive weeks. The spleen extracts were then injected (0.25 cc. each) intraperitoneally, within 4 hours after each irradiation, and then twice weekly for several weeks, a total of 10 to 30 injections. The most striking inhibition (69 per cent) of radiation-induced leukemia was observed following injection of crude spleen homogenates. The supernate resulting from centrifugation of the spleen extracts also had a significant inhibiting effect on the radiation-induced leukemia. Heating of the extracts to 60°C for $\frac{1}{2}$ hour destroyed their inhibiting activity.

The radiation-leukemia protecting factor (RLP) was found to be present not only in normal spleens of sheep, but in bovine spleen as well. In experiments performed by Hodes and his colleagues (1966), extracts prepared from either sheep spleens or from bovine spleens exerted a significant inhibiting effect on radiation-induced leukemia in C57 Black mice, and also in BALB/c mice. Some degree of protective effect was also obtained following injection of bovine gamma globulin.

No Inhibiting Effect of Sheep Spleen Extracts on Spontaneous or Carcinogen-induced Mouse Leukemia. Injection of normal sheep spleen extracts had no inhibiting effect on the development of either spontaneous mouse leukemia, or on the development of leukemia induced by carcinogenic chemicals in mice (Berenblum *et al.*, 1965).

Accordingly, the factor present in normal sheep spleens which protects against radiation-induced leukemia is not a general anti-leukemia agent, but is a factor which specifically inhibits that phase of radiation damage which leads to the development of radiation-induced lymphosarcomas or leukemia in mice.

The Important Role of the Thymus in Radiation-induced Mouse Leukemia

The role of the thymus in the development of spontaneous leukemia in mice has already been discussed in the chapter on Mouse Leukemia of this monograph. Thymectomy was found to reduce considerably the incidence of spontaneous leukemia in mice of high-leukemic strains, such as Ak (McEndy *et al.*, 1944) and C58 (Law and Miller, 1950), and also that of virus-induced leukemia in C3H mice inoculated with the passage A virus (Gross, 1959. Levinthal, Buffett, and Furth, 1959. Miller, 1959).

Removal of thymus also reduced the incidence of radiation-induced leukemia (Kaplan, 1950); only 4 per cent of thymectomized C57 Black mice developed radiation-induced leukemia, as compared with 48 per cent among the non-thymectomized irradiated controls. Furthermore, thymectomy also inhibited the development of leukemia in methylcholanthrene-treated DBA mice (Law and Miller, 1950).

Splenectomy or gonadectomy did not inhibit the development of radiation-induced lymphatic leukemia.

Fractionated total-body X-ray irradiation of mice of strain RF resulted in the development of either myeloid leukemia or thymic lymphomas. *Removal of thymus* prior to irradiation eliminated the induction of thymic lymphomas, but did not prevent the development of lymphomas in extrathymic lymphoid tissues; furthermore, thymectomy did not influence the induction of myeloid leukemia.

On the other hand, *removal of spleen* in RF mice before irradiation lowered the susceptibility to the induction of myeloid leukemia, but did not influence the induction of lymphomas (Upton *et al.*, 1958).

In 1950 Law and Miller reported that subcutaneous implantation of normal autologous or isologous thymic tissue restored the susceptibility of thymectomized mice to either spontaneous or hydrocarbon-induced leukemia. This observation was later applied also to radiation-induced leukemia. Kaplan and his associates reported in 1956 that at least some of the mice of the C57 Black strain, that had been rendered refractory to the development of radiation-induced leukemia by thymectomy performed prior to radiation, developed leukemia nevertheless, when thymus lobes, removed from normal C57 Black mice, were implanted subcutaneously into the thymectomized mice after the completion of irradiation. The thymus could be grafted as late as 8 days after the irradiation of thymectomized hosts; leukemia still developed in such animals. The site of the origin of lymphoid tumors was the thymic implant itself. The age of the donor mice from which thymus had been removed for implantation into thymectomized mice was of considerable importance in determining the degree of restitution of susceptibility of the thymectomized mice to radiation-induced leukemia. When fragments of thymus from 2-day-old mice were grafted subcutaneously into thymectomized C57 Black mice, the incidence of radiation-induced leukemia was 70 per cent. This compared with an incidence of only 22 per cent when thymus from 2-month-old donors was used for grafting (Carnes *et al.*, 1956).

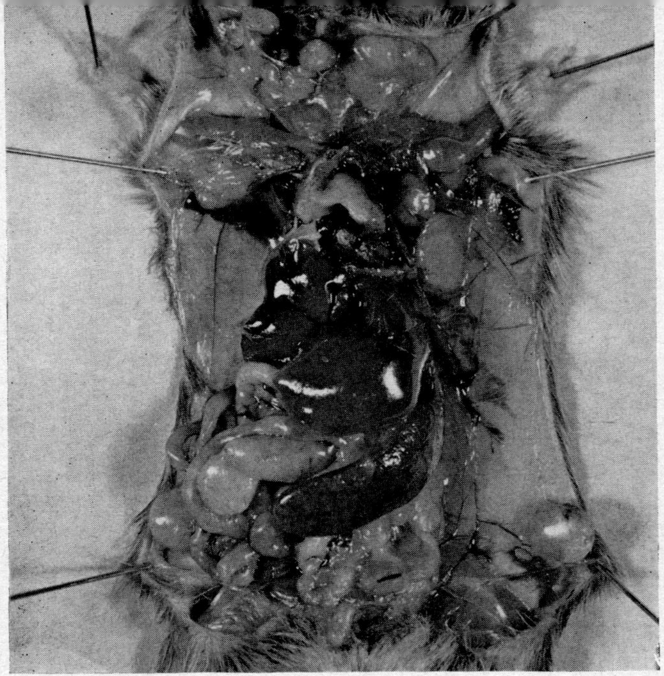

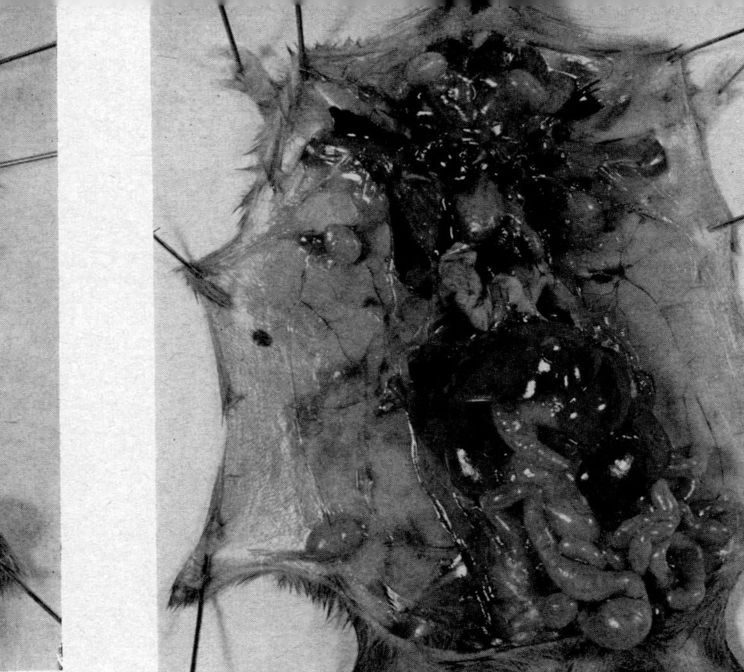

FIG. 45a. RADIATION-INDUCED LEUKEMIA IN A C3H MOUSE.

This C3H male received 5 total-body X-ray irradiations of 150 R each at weekly intervals, starting at age of 2 months. At the age of $8\frac{1}{2}$ months this mouse developed generalized lymphatic leukemia. Note the large spleen and liver, large mediastinal tumor and large tumorous lymph nodes in the mesentery, in the axillary and inguinal pits, and in the submaxillary area. (From: L. Gross, *Acta Haemat.*, **19**: 353, 1953.)

FIG. 45b. RADIATION-INDUCED LEUKEMIA IN A C57 BROWN MOUSE.

This C57 Brown/cd female received 5 total-body X-ray irradiations of 150 R each at weekly intervals, starting at the age of 2 months. At the age of 9 months this mouse developed generalized lymphatic leukemia. Note large spleen and liver, a moderately large mediastinal tumor, and tumorous lymph nodes in the mesentery, in the submaxillary area, and also in the axillary and inguinal pits.

The possible mechanism of the inhibiting effect of thymectomy on the development of radiation-induced leukemia in mice will be discussed again at the end of this chapter when the possible implications of some of the recent electron microscopic observations are reviewed.

What is the Nature of Radiation-induced Leukemia in Mice?

Experiments reviewed in this chapter suggest clearly that leukemia can be readily induced in mice by fractionated total-body X-ray irradiation. It is also apparent, however, as discussed in more detail in the two preceding chapters of this monograph, that leukemia can be induced in mice with carcinogenic chemicals or hormones, and also by inoculation of a transmissible virus isolated from organs of leukemic mice, or from certain other sources, such as transplanted mouse tumors.

Theoretically, one could assume that all these different leukemogenic factors are comparable in their action, since they all induce the same, or a very similar, disease. And yet, a more critical appraisal could lead to another explanation.

The fact that ionizing radiation, hormones, or carcinogenic chemicals may be able to induce tumors or leukemia, does not necessarily imply that these tumor-inducing factors are similar in their pathogenic action on oncogenic viruses. It is possible to speculate that hormones, chemical carcinogens, and ionizing radiation may serve only as inducing triggers, acting on latent oncogenic viruses. The trigger mechanism would thus release the pathogenic potential of a latent virus, already present in the host (Gross, 1954).

There exist certain fundamental differences between the oncogenic potential of ionizing radiation, hormones, or carcinogenic chemicals, and of tumor-inducing viruses.

Ionizing radiation, hormones, and carcinogenic chemicals are able to exert their oncogenic potential on a wide variety of different species of hosts, and cannot be recovered from tumors which they have induced, since they are metabolized, decomposed, and/or excreted. The tumor-inducing viruses, on the other hand, are often limited in their pathogenic potential to one or a few related species. However, significant exceptions exist to this rule, since the mouse leukemia virus may induce leukemia also in rats, the tissue-culture-grown mouse parotid tumor (polyoma) virus may induce tumors in mice, hamsters, and rats, and certain strains of Rous sarcoma virus can induce tumors not only in chickens, but also in rats and several other species, etc.

Furthermore, in many instances, under favorable experimental conditions, oncogenic viruses can be recovered, frequently even with an increased potential, from tumors and leukemias which they induced, and can be transmitted serially from one host to another; oncogenic viruses multiply in susceptible cells on host-to-host passage. However, a reservation is again necessary at this point, since certain oncogenic viruses, such as the parotid tumor (polyoma) virus, the adenovirus, or the SV 40 virus cannot be recovered from tumors which they induce following inoculation into susceptible newborn hosts.

In spite of these reservations, the differences between the oncogenic action of ionizing radiation, of carcinogenic chemicals, or of hormones, on the one hand, and of oncogenic viruses on the other, are of a fundamental nature.

* * *

We have reviewed on the preceding pages the leukemogenic effect of total-body X-ray irradiation on mice of certain low-leukemic inbred strains, such as C57 Black, C3H, or C57 Brown. The remarkable effect of a single, or preferably fractionated, total-body X-ray irradiation was reflected by the development of a high incidence of leukemia in the irradiated mice, as compared with a very low incidence observed in the non-irradiated control animals of the same inbred lines.

It is of considerable interest, therefore, that total-body X-ray irradiation had only a very slight effect on the development of spontaneous leukemia in mice of certain high-leukemic inbred lines, such as the Ak strain, in which the animals develop a very high incidence of spontaneous leukemia without any treatment or laboratory manipulation.

Effect of Irradiation of Mice of the High-leukemic Ak Strain

It is of interest that fractionated, total-body X-ray irradiation of young, adult female mice of the high-leukemic Ak strain had practically no effect on the incidence of spontaneous leukemia. Of 288 irradiated Ak mice, 93 per cent developed leukemia at 7.8 months average age, as compared with an incidence of 90 per cent of leukemia at 8.5 months average age among the 227 non-irradiated litter-mate controls (Gross *et al.*, 1959). Duplan (1962) also observed that X-ray irradiation of young adult (about 70 days old) males and females of the AkR strain with either 460 or 600 R did not influence either the incidence or latency of spontaneous leukemia developing in such mice, as compared with non-irradiated controls. However, in AkR mice which received total-body X-ray irradiation of 800 R, followed by a restorative dose of normal AkR bone marrow given by injection, there was observed a considerable reduction in the incidence of spontaneous leukemia, i.e. 21 per cent in the irradiated mice, as compared with 75 per cent in the controls (Duplan, 1962).

The effect of irradiation was more pronounced when *newborn* AkR mice were exposed to total-body X-ray irradiation. In experiments carried out at the Radium Institute in Paris, Reverdy, Rudali, Duplan, and Latarjet (1958) irradiated AkR mice at birth with a single total-body X-ray dose ranging from 50 to 500 R. The total number of mice employed for this study was 2184.

The results were as follows: the irradiation lowered the incidence of leukemia only slightly among females, and quite markedly among males, this effect increasing with the dose of irradiation. However, the average latency remained unchanged. In a more recent study (Jullien and Rudali, 1964), irradiation of either suckling or young adult Ak mice with a total of 600 R given in fractionated doses reduced the latency period preceding the development of spontaneous leukemia, but did not influence the total incidence of the disease.

ATTEMPT TO TRANSMIT RADIATION-INDUCED LEUKEMIA BY FILTRATES

In an effort to bring some clarification to the fundamental question concerning the nature of radiation-induced leukemia, an attempt was made to determine whether leukemia induced in mice by total-body X-ray irradiation could be transmitted by filtrates. This study was based on the theoretical assumption that radiation-induced leukemia may be the result of an activation, by radiation energy, of a hitherto latent oncogenic agent.

The plan of experiments was as follows: young mice of a low-leukemic strain were to be exposed to fractionated doses of total-body X-ray irradiation. It was anticipated that a certain number of such mice would develop leukemia. From the leukemic donors, filtrates were to be prepared and inoculated into newborn mice of the same strain (Gross, 1957b, 1958a).

Induction of Leukemia in C3H Mice by Total-Body X-ray Irradiation

Young male and female mice, approximately 1 to 3 months old, of the C3H strain (Bittner subline), known in our laboratory to have an incidence of spontaneous leukemia of less than 0.5 per cent, were irradiated with X-rays (150 to 200 R, total-body, at weekly intervals, for 4 to 6 times). Of 154 irradiated C3H mice, 81, or 53 per cent, developed leukemia after an average latency of 9 months. Of 124 brothers and sisters of these mice, not irradiated and kept as controls, none developed spontaneous leukemia, although they lived to an average age of 14 months.

In a similar experiment, mice of the C57 Brown/cd strain, also known to have a very low incidence of spontaneous leukemia, received fractionated total-body X-ray irradiation (150 R, at weekly intervals, for 4 to 5 consecutive weeks). Of 72 irradiated C57 Brown mice, 43, or 60 per cent, developed leukemia at 9 months average age. Of 52 litter-mate, non-treated controls, only one (2 per cent) developed spontaneous leukemia at 22 months of age.

Fractionated total-body X-ray irradiation (150 R, at weekly intervals, for 5 times) of some other strains was also carried out. Of 28 mice of strain A,

10, or 36 per cent, developed leukemia after a latency of 10 months. Of 65 foster-nursed mice of strain A, 29, or 45 per cent, developed leukemia after a latency of 10 months. Of 52 strain I mice, 14, or 27 per cent, developed leukemia after a latency of 10 months (Gross *et al.*, 1959).

Prevention of Radiation-induced Leukemia in C3H Mice by Thymectomy

Thymectomy effectively prevented the development of leukemia in irradiated C3H mice. Of 14 C3H mice that were thymectomized, and then received 5 consecutive total-body irradiations of 150 R each at weekly intervals, none developed leukemia, but 2 developed parotid gland tumors. Of 12 normal, non-thymectomized litter-mate controls irradiated simultaneously, 6 developed leukemia after a latency varying from 6 to 8 months (Gross, 1958). Thymectomy prevented therefore the development of radiation-induced leukemia not only in C57 Black mice (Kaplan, 1950) but also in those of the C3H strain.

Morphology of Radiation-induced Leukemia

Morphology of Radiation-induced Leukemia in C3H Mice. Following total-body fractionated X-ray irradiation, a large number of C3H mice developed generalized leukemia after a latency which varied from 5 to 9 months. Reviewing the general morphology of leukemia induced by fractionated total-body irradiation in a total of 133 C3H mice (Gross *et al.*, 1959), the results were as follows: a large number of the irradiated mice (72 per cent) developed generalized leukemia with enlarged peripheral lymph nodes, large spleens and livers, and large thymic and mesenteric tumors. Among the irradiated mice, however, some (28 per cent) developed only very large thymic lymphosarcomas, with only occasional evidence of other generalized pathology.

Blood Picture. Peripheral (tail) blood counts were made on 42 leukemic mice. The number of white cells varied from 1,250 to 192,400 per mm^3 (average 27,145, as compared with 9,790 in normal C3H mice). Fifty-five per cent of the leukemic blood smears showed the presence of lymphoblasts and smudge cells (average of 3 lymphoblasts and 18 smudge cells per 100 white cells). Thirty-three per cent of the blood smears showed the presence of nucleated red cells in peripheral blood. The dominant white cell was the lymphocyte; most of the lymphocytes appeared normal, but at least 17 per cent could be classified as atypical.

Most of the leukemic mice showed marked to moderate anemia. The hemoglobin ranged from 3.5 to 14 gm, average 11.1 gm, per 100 cc. of blood, as compared with 15.3 gm in normal C3H mice.

Development of Tumors in the Irradiated Mice. Some of the irradiated C3H mice developed also ovarian tumors, and others developed parotid gland carcinomas and/or subcutaneous fibromyxosarcomas. Among the irradiated and non-irradiated C3H mice, several developed pulmonary adenomas, and some of the C3H females developed also mammary carcinomas.

Transplantation of Radiation-induced Leukemia by Cell-Graft. The radiation-induced leukemia proved to be readily transplantable by cell-graft to mice of the same inbred line. Leukemia induced by irradiation of mice of the C3H strain could be transplanted to C3H mice, whereas leukemia induced by irradiation in mice of the C57 Brown line could be transplanted to mice of the C57 Brown strain.

Inoculation of Filtrates Prepared from Radiation-induced Leukemia into Newborn C3H Mice

Leukemic thymic and mesenteric tumors as well as livers and spleens from C3H or C57 Brown donors, in which leukemia was induced by total-body X-ray irradiation, were used for the preparation of either centrifuged (7,000 $\times g$) or filtered (through Selas, porosity 02 or 03, filter candles) extracts.

The filtrates were prepared in the usual manner, described in the preceding chapter; a cell suspension of 20 per cent concentration was prepared from leukemic organs, including spleen and liver, centrifuged at 0°C, first at 3,000 r.p.m. (1,400 $\times g$) for 15 minutes, then at 9,500 r.p.m. (7,000 $\times g$) for 5 minutes; the final supernate, mixed with 1 : 2,000 dilution of *E. coli*, was passed through Selas, porosity 02 or 03, filter candle. All resulting filtrates were bacteriologically sterile. Each extract was prepared from a different donor with primary, radiation-induced leukemia.

Newborn, less than 16-hour-old, C3H mice were then inoculated. Fourteen centrifuged extracts were inoculated into a total of 124 C3H mice, and 15 of them (12 per cent) developed leukemia at an average age of 9 months; in addition, 7 mice developed parotid gland tumors. However, only 6 out of the 14 extracts tested proved to be active on inoculation tests.

Eighteen filtrates were inoculated into a total of 148 C3H mice, and 16 of them (11 per cent) developed leukemia at an average age of 13 months; in addition, 7 mice developed parotid gland tumors. Again, of the 18 filtrates tested, only 11 proved to be leukemogenic.

In a control experiment, centrifuged extracts prepared from normal organs of healthy C3H mice were inoculated into 186 newborn C3H mice, but only one of them (0.5 per cent) developed leukemia; 14 mice, however, (7.5 per cent) developed parotid gland tumors (Gross, 1958a).

Serial, Cell-free Passage of a Radiation-activated Mouse Leukemia Virus

It was evident that leukemia induced by X-ray irradiation could be transmitted by filtrates. The incidence of induced leukemia was relatively low, however, and many of the filtrates tested were found inactive on inoculation tests.

Actually, a similar situation existed when the initial experiments were carried out dealing with cell-free transmission of spontaneous mouse leukemia. The leukemogenic potency of filtrates prepared from Ak donors with spontaneous leukemia was relatively low; moreover, many of the extracts tested were found inactive on inoculation tests (Gross, 1957a). However, by selecting a relatively potent leukemic filtrate derived initially from an Ak donor with spontaneous leukemia, and passing it serially through newborn mice, it was possible to develop eventually a highly potent "passage A" leukemic virus, which induced leukemia consistently in up to 90 per cent of the inoculated C3H mice (Gross, 1957c). Since we were now faced with an apparently similar situation, one of the more potent extracts among those prepared from radiation-induced C3H leukemias was selected and then passed serially through newborn C3H mice. This virus strain was designated "passage X" (Gross, 1959a).

The donor serving for the preparation of the initial filtrate was a C3H female which at the age of $1\frac{1}{2}$ months received a series of total-body X-ray irradiations, 150 R each, at weekly intervals, for 4 consecutive weeks. Five months after the last irradiation, this mouse developed a very large thymic lymphosarcoma, and was then used for the preparation of the initial filtrate.

In the first passage, 8 newborn C3H mice were inoculated with the filtrate, and 3 (37 per cent) developed leukemia after an average latency of 9.3 months. A filtrate was then prepared from one of the leukemic mice of this passage, and inoculated into 7 newborn C3H mice; as a result, 6 of them (86 per cent) developed leukemia after an average latency of 9 months. In the third passage, two filtrates were prepared from leukemic donors of the preceding passage and inoculated into 16 newborn C3H mice; as a result, 14 of them (87 per cent), developed leukemia after an average latency of 7.8 months.

In the fourth serial passage, 30 out of 38 inoculated C3H mice developed leukemia (79 per cent) after an average latency of 7.3 months.

In the fifth passage, 28 out of 34 inoculated C3H mice developed leukemia (82 per cent) after an average latency of 6·7 months.

The incidence of induced leukemia remained approximately the same in the 6th, 7th and 8th passages, but the latency was gradually reduced to about 5 months.

At the present time this virus strain has passed its 27th serial, mouse-to-mouse, filtrate transfer. The incidence of leukemia resulting from inoculation of this virus into suckling C3H(f) or C57 Brown/cd mice varies from 60 to 100 per cent, and the average time of latency elapsing between the inoculation and the development of leukemia varies from $4\frac{1}{2}$ to $6\frac{1}{2}$ months.

The experiments here reviewed demonstrated, therefore, that a filterable leukemogenic virus could be recovered from radiation-induced leukemia in mice. This virus could be passed serially in newborn mice. The potency of the filtrates gradually increased with successive passages, as evidenced by increased incidence of induced leukemia, and gradual decrease of the latency elapsing between the time of inoculation and the development of disease. However, the virus strain which originated from radiation-induced leukemia (passage X) is less potent than that which originated from spontaneous Ak leukemia (passage A).

Forms of Leukemia Developing in C3H(f) Mice as a Result of Inoculation of Passage X Virus. In a group consisting of 40 C3H(f) mice inoculated within 5 days after birth with passage X mouse leukemia virus filtrate, which developed leukemia at an average age of 7 months, the forms of induced leukemia could be classified as follows:

Among mice of this group 24 mice (60 per cent) were "aleukemic," i.e. had essentially no pathologic changes in peripheral blood morphology. These 24 mice were included in the tabulation under the designation of lymphatic leukemia, although a more appropriate term would be that of disseminated lymphosarcomas, since they developed lymphosarcomas in the peripheral and visceral lymph nodes, in spleen, liver, and in most instances also in the thymus.

Of the remaining 16 mice in this sample studied, leukemia could be recognized on the basis of examination of peripheral blood smears which showed an elevation of the white blood cell counts, and the presence of abnormal blood cells. The white blood cell counts in these mice ranged from 23,350 to 162,000 (average 64,950) per mm^3. A moderate anemia was present in most of the leukemic mice examined. In a few, the anemia was pronounced; the lowest hemoglobin level was 5.2 grams per 100 cc. of whole blood. Among the 16 mice with leukemic blood changes, 8 developed lymphatic leukemia, 5 developed stem-cell leukemia, 2 developed myeloid, and one erythro-myeloid leukemia.

Infiltration with leukemic cells of lymph nodes, and of some of the visceral organs, such as liver and spleen, with formation of lymphosarcomas, was present in most of these animals.

To summarize, in a sample of 40 C3H(f) mice inoculated with passage X leukemic filtrates, the forms of leukemia could be classified as lymphatic (including the aleukemic group) in 32 mice (80 per cent), stem-cell in 5 mice (13 per cent), and myeloid or erythro-myeloid in 3 mice (7 per cent).

Transmission, by Filtrates, of Radiation-induced Leukemia in C57 Black Mice

The Experiments of Lieberman and Kaplan. Experiments discussed on the preceding pages of this chapter established the fact that mice of the C3H strain remain essentially free from spontaneous leukemia under normal conditions of life, but develop a high incidence of lymphatic leukemia when exposed to total-body X-ray irradiation; furthermore, the resulting leukemia can be transmitted by inoculation of filtrates prepared from organs of leukemic mouse donors into newborn mice of the same inbred strain (Gross, 1957, 1958, 1959).

A similar observation was made by Lieberman and Kaplan (1959) at the Department of Radiology, Stanford University, in California, on mice of strain C57 Black. The incidence of spontaneous leukemia in untreated mice of the subline of the C57 Black strain of mice (C57BL/Ka), which has been maintained in their laboratory, is negligible. In a sample of 74 C57 Black mice, either untreated or injected with physiological saline solution, and observed for 20 months or longer, only one spontaneous lymphosarcoma was observed (1.3 per cent). When, however, a group of C57 Black mice received fractionated total-body X-ray irradiation (4 weekly doses of 168 R each, starting at approximately one month of age), 80 to 90 per cent of the irradiated mice developed lymphatic leukemia after a latency varying from 6 to 7 months. Filtered extracts prepared from tissues of those C57 Black mice that developed radiation-induced leukemia were inoculated into newborn mice of the same inbred line. Of 59 inoculated mice, 10 developed leukemia (17 per cent) after an average latency varying from 8.4 to 23 months. In another similar experiment, filtrates were prepared from a lymphosarcoma which had been originally also induced by radiation in a C57 Black mouse, but which had been transplanted for the previous 7 years by cell-graft in mice of the same inbred strain. Of 26 newborn C57 Black mice inoculated with these filtrates, 5 mice (19 per cent) developed leukemia after a latency of 15 months.

Filtrates prepared from normal organs removed from healthy, untreated C57 Black mice, and injected into newborn mice of the same strain, induced no leukemias.

An attempt was then made to pass serially a filtrate-induced lymphosarcoma in newborn F_1 hybrid mice (C57 Black $\times$ BALB/c). In the first two passages, leukemia developed in 2 out of 6, and in 9 out of 13 mice, after a latency of 3 to 11 months.

Lieberman and Kaplan obtained therefore results similar to those observed in our laboratory. Using mice of a different inbred line, they also determined that radiation-induced leukemia could be transmitted by cell-free extracts inoculated into newborn mice, and that the potency of the agent thus recovered could be increased by serial cell-free passage.

Isolation of a Leukemogenic Virus from Radiation-induced Mouse Leukemia at the Radium Institute in Paris. The Experiments of Lartarjet and Duplan. In view of the importance of the observation that a filterable leukemogenic virus could be recovered from radiation-induced leukemia (Gross, 1957, 1958, 1959. Lieberman and Kaplan, 1959), Lartarjet and Duplan (1962) repeated and verified these experiments in their laboratory at the Radium Institute in Paris. They employed C57 Black mice for their study; the incidence of spontaneous leukemia developing in untreated mice of their breeding stock was about 4 per cent. However, following four consecutive total-body X-ray irradiations, 175 R each at weekly intervals, of young, less than 2-month-old, C57 Black mice, 17 out of 23 irradiated mice (73 per cent) developed leukemia. Ten centrifuged cell-free extracts prepared from the leukemic mouse donors were inoculated into newborn, and also into young adult, 30-day-old, C57 Black mice. Out of 10 extracts tested, 6 were found to be leukemogenic on bio-assay. The newborn mice received a single injection of the extract, whereas the 30-day-old mice received one or three consecutive injections of the extracts at weekly intervals. Among the 47 mice that were treated at birth, 15 developed leukemia. Among 13 mice which received a single injection of the extract at 30 days of age, none developed leukemia; however, among 16 mice which received three consecutive injections of the extracts, starting at 30 days of age, 8 developed leukemia. The latency time elapsing between the inoculation of the extracts and the development of leukemia varied from 13 to 17 months. The virus recovered from radiation-induced leukemia could be passed serially; its leukemogenic potency increased with host-to-host passage.

Results of these experiments confirmed the fact that cell-free extracts prepared from radiation-induced mouse leukemia contain a virus which may induce leukemia following inoculation into newborn or young adult mice of susceptible strains.

Inoculation of Radiation-induced Lymphoma Extracts Directly into Intrarenal Thymus Implants in C57 Black Mice. In a recent study carried out by Haran-Ghera (1966) at the Weizmann Institute of Science, in Rehovoth, Israel, the leukemogenic activity of cell-free extracts prepared from organs of C57 Black mice with radiation-induced lymphomas was again tested, employing a new bio-assay method. Leukemia was first induced in C57 Black mice by fractionated total-body X-ray irradiation. Twelve centrifuged cell-free extracts were prepared from thymic lymphomas and bone marrow of mouse donors with radiation-induced leukemia. These extracts were then injected directly into several-day-old thymus implants placed beneath the kidney capsules in thymectomized irradiated C57 Black mice. This method, recently described (Haran-Ghera and Kaplan, 1964), was chosen for this study because of its apparent sensitivity as a bio-assay test serving for the detection of leukemogenic agents of relatively low pathogenic potency.

Of the 12 extracts tested, 6 were found to be leukemogenic on bio-assay; they induced a 14 per cent incidence of lymphomas developing after an average latency of $5\frac{1}{2}$ months.

In the same experiment, centrifuged extracts were also prepared from thymuses and bone marrow taken from irradiated donor mice only 5 or 10 days after the completion of the irradiation, i.e. before such donors developed leukemia. Such extracts also demonstrated leukemogenic activity on bio-assay tests, and induced a leukemia incidence of up to 30 per cent.

Centrifuged extracts prepared from organs of mice taken 20, 30, 45 and 60 days after irradiation showed only a slight leukemogenic potency.

Isolation of a Leukemogenic Virus from Mice of the RF Strain

Jenkins and Upton (1963) at the Oak Ridge National Laboratory, Tennessee, were also able to transmit radiation-induced leukemia by filtrates. They carried out their experiments on mice of the RF strain. Only 3 to 5 per cent of these mice develop myeloid leukemia spontaneously; this incidence could be increased to almost 40 per cent following exposure of such animals to 300 R total-body X-ray irradiation early in adult life (Upton, 1959). The radiation-induced myeloid leukemia of the RF mouse was transmitted by inoculation of cell-free filtrates prepared from organs of the leukemic mouse donors into newborn, and also into young adult, RF mice. The incidence of leukemia developing in inoculated mice increased on successive passages to 50 per cent, and the latency gradually decreased to less than 3 months. Although the induced leukemia retained its granulocytic character on serial transmission in adults, a significant number of newborn mice inoculated with the extracts developed thymic lymphomas within 90 days after inoculation.

In a similar study carried out by Irino and his coworkers (1966) at the Department of Internal Medicine, Okayama University Medical School, in Japan, leukemia was induced in mice of the RF strain by a single total-body irradiation with 350 R. The incidence of radiation-induced leukemia was 77 per cent, as compared with a 1 per cent incidence of spontaneous leukemia observed in non-irradiated RF mice in the same laboratory.

Filtered cell-free extracts were then prepared from organs of mice in which leukemia had been induced by irradiation. The extracts were inoculated into 16 newborn RF mice and induced leukemia in 4 of the inoculated animals after a latency varying from 12 to 22 months. The leukemogenic virus was then passed serially in newborn RF mice. Six out of 10 mice in the second passage, and 1 out of 6 mice in the third passage developed leukemia. In a control experiment cell-free extracts prepared from normal non-leukemic RF mice were inoculated into 20 newborn mice of the same strain, but no leukemia developed in the inoculated animals.

Morphologic Changes in Chromosomes Following Inoculation of Radiation-induced Mouse Leukemia in RF Mice. In a study carried out by Wald and his associates (1964), myelogenous leukemia, induced in a mouse of the RF strain by X-ray irradiation, was serially transmitted in newborn RF mice. An extra chromosome, as well as a morphologically unusual chromosome were found in the bone marrow cells of all the leukemic mice that had been injected previously either with leukemic spleen cells or with cell-free centrifuged extracts prepared from organs of leukemic mouse donors. This observation suggested that the changes in the chromosomes were caused by a virus.

Electron Microscopic Studies of Radiation-induced Leukemia in Mice

In the early electron microscopic studies of radiation-induced mouse leukemia, virus particles were found only in organs of C3H(f) mice in which leukemia was induced by inoculation of the passage X virus (Dmochowski, Grey, and Gross, 1959); no virus particles, however, could be found in organs of mice with primary radiation-induced leukemia. In recent studies, virus particles could also be found in organs of C3H(f) mice in which leukemia developed as a result of total-body X-ray irradiation (Gross and Feldman, 1968). Electron microscopic examination of ultrathin sections prepared from organs of 8 C3H(f) mice in which leukemia was induced by fractionated total-body X-ray irradiation revealed the presence of characteristic virus particles in intercellular spaces, or budding from cell membranes, in the thymus, in bone marrow, in the spleen, and in lymph nodes. The particles were morphologically indistinguishable from those observed either in spontaneous Ak mouse leukemia, or in leukemia induced in C3H(f) mice by inoculation of the passage A (Gross) mouse leukemia virus. The particles had a diameter of about 100 mμ; some had the typical doughnut-like form and an electron-lucent center; other particles had an electron-dense nucleoid. They could be classified as type C immature, or mature, virus particles. Their distribution in organs and cells was also very similar to that observed in spontaneous and virus-induced mouse leukemia. However, they were less numerous in organs of mice with radiation-induced leukemia, particularly when compared with organs of mice or rats in which leukemia was induced with the passage A virus.

Of particular interest was the appearance of virus particles in the thymus, in bone marrow, spleen, and in lymph nodes of normal C3H(f) mice only a few days after total-body X-ray irradiation (Gross and Feldman, 1968). Characteristic virus particles were found budding from cell membranes, sometimes in considerable numbers; fully formed type C particles were observed lying singly, or in small clusters, in intercellular spaces. These particles were found in tissues of these mice as early as one or two weeks after the completion of fractionated total-body X-ray irradiation (5 times 150 R at weekly intervals), and in one case only 24 hours after a single total-body irradiation with 250 R. Accordingly, in all these animals the virus particles appeared several months before the development of radiation-induced leukemia. On electron microscopic examination of organs of normal, non-injected and non-irradiated C3H(f) mice very few particles could be found in the thymus; very occasionally isolated particles could be found after prolonged search also in bone marrow (Feldman and Gross, 1966), and in the lymph nodes (Gross and Feldman, 1968) but not in other organs thus far examined.

This observation was consistent with results of experiments recently reported by Haran-Ghera (1966) in which extracts prepared from thymus and bone marrow of C57 Black mice had a leukemogenic activity on bio-assay, even when the organs serving for the preparation of extracts were removed from the donor mice only a few days after irradiation.

The presence of virus particles on electron microscopic examination of organs of non-leukemic mice shortly after total-body X-ray irradiation, and the leukemogenic activity of extracts prepared from such organs, are consistent with the assumption that X-ray irradiation releases and activates a latent virus carried by either C3H(f) or C57 Black mice.

In other laboratories virus particles were also observed on electron microscopic examination of organs of mice in which leukemia was induced with a virus isolated from radiation-induced leukemia. Dalton (1962) observed typical virus particles, indistinguishable from mouse leukemia type C particles, in megakaryocytes in the bone marrow of a C57 Black mouse bearing lymphomas induced by inoculation of a radiation-induced and serially passaged mouse leukemia virus. More recently Carnes and his colleagues also reported presence of type C virus particles in organs of C57 Black mice in which leukemia was induced by inoculation, into grafted thymus fragments, of serially transmitted radiation-activated mouse leukemia virus. These particles were found in the lymphoid tumor cells budding from the cell membranes, and also lying free in cytoplasmic vacuoles in the epithelial cells in the grafted thymus tissue (Carnes *et al.*, 1966. Kaplan, 1966).

Parsons and his colleagues (1962) observed the presence of virus particles in RF mice in which leukemia was induced either by total-body X-ray irradiation or with the passaged radiation-activated virus. Spleen, liver, and bone marrow of nearly all such mice, and in a few animals also thymus and pancreas, revealed on electron microscopic examination the presence of virus particles very similar to those observed in leukemic mice of the Ak strain. Particles of the same morphology were observed by these authors also in tissue culture cells derived from serially passaged radiation-activated mouse leukemia.

Is the Virus Recovered from Radiation-induced Leukemia Different from that Isolated from Spontaneous Mouse Leukemia?

Are the leukemogenic virus strains isolated from radiation-induced leukemia different from the mouse leukemia virus originally isolated from spontaneous Ak mouse leukemia? This problem is essentially similar to that discussed in more detail in the preceding chapter, in which the isolation of leukemogenic virus strains from certain transplanted mouse tumors was reviewed. The disease, usually a disseminated lymphosarcoma, induced with at least some of the virus strains isolated from radiation-induced leukemia, is morphologically indistinguishable from that induced with the passage A virus, originally isolated from spontaneous Ak mouse leukemia. This is true for the passage X virus isolated from radiation-induced leukemia in C3H(f) mice, and also for the virus strains isolated from radiation-induced leukemia in C57 Black mice.

It is of interest that the virus strain isolated from radiation-induced leukemia in RF mice (Jenkins and Upton, 1963) induced only in some of the RF mice thymic lymphomas, particularly when it was inoculated into newborn animals. In most instances, however, following inoculation into adult RF mice, the same virus induced a relatively high incidence of myelogenous leukemia. It remains to be determined whether the ability of this virus strain to induce myelogenous leukemia is an intrinsic virus property, or whether it was related to experimental conditions, and also to the genetic susceptibility of mice of the RF strain of mice employed in this study. The Graffi virus strain was reported to induce usually myelogenous leukemia under experimental conditions employed in Dr. Graffi's laboratory (Graffi, 1960); the same virus, however, induced predominantly lymphatic leukemia when tested on mouse strains employed in our studies (Gross, 1964). Similar observations suggesting that conditions of the recipient host, including genetic susceptibility, influence the form of leukemia induced with the Graffi virus were reported by Fiore-Donati and Chieco-Bianchi (1964).

We are therefore faced with the fact that leukemogenic virus strains could be isolated from different sources, such as from spontaneous mouse leukemia, from certain transplanted mouse tumors, and from radiation-induced leukemia in mice. These virus strains have the same physical and biological properties. When tested by inoculation into newborn mice of certain inbred strains, most of these virus strains induce a very similar disease, usually thymic or disseminated lymphosarcomas, less frequently either lymphatic, stem-cell, or myelogenous leukemias. It is quite possible that all these virus strains actually represent the same virus prototype; however, the possibility must also be considered that at least some of them may represent substrains of the mouse leukemia virus, which may have certain individual characteristic features, including certain pathogenic and antigenic differences. Similar observations have been made in the study of other oncogenic and non-oncogenic viruses.

Attempt to Neutralize the Passage X Mouse Leukemia Virus by Immune Passage A serum. One of the generally accepted methods of identifying viruses is *in vitro* serum neutralization test employing a specific immune serum. Unfortunately, the mouse leukemia virus is only weakly antigenic.

For this reason careful titration of the virus filtrate is required prior to its use in the serum neutralization tests. Specific neutralization with an immune serum can occur only under quantitative experimental conditions; a high-titer virus filtrate may not be neutralized by a relatively weak immune serum, particularly if a heterologous serum is employed for the neutralization test.

In several experiments thus far performed immune rabbit serum prepared with the passage A mouse leukemia virus (Gross) neutralized not only the passage A virus, but also the passage X virus isolated from radiation-induced mouse leukemia. Under quantitative experimental conditions employed in these studies, the leukemogenic virus isolated from radiation-induced leukemia in C3H(f) mice could not be differentiated immunologically by serum neutralization tests from the passage A virus isolated from spontaneous Ak mouse leukemia. Since both virus strains have identical physical, biological, and pathogenic properties, the conclusion may appear justified that both represent the same virus or virus prototype. The only difference between these two virus strains observed in our laboratory was that of the titer. The passage A mouse leukemia virus has a considerably higher titer and is capable of inducing leukemia in higher dilutions than the passage X virus.

In recent studies Kaplan (1967) also reported that the passage A mouse leukemia virus (Gross) and the radiation-activated mouse leukemia virus isolated from C57 Black mice in his laboratory were immunologically indistinguishable; he did note, however, biological differences between these two virus strains reflected in their different host range. The radiation-activated virus isolated from C57 Black mice had a higher leukemogenic potency for C57 Black mice and a relatively lower potency for mice of the C3H(f) strain, whereas the reverse was true for the passage A mouse leukemia virus. However, the host range of the passage A leukemia virus, and presumably also that of other leukemic virus strains, depends to a

---

FIG. 46. VIRUS PARTICLES IN ORGANS OF C3H(F) MICE WITH RADIATION-INDUCED LEUKEMIA, ALSO IN ORGANS OF MICE INJECTED WITH RADIATION-ACTIVATED "PASSAGE X" VIRUS.

(A). An area of lymph node from a C3H(f) mouse with lymphatic leukemia induced by total-body X-ray irradiation (150 R $\times$ 4 at weekly intervals). Budding particles (b) and mature type C particles (C) containing nucleoids are illustrated. Magnification 62,000 $\times$. (From: L. Gross and D. G. Feldman, *Cancer Research*, **28**: 1677, 1968.) (B). Section of lymph node from a C3H(f) mouse with passage X virus-induced lymphatic leukemia. Several particles (b) are shown budding from the cell membrane. Also illustrated in the intercellular space are mature type C particles (C) containing nucleoids, a cylindrical particle (cl), and a particle with a tail-like structure (t). Magnification 33,600 $\times$. (From: L. Gross, *Acta Haemat.*, **32**: 44, 1964.) Electron micrographs prepared by D. G. Feldman in cooperation with the author.

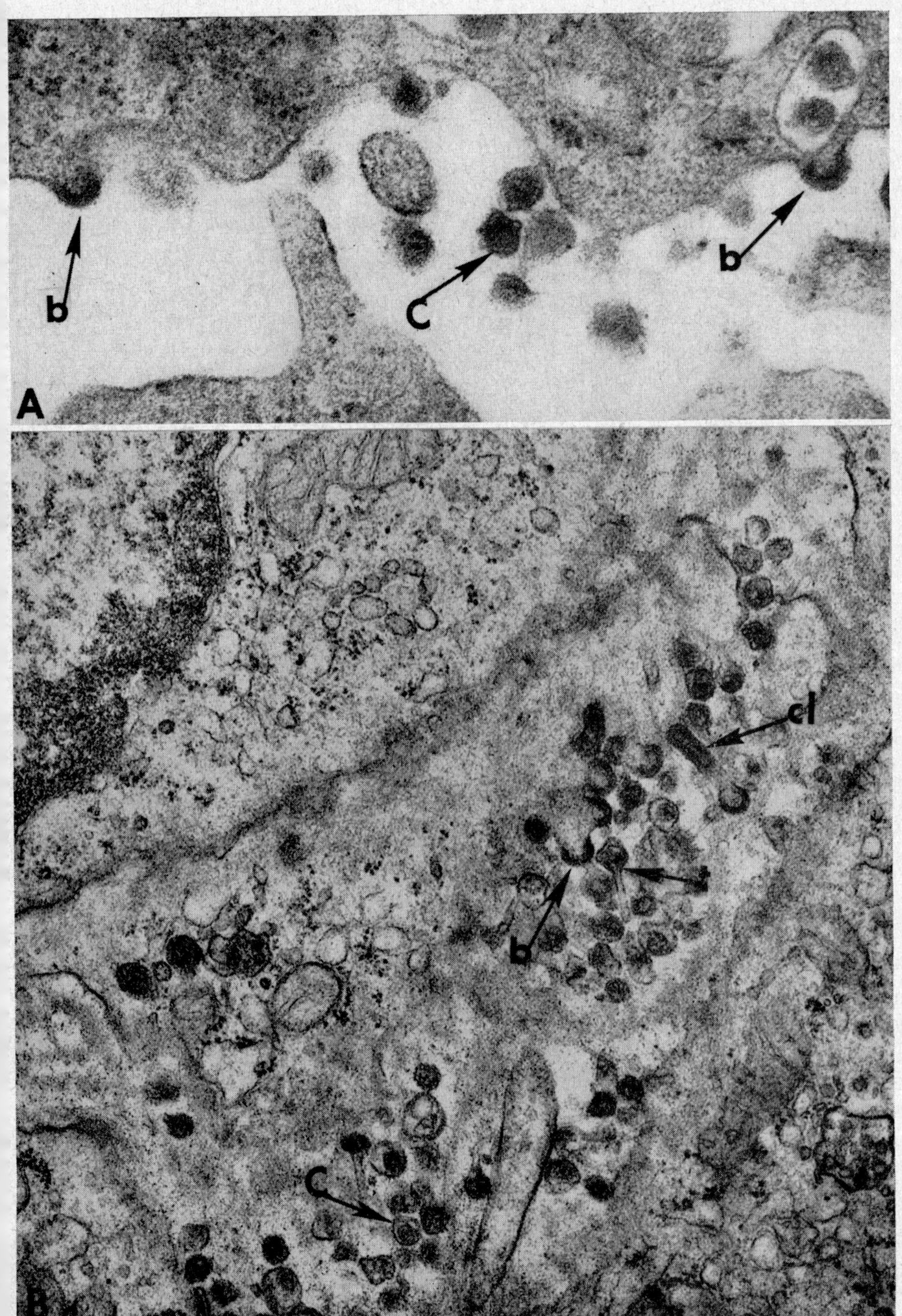

Fig. 46. Virus Particles in Organs of C3H(f) Mice With Radiation-induced Leukemia, also in Organs of Mice Injected with Radiation-activated "Passage X" Virus.

considerable degree on the titer of the virus filtrate employed. Furthermore, a virus passed serially for a considerable number of transfer generations in C3H(f) mice or in C57 Black mice, respectively, will be obviously more adapted to, and leukemogenic for, mice of the particular strain in which the passage has been accomplished, than for mice of other strains. This could explain the fact that the passage A virus which has been maintained for over 40 serial passages in C3H(f) mice is more leukemogenic for mice of that particular strain, whereas radiation-activated virus isolated from, and passaged serially in, C57 Black mice is more leukemogenic for mice of the C57 Black strain. A similar observation was made in our studies in which the mouse leukemia virus was passed serially in rats, and gradually after several rat-to-rat passages became as potent for rats as it had been in the original passage for C3H(f) mice. This is discussed in more detail in the chapter on Mouse Leukemia.

Is Radiation-induced Leukemia in Mice the Result of Activation of a Latent Virus?

Leukemia is a relatively rare disease in the general mouse population. The incidence of leukemia and lymphomas is relatively low in mice, as it is in other species also. It appears, nevertheless, that many normal and healthy mice may carry latent, but potentially leukemogenic viruses.

We have already discussed the fact that by selective inbreeding, strains of mice were developed in which the incidence of spontaneous leukemia is very high. Other inbred lines have a very low or negligible incidence of spontaneous leukemia.

It has been demonstrated that mice of some of the low-leukemic strains may develop a high incidence of leukemia or lymphomas following total-body X-ray irradiation. Although the mechanism of the development of radiation-induced leukemia has not yet been fully clarified, it is quite probable that it is closely related to the release, following application of radiation energy, of a hitherto latent oncogenic virus carried by such animals. This interpretation would be consistent with results of experiments reviewed on the preceding pages of this chapter, in which the isolation of leukemogenic viruses from radiation-induced leukemia was demonstrated experimentally in mice of certain low-leukemic strains, such as C3H(f) (Gross, 1957b, 1958a), C57 Brown (Gross, 1958a, also unpublished), C57 Black (Lieberman and Kaplan, 1959. Latarjet and Duplan, 1962. Haran-Ghera, 1966), and RF (Jenkins and Upton, 1963. Irino *et al.* 1966).

The implications of these observations are of considerable importance. It is possible to assume that the mechanism of radiation-induced leukemia, revealed in experimental studies performed on mice of a few inbred lines, is not necessarily limited to this relatively small group of animals. The results obtained may be interpreted in more general terms, which may include not only the general mouse population, but possibly other species also.

Vertical Transmission of a Latent, Potentially Leukemogenic Virus in Mice.* It appears therefore that normal and healthy mice of certain inbred lines in which leukemia develops only occasionally under natural life conditions may, nevertheless, carry latent, potentially leukemogenic viruses. In such families of mice the leukemogenic viruses are transmitted in a latent form vertically from one generation to another, presumably directly through the ova and sperm of their carriers. Although potentially pathogenic, these viruses usually behave like perfect parasites and remain under favorable life conditions harmless and very well adapted to their carrier hosts. Accordingly, most of the animals which carry such viral agents may live out their normal life span without any manifestation of disease.

Under favorable conditions, however, triggered by certain inducing factors, the hitherto latent viruses may become pathogenic, causing in their carrier hosts the development of leukemia or lymphosarcomas.

After activation, the leukemogenic viruses can then be isolated and under favorable experimental conditions passed by inoculation to other hosts in their infective and pathogenic form.

This concept, first advanced by the author as a working hypothesis (Gross, 1954, 1958a), has been found consistent with experimental observations described in this chapter.

What is the Mechanism of Radiation-induced Leukemia in Mice? Virus-Activation and Release? Recent electron microscopic studies have revealed that virus particles are formed by budding in large numbers in organs of mice of the low-leukemic C3H(f) inbred line only a few days or weeks following total-body X-ray irradiation (Gross and Feldman, 1968). This observation appears to be consistent with the concept of activation, and release, of a hitherto latent leukemogenic virus after total-body X-ray irradiation. Leukemia develops in such animals several months later.

There are other examples suggesting that radiation energy may activate hitherto latent pathogenic agents. The bacteriophage may remain latent and perfectly harmless when carried under normal life conditions by certain strains of lysogenic bacteria. Such latent form of the bacteriophage was designated "prophage" (Lwoff *et al.*, 1950. Lwoff and Gutmann, 1950. Lwoff, 1953). Under the influence of ultraviolet rays (Lwoff *et al.*, 1950), exposure to X-ray

* The term *vertical transmission* was coined by the author and suggested to designate transmission of a latent, but potentially oncogenic virus from one generation to another (Gross, 1944, 1951b, 1954, 1958b) directly through germinal cells, occasionally also though milk of nursing females.

irradiation (Latarjet, 1951), or certain other inducing factors, the prophage may become activated and pathogenic. Once activated, the phage destroys its host by lysis.

Whether radiation-induced leukemia, however, is a phenomenon directly comparable to the induction of bacteriophage, remains to be determined.

Radiation energy may represent only one of the trigger factors which may activate a latent leukemogenic virus carried by the host. Other external or internal inducing factors, including chemical carcinogens or hormones, may also activate latent leukemogenic or other oncogenic viruses carried by the host, and cause the development of either leukemia, lymphomas or other neoplasms.

This concept may not necessarily be limited to mouse leukemia, but may also apply to leukemia, lymphomas, and to other malignant tumors not only in mice but in other species also, including humans. This approach to the problem of the etiology of cancer and allied diseases will be discussed in a more comprehensive manner in the last chapter of this monograph.

ATTEMPT TO INDUCE LEUKEMIA IN RATS BY TOTAL-BODY X-RAY IRRADIATION. DEVELOPMENT OF A VARIETY OF SOLID TUMORS, INSTEAD OF LEUKEMIA, IN THE IRRADIATED RATS

Results of Fractionated Total-Body X-ray Irradiation of Sprague-Dawley Rats. We have attempted to induce leukemia in rats by fractionated total-body X-ray irradiation (Gross, Roswit, Malsky, and Dreyfuss, 1964, unpublished). A group of 38 Sprague-Dawley rats received five consecutive total-body X-ray irradiations, 150 R each, at weekly intervals, starting at ages ranging from 2 to 3 weeks. Out of 38 irradiated rats (23 females and 15 males), 33 rats (21 females and 12 males) developed single or multiple tumors at ages varying from 7 to 16 months (average age 11.3 months). Only five rats remained free from tumors through the time of observation, until they died or were sacrificed at an average age of 16 months.

Most of the tumors which developed in the irradiated rats were malignant. Some tumors could be classified as "benign" on the basis of cell morphology, even though they grew progressively and reached large size; a few of the non-malignant tumors remained encapsulated. Six rats developed multiple tumors, frequently a combination of malignant and non-malignant neoplasms developing in the same animals.

In striking contrast to results of our experiments carried out on mice, no leukemia was induced in the irradiated rats; only one male rat developed a localized reticulum-cell sarcoma in the spleen at 17 months of age.

Among the variety of neoplasms induced in the irradiated rats, the majority of tumors in females developed in the mammary glands. Nine out of 21 females in this group developed mammary carcinomas; some of them in addition also had fibroadenomas of the mammary glands. It is of interest that among the males, one also developed a large fibroadenoma of the mammary gland.

Five males and one female developed progressively growing, large, subcutaneous sarcomas, fibrosarcomas, or myxosarcomas, infiltrating the adjacent tissues, muscles and, in some instances also the peritoneal lining; one male in this group developed ascites.

One male and one female developed malignant mixed tumors of the salivary glands. Two female rats developed ovarian carcinomas, and one developed a renal carcinoma.

The principal observation which impressed us in this study was that leukemia could be readily induced by total-body X-ray irradiation in mice, but only exceptionally in rats, even though a similar technique was employed for both species. Furthermore, we have never seen such a high incidence, multiplicity, and variety of tumors among non-irradiated rats of our colony of Sprague-Dawley rats. This high incidence of tumors developing in the irradiated rats contrasted sharply with the substantially lower incidence of spontaneous tumors recorded in untreated rats of the same strain. In our laboratory we have seen only occasionally spontaneous tumors in untreated Sprague-Dawley males, but we have observed spontaneous mammary carcinomas developing in from 8 to 12 per cent of untreated females (Gross, 1963c).

Results of Fractionated Total-Body X-ray Irradiation of Long-Evans Rats. In a recent experimental series we have also irradiated in our laboratory a group of 37 Long-Evans rats. Thirty-five rats in this group received 5 consecutive total-body X-ray irradiations of 150 R each, at weekly intervals, and 2 rats received only 4 weekly irradiations, starting at 16 to 23 days of age. Among the 37 irradiated rats, only one animal developed leukemia at the age of 12½ months.

This rat developed a large spleen and liver; both organs were infiltrated with irregular, rather bizarre cells which were difficult to classify. There was also a large tumor consisting of similar cells in the mesentery. The difficulty in the classification of the form of leukemia which developed in this rat was increased by the fact that this animal was found dead, and the tissues were not well preserved.

Among the remaining animals, 16 rats developed a variety of solid tumors at ages varying from 6½ to 17 months (average 12.3 months). In this group 2 females developed fibroadenomas of the breast; one of these animals had also carcinoma of the ovary and kidney, and the other had a mixed malignant tumor of the salivary gland. One female developed carcinoma of the breast and 3 other females developed adenomas of the breast. One male developed a large hemorrhagic benign tumor of the mammary gland. Most of the remaining animals in this group developed subcutaneous sarcomas; some were fibrosarcomas, others were difficult to classify; one rat developed a leiomyoma, and another a rhabdomyosarcoma.

Seventeen rats died without evidence of tumors or leukemia at ages ranging from $6\frac{1}{2}$ to 17 months (average 14.3 months). Three animals were still alive and apparently well at 18 months of age, when this experiment was terminated.

Thus, out of a total of 37 rats which received total-body X-ray irradiation, 16 rats (43 per cent) developed tumors, and one rat developed leukemia. In this group also, therefore, total-body X-ray irradiation did not induce the development of a significant incidence of leukemia or lymphomas, but caused instead the development of a high incidence of solid tumors.

We have only preliminary information available concerning the incidence of spontaneous tumors in non-treated Long-Evans rats bred in our laboratory. Our observations suggest that the incidence and variety of tumors in non-treated Long-Evans rats are substantially lower than in the irradiated animals.

Most of the spontaneous tumors observed in the non-treated Long-Evans rats bred in our laboratory were either benign or malignant tumors of the mammary glands or ovaries in females, and occasionally subcutaneous sarcomas in old males or females. The total incidence of such tumors did not exceed 10 per cent in males, and 20 per cent in females.

The development of tumors in rats following irradiation has been observed previously in several laboratories. The interested reader is referred to the publications of Cronkite (1960), Shellabarger (1960), Bond (1960), Rosen (1961), and their associates, as well as to the review by Koletsky and Gustafson (1955). The incidence of tumors in normal rats was reviewed among others by Davis (1956), Thompson (1961), and their associates, by Noble and Cutts (1956), and also by Bullock (1930), Curtis (1931), and their associates.

* * *

Recapitulation of Recent Irradiation Experiments and Some Possible Implications of the Electron Microscopic Studies of Mouse and Rat Leukemia

The possible relationship of the presence of virus particles observed with the electron microscope in organs of normal mice to the induction of leukemia by total-body X-ray irradiation is of considerable interest. The following observations appear of fundamental importance:

Virus Particles Present in Organs of Mice and Rats with Virus-induced Leukemia. We have discussed in the preceding chapter results of electron microscopic studies of mouse and rat leukemia, which revealed the consistent presence of characteristic mature and immature type C virus particles in organs of practically all mice and rats with virus-induced leukemia, and also in the majority of mice with spontaneous leukemia.*

Similar virus particles are also present in organs of mice with radiation-induced leukemia.

On the basis of experimental data thus far accumulated it appears reasonable to assume that all leukemias and lymphomas in mice (and presumably in other species also) are caused by viruses. Accordingly, "spontaneous leukemia" is also of viral origin. However, when speaking of "spontaneous leukemia," we refer to leukemia or lymphomas developing in untreated mice, and caused by a naturally transmitted *wild* or *field* virus. This could be compared with Pasteur's *street virus* of rabies, of unpredictable potency, but responsible for naturally occurring disease.

On the other hand, when speaking of "virus-induced leukemia," we refer to leukemia or lymphomas induced in mice or rats by inoculation of the highly potent, serially passaged, mouse leukemia virus (Gross, 1957c). The passage A mouse leukemia virus, which has a high and stabilized pathogenic potency for mice and rats, can be compared with Pasteur's *fixed virus* of rabies, which is also a serially passaged virus, and has a constant and predictable pathogenic potential (Gross, 1963b).

Virus Particles Present in Thymus of Mice of Low-leukemic Inbred Lines. Electron microscopic examination of ultrathin sections of organs of normal mice of low-leukemic strains, such as C3H, C3H(f), C57 Brown, or Swiss, revealed the presence of characteristic virus particles morphologically indistinguishable from those observed in organs of mice that developed either spontaneous or virus-induced leukemia. However, these particles were very few in number, and, with occasional exceptions, could be found only in the thymus (de Harven, 1964. Feldman and Gross, 1966); in a few instances, after a prolonged search, we found isolated virus particles in the bone marrow (Feldman and Gross, 1966) and, on rare occasions, also in lymph nodes of such mice (Gross and Feldman, 1968).

Virus particles morphologically indistinguishable from type C particles of the mouse leukemia virus have also been found in several organs, such as thymus, spleen, liver, and bone marrow of embryos of normal C3H(f), and BALB/c mice (Feldman, Dreyfuss, and Gross, 1967), and also in the thymus of normal C57 Black embryos (Carnes *et al.*, 1967).

In adult mice of the low-leukemic strains, however, the distribution and

* We have examined with Dr. Feldman ultrathin sections of organs from 10 Ak mice with spontaneous leukemia and found virus particles in a variety of organs in all these animals. For further details see chapter on Mouse Leukemia.

number of virus particles are different. The particles are considerably fewer in number, and they seem to be present principally in the thymus, rarely in other organs.

Total-Body X-ray Irradiation Induces a High Incidence of Leukemia in Mice of Low-leukemic Strains. Mice of several inbred lines commonly employed in several laboratories, such as C3H, C57 Brown, C57 Black, or RF, develop only very occasionally spontaneous leukemia when left undisturbed and allowed to live out their life span without any laboratory manipulation. However, as explained in more detail on the preceding pages of this chapter, the great majority of these mice develop leukemia following total-body X-ray irradiation. The development of radiation-induced leukemia in these animals is apparently caused by activation of a latent, indigenous, but potentially leukemogenic virus harbored by many normal and healthy mice of the low-leukemic inbred lines.

Thymectomy Prevents Radiation-induced Leukemia. As already discussed on the preceding pages of this chapter, removal of thymus usually prevents the development of radiation-induced leukemia in mice. Since in normal mice of low-leukemic strains most of the virus particles can be found in the thymus, it is possible to speculate that removal of thymus eliminates in such animals the principal source of latent leukemogenic virus particles, and may for that reason render these animals refractory to radiation-induced leukemia.

In addition, thymectomy also removes the target organ in which the leukemic virus particles usually may initiate the development of disease. This is true also in spontaneous and in virus-induced leukemia.

No Virus Particles Present in Organs of Normal, Non-injected Rats. No leukemic virus particles could be found on electron microscopic examination in either thymus, spleen, bone marrow, lymph nodes, liver, or other organs of normal Sprague-Dawley rats thus far examined (Dmochowski, Padgett, and Gross, 1961. Feldman and Gross, 1966).

In a more recent study we have also examined organs of a small number of Long-Evans rats, but could not find virus particles in any of the organs examined.

No Leukemia Could be Induced in Rats by X-ray Irradiation. Fractionated total-body X-ray irradiation of 38 Sprague-Dawley rats did not result in the development of leukemia. Only one out of 39 irradiated Long-Evans rats developed leukemia. It would be possible to speculate that the failure of irradiated rats to develop leukemia following exposure to X-rays may be related to the fact that, unlike mice, most of these animals apparently do not harbor indigenous and latent, but potentially leukemogenic, virus particles.

Irradiated Rats Developed Multiple Solid Tumors, Mostly Mammary Carcinomas, and Subcutaneous Sarcomas. The fact that following total-body

X-ray irradiation of rats the majority of irradiated animals developed solid tumors, but no leukemia, does not necessarily imply that such tumors are not caused by a latent virus. However, should the radiation-induced tumors in rats be actually caused by an oncogenic virus, it may be necessary to assume that such a virus exists in the normal rats in a form which has not yet been detected by electron microscopic studies. We have not been able to reveal the presence of virus particles on electron microscopic examination of the radiation-induced rat tumors thus far performed.*

TABLE 11. X-RAYS, VIRUS PARTICLES, AND LEUKEMIA IN MICE AND RATS

	Presence of Virus Particles on Electron Microscopic Exam.		Susceptibility to Radiation-induced Leukemia	Susceptibility to Virus-induced Leukemia
	Normal Animals	Animals with Virus-induced Leukemia†		
Mice	+*	+++	+++	+++
Rats‡	—	+++	—	+++

* Only in thymus; occasionally very few isolated particles also in bone marrow and lymph nodes.

† In all organs examined.

‡ Sprague-Dawley and Long-Evans.

REFERENCES

ARNSTEIN, A., Ueber den sogenannten "Schneeberger Lungenkrebs." *Wiener Klin. Wochenschr.*, **26**: 748–752, 1913.

AUB, J. C., EVANS, R. D., HEMPELMANN, L. H., and MARTLAND, H. S., The main effects of internally deposited radioactive materials in man. *Medicine*, **31**: 221–329, 1952.

BERENBLUM, I., CIVIDALLI, G., HODES, M. E., and TRAININ, N., A factor ('RLP') from sheep spleen which inhibits radiation leukaemogenesis in mice. *Nature*, **202**: 973–974, 1964.

BERENBLUM, I., CIVIDALLI, G., TRAININ, N., and HODES, M. E., Some properties of "RLP"—A factor from sheep spleen capable of inhibiting radiation leukemogenesis in mice. *Blood*, **26**: 8–19, 1965.

BERNHARD, W., and GROSS, L., Présence de particules d'aspect virusal dans les tissus tumoraux de souris atteintes de leucémies induites. *Compt. Rend. Acad. Sci. (Paris)*, **248**: 160–163, 1959.

BIZZOZERO, O. J., JR., JOHNSON, K. G., and CIOCCO, A., Radiation-related leukemia in Hiroshima and Nagasaki, 1946–1964. I. Distribution, incidence and appearance time. *New England J. Med.*, **274**: 1095–1101, 1966.

* Attempts, carried out in our laboratory, to recover an oncogenic, or leukemogenic, virus from radiation-induced tumors in rats, have been thus far unsuccessful.

Bond, V. P., Cronkite, E. P., Lippincott, S. W., and Shellabarger, C. J., Studies on radiation-induced mammary gland neoplasia in the rat. III. Relation of the neoplastic response to dose of total-body radiation. *Radiation Research*, **12**: 276–285, 1960a.

Bond, V. P., Shellabarger, C. J., Cronkite, E. P., and Fliedner, T. M., Studies on radiation-induced mammary gland neoplasia in the rat. V. Induction by localized irradiation. *Radiation Research*, **13**: 318–328, 1960b.

Brues, A. M., Carcinogenic effects of radiation. pp. 171–191 in: *Advances in Biological and Medical Physics*, vol. 2. Academic Press, New York, 1951.

Bullock, F. D., and Curtis, M. R., Spontaneous tumors of the rat. *J. Cancer Research*, **14**: 1–115, 1930.

Carnes, W. H., Radiation leukemia virus in embryonic C57BL mouse thymus. (Abstract). *Fed. Proc.*, **26**: 748, 1967.

Carnes, W. H., Kaplan, H. S., Brown, M. B., and Hirsch, B. B., Indirect induction of lymphomas in irradiated mice. III. Role of the thymic graft. *Cancer Research*, **16**: 429–433, 1956.

Carnes, W. H., Lieberman, M., Marchildon, M., and Kaplan, H. S., Electron micrographic demonstration of C57BL mouse lymphoma virus (RLV). (Abstract). *Fed. Proc.*, **25**: 478, 1966.

Casarett, G. W., Experimental radiation carcinogenesis. *Prog. Exp. Tumor Research*, **7**: 49–82, 1965.

Clark, D. E., Association of irradiation with cancer of the thyroid in children and adolescents. *J. Am. Med. Assoc.*, **159**: 1007–1009, 1955.

Cole, L. J., Fishler, M. C., Ellis, M. E., and Bond, V. P., Protection of mice against X-irradiation by spleen homogenates administered after exposure. *Proc. Soc. Exp. Biol. & Med.*, **80**: 112–117, 1952.

Congdon, C. C., and Lorenz, E., Humoral factor in irradiation protection: Modification of lethal irradiation injury in mice by injection of rat bone marrow. *Am. J. Physiol.*, **176**: 297–300, 1954.

Court-Brown, W. M., and Doll, R., Leukaemia and aplastic anaemia in patients irradiated for ankylosing spondylitis. *Medical Research Council Special Report Series No. 295*, pp. 135. Her Majesty's Stationery Office, London, 1957.

Court-Brown, W. M., and Doll, R., Mortality from cancer and other causes after radiotherapy for ankylosing spondylitis. *Brit. Med. J.*, **2**: 1327–1332, 1965.

Cronkite, E. P., Shellabarger, C. J., Bond, V. P., and Lippincott, S. W., Studies on radiation-induced mammary gland neoplasia in the rat. I. The role of the ovary in the neoplastic response of the breast tissue of total- or partial-body X-irradiation. *Radiation Research*, **12**: 81–93, 1960.

Curtis, M. R., Bullock, F. D., and Dunning, W. F., A statistical study of the occurrence of spontaneous tumors in a large colony of rats. *Am. J. Cancer*, **15**: 67–121, 1931.

Dalton, A. J., Micromorphology of murine tumor viruses and of affected cells. *Fed. Proc.*, **20**: 936–941, 1962.

Davis, R. K., Stevenson, G. T., and Busch, K. A., Tumor incidence in normal Sprague-Dawley female rats. *Cancer Research*, **16**: 194–197, 1956.

de Harven, E., Virus particles in the thymus of conventional and germ-free mice. *J. Exp. Med.*, **120**: 857–868, 1964.

Dmochowski, L., and Grey, C. E., Electron microscopy of tumors of known and suspected viral etiology. *Texas Rep. Biol. & Med.*, **15**: 704–756, 1957.

Dmochowski, L., and Grey, C. E., Subcellular structures of possible viral origin in some mammalian tumors. *Ann. N.Y. Acad. Sci.*, **68**: 559–615, 1957.

DMOCHOWSKI, L., GREY, C. E., and GROSS, L., The role of viruses in X-ray induced leukemia. pp. 382–399 in: Radiation Biology and Cancer. *Twelfth Ann. Symposium on Fundamental Cancer Research*, 1958. M. D. Anderson Hospital and Tumor Inst., Univ. of Texas Press, Austin, 1959.

DMOCHOWSKI, L., PADGETT, F., and GROSS, L., An electron microscopic study of rat leukemia induced with mouse leukemia virus (Gross). *Cancer Research*, **24**: 869–899, 1964.

DUNN, T. B., Normal and pathogenic anatomy of the reticular tissue in laboratory mice, with a classification and discussion of neoplasms. *J. Nat. Cancer Inst.*, **14**: 1281–1433, 1954.

DUPLAN, J. F., Les radioleucémies expérimentales. *La Semaine des Hôpitaux*, **33**: 1559–1578, 1957.

DUPLAN, J. F., Influence de l'irradiation X et de la restauration isologue ou homologue sur la leucémogenèse spontanée dans la lignée AkR. *Nouv. Rev. Franç. Hematol.*, **2**: 551–562, 1962.

ELLINGER, F., Short- and long-term observations concerning the effect of homologous and heterologous cell-free spleen extracts on radiation mortality in mice and guinea pigs. *Atompraxis*, **4**: 439–444, 1958.

ELLINGER, F., Postirradiation treatment of lethal total body irradiation by cell-free spleen extracts. *Am. J. Roentgenol. Radium Ther. and Nuclear Med.*, **87**: 547–554, 1962.

EVANS, R. D., Quantitative aspects of radiation carcinogenesis in humans. *Acta Internat. Union Against Cancer*, **6**: 1229–1237, 1950.

FELDMAN, D. G., and GROSS, L., Electron-microscopic study of the mouse leukemia virus (Gross), and of tissues from mice with virus-induced leukemia. *Cancer Research*, **24**: 1760–1783, 1964.

FELDMAN, D. G., and GROSS, L., Electron microscopic study of the distribution of the mouse leukemia virus (Gross) in organs of mice and rats with virus-induced leukemia. *Cancer Research*, **26** (1): 412–426, 1966.

FELDMAN, D. G., DREYFUSS, Y., and GROSS, L., Electron microscopic study of the mouse leukemia virus (Gross) in organs of mouse embryos from virus-injected and normal C3Hf parents. *Cancer Research*, **27** (1): 1792–1804, 1967.

FINKEL, M. P., BISKIS, B. O., and JINKINS, P. B., Virus induction of osteosarcomas in mice. *Science*, **151**: 698–700, 1966.

FIORE-DONATI, L., and CHIECO-BIANCHI, L., Influence of host factors on development and type of leukemia induced in mice by Graffi virus. *J. Nat. Cancer Inst.*, **32**: 1083–1107, 1964.

FOLLEY, J. H., BORGES, W., and YAMAWAKI, T., Incidence of leukemia in survivors of the atomic bomb in Hiroshima and Nagasaki, Japan. *Am. J. Med.*, **13**: 311–321, 1952.

FORD, C. E., and MICKLEM, H. S., The thymus and lymph-nodes in radiation Chimaeras. *Lancet*, **1**: 359–362, 1963.

FRIEBEN,* Cancroid des rechten Handrücken. *Deutsche med. Wochenschr., Vereins-Beilage No.* 46, p. 335, 1902.

FRIEDLANDER, A., Status lymphaticus and enlargement of the thymus with a report of a case successfully treated by the X-ray. *Arch. Pediat.*, **24**: 490–501, 1907.

FURTH, J., and BUTTERWORTH, J. S., Neoplastic diseases occurring among mice subjected to general irradiation with X-rays. II. Ovarian tumors and associated lesions. *Am. J. Cancer*, **28**: 66–95, 1936.

* No first name initial in original paper.

FURTH, J., and FURTH, O. B., Neoplastic disease produced in mice by general irradiation with X-rays. I. Incidence and types of neoplasms. *Am. J. Cancer*, **28**: 54–65, 1936.

FURTH, J., and LORENZ, E., Carcinogenesis by ionizing radiation. Chapter 18, pp. 1145–1201 in: *Radiation Biology*, vol. 1, part 2. McGraw Hill, New York, 1954.

FURTH, J., and UPTON, A. C., Leukemogenesis by ionizing radiation. *Acta Radiol., Suppl.* 116, pp. 469–476, 1954.

FURTH, J., UPTON, A. C., CHRISTENBERRY, K. W., BENEDICT, W. H., and MOSHMAN, J., Some late effects in mice of ionizing radiation from an experimental nuclear detonation. *Radiol.*, **63**: 562–570, 1954.

GARDNER, W. U., Ovarian and lymphoid tumors in female mice subsequent to roentgen-ray irradiation and hormone treatment. *Proc. Soc. Exp. Biol. & Med.*, **75**: 434–436, 1950.

GRAFFI, A., Neuere Untersuchungen über das Virus der myeloischen Leukämie der Maus. pp. 112–161 in: *Progress in Experimental Tumor Research*. S. Karger, Basel, and J. B. Lippincott, Philadelphia, 1960.

GROSS, L., Is cancer a communicable disease? *Cancer Research*, **4**: 293–303, 1944.

GROSS, L., "Spontaneous" leukemia developing in C3H mice following inoculation, in infancy, with Ak-leukemic extracts, or Ak-embryos. *Proc. Soc. Exp. Biol. & Med.*, **76**: 27–32, 1951a.

GROSS, L., Pathogenic properties, and "vertical" transmission of the mouse leukemia agent. *Proc. Soc. Exp. Biol. & Med.*, **78**: 342–348, 1951b.

GROSS, L., A filterable agent, recovered from Ak leukemic extracts, causing salivary gland carcinomas in C3H mice. *Proc. Soc. Exp. Biol. & Med.*, **83**: 414–421, 1953.

GROSS, L., Is leukemia caused by a transmissible virus? A working hypothesis. *Blood*, **9**: 557–573, 1954.

GROSS, L., Studies on the nature and biological properties of a transmissible agent causing leukemia following inoculation into newborn mice. *Ann. N.Y. Acad. Sci.*, **68**: 501–521, 1957a.

GROSS, L., Attempt to recover filterable agent from X-ray-induced leukemia in C3H and C57 BR mice. (Abstract). *Proc. Am. Assoc. Cancer Research*, **2**: 209, 1957b.

GROSS, L., Development and serial cell-free passage of a highly potent strain of mouse leukemia virus. *Proc. Soc. Exp. Biol. & Med.*, **94**: 767–771, 1957c.

GROSS, L., Attempt to recover filterable agent from X-ray-induced leukemia. *Acta Haemat.*, **19**: 353–361, 1958a.

GROSS, L., The aetiology of cancer and allied diseases. Development of a concept based on recent experiments dealing with a cell-free transmission of mouse leukaemia. *Brit. Med. J.*, **2**: 1–5, 1958b.

GROSS, L., Serial cell-free passage of a radiation-activated mouse leukemia agent. *Proc. Soc. Exp. Biol. & Med.*, **100**: 102–105, 1959a.

GROSS, L., Effect of thymectomy on development of leukemia in C3H mice inoculated with "passage" virus. *Proc. Soc. Exp. Biol. & Med.*, **100**: 325-328, 1959b.

GROSS, L., Viral etiology of mouse leukemia. *Advances in Cancer Research*, **6**: 149–180. Academic Press, New York, 1961.

GROSS, L., Pathogenic potency and host range of the mouse leukemia virus. *Acta Haemat.*, **29**: 1–15, 1963a.

GROSS, L., Properties of a virus isolated from leukemic mice, inducing various forms of leukemia and lymphomas in mice and rats. Bertner Foundation Lecture. pp. 403–426 in: Viruses, Nucleic Acids, and Cancer. *17th Ann.*

Symposium on Fundamental Cancer Research. Univ. of Texas, M.D. Anderson Hospital and Tumor Inst., Williams & Wilkins, Baltimore, Md., 1963b.

GROSS, L., Serial cell-free passage in rats of the mouse leukemia virus. Effect of thymectomy. *Proc. Soc. Exp. Biol. & Med.*, **112**: 939–945, 1963c.

GROSS, L., How many different viruses causing leukemia in mice? *Acta Haemat.*, **32**: 44–62, 1964.

GROSS, L., and FELDMAN, D. G., Electron microscopic studies of radiation-induced leukemia in mice. Virus release following total-body X-ray irradiation. *Cancer Research*, **28**: 1677–1685, 1968.

GROSS, L., ROSWIT, B., MADA, E. R., DREYFUSS, Y., and MOORE, L. A., Studies on radiation-induced leukemia in mice. *Cancer Research*, **19**: 316–320, 1959.

HARAN-GHERA, N., Leukemogenic activity of centrifugates from irradiated mouse thymus and bone marrow. *Internat. J. Cancer*, **1**: 81–87, 1966.

HARAN-GHERA, N., and KAPLAN, H. S., Lymphoma development in intrarenal thymus implants in thymectomized, irradiated mice. (Abstract). *Proc. Am. Assoc. Cancer Research*, **5**: 25, 1964.

HASTERLIK, R. J., FINKEL, A. J., and MILLER, C. E., The late effects of radium deposition in man. pp. 943–946 in: *Radiation Standards, Including Fallout*, part II. Congress of the United States, 87th Congress, second session, 1962.

HASTERLIK, R. J., FINKEL, A. J., and MILLER, C. E., The cancer hazards of industrial and accidental exposure to radioactive isotopes. *Ann. N.Y. Acad. Sci.*, **114**: 832–837, 1964.

HATCHER, C. H., The development of sarcoma in bone subjected to roentgen or radium irradiation. *J. Bone and Joint Surg.*, **27**: 179–195, 1945.

HENSHAW, P. S., Experimental roentgen injury. IV. Effects of repeated small doses of X-rays on blood picture, tissue morphology, and life span in mice. *J. Nat. Cancer Inst.*, **4**: 513–522, 1944.

HENSHAW, P. S., Leukemia in mice following exposure to X-rays. *Radiol.*, **43**: 279–285, 1944.

HENSHAW, P. S., and HAWKINS, J. W., Incidence of leukemia in physicians. *J. Nat. Cancer Inst.*, **4**: 339–346, 1944.

HODES, M. E., CLEWELL, D. B., HUBBARD, D., and YU, P.-L., Prevention of X-ray-induced leukemia in mice. I. Action of a radiation leukemia protection factor in several mouse strains following leukemogenic or sublethal doses of X-ray. *Cancer Research*, **26**: 1780–1786, 1966.

HUEPER, W. C., Leukemoid and leukemic conditions in white mice with spontaneous mammary carcinoma. *Folia Haemat.*, **52**: 167–178, 1934.

International Commission on Radiological Protection. Committee I. The Evaluation of Risks from Radiation. *Health Physics*, **12**: 239–302, 1966.

IRINO, S., SÔTA, S., and HIRAKI, K., The role of virus in radiation leukemogenesis. *Gann*, **57**: 507–511, 1966.

JACOBSON, L. O., Evidence for a humoral factor (or factors) concerned in recovery from radiation injury: A review. *Cancer Research*, **12**: 315–325, 1952.

JACOBSON, L. O., MARKS, E. K., ROBSON, M. J., GASTON, E., and ZIRKLE, R. E., The effect of spleen protection on mortality following X-irradiation. *J. Lab. & Clin. Med.*, **34**: 1538–1543, 1949.

JACOBSON, L. O., SIMMONS, E. L., MARKS, E. K., ROBSON, M. J., BETHARD, W. F., and GASTON, E. O., The role of the spleen in radiation injury and recovery. *J. Lab. & Clin. Med.*, **35**: 746–770, 1950.

JACOBSON, L. O., SIMMONS, E. L., MARKS, E. K., GASTON, E. O., ROBSON, M. J., and ELDREDGE, J. H., Further studies on recovery from radiation injury. *J. Lab. & Clin. Med.*, **37**: 683–697, 1951.

v. JAGIĆ, N., SCHWARTZ, G., and v. SIEBENROCK, L., Blutbefunde bei Röntgenologen. *Berliner klin. Wochenschr.*, **48**: 1220–1222, 1911.

JENKINS, V. K., and UPTON, A. C., Cell-free transmission of radiogenic myeloid leukemia in the mouse. *Cancer Research*, **23**: 1748–1755, 1963.

JULLIEN, P., and RUDALI, G., Leucoses précoces apparaissant chez les souriceaux et les jeunes adultes AkR exposés aux rayons X. *Bull. du Cancer*, **50**: 147–152, 1964.

KAPLAN, H. S., Observations on radiation-induced lymphoid tumors of mice. *Cancer Research*, **7**: 141–147, 1947.

KAPLAN, H. S., Comparative susceptibility of the lymphoid tissues of strain C57 Black mice to the induction of lymphoid tumors by irradiation. *J. Nat. Cancer Inst.*, **8**: 191–197, 1948a.

KAPLAN, H. S., Influence of age on susceptibility of mice to the development of lymphoid tumors after irradiation. *J. Nat. Cancer Inst.*, **9**: 55–56, 1948b.

KAPLAN, H. S., Preliminary studies on the effectiveness of local irradiation in the induction of lymphoid tumors in mice. *J. Nat. Cancer Inst.*, **10**: 267–270, 1949.

KAPLAN, H. S., Influence of thymectomy, splenectomy and gonadectomy on incidence of radiation-induced lymphoid tumors in strain C57 Black mice. *J. Nat. Cancer Inst.*, **11**: 83–90, 1950.

KAPLAN, H. S., The pathogenesis of experimental lymphoid tumors in mice. pp. 127–141 in: *Proc. Second Canadian Cancer Conference*. Academic Press, New York, 1957.

KAPLAN, H. S., On the natural history of the murine leukemias: Presidential address. *Cancer Research*, **27**: 1325-1340, 1967.

KAPLAN, H. S., and BROWN, M. B., Further observations on inhibition of lymphoid tumor development by shielding and partial-body irradiation of mice. *J. Nat. Cancer Inst.*, **12**: 427–436, 1951.

KAPLAN, H. S., and BROWN, M. B., Protection against radiation-induced lymphoma development by shielding and partial-body irradiation of mice. *Cancer Research*, **12**: 441–444, 1952a.

KAPLAN, H. S., and BROWN, M. B., Mortality of mice after total-body irradiation as influenced by alterations in total dose fractionation, and periodicity of treatment. *J. Nat. Cancer Inst.*, **12**: 765–775, 1952b.

KAPLAN, H. S., and BROWN, M. B., A quantitative dose-response study of lymphoid-tumor development in irradiated C57 Black mice. *J. Nat. Cancer Inst.*, **13**: 185–208, 1952c.

KAPLAN, H. S., and BROWN, M. B., Development of lymphoid tumors in nonirradiated thymic grafts in thymectomized irradiated mice. *Science*, **119**: 439–440, 1954.

KAPLAN, H. S., BROWN, M. B., and PAULL, J., Influence of postirradiation thymectomy and of thymic implants on lymphoid tumor incidence in C57BL mice. *Cancer Research*, **13**: 677–680, 1953a.

KAPLAN, H. S., BROWN, M. B., and PAULL, J., Influence of bone-marrow injections on involution and neoplasia of mouse thymus after systemic irradiation. *J. Nat. Cancer Inst.*, **14**: 303–316, 1953b.

KAPLAN, H. S., BROWN, M. B., HIRSCH, B. B., and CARNES, W. H., Indirect induction of lymphomas in irradiated mice. II. Factor of irradiation of the host. *Cancer Research*, **16**: 426–428, 1956.

KAPLAN, H. S., CARNES, W. H., BROWN, M. B., and HIRSCH, B. B., Indirect induction of lymphomas in irradiated mice. I. Tumor incidence and morphology in mice bearing nonirradiated thymic grafts. *Cancer Research*, **16**: 422–425, 1956.

KATZ, S., and ELLINGER, F., Isolation of a radiation-mortality reducing factor from spleen. *Nature*, **197**: 397–399, 1963.

KIRSCHBAUM, A., and MIXER, H. W., Induction of leukemia in eight inbred stocks of mice varying in susceptibility to the spontaneous disease. *J. Lab. & Clin. Med.*, **32**: 720–731, 1947.

KOLETSKY, S., and GUSTAFSON, G. E., Whole-body radiation as a carcinogenic agent. *Cancer Research*, **15**: 100–104, 1955.

KREBS, C., RASK-NIELSEN, H. C., and WAGNER, A., The origin of lymphosarcomatosis and its relation to other forms of leucosis in white mice. *Acta Radiol., Suppl.* 10, pp. 1–53, 1930.

LATARJET, R., Induction, par les rayons X, de la production d'un bactériophage chez *B. Megatherium* lysogène. *Ann. Inst. Pasteur*, **81**: 389–393, 1951.

LATARJET, R., and DUPLAN, J.-F., Experiment and discussion on leukaemogenesis by cell-free extracts of radiation-induced leukaemia in mice. *Internat. J. Radiation Biol.*, **5**: 339–344, 1962.

LAW, L. W., and MILLER, J. H., Observations on the effect of thymectomy on spontaneous leukemias in mice of high leukemia strains RIL and C58. *J. Nat. Cancer Inst.*, **11**: 253–262, 1950a.

LAW, L. W., and MILLER, J. H., The influence of thymectomy on the incidence of carcinogen-induced leukemia in strain DBA mice. *J. Nat. Cancer Inst.*, **11**: 425–437, 1950b.

LEVINTHAL, J. D., BUFFETT, R. F., and FURTH, J., Prevention of viral lymphoid leukemia of mice by thymectomy. *Proc. Soc. Exp. Biol .& Med.*, **100**: 610–614, 1959.

LIEBERMAN, M., and KAPLAN, H. S., Leukemogenic activity of filtrates from radiation-induced lymphoid tumors of mice. *Science*, **130**: 387–388, 1959.

LINDOP, P. J., and ROTBLAT, J., Long-term effects of a single whole-body exposure of mice to ionizing radiations. I. Life-shortening. *Proc. Roy. Soc. B.*, **154**: 332–349, 1961a.

LINDOP, P. J., and ROTBLAT, J., Long-term effects of a single whole-body exposure of mice to ionizing radiations. II. Causes of death. *Proc. Roy. Soc. B.*, **154**: 350–368, 1961b.

LORENZ, E., and CONGDON, C. C., Modification of lethal irradiation injury in mice by injection of homologous or heterologous bone. *J. Nat. Cancer Inst.*, **14**: 955–965, 1954.

LORENZ, E., CONGDON, C. C., and UPHOFF, D., Modification of acute irradiation injury in mice and guinea-pigs by bone marrow injections. *Radiol.*, **58**: 863–877, 1952.

LORENZ, E., CONGDON, C. C., and UPHOFF, D., Prevention of irradiation induced lymphoid tumors in C57BL mice by spleen protection. *J. Nat. Cancer Inst.*, **14**: 291–297, 1953.

LORENZ, E., UPHOFF, D., REID, T. R., and SHELTON, E., Modification of irradiation injury in mice and guinea pigs by bone marrow injections. *J. Nat. Cancer Inst.*, **12**: 197–201, 1951.

LOUTIT, J. F., Protection against ionizing radiation. The "recovery factor" in spleen and bone-marrow. *J. Nuclear Energy*, **1**: 87–91, 1954.

LOUTIT, J. F., Transplantation of haemopoietic tissues. *Brit. Med. Bull.*, **21**: 118–122, 1965.

LWOFF, A., Le bactériophage: L'induction. *Ann. Inst. Pasteur*, **84**: 225–241, 1953.

LWOFF, A., Lysogeny. *Bateriol. Rev.*, **17**: 269–337, 1953.

LWOFF, A., and GUTMANN, A., Recherches sur un *Bacillus megatherium* lysogène. *Ann. Inst. Pasteur*, **78**: 711–739, 1950.

LWOFF, A., SIMINOVITCH, L., and KJELDGAARD, N., Induction de la production de bactériophages chez une bactérie lysogène. *Ann. Inst. Pasteur*, **79**: 815–859, 1950.

MACKENZIE, I., Breast cancer following multiple fluoroscopies. *Brit. J. Cancer*, **19**: 1–8, 1965.

MACMAHON, B., Prenatal X-ray exposure and childhood cancer. *J. Nat. Cancer Inst.*, **28**: 1173–1191, 1962.

MARCH, H. C., Leukemia in radiologists. *Radiol.*, **43**: 275–278, 1944.

MARCH, H. C., Leukemia in radiologists in a 20 year period. *Am. J. Med. Sci.*, **220**: 282–286, 1950.

MARTLAND, H. S., The occurrence of malignancy in radioactive persons. *Am. J. Cancer*, **15**: 2435–2516, 1931.

MCENDY, D. P., BOON, M. C., and FURTH, J., Induction of leukemia in mice by methylcholanthrene and X-rays. *J. Nat. Cancer Inst.*, **3**: 227–247, 1942.

MCENDY, D. P., BOON, M. C., and FURTH, J., On the role of thymus, spleen and gonads in the development of leukemia in a high-leukemia stock of mice. *Cancer Research*, **4**: 377–383, 1944.

MILLER, J. F. A. P., Role of the thymus in murine leukaemia. *Nature*, **183**: 1069, 1959.

MILLER, R. W., Radiation, chromosomes and viruses in the etiology of leukemia. Evidence from epidemiologic research. *New England J. Med.*, **271**: 30–36, 1964.

NOBLE, R. L., and CUTTS, J. H., Mammary tumors of the rat: A review. *Cancer Research*, **19**: 1125–1139, 1959.

PARSONS, D. F., UPTON, A. C., BENDER, M. A., JENKINS, V. K., NELSON, E. S., and JOHNSON, R. R., Electron microscopic observations on primary and serially passaged radiation-induced myeloid leukemias of the RF mouse. *Cancer Research*, **22**: 728–736, 1962.

PELLER, S., Lung cancer among mine workers in Joachimsthal. *Human Biol.*, **11**: 130–143, 1939.

RAJEWSKY, B., SCHRAUB, A., and KAHLAU, G., Experimentelle Geschwulsterzeugung durch Einatmung von Radiumemanation. *Naturwissenschaften*, **31**: 170–171, 1943.

REVERDY, J., RUDALI, G., DUPLAN, J.-F., and LATARJET, R., Leucémogenèse chez des souris AKR irradiées (rayons X) à la naissance. *Le Sang*, **29**: 796–804, 1958.

ROSEN, V. J., CASTANERA, T. J., KIMELDORF, D. F., and JONES, D. C., Renal neopla:sms in the irradiated and nonirradiated Sprague-Dawley rat. *Am. J. Path.*, **38** 359–364, 1961.

RUDALI, G., and REVERDY, J., Action sur la leucémogenèse des souris AkR de très faibles doses (5 r) de rayons X, reçues à la naissance. *Compt. Rend. Acad. Sci. (Paris)*, **248**: 1248–1249, 1959.

SELTSER, R., and SARTWELL, P. E., The influence of occupational exposure to radiation on the mortality of American radiologists and other medical specialists. *Am. J. Epidemiology*, **81**: 2–22, 1965.

SHELLABARGER, C. J., BOND, V. P., and CRONKITE, E. P., Studies on radiation-induced mammary gland neoplasia in the rat. IV. The response of females to a single dose of sublethal total-body gamma radiation as studied until the first appearance of breast neoplasia or death of the animals. *Radiation Research*, **13**: 242–249, 1960.

SHELLABARGER, C. J., LIPPINCOTT, S. W., CRONKITE, E. P., and BOND, V. P., Studies on radiation-induced mammary gland neoplasia in the rat. II. The response of castrate and intact male rats to 400 r of total-body irradiation. *Radiation Research*, **12**: 94–102, 1960.

Simpson, C. L., Hempelmann, L. H., and Fuller, L. M., Neoplasia in children treated with X-rays in infancy for thymic enlargement. *Radiology*, **64**: 840–845, 1955.

Stewart, A., Webb, J., Giles, D., and Hewitt, D., Malignant disease in childhood and diagnostic irradiation in utero. Preliminary communication. *Lancet*, **2**: 447, 1956.

Stewart, A., Webb. J., and Hewitt, D., A survey of childhood malignancies. *Brit. Med. J.*, **1**: 1495–1508, 1958.

Stewart, S. E., Eddy, B. E., and Borgese, N., Neoplasms in mice inoculated with a tumor agent carried in tissue culture. *J. Nat. Cancer Inst.*, **20**: 1223–1243, 1958.

Thompson, S. W., Huseby, R. A., Fox, M. A., Davis, C. L., and Hung, R. D., Spontaneous tumors in the Sprague-Dawley rat. *J. Nat. Cancer Inst.*, **27**: 1037–1057, 1961.

Toch, P., Hirsch, B. B., Brown, M. B., Nagareda, C. S., and Kaplan, H. S., Lymphoid tumor incidence in mice treated with estrogen and X-radiation. *Cancer Research*, **16**: 890–893, 1956.

Ulrich, H., The incidence of leukemia in radiologists. *New England J. Med.*, **234**: 45–46, 1946.

United Nations Scientific Committee on the Effects of Atomic Radiation. *Radiation Carcinogenesis in Man. Annex B*, pp. 81–110 in: General Assembly Official Records, Nineteenth Session, Suppl. No. 14 (A/5814). United Nations, Publ., New York, 1964.

Upton, A. C., Studies on mechanism of leukemogenesis by ionizing radiation. pp. 249–268 in: *CIBA Foundation Symposium on Carcinogenesis: Mechanisms of Action*. Little, Brown & Co., Boston, 1959.

Upton, A. C., Kimball, A. W., Furth, J., Christenberry, K. W., and Benedict, W. H., Some delayed effects of atom-bomb radiations in mice. *Cancer Research*, **20**: 1–60, 1960.

Upton, A. C., Wolff, F. F., Furth, J., and Kimball, A. W., A comparison of the induction of myeloid and lymphoid leukemias in X-radiated RF mice. *Cancer Research*, **18**: 842–848, 1958.

Wald, N., Upton, A. C., Jenkins, V. K., and Borges, W. H., Radiation-induced mouse leukemia: Consistent occurrence of an extra and a marker chromosome. *Science*, **143**: 810–813, 1964.

CHAPTER 14

The Friend Virus

The current difficulties in clarification and classification of the mouse leukemia viruses have been increased by the introduction into the study of experimental mouse leukemia of a progressive disease of the hemato-poietic system developing in mice following inoculation of the Friend virus. This curious syndrome seems to be a true "laboratory disease" and appears to be exceedingly rare under natural life conditions, if it occurs spontaneously at all; however, the disease can be readily induced in the laboratory by inoculating susceptible mice with a virus which was isolated originally from a Swiss mouse by Dr. Charlotte Friend (1956) at the Sloan-Kettering Institute in New York City.

Origin of the Virus

Prior Developments in Experimental Leukemia Research which Led to Its Unexpected Isolation. We have reviewed in one of the preceding chapters the experiments of Graffi and his associates (1955, 1956), in which cell-free extracts prepared from certain transplanted mouse tumors unexpectedly induced leukemia following inoculation into newborn mice. Previous attempts to transmit some of the common transplanted mouse sarcomas and carcinomas by filtrates were not successful, and gradually led to the commonly accepted assumption that these tumors were not caused by filterable viruses, and that they could be transmitted from host-to-host only by cell-graft. The introduction of newborn mice as sensitive test animals for bio-assay of oncogenic viruses (Gross, 1951) provided a new incentive in the search for filterable oncogenic viruses as causative agents responsible for the development of tumors hitherto thought to be of non-viral origin.

Graffi and his colleagues prepared cell-free extracts from several transplanted mouse tumors and inoculated such extracts into newborn mice apparently expecting to reproduce in the inoculated mice the development of tumors essentially similar to those that had served as donors for the preparation of the extracts.* Surprisingly, however, leukemia, instead of tumors, developed in the inoculated mice.

* Graffi, A. Personal communication to the author (1966).

Thus, the introduction of newborn mice as a new experimental bio-assay tool did not reveal in these experiments the viral etiology of transplanted mouse tumors, but led unexpectedly to the isolation of the mouse leukemia virus from such tumors.

A Virus Isolated by Charlotte Friend, Causing a Leukemia-like Disease in Mice

A study, essentially similar to experiments of Graffi, was carried out subsequently by Dr. Charlotte Friend (1956, 1957) at the Sloan-Kettering Institute in New York. In her study, a pathogenic virus causing a leukemia-like disease in mice was unexpectedly isolated from mouse donors which had received inoculation of cell-free extracts prepared from a transplanted mouse carcinoma. As was the case in experiments of Graffi, in this study also, the virus isolated by Friend had no apparent etiological relationship to the tumor which served as donor for the preparation of the extracts. Dr. Friend isolated this virus unexpectedly in the course of her experiments dealing with an attempt to transmit by cell-free extracts one of the common transplanted mouse tumors, the Ehrlich ascites mouse carcinoma. This particular tumor, as was the case with other transplanted mouse tumors, such as those employed for the preparation of extracts in Graffi's experiments, had also been tested before, and was found to be transmissible from mouse to mouse only by cell-graft. However, after the introduction of the newborn mouse as a new tool for bio-assay of oncogenic viruses, an attempt was made by Friend to transmit the Ehrlich ascites mouse carcinoma by cell-free extracts, employing newborn mice as test animals.

Both the Ehrlich ascites carcinoma and the Ehrlich solid carcinoma originated from one of the several transplantable mouse tumors developed half a century ago (Ehrlich, 1907). There exist several distinct strains of these tumor lines (H. L. Stewart *et al.*, 1959). The Ehrlich ascites carcinoma has been transplanted for many years in various laboratories. It grows readily in mice of several strains, causing in most instances a progressive and fatal disease. Following intraperitoneal inoculation of a tumor cell suspension, a general peritoneal carcinomatosis results, with the formation of an ascitic fluid with numerous floating tumor cells. The particular strain of Ehrlich ascites carcinoma employed as a prospective source of virus isolation in Dr. Friend's experiment had been maintained for a number of years by Dr. K. Sugiura at the Sloan-Kettering laboratories by routine biweekly cell-transplantations in Swiss mice.

The Ehrlich ascites carcinoma was employed by Friend for her study not only because it was readily accessible, being carried routinely by cell-graft by one of her colleagues in an adjoining laboratory, but primarily because of the presence of virus-like spherical particles which were found on electron microscopic examination of ultrathin sections prepared from this tumor in 4 out of 70 tumor specimens examined. These particles had an average diameter of approximately 58 mμ, and were found exclusively in the cytoplasm, often aggregated in hexagonal groups (Selby, 1953. Selby *et al.*, 1954). No relation whatever of these particles to the etiology of the tumor was established or claimed; not only were they absent in 66 of 70 other tumor specimens examined, but no adequate control studies of normal tissues were reported. However, in spite of lack of evidence of any causal relationship between the occasional presence of such particles and the origin of the Ehrlich ascites carcinoma, the presence of these particles in some of the tumor cells prompted Dr. Friend's investigation of a possible viral etiology of this tumor (Friend, 1957).

Inoculation of the Initially Prepared Cell-free Extract into Newborn Mice. In the initial experiment carried out by Friend (1957), the ascitic fluid containing tumor cells was collected from a Swiss mouse that had been grafted routinely, 14 days earlier, with the Ehrlich ascites carcinoma.

The tumor cells were ground with sand in a mortar, and suspended in Locke-Ringer's solution. The tumor cell suspension thus obtained was centrifuged in a Spinco Model L Ultracentrifuge at 40,000 r.p.m. for 2 hours. After the centrifugation, the supernatant fluid was removed and inoculated subcutaneously into 30 newborn, less than 24-hour-old, mice of the Swiss strain.*

After 14 months, all inoculated animals were sacrificed. There was no evidence of a tumor in any of these mice, but, unexpectedly, in 6 mice considerably enlarged spleens and livers were noticed.

Transmission by Cell-Graft of the Newly Observed Leukemia-like Disease

An attempt was then made to transplant this leukemia-like condition, by cell-graft, to other mice of the same Swiss strain. Each of the 6 enlarged spleens was removed aseptically and ground in a mortar with Locke-Ringer's solution added. The cell suspensions thus obtained were then inoculated into Swiss mice. Since no newborn mice were immediately available for inoculation, adult Swiss mice were employed. Five mice were inoculated in each of six groups.

* Commercially available albino mice with a relatively low incidence of spontaneous leukemia. Several substrains are available; only some of them are inbred. In a sample of 300 Swiss mice observed over a period of one year by Dr. C. Friend, the incidence of spontaneous leukemia, mostly thymic lymphosarcomas or generalized lymphatic leukemia, varied in different groups, reaching in some of the groups observed 11 per cent (personal communication to the author from Dr. C. Friend, 1960). The reader is also referred to Table 2, on page 234.

Four of the inoculated groups remained negative and were eventually discarded. However, marked enlargement of spleens and livers was noticed in 3 out of 5 inoculated mice in each of the two remaining groups.

Serial passage of the leukemia-like disease that developed in one of the groups was continued. Mice of the other positive group were discarded.

Serial Transmission by Either Cell-Graft or Filtrates

The disease, first observed in the few mice of the Swiss strain that had been inoculated with the Ehrlich carcinoma extracts, could be transmitted serially by inoculating cell suspensions prepared from the affected spleens into adult mice of the same strain. Further experiments demonstrated that the disease could be transmitted readily also by inoculation of filtrates prepared from extracts that had been passed through Selas 03, or Berkefeld N, filter candles.

Following inoculation of either cell suspensions or filtrates, similar results were obtained. The latency and the course of the induced disease, as well as the resulting final incidence, were essentially the same.

The Disease Syndrome Induced with the Friend Virus

Progressive Enlargement of Spleen and Liver, and Characteristic Blood Changes Developing in Mice Following Inoculation of the Friend Virus. Following inoculation of filtrates prepared from spleens and livers of donor mice with Friend virus-induced disease into 3 to 4-week-old mice of several susceptible strains, such as DBA/2, Swiss, BALB/c, or C3H(f), considerable enlargement of spleen and liver is induced after a relatively short latency of only a few weeks; this striking pathologic manifestation represents the principal macroscopic picture of the induced disease. There are no thymic tumors, and the peripheral or internal lymph nodes are not enlarged. This is in sharp contrast to the great majority of the conventional forms of mouse leukemias. It should be emphasized that the disease syndrome induced with the Friend virus has no apparent relation to the presence or absence of thymus.

Thymectomy performed on young adult mice of the Swiss strain did not render these animals resistant to subsequent inoculation of the Friend virus (Gross and Woolley, unpublished experiments, 1959. Metcalf *et al.*, 1959).

Splenectomy performed prior to, or after, inoculation of the Friend virus delayed the development of leukemia in some of the inoculated animals, but did not influence either the total incidence, form, or the eventual outcome of the disease (Friend, 1959. Metcalf *et al.*, 1959).

The peripheral blood smear reveals a characteristic picture; there is evidence of considerable anemia, and nucleated red cells are common;

most striking are innumerable "smudge cells" appearing among various cells of the myeloid series. On microscopic examination of liver and spleen there is considerable infiltration with abnormal segmented and non-segmented leukocytes, as well as nucleated red cells; there are also areas of destruction and necrosis. It is of interest that this infiltration is in most instances limited only to spleen and liver. Other organs only occasionally show infiltration with abnormal cells.

The disease may become chronic, with enlargement of spleen persisting over long periods of time; in rare instances, spontaneous regression of the enlarged spleen has been observed, with resulting recovery. Usually, however, the disease progresses rapidly, and the animals die within 2 or 3 months after inoculation. The latency and survival time depend on the genetic susceptibility of the inoculated mice, and also on age at inoculation and dose of the injected virus.

It is difficult to classify the curious disease syndrome induced with the Friend virus. The terms "erythroblastosis" or "erythroblastosis-like disease" are descriptive, but do not fully reflect all pathologic manifestations. The term "erythro-leukemia" may appear more appropriate, but would also require reservations, since the pathologic features of this syndrome do not entirely fulfil the diagnostic criteria required for an unequivocal classification of the disease induced in mice with the Friend virus as leukemia. We will return to the discussion of this problem and review the classification difficulties again on subsequent pages of this chapter.

Basic Differences between the Conventional Forms of Mouse Leukemia and the Disease Induced in Mice with the Friend Virus

In the conventional form of spontaneous mouse leukemia, which is usually lymphatic, development of thymic tumors is common and occurs in most instances. Thymic tumors are a characteristic feature of either spontaneous or induced mouse leukemia. The relation of this obscure organ to the development of mouse leukemia has not yet been fully clarified, but appears to be of fundamental importance. Surgical removal of thymus may result in delay or actual prevention of the development of virus- or radiation-induced leukemia in mice. Development of not only thymic tumors but generalized lymphosarcomas, replacing peripheral and visceral lymph nodes, and infiltrating spleen, liver, kidneys, and other organs, is a common and characteristic feature of the conventional form of mouse leukemia.

In sharp contrast, in a typical case of disease syndrome induced in susceptible mice with the Friend virus, there is no enlargement of thymus. The characteristic disease induced in mice with the Friend virus is usually manifested by the presence of a very large spleen and liver. In fact, the spleen may become enormously enlarged, like a balloon, and filled with blood. There are no thymic tumors, however, and the peripheral and internal lymph nodes are not enlarged.

We have discussed in the chapter on Mouse Leukemia transmission of leukemia from mouse-to-mouse by cell-graft. Following inoculation of a cell suspension prepared from spontaneous or virus-induced mouse leukemia into susceptible mice, a local tumor usually develops at the site of inoculation. In case of intraperitoneal inoculation, a small tumor develops frequently within the abdominal wall, at the point where the inoculating needle was introduced and pierced the skin and peritoneal lining. This local tumor development is followed rapidly by generalized leukemia. In contrast, following inoculation of a cell suspension prepared from spleens of mouse donors with Friend virus-induced disease, no local tumors usually develop at the site of inoculation. A generalized disease develops in the form of enlargement of spleen and liver, with the characteristic changes in blood morphology. The latency elapsing between the inoculation of the Friend virus and development of disease is similar, regardless of whether the inoculum contains a cell suspension prepared from organs of mice with Friend virus-induced disease or a cell-free virus filtrate. In this respect again there is a basic difference between the conventional forms of mouse leukemia and the Friend disease. Transmission of lymphoid or of another conventional form of mouse leukemia by cell-graft into susceptible mice is characterized by a relatively short latency period, usually of only 2 to 3 weeks, whereas transmission of the same leukemia by filtrates requires a latency which may vary from a few months to one year or more, according to the potency of the injected virus filtrate.

Under certain experimental conditions, however, local tumors may develop at the site of implantation of fragments of spleens or livers from mouse donors with Friend virus-induced disease (Friend and Haddad, 1959, 1960. Buffett and Furth, 1959. Metcalf *et al.*, 1959). Such local tumors are followed subsequently by enlargement of spleen and liver and the characteristic blood picture. Mice of strain DBA/2 are more susceptible to the development of local tumors than mice of the Swiss stock. Friend and Haddad (1960) succeeded in transmitting serially, by tumor grafts, the disease in DBA/2 mice.

Technique of Preparation of Friend Virus Filtrates Employed in Our Laboratory. In our studies carried out with the Friend virus (Gross, 1964), we have prepared filtrates from fragments of spleens and livers, removed aseptically from mice with Friend virus-induced disease, employing our routine method of preparation of leukemic filtrates described in the chapter on Mouse Leukemia. The tissue fragments were cut with scissors and ground by hand in a mortar, physiological saline solution being added to obtain a 10 per cent concentration. The cell suspensions were centrifuged at 3000 r.p.m. for 15 minutes; the supernate was removed and centrifuged at 9500 r.p.m. for 5 minutes. The second supernate was passed through Selas 02 filter candles. The filtrate was diluted with an equal amount of physiological saline solution to obtain a final 5 per cent concentration, and was then inoculated (0.3 cc., i.p.) into 3 to 4-week-old mice of either C3H(f) or BALB/c strain. At that age, mice of both strains were found to be uniformly susceptible to the Friend virus. As a routine procedure, part of the freshly prepared filtrate was placed in glass ampoules, sealed, and frozen at − 70°C. We have kept such filtrates frozen for over a year at −70°C in a Revco freezer, and have used them later for inoculation without noticing any apparent loss in their infectivity.

Host Range and Importance of Age at Inoculation. In the initial experiments Friend reported (1957) that among adult mice of several strains tested, only Swiss mice and those of strain DBA/2 were found to be susceptible. For routine passage of the virus, mice approximately 2 months old were employed. Adult mice of several other strains tested, including those of strains C3H and A, were found to be resistant.

In our studies (Gross, 1964) we found mice of several strains tested, such as C3H(f)/Bi (Bittner subline of foster-nursed C3H mice raised in our laboratory), as well as BALB/c and Swiss, to be uniformly susceptible to the Friend virus, provided that mice of proper age were employed for inoculation. The optimum age was found to be about 3 to 5 weeks with an average around 4 weeks. At that age male and female mice of all three strains were found to be consistently susceptible to intraperitoneal inoculation of the virus filtrate. Characteristic symptoms of disease developed usually within 2 to 3 weeks following inoculation.

When newborn or suckling mice were inoculated, the immediate mortality was high; in surviving animals the disease developed after a short latency and had a rapid course.

On the other hand, when 2 to 4-month-old mice were inoculated with the virus filtrate, the disease was not always induced; some remained in good health. Others in such groups developed disease only after a prolonged delay; furthermore, at least in some of them the resulting disease had a slow and chronic course.

Development of Lymphatic Leukemia Following Inoculation of the Friend Virus

Inoculation of the Friend Virus Filtrate into C57 Brown Mice. When suckling mice of the C57 Brown strain were inoculated with Friend virus filtrate, some of them developed the characteristic erythroblastosis syndrome. Unexpectedly, however, other mice in this group developed lymphatic leukemia (Gross, 1964). The induction of lymphatic leukemia was even more striking when 3 to 4-week-old mice of the C57 Brown strain were inoculated with the Friend virus filtrate; most of the C57 Brown mice of this age were found to be resistant to the induction of the Friend disease, but they developed instead typical lymphatic leukemia, with characteristic thymic tumors and multiple lymphosarcomas (Gross, 1964).

Thus, it was determined that under certain experimental conditions, inoculation of the Friend virus filtrate resulted in the development of lymphatic leukemia in mice of a strain relatively resistant to the induction of the Friend disease.

Inoculation of the Friend Virus Filtrate into Suckling Rats. Rats do not develop the characteristic hepato-splenomegaly syndrome observed in mice following inoculation of the Friend virus. However, following inoculation of the Friend virus filtrate into suckling rats, development of typical lymphatic, stem-cell, or myeloid leukemia was observed, accompanied frequently by development of thymic tumors and multiple lymphosarcomas (Mirand and Grace, 1962. Gross, 1964).

Since rats do not develop the characteristic erythroblastosis-like disease observed in mice, following inoculation of the Friend virus, but develop, instead, one of the conventional forms of leukemia, it appeared of interest to pass the Friend virus serially through rats. An attempt was then made to determine whether the rat-adapted Friend virus still retained its ability to induce the typical syndrome similar to erythroblastosis when inoculated back into mice (Gross, 1966). Thus far only 6 consecutive rat-to-rat passages have been performed, and the inoculated rats have developed large thymic lymphosarcomas. The rat-adapted Friend virus, harvested from leukemic rats after only 2 consecutive passages in that species, was inoculated back into 3 to 4-week-old C3H(f) mice; out of 20 inoculated mice, 4 developed typical lymphatic leukemia, and 16 remained in good health. The original Friend virus, carried in our laboratory in mouse-to-mouse passage, induces a 100 per cent incidence of the characteristic erythroblastosis-like syndrome following inoculation into less than 4-week-old C3H(f) mice.

Further rat-to-rat passages of Friend virus will be carried out; however, results of these preliminary experiments suggest that the Friend virus could be eliminated from Friend virus filtrate by serial passage through rats, leaving the conventional mouse leukemia virus (Gross) component.

Friend Virus Filtrate: A Mixture of the Friend Virus and of the Conventional Mouse Leukemia Virus (Gross)?

It would be possible to explain this dual pathogenic effect of the Friend virus filtrate by assuming that the Friend virus is capable of inducing in mice either the peculiar syndrome similar to erythroblastosis, or one of the conventional forms of mouse or rat leukemia such as thymic lymphosarcomas, lymphatic or stem-cell leukemia, i.e. forms induced usually by the mouse leukemia virus (Gross). On the other hand, it also may be possible to assume that what is now considered to be the Friend virus may actually be a mixture of two distinct viruses. It is conceivable that a filtrate prepared from spleens and livers of mouse donors with Friend virus-induced disease may contain two distinct viruses, the Friend virus and also the conventional mouse leukemia virus (Gross). Following inoculation of such a filtrate into susceptible animals, either form of disease could be induced. However, the Friend virus induces the erythroblastic disease after a relatively short latency, and for that reason, when susceptible mice are inoculated, they usually develop and die from the characteristic erythroblastosis-like syndrome before they have an opportunity to develop lymphatic leukemia or another form of leukemia caused by the conventional mouse leukemia virus (Gross).

The possibility that the Friend virus filtrate may actually consist of a mixture of the Friend virus and of the Gross mouse leukemia virus will be discussed in more detail in the next section of this chapter, dealing with the Rauscher virus strain.

Properties of the Friend Virus

The Friend virus is *filterable* and passes readily through bacterial filters, such as Berkefeld N, or Selas 02, or 03.

The virus is *thermolabile* and can be inactivated by heating for 30 minutes to 56°C (Friend, 1957), or even to only 50°C for 30 minutes (Gross, 1965, unpublished).

The virus was also found to be *sensitive to ether*. Exposure of the filtrate to *in vitro* exposure to ethyl ether inactivated its pathogenic potency (Friend, 1957).

The virus could be preserved without loss of infectivity for 6 months at −70°C in carbon dioxide dry ice; furthermore, it resisted freeze-drying, and could be preserved by lyophilization (Friend, 1957).

Titration of the Virus Filtrate. The infectivity of the Friend virus filtrate prepared from spleens of mice with virus-induced disease was consistent only when relatively high concentrations were employed for bio-assay experiments. This observation was made by Friend in her early titration studies (1957), carried out on a relatively small number of animals, in which she noticed that only a 10^{-2} dilution of the filtrate induced disease in all inoculated mice, whereas 10^{-3} dilution induced disease in only 3 out of 5 injected mice, and no disease resulted following inoculation of either 10^{-4} or 10^{-5} dilutions. In our more recent studies (Gross, 1965, unpublished), we have observed development of the characteristic hepatosplenomegaly syndrome in all mice following inoculation of 10^{-2}, 10^{-3}, or 10^{-4} dilutions of the Friend virus filtrate into 3 to 4-week-old C3H(f) mice. We noticed, however, that at least in some of the injected mice the latency was considerably prolonged following inoculation of 10^{-3}, and particularly 10^{-4} dilutions of the filtrate. Thus, the average latency was about 38 days following inoculation of the 10^{-2} dilution, as compared with 64 and 112 days, following inoculations of 10^{-3} and 10^{-4} dilutions, respectively. No disease resulted following inoculation of a 10^{-5} dilution of the filtrate.

The Friend virus is *antigenic* (Friend, 1959). Serum from rabbits that had been immunized with the virus neutralized the pathogenic potency of the filtrates *in vitro*. In our studies (Gross, 1964) we also found that an immune serum obtained from rabbits that received several injections of the Friend virus inactivated the Friend virus *in vitro*. No neutralization of the virus occurred when the virus filtrate was mixed with a control serum obtained from rabbits that received injections of normal mouse organ extracts. In another experiment neutralization did not occur when the Friend virus was mixed with immune serum obtained from rabbits that received several consecutive injections of the passage A (Gross) mouse leukemia virus.

Friend reported (1959) that a vaccine could be prepared by adding formaldehyde (1 : 500) to the virus filtrate; the mixture was kept at 4°C for 21 days prior to its use. Three immunizing intraperitoneal injections were given at weekly intervals, followed at intervals varying from 7 to 21 days by a challenging inoculation of an active filtrate. Approximately 80 per cent of immunized mice in each of the challenged group survived, as compared with only 14 per cent among the controls.

Propagation of the Friend Virus in Tissue Culture

The Friend virus could be propagated in tissue culture on mouse embryo cells, but only with moderate success (Moore and Friend, 1958. Moore, 1960, 1963. Vigier and Goldé, 1962. Chamorro *et al.*, 1962. Osato *et al.*, 1964). No cytopathic effect of the virus on normal mouse cells was noticed. However, the virus could be maintained through successive tissue culture passages, as evidenced by positive results of animal bio-assay tests.

Mouse-embryo cell cultures that had been seeded with leukemic *cells* obtained from mice inoculated with Friend virus continued to produce small amounts of infective virus for periods up to 633 days (Moore, 1963).

Mouse embryo cells exposed to Friend virus *filtrates*, and passed up to 30 times at weekly intervals, induced only occasionally the characteristic syndrome of Friend disease following inoculation into mice. Different culture methods used to increase the virus yield were unsuccessful (Moore,

1963). Even under optimal experimental conditions thus far employed, the growth of the virus *in vitro* was only slight. The inoculation of susceptible mice with the harvested tissue culture fluids resulted only now and then in the induction of the characteristic erythroblastosis-like syndrome; the incidence of induced disease was low and unpredictable.

Thus, for routine maintenance of the Friend virus, propagation of the virus in susceptible mice, instead of tissue cultures, still remains the method of choice.

Relative Resistance of the Friend Virus to In Vitro Gamma Irradiation

The Friend virus (10 per cent filtrate) was exposed in sealed ampoules to gamma irradiation in doses equivalent to 1,100,000, 2,300,000, 3,200,000, 4,500,000, and 6,000,000 R. This was performed using fresh spent radioactive fuel elements from nuclear reactor at Industrial Reactor Laboratories, AMF Atomics, Plainsboro, New Jersey (Gross *et al.*, 1968b). Following irradiation *in vitro*, the filtrates were inoculated intraperitoneally (0.5 cc. each) into weanling 3 to 4-week-old C3H(f) mice. Irradiation of up to 3,200,000 R had no significant effect on the infectivity of the virus. Seven mice were inoculated with virus filtrate that had been exposed to 1,100,000 R, and all developed the characteristic erythroblastosis-like syndrome after a latency of 3 weeks; nine mice were inoculated with the virus filtrate that had been exposed to 2,300,000 R, and 7 of them developed the erythroblastosis-like syndrome after an average latency of 2 months; eight mice received the virus filtrate that had been exposed to 3,200,000 R and 6 of them developed the characteristic hepato-splenomegaly syndrome after an average latency of 3 months. However, none of the 18 mice inoculated with virus filtrate that received *in vitro* either 4,500,000 or 6,000,000 R developed either the erythroblastosis-like syndrome, or any other form of leukemia, or leukemia-like disease.* These animals were observed and remained well until they reached an average age of 14 months. Six control mice were inoculated with non-irradiated virus filtrate, and all developed the characteristic hepato-splenomegaly syndrome after an average latency of 3 weeks.

Electron Microscopic Studies of the Friend Virus

Electron microscopic studies of ultrathin sections prepared from organs of mice in which the characteristic leukemia-like disease syndrome was induced with the Friend virus revealed the presence of spherical virus

* It is of interest that the passage A mouse leukemia virus (Gross) was also found to be inactivated *in vitro* by 4,500,000 R gamma irradiation (Gross *et al.*, 1968a). This was discussed in more detail in the chapter on Mouse Leukemia.

particles in some of the organs, particularly in liver, spleen, bone marrow, and also in blood plasma. In the white blood cells infiltrating liver and spleen of such animals, particles were found frequently budding from the edges of cellular membranes; numerous particles were also found in the intercellular spaces (de Harven and Friend, 1958, 1960). In the bone marrow, the particles were found in megakaryocytes within the cytoplasmic vacuoles; they were also formed by budding from vacuolar membrane into the lumen of the vacuoles (de Harven and Friend, 1960. Dalton *et al.*, 1961).

The virus particles were found to be spherical, with one or two external membranes. Two typical forms of the particles could be observed: The doughnut-like, considered to be the immature type C virus particle, has two external membranes, but no internal nucleoid; a third membrane was frequently observed between the outer and the inner shells (de Harven and Friend, 1960). The other form, considered to be the mature type C virus particle, has usually one, or occasionally two external membranes, and a centrally located electron-dense nucleoid.* The average external diameter of the virus particles is probably somewhere between 87 mμ and slightly over 100 mμ; the particles with nucleoids are larger than the doughnut-like particles (de Harven and Friend, 1960. Dalton *et al.*, 1961. de Harven, 1962. Feldman and Gross, 1965, unpublished. Yumoto *et al.*, 1966).

Large numbers of virus particles could also be found in the blood plasma of mice in which the disease was induced with the Friend virus. Following ultracentrifugation of blood plasma, electron microscopic examination of ultrathin sections prepared from the sedimented pellet revealed a very high concentration of virus particles (de Harven and Friend, 1964).

The virus particles observed on electron microscopic studies of ultrathin sections of organs from mice with Friend virus-induced disease were morphologically indistinguishable from those found in organs of mice with spontaneous leukemia, as well as from those found in organs of mice and rats in which one of the conventional forms of leukemia, such as lymphatic, stem-cell, or myeloid leukemia, was induced with the mouse leukemia virus (Gross). Thus, the differentiation of the Friend virus from the conventional mouse leukemia virus was not possible on the basis of electron microscopic studies (de Harven, 1962. Dalton *et al.*, 1964.

* In more recent electron microscopic studies (Feldman and Gross, 1966, 1967, unpublished) employing improved technique in the preparation of specimens, and with better resolution of the electron microscope, the immature type C virus particles were more consistently found to have 3 concentric membranes and an electron-lucent center, and the mature virus particles were found to have 2 outer membranes and an electron-dense nucleoid. In this respect, therefore, both the immature and the mature Friend virus particles were found to be indistinguishable from the mouse leukemia virus (Gross).

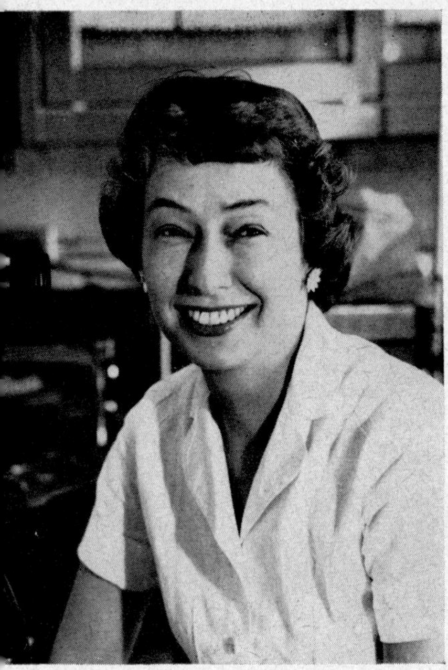

Charlotte Friend

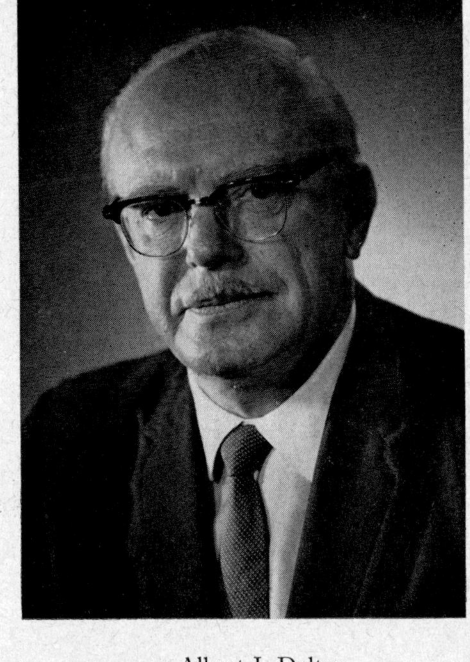

Albert J. Dalton

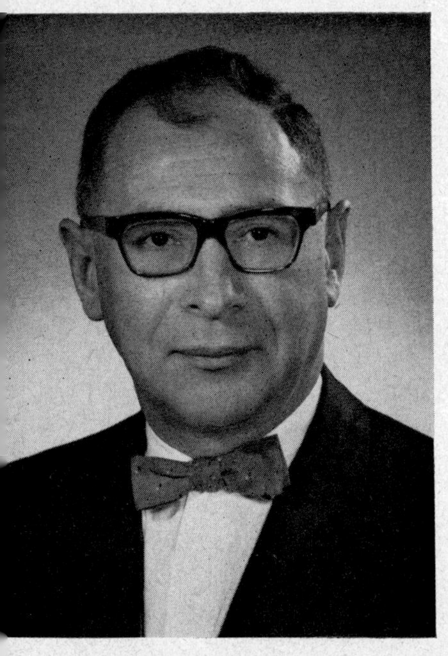

Henry S. Kaplan

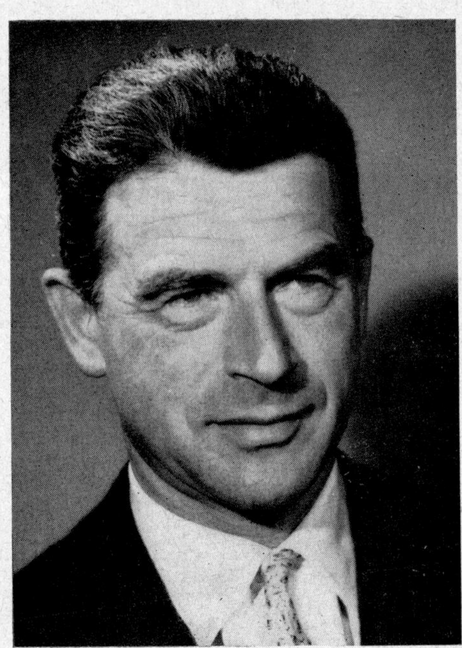

Raymond Latarjet

Fig. 47.

Dmochowski, 1963. Gross, 1964. Feldman and Gross, 1965, unpublished. Yumoto *et al.*, 1966).

In previous electron microscopic studies reported by Selby and his associates (1954), and discussed at the beginning of this chapter, examination of ultrathin sections prepared from some of the Ehrlich carcinoma specimens revealed presence of small spherical particles about 58 mμ in diameter in the cytoplasm, often aggregated in hexagonal groups. However, no similar particles could be found in any of the mice with Friend virus-induced syndrome; accordingly, the particles found by Selby, which actually prompted Dr. Friend's study, had no apparent relation to the Friend virus.

What is the Nature of the Disease Induced with the Friend Virus?

The identification of the curious disease syndrome induced with the Friend virus, and diagnosed at first as a "leukemia-like disease" (Friend, 1957), encountered initial difficulties and was a matter of prolonged discussions. There is little doubt that the disease described by Friend belongs to the broad group of leukemias. It is also apparent, however, that the peculiar disease syndrome induced in susceptible mice with the Friend virus is quite different from spontaneous leukemia that develops in untreated mice of various high-leukemic strains. The Friend disease syndrome is also different from those leukemias that can be induced in mice of different strains with carcinogenic chemicals, hormones, or ionizing radiation. Metcalf, Furth and Buffett stated (1959) that leukemia induced with the Friend virus "is unlike any spontaneous leukemia of the mouse thus far encountered by us." We can make the same statement, since we have not seen a similar form of leukemia in mice or, as a matter of fact, in any other species. Furthermore, as we already stressed at the beginning of this chapter, the disease induced with the Friend virus has not been thus far reported to occur spontaneously. It is a curious laboratory disease.

In certain respects this syndrome is similar to erythroblastosis. The large number of nucleated red cells in peripheral blood with marked anemia, and the presence of nucleated red cells in liver and spleen infiltrations, would be consistent with such a designation. On the other hand, some of the morphologic features would indicate that this disease may be a form of leukemia. The large number of smudge cells in peripheral blood is striking; although it is almost impossible to identify the nature of the smudge cells, one can assume that at least some of them may be blast cells. Smudge cells are very often seen in leukemic, but not in normal blood. The presence of abnormal leukocytes in spleen and liver, and in certain instances presence of abnormal white cells of the myeloid series in peripheral blood of some animals, would also be consistent with the assumption that this disease syndrome represents a form of leukemia. Against the diagnosis of leukemia would be the fact that infiltration of internal organs is virtually limited to liver and spleen only, and, furthermore, that there is no involvement of thymus or lymph nodes, and no formation of lymphoid tumors. With certain reservations, this disease could be designated as "erythro-leukemia" although the pathological features of the disease syndrome induced with the Friend virus do not entirely fulfill the criteria required for such terminology. The terms "erythroblastosis" or "erythroblastosis-like" are descriptive, but do not reflect precisely all pathologic manifestations induced with the Friend virus.

What is the Origin of the Friend Virus?

We have described in more detail at the beginning of this chapter the original isolation by Dr. Friend of a virus capable of inducing a leukemia-like disease in mice. This virus was isolated from a few Swiss mice which developed enlargement of spleen and liver, following inoculation shortly after birth of Ehrlich ascites carcinoma extracts.

Theoretically, it would be possible to assume that the characteristic enlargement of spleen and liver observed in the original mouse donors from which the virus was first isolated by Dr. Friend, developed spontaneously, and that inoculation of the Ehrlich tumor extracts into these mice had no causal relation to subsequent development of the characteristic leukemia-like disease.

It would be rather difficult, however, to assume that spontaneous development of the characteristic disease syndrome in mice of the Swiss strain was a unique incident. Rather, it should have been possible to find again mice of the same Swiss strain with a similar form of disease developing either in Dr. Friend's laboratory, or in another laboratory where such mice have been observed for prolonged periods of time. This has not been the case. It is, therefore, quite possible that the inoculation of the Ehrlich ascites carcinoma extracts into newborn Swiss mice was responsible for the induction of the hepato-splenomegaly syndrome in some of the inoculated animals. However, this disease could not be induced at will by injection of the Ehrlich carcinoma extracts into newborn Swiss mice. Some 40 unsuccessful attempts had been made by Dr. Friend to recover filterable oncogenic agents from the same transplantable Ehrlich ascites carcinoma, prior to the initial observation of the development of splenomegaly in the six inoculated mice.* It is possible to speculate, nevertheless, that additional attempts to extract a similar virus from that strain of the Ehrlich mouse carcinoma which was carried at the Sloan-Kettering Institute, might have met with success, particularly if presumably more favorable experimental conditions were applied for the preparation of the extracts, such as concentration of the virus by differential ultracentrifugation, and the use of newborn mice of a variety of inbred strains for the bio-assay.

* Personal communication from Dr. Charlotte Friend to the author (1959).

It is quite apparent that many viruses, including those potentially capable of inducing tumors and leukemia, are carried in a latent and non-pathogenic form in different animal species, including mice. As discussed in more detail in a separate chapter of this monograph, the polyoma, i.e. parotid tumor virus is as a rule non-pathogenic under natural life conditions, and is carried in a latent form not only in laboratory mice of different inbred strains, but also in wild mice. The same is true for many other potentially oncogenic, as well as non-oncogenic, viruses carried not only in mice, but in many other animal species, including humans. It is therefore quite possible that the virus originally isolated by Friend is carried in a latent form in many normal mice. This virus apparently remains perfectly harmless under natural life conditions. Only under certain experimental conditions can it be isolated and altered in its pathogenic potential, so that it may then induce the characteristic disease syndrome following inoculation into susceptible mice.

The experimental conditions which may favor isolation of this, or of another latent but potentially pathogenic virus may require initial passage of the virus from host-to-host. Such passage may be accomplished by inoculation of transplanted tumor extracts (etiologically unrelated to the virus, but carrying the virus as a "passenger") into newborn hosts.

Dr. Friend isolated the virus from mice that had been inoculated previously with a cell-free extract prepared from Ehrlich ascites carcinoma. It is quite possible that this transplanted mouse tumor carried a latent "passenger virus" which was transmitted by inoculation into newborn Swiss mice employed in the initial experiment. Such mouse-to-mouse passage of the virus might have been sufficient to activate its pathogenic potential and to induce disease in some of the inoculated hosts.

However, it appears that under certain experimental conditions, the host-to-host passage, leading to increased potency of the virus, may also be accomplished by inoculation of newborn mice with normal mouse organ extracts containing a latent virus ("blind passage"). This was the case in the experiments of Pope (1961) who in this manner isolated from a wild mouse a virus which was capable of inducing splenomegaly and erythroblastosis following inoculation into newborn mice.

Isolation of Virus Strains Similar to the Friend Virus in Other Laboratories

The Experiments of Pope, Franks, and Bather. The virus isolated by Pope (1961) at the Queensland Institute of Medical Research in Brisbane, Australia, and designated WM1, induced general enlargement of lymph nodes and moderate splenomegaly following inoculation into newborn or weanling mice.

> A wild male house mouse, *Mus musculus*, weighing 10 gm, was captured in Brisbane, and sacrificed on January 3, 1952. No abnormalities were found on examination. A saline cell suspension was prepared from liver and spleen, and was inoculated into suckling, less than 48-hour-old, and into weanling mice; serial intraperitoneal passages were made. It was evident from the incidence of splenomegaly induced in the first seven passages, that an agent inducing splenomegaly was being transmitted. This virus was named the Wild Mouse 1 (WM1) strain, after the mouse of origin (Pope, 1961). Several lines were subsequently maintained in serial passages, made usually at 14 to 21-day-intervals; the only indication of the presence of the transmitted virus was the occurrence of moderate splenomegaly induced in the inoculated mice.

In his further studies Pope noticed (1962) that another virus could be isolated from mice that had been injected with the WM1 virus. This second virus strain, designated by Pope WM1-B, proved to be very similar to the Friend virus, inducing a disease strikingly similar to that induced with the Friend virus, i.e. considerable enlargement of spleen and liver with presence of erythroblasts in peripheral blood. Furthermore, the WM1-B virus could be neutralized by an immune rabbit serum prepared against the Friend virus.

Later on, Pope (1963) detected another virus apparently related to the Friend virus, but of a non-pathogenic form. This avirulent virus was found to occur in wild mice trapped in various parts of Brisbane, in Queensland, Australia.

Franks and his colleagues (1957, 1959), in Toronto, isolated a virus similar to the Friend virus from some of the Swiss mice which they inoculated with Sarcoma 37. Bather (1961) obtained the virus from Franks for his studies, and noticed its similarity to the Friend virus.

Fey and Graffi reported (1965) that in the course of serial passage of their virus strain, which usually induced myelogenous leukemia, one of the inoculated mice unexpectedly developed erythroblastosis. The principal morphologic manifestation consisted of a very large spleen and liver, which developed after a relatively short incubation period. The lymph nodes were not enlarged. There was a large number of erythroblasts in the peripheral blood of this animal, and erythroblasts were also present among the white cells infiltrating spleen and liver.

A cell-free extract was then prepared from spleen and liver of this animal, and inoculated into newborn mice. A variety of forms of leukemia developed in the inoculated animals; some inoculated mice developed erythroblastosis (26 per cent); most of the remaining mice developed erythro-myeloid leukemia, myeloid leukemia, or chloroleukemia.

Whether the erythroblastosis-like syndrome observed by Fey and Graffi was similar to that observed in mice inoculated with either the Friend virus, or with the Rauscher virus strain, remains to be determined.

Thus, the original isolation by Charlotte Friend in 1956 of a virus causing erythroblastosis-like syndrome in mice might not have been a unique phenomenon. The same or a closely related virus, or viruses, may be present in a latent form in other laboratory mice, in certain transplanted mouse tumors, and perhaps also in wild mice not only in America, but also on distant continents.

THE RAUSCHER VIRUS STRAIN

A few years ago, Frank J. Rauscher at the National Cancer Institute in Bethesda, Maryland, isolated a virus capable of inducing in mice either the characteristic erythroblastosis-like syndrome of hepato-splenomegaly, described in more detail on the preceding pages of this chapter, or one of the conventional forms of mouse leukemia, such as lymphoid leukemia, including development of characteristic thymic lymphosarcomas.

The virus strain isolated by Rauscher has been employed extensively during the past several years in studies dealing with experimental mouse leukemia; for that reason a more detailed description of its properties appears to be of interest, even though this virus strain may actually represent a mixture of the Friend virus and of the conventional mouse leukemia virus (Gross).

Origin of the Virus. The origin of the virus strain isolated by Rauscher is not clear. According to the original report of Rauscher (1962), his initial studies were carried out on a "virus-induced leukemia of adult Swiss mice" previously reported by Schoolman and his associates (1957) at the Hektoen Institute, Cook County Hospital, Chicago, Illinois. "Tumor-bearing Swiss mice" received from Dr. Steven O. Schwartz were employed by Dr. Rauscher as donors for the preparation of the extracts. Twenty-eight biweekly serial intraperitoneal passages of "ascites tumor cells" were made in adult Swiss mice, and subsequently in weanling mice of the BALB/c strain. After six transplantations of the ascites tumor cells in BALB/c mice, unfiltered extracts were prepared and inoculated by different routes into BALB/c and Swiss mice of various ages.

One of the injected BALB/c mice developed a "lymphoblastoma" at the site of inoculation. This tumor grew well in ascites form on intraperitoneal transplantation in BALB/c mice. Fragments of spleens, thymuses, and lymph nodes, pooled from several leukemic BALB/c mouse donors of the ninth serial transplant generation, were employed for the preparation of an extract which was filtered and then inoculated into newborn BALB/c mice. After $5\frac{1}{2}$ months, 4 out of 39 mice developed leukemia. An extract was then prepared from spleens, lymph nodes, and thymuses of the leukemic donor mice, and centrifuged in Spinco Model L Ultracentrifuge at $105{,}000 \times g$. The pellet was resuspended in a small amount of physiological saline solution, and inoculated into 53 suckling

(4 to 12-day-old) BALB/c mice. After a short latency of only 4 weeks, 67 per cent of the inoculated mice developed considerably enlarged spleens and a moderate enlargement of inguinal lymph nodes. Serial passage of the virus through suckling BALB/c mice was then made, leading to a gradual increase in its potency, and resulting eventually in the development of a potent virus strain. The incidence of leukemia induced with this virus exceeded 95 per cent; the latency period elapsing between the time of inoculation and the development of a large palpable spleen decreased to only 3 to 4 weeks.

Following inoculation of this virus into suckling, or 3-week-old, BALB/c mice, practically all inoculated animals developed, after a short latency of 2 to 3 weeks, enormous spleens and very large livers; other organs were normal in macroscopic appearance. The injected mice died within 28 to 37 days after inoculation, some of them with hemorrhagic and ruptured spleens. The number of mice developing this form of disease depended on the age at inoculation and the amount of injected virus. When smaller quantities of the virus or older animals were inoculated, some of the mice survived the early phase of the disease, and did not develop the characteristic hepato-splenomegaly syndrome, but developed instead, a few months after inoculation, large but firm spleens, significantly enlarged peripheral lymph nodes, and also large thymic tumors.

Mice of certain strains, such as C57 Black, were found to develop consistently lymphatic leukemia, greatly enlarged lymph nodes, and thymic tumors following inoculation of the virus, instead of developing the characteristic hepato-splenomegaly syndrome. Furthermore, lymphatic leukemia was also induced in rats following inoculation of the Rauscher virus strain.

Pathogenic Properties of the Rauscher Virus Strain. It is clear from the foregoing description of the results of inoculation of the Rauscher virus strain into mice and rats, that the Rauscher virus strain has two principal pathogenic properties: (a) it can induce in susceptible mice the characteristic syndrome of erythroblastosis, described in more detail on preceding pages of this chapter. It is of considerable interest, however, that (b) under certain experimental conditions, the same virus strain can also induce lymphatic leukemia, including thymic and generalized lymphosarcomas; this occurs when mice of certain strains, or when newborn rats, are inoculated.

Development of Erythroblastosis-like Disease in Mice Following Inoculation of the Rauscher Virus

When inoculated into either suckling or young adult (3 to 4-week-old) mice of susceptible strains, such as C3H, BALB/c, or Swiss, the Rauscher virus induces, after a short latency of only a few weeks, a characteristic syndrome very similar to that induced with the Friend virus. Considerable enlargement of spleen and liver represent the most striking macroscopic feature of the induced disease. Characteristically, and within a relatively short time, the spleen may become enormously enlarged, and filled with fragments of destroyed cells and altered blood. There are no thymic tumors, and the peripheral lymph nodes are not enlarged. This is in striking contrast to the great majority of the conventional forms of mouse leukemia. The white blood cell count is considerably increased, and the peripheral blood smears show evidence of pronounced anemia, presence of many nucleated red cells, and characteristically also a very large number of "smudge" cells, among a variety of cells of the myeloid series in different phases of maturation. Microscopic examination of liver and spleen reveals considerable infiltration with abnormal white cells, as well as with nucleated red cells; there are also areas of destruction and necrosis. This characteristic infiltration is usually limited to spleen and liver. In most instances the disease progresses rapidly, and the animals die within 2 or 3 months after inoculation.

This macroscopic and microscopic picture of the erythroblastosis-like syndrome induced in mice with the Rauscher virus is indistinguishable from that resulting from inoculation of the Friend virus (Gross, 1964, 1966).

Development of Thymic Lymphosarcomas and other Conventional Forms of Mouse Leukemia in Mice and Rats Following Inoculation of the Rauscher Virus

Under certain experimental conditions, inoculation of the Rauscher virus filtrate may induce lymphatic leukemia with the characteristic development of thymic and generalized lymphosarcomas. This may take place when suckling or weanling (3 to 4-week-old) mice of certain strains, such as C57 Black or C57 Brown, relatively resistant to the Friend virus, or when suckling rats, are inoculated with the Rauscher virus filtrate (Rauscher, 1962).

The natural resistance of mice of certain strains, such as C57 Brown, to the induction of erythroblastosis following inoculation of the Rauscher virus is only relative, and is apparent when weanling mice are employed for bio-assay. When newborn or suckling C57 Brown mice are inoculated with the Rauscher virus filtrate, some develop, after a short incubation period, acute enlargement of spleen and liver, with the characteristic blood picture of erythroblastosis-like syndrome; other mice in such groups survive, but develop, after a prolonged latency, lymphoid leukemia with thymic and generalized lymphosarcomas; a few develop a "mixed" form, i.e. thymic and generalized lymphosarcomas with blood morphology similar to that observed in erythroblastosis induced with the Friend virus (Gross, 1964, 1966).

It should be pointed out that similar results can be obtained by employing the Friend virus filtrate for inoculation of suckling and 3 to 4-week-old mice. Furthermore, the Friend virus can also induce thymic lymphosarcomas, as well as lymphatic, stem-cell, or myeloid leukemia, following inoculation into suckling rats. Inoculation of the Friend virus filtrate into mice of certain strains, such as C57 Brown, and also into rats, may result in the development of lymphatic leukemia, including the characteristic development of thymic lymphosarcomas. In this respect, therefore, the Friend virus filtrate is essentially similar to the Rauscher virus strain. This pathogenic action of the Friend virus may be due to the presence in the Friend virus filtrate of the conventional mouse leukemia virus component (Gross, 1964).

The interesting ability of the Rauscher virus to induce either the erythroblastosis-like syndrome, with its characteristic pathologic features and striking blood picture, or one of the conventional forms of mouse leukemia, frequently associated with the development of a thymic lymphosarcoma, such as lymphatic, stem-cell, or myeloid leukemia, could be explained by an assumption that a single virus, present in the Rauscher filtrate, has a wide range of pathogenic potential, and is capable of inducing both erythroblastosis and one of the conventional forms of mouse leukemia, such as thymic lymphosarcomas.

On the other hand, it would be also possible to assume that what is now considered to be the "Rauscher virus" may actually represent a mixture of two distinct viruses, the Friend virus and, in addition, the conventional mouse leukemia virus (Gross). Such an explanation (Gross, 1966) would be consistent with the observation that inoculation of the Rauscher virus can induce two phases of pathologic manifestations, the early phase identical with the erythroblastosis-like syndrome induced with the Friend virus, and the second phase usually represented by the development of lymphatic leukemia. However, under present conditions in many laboratories the Rauscher virus is considered to be a single virus and is being studied as such in its physical, morphological, and biological properties.

It should be emphasized that the Rauscher virus could not be differentiated on the basis of either physical properties or its morphology from other leukemogenic viruses described in mice. The Rauscher virus was found to have physical properties similar to those of the mouse leukemia virus (Gross), as well as those of the Friend virus.

Propagation in Tissue Culture. The Rauscher virus could be propagated in tissue culture on normal mouse embryo cells. No cytopathic effect of the virus on the cells on which it was grown could be observed; however, the virus multiplied, as determined on animal bio-assay. The virus was grown for up to 71 days. The fluid harvested from tissue culture cells induced leukemia following inoculation into newborn BALB/c mice after a latency varying from $2\frac{1}{2}$ to 4 months (Peries *et al.*, 1964).

Electron Microscopic Studies were carried out employing either the negative staining technique (Zeigel and Rauscher, 1963, 1964. Lévy *et al.*, 1966) or examining ultrathin sections prepared from organs of mice with virus-induced leukemia (Feldman and Gross, 1965, unpublished. Yumoto *et al.*, 1966). The electron microscopic studies of ultrathin sections of organs of mice with virus-induced leukemia and of tissue culture cells in which the virus was propagated (Zeigel *et al.*, 1966) demonstrated that the size, general morphology, and location in organs and within the cell, and the manner of development of the Rauscher virus strain were essentially the same as those described for either the mouse leukemia passage A virus (Gross), for the Moloney or Graffi virus strains, or for the Friend virus (Feldman and Gross, 1965, unpublished. Yumoto *et al.*, 1966. Gross, 1966).

What is the Nature of the Rauscher Virus? A Single Virus, or a Mixture of Friend Virus and of the Mouse Leukemia Virus (Gross)?

Let us consider the possibility that the Rauscher virus strain consists of a mixture of the Friend virus and of the Gross mouse leukemia virus (Gross, 1964, 1966). Following inoculation of such a filtrate into animals susceptible to both viruses, either form of disease can be induced. However, the Friend virus, presumably present in the Rauscher virus filtrate, induces disease after a relatively shorter latency, and for that reason when susceptible mice are inoculated they usually develop the erythroblastosis-like syndrome before they have an opportunity to develop lymphatic leukemia; the latter requires a considerably longer latency period.

On the other hand, if the Rauscher filtrate is inoculated into mice of certain inbred strains, such as C57 Black or C57 Brown, or into suckling rats which are relatively resistant to the induction of the Friend syndrome, lymphatic leukemia may develop as a result of the pathogenic action of the Gross mouse leukemia virus present in the Rauscher filtrate. Characteristically, most of these animals develop thymic lymphosarcomas, as a rule absent in mice with Friend virus-induced syndrome.

Attempt to Inhibit the Friend Virus Component of the Rauscher Virus Filtrate by Serum Neutralization. An attempt was made to neutralize *in vitro* the Friend virus component, present in the Rauscher virus filtrate, by a specific immune serum. The Rauscher virus was mixed with immune serum obtained from rabbits that had received several injections of Friend virus filtrates. The mixture was then inoculated into suckling and also into 3-week-old C3H(f) mice. After neutralization with anti-Friend serum, the Rauscher virus strain filtrate was still able to induce lymphatic leukemia; however, its potency to induce erythroblastosis-like disease was considerably diminished (Gross, 1964).

Elimination from the Rauscher Virus Filtrate of the Friend Virus Component by Serial Passage Through Rats

Rats do not develop the typical erythroblastosis syndrome seen in mice, but usually develop lymphatic leukemia following inoculation of the Rauscher virus strain. It appeared of interest, therefore, to pass the Rauscher virus serially through rats, in an attempt to determine whether such rat-adapted Rauscher virus would still retain its ability to induce the typical Friend syndrome when inoculated back into mice (Gross, 1966).

Accordingly, the Rauscher virus, harvested from mice, was inoculated into suckling, less than 6-day-old, Sprague-Dawley rats. As soon as the inoculated rats developed leukemia, they were sacrificed; the virus was harvested from the leukemic rat donors, and inoculated again into newborn rats. This procedure was repeated serially, and the Rauscher virus was passed through 10 consecutive rat-to-rat passages, inducing in practically all inoculated animals thymic tumors and disseminated lymphosarcomas, occasionally stem-cell or myelogenous leukemia, very similar to forms induced with the Gross passage A virus. From each consecutive rat-to-rat passage, an attempt was made to inoculate the rat-adapted virus back into suckling, or 3 to 4-week-old, C3H(f) mice, known to be uniformly susceptible to the induction of the erythroblastosis-like syndrome.

After the initial 2 or 3 consecutive rat-to-rat passages, the Rauscher virus lost much of its ability to induce erythroblastosis. Following inoculation into either suckling, or 3-week-old, C3H(f) mice, the rat-adapted virus induced either lymphatic leukemia or a "mixed" form, manifested by the development of thymic lymphosarcomas and also some of the features, such as a very large spleen or the characteristic blood picture, of the erythroblastosis syndrome.

FIG. 48a. ERYTHROBLASTOSIS-LIKE SYNDROME INDUCED IN A MOUSE WITH THE FRIEND VIRUS.

This C3H(f) female mouse was inoculated when 25 days old with Friend virus filtrate, developed the characteristic erythroblastosis-like syndrome, and was sacrificed 30 days after inoculation. Note the very large spleen and liver. The peripheral lymph nodes are not enlarged and there is no thymic tumor. WBC 224,400 per mm^3 with 85% smudge cells, and many nucleated red cells. Hb 2 gm per 100 cc. of blood.

FIG. 48b. ERYTHROBLASTOSIS-LIKE SYNDROME INDUCED IN A MOUSE WITH THE RAUSCHER VIRUS STRAIN.

This C3H(f) female was inoculated when 5 weeks old with the Rauscher virus strain, developed the characteristic erythroblastosis-like syndrome within 2 to 3 weeks, and was sacrificed 25 days after inoculation. Note the considerably enlarged spleen and liver. The peripheral lymph nodes are not enlarged, and there is no thymic tumor. WBC 138,200 per mm^3 with 78% smudge cells and many nucleated red cells. Hb 7.2 gm per 100 cc. of blood.

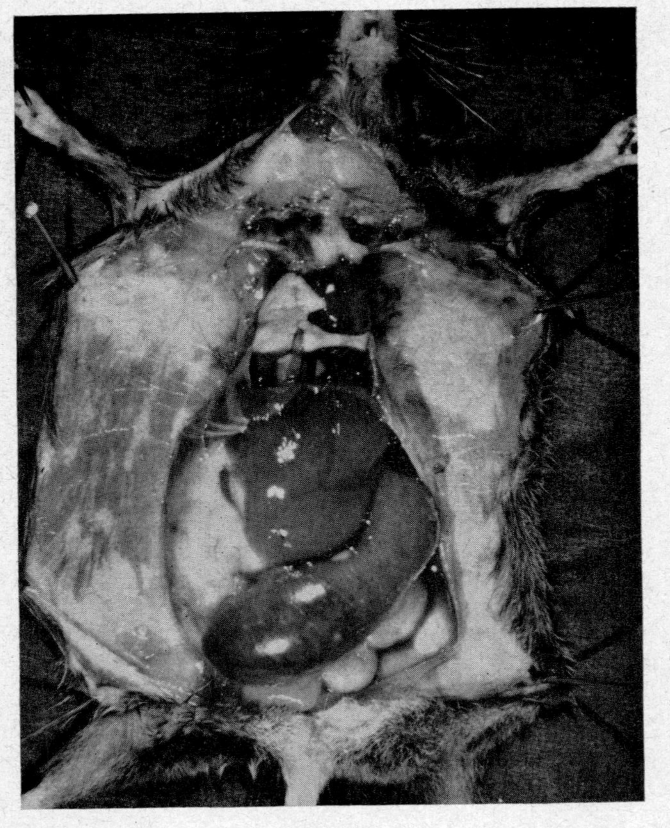

Fig. 48a. Erythroblastosis-like Syndrome Induced in a Mouse with the Friend Virus.

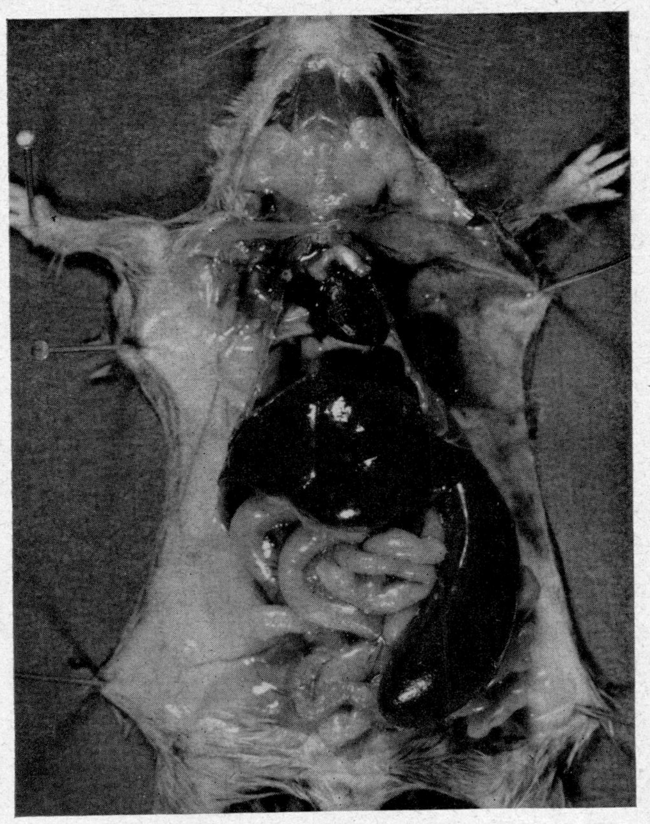

Fig. 48b. Erythroblastosis-like Syndrome Induced in a Mouse with the Rauscher Virus Strain.

After 7 to 8 consecutive rat-to-rat passages, the Rauscher virus lost its characteristic potency to induce erythroblastosis in susceptible mice, but retained nevertheless its ability to induce lymphatic leukemia in either mice or rats. Thus, when after 7 to 10 rat-to-rat passages, the Rauscher virus, harvested from leukemic rat donors, was inoculated into suckling, or 4 to 5-week-old, C3H(f) mice, none developed the characteristic acute enlargement of spleen and liver, as well as the peculiar blood picture typical for the Friend virus syndrome. It appeared, therefore, that after several consecutive rat-to-rat passages, the Rauscher virus lost its Friend virus component. The same rat-adapted virus inoculated into suckling C3H(f) mice induced in all of them thymic and generalized lymphosarcomas, presumably caused by the mouse leukemia virus (Gross) component remaining in the filtrate (Gross, 1966).

Results of Serial Rat-to-Rat Passage of the Mouse Leukemia Virus (Gross)

As a comparison, it is of interest to stress at this point that serial passage through rats of the passage A mouse leukemia virus did not alter its pathogenic potential determining the form of induced disease. Thus, the mouse leukemia virus (Gross) isolated originally from spontaneous mouse leukemia was found to be pathogenic not only for mice, but also for rats, inducing in that species forms of leukemia and lymphomas essentially similar to those induced in mice. The virus has been passed serially through over 21 consecutive rat-to-rat passages, inducing predominantly thymic and disseminated lymphosarcomas, but also lymphatic, stem-cell, and myelogenous leukemia.

At several passage intervals, i.e. after 8, 10, 13, 17, 18, 20, etc. consecutive rat-to-rat passages, the mouse leukemia virus, harvested from leukemic rats, was inoculated back into suckling C3H(f) mice, inducing the same forms of leukemia and lymphomas as did the original virus that had been harvested from leukemic mice. Thus, serial passage through rats might have increased the titer of the virus for the rat species, but did not alter the intrinsic pathogenic property of the virus, expressed by the form of leukemias and lymphomas induced on inoculation tests in the host of origin, i.e. in mice (Gross, 1966).

Neutralization in Vitro of the Lymphatic Leukemia Virus Component of the Rauscher Virus Filtrate with Immune Mouse Leukemia (Passage A, Gross) Virus Serum

Since the "rat-adapted" Rauscher virus strain retained its potency to induce in rats thymic and generalized lymphosarcomas, after several serial passages through rats an attempt was made to determine whether this pathogenic potency of the Rauscher virus strain could be inhibited by an immune serum obtained from rabbits immunized with the passage A virus (Gross). The Rauscher virus strain, that had been passed through

8 consecutive rat-to-rat passages, was employed. The virus filtrate was prepared from thymic tumors and spleens of leukemic rat donors, employing our method used routinely for the preparation of passage A filtrates. A 10^{-3} dilution of the rat-adapted Rauscher virus strain filtrate was then mixed *in vitro* with an equal amount of undiluted immune serum obtained from rabbits that had received several consecutive injections of passage A virus, harvested from leukemic C3H(f) mice, with Freund adjuvant. In a

TABLE 12. NEUTRALIZATION *In Vitro* OF LYMPHATIC LEUKEMIA COMPONENT OF RAUSCHER VIRUS STRAIN* WITH IMMUNE PASSAGE A (GROSS) VIRUS SERUM†

Serum from rabbits immunized with	Virus fil. dil.	No. of rats inoc.‡	No. dev. leuk.**	Leuk. incid. per cent	Avg. age leuk. dev. mos.††
Exp. 1					
Passage A virus harvested from mice (with adjuvant)	10^{-3}	5	0	—	—
Normal mouse organs (with adjuvant)	10^{-3}	6	6	100	4.9
Saline controls	10^{-3}	6	6	100	3.6
Exp. 2					
Passage A virus harvested from mice (with adjuvant)	10^{-3}	7	1	14	8.0
Normal mouse organs (with adjuvant)	10^{-3}	6	5	83	4.4
Saline controls	10^{-3}	4	4	100	4.0

* Rauscher virus strain after 8 consecutive rat-to-rat passages harvested from thymic tumors and spleens of leukemic rat donors. Virus filtrate mixed 1 : 1 with undiluted serum, and incubated in the first experiment at room temperature for 30 minutes, then at +4°C for $3\frac{1}{2}$ hours; in the second experiment the virus-serum mixtures were incubated at room temperature for 30 minutes, followed by incubation at 37°C for 30 minutes, and then at +4°C for $3\frac{1}{2}$ hours.

† Serum inactivated at 56°C for 30 minutes.

‡ Less than 7-day-old suckling Sprague-Dawley rats were inoculated intraperitoneally (0.6 to 0.8 cc. each).

** Lymphatic leukemia with development of large thymic lymphoid tumors and generalized lymphosarcomas involving spleen, liver, and lymph nodes.

†† Surviving non-leukemic animals observed 9 to 10 months for development of leukemia.

simultaneous control experiment, a 10^{-3} dilution of the virus filtrate was mixed with equal amount of undiluted serum obtained from rabbits that had received several injections of normal C3H(f) mouse organs, with Freund adjuvant. All sera were inactivated at 56°C for $\frac{1}{2}$ hour prior to neutralization tests. In a third group, as an additional control, the 10^{-3} virus filtrate dilution was mixed with an equal amount of physiological saline solution. The virus-serum mixtures, as well as the virus-saline controls, were incubated at room temperature for 30 minutes, followed by incubation at +4°C for $3\frac{1}{2}$ hours, and were then inoculated into suckling Sprague-Dawley rats.

The passage A immune rabbit serum inhibited completely the ability of the Rauscher virus strain to induce lymphatic leukemia, following inoculation into suckling rats. There was no inhibiting effect whatever of the normal mouse organ serum. Virus filtrate mixed with normal mouse organ serum, as well as the virus filtrate diluted only, as a control, with equal amount of physiological saline solution, induced in all inoculated rats lymphatic leukemia with characteristic large thymic lymphosarcomas, and also generalized lymphosarcomas in spleens, livers, and other organs (Gross, 1966).

Mixture of Two Oncogenic Viruses in One Filtrate *A Common Difficulty in Experimental Mouse Leukemia Studies*

It would not be the first time that a filtrate prepared from leukemic mouse tissues was found to contain a mixture of two distinct oncogenic viruses. It may be of interest to recall at this point the early studies on mouse leukemia. In the initial experiments, when the mouse leukemia virus was first isolated from organs of Ak mice with spontaneous leukemia, some of the extracts, prepared from such organs, inoculated into newborn C3H mice induced parotid gland tumors instead of leukemia (Gross, 1953). A few animals developed both leukemia and parotid tumors (Gross, unpublished experiments, 1953, 1955). The possibility had to be considered that a single virus was responsible for the induction of either leukemia or parotid gland tumors. It was soon realized, however, that extracts prepared from leukemic mouse tissues contained two different viruses, one causing leukemia and another causing parotid, and other salivary gland tumors. The mouse leukemia virus and the parotid tumor virus, even though initially present simultaneously in the same filtrates, could readily be separated by ultracentrifugation, or by differential heating, since the mouse leukemia virus was found to be larger and more susceptible to heat (Gross, 1953). In general, however, the separation of two different viruses present in the same filtrate may be difficult, particularly if such viruses have similar physical and biological properties.

ISOLATION FROM SPONTANEOUS MOUSE LYMPHOMAS OF A VIRUS CAUSING ERYTHROBLASTOSIS-LIKE DISEASE IN MICE AND RATS

W. H. Kirsten and his colleagues at the Department of Pathology and Pediatrics, University of Chicago (1967b), recently isolated a virus causing erythroblastosis-like* disease in mice and rats. The virus was recovered unexpectedly in the course of serial cell-free passage of thymic lymphomas which arose spontaneously in old mice of the C3H(f) strain.

Preliminary Experiments. Inoculation of Human Leukemic Extracts into Newborn Mice. In extensive experimental studies, in which more than 2,500 mice were employed, filtrates prepared from human leukemic tissues (spleen, liver, brain, and lymph nodes) of 24 children with acute stem-cell leukemia were inoculated into newborn C3H(f) mice.

Development of Lymphomas in the Experimental and also in the Control Group. Development of lymphomas, mostly thymic lymphosarcomas, was observed in some of the inoculated mice following inoculation of extracts of human leukemic tissues. However, the development of lymphosarcomas in these mice had apparently no relation to the injection of the human leukemic extracts, since similar lymphomas developed also in a control group which received inoculation of normal tissue extracts. The overall tumor incidence observed in the inoculated mice after 18 to 26 months of observation was not significantly different from that observed in control animals which received tissue extracts from children that had died from congenital heart disease, neuroblastoma, or non-leukemic hematological disorders. Untreated control mice were also observed.

When the frequency of the lymphomas developing in the injected mice was analyzed, more lymphomas (9 per cent) developed in mice given injections of extracts from 5 of the 24 leukemic children than in recipients of tissues prepared from the other 19 children (2.9 per cent) or the combined control groups (2 per cent). Most of the lymphomas were histologically thymic lymphomas; a few were reticulum-cell sarcomas.

Transmission of Lymphomas in Mice with Cell-free Extracts. Cell-free filtered extracts prepared from thymic lymphomas which developed in some of the injected C3H(f) mice were inoculated into newborn mice of the same inbred line. Among the inoculated mice, those which developed

* The term "erythroblastosis" was suggested as a descriptive term by Kirsten and his coworkers to designate the disease induced in mice and rats with the virus isolated in their laboratory. They emphasized, however, that the use of this term did not imply a generalized or systemic proliferation of malignant erythroblasts (Kirsten *et al.*, 1967).

lymphomas were again used as donors for the preparation of new extracts which were inoculated into another group of newborn mice. This procedure was repeated.

Development of Splenomegaly in Three Inoculated Mice. Isolation of the Erythroblastosis Virus. In the course of the third consecutive mouse-to-mouse passage, out of 206 mice, 60 developed thymic lymphomas, and 3 mice were found with greatly enlarged spleens as the only pathological manifestation. Microscopic examination of tissues of these 3 mice revealed numerous erythroblasts in the spleen, liver, and bone marrow; the thymus and lymph nodes of these animals were normal. The erythroblastosis which developed in these mice was accompanied by a severe, probably hemolytic, anemia. Morphologically, this disease was very similar to the erythroblastosis-like syndrome induced with the Friend virus, or with the Rauscher virus strain.

Some months later, in the control group which had also received extracts from spontaneous mouse lymphomas, 3 out of 71 mice, in a third consecutive mouse-to-mouse filtrate passage, developed similar enlargement of spleen, with the same histological changes as those observed in mice of the experimental group. Thus, it was apparent that the isolation of erythroblastosis virus from mice in the experimental group had no relation to the prior injection of the original donor mice with human leukemia extracts, since similar erythroblastic disease developed also in the control group whose original donors had received extracts from normal or non-leukemic tissues.

Further Passage of the Erythroblastosis Virus in Mice. Cell-free extracts were prepared from the pooled spleens of mice of the experimental group, and were inoculated into newborn mice. In each passage, mice which first developed splenomegaly were used as donors for the preparation of extracts for the next passage. The incidence of induced erythroblastosis gradually increased to 100 per cent, and the latency and survival time decreased to 2.4 months. Among the inoculated mice some survived without spleen enlargement for several months, but later developed thymic lymphomas at 4 to 9 months of age.

Inoculation of the Erythroblastosis Virus into Newborn Rats and Induction of Lymphosarcomas. When the erythroblastosis virus was inoculated into suckling 3-day-old Wistar/Fu rats, generalized lymphomas developed in the inoculated animals after a latency of 6 to 7 months.

In a second rat-to-rat passage, cell-free extracts, prepared from rat lymphomas and inoculated into newborn rats, induced in less than 20 per cent of the inoculated animals erythroblastosis after a short latency of only 4 weeks; the surviving animals remained well for several months, but later, at 4 to 6 months of age, they developed generalized lymphosarcomas.

Inoculation of Extracts from Rat Lymphomas into Newborn Mice and Induction of Lymphosarcomas. Inoculation of rat lymphoma extracts into newborn C3H(f) mice induced generalized lymphosarcomas. The lymphomas induced in mice and rats were indistinguishable from thymic and generalized lymphosarcomas induced in both species by the Gross mouse leukemia virus (Kirsten and Mayer, 1967).

Inoculation of Extracts Prepared from Spleens and Plasma of Rats with Erythroblastosis into Newborn Rats and Mice. Induction of Erythroblastosis, Sarcomas, and Osteolytic Lesions. In another virus passage, cell-free extracts prepared from spleens or plasma of rats with erythroblastosis were inoculated into newborn mice and rats. The inoculated mice and rats developed erythroblastosis and multiple pleomorphic sarcomas; some of the inoculated rats also developed multiple osteolytic lesions (Kirsten and Mayer, 1967).

Is the Virus Isolated by Kirsten a Variant of the Friend Virus?

The pathologic manifestations induced in mice following inoculation of the virus isolated by Kirsten and his colleagues (1967) are very similar to those observed in mice inoculated with either the Friend virus (1957) or with the virus strains isolated by Pope (1961) or Rauscher (1962). Accordingly, it appears that Kirsten and his coworkers isolated yet another murine leukemia virus which induces an erythroblastosis-like syndrome in susceptible mice. Under certain conditions this virus can also induce disseminated lymphosarcomas, including thymic lymphosarcomas. In this respect also this virus is similar to the Friend virus, and perhaps more so to the Rauscher virus strain which induces more readily lymphosarcomas than the Friend virus. However, unlike the Friend or Rauscher virus, the virus isolated by Kirsten and his colleagues induced also typical erythroblastosis in some of the inoculated rats. Furthermore, after passage in rats, when harvested from spleens or plasma of the rat donors, the virus induced in either mice or rats erythroblastosis and multiple pleomorphic sarcomas, and in rats also osteolytic lesions.

It remains to be determined whether these differences in pathogenic potential between the virus isolated by Kirsten and the Friend or Rauscher virus strains are permanent and characteristic for the virus isolated by Kirsten, or whether they are due to the titer of the virus employed, to the different passage history of the virus, or to a particular host response of animals employed for the inoculation tests. The virus isolated by Kirsten and his colleagues may be a variant of the Friend virus. It is also possible that, like the Rauscher virus strain, the virus isolated by Kirsten represents a mixture of an erythroblastosis virus, closely related to the Friend virus, and of the conventional mouse leukemia virus (Gross).

REFERENCES

BATHER, R., Observations on murine monocytic leukaemia induced by a virus isolated from S37 sarcoma. *Brit. J. Cancer*, **15**: 114–119, 1961.

BOIRON, M., LEVY, J.-P., LASNERET, J., OPPENHEIM, S., and BERNARD, J., Pathogenesis of Rauscher leukemia. *J. Nat. Cancer Inst.*, **34**: 865–884, 1965.

BUFFETT, R. F., and FURTH, J., A transplantable reticulum-cell sarcoma variant of Friend's viral leukemia. *Cancer Research*, **19**: 1063–1069, 1959.

CHAMORRO, A., LATARJET, R., VIGIER, P., and ZAJDELA, F., New investigations on the Friend disease. pp. 176–184, in: *CIBA Foundation Symposium on Tumour Viruses of Murine Origin*. J. & A. Churchill Ltd., London, 1962.

DALTON, A. J., HAGUENAU, F., and MOLONEY, J. B., Further electron microscopic studies on the morphology of the Moloney agent. *J. Nat. Cancer Inst.*, **33**: 255–275, 1964.

DALTON, A. J., LAW, L. W., MOLONEY, J. B., and MANAKER, R. A., An electron microscopic study of a series of murine lymphoid neoplasms. *J. Nat. Cancer Inst.*, **27**: 747–791, 1961.

DE HARVEN, E., Ultrastructural studies on three different types of mouse leukemia; A review. pp. 183–206 in: *Tumors Induced by Viruses: Ultrastructural Studies*. Academic Press, New York and London, 1962.

DE HARVEN, E., and FRIEND, C., Electron microscope study of a cell-free induced leukemia of the mouse: A preliminary report. *J. Biophys. and Biochem. Cytol.*, **4**: 151–156, 1958.

DE HARVEN, E., and FRIEND, C., Further electron microscope studies of a mouse leukemia induced by cell-free filtrates. *J. Biophys. and Biochem. Cytol.*, **7**: 747–752, 1960.

DE HARVEN, E., and FRIEND, C., Structure of virus particles partially purified from the blood of leukemic mice. *Virology*, **23**: 119–124, 1964.

DMOCHOWSKI, L., The electron microscopic view of virus-host relationship in neoplasia. *Prog. Exp. Tumor Research*, **3**: 35–147, S. Karger, Basel and New York, 1963.

EHRLICH, P., Experimentelle Studien an Mäusetumoren. *Zeitschr. f. Krebsforsch.*, **5**: 59–81, 1907.

FEY, F., and GRAFFI, A., Erythroblasten-Leukämie nach Injektion von Virus der myeloischen Leukämie der Maus. *Zeitschr. f. Krebsforsch.*, **67**: 145–151, 1965.

FRANKS, W. R., MCGREGOR, A., SHAW, M. M., and SKUBLICS, J., Immunoselection of a latent lymphomatosis from sarcoma 37 in immune Swiss strain mice. (Abstract.) *Proc. Am. Assoc. Cancer Research*, **2**: 202, 1957.

FRANKS, W. R., MCGREGOR, A., SHAW, M. M., and SKUBLICS, J., Development of leukosis by cell-free filtrates of solid tumors or in mice surviving immune to these tumors. (Abstract.) *Proc. Am. Assoc. Cancer Research*, **3**: 19–20, 1959.

FRIEND, C., The isolation of a virus causing a malignant disease of the hematopoietic system in adult Swiss mice. (Abstract.) *Proc. Am. Assoc. Cancer Research*, **2**: 106, 1956.

FRIEND, C., Cell-free transmission in adult Swiss mice of a disease having the character of a leukemia. *J. Exp. Med.*, **105**: 307–318, 1957.

FRIEND, C., Leukemia of adult mice caused by a transmissible agent. *Ann. N.Y. Acad. Sci.*, **68**: 522–532, 1957.

FRIEND, C., Immunological relationships of a filterable agent causing a leukemia in adult mice. *J. Exp. Med.*, **109**: 217–228, 1959.

FRIEND, C., and HADDAD, J., Local tumor formation with transplants of spleen or liver of mice with a virus-induced leukemia. (Abstract.) *Proc. Am. Assoc. Cancer Research*, **3**: 21, 1959.

FRIEND, C., and HADDAD, J. R., Tumor formation with transplants of spleen or liver from mice with virus-induced leukemia. *J. Nat. Cancer Inst.*, **25**: 1279–1289, 1960.

GRAFFI, A., BIELKA, H., and FEY, F., Leukämieerzeugung durch ein filtrierbares Agens aus malignen Tumoren. *Acta Haemat.*, **15**: 145–174, 1956.

GRAFFI, A., BIELKA, H., FEY, F., SCHARSACH, F., and WEISS, R., Gehäuftes Auftreten von Leukämien nach Injektion von Sarkom-Filtraten. *Wiener med. Wochenschr.*, **105**: 61–64, 1955.

GROSS, L., Pathogenic properties, and "vertical" transmission of the mouse leukemia agent. *Proc. Soc. Exp. Biol. & Med.*, **78**: 342–348, 1951.

GROSS, L., A filterable agent, recovered from Ak leukemic extracts, causing salivary gland carcinomas in C3H mice. *Proc. Soc. Exp. Biol. & Med.*, **83**: 414–421, 1953.

GROSS, L., Development and serial cell-free passage of a highly potent strain of mouse leukemia virus. *Proc. Soc. Exp. Biol. & Med.*, **94**: 767–771, 1957.

GROSS, L., Attempt at classification of mouse leukemia viruses. *Acta Haemat.*, **32**: 81–88, 1964.

GROSS, L., Are the common forms of spontaneous and induced leukemia and lymphomas in mice caused by a single virus? pp. 407–424 in: *Conference on Murine Leukemia. Nat. Cancer Inst. Monograph No. 22*, U.S. Publ. Health Service, Bethesda, Md., 1966.

GROSS, L., The Rauscher virus: A mixture of the Friend virus and of the mouse leukemia virus (Gross)? *Acta Haemat.*, **35**: 200–213, 1966.

GROSS, L., ROSWIT, B., MALSKY, S. J., DREYFUSS, Y., and AMATO, C. G., Inactivation of the mouse leukemia virus (Gross) with 4,500,000 R gamma irradiation. (Abstract.) *Proc. Am. Assoc. Cancer Research*, **9**: 26, 1968a.

GROSS, L., ROSWIT, B., MALSKY, S. J., DREYFUSS, Y., and AMATO, C. G., Inactivation of the Friend virus with 4,500,000 R gamma irradiation. Unpublished data, 1968b.

KIRSTEN, W. H., and MAYER, L. A., Morphologic responses to a murine erythroblastosis virus. *J. Nat. Cancer Inst.*, **39**: 311–335, 1967a.

KIRSTEN, W. H., MAYER, L. A., WOLLMANN, R. L., and PIERCE, M. I., Studies on a murine erythroblastosis virus. *J. Nat. Cancer Inst.*, **38**: 117–139, 1967b.

LEVY, J. P., BOIRON, M., SILVESTRE, D., and BERNARD, J., The ultrastructure of Rauscher virus. *Virology*, **26**: 146–150, 1965.

METCALF, D., FURTH, J., and BUFFETT, R. F., Pathogenesis of mouse leukemia caused by Friend virus. *Cancer Research*, **19**: 52–58, 1959.

MIRAND, E. A., and GRACE, J. T., JR., Induction of leukemia in rats with Friend virus. *Virology*, **17**: 364–366, 1962.

MOORE, A. E., Discussion. p. 163 in: *Symposium, Phenomena of the Tumor Viruses. Nat. Cancer Inst. Monograph No. 4*, U.S. Publ. Health Service, Bethesda, Md., 1960.

MOORE, A. E., Growth and persistence of Friend leukemia virus in tissue culture. *J. Nat. Cancer Inst.*, **30**: 885–895, 1963.

MOORE, A. E., and FRIEND, C., Attempts at growing the mouse leukemia virus in tissue culture. (Abstract.) *Proc. Am. Assoc. Cancer Research*, **2**: 328, 1958.

OSATO, T., MIRAND, E. A., and GRACE, J. T., JUN., Propagation and immunofluorescent investigations of Friend virus in tissue culture. *Nature*, **201**: 52–54, 1964.

PERIES, J., LEVY, J. P., BOIRON, M., and BERNARD, J., Multiplication of Rauscher virus in cultures of mouse kidney cells. *Nature*, **203**: 672–673, 1964.

POPE, J. H., Studies of a virus isolated from a wild house mouse, *Mus musculus*, and producing splenomegaly and lymph node enlargement in mice. *Australian J. Exp. Biol. & Med. Sci.*, **39**: 521–536, 1961.

POPE, J. H., The isolation of a mouse leukemia virus resembling Friend virus. *Australian J. Exp. Biol. & Med. Sci.*, **40**: 263–276, 1962.

POPE, J. H., Detection of an avirulent virus apparently related to Friend virus. *Australian J. Exp. Biol. & Med. Sci.*, **41**: 349–362, 1963.

RAUSCHER, F. J., A virus-induced disease of mice characterized by erythrocytopoiesis and lymphoid leukemia. *J. Nat. Cancer Inst.*, **29**: 515–543, 1962.

SCHOOLMAN, H. M., SPURRIER, W., SCHWARTZ, S. O., and SZANTO, P. B., Studies in leukemia. VII. The induction of leukemia in Swiss mice by means of cell-free filtrates of leukemic mouse brain. *Blood*, **12**: 694–700, 1957.

SELBY, C. C., The electron microscopy of normal and neoplastic cells. *Texas Rep. Biol. & Med.*, **4**: 728–744, 1953.

SELBY, C. C., GREY, C. E., LICHTENBERG, S., FRIEND, C., MOORE, A. E., and BIESELE, J. J., Submicroscopic cytoplasmic particles occasionally found in the Ehrlich mouse ascites tumor. *Cancer Research*, **14**: 790–794, 1954.

STEWART, H. L., SNELL, K. C., DUNHAM, L. J., and SCHLYEN, S. M., Transplantable and transmissible tumors of animals. *Atlas of Tumor Pathology*. Sect. 12. Fasc. 40, pp. 378. Am. Reg. Path., Armed Forces Inst. of Path., Washington, D.C., 1959.

VIGIER, P., and GOLDÉ, A., Culture *in vitro* du virus de Friend. *Bull. du Cancer*, **49**: 374–381, 1962.

YUMOTO, T., RECHER, L., SYKES, J. A., and DMOCHOWSKI, L., Morphology and development of some murine leukemia viruses. pp. 107–137 in: *Conference on Murine Leukemia. Nat. Cancer Inst. Monograph No. 22*, U.S. Publ. Health Service, Bethesda, Md., 1966.

ZEIGEL, R. F., and RAUSCHER, F. J., Electron microscopic and bioassay studies on a murine leukemia virus (Rauscher): Preliminary report. *J. Nat. Cancer Inst.*, **30**: 207–219, 1963.

ZEIGEL, R. F., and RAUSCHER, F. J., Electron microscopic and bioassay studies on a murine leukemia virus (Rauscher). I. Effects of physiochemical treatments on the morphology and biological activity of the virus. *J. Nat. Cancer Inst.*, **32**: 1277–1307, 1964.

ZEIGEL, R. F., TYNDALL, R. L., O'CONNOR, E., TEETER, E., and ALLEN, B. V., Observations on the morphology of a murine leukemia virus (Rauscher) propagated in tissue culture. pp. 237–263 in: *Conference on Murine Leukemia. Nat. Cancer Inst. Monograph No. 22*, U.S. Publ. Health Service, Bethesda, Md., 1966.

CHAPTER 15

The Murine Sarcoma Virus

A Virus Isolated from Rat and Mouse Leukemia which Induces Pleomorphic Sarcomas in Mice, Rats, and Hamsters.

In the course of routine passage of the mouse leukemia virus in rats, Dr. Jennifer J. Harvey (1964), at the Department of Cancer Research of the London Hospital Medical College, observed unexpectedly that newborn BALB/c mice inoculated, as a test of the potency of the passaged virus, with plasma harvested from leukemic rats developed, after a short latency of only one month, instead of leukemia, pleomorphic sarcomas at or near the injection site.

The blood plasma used for inoculation was harvested from a rat which developed leukemia following inoculation of the mouse leukemia virus (Moloney strain*). The blood plasma of this rat was stored at −70°C for 3 months. After storage the plasma was diluted (1 to 30 with Hanks' saline), passed through a Selas 02 filter candle, and inoculated into 15 newborn BALB/c mice. Only 6 mice survived until weaning. On the 32nd day, 5 mice had tumors at or near the site of injection, and all had grossly enlarged spleens. Additional samples of the same stored plasma filtrate were injected into newborn BALB/c mice, and into newborn rats. Twenty-eight of the 35 inoculated mice and one of the 13 rats developed tumors, and all developed also enlarged spleens.

Morphology of the Induced Tumors. The tumors were either solid and firm or cystic and filled with blood. The solid tumors developed in the subcutaneous tissues, and in the peritoneum near the site of inoculation; they were sometimes attached to the muscles of the abdominal wall, thorax, or diaphragm.

On microscopic examination, the morphology of the induced solid tumors was that of anaplastic sarcomas, consisting of pleomorphic or spindle cells, and invading the adjacent tissues. The cystic angiomatous tumors, consisting of multiple dilated sinuses filled with blood cells and

* The strain of mouse leukemia virus, isolated by Moloney (1960) from sarcoma S.37, following the method suggested by Graffi and his colleagues (1956), is essentially identical with the prototype of the mouse leukemia virus isolated originally in the author's laboratory (Gross, 1951, 1957, 1964, 1965). See also p. 485.

debris, developed in subcutaneous spaces or in the peritoneal cavity, and were often related to the lymph nodes. *All animals also had very large spleens*, and many died from splenic rupture. The microscopic morphology of the spleen and also of blood smears was very similar to the erythroblastosis syndrome induced in mice with the Friend virus.

Importance of Age at Inoculation. Tumor extracts or blood plasma, filtered through Selas 02 filter candles, induced rapid development of tumors and splenomegaly in mice inoculated when 1 to 7 days old, in some cases as early as 12 days after injection. As the age at the time of injection increased, the incidence of induced tumors declined, but that of spleen enlargement and erythroblastosis remained high. Fifteen mice inoculated at the age of $3\frac{1}{2}$ months all developed splenomegaly, but only two developed tumors.

One to 2-day-old Chester Beatty albino rats were injected with the original plasma filtrate. Their plasma was collected at 8, 30, and 54 days and injected into less than 3-day-old BALB/c mice. As a result, mice which received the 30 and 54-day samples developed tumors and splenomegaly in 12 to 15 days. Those which received the 8-day sample remained healthy at first for about 70 days, but then developed typical lymphatic leukemia.

Susceptibility of Newborn Mice and Rats to Inoculation of the Sarcoma Virus. In an extensive series of experiments (Harvey *et al.*, 1964, 1965, also personal communication to the author, 1967), newborn mice, rats, and hamsters were inoculated with extracts prepared from the sarcomas and also from spleens and from blood plasma of the tumor-bearing mice or rats.

Mice of several strains, such as BALB/c, C3H, Ak, NZB, C57 Black, C57 Brown, as well as non-inbred mice, were inoculated when newborn, and all were found susceptible.

Among the rats tested were Sprague-Dawley, Chester Beatty hooded, and August rats. These animals were also found susceptible. Out of 46 CB hooded rats inoculated when newborn with the sarcoma virus, 30 developed enlarged spleens, and 16 developed sarcomas at the diaphragm or at other sites. Many of the rats also had large thin-walled cysts containing clear or blood-stained fluid at the site of lymph nodes.

When newborn mice or rats were inoculated, tumors developed usually at the site of inoculation within 3 weeks; in addition, the spleen in these animals became considerably enlarged; this spleen enlargement was similar to that observed in susceptible mice following inoculation of the Friend virus.

Among those mice and rats which did not develop the early lesions, and survived for at least 8 weeks, some later developed lymphocytic leukemia.

Development of Splenomegaly. Splenomegaly was a frequent finding in both mice and rats injected with the virus. In the spleen, particularly in mice, there were sometimes localized cystic nodules which were found to be filled with blood. There was proliferation of reticulum cells with associated erythroblastosis, replacing the normal follicular pattern (Chesterman *et al.*, 1966). These changes, as well as the peripheral blood morphology, were very similar to those observed in the Friend virus-induced disease syndrome.

It has never been possible to separate the mouse sarcoma virus into two distinct components, one of which would produce only tumors, and the other only splenomegaly. In certain instances, the inoculated mice or rats developed an enlarged spleen without evidence of development of any tumors; however, the tissues of these animals always contained a virus which produced tumors when injected back into newborn mice.

Induction of Plasmocytomas in Rats Injected Intracerebrally with the Mouse Sarcoma Virus. Plasmocytomas are rare tumors in rats. It was therefore surprising to observe that following intracerebral inoculation of the murine sarcoma virus into newborn rats, some of the inoculated animals developed not only intracranial tumors but also multiple plasmocytomas, most of them located on the legs and paws (Ribacchi and Giraldo, 1966).

One to 3-day-old CB, Sprague-Dawley, and Osborne-Mendel rats were injected intracerebrally with the Moloney strain of the murine sarcoma virus.* Intracranial tumors developed in all rats of the CB strain, and in 90 per cent of Sprague-Dawley and Osborne-Mendel rats, at the average age of 18, 26 and 27 days, respectively. Plasmocytomas were observed only in Sprague-Dawley and Osborne-Mendel rats, with an incidence of 20 per cent at the average age of 30 and 28 days.

The primary bone plasmocytomas always developed in animals which also had intracranial tumors. They were often multiple. The plasmocytomas could be transplanted subcutaneously or intraperitoneally in newborn rats of the same strain.

Susceptibility of Newborn Hamsters to the Mouse Sarcoma Virus. Inoculation of the virus into either golden or cream colored newborn hamsters produced as an early effect, occurring within the first 3 weeks after inoculation, pleural effusions or multiple cystic lesions containing clear or blood-stained fluid. This was followed by the development of pleomorphic or spindle-cell sarcomas within 5 weeks after inoculation. Out of 28 hamsters inoculated intraperitoneally, when newborn, 9 developed sarcomas situated mainly on or near the diaphragm.

None of the hamsters developed erythroblastosis, and none developed leukemia (Harvey *et al.*, 1964, 1965. Harvey, 1968a).

* Following the original report by Harvey (1964), a murine sarcoma virus was subsequently also isolated by Moloney (1966). Both represent most probably the same virus or closely related virus strains. Isolation of the murine sarcoma virus from different sources is discussed in more detail on subsequent pages of this chapter.

Susceptibility of Newborn Mastomys. The virus also induced sarcomas and splenomegaly following inoculation into newborn *Rattus* (*Mastomys*) *natalensis** (Harvey, 1968b).

Transplantation of Tumors Induced with the Murine Sarcoma Virus in Mice, Rats, and Hamsters. The tumors which were induced in mice could be transplanted by cell-graft in mice of the same inbred lines. All inoculated animals developed not only tumors, but also erythroblastic splenomegaly. One of the tumors was transplanted by cell-graft through 17 serial generations in mice. The tumors induced in rats could also be transplanted by cell-graft to other rats of the same strain.

In a similar experiment, a sarcoma induced in a hamster was transplanted by cell-graft through 16 serial cell passages in hamsters.

Attempts to Recover the Virus from Induced Tumors and from Blood Plasma of the Inoculated Animals. The murine sarcoma virus could be readily recovered from the sarcomas, or from blood plasma, of either mice or rats in which the tumors had been induced. The titer of the virus isolated from plasma was lower than that isolated from tumors.

No virus could be demonstrated in plasma of tumor-bearing hamsters when newborn mice were used as test animals; however, similar filtrates induced characteristic cystic lesions and sarcomas, when inoculated into newborn hamsters (Harvey *et al.*, 1964. Harvey, 1968a).

Titration Experiments in Newborn Mice. Serial dilutions of the virus were inoculated into newborn, less than 3-day-old, BALB/c mice. The results of these experiments demonstrated clearly that tumors and erythroblastic splenomegaly could be induced after a short latency only with relatively high concentrations of the virus, i.e., with undiluted extracts, or with a 10 per cent dilution of the virus filtrate. The pathologic manifestations appeared after a short average latency of 19 or 28 days, respectively. A virus filtrate dilution of 10^{-2} induced, on bio-assay, erythroblastic splenomegaly but no tumors, after an average latency of 43 days. Inoculation of a 10^{-3} dilution resulted in the development of lymphocytic leukemia after a latency of $4\frac{1}{2}$ months or more.

The lymphatic leukemia which developed as a delayed reaction in these animals could be transmitted in its original form by filtrate passage. The sarcoma virus could not be recovered, however, from the leukemic tissues of such animals. This development was significant and similar to results of recent experiments carried out with the Rauscher virus strain (Gross, 1966) suggesting the possibility that the prototype of the conventional mouse leukemia virus was present in the original filtrate employed for inoculation.

Titration Experiments in Newborn Rats. In newborn Sprague-Dawley

* See p. 804 for more information about *Mastomys*.

rats, undiluted extracts, or a 10 per cent dilution of the filtrate, induced erythroblastic splenomegaly and sarcomas, but no leukemia, after a short latency of 19 or 30 days, respectively. Lower doses of virus, i.e., 10^{-2} and 10^{-3} filtrate dilutions, induced either erythroblastic splenomegaly or a delayed development of lymphatic leukemia, after a latency of 2 to 3 months; however, rarely did the animals inoculated with such low doses of virus develop sarcomas (Mahy *et al.*, 1966. Harvey, personal communication to the author, 1967).

Physical Properties of the Virus. The size of the virus particles determined by filtration procedure was similar to that of the Friend virus tested simultaneously as a control in the same experiment; the diameter of the virus was considered on this basis to be 100 to 150 mμ. (The morphology and diameter of the Friend virus are identical with those of the Gross mouse leukemia virus). Electron microscopic studies revealed that the type C virus particles observed in murine sarcoma were similar to those observed in mouse leukemia, i.e., had an average diameter of about 100 mμ.

The virus could be preserved without apparent loss of infectivity for at least 2 months at −60°C. Samples of the virus survived storage at −70°C for 2 years, but some loss of potency was noted under such conditions.

The murine sarcoma virus could be inactivated by heating to 56°C for ½ hour. The virus was also sensitive to ether; it was almost completely inactivated by overnight *in vitro* exposure to 20 per cent volume of ethyl ether (Harvey *et al.*, 1965. Mahy *et al.*, 1966).

Accordingly, on the basis of physical properties tested, the murine sarcoma virus could not be differentiated from the mouse leukemia virus which is also inactivated by heating to 56°C for ½ hour and is similarly inactivated by ether.

Propagation of the Murine Sarcoma Virus in Tissue Culture.

Replication of Virus in Tumor Cells Grown in Vitro

The virus could be readily propagated in tumor cell lines. Trypsinized cells of the virus-induced mouse sarcomas were cultivated for two months; they grew very slowly. The final supernate was injected into newborn mice and induced erythroblastic splenomegaly but no tumors; however, the plasma of these mice injected into newborn rats induced both splenomegaly and tumors (Harvey *et al.*, 1964. Chesterman *et al.*, 1966).

In another more recent experiment (Harvey, personal communication to the author, 1967), fragments of virus-induced tumors from mice and rats were trypsinized and established as cell lines *in vitro*. They readily replicated the virus. The tissue-culture-grown virus behaved as the animal-passaged mouse sarcoma virus; newborn mice inoculated with supernatant fluid harvested from tissue cultures in which the virus was propagated developed early tumors and erythroblastic splenomegaly; inoculation of higher dilution of the supernate induced the development of lymphocytic leukemia.

However, when the murine sarcoma virus was harvested from hamster tumor cell lines it was not pathogenic for mice, but induced sarcomas when inoculated into newborn hamsters (Bassin *et al.*, 1968. Harvey, 1968a).

Propagation of the Murine Sarcoma Virus on Normal Mouse, Rat, and Hamster Embryo Cells. Transformation of Cells Infected with the Virus. The murine sarcoma virus could be propagated on normal mouse embryo cells, and induced under such conditions characteristic changes in the cell morphology. In a study in which the murine sarcoma virus isolated by Moloney was employed (Hartley and Rowe, 1966), extracts from mouse tumors, and also from organs (liver, spleen, or salivary glands) of virus-infected tumor-bearing mice, induced characteristic focal lesions in both Swiss mouse embryo cells and in a continuous (CL-1) line of BALB/c mouse embryo cell cultures. The foci, which became apparent within 5 days, contained two types of altered cells, i.e., round cells and spindle-shaped cells. Culture fluid of cell extracts produced similar changes on serial passage.

In another series of experiments (Simons *et al.*, 1967c), in which the murine sarcoma virus originally isolated by Harvey was employed, similar morphological changes were induced following inoculation of cultures of C57 Black mouse embryo cells with the virus. Again, some of the infected cells became spindle-shaped and vividly stained with acridine orange. The transformed cells continuously produced virus *in vitro* and induced tumors on inoculation into adult C57 Black mice.

The mouse embryo cells transformed by the virus grew vigorously for more than 4 months and continuously released virus into the medium. When the fluid from transformed cultures was filtered through 0.45 μ Millipore membranes, and was then passed in new mouse embryo cell cultures, it again produced morphological transformation of the cells in which it was propagated.

The tissue-culture-grown virus behaved exactly like the virus which was passed in animals; thus, mice injected with fluid harvested from cultures in which the virus had been propagated developed, after a short latency, both tumors and erythroblastic splenomegaly; those animals which received higher dilutions of the tissue culture fluid, i.e., lower doses of the virus, did not develop the early pathological manifestations, such as splenomegaly or tumors; however, they later developed lymphatic leukemia (Harvey, personal communication to the author, 1967).

The sarcoma virus could also be propagated in rat embryo cells, and induced morphological transformation of such cells into neoplastic cells (Ting, 1966. Bernard *et al.*, 1967).

Hamster embryo cells injected with high concentrations of the murine sarcoma virus were also rapidly transformed, showing foci of spindle-shaped cells. Induction of splenomegaly and sarcomas with filtered fluid harvested from such cultures and inoculated into newborn mice was reported (Simons *et al.*, 1967a,b), but could not be reproduced in more recent experiments (Bassin *et al.*, 1968. Harvey, 1968a).

Electron Microscopic Studies. Electron microscopic studies of ultrathin sections prepared from fragments of virus-induced sarcomas revealed presence of spherical virus particles which resembled type C particles observed in mouse leukemia. Similar virus particles could be found also in the cytoplasmic vacuoles of megakaryocytes in the spleen of a BALB/c mouse that had been inoculated with the murine sarcoma virus (Chesterman *et al.*, 1966).

In a study carried out by Dalton (1966), ultrathin sections of fragments of virus-induced mouse sarcomas, and also of pellets of blood plasma prepared from tumor-carrying BALB/c mice, were examined. Spherical particles, about 100 mμ in diameter, indistinguishable from mouse leukemia virus particles, were observed in small numbers budding from tumor cells or fully formed in intercellular spaces; similar particles were also found in plasma pellets.

Cells and media from tissue culture passages of the murine sarcoma virus grown on mouse embryo cells also revealed large numbers of type C virus particles in extracellular spaces and also budding from the cell membranes (Dourmashkin and Simons, 1966). A pellet of the medium from the infected culture was obtained by ultracentrifugation; ultrathin sections prepared from a fixed embedded fragment of the pellet showed that it was almost entirely composed of similar type C particles. Control cultures did not show any particles. Particles of similar morphology were seen also in both mouse and rat tumor cell lines carried in tissue culture.

In another experiment (Dourmashkin and Simons, 1966), mouse embryo cells were infected with 10-fold dilutions of murine sarcoma virus; after repeated transfers, ultrathin sections of the cells were examined in the electron microscope. Virus particles were seen only in transformed cultures. No particles were seen in cultures inoculated with the dilution immediately after the last one inducing transformation.

Examination of mouse tumors induced by tissue-culture-grown preparations of the murine sarcoma virus showed large numbers of type C particles budding from the surface of tumor cells.

* * *

The interpretation of the results of electron microscopic studies thus far performed on the mouse sarcoma virus is difficult. There is no clear evidence that the type C particles observed in mouse sarcoma, and also in organs of tumor-bearing mice, actually represent the murine sarcoma virus.

It must be kept in mind that, under certain experimental conditions, extracts prepared from the sarcomas and from organs of tumor-bearing mice induced typical leukemia or lymphosarcomas following inoculation into newborn mice or rats. The question remains open whether the type C particles observed in sarcomas, spleens, or plasma pellets of tumor-bearing mice or rats do not after all represent the mouse leukemia virus.

It is also possible, however, that both the murine sarcoma virus and the mouse leukemia virus have identical morphology and are indistinguishable on electron microscopic examination. The murine sarcoma virus may be a variant of the mouse leukemia virus; its differentiation may not be possible on the basis of morphological features.

ISOLATION OF THE MURINE SARCOMA VIRUS FROM DIFFERENT SOURCES IN OTHER LABORATORIES

Following the initial report by Harvey, induction of pleomorphic sarcomas in mice or rats with extracts prepared from either mouse or rat donors with virus-induced leukemia, or erythroblastosis, has been reported from several laboratories.

Induction of Rhabdomyosarcomas in Mice with High Doses of Mouse Leukemia Virus. Moloney (1966a,b) described development of multiple rhabdomyosarcomas following inoculation of high doses of mouse leukemia virus (Moloney strain*) into newborn BALB/c mice. An extract containing the mouse leukemia virus, harvested from plasma of leukemic mice and concentrated by ultracentrifugation, was inoculated into newborn BALB/c mice; as a result, rhabdomyosarcomas developed after a short latency at the site of virus inoculation.

Cell-free extracts prepared from the induced sarcomas were then passed serially in newborn mice, inducing after a short latency of less than 2 weeks pleomorphic sarcomas and rhabdomyosarcomas. The virus was found to be infectious for newborn mice of several strains tested, such as BALB/c, C57 Black, DBA/2 and Swiss. However, the virus was not pathogenic for rats. Inoculation of the same virus into thymectomized rats, or into rats treated with cortisone, did not induce sarcomas.

In contrast to observations repeatedly made by Harvey and her colleagues, no development of leukemia was observed by Moloney in mice inoculated with the murine sarcoma virus. However, the observation period

* See footnote on p. 588.

of the inoculated animals was very short, and this could have accounted for the failure to observe a late development of leukemia in these mice.

Induction by Kirsten and his Colleagues of Pleomorphic Sarcomas in Mice and Rats with Filtrates Prepared from Rat Donors with Virus-induced Erythroblastosis. In the preceding chapter we have described the isolation by Kirsten and his colleagues (1967a), at the Department of Pathology and Pediatrics, University of Chicago, of a transmissible agent causing erythroblastosis in mice and rats.

> The virus was isolated during cell-free passages of thymic lymphomas which arose spontaneously in old C3H(f) mice. Inoculation of the virus into newborn mice caused the development of erythroblastosis after a short latency of 25 days; inoculation of the virus into newborn rats induced the development of thymic lymphomas after 8 to 16 months.
>
> In further passage of the virus (Kirsten and Mayer, 1967b. Kirsten *et al.*, 1968), extracts prepared from rat lymphomas and inoculated into newborn rats induced either erythroblastosis or disseminated lymphosarcomas; however, when spleen extracts or plasma from rats with erythroblastosis were injected into newborn Wistar/Fu rats, or C3H(f) mice, the inoculated animals of both species developed erythroblastosis and multiple pleomorphic sarcomas. In addition, many of the inoculated rats developed also polyostotic osteolytic lesions.

The sarcomas developed in multiple sites in both rats and mice; they presented themselves as small gray-white nodules, attached to the inner sternum, or scattered through the diaphragm; once recognized as distinct lesions, similar nodules were also detected in the muscles of the neck and back, in the retroperitoneal fat, in the subcutis of the abdomen, and in other sites. The individual tumor nodules usually did not exceed 5 mm in diameter.

Microscopic morphology of the induced sarcomas was quite variable, depending on the site of origin; some were similar to fibrosarcomas, others suggested angiomatous growths, still others, presumably arising in striated muscle fibers, contained giant cells, and the possibility of rhabdomyosarcomas was considered. However, no single differentiated pattern prevailed, and the tumors were interpreted as primitive and essentially undifferentiated sarcomas.

The osteolytic lesions were observed only in the inoculated rats; these lesions were also multicentric in origin, affecting particularly the vertebrae and long bones, but were also present in the ribs and skull.

In summary, a transmissible virus originally isolated from mouse lymphomas, and passed through rats, induced in subsequent cell-free passages in mice and rats either erythroblastosis or lymphomas. Filtrates prepared from spleens or plasma of rats with erythroblastosis induced in mice and rats multiple undifferentiated, pleomorphic sarcomas. All mice and rats which developed sarcomas also had large erythroblastic spleens. The rats also had multiple osteolytic lesions.

Induction of Pleomorphic Sarcomas, Rhabdomyosarcomas, and Myxomatous Tumors with Filtrates from Organs of Rats with Passage A Virus-induced Leukemia. In the course of routine cell-free transmission of the passage A (Gross) mouse leukemia virus in newborn rats, the development of myxomatous tumors was repeatedly observed in the inoculated rats (Gross, 1963). The tumors presented themselves as gelatinous masses developing usually in the subcutaneous tissues of the back and abdomen, in the inguinal and axillary pits, and also in the cervical region; all animals that developed myxomatous tumors also had thymic and generalized lymphosarcomas.

More recently, in a study dealing with exposure *in vitro* of the mouse leukemia virus to high doses of gamma irradiation (Gross *et al.*, 1965), a rat litter was inoculated at 5 days of age with rat-passaged mouse leukemia virus which had received 750,000 R *in vitro*. It was unexpectedly observed in this experiment that among 6 inoculated rats, 3 developed, after a short latency of 18 days only, enlarged spleens and multiple intraperitoneal sarcomas (Gross, unpublished data). The tumors were disseminated, white, soft masses present predominantly in the peritoneal cavity, on the posterior wall of the abdomen, around the kidneys and vertebral column, on the diaphragm, and also in subcutaneous tissues. On microscopic examination, they were pleomorphic undifferentiated sarcomas; some had a distinct structure of rhabdomyosarcomas. A third animal was found dead when 3½ months old, with multiple, small, soft caseous tumors in peritoneal cavity; however, no microscopic examination of tumors was made in this animal. The remaining 3 rats of the original litter all died after 4 to 4½ months with disseminated lymphosarcomas, and also with large spleens and livers, but did not develop sarcomas; one of these rats, however, had an extensive myxomatous tumor of gelatinous consistency in the cervical and axillary areas in addition to a thymic lymphoma.

When extracts were made from spleens and tumors of these animals and inoculated into newborn rats, thymic and disseminated lymphosarcomas were induced after a latency varying from 6 to 8½ months. However, no sarcomas developed in the inoculated animals.

What is the Nature of the Murine Sarcoma Virus? A Distinct Viral Entity, or a Variant of the Mouse Leukemia Virus?

The induction of pleomorphic sarcomas in mice and rats with cell-free extracts prepared from leukemic mouse and rat donors raises several important questions: are these tumors related to either mouse leukemia or mouse erythroblastosis, or are they caused by a distinct virus?

The possibility that the sarcomas were caused by the parotid tumor, i.e., polyoma virus, which is so often present in extracts prepared from leukemic mouse organs, could be excluded; the polyoma virus induces different types of tumors including the characteristic tumors of the salivary glands in mice. The polyoma virus is not inactivated after heating to 56°C for ½ hour, and is resistant to *in vitro* exposure to ether, whereas the sarcoma-inducing virus is inactivated under such experimental conditions. Furthermore, the murine sarcoma virus did not agglutinate guinea pig erythrocytes *in vitro*, and mice bearing the virus-induced sarcoma did not show in their blood serum presence of antibodies inhibiting the ability of the polyoma virus to agglutinate red blood cells (Harvey, 1964).

Thus far it has not been possible to differentiate the murine sarcoma virus from the mouse leukemia virus on the basis of physical or morphological properties.

In contrast, in previous studies, the parotid tumor, i.e., polyoma virus, which was also originally isolated from organs of leukemic mice (Gross, 1953), could be readily differentiated from the mouse leukemia virus. It is more resistant to heat; it is not inactivated by ethyl ether *in vitro*, and it has a different size and morphology.

Once more, the study of mouse leukemia has revealed interesting observations similar to those reported in studies of the chicken leukosis complex. Generalized visceral lymphosarcomas and leukemia are not the only pathological manifestations observed in chickens inoculated with the lymphomatosis virus. The development of different forms of sarcomas, of kidney tumors (nephroblastomas), and osteopetrosis has been also observed and was discussed in detail in the chapter on the Chicken Leukosis Complex in this monograph.

There are, nevertheless, certain fundamental biological features which distinguish the murine sarcoma agent from the virus of mouse leukemia. The principal characteristic of the murine sarcoma virus is its ability to cause the development of pleomorphic sarcomas, such as rhabdomyosarcomas, spindle-cell sarcomas, or undifferentiated sarcomas in mice or rats, and spindle-cell sarcomas in hamsters. The mouse leukemia virus is capable of inducing the various forms of leukemia and lymphomas in mice and rats, but it does not induce pleomorphic sarcomas, and it is not pathogenic for hamsters.

Furthermore, the murine sarcoma virus can be readily propagated in tissue culture. It replicates well on normal mouse or rat embryo cells, causing characteristic foci of transformed cells. The transformed cells continuously produce virus *in vitro*; as a result, the virus can be consistently harvested from the tissue culture fluid, and induces tumors following inoculation into mice or rats. On the other hand, although the mouse leukemia virus can be propagated in tissue culture on normal mouse embryo cells, it does not produce foci of altered cells under such conditions. More recently, however, it was found that the mouse leukemia virus can also be maintained in long-term cultures of normal rat embryo thymus cells *in vitro*; the virus replicates under such conditions abundantly and induces cellular neoplastic transformation (Ioachim and Berwick, 1968).

If the murine sarcoma virus is a separate entity, it cannot be separated from either the mouse leukemia (Gross) virus or from the Friend virus on the basis of its physical or morphological properties. It is indistinguishable in sensitivity to heat and ether, and also in size and morphology.

Up to the present time, however, it has not been possible to separate the sarcoma-inducing property of the virus from its ability to induce erythroblastic splenomegaly in the inoculated mice or rats (Harvey, 1966; also personal communication to the author, 1967). Furthermore, typical lymphatic leukemia could frequently be induced following inoculation of the murine sarcoma virus into newborn mice and rats, particularly if higher dilutions of virus were employed. In all probability, the murine sarcoma virus filtrates contain a mixture of the murine sarcoma virus and of the conventional mouse leukemia virus (Harvey, 1969). It appears that the murine sarcoma virus is a "defective" or incomplete virus which requires the presence of the mouse leukemia virus, the latter acting as a "helper" virus, in order to reveal its pathogenic potential for mice and rats (Hartley and Rowe, 1966. Huebner *et al.*, 1966. Huebner, 1967. Harvey and East, 1969).

REFERENCES

Bernard, C., Boiron, M., and Lasneret, J., Transformation et infection chronique de cellules embryonnaires de rat par le virus du sarcome de Moloney. *Compt. Rend. Acad. Sci.* (*Paris*), **264**: 2170–2173, 1967.

Bassin, R. H., Simons, P. J., Chesterman, F. C., and Harvey, J. J., Murine sarcoma virus (Harvey): characteristics of focus formation in mouse embryo cells cultures, and virus production by hamster tumor cells. *Int. J. Cancer*, **3**: 265–272, 1968.

Chesterman, F. C., Harvey, J. J., Dourmashkin, R. R., and Salaman, M. H., The pathology of tumors and other lesions induced in rodents by virus derived from a rat with Moloney leukemia. *Cancer Research*, **26**: 1759–1768, 1966.

Dalton, A. J., An electron microscopic study of a virus-induced murine sarcoma (Moloney). pp. 143–168 in: *Conference on Murine Leukemia. Nat. Cancer Inst. Monograph No. 22.* U.S. Publ. Health Service, Bethesda, Md., 1966.

Dourmashkin, R. R., and Simons, P., Electron microscopy of MSV., in: Murine sarcoma virus (Harvey), pp. 63–66. *Imperial Cancer Research Fund 64th Annual Report for 1965–1966.*

Graffi, A., Bielka, H., and Fey, F., Leukämieerzeugung durch ein filtrierbares Agens aus malignen Tumoren. *Acta Haemat.*, **15**: 145–174, 1956.

Gross, L., Pathogenic properties, and "vertical" transmission of the mouse leukemia agent. *Proc. Soc. Exp. Biol. & Med.*, **78**: 342–348, 1951.

Gross, L., A filterable agent, recovered from Ak leukemic extracts, causing salivary gland carcinomas in C3H mice. *Proc. Soc. Biol. & Med.*, **83**: 414–421, 1953.

Gross, L., Development and serial cell-free passage of a highly potent strain of mouse leukemia virus. *Proc. Soc. Exp. Biol. & Med.*, **94**: 767–771, 1957.

Gross, L., Serial cell-free passage in rats of the mouse leukemia virus. Effect of thymectomy. *Proc. Soc. Exp. Biol. & Med.*, **112**: 939–945, 1963.

Gross, L., How many different viruses causing leukemia in mice? *Acta Haemat.*, **32**: 44–62, 1964.

Gross, L., Neutralization *in vitro* of mouse leukemia virus by specific immune serum. Importance of virus titration. *Proc. Soc. Exp. Biol. & Med.*, **119**: 420–427, 1965.

Gross, L., The Rauscher virus: A mixture of the Friend virus and of the mouse leukemia virus (Gross)? *Acta Haemat.*, **35**: 200–213, 1966.

Gross, L., Roswit, B., Malsky, S. J., Dreyfuss, Y., and Amato, C. G., Resistance of mouse leukemia virus to *in vitro* gamma rays irradiation. (Abstract). *Proc. Am. Assoc. Cancer Research*, **6**: 24, 1965.

Hartley, J. W., and Rowe, W. P., Production of altered cell foci in tissue culture by defective Moloney sarcoma virus particles. *Proc. Nat. Acad. Sci., USA*, **55**: 780–786, 1966.

Harvey, J. J., An unidentified virus which causes the rapid production of tumours in mice. *Nature*, **204**: 1104–1105, 1964.

Harvey, J. J., Discussion following presentation of paper "A virus-induced rhabdomyosarcoma of mice" by J. B. Moloney. pp. 141–142 in: *Conference on Murine Leukemia, Nat. Cancer Inst. Monograph No. 22.* U.S. Publ. Health Service, Bethesda, Md., 1966.

Harvey, J. J., Replication of murine sarcoma virus–Harvey (MSV–H) in tissue culture of virus-induced sarcomas. *J. Gen. Virol.*, **3**: 327–336, 1968a.

Harvey, J. J., Susceptibility of *Praomys* (*Mastomys*) *natalensis* to the murine sarcoma virus–Harvey (MSV–H). *Int. J. Cancer*, **3**: 634–643, 1968b.

Harvey, J. J., and East, J., Biological activity and separation of a leukaemogenic virus from murine sarcoma virus–Harvey (MSV–H). *Int. J. Cancer*, **4**: 655–665, 1969.

Harvey, J. J., Mahy, B. W. J., Gillespie, A. V., Salaman, M. H., Chesterman, F. C., and Dourmashkin, R. R., Further studies on a murine sarcoma virus (MSV). *Brit. Empire Cancer Campaign for Research, 43rd Annual Report* (*Part II*), pp. 169–170, 1965.

Harvey, J. J., Salaman, M. H., Chesterman, F. C., Gillespie, A. V., Harris, R. J. C., Evans, R., and Mahy, B. W. J., Studies on a murine sarcoma virus (MSV). *Brit. Empire Cancer Campaign for Research, 42nd Annual Report* (*Part II*), pp. 185–189, 1964.

Huebner, R. J., The murine leukemia-sarcoma virus complex. *Proc. Nat. Acad. Sci., USA*, **58**: 835–842, 1967.

Huebner, R. J., Hartley, J. W., Rowe, W. P., Lane, W. T., and Capps, W. I., Rescue of the defective genome of Moloney sarcoma virus from a noninfectious hamster tumor and the production of pseudotype sarcoma viruses with various murine leukemia viruses. *Proc. Nat. Acad. Sci., USA*, **56**: 1164–1169, 1966.

Ioachim, H. L., and Berwick, L., Continuous viral replication and cellular neoplastic transformation in cultures of normal rat thymus infected with Gross leukemia virus. *Int. J. Cancer*, **3**: 61–73, 1968.

Kirsten, W. H., and Mayer, L. A., Morphologic responses to a murine erythroblastosis virus. *J. Nat. Cancer Inst.*, **39**: 311–335, 1967a.

Kirsten, W. H., Mayer, L. A., Wollmann, R. L., and Pierce, M. I., Studies on a murine erythroblastosis virus. *J. Nat. Cancer Inst.*, **38**: 117–139, 1967b.

Kirsten, W. H., Somers, K. D., and Mayer, L. A., Multiplicity of cell response to a murine erythroblastosis virus. pp. 64–65, in: *Proc. 3rd Internat. Symp. on Comparative Leukemia Research, Paris* (July, 1967), Bibl. Haemat. No. 30, S. Karger, Basel and New York, 1968.

Mahy, B. W. J., Harvey, J. J., and Rowson, K. E. K., Some physical properties of a murine sarcoma virus (Harvey). *Texas Rep. Biol. & Med.*, **24**: 620–628, 1966.

Mitchiner, M. B., Ultrastructural observations on the Harvey mouse leukemia-sarcoma virus. *J. Path. and Bact.*, **93**: 593–600, 1967.

Moloney, J. B., Biological studies on a lymphoid leukemia virus extracted from sarcoma S.37. I. Origin and introductory investigations. *J. Nat. Cancer Inst.*, **24**: 933–951, 1960.

Moloney, J. B., A virus-induced rhabdomyosarcoma of mice. pp. 139–142 in: *Conference on Murine Leukemia, Nat. Cancer Inst. Monograph No. 22.* U.S. Publ. Health Service, Bethesda, Md., 1966a.

Moloney, J. B., The application of studies in murine leukemia to the problems of human neoplasia. pp. 251–258 in: Some Recent Developments in Comparative Medicine, *Symposia of the Zoological Soc. of London*, No. 17. Academic Press, London and New York, 1966b.

Perk, K., and Moloney, J. B., Pathogenesis of a virus-induced rhabdomyosarcoma in mice. *J. Nat. Cancer Inst.*, **37**: 581–599, 1966.

Perk, K., Moloney, J. B., and Jenkins, E. G., Further studies on the relationship of a rhabdomyosarcoma virus to muscle tissue. *Internat. J. Cancer*, **2**: 43–51, 1967.

Ribacchi, R., and Giraldo, G., Plasmacytomas occurring in the bones of rats injected intracerebrally with murine sarcoma virus (MSV), Moloney's strain. Preliminary report. *Lav. Anat. Pat. Perugia*, **26**: 149–156, 1966.

Simons, P. J., Bassin, R. H., and Harvey, J. J., Transformation of hamster embryo cells *in vitro* by murine sarcoma virus (Harvey). *Proc. Soc. Exp. Biol. & Med.*, **125**: 1242–1246, 1967a.

Simons, P. J., Chesterman, F. C., Dourmashkin, R. R., Phillips, D. E. H., and Turano, A., Murine sarcoma virus (Harvey). *Imperial Cancer Research Fund 64th Annual Report for 1965–1966*, pp. 63–66, 1967b.

Simons, P. J., Dourmashkin, R. R., Turano, A., Phillips, D. E. H., and Chesterman, F. C., Morphological transformation of mouse embryo cells *in vitro* by murine sarcoma virus (Harvey). *Nature*, **214**: 897–898, 1967c.

Ting, R. C., *In vitro* transformation of rat embryo cells by a murine sarcoma virus. *Virology*, **28**: 783–785, 1966.

CHAPTER 16

Leukemia and Lymphosarcoma in Cats, Dogs and Guinea Pigs

LEUKEMIA AND LYMPHOSARCOMA IN CATS

Lymphosarcoma is quite common in cats. It has been estimated that leukemia, lymphosarcoma, and related tumors of the hematopoietic system represent about 9 to 15 per cent of the total of all malignant tumors in that species (Cotchin, 1952, 1957. Jarrett, 1966). The disease presents itself usually as a disseminated lymphosarcoma, frequently involving also the thymus. Leukemia involving peripheral blood may also occur, particularly in the more advanced and terminal phases of the disease; however, as in dogs, mice, or cattle, most cases are not accompanied by frank leukemia. Moderate to severe anemia is more common and occurs in the majority of cases, particularly in advanced periods of the disease.

Transmission by Centrifuged Extracts. Jarrett and his colleagues (1964b), at the Veterinary Hospital, University of Glasgow, first reported successful transmission of lymphosarcoma in cats by a centrifuged, presumably cell-free extract. The extract was prepared from a field case of spontaneous lymphosarcoma which developed in an 8½-year-old female cat. The donor animal had a large thymic tumor, a large spleen, and multicentric enlargement of lymph nodes. Tissue fragments from the mediastinal tumor were removed aseptically, stored first at $-40°C$ for 5 days, then placed in 50 per cent glycerin at $-10°C$ for 66 days. The extract was prepared from the stored tissues by grinding in a mortar, and then centrifuged at $2,000 \times g$ for 20 minutes.

The supernatant fluid was inoculated subcutaneously into 4 kittens of a litter less than 12 hours old. Six months after inoculation, the inoculated cats had palpable lymph nodes, and 2 of them also developed large spleens. All 4 cats died, or were sacrificed, when in terminal phase of the disease 9 to 18 months after inoculation; all had disseminated lymphosarcoma, including large thymic tumors, large spleens, and large mesenteric tumors. The predominant leukemic cell, revealed on microscopic examination of the infiltrated organs, was of the primitive stem-cell type.

A second cell-free passage was then made with a tumor removed from one of the experimental animals in which lymphosarcoma had been induced. In the second passage, the centrifuged extract induced lymphosarcoma in the inoculated kittens after 8 weeks (Jarrett, 1966). A further primary passage was obtained with the original field material using a centrifuged cell-free extract; in this transmission experiment, 2 inoculated kittens developed, and died from, acute blast-cell leukemia after a latency of 6 months (Jarrett, 1966).

In another similar study, Rickard and his colleagues (1967), at the New York State Veterinary College, Cornell University, in Ithaca, prepared a leukemic cell suspension from a large mediastinal lymphosarcoma which developed spontaneously in a one-year-old male Siamese cat. The cell suspension and also blood of this animal were inoculated intraperitoneally into three kittens of a litter which was three days old. All inoculated kittens developed mediastinal lymphosarcomas 9 to 12 months after inoculation. The spleens and livers were also enlarged, and there was enlargement of mesenteric and other lymph nodes. Lymphoblasts were also present in peripheral blood of one of the animals examined. More recently Rickard and his colleagues (personal communication to the author, 1968) succeeded in transmitting cat leukemia by centrifuged cell-free extracts.

Kawakami and his colleagues (1967) at the School of Veterinary Medicine, University of California, Davis, also demonstrated transmission of leukemia in cats by cellular, and also by cell-free, extracts.

The donor animal was a 3-year-old castrated male Persian cat with a spontaneous generalized lymphosarcoma which involved primarily the thymus and mediastinal lymph nodes. Infiltration with leukemic cells was also evident on microscopic examination of other organs. Cell suspensions prepared from lymphoid tumors of this cat were inoculated into five 4-day-old kittens; as a result, 3 of the inoculated animals developed lymphosarcomas. In another experiment, a centrifuged, presumably cell-free, extract was prepared from leukemic organs of the donor animal and was inoculated into four kittens less than one day old. As a result, two of the inoculated cats developed disseminated lymphosarcomas after a latency of 7 to 8 weeks. A third animal died earlier, 5 weeks after inoculation, with early lesions of lymphosarcoma in some of the lymph nodes. There were no tumors at the site of inoculation (personal communication to the author from Dr. G. H. Theilen, 1967).

It is apparent, therefore, that cat lymphosarcoma could be readily transmitted by cell-graft, or by cell-free centrifuged extracts, to newborn cat (see also *Transmissible Cat Fibrosarcoma* on p. 622).

Electron Microscopic Studies

In the initial electron microscopic studies carried out by Jarrett and his colleagues, ultrathin sections were prepared from mesenteric tumor, spleen, and thymus of a leukemic cat with spontaneous leukemia, as well as from organs of a cat in which leukemia was induced by inoculation of cell-free extracts. No virus particles were found in organs of the cat which developed spontaneous leukemia; however, examination of organs of the cat with induced leukemia revealed presence of virus-like particles, about 100 mμ in diameter, often in groups, in vacuoles in the cell cytoplasm; none of the particles had electron-dense nucleoids. Similar particles were found also in cultured leukemic cells after second tissue culture passage. Examination of lymph nodes from 14 apparently normal cats did not reveal presence of similar particles (Jarrett *et al.*, 1964a. Jarrett, 1966). In more recent studies, Helen M. Laird in Dr. Jarrett's laboratory observed the presence of characteristic virus particles not only in induced, but also in spontaneous cat lymphosarcoma (Laird *et al.*, 1968a,b. See also Fig. 49 on opposite page).

A similar observation was reported recently by Rickard and his colleagues (1967, 1968a,b). In this study, electron microscopic examination was made of ultrathin sections of neoplastic tissues and bone marrow from two cats with spontaneous lymphocytic leukemia. One of the cats was a one-year-old domestic, short-hair male; the other was a five-year-old castrated male. Both had peripheral blood morphology characteristic for lymphatic leukemia, as well as infiltration of thymus, spleen, liver, bone marrow and lymph nodes, with leukemic cells. Rickard and his coworkers (personal communication to the author, 1968) examined ultrathin sections of tissues from 8 cats with lymphatic leukemia and lymphosarcomas, and found presence of virus particles in tissues from 5 of the 8 animals examined (see also Fig. 50, on page 615).

The neoplastic lymph nodes, thymus, and bone marrow contained scattered virus-like particles which were located predominantly in intercellular spaces; two or three particles were usually together in groups. The average diameter of these particles was about 110 mμ. The typical

---

FIG. 49. CAT LEUKEMIA VIRUS PARTICLES.

(A). Section of a fragment of a lymphoid cell from bone marrow of a cat with spontaneous lymphosarcoma. Virus particle budding from edge of cell membrane (arrow). Magnification 75,000 ×. (B). Section of a fragment of a lymphoid cell from spleen of a cat with spontaneous lymphosarcoma. Virus particle (arrow) in intercellular space. Magnification 100,000 ×. (C). Section of a platelet from a kitten that had been inoculated 28 days previously with a high-speed centrifuged extract prepared from a spontaneous cat lymphosarcoma. Virus particle budding from outer membrane (arrow). Magnification 75,000 ×. (D). Section of a fragment of megakaryocyte from spleen of a kitten that had been inoculated 28 days earlier with centrifuged extract prepared from a spontaneous cat lymphosarcoma, the same as that described in C. Two immature type C virus particles (arrow). Magnification 62,500 ×. Electron micrographs prepared by Helen M. Laird, Animal Leukemia Research Unit, University of Glasgow, Scotland.

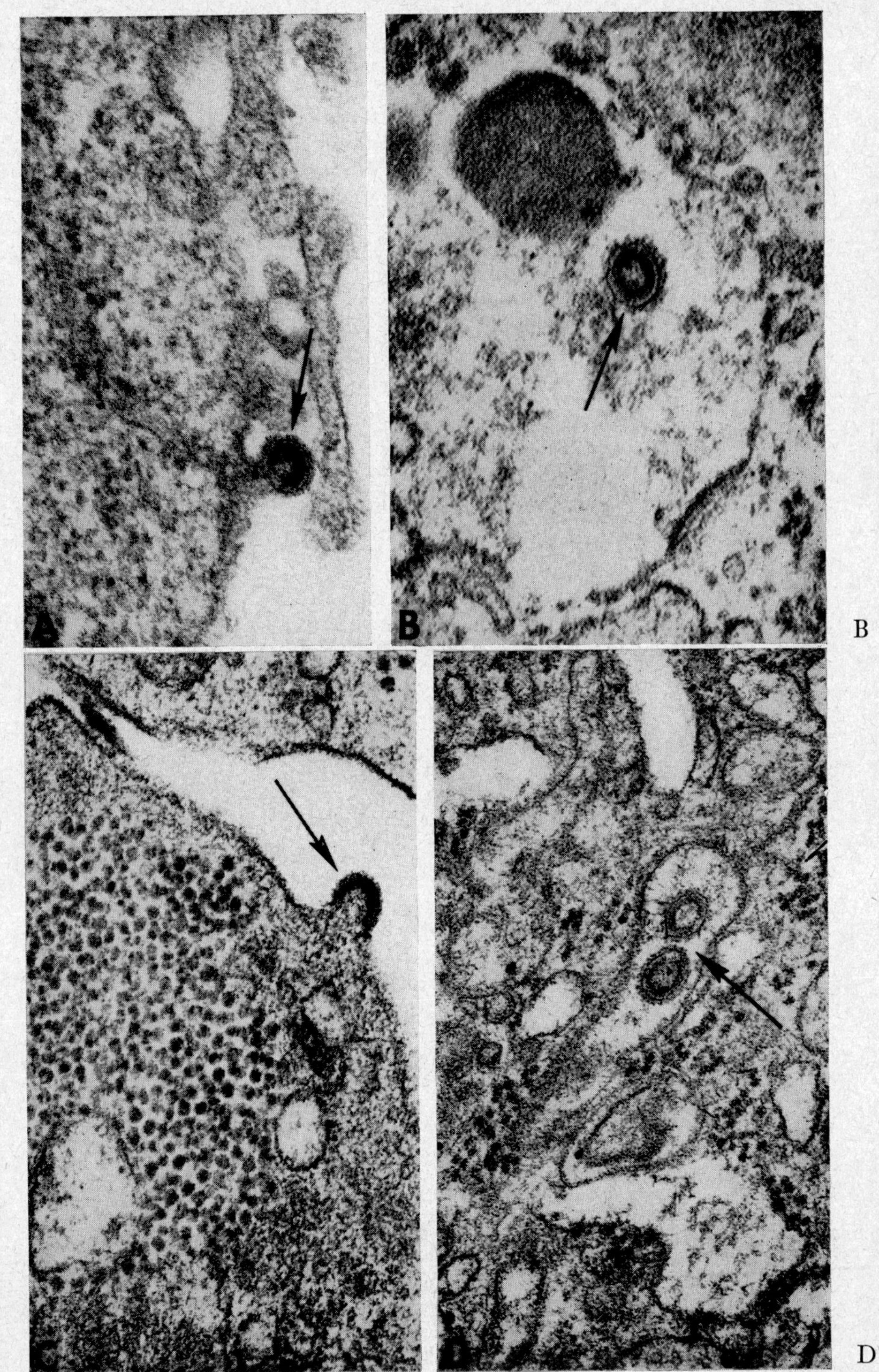

FIG. 49. CAT LEUKEMIA VIRUS PARTICLES.

particle contained an electron-dense nucleoid. The particles resembled the characteristic type C particles found in mouse leukemia.

Budding particles, as many as three on the surface of one cell section, could be observed extending into the intercellular spaces. Early buds were semicircular, showing continuity of the plasma membrane of the cell with the limiting membrane of the emerging virus particle. Later, buds were attached to the cell surface by a thin stalk. Virus particles were observed in the cytoplasmic vesicles of megakaryocytes in the bone marrow, as well as budding from plasma membranes.

Similar virus-like particles and buds were present in tissue cultures of the lymphosarcoma cells after three culture passages (Rickard *et al.*, 1967b).

Virus-like particles, about 115 mμ in diameter, were also observed by Kawakami and his colleagues (1967) in blood plasma, and in leukemic organs of a cat with spontaneous leukemia, and also in organs of kittens with experimentally transmitted disease. Particles observed in their study were predominantly of the mature type C form with an outer envelope, and a uniform electron-dense nucleoid. Immature particles, also present, were of the same diameter and consisted of an outer envelope and two additional concentric inner shells.

LEUKEMIA AND LYMPHOSARCOMA IN DOGS

Lymphosarcoma and related neoplasms, such as mastocytoma, develop occasionally in middle-aged dogs of different breeds. True leukemia, with peripheral blood involvement, is less common but has been observed also. Jarrett and his colleagues (1966) estimated that among 10,000 canine admissions to the Veterinary Hospital at the University of Glasgow Veterinary School, the incidence of lymphosarcoma among adult dogs was 2 per cent.

Transmission of Lymphosarcoma in Dogs by Cell-Graft. Transmission of lymphosarcoma by cell-graft to irradiated puppies was recently reported (Moldovanu *et al.*, 1966). All three recipients were newborn mongrel dogs of unknown origin. As a preliminary treatment, the dogs received 85 to 128 R total body irradiation. Repeated inoculations of leukemic cell suspensions were made after the irradiation.

Progressively growing disseminated lymphosarcomas developed in the inoculated dogs after a latency varying from 1 to 3 months. One inoculated dog developed generalized lymphosarcomas after 26 days, and the second dog after 90 days, following inoculation of cell suspensions prepared from donor dogs with spontaneous lymphosarcomas. The third animal developed generalized lymphosarcomas after 44 days, following inoculation of a canine lymphosarcoma cell line, LS No. 30, which had been carried in tissue culture for almost one year. The authors noted that in previous attempts, 35 adult dogs had been inoculated with dog lymphosarcoma cells, and none developed symptoms of disease.

In more recent studies, two lymphosarcomas, which developed spontaneously in adult dogs, were carried serially through 6 transplantations in irradiated newborn pups (Moldovanu *et al.*, 1968). The inoculated dogs developed lymphosarcomas at the site of inoculation after a short latency of only 2 weeks. Most of these tumors grew progressively and killed their hosts; some tumors, however, regressed spontaneously after a temporary growth. Beginning with the third passage, up to 40 per cent of the transplanted lymphosarcomas eventually regressed.

Kakuk and his coworkers (1968) also reported recently two serial passages by cell-graft of a malignant lymphoma in dogs. Cell suspensions prepared from a spontaneous lymphoma which developed in a 20-month old Doberman Pinscher female were inoculated into 2 litters of newborn Beagles. Three out of 15 inoculated dogs developed lymphomas 2 to 3 months after inoculation.

Transmission of Mastocytoma in Dogs by Cell-Graft and by Cell-free Extracts

Mastocytoma (mast cell tumor) occurs occasionally in dogs. This tumor belongs to the general group of lymphomas; it frequently affects the skin, but also spleen, liver, and lymph nodes, and is often associated with leukemic manifestations, i.e., increased number of white blood cells and presence of neoplastic mast cells and anemia in peripheral blood. It has been estimated that mastocytoma accounts for approximately 6 per cent of all tumors observed in dogs (Mulligan, 1949. Smith and Jones, 1957. Moulton, 1961).

A previous attempt to transplant mastocytoma by cell-graft did not succeed (Nielsen and Cole, 1961). However, more recently, Lombard and her colleagues reported (1963) that a spontaneous mastocytoma could be successfully transmitted by cell-free extracts to mixed-breed and Beagle puppies.

The original tumor developed in an eleven-year-old female Doberman Pinscher. The animal had multiple skin tumors, markedly enlarged spleen, liver, and peripheral lymph nodes; neoplastic mast cells were also present in peripheral blood. The tumor could be transmitted to newborn puppies by cell-graft, and also by centrifuged and filtered extracts.

Following inoculation of leukemic cell suspensions, tumors developed after a latency varying from 14 days to 5 months. In some litters, only a few animals developed tumors; in other litters, all inoculated puppies developed disseminated mastocytomas; in advanced phases of the disease, pleomorphic mast cells appeared in peripheral blood, and eventually constituted 6 to 30 per cent of the total number of white blood cells. The tumors could be transmitted serially, through several transplant generations. Some of the tumors regressed, but most grew progressively.

Transmission by Filtrates. The mastocytoma could be successfully transmitted also by means of filtrates. The extracts were prepared from subcutaneous tumors resulting from transplantation of the original tumor cell suspensions. The cell extracts were homogenized and centrifuged at 2,300 $\times g$ for 20 minutes. The supernatant fluid was then passed through No. 12 Mandler, or through Millipore 0.45 μ, filter candles. The filtrates thus obtained were concentrated by ultracentrifugation and then inoculated into newborn puppies.

Four of 12 puppies inoculated with the Mandler filtrates, and 17 out of 38 puppies inoculated with the Millipore filtrates, developed tumors. Two animals developed mastocytomas after only 2 to 3 weeks; all others after an average latency varying from 2 to over 3 months. The mast cell tumors could be passed serially, by inoculation of filtrates, through three successive generations of dogs.

Transmission of Another Case of Mast Cell Leukemia in Dogs by Cell-free Extracts. In a similar more recent study, Rickard and Post (1967) were also able to transmit serially mast cell leukemia in dogs, either by cell-graft or by centrifuged cell-free extracts. The disease originated spontaneously in a nine-year-old male Beagle dog. This animal had a large tumor in the mesentery, also an extensive infiltration by neoplastic mast cells of spleen, liver, and several mesenteric lymph nodes. Mast cells were also present in peripheral blood. No tumors were present in the skin.

A suspension of tumor cells, prepared from tumors and liver of the donor animal, was inoculated into 2-week-old puppies. Three out of 5 inoculated puppies developed mast cell leukemia after 1 to 3 months. Additional serial passages by cell-graft were made using 1 to 7-day-old puppies for inoculation. One-half or more of the inoculated animals at each passage level, and all injected puppies in the more recent passages, developed mast cell tumors. The latent period gradually declined to only one week.

Cell-free, centrifuged extracts were also prepared and injected at several cell passage levels; however, no cell-free transmission succeeded before the eighth serial cellular transfer. From the eighth to thirteenth passages, a total of 6 puppies, out of 45 inoculated, developed the disease. Subsequently, however, all 13 puppies inoculated at passage levels 14 and 15 developed mast cell leukemia.

The disease induced in the inoculated puppies was characterized by marked infiltration of spleen, liver, lymph nodes, and bone marrow, with leukemic cells, and also by the development of mast cell leukemia with increased white cell count, and presence of over 50 per cent of neoplastic mast cells in peripheral blood. Mast cell tumors developed in most of the inoculated animals, either at the site of inoculation or in internal organs. No skin tumors, however, developed in the inoculated animals; it is of interest that no skin lesions were observed in the original spontaneous case which served as donor source for this tumor line. On the other hand, in experiments described by Lombard and her coworkers (1963), skin lesions were observed in the original donor and also in the inoculated animals.

Electron Microscopic Studies

Electron Microscopic Studies of Mastocytoma. In the initial electron microscopic studies of dog mastocytoma, Lombard and her coworkers reported (1963) the presence of "round particles with an electron-dense membrane and a less dense core," measuring about 109 mμ in diameter, some in intercellular spaces and others within cytoplasmic vacuoles. The authors suggested that these round bodies within vacuoles might represent viral particles. However, the quality and resolution of electron micrographs of ultrathin sections published in the original paper were not satisfactory, and in retrospect it seems that identification of virus particles on the basis of photographs published at that time would not be justified.

Electron Microscopic Studies of Reticulum-Cell Sarcomas in Dogs. In a recent study, Chapman and his coworkers (1967) examined ultrathin sections of fragments of spleens, lymph nodes, bone marrow and other tissues from two dogs with reticulum-cell sarcomas. One of the spontaneous tumors employed in this study developed in a male German Shepherd dog aged 3 years; the other tumor developed in a male Weimaraner aged 8 years. In both animals there was an enlargement of liver, spleen and lymph nodes, due to infiltration with leukemic cells. On electron microscopic examination, virus particles were found in some of the tissues examined; a few particles were found budding from the cell membranes; other particles were found within the cytoplasmic matrix. Budding of virus-like particles from endoplasmic reticulum into the cytoplasmic matrix was also observed.

However, the fact that some of the virus particles were found in the cytoplasmic matrix and that other particles were budding from the cytoplasmic vacuoles into the matrix, instead of budding in reverse direction into the vacuoles, was rather puzzling and did not have a parallel in electron microscopic observations dealing with mouse or rat leukemia.

In the same study Chapman and his colleagues (1967) examined cell cultures derived from both leukemic dogs. One culture was derived from pleural cells of one of the leukemic dogs. After a few passages the cells assumed epithelioid character; in these cells numerous virus particles could be found not only within cytoplasmic vacuoles, but also in extracellular spaces; some of these particles contained nucleoids, and were morphologically similar to mature type C mouse leukemia virus particles. However, on bio-assay, extracts prepared from this cell culture readily induced leukemia when inoculated into newborn mice, but failed to induce leukemia following inoculation into newborn dogs (personal communication to the author from Dr. A. L. Chapman, 1968). For that reason results of the electron microscopic observation of virus particles in this tissue culture cell line must be accepted with reservations.

Other Electron Microscopic Studies of Dog Lymphosarcoma. In general, electron microscopic studies of dog lymphosarcoma did not bring convincing and satisfactory results. Occasionally, virus-like particles could be detected in only some of the animals examined; however, the possible relation of such particles to the etiology of the lymphosarcomas remained undetermined.

Chapman and his coworkers (personal communication to the author, 1968) examined 21 field cases of canine lymphoma; only 3 had small numbers of structures resembling virus particles; in addition, 4 cases of transplanted lymphomas were examined, but none revealed presence of virus-like particles.

We have examined recently with Dr. D. G. Feldman (1968) ultrathin sections of organs of six dogs with spontaneous lymphomas and found in one of them crystalline arrays of very small virus-like particles about 20 mμ in diameter in the tumor cell cytoplasm; similar intracytoplasmic crystalline arrays of small particles, about 18 to 20 mμ in diameter, were observed recently by Kakuk and his coworkers (1968) in three Beagle dogs which developed tumors as a result of implantation of lymphoma cells from a spontaneous dog lymphosarcoma. Whether these small particles have any causal relationship to the etiology of dog lymphosarcoma remains to be determined, and appears rather doubtful.

LEUKEMIA IN GUINEA PIGS

Leukemia and lymphosarcoma have long been observed to develop occasionally in middle-aged guinea pigs. The leukemic tumors could be transmitted by cell-graft in guinea pigs, inducing disseminated lymphosarcomas and generalized leukemia (Miguez, 1918. Snijders, 1926, 1927). In these early studies some of the leukemias and lymphosarcomas could be transmitted serially in guinea pigs for over 50 successive transplant generations. The guinea pig lymphosarcoma maintained in serial transplantations in guinea pigs by Miguez could also be transplanted to a closely related species *Cavia Pallas Caviidae*, i.e., "cuis," closely resembling the guinea pig (Fischer and Kantor, 1919).

In fact, serial transmission by cell-graft of lymphosarcoma in guinea pigs had been reported prior to successful transplantation of mouse leukemia. However, experimental studies on leukemia and lymphosarcoma in guinea pigs have been carried out only on a very limited basis. Following the early transplantation experiments referred to above, there were no other significant reports on guinea pig leukemia until the relatively recent studies described below.

Spontaneous Leukemia in Inbred and Non-inbred Guinea Pigs. In 1954, Congdon and Lorenz reported that they observed several cases of spontaneous lymphatic leukemia among guinea pigs at the National Cancer Institute in Bethesda, Md. The disease developed in animals which were over one year old; these animals developed generalized lymphatic leukemia with formation of disseminated lymphosarcoma, infiltration of internal organs with leukemic cells, and also involvement of blood morphology; the peripheral white blood cell count was increased, with predominance of lymphocytes and presence of many immature blast cells. Some of the guinea pigs were irradiated; however, the incidence of spontaneous leukemia was about equally distributed in irradiated and non-irradiated animals.

Among a total of 303 guinea pigs observed, 10 animals developed leukemia, an incidence of 3.3 per cent. The disease developed in three different groups of animals, as follows: among 112 "strain 2" guinea pigs, 4 animals (3.6 per cent) developed leukemia; among 30 "strain 13" guinea pigs, 2 developed leukemia (6.7 per cent); and finally, among 161 heterogeneous hybrid guinea pigs, 4 animals (2.5 per cent) developed leukemia.

Transplantation by Cell-Graft to Inbred Guinea Pigs. Transplantation by cell-graft was accomplished in young guinea pigs of the same strain. Four primary leukemias were transplanted successfully. In these initial experiments, successful transplantation by cell-graft was accomplished only in animals of the same inbred strain in which leukemia had originally developed (Congdon and Lorenz, 1954). The latency period was rather long in first transplantation, and lasted up to several months, but became shorter with each successive transplantation; eventually the latency was reduced to only 2 weeks in some instances, and to 1 to 2 months in other cases. One of the leukemias was transmitted through 32 consecutive serial transplantations. In some of the animals with induced leukemia the number of white cells, including primitive blast cells, in peripheral blood was very high and exceeded 500,000 per mm^3.

Transplantation by Cell-Graft to Non-inbred Guinea Pigs. Importance of Age at Inoculation. More recently it was realized that leukemia could also be transmitted by cell-graft from inbred "strain 2" to non-inbred guinea pigs, provided that suckling, less than 7-day-old, guinea pigs were used for inoculation. In the study carried out by Nadel (1954, 1957), the lymphatic leukemia strain (L2B), which was employed for cell transfer, developed originally in a "strain 2" female guinea pig. Cell suspensions prepared from leukemic tumors and from the spleen of the donor animal were inoculated into less than 7-day-old guinea pigs of non-inbred Hartley and Beltsville stocks. The implanted cells grew progressively and induced generalized leukemia in every inoculated animal. Leukemia could be passed serially in such very young non-inbred guinea pigs for over 18 transplant generations. Slightly older, 7 to 10-day-old, guinea pigs were also susceptible, but to a lesser degree than younger animals. The susceptibility decreased rapidly with increasing age, and no positive results were observed in animals that were inoculated at 8 weeks of age.

This observation followed similar earlier studies on mouse leukemia in which it was demonstrated that leukemia could be transplanted by cell-graft from one strain of mice to another, provided that either newborn, or suckling, less than 7-day-old mice were used for inoculation (Gross, 1950).

However, transmission to non-inbred stock guinea pigs did not always succeed, even if young animals were employed for inoculation (Jungeblut and Kodza, 1960). For that reason in subsequent studies dealing with experimental transmission of leukemia L2B and L2C, which originated in "strain 2" guinea pigs, Jungeblut and Kodza employed either young adult guinea pigs of the inbred "strain 2," or first generation hybrids born to "strain 2" males and Hartley stock (non-inbred) females. Both "strain 2" and first generation hybrid guinea pigs were highly susceptible to inoculation of either L2B or L2C leukemia.

Transmission Experiments and Some Properties of the Leukemogenic Agent. In experiments reported by Jungeblut and Kodza (1962), transmission was accomplished by inoculation of either blood, plasma, serum, or leukemic cell suspensions prepared from leukemic spleens. The inoculated animals ranged in age from 1 to 3 months. Leukemia developed in the inoculated animals after a short latency of 2 to 3 weeks. The induced disease was manifested by the development of disseminated lymphosarcomas; in most animals there was also a considerable increase in the number of white cells of the lymphocytic series in peripheral blood, with presence of many abnormal cells and also primitive blast cells. From the description of the morphologic findings, it appears that the disease could be classified as either lymphatic or stem-cell leukemia.

Titration of leukemic spleen extracts and plasma revealed that the disease could be induced with 1 : 100 and 1 : 500 dilutions.

Cell suspensions prepared from leukemic spleens could be frozen and stored at – 70°C for up to 6 months without losing their leukemogenic potency. However, frozen plasma did not retain its leukemogenic potency for more than 10 days.

The active leukemogenic factor present in the leukemic extracts could be inactivated by heating to 56° for 30 minutes, or by exposure *in vitro* to ethyl ether.

Attempt to transmit leukemia by centrifuged extracts, and by filtrates. Jungeblut and Kodza (1962) reported that they were able to transmit leukemia in guinea pigs by centrifuged, presumably cell-free, extracts. The extracts were prepared from leukemic spleens; they were then centrifuged 1 to 3 consecutive times (5,500 to 16,000 r.p.m.). The final supernate was then inoculated, and induced leukemia after a short latency of only 15 to 21 days. Blood plasma was also harvested from leukemic animals, centrifuged, and inoculated; leukemia developed in the inoculated animals after a short latency of only 15 to 30 days.

In another experiment, extracts were passed through either Berkefeld N filters, or Millipore 0.45 μ membranes, or through Seitz EK asbestos disks; the filtrates were then inoculated into young guinea pigs, and induced leukemia after a latency of 3 to 4 weeks in 11 out of 43 filtration experiments (Jungeblut and Kodza, 1962).

In more recent studies (personal communication to the author from Dr. C. W. Jungeblut, 1968), leukemia in guinea pigs could be transmitted by filtrates, but with considerable difficulties and only in some instances. Relatively large quantities (5 to 15 cm^3) of the filtrates were inoculated into young adult first generation hybrids, born to "strain 2" males and Hartley stock female guinea pigs; these animals are highly susceptible to the guinea pig leukemia agent. Nine extracts prepared from either plasma or organs of leukemic donors were passed through Selas 02 or 03 filter candles; only one of these 9 filtrates proved leukemogenic. In another series, 15 extracts were passed through either 0.8, 0.45, or 0.2 μ Millipore membranes; only 4 out of the 15 filtrates tested proved leukemogenic on inoculation tests.

FIG. 50. CAT LEUKEMIA VIRUS PARTICLES.

(A). Ultrathin section of a thymic lymphoid tumor cell from a 5-year-old male cat with spontaneous lymphatic leukemia. Two budding particles at the edge of cell membrane. Magnification 92,750×. (B). Doughnut-like virus particles in a thymic tumor cell from the same animal as that described in (A). Magnification 92,750×. (C). Virus particles in a cytoplasmic vacuole in a thymic tumor cell, same animal as in (A). Some of the virus particles have internal nucleoids. Magnification 92,750×. (D). Fourth passage of the virus isolated from spontaneous lymphatic leukemia described in (A). A centrifuged cell-free extract prepared from organs of a leukemic cat was inoculated into a newborn male kitten; the inoculated animal developed stem-cell leukemia and died after 4 months. Ultrathin section of a bone marrow fragment showing characteristic mature type C virus particles about 110 mμ in diameter, with internal electron-dense nucleoids. Magnification 90,000×. Electron micrographs prepared by C. G. Rickard, New York State Veterinary College, Cornell University, Ithaca.

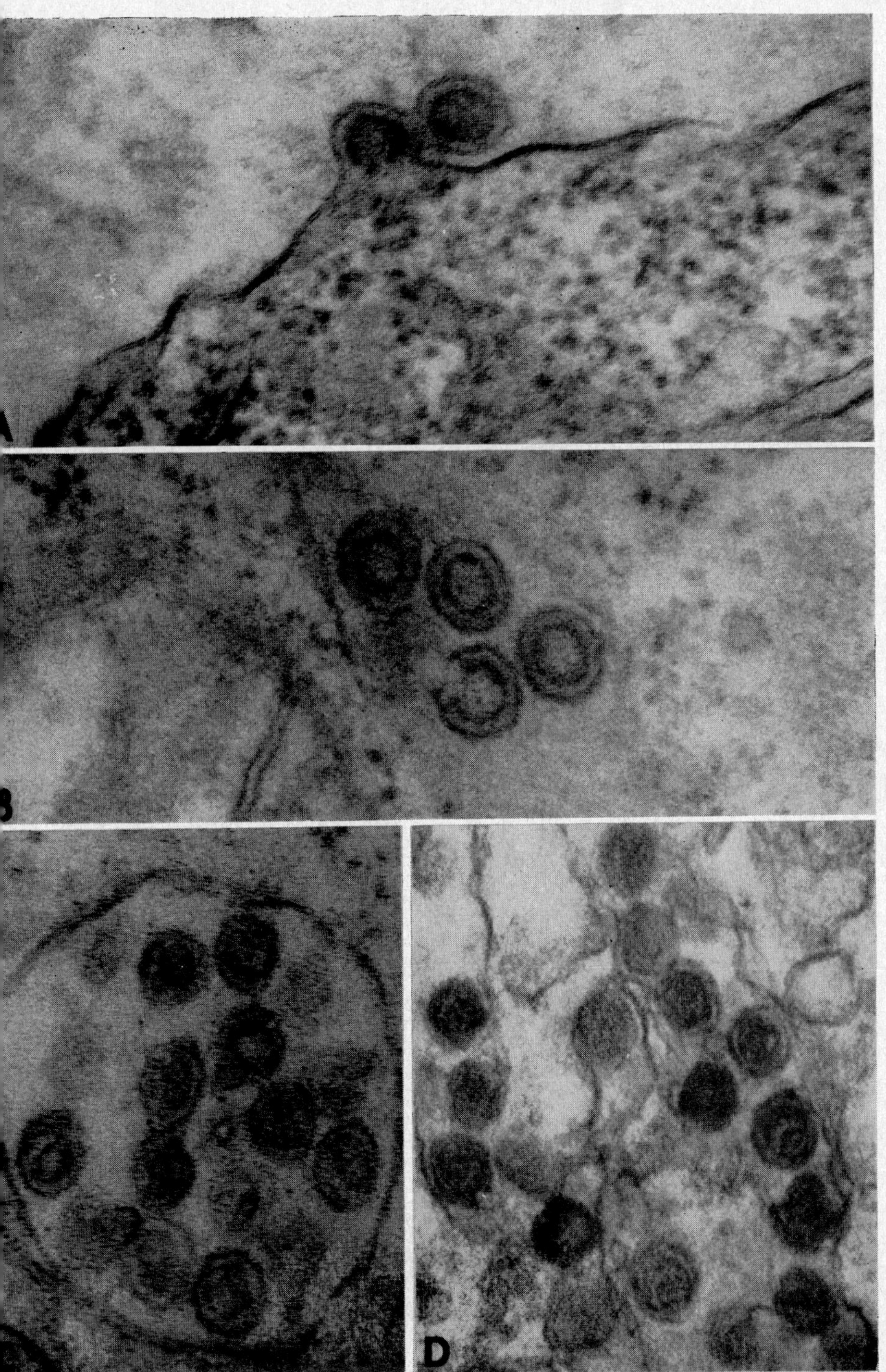

Fig. 50. Cat Leukemia Virus Particles.

In a similar study, carried out in another laboratory, guinea pig leukemia could not be transmitted by filtrates; the leukemic extracts passed through either Seitz filter pads or through Millipore filters were inactive on inoculation tests (E. M. Nadel, personal communication to the author, 1967). In spite of this difficulty, in the same study, transmission by presumably cell-free centrifuged, but not filtered, extracts was successful; blood plasma that had been centrifuged several times at slow speeds, followed by high speed centrifugation at 35,000 r.p.m., was also leukemogenic on inoculation tests.

Experimental data referring to the transmission of leukemia in guinea pigs by filtrates require confirmation in more extensive experiments. It may be of interest to inoculate with the filtrates newborn or suckling, less than 7-day-old, inbred or non-inbred guinea pigs; the observation time should be extended to at least 18 months. In experiments thus far reported, the inoculated animals were observed for only 3 to 4 months (Jungeblut and Kodza, 1960, 1962). Such a short observation period would be insufficient in experiments dealing with mouse or rat leukemia.

Current Experiments on the Transmission of Guinea Pig Leukemia. We have transmitted recently in our laboratory guinea pig leukemia in "strain 2" young adult guinea pigs by cell-graft; the average latency was 23 days. Centrifuged plasma supernate was also inoculated into 4 young adult guinea pigs and induced leukemia in 2 animals after a latency of 45 days. However, we have not been able, thus far, to transmit guinea pig leukemia by filtered extracts prepared from plasma or from spleen and lymphoid tumors. These experiments, still in progress, include attempts to transmit leukemia by filtrates to newborn guinea pigs; a long observation period may be required (Gross, to be published).

In Vitro Adsorption of the Virus on Blood Cells

The leukemogenic agent present in plasma of leukemic guinea pigs could be adsorbed *in vitro* by either guinea pig, rabbit or human blood cells (Jungeblut and Kodza, 1962. Jungeblut and Opler, 1967). Adsorption was incomplete with large doses of the agent; however, smaller doses were completely adsorbed after standing for 30 minutes at 37°C, or at room temperature, on a rocking table, leaving no detectable trace of the agent in the supernatant fluid.

Electron Microscopic Studies

Recently reported preliminary electron microscopic studies of ultrathin sections of blood plasma pellets, and fragments of bone marrow, spleen and lymph nodes from leukemic guinea pigs revealed the presence of spherical virus-like particles (Opler, 1967. Nadel *et al.*, 1967). The particles, which had a diameter of about 70 to 90 mμ, were found in the perinuclear cisternae, as well as in the cisternae of the endoplasmic reticulum in the leukemic cells; some of the particles were found budding into the cisternae.

These particles were of a doughnut-like form, and had a "fuzzy" outer coat (Nadel *et al.*, 1967). Among the particles found in the blood plasma pellets, a few appeared to have electron-dense nucleoids (Opler, 1967).

In our current experiments (Gross and Feldman, 1969, to be published), a guinea pig leukemia strain, which we obtained through the courtesy of Dr. C. W. Jungeblut from Lenox Hill Hospital in New York City, was carried in serial cell-graft passage in "strain 2" guinea pigs. Examination of ultrathin sections prepared from organs of 10 leukemic guinea pigs revealed, in the cisternae of the endoplasmic reticulum in the leukemic cells, the presence of previously reported doughnut-like virus particles. These particles consisted of 2 concentric membranes, had relatively electron-lucent centers and measured about 90 to 100 mμ in diameter; they appeared to be formed by budding from the membranes of the endoplasmic reticulum into the cisternae.

In addition, spherical particles about 100 mμ in diameter, with thick outer envelopes and centrally located electron-dense nucleoids, were found in intercellular spaces.

Both the doughnut-like particles and the particles with nucleoids were found in all 10 animals examined; they were observed in a variety of tissues, such as subcutaneous and visceral lymphoid tumors, spleen, thymus, lymph nodes, bone marrow and ovaries.

In a control study, no virus particles were found either in the endoplasmic reticulum or in the intercellular spaces of tissue fragments of spleen, liver, thymus, lymph nodes or bone marrow from 9 normal, healthy, "strain 2" guinea pigs examined.

REFERENCES

Chapman, A. L., Bopp, W. J., Brightwell, A. S., Cohen, H., Nielsen, A. H., Gravelle, C. R., and Werder, A. A., Preliminary report on virus-like particles in canine leukemia and derived cell cultures. *Cancer Research*, **27**: 18–25, 1967.

Congdon, C. C., and Lorenz, E., Leukemia in guinea-pigs. *Am. J. Path.*, **30**: 337–359, 1954.

Cotchin, E., Neoplasms in cats. *Proc. Roy. Soc. Med.*, **45**: 671–674 (Sect. Comp. Med., pp. 17–20), 1952.

Fig. 51a. Virus Particles in Guinea Pig Leukemia.

Ultrathin sections of a fragment of bone marrow obtained from a leukemic "strain 2" guinea pig. This male was inoculated subcutaneously, when about 6 weeks old, with a cell suspension prepared from a transplantable strain of guinea pig leukemia, and developed a local lymphoid tumor at the site of inoculation and a generalized stem-cell leukemia. Sacrificed 19 days after inoculation. WBC 344,000 per mm^3, with 89 per cent of blast cells. Hb. 4.4 gm per 100 cc. of blood. (A). Intracisternal doughnut-like virus particles. Magnification 84,800 ×. (B). Spherical virus particles with electron-dense nucleoids in an intercellular space. Magnification 122,000 ×. (L. Gross and D. G. Feldman, to be published).

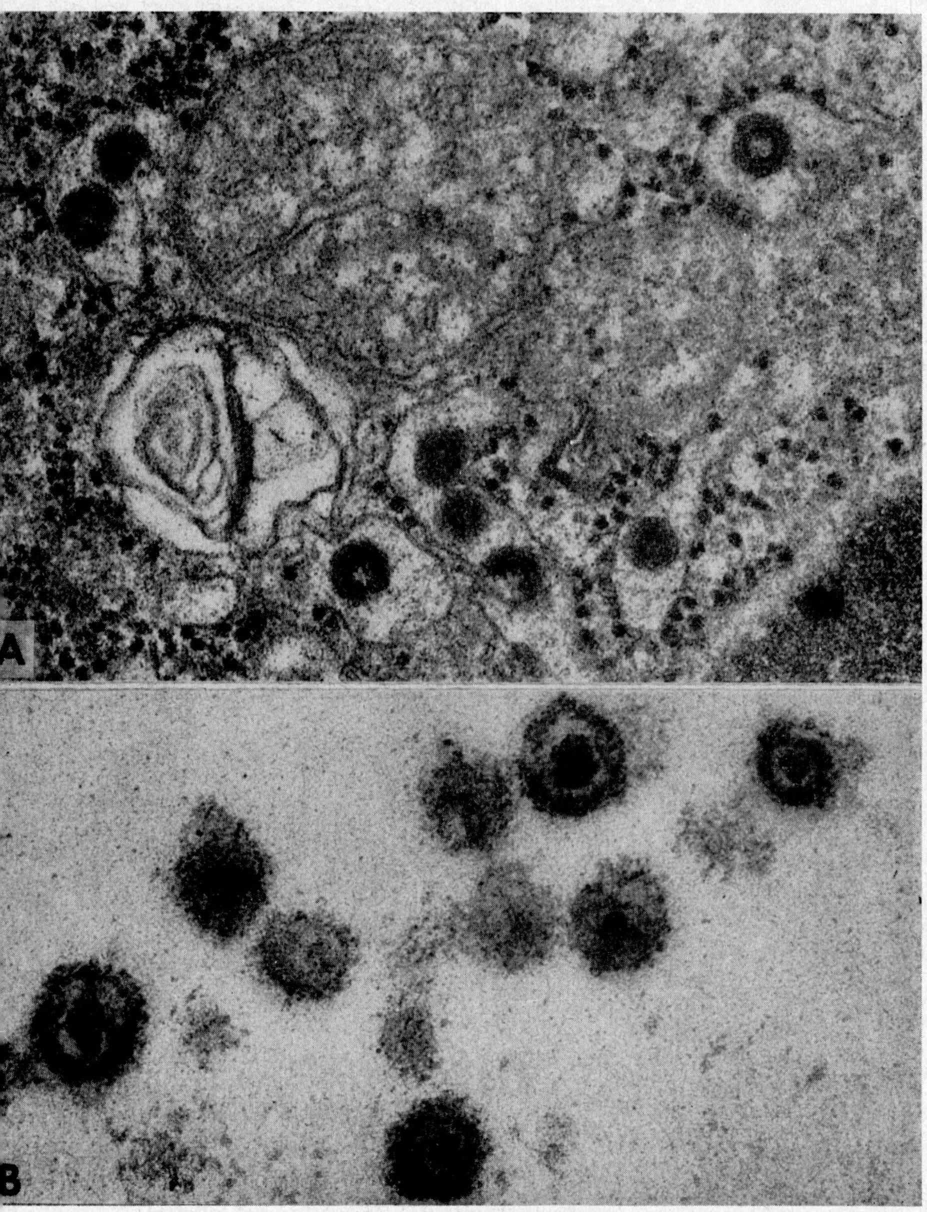

Fig. 51a. Virus Particles in Guinea Pig Leukemia.

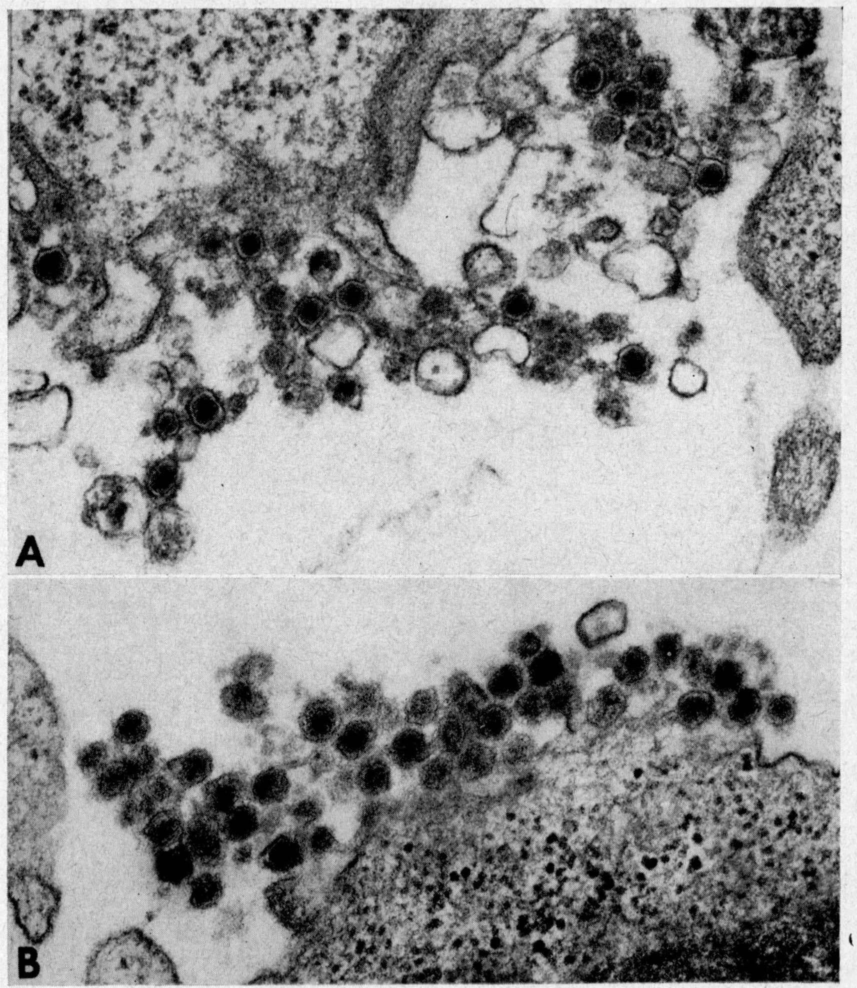

FIG. 51b. VIRUS PARTICLES IN BOVINE LYMPHOSARCOMA

(A). Ultrathin section of a lymphocyte culture from peripheral blood of a cow with lymphosarcoma; this culture was stimulated with phytohemagglutinin, and incubated at 37°C for 72 hours. Numerous extracellular, mature, type C, virus particles 90 to 120 mμ in diameter, with electron-dense nucleoids. Magnification 69,000 ×. (B). Ultrathin section of a lymphocyte from a 24 hour culture of a tumor explant from a cow with lymphosarcoma; this culture was not exposed to phytohemagglutinin. Numerous extracellular virus particles clustered at the cell surface. Magnification 66,000 ×. Electron micrographs received from J. M. Miller, L. D. Miller, C. Olson and K. G. Gilletta, Dept. of Veterinary Science, University of Wisconsin, Madison (*J. Nat. Cancer Inst.*, in press, 1969). (See *Addendum* on p. 650.)

COTCHIN, E., Neoplasia in the cat. *Vet. Rec.*, **69**: 425–434, 1957.

FISCHER, G., and KANTOR, L., Contribución al estudio del parentesco entre especies animals por métodos biológicos. *Rev. Inst. Bact., Buenos Aires*, **2**: 303–308, 1919.

GROSS, L., Susceptibility of newborn mice of an otherwise apparently "resistant" strain to inoculation with leukemia. *Proc. Soc. Exp. Biol. & Med.*, **73**: 246-248, 1950.

GROSS, L., Susceptibility of suckling-infant and resistance of adult mice of the C3H and of the C57 lines to inoculation with Ak leukemia. *Cancer*, **3**: 1073–1087, 1950.

JARRETT, W. F. H., Experimental studies of feline and bovine leukaemia. *Proc. Roy. Soc. Med.*, **59**: 661–662, (Sect. Comp. Med., pp. 21–22), 1966.

JARRETT, W. F. H., CRIGHTON, G. W., and DALTON, R. G., Leukaemia and lymphosarcoma in animals and man. I. Lymphosarcoma or leukaemia in the domestic animals. *Vet. Rec.*, **79**: 693–699, 1966.

JARRETT, W. F. H., CRAWFORD, E. M., MARTIN, W. B., and DAVIE, F., Leukaemia in the cat. A virus-like particle associated with leukaemia (lymphosarcoma). *Nature*, **202**: 567–568, 1964a.

JARRETT, W. F. H., MARTIN, W. B., CRIGHTON, G. W., DALTON, R. G., and STEWART, M. F., Leukaemia in the cat: Transmission experiments with leukaemia (lymphosarcoma). *Nature*, **202**: 566–567, 1964b.

JUNGEBLUT, C. W., and KODZA, H., Attempts to adapt leukemia L_2C from inbred to noninbred guinea pigs. *Am. J. Path.*, **37**: 191–201, 1960.

JUNGEBLUT, C. W., and KODZA, H., Studies of leukemia L_2C in guinea pigs. *Arch. Ges. Virusforsch.*, **12**: 537–551, 1962.

JUNGEBLUT, C. W., and OPLER, S. R., In-vitro adsorption of cavian leukemia virus on blood cells. *Am. J. Path.*, **51**: 1161–1166, 1967.

KAKUK, T. J., HINZ, R. W., LANGHAM, R. F., and CONNER, G. H., Experimental transmission of canine malignant lymphoma to the Beagle neonate. *Cancer Research*, **28**: 716–723, 1968.

KAWAKAMI, T. G., THEILEN, G. H., DUNGWORTH, D. L., BEALL, S. G., and MUNN, R. J., "C"-type viral particles in plasma of feline leukemia. *Science*, **158**: 1049–1050, 1967.

LAIRD, H. M., JARRETT, O., CRIGHTON, G. W., and JARRETT, W. F. H., An electron microscopic study of virus particles in spontaneous leukemia in the cat. *J. Nat. Cancer Inst.*, **41**: 867–878, 1968a.

LAIRD, H. M., JARRETT, O., CRIGHTON, G. W., JARRETT, W. F. H., and HAY, D., Replication of leukemogenic-type virus in cats inoculated with feline lymphosarcoma extracts. *J. Nat. Cancer Inst.*, **41**: 879–893, 1968b.

LOMBARD, L. S., MOLONEY, J. B., RICKARD, C. G., Transmissible canine mastocytoma. *Ann. N.Y. Acad. Sci.*, **108**: 1086–1105, 1963.

MIGUEZ, C., Sarcoma espontáneo transplantable en el cobayo. *Rev. Inst. Bact., Buenos Aires*, **1**: 147–154, 1918.

MOLDOVANU, G., MOORE, A. E., FRIEDMAN, M., and MILLER, D. G., Cellular transmission of lymphosarcoma in dogs. *Nature*, **210**: 1342–1343, 1966.

MOLDOVANU, G., MOORE, A. E., FRIEDMAN, M., and MILLER, D. G., Canine lymphosarcoma maintained in serial passage. pp. 276–278, in: *Proc. 3rd Internat. Symp. on Comparative Leukemia Research, Paris* (July, 1967), Bibl. Haemat. No. 30, S. Karger, Basel and New York, 1968.

MOULTON, J. E., *Tumors in Domestic Animals*. p. 279. Univ. of California Press, Berkeley and Los Angeles, 1961.

MULLIGAN, R. M., *Neoplasms of the Dog*. p. 135. Williams & Wilkins, Co., Baltimore, Md., 1949.

NADEL, E. M., An influence of age on transplantation of leukemia from inbred to noninbred guinea pigs. (Abstract.) *Fed. Proc.*, **13**: 439–440, 1954.

NADEL, E. M., Transplantation of leukemia from inbred to noninbred guinea pigs. *J. Nat. Cancer Inst.*, **19**: 351–359, 1957.

NADEL, E., BANFIELD, W., BURSTEIN, S., and TOUSIMIS, A. J., Virus particles associated with strain 2 guinea pig leukemia (L2C/N-B). *J. Nat. Cancer Inst.*, **38**: 979–981, 1967.

NIELSEN, S. W., and COLE, C. R., Homologous transplantation of canine neoplasms. *Am. J. Vet. Research*, **22**: 663–672, 1961.

OPLER, S. R., Observations on a new virus associated with guinea pig leukemia: Preliminary note. *J. Nat. Cancer Inst.*, **38**: 797–800, 1967.

RICKARD, C. G., BARR, L. M., NORONHA, F., DOUGHERTY, E., 3rd, and POST, J. E., C-type virus particles in spontaneous lymphocytic leukemia in a cat. *Cornell Vet.*, **57**: 302–307, 1967.

RICKARD, C. G., and POST, J. E., Cellular and cell-free transmission of a canine mast cell leukemia. pp. 279–281, in: *Proc. 3rd Internat. Symp. on Comparative Leukemia Research, Paris* (July, 1967), Bibl. Haemat. No. 30, S. Karger, Basel and New York, 1968a.

RICKARD, C. G., GILLESPIE, J. H., LEE, K. M., NORONHA, F., POST, J. E., and SAVAGE, E. L., Transmission and electron microscopy of lymphocytic leukemia in the cat. pp. 282–284, in: *Proc. 3rd Internat. Symp. on Comparative Leukemia Research, Paris* (July, 1967), Bibl. Haemat. No. 30, S. Karger, Basel and New York, 1968b.

SMITH, H. A., and JONES, T. C., Neoplasia. Chapter 7, pp. 154–233 in: *Veterinary Pathology*, p. 959. Lea and Febiger, Philadelphia, 1957.

SNIJDERS, E. P., Over een overentbare leukaemie bij cavia's. *Nederland. T. Geneesk.*, **70**: 1256–1262, 1926.

SNIJDERS, E. P., Eenige resultaten van proefnemingen mit een overentbare cavia leukose. pp. 160–164 in: *Handel. van het Nederland. Natuur-en Geneesk. Congr. 21, Amsterdam*, 1927.

ADDENDUM: TRANSMISSIBLE CAT FIBROSARCOMA

In a recent study carried out at the School of Veterinary Medicine, University of California, in Davis, S. P. Snyder and G. H. Theilen (*Nature*, **21**: 1074–1075, 1969) observed multiple subcutaneous fibrosarcomas in a 2-year-old Siamese female cat. The tumor could be transmitted serially by filtrates to newborn cats, inducing fibrosarcomas after a short latency period of 2 to 3 weeks. Electron microscopic examination of tumor tissues from the donor cat and also from the inoculated animals revealed large numbers of type C spherical virus particles about 110 to 120 mμ in diameter, many of them with electron-dense nucleoids. This observation was promptly confirmed in other laboratories. Several similar tumors were found in cats and transmitted experimentally. The cat fibrosarcoma was transmitted to other species. Theilen and Deinhardt at the Presbyterian–St. Luke's Hospital in Chicago inoculated intraperitoneally 2 marmosets, small South American monkeys, with centrifuged cell-free extracts prepared from cat fibrosarcoma; both developed multiple progressively growing fibrosarcomas after a short latency of only 2 to 4 weeks. However, attempts, in other laboratories, to transmit cat fibrosarcoma to dogs, rabbits, or rhesus monkeys, were only partially successful: fibrosarcomas induced in these animals grew only temporarily and eventually regressed (IVth Int. Symp. Comp. Leuk. Research, 1969).

CHAPTER 17

Bovine Leukosis
Leukemia and Lymphosarcoma in Cattle

Leukemia and lymphosarcoma occur in cattle of all ages, but predominantly in the five to eight-year-old age group. The disease in cattle is very similar to that occurring in other animal species, such as chickens, mice, rats, cats, horses, etc., and also in humans. The principal pathologic manifestation of this neoplastic condition of the hematopoietic system consists of proliferation of white blood cells, particularly of the lymphatic series, which eventually results in the development of solid tumor masses forming local or, more often, generalized lymphosarcomas, involving peripheral lymph nodes, spleen, thymus, and other organs. There is also frequently diffuse infiltration of tissues and organs with lymphoid cells.

Pathologic manifestations. Among general symptoms, weakness, pallor, and progressive weight loss are common in the more advanced phases of the disease. Anemia is also common and represents a characteristic feature of the disease syndrome. Hemoglobin levels below 5 grams per 100 cc. of blood are not unusual, particularly in terminal phases of the disease.

Enlargement of peripheral lymph nodes is an outstanding feature present in most of the cases. Involvement of the lymph nodes is often, but not always, symmetrical; some of the lymph nodes may become enlarged to a considerable extent, forming large tumor masses. Thymic lymphosarcomas are common, particularly in younger animals (Dungworth *et al.*, 1964). Out of 92 cases of bovine lymphosarcoma described by Jarrett (1966), 53 (58 per cent) were of the thymic type; in another series described by Cotchin (1960), 14 out of 22 (63 per cent) were thymic. In the United States, Theilen and his colleagues (1964) described 14 thymic lymphosarcomas among 72 animals (19 per cent) suffering from leukosis. Liver and spleen enlargement is also common and occurs in at least one third of all cases of leukemia and lymphosarcoma in cattle.

Cardiac involvement is a characteristic feature of bovine leukemia. In certain series of leukotic animals examined, the heart was found to be one of the sites of tumor development in from 50 to over 85 per cent of cases of bovine lymphosarcoma (Bendixen, 1958. Marshak *et al.*, 1962). Infiltration of the heart, particularly of the right atrium, with leukemic cells leads to a considerable increase in the thickness of the atrial wall and frequently involves also the pericardium. The involvement of heart may lead to clinical symptoms of cardiovascular disease and eventually to cardiac failure.

In certain animals a wide-spread intradermal infiltration with lymphoid cells leads to the development of characteristic, multiple nodular skin lesions (Bendixen, 1958, 1963. Bendixen and Friis, 1965. Lombard, 1965. Clegg and Moss, 1965. Jarrett *et al.*, 1966). The cutaneous form of bovine lymphosarcoma is very rare in the United States, but a few cases have been described (Marshak *et al.*, 1966).

Blood Picture. The blood and bone marrow may not always reveal the true nature of this disease. In fact, in at least 50 per cent of cases involving localized or generalized lymphosarcomas, the peripheral blood picture remains essentially within normal limits, except for anemia, occasional presence of abnormal lymphocytes, and possibly a relative lymphocytosis. Weber (1963) found a true leukemic picture in peripheral blood morphology (50,000 to 600,000 WBC per mm^3) in only about 10 per cent of animals with lymphosarcoma; in 55 per cent, there was only a moderate leukocytosis, with a relative increase in the lymphocyte number; in from 10 to 30 per cent, the blood picture was practically normal. Marshak and his coworkers (1962) reported results of blood counts made on 19 animals with lymphosarcomas; in 4 animals the total white blood cell counts ranged from 81,500 to 293,000 per mm^3 with over 90 per cent of lymphocytes; in the remaining animals the peripheral white blood cell counts were only moderately increased or were normal; in some animals in which the initial counts were normal, the blood picture became leukemic in advanced phases of the disease. Ritter (1964) found that some 30 per cent of cattle with lymphosarcomas had essentially a normal blood morphology; in about 20 per cent of animals, the examination of peripheral blood was inconclusive, and some 40 per cent had a peripheral blood morphology diagnostic for leukemia. Winqvist (1958) noted that 25 per cent of cattle with lymphosarcoma included in his study had a normal peripheral blood morphology.

There is also a certain influence of age on the involvement of blood in general manifestations of the disease. In older animals with advanced generalized lymphosarcoma, leukemic manifestations in peripheral blood morphology, or at least a distinct lymphocytosis, are rather common; however, in juvenile leukosis developing in very young animals up to 2 years old, about 50 per cent of animals in that age group have no pathologic changes in peripheral blood morphology.

Disseminated Lymphosarcomatosis or Leukemia? It is quite apparent that pathologic changes in peripheral blood morphology in bovine leukemia are essentially comparable to those observed in cases of this disease developing in certain other animal species, particularly in mice. The blood involvement is far from common. It appears that a more exact term describing this condition in cattle, as is the case in mice or chickens, should be lymphosarcoma or a disseminated lymphosarcomatosis rather than leukemia, unless the term leukemia is used in a more general manner.

The term "leukemia" was adopted at a recent World Health Organization Conference on Comparative Studies in Leukemia held on February 27–March 4, 1961, in Philadelphia, to include all proliferative diseases of the hematopoietic system, including true leukemias and localized or generalized lymphosarcomas in cattle.

More recently an International "Bovine Leukemia Criteria Committee" was organized by Dr. R. R. Marshak under the terms of a United States Public Health Service research contract. A meeting of the Committee was held on August 29–31, 1966, at University of Pennsylvania School of Veterinary Medicine, in New Bolton Center, near Philadelphia. Among other questions the terminology employed by various workers in this field was also discussed. The majority, and particularly the European investigators, favored the term "leukosis" to designate the various forms of leukemia and lymphosarcoma in cattle. (The term "leukosis" was originally suggested by Ellermann and Bang (1908) in their studies on chicken leukemia.)

The term "*disseminated lymphosarcomatosis*" would probably be more descriptive and accurate for the majority of cases of this disease in cattle, as it would be also in mouse leukemia. The disease may involve, as a part of its manifestation, the peripheral blood and also the bone marrow; however, the peripheral blood involvement is not common in the early phases of the disease and is more frequently observed in advanced or terminal phases.

The form of leukemia observed in cattle is almost exclusively lymphatic. Cases of myelogenous leukemia in cattle are rare but have been reported (Hyde *et al.*, 1958. Bendixen, 1966*). In this respect cattle leukemia is quite similar to this disease observed in certain other animal species, such as mice, rats, or chickens.

Incidence of Leukemia and Lymphosarcoma in Cattle

Leukemia and lymphosarcoma represent probably the most common malignant tumors occurring in cattle. It is difficult to evaluate the general incidence of leukemia in cattle, since not many animals live their full life span and reach the age at which leukemia or lymphosarcoma usually develop. Accurate statistics are difficult to obtain, but it is quite apparent that this disease is widely prevalent among cattle, and that it has a tendency to occur more frequently in certain districts, and particularly in certain herds and families of cattle.

A considerable increase in the incidence of lymphosarcoma and leukemia

* Personal communication to the author from Dr. H. J. Bendixen, 1966.

in cattle has been observed in several countries during the past two decades. The incidence actually doubled in eastern Germany in the years between 1950 and 1960, and more than doubled in certain parts of Sweden; it also increased considerably in the United States and in Denmark.

It may be of interest to quote, as an example, the report by Johansson* who observed that in one slaughter house in Eksjo in Sweden, the average incidence of leukosis observed in slaughtered cattle rose from 0.1 per cent in 1939–1941 to 3.7 per cent in 1950–1952.

The overall incidence of leukemia and lymphosarcoma in cattle varies, and averages approximately 17 to 18 cases of lymphosarcoma per 100,000 head of cattle annually in the United States (Sorensen, 1961. Theilen *et al.*, 1961. Smith, 1962). This figure represents the total average incidence; actually the incidence varies in different parts of the country from a low, varying from 0 to 7 (average 3) per 100,000 in the arid Rocky Mountains and in Pacific regions (Smith, 1962), or about 2.5 per 100,000 in California (Theilen *et al.*, 1963), to a relative high, varying from 29 to 91 (average 60) per 100,000 in the Southern Plains, reaching from southeastern Kansas through Oklahoma and the eastern part of Texas. In Minnesota, Western Great Lakes regions, Kentucky, Tennessee, and Mississippi, the incidence averages from 42.5 to 46 per 100,000 (Smith, 1962).

Theilen and his colleagues (1963) reported that during the period of one year following July, 1961, at which time bovine lymphosarcoma became a reportable disease in the state of California, 108 animals in California were diagnosed as having lymphosarcoma. Only 90 of those were confirmed histologically as having this disease. Since California cattle population exceeds 4,200,000 animals, the overall incidence of leukemia and lymphosarcoma in California would be slightly over 2 per 100,000 of the total cattle population. About 40 per cent of all the leukosis cases in this survey could be traced to multiple-incidence herds. It also appeared of interest that the incidence was higher among dairy cows than among beef cattle.

Similar figures, with some variations, have been reported from other countries. Fortner (1953) reported that according to a review of data obtained from 28 slaughterhouses in Germany for the years 1938 through 1942, 0.2 per cent of all slaughtered cattle, i.e. 200 per 100,000, were condemned because of leukosis. A more detailed study of his report indicates that the incidence varied from a low of 7 to 9 per 100,000 slaughtered cattle in Frankfurt and Cologne in the western part of Germany to as much as 300 per 100,000 in Koenigsberg, and 1,500 per 100,000 in Tilsit, in the eastern part of the country. Dobberstein and Seifried (1938) reported an incidence of leukemia and lymphosarcoma varying from 150 to 400 per 100,000 cattle slaughtered annually in East Germany.

* Johansson, S., *Medlemsbl. Sveriges Vet. Förb.* **5**: 300, 1953.

Jarrett and his colleagues (1966) estimated the incidence of this disease in Scotland to be about 20 per 100,000 cattle slaughtered annually. In Sweden, Olson (1961) reported that during the years 1932 through 1958 the average annual incidence of leukemia and lymphosarcoma in the total area of Sweden varied from a low of 40 per 100,000 to a high of 170 per 100,000 of cattle slaughtered annually. In the southeastern part of the country, however, the incidence was much higher, exceeding one per cent of slaughtered animals, i.e. 1,000 per 100,000 head of cattle, as compared with a very low incidence in the northern provinces of Sweden (Svanberg and Aberg, 1955. Hjärre, 1956. Olson, 1961).

Leukemic Herds and Families. The most striking observation concerning the occurrence of bovine leukemia and lymphosarcoma has been the accumulation of cases of this disease in certain herds, and particularly in certain families of cattle.

The Danish cattle population consists of about 3.5 million animals. The total incidence of bovine leukemia and lymphosarcoma in Denmark is approximately 4.1 per 100,000, but it varies considerably in different parts of the country. The lymphosarcoma incidence is particularly high on the islands of Sjaelland and Lolland-Falster where the annual incidence is about 15 per 100,000 among 0.5 million cattle living on these islands (Bendixen, 1963). In a few leukotic herds consisting of 30 to 40 cows each, as many as two to five per cent of the adult animals develop lymphosarcoma every year. On the other hand, in the remaining part of Denmark where 80 per cent of the cattle population lives, the lymphosarcoma incidence is very low, averaging only about one per 100,000 animals.

The occurrence of lymphosarcoma in certain cattle families, or herds, has long been observed by European veterinarians (Hartenstein, 1897. Knuth and Volkmann, 1916). Schäper (1938) collected 23 cases of leukemia developing in a cow and its offspring; in one instance a cow and a bull had 2 calves; both parents and their 2 offspring died from leukemia; one of the offspring, a bull, was, in turn, the father of 3 calves all of which also died from leukemia. Similar reports were published by several observers (P.T.F., 1927. Lockau, 1933. Henricson and Olson, 1961). Czymoch (1937) observed 8 cases of leukemic cows with leukemic offspring, one of which concerned 2 leukemic calves from the same cow; in another instance there were 3 cases of leukemic cows in two successive generations of the same family; most of these animals developed leukemia at the age of 6 years. His observation that 16 out of 20 leukemic cows bred in a particular district were the offspring of one and the same bull "G," which eventually also died from leukemia at the age of 4 years, was striking. Both Czymoch and Schäper observed many cases of leukemia in herds of cattle in which a particular bull was used for breeding purposes, the occurrence of the disease ceasing on removal of the bull. Czymoch also reported a family case where a breeding bull "Kanzler" and his son "Nero" both died from lymphosarcoma at the age of 4 and 3 years, respectively.

Böttger (1954, 1955) in Germany described dramatically, quoting interesting details of case histories obtained from farmers, several remarkable families and herds of cattle with an unusually high incidence of lymphosarcoma; in most instances, each case of lymphosarcoma could be traced to another case of lymphosarcoma in either one of the parents or in a sibling; among many cases quoted was a case history of lymphosarcoma in a cow, her sister, her daughter, and her granddaughter. A number of impressive case reports were given in which a bull used for breeding spread the disease among its offspring, and then eventually also died from lymphosarcoma. One outstanding history refers to bull No. 21527 and his many offspring with a remarkably high incidence of lymphosarcoma. In another case, farmer "J" complained that during the years 1943 to 1951 he lost on his farm 13 cows from lymphosarcoma; eight of them were daughters of the same bull "L."

Karlson (1942) at the University of Minnesota reported that in an Aberdeen-Angus beef herd at the University Farm, three lymphosarcoma cases were diagnosed; two of these cases were in sisters, and one was in a daughter of one of the sisters. Karlson also described a pure-bred Jersey herd in which six cases of lymphosarcoma occurred in a single family during a ten-year period; each of the six cases was closely related to at least one other case, and all had common ancestors only a few generations back.

Familial aggregations of lymphosarcoma cases were also reported by Starr and Young (1941) who studied a Holstein family in which two daughters, one granddaughter, and one grandson of a normal cow developed lymphosarcoma, and a Guernsey family in which four successive female generations succumbed to this disease.

Fortner (1953) at the Robert Koch Institute in Berlin-Dahlem reported a cattle family No. 1 in which one bull, named Emil, had 28 offspring, among which 7 developed leukosis; his son, Emir, had 13 offspring, 3 of which developed leukosis; the grandson, Emilius, had 9 offspring, one of which developed leukosis. Thus, in this single family, among 50 offspring of 3 directly related bulls, 11 developed leukosis (22 per cent).

As a comparison, Fortner quoted another family of cattle in which the father-bull, his son, and grandson had a total of 120 offspring; among these only one animal developed leukosis.

In recent studies carried out at the School of Veterinary Medicine, University of Pennsylvania in Philadelphia, and in New Bolton Center, by Marshak (1962), Croshaw (1963), and their colleagues, several striking examples of familial incidence of leukemia and lymphosarcoma in cattle have been observed. In one Jersey family (Herd No. 2), bull "Y" had 4 daughters; all developed lymphosarcoma at ages varying from 7½ to 9 years; two female offspring of these cows also developed lymphosarcoma. Furthermore, a son of bull "Y," known as "Sire Luke," had 2 daughters which developed leukemia at 6½ and 7 years of age. Bull "Y" died when 7 years old with no evidence of leukemia. His son "Luke" was slaughtered at young age in good health. In another Jersey family (herd No. 1), lymphosarcoma developed in two daughters and one granddaughter. These observations were striking, since most of the other families appeared to be free from this disease. In another case report (Croshaw *et al.*, 1963), 15 animals were observed to develop lymphosarcoma within six years in Jersey herd BF. All the affected animals, with one exception only, were descendants of sire H. In another example, in a Holstein herd AG, six cases of lymphosarcoma were diagnosed in a period of approximately 18 months. Five of the affected animals were daughters of sire R, and one was a young granddaughter of sire R.

It is quite apparent from the examples quoted that multiple-case lymphosarcoma herds and families are quite common, and that significant accumulations of lymphosarcoma developing in members of certain families of cattle can be observed in spite of the difficulty caused by the time factor, and frequently also by lack of accurate records affecting several successive generations.

It is of considerable interest that either parent can be responsible for transmission of the disease. The disease can be transmitted through the mother, but very often, and in a rather striking manner, the father may be responsible for the transmission of the causative factor. Certain case reports dealing with the transmission of leukemia or lymphosarcoma through the male are particularly impressive and may be interpreted as a serious public health warning. Most of the modern cattle breeding is now carried out with the aid of artificial insemination. It is therefore quite apparent that under certain conditions the semen of a potentially leukemic bull may disseminate the seeds of the disease among thousands of his progeny.

The Significance of Increased Number of Lymphocytes in Peripheral Blood

The blood of normal adult cattle is characterized by a predominance of lymphocytes. The total white blood cell counts in cattle range from 4,000 to 10,000 cells per mm³; it should be stressed that in animals below 2 years of age the counts are usually higher. The relative percentage of lymphocytes in cattle of all ages is rather high, ranging from 45 to 60 per cent in normal animals; in the younger age group the percentage of lymphocytes may be even higher, and may reach or even exceed 80 per cent

(Knuth and Volkmann, 1916. du Toit, 1917, 1920. Marshak *et al.*, 1962. Weber, 1963. Schalm, 1965). In a statistical calculation of normal leukocyte counts in cattle of different ages, based on examination of a total of 171 samples, Bendixen reported (1963) that the average number of leukocytes per mm^3 in peripheral blood in normal cattle drops from 9,200 to 7,500 within the first four years of life, and that the corresponding average values of lymphocytes decrease during the same period from 79 to 52 per cent.

It has been observed for a long time that lymphocytosis may occur among apparently healthy cows in herds where cases of manifest leukosis develop from time to time. Several authors described hematological changes in the peripheral white blood cell picture among apparently normal animals in herds in which leukotic tumor cases were found (Knuth and Volkmann, 1916. du Toit, 1920. Götze *et al.*, 1953, 1954). These changes, consisting essentially of an increase in the total number of peripheral white blood cells and a relative increase in the number of lymphocytes, revealing also an occasional presence of atypical lymphocytes, were interpreted as symptoms of an early, precancerous phase of bovine leukemia. On the basis of this assumption, systematic blood examinations of cattle herds were suggested as a method aiming at the detection of animals susceptible to the development of lymphosarcoma.

The Leukosis Key

A standard table designated "Leukosis Key" was proposed by Götze and his coworkers (1953, 1954) as an aid in detecting potentially leukemic animals; this table listed average total white blood cell counts and percentage of lymphocytes in peripheral blood of cattle. Briefly, those having total white blood cell counts up to 10,000 per mm^3 with up to 60 per cent of lymphocytes were considered to be within normal limits. Those having total white blood cell counts exceeding 10,000 per mm^3 and a relative number of lymphocytes exceeding 60 per cent were considered "suspicious" for eventual development of leukemia. The table was rather complicated in its details, and the animals tested were divided into four successive groups, the first one normal, and three subsequent groups with a gradually increased degree of suspicion for potential development of disease.

Winqvist (1958, 1960) in Stockholm suggested a simplification of the original "Leukosis Key." In view of the fact that in normal cattle over 3 years old the average number of lymphocytes per mm^3 is below 6,000 in the peripheral blood, he suggested that among animals at least 3 years old, those with a lymphocyte count of less than 6,000 per mm^3 in the peripheral blood could be considered as "normal"; those within the

6,000 to 12,000 lymphocyte range as "suspicious," and, finally, those having over 12,000 lymphocytes per mm³ should be considered "strongly suspicious" for the eventual development of leukemia. Winqvist stressed, however, the difficulties in accepting without reservations the value of the "Leukosis Key," since lymphocytosis could be observed in cattle following piroplasmosis infection (Winqvist, 1961), and also in certain other conditions unrelated to leukemia; on the other hand, he also stressed that in his own studies, 25 per cent of cattle with manifest lymphosarcoma had normal blood morphology.

Bendixen (1958, 1959) further modified and simplified the original "Leukosis Key" (a) stressing the influence of age on the level of lymphocytes in peripheral blood and evaluating the results of lymphocyte counts according to age groups examined; and (b) tabulating the results of blood examinations in the form of "absolute lymphocyte numbers per mm³," arrived at by multiplying the total number of white blood cells by percentage of lymphocytes, divided by 100.* The table suggested by Bendixen, and designated the "Leukosis Evaluation Guide," listed the upper limits of lymphocytes in peripheral blood for different age groups of cattle. Animals having lymphocyte counts above certain levels indicated in the guide, and retaining such high lymphocyte counts on several successive examinations, are considered either "questionable" or "potentially leukemic" under local conditions existing in Denmark (Bendixen, 1963). Such animals cannot be sold, except for slaughter.

The "Leukosis Key" or, as it is called in Denmark, the "Leukosis Evaluation Guide," therefore consists essentially of a series of upper limits for the lymphocyte counts of normal cattle, depending on age. There are significant variations in different age groups, and these have to be con-

TABLE 13. THE LEUKOSIS EVALUATION GUIDE EMPLOYED IN DENMARK (BENDIXEN, 1959). GROUPS IN WHICH ANIMALS ARE DIVIDED ACCORDING TO AGE AND THE NUMBER OF LYMPHOCYTES PER mm³.

Age in years	Group I normal	Group II questionable	Group III potentially leukemic
0–1	<10,000	10,000–12,000	>12,000
1–2	<9,000	9,000–11,000	>11,000
2–3	<7,500	7,500– 9,500	>9,500
3–4	<6,500	6,500– 8,500	>8,500
>4	<5,000	5,000– 7,000	>7,000

* $\frac{\text{WBC} \times \text{per cent of lymphocytes}}{100}$

sidered. Counts above these limits have been designated as "lymphocytosis" and are believed to occur in a proportion of apparently normal animals in herds having a multiple incidence of lymphosarcoma (multiple incidence, or "M.I." herds). This contrasts with normal herds which have no apparent incidence of lymphosarcoma or in which only occasionally single cases of leukotic tumors develop (single incidence, or "S.I." herds).

According to Götze and his coworkers (1954), 5 to 10 per cent of cattle with significantly increased lymphocyte counts in peripheral blood eventually develop lymphosarcoma. More recently (1963) Bendixen estimated that two to five per cent of cattle in the "multiple incidence" herds with high lymphocyte counts develop leukemia or lymphosarcoma every year.

Attempt to Eradicate Cattle Leukemia in Denmark

On the basis of the assumption that leukemia in cattle is caused by a transmissible virus, and that a relative lymphocytosis in peripheral blood can be interpreted as an early, preclinical manifestation of the virus infection, a rather extensive program aiming at the eradication of this disease in cattle was introduced in Denmark in 1959.

All leukemia and lymphosarcoma cases are reportable in clinical work and in meat inspection. When the diagnosis is confirmed, the herd is examined hematologically, and if this procedure reveals suspect preleukotic cases, the herd is placed under governmental supervision as a so-called "leukosis herd." If only one tumor case is demonstrated, but no blood changes are present, then the herd is regarded as an "observation herd," requiring repeated hematologic examinations during at least two years. Herds having had contact with animals from leukotic herds are also regarded as observation herds. The measures in the leukosis herds introduced in Denmark in 1959 include ear-tagging, prohibition of selling animals except for slaughter, and economic aid to cattle owners after slaughter. At the present time about 2,000 adult and 2,000 young animals in about 60 herds are under public supervision (Bendixen, 1963).

Bendixen reported recently (1965a,b) that the results so far have shown a relative drop in tumor incidence since 1960. In the most heavily affected part of Denmark the incidence thus far has dropped from 29 cases in 1960 to 10 cases per 100,000 head of cattle in 1963.

> There are about 145 cases of bovine leukosis each year in Denmark. Among these, 100 occur in adult cattle, 35 in young animals up to 2 years old (juvenile form of leukosis), and, in addition, there are about 10 cases of skin leukosis. More than half of all cases of leukosis occur on the island of Sjaelland, a limited province area in Denmark.

Attempt to Eradicate Cattle Leukemia in West Germany

A program similar to that used in Denmark was also introduced in West Germany (Rosenberger, 1964. Tolle, 1965); however, reporting of lymphosarcoma in cattle is not compulsory, and the participation of cattle owners is voluntary. The owners of cattle herds in which the disease has been demonstrated, either by finding animals with lymphosarcoma or following detection of hematologic changes, receive economic aid for the slaughtering of such animals. Partial elimination of the disease from a given herd of cattle is considered to be completed if no animals with positive or suspicious hematologic changes can be demonstrated by blood examinations repeated at 6-month-intervals for 2 years.

Recently, some of the federal states in Germany stopped importation of cattle, unless they are certified to come from herds in which no symptoms of bovine leukosis can be demonstrated. A herd is considered as not suspicious with regard to leukemia if no tumor cases have been found within the last 5 years, and if blood examination of all animals above 2 years of age performed within the last 12 months has shown that no significant lymphocytosis exists. Since 1964 the evaluation of the changes has been based, as it is also in Denmark, on total number of lymphocytes per mm^3. An official "key," very similar to that employed in Denmark, has been used in the evaluation of the hematologic changes (Rosenberger, 1964). The hematologic examination of cattle, employing a modified "Leukosis Key" as a guide, is considered by several German veterinarians to be a reliable method for the control of leukemia and lymphosarcoma (Götze *et al.*, 1953. Rosenberger, 1964. Tolle *et al.*, 1963. Tolle, 1965). The official table, designated the "Göttingen Leukosis Key," listing standard values of total white blood cell counts and relative numbers of

TABLE 14. OFFICIAL "GÖTTINGEN" LEUKOSIS KEY EMPLOYED IN WEST GERMANY (TOLLE, 1965). GROUPS IN WHICH ANIMALS ARE DIVIDED ACCORDING TO AGE AND THE NUMBER OF LYMPHOCYTES PER mm^3

Age in years	Group I normal	Group II questionable	Group III pathologically increased
0–1	<10,000	10,000–13,000	>13,000
1–2	<9,000	9,000–12,000	>12,000
2–3	<7,500	7,500–10,000	>10,000
3–6	<6,500	6,500– 9,000	>9,000
>6	<5,500	5,500– 7,500	>7,500

lymphocytes in "normal," "questionable," and "pathologically increased" groups of cattle varying for different ages, employed in West Germany, is essentially very similar to the "Leukosis Evaluation Guide" employed for the same purpose in Denmark.

Some Questions About the Justification of Use of the "Leukosis Key" as a Guide for the Eradication Program of Leukemia and Lymphosarcoma in Cattle

The eradication program of bovine lymphosarcoma, based on repeated blood examinations of large numbers of animals, and on the determination of relative lymphocytosis in certain herds, has now been in progress for several years in Denmark, and also in West Germany. This program requires not only the cooperation of farmers and cattle owners, but also a considerable effort on the part of trained personnel scheduled to perform repeated blood counts on large numbers of animals; the program is costly to the government, since farmers are subsidized for the slaughter of cattle designated as carriers of a subclinical form of disease. The ultimate results of this interesting and important program will become apparent in the future.

The empirical observations based on statistical studies on relative lymphocytosis occurring in certain herds of cattle susceptible to development of leukemia were originally made at a time when the viral etiology of this disease was only suspected; hereditary factors, other than viral agents, had to be considered. Gradually, however, the viral etiology of bovine leukemia has gained more acceptance, even though no experimental proof has yet been furnished to substantiate such a concept. At present, those advocating the introduction of the "Leukosis Key" and of the leukosis eradication program speak freely of a transmissible leukemogenic agent present in certain herds of cattle, and base their program on an epidemiological pattern employed in other communicable diseases, such as isolation and eradication of animal-carriers, prevention of the spread of disease, etc. (Bendixen, 1963, 1965a). Thus, at the present time at least, the eradication program of bovine leukemia and lymphosarcoma is obviously based on the assumption that this disease in cattle is caused by a transmissible virus, as it is also in mice, rats, and chickens. We are not questioning this assumption, and we are convinced that time will prove that the concept of viral etiology of leukemia and lymphomas is correct for bovine leukemia, and, as a matter of fact, for other species also, including humans.

However, the eradication program of cattle lymphosarcoma is also based on the assumption that examination of peripheral blood of cattle carrying the virus may reveal a relative lymphocytosis, and that this lymphocytosis represents a preclinical phase of the disease. Lymphocytosis is apparently considered to be an indicator of the presence of a latent infection with the leukemic virus, and is thought to occur not only in herds of cattle having a high incidence of lymphosarcomas, but also in normal herds which have been exposed to cattle brought for breeding, or for other purposes, from "multiple-incidence" herds; such exposure presumably might have introduced the virus to animals of the normal, not infected herds.

It should be emphasized, however, that it has never been determined experimentally that clinical manifestations of leukemia or lymphomas are preceded in either cattle or in any other species by the development of lymphocytosis, or that lymphocytosis represents a symptom indicating presence of a latent infection with the leukemogenic virus.

In mice, at least, in which the viral etiology of leukemia and lymphomas has been established experimentally, and in which the relative frequency of lymphatic form of leukemia and lymphosarcoma is very high as compared with other forms of this disease, just as it is in cattle, we have not been able thus far to observe the development of lymphocytosis prior to the actual development of either leukemia or lymphosarcoma (Gross, 1965, 1966, unpublished). Moreover, the blood may remain perfectly normal in mice or in cattle that have developed localized or generalized lymphosarcoma.

On the other hand, it should be emphasized that transient or recurrent lymphocytosis may occur in many different conditions not necessarily related to either leukemia or lymphoma. This is true for several species, including humans, and presumably also for cattle. Among the conditions, other than leukemia or lymphosarcoma, that may cause lymphocytosis in peripheral blood in cattle are certain protozoal, bacterial, and viral infections unrelated to leukosis, recent vaccinations, etc. To give only a few examples, lymphocytosis may occur in mastitis, and other localized and generalized infections, in viral pneumonia, in "piroplasmosis," etc. Even those who introduced the leukosis key as a basis for the eradication program realize the difficulties and pitfalls of this method, and stress that breed, environmental conditions, and certain diseases unrelated to lymphosarcoma may exert an influence on the value of lymphocyte counts in peripheral blood, and may cause diagnostic difficulties.

Field Reports and Difficulty in Reaching a Tentative Conclusion Concerning the True Value of the Leukosis Key

Some observers (Bendixen, 1963. Tolle *et al.*, 1963, 1965. Rosenberger, 1964) have been quite satisfied with the results thus far obtained, and consider the leukosis key to be a dependable means of detecting animals susceptible to the development of lymphosarcoma. Theilen and his coworkers (1964) reported that with one exception all of his "multiple incidence" herds in California (where leukemia and lymphosarcoma became a reportable disease in 1963) could be recognized by the pattern of lymphocytosis.

Other observers, however, have expressed doubts as to the validity of the leukosis key employed as a basis for detecting leukotic herds, and have stressed the fact that bovine leukemia may often occur without concomitant peripheral blood manifestations (Dobberstein, 1953. Fortner, 1953. Niepage, 1953, 1954. Böttger, 1954, 1955. Wiesner, 1961. Marshak *et al.*, 1963, 1966, 1967. Hare *et al.*, 1964. Jarrett *et al.*, 1966).

It should be emphasized that generalized lymphocytosis may occur also in leukemia-free herds; on the other hand, many affected herds in which lymphosarcomas develop may not show a generalized lymphocytosis. In Denmark, Bendixen (1965a) recorded generalized lymphocytosis in 85 single-case herds and in 8 leukemia-free herds. Some multiple-case herds do not show lymphocytosis (Hare *et al.*, 1964. Theilen *et al.*, 1964. Marshak *et al.*, 1963), and individual animals in such herds may show lymphocytosis at one time and not at another. Jarrett (1966) reported from Scotland that in an investigation of over 100 farms, only one farm was found in which more than one case of lymphosarcoma occurred; the affected animals in that case were two calves with a common grandmother. In no case was there any lymphocytosis in a herd.

A random sampling of 10 per cent of the cattle population in 3 Minnesota counties showed that from 24 to 54 per cent of the herds had generalized lymphocytosis (Sorensen *et al.*, 1964). In the eastern United States a majority of multiple-case herds tested was free from lymphocytosis (Marshak *et al.*, 1963). Moreover, the lymphocytosis level of carefully studied American herds was observed to change with yearly samplings (Marshak *et al.*, 1966). Studies of 11 contact herds, i.e. stocks introduced from known multiple-case herds, in the United States have also shown inconsistent results. Even the very carefully selected leukemia-free control herds, representing the major cattle breeds, do not maintain constant absolute lymphocyte counts over a period of years (Marshak *et al.*, 1963).

Bendixen (1963) gave several examples of hematologic studies carried out on multiple tumor case herds with a follow-up tracing the development of lymphosarcomas through periods of several years. In one example a survey was given of changes found in 156 sets of mothers and daughters. Most of these animals have been followed by blood examinations through several years. All daughters were more than two years old at the time of the survey. Within the control period, 22 mother-cows developed tumors. Eleven daughters of these cows developed lymphocytosis, and five daughters became leukotic within the observation period. Eighty-three mother-cows developed lymphocytosis; 45 of the daughters of these cows also developed lymphocytosis, and eight of the daughters developed leukotic tumors. Lymphocytosis and leukotic tumors developed, however, also among daughters of apparently normal mother-cows, although in a smaller number of animals.

In another series of studies (Hare *et al.*, 1964), the results were as follows: of 18 multiple-case herds studied, 6 showed generalized lymphocytosis, 3 showed partial lymphocytosis, and 9 showed no lymphocytosis. Of 9 leukemia-free herds which had contact with multiple-case herds, 2 showed generalized lymphocytosis, and 7 showed no lymphocytosis. Of 13 leukemia-free herds, which had no known contact with multiple-case herds, one showed general lymphocytosis, and 12 (which comprised "normal" herds) showed no lymphocytosis. On the basis of these data, Hare and his colleagues concluded that generalized lymphocytosis cannot be regarded as a universal phenomenon in multiple-case lymphosarcoma herds in the Eastern United States.

In summary, therefore, opinions concerning the justification of the leukosis key as a guide in a massive eradication program of this disease in cattle have been divided, and the problem of its justification is far from being resolved at this time.

In 1962 a World Health Organization report* summarizing this position stated: "On the whole, American studies seem to confirm European observations of high absolute lymphocyte numbers in cattle from herds with multiple cases of lymphosarcoma. However, as our statistical analyses indicate so much variability, we are hesitant to develop any sort of generalization from these data."

In more recent studies carried out in the eastern United States the majority of "multiple case herds" did not show consistent lymphocytosis (Marshak *et al.*, 1966. Marshak and Abt, 1968). In the course of consecutive samplings the lymphocytosis levels did not show any persistent pattern, but varied considerably within the same herds. In certain cattle families there were higher values of lymphocyte counts than in others; these values had no relation, however, to the incidence of leukemia or lymphosarcoma. The survey suggested that some families of cattle may have a relatively high lymphocytosis and at the same time a very low incidence of lymphosarcoma; in other families the white blood cell counts and the relative percentage of lymphocytes may be within normal limits, and yet one or several members of such families may develop lymphosarcoma.

Viral Etiology of Bovine Leukemia?

The development of leukemia or lymphosarcoma in several members of the same family in cattle, within the same generation, i.e. among

* Internat. Symposium, Comparative Leukemia Research, Davis, California, 1962.

brothers, sisters, or cousins, or in successive generations, such as in one or both parents and their offspring, etc., is striking and reminiscent of similar observations made in mice and other species, occasionally also in humans. An explanation of familial susceptibility to this disease on the basis of genetic inheritance encounters considerable difficulties. Development of leukemia or lymphomas in individual members of certain families within the same or in successive generations cannot be explained in a satisfactory manner on the basis of inheritance of either a dominant or a recessive disease-inducing factor; leukemia or lymphosarcoma develop rather in an unpredictable "hit-or-miss" manner in some members of certain families, sparing others which should be equally susceptible on the basis of their genetic make-up.

Familial incidence of bovine leukemia could be explained in a more rational manner by an assumption that this disease is caused, as was the case demonstrated experimentally in mice, by an oncogenic virus transmitted in certain families "vertically" from one generation to another.* It would be necessary to assume further that such a virus is usually latent and harmless for the carrier hosts, causing no disease unless activated. When triggered into action by a variety of either intrinsic or extrinsic factors, the virus would become pathogenic, causing uncontrolled multiplication of cells harboring it, and leading thereby to the development of leukemia or lymphosarcomas.†

It is of particular importance that the transmission of the leukemic virus in cattle seems to occur as readily through the female as it does through the male. Observations reporting the development of multiple cases of leukemia and lymphosarcoma in progeny of certain cows, as well as in those of certain bulls, which eventually also developed this disease, are common; a few typical examples have been quoted on the preceding pages of this chapter. Some of the reports of transmission of the disease through the male are particularly striking, and are of considerable importance, since artificial insemination has been generally employed in recent years for breeding of cattle. Under such conditions, a single stud bull carrying the leukemic virus may be responsible for dissemination of seeds of the disease among a very large number of his progeny.

Circumstantial Evidence for the Existence of a Leukemogenic Virus in Cattle

Even though the existence of a leukemogenic virus in cattle has not yet been determined experimentally, there is sufficient circumstantial evidence

* The term "vertical transmission" designates the passage of a potentially pathogenic virus from one generation to another (Gross, 1944, 1951). See p. 915.

† The interested reader is referred to the chapter on Mouse Leukemia in this monograph for a more detailed discussion of this concept of the etiology of leukemia and lymphomas (Gross, 1954).

to suggest that bovine leukemia is caused by a transmissible virus. From a morphological and clinical point of view, leukemia and lymphosarcoma in cattle do not seem to be different from the same disease observed in mice; the latter is known to be caused by a filterable virus. The striking accumulation of leukemia and lymphosarcoma cases in certain families of cattle would also be consistent with the assumption that this disease is caused by an oncogenic virus transmitted "vertically" from one generation to another.

There are only limited means available to determine the viral nature of an obscure disease; as discussed in more detail in the introductory chapter of this monograph, experimental transmission of a disease from one host to another by a filtered extract is a rather unsophisticated but quite dependable method employed in order to determine the viral nature of an investigated disease. It is possible to anticipate that, unless determined earlier by another equally satisfactory method, the proof of the viral etiology of bovine leukemia will be forthcoming as soon as transmission of this disease by filtrates succeeds. There is little doubt that experimental transmission of bovine leukemia by inoculation of filtrates prepared from tissues of leukotic cattle will be accomplished eventually; preliminary experiments along this line are now in progress in several laboratories. The difficulties are increased by the relatively long life span of cattle. In mice or rats the period of time elapsing between the time of inoculation of the mouse leukemia virus into newborn hosts and the subsequent development of leukemia may usually vary from 3 to 12, and rarely up to 16 months. It can be anticipated that in similar experiments carried out in cattle, the latency period elapsing between the inoculation of a bovine leukemia virus into newborn calves and the development of leukemia or lymphosarcoma may extend over a period of several years. This anticipation is based theoretically on the relatively much longer life span of cattle as compared with that of mice or rats, and on the observation that the most frequently observed age at which leukemia and lymphosarcoma develop spontaneously in cattle varies from 5 to 7 years. The long latency period anticipated in the experimental transmission of bovine leukemia by virus filtrate may add considerably to the difficulty in carrying out these fundamental experiments.

Preliminary Attempts to Transmit Leukemia in Cattle Experimentally

Attempts have been made recently to transmit lymphosarcoma in cattle by either cell-graft or filtrates.

Olson, Thorell and Winqvist (1963) inoculated intravenously 2 calves, 2 and 7 days old, with leukemic cell suspensions prepared from organs of cattle with lymphosarcoma. After a period of 4 years, one of the inoculated animals died with a lymphosarcoma involving the mediastinal lymph nodes, the heart base, pericardium, and the diaphragm. About one year later, the second animal also developed and died from a typical generalized lymphosarcoma (Thorell, personal communication to the author, 1966). This positive result is interesting and may represent the first successful transmission of bovine lymphosarcoma by cell-graft. However, the very long latency period elapsing between the inoculation of the cell suspension and the development of lymphosarcoma adds to the difficulty in evaluating the results of this experiment; the development of lymphosarcoma in 4 or 5-year-old animals could be interpreted as being unrelated to the inoculation of the cells, since spontaneous lymphosarcomas usually develop at this age. The results would be more significant if more than two animals had been inoculated and had developed lymphosarcoma, and also if the incubation period had been shorter.

More recently Marshak and his colleagues (1967), at the School of Veterinary Medicine in Philadelphia, also reported successful transplantation of bovine lymphosarcoma into newborn irradiated calves. Six calves (1 female and 5 males) received, when less than 2 days old, a single total-body irradiation with 200 rads. Approximately 24 hours after irradiation each calf was inoculated with a freshly prepared leukemic cell suspension. These cell suspensions were prepared from fragments of lymphosarcomatous lymph nodes removed aseptically from 3 cow donors in advanced phases of generalized lymphosarcoma. One of the injected calves (male BF0997) was injected with leukemic cells from his own mother.

The cell suspensions were injected into the jugular vein of each calf, and in addition also intraperitoneally, and subcutaneously in the areas of the prefemoral and prescapular lymph nodes. In all inoculated calves, small subcutaneous tumor masses involving one or several prefemoral or prescapular lymph nodes developed within two weeks after inoculation. In each instance it was possible to make a histological diagnosis of lymphosarcoma, and the growing cells were indistinguishable from the lymphosarcomatous donor cells. In five calves chromosome analysis also showed that the cells growing in the inoculated calves were of donor origin.

In four calves the transplanted lymphosarcomas gradually regressed. Disseminated growth of transplanted lymphosarcomas was progressive in two calves and appeared to be responsible for the moribund condition of at least one calf (male BF0997) which was injected with its own mother's cells, and for the poor condition of another calf (male BF0857) with generalized disease. These two calves were sacrificed at 2 months of age, as were also 2 others in which the tumors were regressing. In the remaining 2 calves the tumors regressed completely; these 2 calves remained alive and apparently in good health.

In a more recent experiment carried out by W. J. Donawick, R. R. Marshak and their coworkers (personal communication to the author, 1968), two calves, about two weeks old, received several consecutive injections of anti-bovine-lymphocyte horse serum; a few days later they received a subcutaneous inoculation of a cell suspension prepared from bovine lymphosarcoma. Following a latency of about 5 to 6 weeks, small tumors developed at the site of inoculation concurrently with a generalized lymphadenopathy in both animals. One month later both calves were sacrificed; they had very advanced generalized lymphosarcomas with diffuse leukemic infiltration of internal organs, and leukemic changes in peripheral blood morphology.

* * *

The observation that bovine lymphosarcoma could be transplanted in cattle by cell-graft is of considerable interest, but actually should not be surprising. Leukemia and lymphosarcomas in mice, rats, or chickens are readily transplantable by cell-graft within the same species.

In earlier studies there were difficulties in transmitting mouse leukemia by cell-graft, unless the transplantation was made in homozygous mice of the same inbred line in which the donor's leukemia had developed (Richter and MacDowell, 1929); occasionally, however, success could also be observed using non-inbred mice for inoculation (Korteweg, 1929), or employing mice of a non-inbred stock in which the host's resistance had been lowered by a prior total-body X-ray irradiation (Krebs *et al.*, 1930). Transmission of mouse leukemia by cell-graft in mice of different inbred lines from those in which the donor's leukemia originated became readily accomplished when newborn hosts were used for inoculation (Gross, 1950a,b).

Attempt to Transmit Bovine Leukemia by Filtrates

Transmission of bovine lymphosarcoma by cell-graft which was recently accomplished, is of considerable interest, but does not necessarily prove that this disease is caused by a virus. In order to determine the viral etiology of bovine leukemia, the transmission of this disease would have to be accomplished not by cell-graft, but by means of a cell-free filtrate. The following experiment may represent an initial step in this direction:

In an attempt to transmit bovine lymphatic leukemia by filtrate (Hoflund, Thorell and Winqvist, 1963), tumor fragments were obtained from a cow with typical lymphosarcoma in the final stage of the disease. The extract, prepared by ultra-filtration of tumor homogenate of 5 to 10 per cent concentration on silica columns (Thorell and Yamada, 1959), was subsequently concentrated by high-speed ultracentrifugation. A suspension of the sediment was then inoculated intravenously or subcutaneously, or by both routes, into 12 newborn calves. The experimental animals were obtained from, and housed in, an area of Sweden hitherto relatively free from bovine leukosis (Olson, 1961). Related calves from the same area of the country were kept as untreated controls. The inoculated animals did not develop clinical signs of disease during the observation time reported by the authors.

In another experiment the ultra-filtrate described above was inoculated into 7 to 8-month-old calf fetuses. Five of such animals inoculated *in utero* were normally delivered. Five years after inoculation of the tumor filtrate at the fetal stage, one of the 5 experimental animals (#111) began to lose weight and developed a high peripheral lymphocyte count and an abnormal bone marrow morphology; later on this animal developed a typical clinical picture of lymphosarcoma (B. Thorell, personal communication to the author, 1966); in addition, 2 animals in this group developed abnormally high lymphocyte counts in peripheral blood; one of these died from an intercurrent disease, without evidence of lymphosarcoma. The remaining animals did not develop any clinical signs of the disease and appeared to be in good health at the time this experiment was reported.

This single positive result is encouraging but not convincing. The fact that following injection of the filtrate one out of five animals developed lymphosarcoma at the age of 5 years does not necessarily suggest that the disease was induced by inoculation; lymphosarcoma could have developed spontaneously in this single animal. Additional results are needed in order to prove unequivocally that bovine lymphosarcoma can be transmitted by filtrates.

Several attempts have been made during the past decade to transmit lymphosarcoma in cattle by means of tumor filtrates, blood, milk, or urine (Götze, 1956. Rosenberger, 1963. Bederke and Tolle, 1964). Following inoculation of the filtrates, or of other extracts tested, into newborn calves, some of the animals developed a transient or persistent lymphocytosis, i.e. values of lymphocyte counts in peripheral blood exceeding those considered to be "normal" by standards defined in the "Leukosis Key." However, in these experiments only very few animals among the inoculated groups actually developed lymphosarcoma; the small number of these very occasional positive cases was well within the range of spontaneous incidence of this disease. Furthermore, no adequate controls were provided. Accordingly, the results of these experiments were inconclusive and cannot be accepted without serious reservations.

In a similar category could be included experiments dealing with the isolation of a transmissible virus from bovine leukemia (Montemagno *et al.*, 1957). Following inoculation of chick embryos with a filtrate prepared from a lymph node removed from a calf affected with lymphatic leukemia, generalized hemorrhagic and parenchymal lesions were induced in the inoculated embryos, resulting in an average mortality of about 40 per cent. The virus causing these changes was found to be thermolabile and could be passed serially in chicken embryos (Papparella *et al.*, 1963). However, no convincing evidence was presented to suggest that the isolated virus was directly or indirectly related to the etiology of bovine lymphosarcoma. An attempt to induce lymphosarcoma with tissue culture fluid containing the virus and inoculated into two young calves (Montemagno, 1958) was inconclusive.

It should be emphasized that the isolation of an undefined virus from normal or diseased tissues is a common laboratory finding when the etiology of an obscure disease is studied. It remains to be determined in such cases whether the isolated virus has a causative relation to the investigated disease.

Electron Microscopic Studies

In view of the success accomplished in electron microscopic studies of viruses causing leukemia and lymphosarcoma in several species, such as chickens, mice, or rats, attempts have also been made in a few laboratories to employ the electron microscope in the study of bovine leukemia. However, electron microscopic studies of bovine leukemia have not yet been carried out on a sufficient scale, and at the present time only preliminary and inconclusive results are available.

In electron microscopic studies of milk obtained from cows from herds having a high incidence of lymphosarcoma, the presence of particles having a diameter of 60 to 110 mμ, some of them with tail-like structures, was reported (Dutcher *et al.*, 1964). Negative staining method with phosphotungstic acid was employed in these studies. The morphology of particles thus revealed does not necessarily suggest that they represent a virus; similar particles were also found in normal milk obtained from healthy cows (Jensen and Schidlovsky, 1964). We have already emphasized in one of the preceding chapters of this monograph that the use of the negative staining method in electron microscopic studies may lead to difficulties, since the electron micrographs obtained with this method can be readily misinterpreted. Virus particles may be confused with normal cell components of similar morphology. On electron microscopic studies of biological samples prepared by the negative staining technique, some of the non-viral particles, such as pleuropneumonia-like organisms (PPLO), may show a morphology similar to that representing viral agents. The negative staining technique is useful when dealing with the examination of virus particles that have been sufficiently purified to allow study and identification by this method. Much more dependable are results of electron microscopic examination of ultrathin sections of tissues embedded in Epon and stained by one of the standard methods employed in electron microscopy, such as uranyl or lead-acetate. In ultrathin sections examined in the electron microscope, virus particles will usually show a characteristic internal structure, such as, for example, the presence of a double membrane, of an electron-dense nucleoid, etc., whereas the PPLO particles, even though they may be of a similar external shape and overall size, show a lack of internal structure comparable to that observed in virus particles.

Examination of Ultrathin Sections. In electron microscopic studies of bovine leukemia, ultrathin sections of either milk pellets, or of fragments of lymph nodes, or of other tissues with lymphosarcomatous infiltration obtained from leukemic cattle donors, were also examined. Ultrathin sections of milk pellets obtained from cattle from a herd with a high incidence of lymphosarcoma were reported to contain particles with double membranes and nucleoids (Dutcher *et al.*, 1964). However, the resolution and clarity of these preliminary electron micrographs were not entirely satisfactory. The particles were isolated, and poorly defined, and the assumption that they represent virus particles could not be accepted without certain reservations; they could as well represent normal milk components, or some other unidentified submicroscopic structures not necessarily related to the presence of an oncogenic virus.

On electron microscopic examination of ultrathin sections of tissues, such as lymph nodes and other organs from leukemic cattle, rather poorly defined small spherical particles, having a diameter of about 50 mμ, were found, either isolated or in clusters, in the cytoplasm of some of the cells examined in one animal only (Sorenson and Theilen, 1963).

We have also carried out preliminary studies on bovine leukemia in co-operation with D. G. Feldman and H. J. Bendixen, and more recently also with R. R. Marshak. Thus far ultrathin sections of organs from 13 cows with lymphosarcomas have been examined in the electron microscope; in the lymph nodes of 3 animals, and in one additional animal in lymphoid cells infiltrating the liver, small particles were found, accumulated in clusters either in vacuoles in the cytoplasm, or in the cytoplasmic matrix. These particles were homogenous, spherical, had a diameter of approximately 35 mμ, and had no external membrane. They appeared to be similar to those observed by Sorenson and Theilen (1963). There is no evidence, however, to suggest that these particles are related to the development of lymphosarcoma in the animals studied, or that they actually represent a virus; they may represent normal cell components.

At this point, it is rather difficult to explain why a search in our studies for virus particles in a variety of organs, particularly in lymphoid tumors and spleens, from 13 cows with lymphosarcoma failed to detect the presence of particles or related structures resembling the virus particles so readily found in mouse leukemia. This striking and rather unexpected difficulty contrasts sharply with the relative ease of finding characteristic virus particles in leukemia and lymphosarcoma occurring in chickens, mice, rats or cats.

We do not doubt that the etiology of bovine lymphosarcoma is similar to the etiology of the same disease occurring in other species, such as chickens, mice or rats, and that oncogenic viruses are responsible for the induction of leukemia and allied diseases in all animal species, including humans. However, for some as yet unexplained reasons, difficulties appear to exist in demonstrating the presence of virus particles in leukemia and lymphosarcoma occurring in certain species, such as cattle, and also in humans. This difficulty does not necessarily imply that in these species the disease is not caused by a transmissible virus. In many other instances, electron microscopic examination of virus-induced tumors failed to reveal the presence of the causative agents. (See also *Addendum* on p. 650, and Fig. 51b on p. 620.)

REFERENCES

Bederke, G., and Tolle, A., Zur Übertragbarkeit der Rinderleukose durch das Blut und den Kontakt mit experimentell behandelten Tieren. *Zentralbl. f. Vet. Med.*, **11**: 433–445, 1964.

Bendixen, H. J., Studies on bovine leukosis. 2. Clinical diagnosis of bovine leukosis. *Nord. Vet.-Med.*, **10**: 273–301, 1958.

Bendixen, H. J., Undersøgelser over Kvaegers Leukose. 3. Om Kontrollen med Leukose Besaetinger ved haematologuske Undersøgelsesmetoder. *Nord. Vet.-Med.*, **11**: 733–758, 1959.

Bendixen, H. J., Untersuchungen über die Rinderleukose in Dänemark. I. Vorkommen und Verbreitungsweise. *Deutsche tierärztl. Wochenschr.*, **67**: 4–7, 1960.

Bendixen, H. J., Untersuchungen über die Rinderleukose in Dänemark. II. Pathogenese und Enzootologie der übertragbaren Rinderleukose. *Deutsche tierärztl. Wochenschr.*, **67**: 57–63, 1960.

Bendixen, H. J., Untersuchungen über die Rinderleukose in Dänemark. III. Die klinischen Erscheinungen der übertragbaren enzootisch auftretenden und der sporadisch vorkommenden Krankheitsformen. *Deutsche tierärztl. Wochenschr.*, **67**: 169–173, 1960.

Bendixen, H. J., Untersuchungen über die Rinderleukose in Dänemark. IV. Das derzeit angewandte Bekämpfungsverfahren. *Deutsche tierärztl. Wochenschr.*, **67**: 257–262, 1960.

Bendixen, H. J., Preventive measures in cattle leukemia: Leukosis Enzootica Bovis. *Ann. N.Y. Acad. Sci.*, **108**: 1241–1267, 1963.

Bendixen, H. J., *Studies of Leukosis Enzootica Bovis. With special regard to diagnosis, epidemiology and eradication.* (Leukosis Enzootica Bovis, Copenhagen, Carl Fr. Mortensen, 1963, translated for the National Cancer Institute) U.S. Department of Health, Education and Welfare, Public Health Service Publication No. 1422, p. 149, 1965a.

Bendixen, H. J., Bovine Enzootic Leukosis. *Advances in Veterinary Science*, **10**: 129–204, 1965. Academic Press, New York, 1965b.

Bendixen, H. J., and Friis, N. F., Die Hautleukose bei Rindern in Dänemark. *Wien. tierärztl. Mschr.*, **52**: 496–505, 1965.

Bodin, S., Enhörning, G., Olson, H., and Winqvist, G., Die Anzahl der Lymphozyten im Blut von Rindern bei Lymphatischer Leukose und Piroplasmose. *Acta Vet. Scand.*, *Suppl. 2*, **2**: 47–54, 1961.

Böttger, T., Beobachtungen über das Auftreten und die Erblichkeit der tumorösen Form der Rinderleukose. *Zeitschr. f. Tierzücht. u. Züchtungsbiol.*, **63**: 223–238, 1954.

Böttger, T., Weitere Ermittlungen über das Auftreten und die Erblichkeit der tumorösen Form der Rinderleukose. *Zeitschr. f. Tierzücht. u. Züchtungsbiol.*, **65**: 243–252, 1955.

Clegg, F. G., and Moss, B., Skin leukosis in a heifer: An unusual clinical history. *Vet. Rec.*, **77**: 271–272, 1965.

Cotchin, E., Tumours of farm animals: A survey of tumours examined at the Royal Veterinary College, London, during 1950–60. *Vet. Rec.*, **72**: 816–822, 1960.

Croshaw, J. E., Jr., Abt, D. A., Marshak, R. R., Hare, W. C. D., Switzer, J., Ipsen, I., and Dutcher, R. M., Pedigree studies in bovine lymphosarcoma. *Ann. N.Y. Acad. Sci.*, **108**: 1193–1202, 1963.

Czymoch, O., Beitrag zur Aetiologie der Rinderleukose in Ostpreussen. *Zeitschr. f. Infektionskr., parasitäre Krankheiten und Hygiene der Haustiere*, **52**: 187–220, 1937.

Dobberstein, J., Zur vergleichenden Pathologie der Leukosen. *Folia Haemat.*, **71**: 591–597, 1953.

Dobberstein, J., and Seifried, O., Leukosen der Haustiere. *13th Internat. Vet. Cong.*, **1**: 571–587, 1938.

Drieux, H., Les leucoses bovines. *Reç. Med. Vet.*, **131**: 887–915, 1955.

Dungworth, D. L., Theilen, G. H., and Lengyel, J., Bovine lymphosarcoma in California. II. The thymic form. *Path. Vet.*, **1**: 323–350, 1964.

Dutcher, R. M., Larkin, E. P., and Marshak, R. R., Virus-like particles in cow's milk from a herd with a high incidence of lymphosarcoma. *J. Nat. Cancer Inst.*, **33**: 1055–1064, 1964.

du Toit, P. J., Beitrag zur Morphologie des normalen und des leukämischen Rinderblutes. *Arch. f. Wissenschaft. und Praktische Tierheilk.*, **43**: 145–202, 1917.

du Toit, P. J., Weitere Untersuchungen über die Lymphozytomatose des Rindes. III. Mitteilung. *Zeitschr. f. Infektionskr., parasitäre Krankheiten und Hygiene der Haustiere*, **20**: 320–350, 1920.

Ellermann, V., and Bang, O., Experimentelle Leukämie bei Hühnern. *Centralbl. f. Bakt., Abt. I*, (Orig.), **46**: 595–609, 1908.

Fortner, J., Die Leukose der Rinder. *Mh. f. Tierheilk., Zeitschr. f. tierärztl. Forschung und Praxis*, **5**: 184–188, 1953.

Götze, R., Über Ursachen und Bekämpfung der Leukose des Rindes. *Mh. Vet. Med.*, **11**: 169–173, 1956.

Götze, R., and Ziegenhagen, G., Zur Frage der Ursachen und der Bekämpfung der Rinderleukose. I. Erblichkeit, züchterische Massnahmen. *Deutsche tierärztl. Wochenschr., Beilage Fortpfl. u. Besam. Haustiere*, **3**: 55, 1953.

Götze, R., Rosenberger, G., and Ziegenhagen, G., Die Leukose des Rindes, ihre hämatologische und klinische Diagnose. *Mh. Vet. Med.*, **9**: 517, 1954.

Götze, R., Rosenberger, G., and Ziegenhagen, G., Über Ursachen und Bekämpfung der Rinderleukose. IV. Übertragbarkeit. *Deutsche tierärztl. Wochenschr.*, **63**: 105–108, 1956.

Götze, R., Rosenberger, G., and Ziegenhagen, G., Über Ursachen und Bekämpfung der Rinderleukose. V. Übertragungswege und Bekämpfungsvorschlag. *Deutsche tierärztl. Wochenschr.*, **63**: 108–114, 1956.

Götze, R., Ziegenhagen, G., and Merkt, H., Zur Diagnose der Leukose des Rindes. *Mh. f. Tierheilk.*, **5**: 201–211, 1953.

Gross, L., Is cancer a communicable disease? *Cancer Research*, **4**: 293–303, 1944.

GROSS, L., Susceptibility of newborn mice of an otherwise apparently "resistant" strain to inoculation with leukemia. *Proc. Soc. Exp. Biol. & Med.*, **73**: 246–248, 1950a.

GROSS, L., Susceptibility of suckling-infant and resistance of adult mice of the C3H and of the C57 lines to inoculation with Ak leukemia. *Cancer*, **3**: 1073–1087, 1950b.

GROSS, L., Pathogenic properties, and "vertical" transmission of the mouse leukemia agent. *Proc. Soc. Exp. Biol. & Med.*, **78**: 342–348, 1951.

GROSS, L., Is leukemia caused by a transmissible virus? A working hypothesis. *Blood*, **9**: 557–573, 1954.

GROSS, L., Unpublished data, 1961.

HANSEN, H.-J., Die schwedischen Untersuchungen der Rinderleukose. *Acta Vet. Scand., Suppl. 2*, **2**: 5–12, 1961.

HARE, W. C. D., MARSHAK, R. R., ABT, D. A., DUTCHER, R. M., and CROWSHAW, J. E., JR., Bovine lymphosarcoma. A review of studies on cattle in the eastern United States. *Canadian Vet. J.*, **5**: 180–198, 1964.

HARTENSTEIN, A., Leukämie. *Bericht über das Veterinärwesen im Freistaat Sachsen*, **41**: 141, 1897.

HENRICSON, B., and OLSON, H., Statistiche Untersuchungen über die Rinderleukose. *Acta Vet. Scand., Suppl. 2*, **2**: 55–62, 1961.

HJÄRRE, A., Über Leukosen bei Tieren mit besonderer Berücksichtigung der Verhältnisse beim Rind. *Berlin. Münch. tierärztl. Wochenschr.*, **69**: 125–129, 1956.

HOFLUND, S., THORELL, B., and WINQVIST, G., Experimental transmission of bovine leukosis. (Abstract.) *Proc. Internat. Symposium on Comparative Leukemia Research*, Doc. III, 2, Hannover, Germany, August, 1963.

HYDE, J. L., KING, J. M., and BENTINCK-SMITH, J., A case of bovine myelogenous leukemia. *Cornell Vet.*, **48**: 269–276, 1958.

JARRETT, W. F. H., Progress report on the status of lymphosarcoma in animals in Great Britain. *Bull. Off. int. Epiz.*, **62**: 727–734, 1964.

JARRETT, W. F. H., Experimental studies of feline and bovine leukemia. *Proc. Royal Soc. Med.*, **59**: 661–662 (Section of Comparative Med., pp. 21–22), 1966.

JARRETT, W. F. H., CRIGHTON, G. W., and DALTON, R. G., Leukaemia and lymphosarcoma in animals and man. I. Lymphosarcoma or leukaemia in the domestic animals. *Vet. Rec.*, **79**: 693–699, 1966.

JENSEN, E. M., and SCHIDLOVSKY, G., Submicroscopic particles in normal bovine and human milks: A preliminary morphological survey. *J. Nat. Cancer Inst.*, **33**: 1029–1053, 1964.

KARLSON, A. G., Clinical and postmortem observations on lymphoblastoma of cattle. Doctoral Thesis. Graduate College, University of Minnesota, Minneapolis, 1942.

KNUTH, P., and VOLKMANN, O., Untersuchungen über die Lymphozytomatose des Rindes. (Lymphosarkomatosis Kundrat, Leukosarkomatosis Sternberg.) *Zeitschr. f. Infektionskr., parasitäre Krankheiten und Hygiene der Haustiere*, **17**: 393–467, 1916.

KORTEWEG, R., Eine überimpfbare Leukosarkomatose bei der Maus. *Zeitschr. f. Krebsforsch.*, **29**: 455–476, 1929.

KREBS, C., RASK-NIELSEN, H. C., and WAGNER, A., The origin of lymphosarcomatosis and its relation to other forms of leukosis in white mice.—Lymphomatosis infiltrans leucemica et aleucemica. *Acta Radiologica*, Suppl. 10, 1–53, 1930.

LOCKAU, N., Die Lymphadenose des Rindes. *Berlin. tierärztl. Wochenschr.*, **49**: 177–180, 1933.

LOMBARD, C., La leucose des bovidés. *Bull. du Cancer*, **51**: 301–308, 1964.

LOMBARD, C., Leucémie, lymphosarcome et leucose lymphoïde des bovidés. *Bull. Off. int. Epiz.*, **63**: 825–881, 1965.

MARSHAK, R. R., and ABT, D. A., Epidemiology of bovine leukosis. pp. 166–182, in: *Proc. 3rd Internat. Symposium on Comparative Leukemia Research, Paris* (July, 1967), Bibl. Haemat. No. 30, S. Karger, Basel and New York, 1968.

MARSHAK, R. R., ABT, D. A., and COHEN, D., Epidemiological aspects of leukemia in mammals, pp. 181–207, in: *Proc. Internat. Symposium on Comparative Leukaemia Research, Stockholm*, September, 1965. Pergamon Press, Oxford and New York, 1966.

MARSHAK, R. R., CORIELL, L. L., LAWRENCE, W. C., CROSHAW, J. E., JR., SCHRYVER, H. F., ALTERA, K. P., and NICHOLS, W. W., Studies on bovine lymphosarcoma. I. Clinical aspects, pathological alterations, and herd studies. *Cancer Research*, **22**: 202–217, 1962.

MARSHAK, R. R., HARE, W. C. D., ABT, D. A., CROSHAW, J. E., JR., SWITZER, J. W., IPSEN, I., DUTCHER, R. M., and MARTIN, J. E., Occurrence of lymphocytosis in dairy cattle herds with high incidence of lymphosarcoma. *Ann. N.Y. Acad. Sci.*, **3**: 1284–1300, 1963.

MARSHAK, R. R., HARE, W. C. D., DUTCHER, R. M., SCHWARTZMAN, R. M., SWITZER, J. W., and HUBBEN, K., Observations on a heifer with cutaneous lymphosarcoma. *Cancer*, **19**: 724–734, 1966.

MARSHAK, R. R., HARE, W. C. D., DODD, D. C., MCFEELY, R. A., MARTIN, J. E., and DUTCHER, R. M., Transplantation of lymphosarcoma in calves. *Cancer Research*, **27**: 498–504, 1967.

MONTEMAGNO, F., Contributo allo studio dell'eziologia virale della leucosi linfatica dei bovini. Nota I.—Trasmissione sperimentale in vitelli inoculati con materiale di coltura. *Acta Med. Vet.*, **4**: 301–310, 1958.

MONTEMAGNO, F., PAPPARELLA, V., and CATELLANI, G., Contributo allo studio dell' eziologia della leucosi linfatica dei bovini. *Acta Med. Vet.*, **3**: 185–187, 1957.

NIEPAGE, H., Der gegenwärtige Stand der Leukoseforschung beim Rinde. *Mh. Vet. Med.*, **8**: 396–398, 1953.

NIEPAGE, H., Zur Diagnose der Rinderleukose durch den Leukoseschlüssel. *Berlin. Münch. tierärztl. Wochenschr.*, **67**: 253–255, 1954.

OLSON, H., Studien über das Autfreten und die Verbreitung der Rinderleukose in Schweden. *Acta Vet. Scand.*, Suppl. 2, **2**: 13–46, 1961.

OLSON, H., THORELL, B., and WINQVIST, G., Experiments quoted in the paper reported by Hoflund, Thorell, and Winqvist (1963) and included in this list of references.

P.T.F., Cow and daughter suffer from leukemia. *Vet. Med.*, **22**: 80, 1927.

PAPPARELLA, V., CALI, A., ROSSI, G. B., and IACOBELLI, A., Researches on a virus isolated from a calf affected with lymphatic leukemia. *Ann. N.Y. Acad. Sci.*, **108**: 1173–1192, 1963.

REISINGER, R. C., Epizootiology of spontaneous cancer in cattle with particular reference to malignant lymphoma. *Ann. N.Y. Acad. Sci.*, **108**: 855–871, 1963.

RICHTER, M. N., and MACDOWELL, E. C., The experimental transmission of leukemia in mice. *Proc. Soc. Exp. Biol. & Med.*, **26**: 362–364, 1929.

RITTER, H., Beobachtungen über epidemische und endemische Ausbreitung der enzootischen Rinderleukose. *Deutsche tierärztl. Wochenschr.*, **71**: 518–522, 1964.

RITTER, H., Die haematologische Diagnose bei der tumorösen Leukose des Rindes. *Berlin. Münch. tierärztl. Wochenschr.*, **78**: 166–169, 1965.

RITTER, H., Studien über die Übertragungswege bei der enzootischen Rinderleukose. *Deutsche tierärztl. Wochenschr.*, **72**: 56–60, 1965.

ROSENBERGER, G., Studies on bovine leukosis in Germany: III. Transmission experiments. *WHO Conference on Comparative Studies in Leukemias.* Philadelphia, February–March, 1961.

ROSENBERGER, G., Ergebnisse zwölfjähriger Leukose-Untersuchungen an der Rinderklinik Hannover. *Deutsche tierärztl. Wochenschr.*, **70**: 410–417, 1963.

ROSENBERGER, G., Public measures for combating of bovine leukosis in West Germany. *Newsletter, Internat. Committee for Comparative Leukemia Research*, 5–6, 1964.

SCHÄPER, W., Entstehung und Bekämpfung der Rinderleukose im Lichte der Konstitutionsforschung. *Deutsche tierärztl. Wochenschr.*, **46**: 833–837, 1938.

SCHALM, O. W., *Veterinary Hematology.* Second Edition, Lea & Febiger, Philadelphia, p. 664, 1965.

SMITH, H. A., Malignant lymphoma in animals. A survey of present knowledge. *Am. J. Clin. Path.*, **38**: 75–87, 1962.

SORENSEN, D. K., ANDERSON, R. K., PERMAN, V., and SAUTTER, J. H., Bovine lymphocytic leukemia. Epidemiological studies. *WHO Conference on Comparative Studies in Leukemias.* Philadelphia, February–March, 1961. Rep. No. 26 (pp. 1–51).

SORENSEN, D. K., ANDERSON, R. K., PERMAN, V., and SAUTTER, J. H., Studies of bovine leukemia in Minnesota. *Nord. Vet. Med., Suppl.* 1, **16**: 562–572, 1964.

SORENSON, G. D., and THEILEN, G. H., Electron microscopic observations of bovine lymphosarcoma. *Ann. N.Y. Acad. Sci.*, **108**: 1231–1240, 1963.

STARR, L. S., and YOUNG, T., Lymphoblastoma in dairy cattle. *Vet. Med.*, **36**: 406–409, 1941.

STÖBER, M., Zytomorphologische und zytochemische Blutuntersuchungen beim Rind im Hinblick auf ihre Brauchbarkeit für die Diagnose der lymphatischen Leukose. p. 194. *Habilitationsschrift*, Tierärztliche Hochschule Hannover, Germany, 1965.

SVANBERG, O., and ABERG, E., Milieubedingte Voraussetzungen der Lymphadenose des Rindes. *Schweiz. Arch. Tierheilk.*, **97**: 294–296, 1955.

SVANBERG, O., ABERG, E., and NORDSTRÖM, G., Influence des conditions du milieu sur la leucose des vaches laitières. Méthodes de recherches, observations et conclusions de quelques travaux suédois. *Reç. Méd. Vét.*, **132**: 285–297, 1956.

THEILEN, G. H., and DUNGWORTH, D. L., Bovine lymphosarcoma in California. III. The calf form. *Am. J. Vet. Research*, **26**: 696–709, 1964.

THEILEN, G. H., APPLEMAN, R. D., and WIXOM, H. G., Epizootiology of lymphosarcoma in California cattle. *Ann. N.Y. Acad. Sci.*, **108**: 1203–1213, 1963.

THEILEN, G. H., DUNGWORTH, D. L., LENGYEL, J., and ROSENBLATT, L. S., Bovine lymphosarcoma in California. I. Epizootiologic and hematologic aspects. *Health Lab. Sci.*, **1**: 96–106, 1964.

THEILEN, G. H., SCHALM, O. W., and GILMORE, V., Clinical and hematologic studies of lymphosarcoma in a herd of cattle. *Am. J. Vet. Research*, **22**: 23–31, 1961.

THORELL, B., and YAMADA, E., The distribution of adenosintriphosphatase activity and virus-induced leukemia cells. *Acta Biochim. and Biophys.*, **31**: 104–114, 1959.

TOLLE, A., Zur Beurteilung quantitativer hämatologischer Befunde im Rahmen der Leukose-Diagnostik beim Rind. *Zentralbl. Vet. Med.*, **12**: 281–290, 1965.

TOLLE, A., ROJAHN, A., and HASSE, G., Reihenuntersuchungen auf Rinderleukose in einem geschlossenen südniedersächsischen Gebiet. *Mh. f. Tierheilk.*, **15**: 192–200, 1963.

UEBERSCHÄR, S., Electronenoptische Untersuchungen an den Zellen der tumorösen Form der Leukose des Rindes. *Deutsche tierärztl. Wochenschr.*, **70**: 417–422, 1963.

WEBER, W. T., Hematologic aspects of bovine lymphosarcoma. *Ann. N.Y. Acad. Sci.*, **108**: 1270–1283, 1963.

WEISCHER, F., Erbbedingtheit und Bekämpfung der Rinderleukose. *Deutsche tierärztl. Wochenschr.*, **52**: 83–84, 1944.

WIESNER, E., *Die Leukose des Rindes*. Gustav Fischer. Jena. p. 97, 1961.

WINQVIST, G., Die Hämatologie der Tierleukosen. *Mh. Vet. Med.*, **13**: 161–164, 1958.

WINQVIST, G., The haematology of bovine leucosis. *Proc. 7th Cong. Europ. Soc. Haemat., London, 1959*. part II, pp. 291–293, 1960.

WINQVIST, G., A transferrable lymphocytosis in cattle. *Proc. 8th Cong. Europ. Soc. Haemat., Vienna, 1961*. p. 128, 1962.

ADDENDUM: VIRUS PARTICLES IN BOVINE LYMPHOSARCOMA

In a recent study carried out in Dr. Olson's laboratory, at the Department of Veterinary Science, University of Wisconsin, in Madison, virus-like particles were found in short-term peripheral blood lymphocyte cultures obtained from cows with lymphosarcoma. Most of the lymphocyte cultures were stimulated with phytohemagglutinin. Virus-like particles were observed in cultures from 9 out of 12 cattle with lymphosarcoma. Particles of the same type were also present in cultures from 15 out of 24 cattle of a multiple case herd, in 15 out of 26 cattle which had been inoculated with bovine lymphosarcoma extracts, and in 2 out of 16 aged cows from herds with no history of lymphosarcoma. Most of the particles were located in the intercellular spaces; the particles were spherical and had a diameter varying from 90 to 120 mμ; many of them had centrally located electron-dense nucleoids 60 to 90 mμ in diameter. In their morphology and size, these particles were similar to mature type C virus particles observed in mouse and cat leukemia (MILLER, J. M., MILLER, L. D., OLSON, C., and GILLETTA, K. G., Virus-like particles in phytohemagglutinin-stimulated lymphocyte cultures with reference to bovine lymphosarcoma. *J. Nat. Cancer Inst.*, 1969, in press). (Fig. 51b, p. 620.)

This important observation* was promptly confirmed by T. G. Kawakami, A. Moore and G. H. Theilen at the School of Veterinary Medicine, Univ. of California, Davis, and also by S. K. Dutta, D. K. Sorensen, V. Perman and their associates at the College of Veterinary Medicine, Univ. of Minnesota. St. Paul. (IVth Internat. Symp. Comp. Leukemia Research, Sept. 21–25, 1969, Cherry Hill, N. J., to be published.)

*Dr. J. M. Miller, studying nuclear membrane projections in bovine lymphosarcoma, added phytohemagglutinin to short-term cultures of peripheral blood lymphocytes, anticipating an intensification of nuclear membrane projections; unexpectedly, virus particles appeared in the cultures examined. (Personal communication from Dr. C. Olson, 1969.)

CHAPTER 18

The Parotid Tumor (Polyoma*) Virus

ISOLATION OF THE PAROTID TUMOR VIRUS FROM LEUKEMIC FILTRATES AND ITS DIFFERENTIATION FROM THE LEUKEMIC AGENT

In the course of experiments dealing with cell-free transmission of mouse leukemia carried out in our laboratory in 1951, filtrates prepared from spontaneous Ak leukemia were inoculated into newborn, less than 16-hour-old, mice of the C3H strain. The unexpected and puzzling observation was then made that among the inoculated mice some, instead of leukemia, developed tumors on one or both sides of the neck. At first, these tumors were barely noticeable; the necks merely had a somewhat swollen appearance. Gradually, however, the tumors increased in size, growing slowly but progressively. Eventually, they formed large collars enveloping in a grotesque manner the necks of these animals (Gross, 1953).

Filterable Agent, Recovered from Leukemic Mouse Tissues, Causing "Neck Tumors." Initial Observations

In our records the first notes concerning the development of "neck tumors" in some of the C3H mice that had been inoculated, when newborn, with cell-free ultracentrifuged (144,000 $\times g$) Ak leukemic extracts, were entered on November 9, 1951. In a litter of C3H(f) mice inoculated with such a cell-free extract shortly after birth, one mouse was noticed to have developed, when 3 months old, small tumors on both sides of the neck; this mouse was found to have a normal blood count and no enlargement of either peripheral lymph nodes or that of spleen or liver, suggesting thereby that the development of these tumors was not a sign of incipient leukemia. Within a week or two, additional 2 mice in this litter, inoculated with the same extract, were found with similar neck tumors. These tumors gradually increased in size. Eventually, all 3 mice had large tumorous masses sur-

* The terms "polyoma virus" and "parotid tumor virus" are synonymous. See page 696. The terms "virus" and "agent" are used interchangeably and have the same meaning.

rounding their necks. Within a few weeks, several other mice that had also been inoculated shortly after birth with cell-free leukemic extracts developed similar neck tumors. Some of these animals subsequently developed also tumors in the inguinal or axillary pits, or under the skin of the back or flank, or on the abdomen.

On dissection, the neck tumors were found to have a characteristic appearance; they formed clusters of small, individual tumor nodules varying in size from that of a head of a pin to a small pea. A typical neck tumor had thus the appearance of a grape-like cluster consisting of innumerable, and varying in size, small, shiny, colorless or rather white nodules, located on one or both sides of the neck. Frequently, the tumor on one side of the neck was larger than that on the opposite side (Fig. 52, p. 657).

This macroscopic picture was striking and quite different from that of any other tumors previously described in the mouse.* In fact, the gross appearance of these neck tumors was so characteristic that once seen they could be recognized *in situ* at once with the naked eye or with the aid of a magnifying glass.

Initial Diagnostic Difficulties

The appearance of tumorous swellings on the necks of mice that had been inoculated with cell-free leukemic extracts was a surprise. It was only logical to expect that leukemic extracts would necessarily induce either leukemia or some form of a lymphoma. The first impression was therefore that the tumorous swellings developing around the necks of the inoculated mice might possibly represent some form of leukemia. It was soon realized, however, that this was not the case. Mice carrying the neck tumors remained free from any signs of leukemia. Their blood and bone marrow showed no pathological changes. The peripheral lymph nodes, spleens, and livers were not enlarged. Even though we realized, however, that these tumors were of a non-leukemic nature, their proper classification encountered some difficulties which were only subsequently clarified.

* Spontaneous tumors of the salivary glands, and particularly those of the parotid glands, are exceedingly rare in the mouse. Guérin (1954) surveyed some 9,000 mice and reported only a single spontaneous tumor of the salivary gland, a myxosarcoma.

Lippincott and his colleagues (1942) observed a few spontaneous tumors of the salivary glands in albino mice of strains C and A. Some of these tumors were solid with a tendency toward keratinization and pearl formation. Others were cystic and contained mucus-like fluid. It was suggested that these tumors were myo-epitheliomas. None of these neoplasms was similar to those observed in our experiments.

The interested reader is referred for further information and more detailed morphological descriptions to previous publications (Gross, 1953–1957. Law *et al.*, 1955), and to the *Atlas of Tumor Pathology* (Stewart, H. L. *et al.*, 1959).

The Identification of "Neck Tumors" as Carcinomas Arising in Multiple Centers Within the Parotid Glands

In February, 1952, several microscopic slides of the neck tumors that had been induced with leukemic filtrates in C3H mice were submitted for examination to Dr. T. Ehrenreich, pathologist of our hospital staff. His diagnosis returned with the slides was that of "anaplastic carcinoma." This diagnosis, which was firm and had no reservations, made it clear already at that time that these tumors were unrelated to leukemia, even though they resulted from inoculation of cell-free leukemic extracts. Later on (February, 1953), a series of microscopic slides prepared from neck tumors in various phases of development, including a few very early and small neoplasms, was studied by Dr. B. Gordon, Chief of the Clinical Laboratory of our hospital. Dr. Gordon's diagnosis was that of "salivary gland carcinomas arising in multiple centers within the parotid glands of the mouse." A similar diagnosis was made independently by Dr. Maurice N. Richter of New York University (February, 1953) and Dr. Jacob Furth, then at Oak Ridge National Laboratory (May, 1953), who were both invited for consultations to our laboratory, and studied gross pathology as well as microscopic sections of these tumors (Gross, 1953).

Microscopic studies of early tumors were particularly revealing. Multiple focal centers of epithelial tumors could be found, arising within the parotid gland. The tumor cells, rounded or elongated, often formed cell accumulations around small glands or ducts, eventually displacing most of the glandular tissue of the parotid glands. The early focal lesions resembled typical adenocarcinomas. Parts of the tumor sections resembled sarcomas, however, particularly those taken from the more advanced and larger tumors. For that reason the term "pleomorphic neoplasms" was suggested by Law, Dunn, and Boyle (1955). Curiously, the neoplastic involvement was in most instances limited to the parotid glands. The lesions extended occasionally to the submaxillary glands, but the latter were usually free from tumors.

Development of Subcutaneous Sarcomas, Occasionally also Mammary Carcinomas and Medullary Adrenal Tumors

Mice carrying the parotid tumors frequently developed later on also subcutaneous tumors in the axillary or inguinal pits, or under the skin of the abdomen. These tumors were usually flat and hard; they infiltrated the adjacent tissues, such as the skin or the peritoneal lining. On microscopic examination they proved to be fibrosarcomas or fibromyxosarcomas (Gross, 1953, 1955).

Some of the sarcomatous tumors developed from the peritoneum or in muscular or perineural fascia; a few originated from uterine muscles. Some of them had a morphology similar to rhabdomyosarcomas. Others had a bizarre appearance which was difficult to classify.

Other tumors developed in the area of the mammary glands; these tumors were also solid, but soft on dissection. They were adenocarcinomas. Both forms of neoplasms appeared in either sex, frequently as early as $2\frac{1}{2}$ to 3 months after inoculation; some of them, however, particularly the subcutaneous sarcomas, appeared later in life (Gross, 1953). Medullary adrenal tumors were also observed (Gross, 1955).

The Leukemic Filtrates Apparently Contained at Least Two Distinct Oncogenic Agents

It was already apparent early in 1953 (Gross) that the parotid gland tumors and the subcutaneous sarcomas and carcinomas had been induced with an agent (or agents) distinct from the leukemic virus, even though they appeared in mice that had been inoculated with leukemic filtrates. The filtrates prepared from leukemic donors presumably contained one agent responsible for the development of leukemia in some of the inoculated mice, and another oncogenic agent causing parotid gland carcinomas and possibly also other tumors, such as sarcomas or carcinomas.

The latter point was still obscure: the subcutaneous sarcomas and carcinomas might have been primary tumors caused by the parotid tumor agent, they might have been secondary tumors developing in mice carrying primary parotid neoplasms, or they might have been caused by a still different oncogenic agent. It was quite clear, nevertheless, that the leukemic filtrates contained at least two distinct oncogenic viruses, i.e. a leukemic agent and an agent causing parotid tumors and possibly also other neoplasms. This assumption was based on the following experimental evidence (Gross, 1953):

(a) When extracts prepared from Ak leukemic donors were passed through filter candles of larger porosity (Selas 02) and were then used for inoculation of newborn C3H mice, leukemia usually resulted. The incidence of induced parotid tumors was higher when extracts were passed through filter candles of smaller porosity (Selas 03) which retained the larger particles.

(b) When the leukemic extracts were centrifuged at a very high speed ($144{,}000 \times g$) in Spinco Model L Ultracentrifuge, the leukemogenic activity was readily sedimented, whereas the supernate still retained its potency to induce parotid gland tumors and subcutaneous sarcomas.

The filtration and the ultracentrifugation experiments suggested that the extracts prepared from leukemic donors contained two separate oncogenic agents: the leukemogenic agent was larger and heavier, since it was often retained by filter candles of smaller porosity, and was also readily sedimented in the ultracentrifuge. The agent causing parotid gland tumors was smaller, since it could pass smaller porosity filter candles, and since it also remained longer in the supernate, following ultracentrifugation.

(c) When cell-free extracts prepared from leukemic donors were heated in a waterbath at 63°C to 64°C for 30 minutes, their leukemogenic potency was abolished. However, such extracts still retained their ability to induce parotid tumors. Heating to a temperature of 70°C for 30 minutes was necessary to inactivate the ability of the extracts to induce not only leukemia but also parotid tumors. This observation suggested that the leukemic agent was more sensitive and could be inactivated by heating for 30 minutes to a relatively lower temperature (63° to 64°C),* whereas the parotid tumor agent was more resistant and required a higher temperature (70°C) for inactivation.

Thus, as early as 1953, i.e. shortly after the initial observation of the parotid gland carcinomas and the identification of their causative agent, the differentiation of the parotid tumor virus from that causing leukemia was accomplished. The separation of these two viruses was based fundamentally on differences in their size and in their sensitivity to heat (Gross, 1953).

Dr. Sarah E. Stewart, working then at the U.S. Public Health Service Hospital in Baltimore, Md., attempted to reproduce our observations dealing with cell-free transmission of mouse leukemia (Gross, 1951). Employing the bio-assay method suggested in our initial report, she inoculated filtrates prepared from leukemic Ak donors into newborn C3H mice, and also into (C3H × AKR) F_1 hybrids. In an abstract entitled "Leukemia in Mice Produced by a Filterable Agent Present in AKR Leukemic Tissues with Notes on a Sarcoma Produced by the Same Agent," which appeared in November, 1953, in the *Anatomical Record*, she reported that some of the injected hybrids, but only a few of the C3H mice, developed leukemia. She observed, however, that "some of the C3H mice inoculated with the filtrate or extracts developed sarcoma of the parotid gland." No figures referring to the number of inoculated animals, or those developing leukemia or tumors, were included. Dr. Stewart concluded, emphasizing the statement expressed in the title of her abstract, that "From these results it would appear that the same filterable agent is capable of producing two different neoplasms, the one produced depending on the strain of mouse used" (Stewart, 1953).

In the meantime, the isolation of the parotid tumor virus from leukemic mouse tissues and its differentiation from the mouse leukemia virus by filtration, ultracentrifugation, or heating to different temperatures, had been accomplished, and was reported (Gross, June, 1953) prior to the appearance of Dr. Stewart's abstract (see also Editorial, *J. Am. Med. Assoc.*, Sept. 12, 1953).

* Subsequent studies demonstrated (Gross, 1959, 1960) that the mouse leukemia virus was inactivated when heated to a temperature of 50° to 56°C for 30 minutes.

Preliminary Studies of Some of the Properties of the Newly Isolated Oncogenic Virus Causing Parotid Tumors and Sarcomas in Mice

The induction of parotid gland carcinomas with leukemic filtrates inoculated into newborn mice attracted the interest of a large number of investigators. No similar tumors had been previously observed in the mouse. Salivary gland tumors had been on rare occasions observed in the submaxillary region of old albino mice of strains A or C (Lippincott *et al.*, 1942). These tumors were, however, myo-epitheliomas, occasionally cystic, with mucus-like fluid content, or with a tendency toward keratinization and pearl formation. They could be readily differentiated macroscopically and microscopically from the virus-induced parotid gland carcinomas. The latter, particularly in their early phases, revealed a multicentric origin within the parotid gland, with a clearly discernible glandular pattern. They later changed into pleomorphic tumors resembling then partly carcinomas, and partly sarcomas.

The induction of parotid tumors with leukemic filtrates, first reported in June, 1953 (Gross), was promptly confirmed that same year by Law* and was shortly thereafter reported also by Stewart.† Additional reports dealing with the induction of parotid tumors, and also of subcutaneous sarcomas, with the leukemic filtrates appeared during the next several years (Gross, 1954–1957. Stewart, 1955. Law *et al.*, 1955. Woolley, 1954. Woolley and Small, 1956. Schmidt, 1956. Dulaney, 1956. Dulaney *et al.*, 1957. Rogel

* Ciba Foundation Symposium, Nov. 16–19, 1953 (Law, 1954).
† See also preceding page.

FIG. 52a. PAROTID TUMORS INDUCED IN A C3H MOUSE.
This C3H(f) male was inoculated when less than 14 hours old with a centrifuged cell-free extract prepared from organs of a leukemic Ak mouse, containing the parotid tumor virus. At the age of 4 months this mouse developed bilateral parotid gland tumors. (From: L. Gross, *Cancer*, **6**: 948, 1953.)

FIG. 52b. PAROTID TUMORS INDUCED IN A C3H MOUSE.
This C3H female was inoculated when less than 7 hours old with a filtrate (Selas 03) prepared from organs of a leukemic Ak mouse, containing the parotid tumor virus. Three months later this mouse developed bilateral parotid tumors.

FIG. 52c. PAROTID AND SUBMAXILLARY GLAND TUMORS INDUCED IN A C3H MOUSE.
This C3H female was inoculated when 15 hours old with a cell-free centrifuged Ak leukemic extract containing the parotid tumor virus, and developed after 4 months bilateral parotid and submaxillary gland tumors. Note on each side of neck grape-like clusters consisting of innumerable and varying in size small tumor nodules reflecting the multicentric origin of this neoplasm.

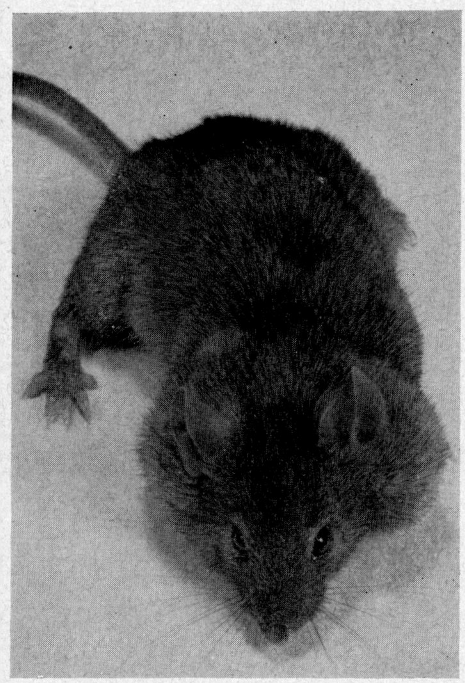

Fig. 52a. Parotid Tumors Induced in a C3H Mouse.

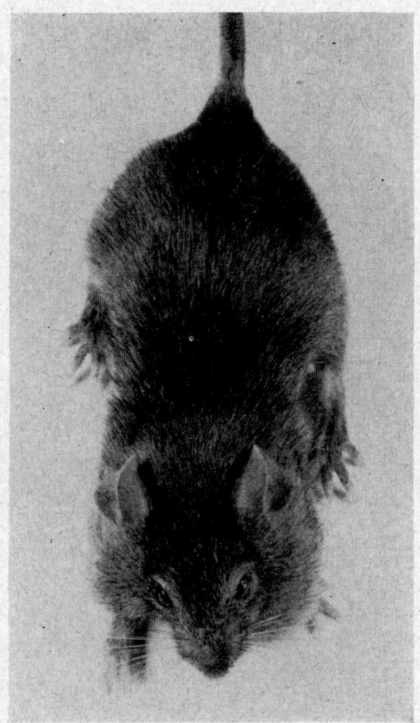

Fig. 52b. Parotid Tumors Induced in a C3H Mouse.

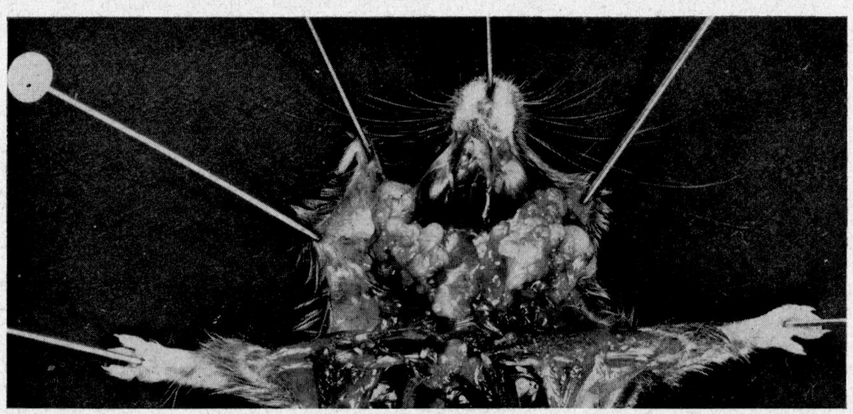

Fig. 52c. Parotid and Submaxillary Gland Tumors Induced in a C3H Mouse.

and Rudali, 1957. Hays *et al.*, 1958. Latarjet *et al.*, 1958. Buffett *et al.*, 1958. Kassel *et al.*, 1959. Salaman, 1959).

During the 3 years which followed the isolation of the parotid tumor virus from leukemic filtrates, experiments were carried out in our laboratory in an attempt to determine general characteristics of the induced tumors, such as the course of their development in the host, their transplantability, etc. Attempts were made to recover the parotid tumor virus directly from the virus-induced parotid and subcutaneous tumors, instead of using the leukemic tissues as a source of the oncogenic agent. General physical, biological, and pathogenic properties of the parotid tumor virus were also studied.

The Course of the Development of Virus-induced Parotid Tumors in the Mouse. The parotid gland tumors appeared frequently as early as 2 or 2½ months after inoculation. In some instances they developed later, occasionally in mice 6 to 8 months old. Early development of these tumors was more frequent, however, and contrasted sharply with the usually delayed development of leukemia in other mice among those that had been inoculated with filtrates prepared from spontaneous Ak leukemia.

There was a difference in susceptibility among the individual litters inoculated with the same filtrate. If, in a litter consisting of several mice, and inoculated with the leukemic filtrate, one mouse developed parotid tumors, sooner or later all remaining mice of the same litter, inoculated with the same filtrate, also developed parotid tumors (Gross, 1953–1955, also unpublished. Law *et al.*, 1955, 1959). Other litters, inoculated simultaneously with the same filtrate, remained in good health or developed leukemia. Only exceptionally did we observe within the same inoculated litter some mice developing parotid tumors and others leukemia. The development of both parotid tumors and leukemia in the same mouse occurred also (Fig. 62, p. 737), but was most unusual and did not exceed one or possibly two per cent of all mice that developed leukemia following inoculation of the filtrates (Gross, 1955–1957).

The parotid tumors appeared first as a slight but firm swelling on one or both sides of the neck; in this early phase they could be scarcely detected by palpation. After one or two weeks, these tumors could be detected by careful inspection. They increased slowly in size and eventually formed enormous tumorous collars surrounding the necks of the animals. The growth was progressive. Among the many hundreds of parotid tumors observed, we have seen only one or two that grew temporarily to a size not exceeding the volume of a small pea, and then regressed (Gross, 1956); the microscopic diagnosis of these two tumors was not confirmed, however. In all other instances the tumors grew progressively, killing their hosts. In many instances, mice bearing parotid tumors subsequently developed also soft tissue sarcomas (fibromyxosarcomas or fibrosarcomas) in the subcutaneous tissues, usually located in inguinal or axillary pits, and some also developed subcutaneous carcinomas. All these tumors grew progressively; none regressed.

The development of subcutaneous sarcomas in some of the inoculated mice, without preceding or concurrent development of parotid tumors, was also observed occasionally.* We have never seen, however, a concurrent development of leukemia and a subcutaneous fibrosarcoma in the same animal.

Transplantation of Parotid Tumors and Subcutaneous Sarcomas by Cell-Graft

The parotid tumors that had been induced in C3H mice with cell-free Ak leukemic filtrates could be transplanted, by cell-graft, to mice of the same strain. Tumor cell suspensions prepared from virus-induced parotid tumors were inoculated under the skin of young adult C3H mice. After a latency varying from several weeks to as long as 3 months, subcutaneous tumors developed in some of the inoculated C3H mice at the site of inoculation. Only a few of the inoculated mice developed tumors, however. The incidence of successful transplantations did not exceed 20 to 25 per cent (Gross, 1953. Law, 1954). The incidence of "takes" was higher when newborn C3H mice were used for the inoculation of the parotid tumor cell suspensions (Gross, 1953, unpublished). The transplanted tumors retained their morphology as undifferentiated, anaplastic carcinomas, or, in some instances, as mixed tumors resembling carcinomas and sarcomas. They grew progressively, infiltrating the surrounding tissues, and eventually formed large tumor masses; they never regressed.

Some of these tumors could be transplanted serially, from one host to another. With each successive transplantation the latency period was shortened, and the incidence of successful "takes" increased.

A few tumor lines could thus be established and carried through over 18 consecutive transplant generations (Gross, 1955) in young adult C3H mice.

Attempts to transplant the parotid tumors from C3H mice to young adult Ak mice by cell-graft failed. These tumors could be transplanted, however, to newborn Ak mice, growing at the site of subcutaneous implantation, then spreading rapidly and forming metastatic tumors in the lungs (Gross, 1953–1955, also unpublished).

The subcutaneous sarcomas induced with leukemic filtrates in C3H mice could also be transplanted by cell-graft into young adult mice of the

* No serial sections of the parotid glands were made, however, in these animals, and the possibility was not excluded that small primary tumor nodules might have been present in the parotid glands of such mice.

same strain. When cell suspensions were used for the transplantation of 28 sarcomas, only 10 grew at the site of inoculation after a latency varying from 2 weeks to 5 months. When, however, large fragments from 6 sarcomatous tumor tissues were implanted surgically, through a skin incision, under the skin of 11 young adult C3H mice, all grew in their new hosts (Gross, 1955–1957).

Attempt to Recover an Oncogenic Virus from Parotid Tumors or Sarcomas

In previous experiments, the source of the oncogenic virus capable of inducing parotid tumors and/or subcutaneous sarcomas was the leukemic extract. Such extracts prepared from leukemic Ak or C58 donors were used for inoculation of newborn mice. The question remained to be answered, however, whether it would also be possible to recover the parotid tumor virus directly from either parotid carcinomas or from subcutaneous sarcomas that had been induced with the parotid tumor virus.

Accordingly, leukemic-filtrate-induced parotid tumors were removed aseptically from C3H mice, ground with sterile saline solution, and the resulting cell suspensions were centrifuged (3,000 r.p.m. for 15 minutes, then 9,500 r.p.m. for 5 to 10 minutes). The final cell-free supernate was either used without any further treatment for inoculation, or was passed first through Berkefeld N, or Selas 02, or 03, filter candles, and then inoculated. Newborn, less than 16-hour-old, C3H or foster-nursed C3H(f) mice were used for inoculation.

Similarly, cell-free, centrifuged or filtered extracts, prepared from filtrate-induced subcutaneous fibrosarcomas and fibromyxosarcomas, were also inoculated into newborn C3H mice.

Among the C3H mice inoculated shortly after birth with cell-free extracts prepared from either parotid tumors or subcutaneous sarcomas, some unexpectedly developed leukemia. Others developed either parotid tumors or subcutaneous sarcomas, or a combination of both. Cell-free extracts prepared from parotid tumors were more active on inoculation tests than those prepared from the subcutaneous sarcomas (Gross, 1955, 1957). The sarcomas, however, were fibrous, hard tumors, very difficult to cut; it was very difficult to prepare a homogenous extract from these rubber-like tumors, and this technical difficulty might have been partially responsible for the low activity of sarcomatous extracts. The parotid tumors were softer and offered no difficulty in the preparation of extracts.

In a large number of experiments in which extracts were prepared from parotid tumors and used for bio-assay, only 7 per cent of the inoculated mice developed parotid tumors (Gross, 1955). Other mice developed leukemia or subcutaneous fibrosarcomas. Concurrent development of parotid tumors and subcutaneous fibrosarcomas in the same mice was also noticed. A few animals developed carcinomas in the submaxillary salivary glands and also medullary adrenal tumors (Gross, 1955). Thus, the incidence of parotid tumors which could be induced with cell-free extracts prepared from parotid tumors was relatively low, but significant and reproducible (Gross, 1957).

In parallel experiments carried out in our laboratory at the same time, up to 11 per cent of C3H mice that had been inoculated with Ak leukemic filtrates developed parotid tumors (Gross, 1955, 1957).

Thus, the surprising observation was made that the virus-induced parotid tumors were not as good a source of the oncogenic agent as were filtrates prepared from Ak leukemic tissues. The same was true for the subcutaneous fibrosarcomas. It was apparent that either these tumors contained the oncogenic agent in relatively small quantities, or that the virus was present but inhibited by specific antibodies or a non-specific inhibitor. Dulaney and Goss observed (1960) that cell-free extracts prepared from parotid tumors, and inoculated into newborn mice of strains C3H, AkR, or Swiss, induced parotid tumors in mice of strain AkR, but only occasionally sarcomas or mammary tumors in C3H or Swiss mice.

The induction of parotid tumors with extracts containing the parotid tumor virus, and inoculated into newborn mice, depended not only on the genetic susceptibility of the strain employed for bio-assay, but also on the presence of specific antibodies in the inoculated animals. The presence of such naturally acquired antibodies might have prevented the development of parotid tumors, even if newborn mice of a susceptible strain, such as C3H or AkR, were inoculated. This will be further discussed in the latter part of this chapter.

The observation that cell-free extracts prepared from solid tumors, such as parotid carcinomas or subcutaneous fibrosarcomas, could induce on bio-assay generalized leukemia was of fundamental importance (Gross, 1955). This observation was similar to that reported at about the same time by Graffi and his associates (1955, 1956). Employing newborn mice for the inoculation of filtrates prepared from transplanted mouse tumors, Graffi was able to demonstrate the presence of a leukemogenic agent in such extracts.*

Biological and Pathogenic Properties of the Parotid Tumor Virus

Extracts prepared from leukemic tissues were thus actually a better source of the parotid tumor agent than those prepared from the parotid tumors (Gross, 1955). Leukemic mice of the Ak or C58 strains, that had

* See also chapter 12 on the Isolation of Mouse Leukemia Virus from Transplanted Mouse Tumors.

developed either spontaneous or transplanted leukemia, were readily available in our laboratory. Such leukemic donors were therefore a convenient source serving for the preparation of extracts containing the parotid tumor agent. It was realized that such extracts also contained the leukemic agent. Gradually, however, experimental conditions were determined which favored the induction, with such extracts, of either parotid tumors or leukemia. When freshly prepared centrifuged extracts of 20 per cent concentration were inoculated into newborn C3H mice, leukemia usually resulted. It was relatively easy, however, to eliminate the leukemogenic action of such extracts, but retain their ability to induce parotid tumors and subcutaneous sarcomas. A simple storage of the extracts in the refrigerator (at +4°C) for several days reduced the leukemogenic potency of such extracts, but did not inhibit their ability to induce parotid tumors and sarcomas. A simple dilution of the extracts with physiological saline solution to 1 : 100 or 1 : 1000 had a similar effect. Passing the extracts through filter candles of relatively small porosity (Selas 03) also decreased, but did not entirely eliminate, their leukemogenic potency, while it did not affect their ability to induce parotid tumors and sarcomas. Heating to 63°C for 30 minutes completely inactivated the leukemic agent* but did not destroy the parotid tumor component (Fig. 57, p. 697). Finally, the leukemogenic agent could be sedimented by ultracentrifugation earlier than the parotid tumor virus.

In the initial experiments (Gross, 1953–1955) the activity of the leukemic extracts used was only moderate. Some extracts were more active than others; frequently, however, neither leukemia nor tumors resulted from inoculation of extracts prepared from leukemic donors under conditions of experiments apparently similar to those yielding active filtrates in other tests. This was due to the low content of virus in the extracts prepared, and probably in part also to the presence of antibodies and non-specific inhibitors. However, carrying out a sufficient number of tests on relatively large numbers of animals, using leukemic filtrates (or centrifuged extracts) as a source of the agent, and newborn C3H mice for bio-assay, some of the principal biological and pathogenic properties of the parotid tumor agent could eventually be determined (Gross, 1953–1957).

Stability of the Virus

The parotid tumor virus was found to be remarkably stable. It could be preserved in a refrigerator at +4°C in physiological saline solution (as leukemic filtrate) for at least several days (Gross, 1953–1957). Subsequent

* It was determined subsequently that heating of the leukemic virus to a temperature not exceeding 50°C for 30 minutes was sufficient for its inactivation (Gross, 1960).

studies, carried out with the tissue-culture-grown parotid tumor virus, demonstrated that this virus could be stored at +4°C, without any apparent loss of infectivity, for at least 8 weeks (Eddy *et al.*, 1958. Brodsky *et al.*, 1959), and probably longer, since samples that had been stored at that temperature for over 5 months were still infectious on bio-assay (Eddy *et al.*, 1958); gradual loss of potency occurred, however, after prolonged storage under such conditions.

At −70°C, in carbon dioxide dry ice, the parotid tumor virus could be preserved in the form of a frozen leukemic filtrate in sealed glass ampoules for at least 4½ months without any apparent loss of potency (Gross, 1957). Subsequent experiments, carried out with the tissue-culture-grown parotid tumor virus, demonstrated that at −70°C, in dry ice, this virus could be preserved, without loss of infectivity, for over one year (Eddy *et al.*, 1958).

When lyophilized, the virus could be preserved without loss of infectivity for 13 months at refrigerator (+4°C) temperature (Gross, 1953).

Furthermore, the parotid tumor virus could be recovered without any apparent loss of infectivity from leukemic tissues that had been preserved in 50 per cent glycerin for periods of time varying from 2 to 15 months (Gross, 1956).

The parotid tumor virus resisted heating to 56°C or 63°C, but was inactivated after heating for 30 minutes to a temperature of 70°C in an electric waterbath (Gross, 1953).

When leukemic extracts were mixed with an equal volume of ethyl ether, and left in a refrigerator (at +4°C) for 23 hours, the parotid tumor virus present in such extracts remained unaffected, whereas the leukemic virus was inactivated (Gross, 1956). This experiment demonstrated that the parotid tumor agent belongs to the group of ether-resistant viruses.*

Relatively Narrow Host Range of the Parotid Tumor Virus in Mice

In these early and preliminary studies, Ak leukemic extracts were employed as a source of the parotid tumor virus. The titer of the virus was relatively low in such extracts; furthermore, it is also possible that some of such extracts, harvested from organs of leukemic mice, contained specific antibodies which could have partially neutralized the parotid tumor virus. As a result, the induction of parotid tumors with extracts prepared from leukemic mouse tissues was not always readily accomplished; frequently such extracts had only a relatively low tumor-inducing potency.

Under such experimental conditions, the genetic susceptibility of mice favoring the induction of salivary gland tumors was of considerable importance. The more recently developed tissue-culture-grown parotid

* For classification of viruses according to susceptibility to ethyl ether, see Andrewes and Horstmann (1949).

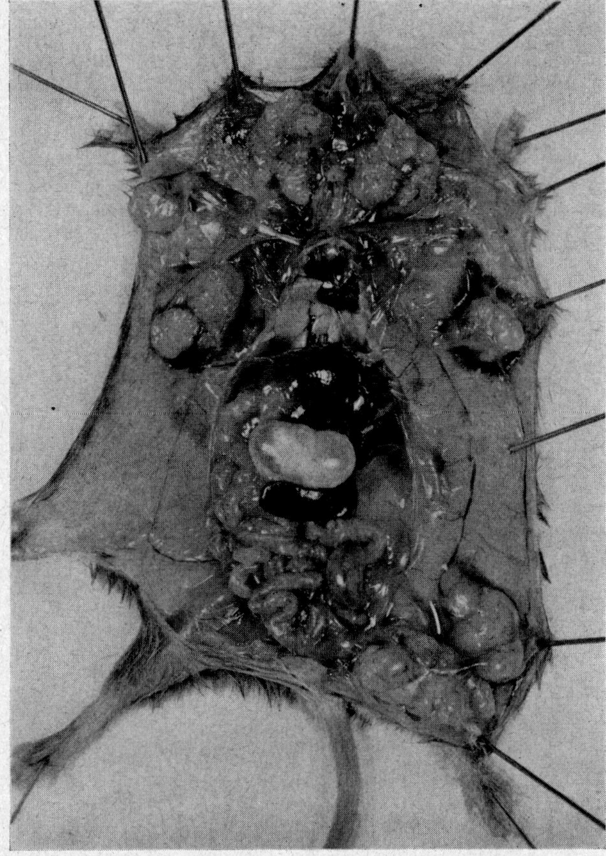

Fig. 53. Salivary Gland Tumors and Multiple Neoplasms Induced in a C3H Mouse with a Cell-free Ak Extract Containing the Parotid Tumor Virus.

This C3H(f) female was inoculated on Feb. 4, 1953, when less than 16 hours old, with a cell-free centrifuged extract prepared from normal Ak embryos; the extract contained the parotid tumor virus. About 3 months after inoculation this mouse developed bilateral multicentric carcinomas in the parotid glands, carcinomas of the submaxillary glands, subcutaneous fibrosarcoma in the left groin, anaplastic carcinomas in the left and right axillary pits, and a medullary adrenal tumor. This was the first published observation of bilateral salivary gland tumors and multiple neoplasms induced in a mouse following inoculation of the parotid tumor virus. (From: L. Gross, *Proc. Soc. Exp. Biol. & Med.*, **83**: 414, 1953.)

tumor virus was found to be more potent, with a wider host range, which included not only several inbred strains of mice but also other animal species, such as hamsters and rats.

Mice of the C3H inbred line (or of the foster-nursed C3H(f) strain) were found to be particularly susceptible to the induction of the salivary gland tumors, whereas mice of strain C57 Brown were found to be relatively resistant. When a large number of newborn mice of the C57 Brown/cd strain was inoculated with cell-free centrifuged extracts or filtrates, prepared from either Ak or C58 leukemic donors, a high incidence of leukemia resulted (Gross, 1954, 1956); none of the inoculated mice, however, developed parotid gland tumors. Only a single animal with parotid tumors was found among a group of C57 Brown mice that had been inoculated shortly after birth with cell-free extracts prepared from normal C58 embryos, which often also carry the virus (Gross, 1956).

Mice of several other inbred strains were also tested, such as those of strains A, DBA/2, C57 Black, and also of the non-inbred Swiss (NIH) stock. Inoculation of newborn mice of these strains with Ak leukemic filtrates resulted in the development of leukemia in some of the inoculated animals; none, however, developed parotid gland tumors (Gross, 1955, 1956, unpublished).

In these experiments, as in the preceding ones, the extracts used for inoculation were prepared from Ak leukemic tissues. Such extracts contained the parotid tumor virus, but were only moderately active on bio-assay. Furthermore, some of the inoculated newborn mice might have carried specific antibodies against the parotid tumor virus, ingested with the milk of their mothers, and this could have rendered such mice resistant to experimental inoculation of the parotid tumor virus.

*Induction of Parotid Tumors in Mice of the Ak Strain**

Among the other strains tested, mice of the Ak strain, even though serving as donors of organs from which the parotid tumor virus was harvested, were at first thought to be relatively resistant to the induction of such tumors (Gross, 1953, 1954). In our preliminary experiments dealing with the induction of parotid gland tumors in C3H mice with Ak leukemic extracts, we were impressed by the fact that mice of the Ak strain, whose tissues provided an excellent source of the parotid tumor virus, had never been observed in our laboratory to develop such tumors spontaneously.† We wondered whether mice of that particular inbred line

* Parotid tumors could also be induced with cortisone in mice of the high-leukemic C58 strain, or in (C58 × Ak) F_1 hybrids. This observation (Woolley, 1954) is discussed on page 672 in this chapter.

† Rogel and Rudali (1957) observed a spontaneous parotid tumor in one of the untreated AkR mice in their laboratory.

might not be naturally resistant to the pathogenic potential of the parotid tumor virus, even though they carried this agent. It became apparent only later (Gross, 1955), however, that mice of other strains, such as C3H, known to be susceptible to experimental induction of parotid tumors, may also carry this virus naturally, even though, with very rare exceptions, they do not develop parotid tumors spontaneously.

In subsequent studies it was observed that under certain experimental conditions parotid tumors could also be induced in Ak mice.

Dr. Anna D. Dulaney (1956) at the Institute of Pathology in Memphis, Tennessee, demonstrated that parotid gland carcinomas could be induced without difficulty in mice of the Ak strain by inoculating newborn, less than 15-hour-old, Ak mice with cell-free leukemic extracts. Of 61 newborn AkR mice inoculated with centrifuged cell-free extracts prepared from leukemic Ak-n or AkR donor mice, 16 animals (26 per cent) developed parotid gland carcinomas, appearing in most instances at 2½ to 3 months of age. A parotid tumor was also observed in a C58 mouse that had received, when newborn, a leukemic extract.

Parotid gland tumors and other neoplasms, such as subcutaneous sarcomas and mammary carcinomas, could also be induced with cell-free extracts prepared from organs of leukemic Ak mice and inoculated into newborn mice of the same strain (Rogel and Rudali, 1957).

A similar observation was also made in our laboratory (Gross, 1954, and 1955, unpublished. Details of these experiments were given on pages 293 and 294 of the first edition of this monograph).

Importance of Age at Inoculation. Susceptibility of Newborn Hosts

The age of the animal at the time of the inoculation of leukemic filtrates was one of the most important factors determining the eventual outcome of the bio-assay. Newborn, less than 16-hour-old, C3H mice were susceptible to the parotid tumor virus, and to the leukemic virus as well. With each passing hour the susceptibility to the parotid tumor virus declined, whereas susceptibility to the leukemic agent decreased much more gradually. Mice more than one day old were, with only few exceptions, already resistant to the parotid tumor virus, whereas they were still susceptible to the leukemogenic action of the filtrates. Thus, the importance of the early age of the host at the time of inoculation of the leukemic filtrates was much more critical for the parotid tumor virus than for that causing leukemia.

Some of the filtrates prepared from spontaneous Ak leukemias had a sufficiently high virus content to induce leukemia following inoculation into suckling, more than one-day-old, C3H mice (Gross, 1953, and unpublished). No parotid tumors, however, developed in such animals. When the same extracts were inoculated into newborn, less than 16-hour-old, C3H mice, either leukemia or parotid tumors resulted.

This phenomenon became particularly apparent in subsequent experiments in which a highly potent leukemic virus was developed (Gross, 1957–1958), capable of inducing leukemia in up to 100 per cent of C3H mice following inoculation into suckling, less than 10-day-old animals. The passage A filtrates also contained the parotid tumor virus. The age of the inoculated animals served, however, as a biological sieve, determining the type of tumors resulting from the inoculation of the extracts. If the filtrate was inoculated into C3H mice less than 16 hours old, in most instances leukemia, occasionally parotid tumors, and in few, rare instances both neoplasms resulted. When, however, the same leukemic filtrates were inoculated into suckling mice 2 to 10 days old, only leukemia resulted (Gross, 1958). The development of parotid tumors following inoculation with the leukemic filtrates of suckling, more than one-day-old mice was most unusual, although it did occur in isolated instances (Gross, 1958, 1959, unpublished).

These preliminary experiments (Gross, 1953–1957) were carried out with cell-free extracts prepared from leukemic Ak or C3H mice. The tissue-culture-grown parotid tumor virus was not yet available at that time. Leukemic tissue extracts provided therefore the best available source of the parotid tumor virus, even though they contained at best only relatively small quantities of this agent. Under such circumstances, it was usually possible to induce the development of parotid tumors only when newborn mice of a particularly susceptible strain, such as C3H, were employed for inoculation.

This situation changed when the tissue-culture-grown parotid tumor virus, with its considerably increased potency, became available. Parotid tumors and related neoplasms could now be induced without difficulty, employing for inoculation not only newborn but also one or several-day-old suckling mice of several inbred strains. This will be discussed later on in this chapter.

Induction of Parotid Tumors and Related Neoplasms with Heated (56°C for ½ hour) Passage A Leukemic Extracts. Passage A leukemic filtrates often contain the leukemic virus and also the parotid tumor agent; however, the leukemic virus can be destroyed in such extracts by heating for 30 minutes to 56°C (Gross, 1959) or even only to 50°C (Gross, 1960). The parotid tumor virus requires a higher temperature for inactivation and is not affected by this procedure.

The curious observation was made that heated (56°C ½ hour) passage A leukemic filtrates have a considerable oncogenic potency when inoculated into newborn, less than 16-hour-old, C3H mice (Gross, 1960). Multiple tumors of parotid and submaxillary glands and subcutaneous fibrosarcomas could be induced with such extracts. In some instances the inoculated mice developed an impressive variety of tumors, including neoplasms of the salivary glands, subcutaneous sarcomas and carcinomas, and multiple epidermoid carcinomas (Gross, 1960), thus reproducing a spectrum of tumors observed in mice inoculated with the tissue-culture-grown parotid tumor (polyoma) virus.

Only very rarely did we see the induction of a variety of tumors with fresh leukemic tissue extracts (Gross, 1953). The oncogenic (but not leukemogenic) potency of heated leukemic extracts appeared to be increased. When older, one to 4-day-old, C3H mice were inoculated with the heated extracts, only very few developed parotid tumors, and now and then also subcutaneous sarcomas. The latency was prolonged, however, and the tumors were few and growing slowly.

The impressive oncogenic potency of heated (56°C ½ hour) passage A leukemic extracts could be explained by assuming that the inactivation of the leukemic virus in filtrates employed for inoculation prevented only the development of leukemia in the inoculated animals. The parotid tumor virus unaffected by the moderate heating, and present in such extracts, was then able to act. This reasoning could not explain the curious fact, however, that many of the parotid tumors and related neoplasms developed in animals inoculated with the heated extracts after a relatively short latency interval of only 2 to 2½ months, i.e. at a time when a certain number of them would still have remained free from leukemia even if they had been inoculated with fresh, unheated extracts. And yet, we have not seen such a variety of tumors induced with unheated passage A filtrates inoculated into newborn mice.

It is therefore possible that there exists some interference between the leukemic virus and that causing parotid gland tumors, if both are present in the same filtrate. It is also possible, however, that heating to 56°C for ½ hour inactivates other inhibiting factors present in such filtrates (Fig. 57, p. 697).

Presence of the Parotid Tumor Virus in Tissues of Normal, Healthy Mice of High-leukemic Strains Ak and C58

Both the leukemic and the parotid tumor agents were present not only in filtrates prepared from leukemic tissues of Ak or C58 mice, but also in normal organ extracts prepared from young healthy animals of these inbred lines (Gross, 1945–1956). When cell-free extracts prepared from normal Ak or C58 embryos were inoculated into newborn C3H mice, leukemia or parotid gland tumors developed in some of the inoculated animals. The incidence of induced leukemia or tumors varied in different experiments.

In a sample of 35 C3H mice inoculated shortly after birth with cell-free extracts prepared from normal Ak embryos, 2 developed leukemia, and 10 mice developed parotid gland carcinomas (Gross, 1955). In another series, cell-free extracts prepared from normal healthy embryos of the high-leukemic C58 strain were inoculated into 63 newborn C3H mice; as a result, 6 developed leukemia, and 7 developed parotid gland carcinomas (Gross, 1956).

It was thus apparent that both oncogenic viruses, i.e. the leukemogenic agent and also the virus causing parotid gland carcinomas, were not only present in extracts prepared from leukemic Ak or C58 donors, but that they could also be found in normal embryos carried by female mice of both Ak and C58 inbred lines.

Presence of Parotid Tumor Virus in Normal Organs of Mice of Low-leukemic Strains

In 1955 the unexpected observation was made in our laboratory that the parotid tumor agent may also be carried in a latent form by young, healthy mice of inbred lines essentially free from spontaneous leukemia, such as C3H or C57 Brown.

In one of our control experiments related to the cell-free transmission of mouse leukemia, young C3H females were mated to their brothers; after the females became pregnant, their embryos were removed aseptically. Cell-free extracts were then prepared in the usual manner from several pooled C3H embryos, and inoculated into 103 newborn C3H mice. None developed leukemia, but unexpectedly 3 mice developed typical parotid gland carcinomas (Gross 1955). In another small group, 9 newborn C3H mice were inoculated with cell-free extracts prepared from normal embryos that had been removed from pregnant female mice of the C57 Brown/cd strain; as a result, 1 mouse developed parotid gland carcinoma (Gross, 1955).

In a third experiment, 74 newborn C3H mice were inoculated with cell-free extracts prepared from pooled normal organs (such as livers, spleens, kidneys etc.) from young, adult, healthy C3H mice. None of the inoculated animals developed leukemia, but 10 of them (14 per cent) developed parotid gland carcinomas (Gross, 1955).

These and other similar experiments clearly indicated that the parotid tumor agent is carried in a latent form by many normal, healthy mice of different inbred lines, such as Ak, C58, C3H, C3H(f) , C57 Brown/cd, etc. This was a wide assortment of strains, some of them with a high incidence of spontaneous leukemia (Ak and C58), or a high incidence of spontaneous mammary carcinoma but a low incidence of spontaneous leukemia (C3H), and others with a low incidence of either spontaneous mammary carcinoma or spontaneous leukemia (C3H(f) or C57 Brown/cd). It was thus quite apparent that the parotid tumor agent may be widely prevalent in perfectly healthy mice of different strains. Under natural conditions of life it may never cause the development of tumors.

Spontaneous development of parotid gland carcinomas is exceedingly rare.* We have seen only a single spontaneous parotid gland carcinoma in one out of more than 10,000 untreated C3H mice observed in our laboratory (Gross, 1955) and none among untreated mice of either the Ak, C58, or C57 Brown/cd strains. Rudali observed a single spontaneous parotid tumor among 1,500 untreated mice of the AKR strain raised in his laboratory (Rogel and Rudali, 1957). Law reported spontaneous development of parotid gland tumors in a single family of C3H mice of the Bittner subline (Law, 1957).

It is quite apparent that spontaneous development of these tumors is

* See also footnote on page 652 of this chapter.

exceedingly rare, and that it occurs only in isolated instances. In many leading laboratories in which large numbers of normal mice of different inbred lines, including those of strains Ak, C58, C3H, etc., have been observed during the past two decades, spontaneous development of parotid tumors has never been recorded.

Activation of the Parotid Tumor Virus in the Carrier Host

If left undisturbed, under normal conditions of life, the parotid tumor virus remains in the great majority of cases perfectly harmless in its natural carrier host. Yet, it may be prompted to induce the development of tumors.

The simplest activating method consists of transferring, by inoculation, a cell-free extract, prepared from normal healthy mouse organs, from one animal to another, using newborn mice of a susceptible strain for the bio-assay. Such a "blind transfer" may result in the development of parotid tumors in some of the inoculated animals, as already described on preceding pages of this chapter (Gross, 1955). In a few instances, parotid tumors could also be induced following inoculation of cell-free extracts prepared from normal guinea pig organs into newborn C3H mice (Gross, 1956).

The development of parotid tumors in otherwise normal mice, carrying the parotid tumor virus naturally, could also be induced by a prolonged treatment with cortisone. Mice of the C58 strain, or (C58 × Ak) F_1 hybrids, received 1 mg daily of Cortone (Merck) subcutaneously, 3 successive days each month throughout life. Parotid tumors developed in some of the treated mice (Woolley, 1954).

Parotid tumors (or generalized leukemia)* could also be induced in normal non-injected C3H mice by fractionated total-body X-ray irradia-

* The induction of leukemia in C3H and C57 Brown/cd mice following fractionated total-body X-ray irradiation has already been discussed in Chapter 13 on Radiation-Induced Leukemia in Mice.

FIG. 54a. PHOTOMICROGRAPH OF A PAROTID TUMOR.

Photomicrograph of a parotid gland tumor which developed bilaterally in a 7-month-old C3H(f) male. This mouse was inoculated when less than 14 hours old with a centrifuged extract prepared from normal Ak embryos containing the parotid tumor virus. Note multicentric origin of the tumor within the parotid gland. Magnification 115× (H. & E.).

FIG. 54b. PHOTOMICROGRAPH OF A PAROTID TUMOR.

Photomicrograph of a parotid gland tumor which developed bilaterally in a 3-month-old C3H female. This mouse was inoculated when less than 3 hours old with a filtrate prepared from organs of a leukemic C58 mouse containing the parotid tumor virus. Note multicentric origin of the tumor and the transition from normal parotid gland into carcinoma. Magnification 260× (H. & E.). (From: L. Gross, *Cancer*, **9**: 778, 1956.)

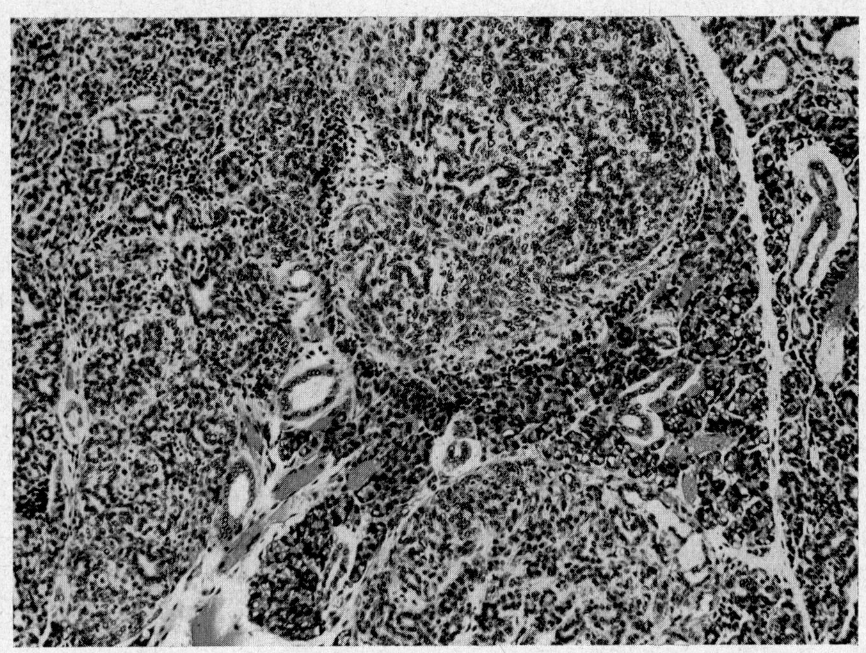

Fig. 54a. Photomicrograph of a Parotid Tumor.

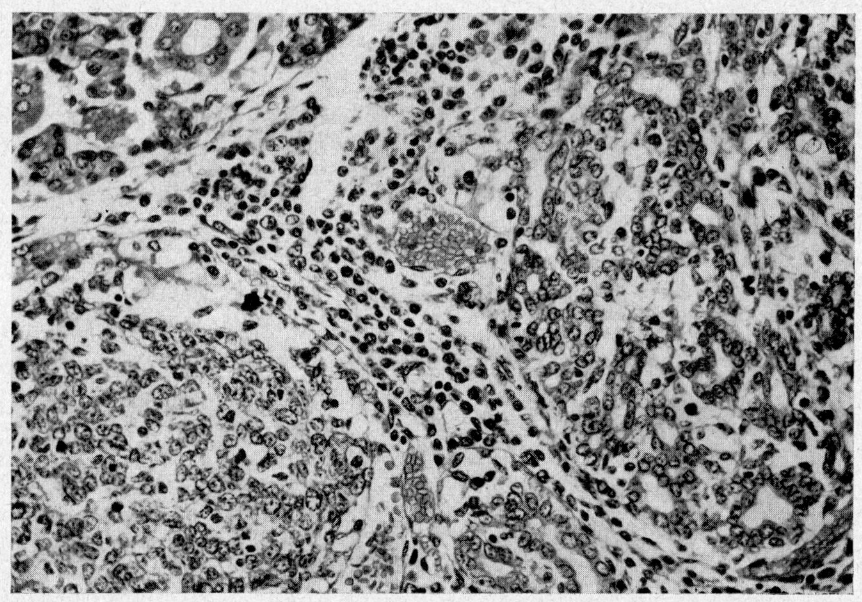

Fig. 54b. Photomicrograph of a Parotid Tumor.

tion (Gross, 1958. Gross *et al.*, 1959). A concurrent development of parotid gland carcinomas and of generalized lymphatic leukemia, following fractionated total-body X-ray irradiation of normal C3H mice, was also observed, but occurred only exceptionally (Gross, unpublished).

In a few instances, fractionated total-body X-ray irradiation of normal C3H mice resulted in the development of a spectrum of parotid and related tumors, i.e. of multiple tumors of the salivary glands (parotid and submaxillary), subcutaneous sarcomas and carcinomas, multiple epidermoid skin carcinomas, etc. (Gross, 1959 and 1960, unpublished). This picture was very similar to that observed in mice inoculated with the tissue-culture-grown parotid tumor virus, as will be discussed later in this chapter. It was thus apparent that under certain, not yet fully defined, experimental conditions, total-body X-ray irradiation could cause an activation of a naturally carried, latent parotid tumor (polyoma) virus. More frequently, however, such activation resulted in the development of well defined unilateral or bilateral parotid gland carcinomas, without a concurrent development of other tumors. The development of a spectrum of tumors in the irradiated animals was rare, but it did occur (Fig. 59, p. 713).

Interference Phenomenon Between the Leukemic Virus and the Parotid Tumor Agent

Although among the C3H mice that had been inoculated shortly after birth with Ak or C58 leukemic filtrates, some developed leukemia and others parotid tumors and/or subcutaneous fibrosarcomas, a concurrent development of both leukemia and parotid tumors in the same animal was observed only exceptionally. We have never seen leukemia and subcutaneous fibrosarcomas in the same animal, although a concurrent development of parotid carcinomas and subcutaneous fibrosarcomas in the same animal was rather frequent. Thus, it is quite possible that there may exist a certain degree of interference between the leukemic virus and the parotid tumor virus present in the inoculated filtrates. This possibility has already been discussed in reference to the increased oncogenic (but not leukemogenic) potency of heated (56°C $\frac{1}{2}$ hour) leukemic filtrates (Gross, 1960).

A slight but noticeable interference has been observed between the leukemic virus and that causing mouse mammary carcinoma. When Ak leukemic filtrates were inoculated into newborn C3H and C3H(f) mice, the incidence of induced leukemia was higher among the C3H(f) mice free from the mammary carcinoma virus than among those mice of the C3H strain which carry the Bittner virus (Gross, 1957). (See also p. 340.)

It is thus quite possible that a similar slight interference may also exist between the leukemic virus and the parotid tumor agent.

THE TISSUE-CULTURE-GROWN PAROTID TUMOR (POLYOMA) VIRUS. ITS ENHANCED POTENCY

Previous Attempts to Grow Oncogenic Viruses in Tissue Culture. Carrel carried out a series of experiments in 1926 in which he demonstrated that the virus of Rous sarcoma could be maintained and propagated *in vitro*, provided that the medium, which was composed chiefly of chicken serum and Tyrode solution, contained also normal leukocytes or fragments of normal chicken spleen or embryonic pulp. If the added tissue fragments were small, the virus disappeared rapidly. When, however, the fragments of normal tissues were sufficiently large, an abundant production of virus resulted. When fragments of spleen or normal leukocytes were added to the medium from time to time, and when the cultures were transferred into new flasks every 2 to 3 weeks, the Rous sarcoma virus maintained its virulence. Cultures that had been kept for 2 months produced at least 1 cm^3 of highly virulent fluid every day. When inoculated into susceptible chickens, tumors were induced within 15 or 16 days.

In Carrel's experiments, the Rous virus did not multiply in the presence of fibroblasts. Ludford (1937), on the other hand, succeeded in propagating the Rous sarcoma virus, or the Fujinami chicken sarcoma virus, in cultures of normal chicken fibroblasts from the pectoral muscle, or from the heart of young chicks.

Furth and his coworkers (1934, 1937) tried to determine whether a chicken leukosis virus (strain 13) capable of inducing sarcoma and leukemia could be propagated in tumor cells. They were able to show that this virus could be readily maintained *in vitro* in tumor cell cultures. After cultivation *in vitro* for 2 to 5 months, the tumor cells still produced a virus which was able to induce either sarcoma or leukosis.

Verne and his associates observed (1936) that bone marrow from leukemic chickens could be maintained in tissue culture, and the virus survived if fragments of normal bone marrow were added to such cultures.

Ruffilli (1937, 1938) showed that cells derived from myocardium of leukemic chickens could be passed in tissue culture repeatedly; after 44 passages (122 days) they still retained their infectivity. Doljanski and Pikovski (1941) were able to maintain in tissue culture cells from leukemic chickens for up to 181 days; such cultures still remained infectious, reproducing leukemia on bio-assay.

In 1942 Doljanski and Pikovski reported that the virus of chicken leukosis could be propagated *in vitro* in the presence of normal fibroblasts, normal bone marrow cells, or normal myocardium. In the absence of living cells the agent of fowl leukosis lost its activity within 24 hours. By serial cultivation of fibroblasts infected with the leukosis agent, the latter could be maintained *in vitro* for 178 days. The transformation of normal fibroblasts into tumor cells *in vitro* under the influence of the Rous sarcoma virus was observed by Halberstaedter and his associates (1941).

The rabbit fibroma virus could be propagated through 14 or 15 successive serial passages, *in vitro*, on normal cottontail rabbit testes cells (Kilham, 1956). No cytopathogenic effect was noted, but the virus increased in its titer in each passage. Bauer, Constantin, and their associates (1956) also were able to maintain and propagate the rabbit fibroma virus in tissue culture. Later on, Kilham (1958) was also able to grow in tissue culture the rabbit myxoma virus on normal rabbit cells or on monkey kidney cells, and the squirrel fibroma virus on normal squirrel or rabbit kidney cells.

Oncogenic viruses could be maintained in tissue culture in heterologous cells; Pikovski (1953) propagated mouse mammary carcinoma virus in chick fibroblast tissue culture for several successive passages.

Lasfargues and his colleagues (1958) were able to maintain the mouse mammary carcinoma agent in cultures of normal mouse mammary epithelium. After 4 passages and 35 days *in vitro* the agent still induced mammary tumors when inoculated into susceptible mice.

Manaker and his associates at the National Cancer Institute (1960) were able to propagate the Moloney strain of mouse leukemia virus on normal mouse spleen cells in tissue culture. No cytopathogenic effect was noticed, but the virus multiplied and could be passed serially.

In these and other experiments carried out with several different oncogenic viruses, it was possible to demonstrate that such viruses survived in tissue culture and that they multiplied to a sufficient extent so that their presence in the tissue culture fluid could be demonstrated by bio-assay even after a number of consecutive serial passages *in vitro*. In none of these studies, however, has there been any evidence that after passage in tissue culture, an oncogenic virus acquired a strikingly higher tumor-inducing potency, as compared with the oncogenic potential of filtrates prepared directly from tumors. Propagation of oncogenic viruses in susceptible animal hosts was still the method of choice, not only because of its simplicity, but mainly because extracts prepared directly from tumors were in most instances more potent on bio-assay than were tissue culture fluids collected after the cultivation of the tumor agents *in vitro*.

Attempt to Grow the Parotid Tumor Virus in Tissue Culture. As in the case of other, previously observed, tumor viruses, it was obviously of interest to determine whether the recently isolated parotid tumor virus could be propagated in tissue culture. Cell-free extracts, prepared either from Ak leukemic donors or from leukemic-filtrate-induced parotid tumors, were placed in tubes containing monkey kidney (*M. rhesus*) cells, i.e. tissue culture cells routinely employed for the propagation of the virus of poliomyelitis and of other human and animal viruses.

The results of these experiments carried out at the National Institute of Health in Bethesda, Md. (Stewart, Eddy *et al.*, 1957) were of considerable interest. At least one of the oncogenic viruses present in the extracts was found to grow and multiply actively in the normal monkey kidney cells *in vitro*. The leukemic extracts prepared from Ak leukemic donors and used for the inoculation of the monkey kidney cells *in vitro* contained the parotid tumor virus (Gross, 1953) and also the leukemic virus (Gross, 1951). The leukemic virus did not grow in tissue culture under the conditions employed. However, the parotid tumor virus grew actively and multiplied on heterologous (monkey) kidney cells. Later on mouse embryo cells were substituted (Stewart *et al.*, 1958) and were found more suitable.

The parotid tumor virus grew in tissue culture with such a vigor that fluids harvested after several serial passages were found to be considerably more potent on bio-assay than extracts prepared directly from either Ak leukemic tissues or from parotid tumors initially employed for the inoculation of the tissue cultures (Stewart *et al.*, 1957).

When cell-free extracts prepared directly from parotid tumors were inoculated into 175 newborn C3H/He mice or (C3H $\times$ AKR) F_1 hybrids, none developed parotid gland tumors or related neoplasms.* When, on the other hand, extracts prepared from parotid tumors, or from spontaneous Ak leukemia, were first used for the inoculation of monkey kidney cells in tissue culture, then passed serially *in vitro*, and the tissue culture fluid subsequently harvested was inoculated into 66 newborn (C3H $\times$ AKR) F_1 hybrids, 34 (51 per cent) of them developed parotid gland tumors. All mice that developed tumors as a result of inoculation of the tissue culture fluid had parotid neoplasms. Some, in addition, had submaxillary tumors; several developed also medullary adrenal tumors, mammary gland carcinomas, and/or epithelial thymic tumors. In a control series, 71 newborn mice were injected with fluids from normal, uninoculated tissue cultures, and none developed tumors.

A similar variety of tumors could be induced in previous experiments, carried out in our laboratory, with filtrates prepared directly from Ak leukemic tissues and inoculated into newborn C3H mice (Gross, 1953). The incidence of tumors induced with leukemic extracts was, however, lower than that which could be induced with the tissue-culture-grown parotid tumor virus.

* In our previous experiments, parotid and submaxillary gland tumors, subcutaneous fibrosarcomas, medullary adrenal tumors, and even leukemia could also be induced with extracts prepared directly from parotid gland tumors (Gross, 1955, 1957). It is quite possible that extracts prepared from parotid tumors in our experiments had a higher content of virus than those prepared from parotid tumors in Dr. Stewart's study. Furthermore, the susceptibility of mice of the C3H/Bi strain employed in our studies for the bio-assay was higher than that of the C3H/He subline used in experiments reported by Stewart.

It was quite apparent, therefore, that the oncogenic potential of the parotid tumor virus was considerably increased after tissue culture passage.

The tumor virus, grown in tissue culture, required a certain incubation period in order to become oncogenic on bio-assay. Thus, after the monkey kidney cells were inoculated with the parotid tumor virus, the tissue culture fluid became pathogenic only after an incubation, at 36°C, for about 2 weeks. Tissue culture fluids harvested only one week after first passage seeding with the virus were usually inactive on inoculation tests. A longer incubation period or several successive passages were essential in order to harvest an amount of virus sufficient to induce tumors on bio-assay (Stewart *et al.*, 1957, 1958).

A limited series of experiments suggested that chick chorioallantoic membrane cells were also suitable for the culture of the virus. More suitable, however, for the *in vitro* propagation of the parotid tumor virus were mouse embryo cells maintained in tissue culture (Stewart *et al.*, 1958).

Serial Passage of the Parotid Tumor, i.e. Polyoma Virus in Mouse Embryo Cells and Gradual Increase of its Potency

Embryos, removed aseptically from randomly bred Swiss mice (of the National Health Institute's "general purpose" stock) in the 14th to 18th day of gestation, were minced, treated with 0.25 per cent trypsin, and suspended in nutrient fluid, usually mixture 199* with inactivated calf serum (1 to 2 per cent) and antibiotics (penicillin and streptomycin) added. The cultures were kept at 36°C. The parotid tumor virus was passed serially after having been maintained in such cultures for 2 weeks or longer. Passages were made from culture to culture, with intervening passages through newborn mice.

The mouse embryo cells were found to be more suitable for the culture of the parotid tumor agent than the monkey kidney cells. This was shown by a greater frequency and variety of tumors induced with the harvested tissue culture fluid, a shorter latency time required for the induction of tumors, and a higher titer of the virus (Stewart *et al.*, 1958).

The tumor virus grown under such conditions induced on bio-assay parotid gland tumors, as well as a variety of other tumors, in the great majority of either (C3H × AKR) F_1 hybrids or mice of the randomly bred Swiss stock. Of 112 hybrids, inoculated when less than 1 day old with the tissue-culture-grown parotid tumor virus, 77 (69 per cent) developed tumors at 4 to 8 months of age. Of 67 Swiss mice, inoculated when less than 1 day old, 62 (92.5 per cent) developed tumors at 3 to 4 months of age. All mice that developed tumors had parotid neoplasms. In addition, about one-third of these mice had also submaxillary gland tumors, and a

* Commercially available, synthetic nutrient medium.

few developed also sublingual gland neoplasms. Over 40 per cent of these mice had also thymic epithelial tumors. About 30 per cent had mammary carcinomas, and some 20 per cent had renal sarcomas. A few mice developed also bone sarcomas, epidermoid carcinomas of the skin or digestive tube, adrenal medullary tumors, liver hemangiomas, and a few other odd tumors. A total of 23 different neoplastic lesions were listed (Stewart *et al.*, 1958a); many of them, however, developed only in very few mice. The primary neoplastic manifestation was the consistent development of parotid gland tumors in all mice that developed neoplasms as a result of the inoculation of the tissue-culture-grown virus.

As controls, 420 Swiss mice and 200 (C3H × AKR) F_1 hybrids were inoculated when less than one-day-old with supernatant fluids from mouse embryo tissue cultures that had not been seeded with the parotid tumor virus. None of the control mice developed parotid gland tumors.

Many of the mice inoculated with the tissue-culture-grown virus were dwarfed. A similar observation was made previously when extracts prepared directly from Ak leukemic tissues or from parotid tumors were inoculated into newborn C3H mice (Gross, 1953, unpublished).

The parotid tumor virus grown on mouse embryo cells required an incubation period similar to that observed in previous experiments in which this agent had been grown on monkey kidney cells. Only fluids from cultures which had been maintained for approximately 2 weeks or longer at 36°C were oncogenic on inoculation tests. In some instances tissue culture fluid became oncogenic earlier, particularly if an agent that had been passed serially was used for the seeding of the tissue cultures. A high oncogenic potency of the tissue culture fluids was usually attained, however, only after 2 or even 3 weeks. Gradually, after several successive passages through tissue culture cells, and also through animals, the virus acquired an increased potency and grew faster in tissue culture. Frequently, cytopathogenic effect could be observed after less than 10 days, occasionally even earlier. Tissue culture fluid collected from such tubes readily induced parotid tumors and related neoplasms on bio-assay.

Fig. 55a. Photomicrograph of a Parotid Tumor.

A C3H(f) male was inoculated when less than 14 hours old with a centrifuged extract prepared from normal Ak embryos containing the parotid tumor virus, and developed at the age of 7 months bilateral parotid gland tumors. A photomicrograph of a section of a small, apparently newly developed tumor nodule was reproduced in Fig. 54a on page 673. This photomicrograph represents a section of a larger and more undifferentiated nodule of the parotid tumor from the same mouse. Magnification 290 × (H. & E.).

Fig. 55b. Photomicrograph of a Virus-induced Subcutaneous Sarcoma.

Spindle and giant-cell sarcoma. This C3H male was inoculated when less than 9 hours old with a cell-free centrifuged (7,000 × g) mouse parotid tumor extract, and developed at 8½ months a rapidly growing subcutaneous tumor infiltrating the right front leg in the vicinity of the axillary pit. This tumor could be readily transplanted to C3H mice, retaining its peculiar morphology. Magnification 330 × (H. & E.). (From: L. Gross, *Proc. Soc. Exp. Biol. & Med.*, **88**: 362, 1955.)

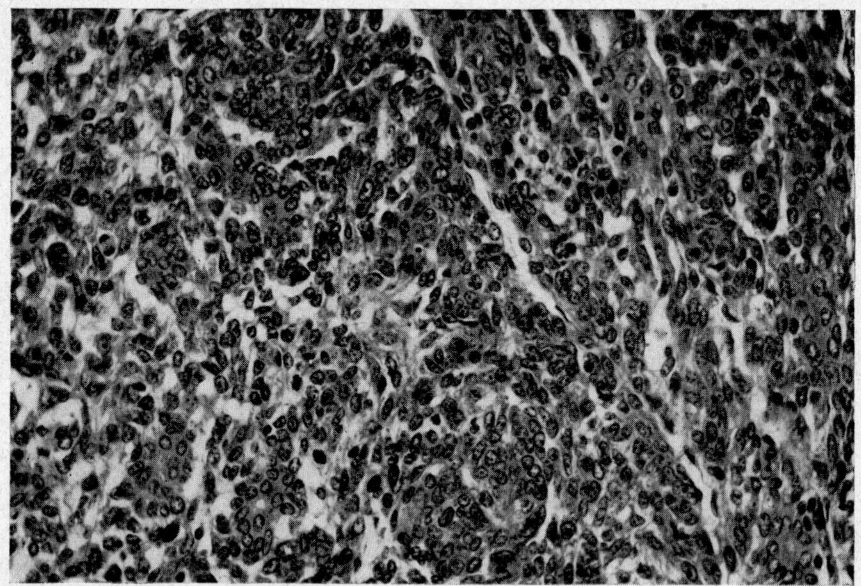

Fig. 55a. Photomicrograph of a Parotid Tumor.

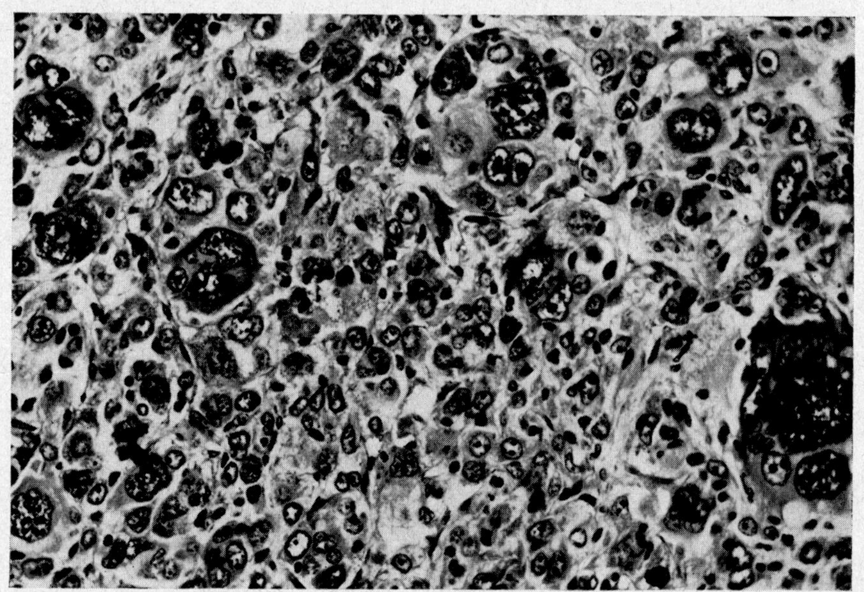

Fig. 55b. Photomicrograph of a Virus-induced Subcutaneous Sarcoma.

Cytopathogenic Effect of the Parotid Tumor, i.e., Polyoma Virus on Mouse Embryo Cells

During the early tissue culture passages of the parotid tumor virus the infected cells did not differ much from the uninfected controls. Gradually, however, as the passages were continued, changes could be noticed in the morphology of the cells. Patches of small dark cells appeared within 4 to 7 days after the inoculation of the virus; the numbers of such pyknotic cells increased gradually within the next week until most of the cells were affected; eventually, many of the damaged cells fell from the glass. These changes were particularly pronounced when the tissue culture virus was grown on mouse embryo cells. When cultured on monkey kidney cells, the virus either did not induce cytopathogenic changes at all, or induced changes which were not very pronounced.

The infectivity of the virus, as determined on bio-assay, appeared to be correlated with the degree of cytopathogenic effect induced in tissue culture (Eddy *et al.*, 1958). The tumor-inducing potency was determined by the ability of the tissue culture fluid to induce tumors following inoculation into newborn hamsters. When the cells in which the virus was grown showed a pronounced cytopathogenic effect, all animals inoculated with the harvested tissue culture fluid developed tumors after a relatively short incubation time. On the other hand, when the cells in which the virus was grown showed only little or no cytopathogenic effect, the fluid harvested from such cultures produced only a few tumors on bio-assay, after a relatively long latency interval.

The bio-assay was, however, a more sensitive test for the demonstration of the presence of the oncogenic virus than the cytopathogenic effect observed in tissue culture.

Susceptibility of Mice of Different Strains

When the parotid tumor virus was initially recovered directly from Ak leukemic extracts (Gross, 1953), it had only a moderate tumor-inducing potency and a rather narrow host specificity. It induced parotid tumors and occasionally also a few related neoplasms, following inoculation into newborn C3H mice, into newborn (C3H × AKR) F_1 hybrids (Stewart, 1955. Law *et al.*, 1955), and also into newborn Ak or AKR mice (Rogel and Rudali, 1957. Latarjet *et al.*, 1958. Dulaney and Goss, 1960).

Following passage through tissue culture, the same virus acquired a substantially higher potency, inducing parotid neoplasms and a wide variety of tumors following inoculation into newborn mice. The tumors induced included salivary gland tumors, subcutaneous and kidney sarcomas, mammary carcinomas, skin tumors, osteosarcomas, etc. Furthermore, the host specificity of the virus became broader. The tissue-culture-grown virus induced tumors not only in mice of the C3H strain or in (C3H × AKR) F_1 hybrids, but also in mice of the Swiss stock (Stewart *et al.*, 1958). Additional experiments carried out subsequently in several laboratories, employing the tissue-culture-grown parotid tumor (polyoma) virus for inoculation of newborn mice, revealed that parotid gland tumors, and in certain instances also related neoplasms, such as subcutaneous sarcomas, etc., could be induced readily in mice of several different inbred strains (Mirand *et al.*, 1958, 1960. Dawe *et al.*, 1959b). Particularly susceptible were mice of strains C3H, Ak or AKR, (C3H × AKR) F_1 hybrids, and DBA/2. Relatively susceptible also were mice of strains SWR (Swiss), RFM, DB/1, StoLi, and C58. Quite resistant were mice of strains C57 Black and C57 Brown, although now and then parotid tumors could also be induced in such animals. These studies established the curious fact that the tissue-culture-grown parotid tumor (polyoma) virus retained its strain specificity in mice even though it was pathogenic also for other species such as rats and hamsters. The possible presence of specific antibodies in mice of certain litters employed for inoculation also had to be considered. Presence of such antibodies in mice of otherwise susceptible strains inhibited the oncogenic potential of the inoculated virus.

Importance of Age at Inoculation

In previous experiments in which the parotid tumor virus recovered directly from leukemic extracts was used for inoculation, only newborn, less than one-day-old, mice were found to be susceptible to the induction of parotid tumors (Gross, 1953, 1958). When suckling mice, more than one day but less than 5 days old, were inoculated, parotid tumors or related neoplasms, such as subcutaneous sarcomas, developed only very occasionally and after a long latency interval (Gross, 1957, 1958, unpublished). After the parotid tumor virus was passed through several tissue culture passages, its potency and host range increased. Moreover the virus was now able to induce tumors following inoculation into suckling, more than one-day-old, mice. This was demonstrated in experiments carried out by Dawe and his associates (1959) at the National Cancer Institute, in which one to 5-day-old C3H mice, and also (C3H × AKR) F_1 hybrids, were found to be susceptible to the induction of tumors with the tissue-culture-grown parotid tumor virus.

We have also observed occasional development of parotid tumors following inoculation of leukemic-tissue-derived parotid tumor virus into one to 5-day-old C3H mice. The latency was prolonged, however, in these cases, and the tumors were more localized and appeared rather as single nodules than multiple clusters; they also grew more slowly.

The use of newborn, less than 16-hour-old, mice for the inoculation of the tissue-culture-grown (or mouse-tissue-derived) parotid tumor virus still remains the method of choice, since newborn mice are more sensitive to the oncogenic potency of this virus than older suckling animals.

Suckling mice 13 to 14 days old were also inoculated, but were found to be considerably more resistant. Only very few tumors could be induced when suckling mice 17 to 21 days old were inoculated (Dawe *et al.*, 1959b). In a few instances, however, even young adult C3H mice 30 to 40 days old were found susceptible, provided that they received massive doses of the parotid tumor virus by intravenous route or had been irradiated (300 R total-body) prior to the inoculation of the virus.

Effect of Thymectomy

In recent experiments in which the tissue-culture-grown parotid tumor (polyoma) virus was employed for inoculation, it was demonstrated that C57 Black mice, which are highly resistant to the induction of parotid tumors, became susceptible following complete thymectomy performed within 24 hours after birth (Miller *et al.*, 1964. Malmgren *et al.*, 1964. Law, 1965). The susceptibility to the oncogenic potency of the polyoma virus could be inhibited in thymectomized mice by implantation of normal spleen cells (Law, 1965).

Thymectomy performed shortly after birth in rats also increased the susceptibility of animals of that species to the oncogenic potency of the polyoma virus (Vandeputte *et al.*, 1963. Vandeputte and De Somer, 1965).

Salivary Gland Tumors and a Variety of Other Neoplasms Developing in Mice Following Inoculation of the Tissue-culture-grown Parotid Tumor (Polyoma) Virus

When newborn mice were inoculated with the tissue-culture-grown parotid tumor (polyoma) virus, most of them developed tumors. The incidence of induced tumors ranged from 80 to 100 per cent. The latent periods varied from 6 weeks to 12 months; the majority of tumors developed after 2 to 5 months. The following is a brief survey of tumors induced in mice with the tissue-culture-grown parotid tumor (polyoma) virus (Stewart *et al.*, 1957, 1958a. Stewart, 1960).

The neoplasms consistently induced in mice with the tissue-culture-grown virus were tumors of the parotid glands; they were present in all mice that developed tumors following inoculation of the virus; in addition to salivary gland tumors, many of these mice developed also a variety of other neoplasms similar to those previously described (Gross, 1953, 1955. Stewart *et al.*, 1957).

Salivary Gland Tumors. The parotid gland was found to be most susceptible to the oncogenic effect of the virus. All mice that developed tumors following inoculation of the tissue-culture-grown polyoma virus developed also parotid gland neoplasms. The parotid tumors were usually multilobular and bilateral. Those mice that received virus of low potency developed only parotid gland tumors. More active virus preparations induced also tumors of the submaxillary and sublingual salivary glands. Still stronger virus cultures induced also tumors of the accessory mucous and serous glands of the head and neck. Metastatic tumors in the lungs were common, particularly in young mice.

Renal Sarcomas and Renal Cortical Lesions. About one-half of the Swiss mice which received tissue-culture-grown polyoma virus developed lesions of the renal convoluted tubules with varying degrees of cellular hyperplasia. In some animals the hyperplasia resulted in a papillary infolding of the epithelium into the lumens of the dilated tubules, resembling early adenocarcinomas (Stewart, 1960). About one-third of the Swiss mice with the renal cortical lesions also developed diffuse kidney sarcomas which arose presumably in the mesenchymal tissues of the pyramids. Frequently several foci of early sarcomas were found in one kidney. In several mice the renal tumors were bilateral.

Epithelial Thymomas. About 26 per cent of the Swiss mice inoculated with the tissue-culture-grown polyoma virus developed circumscribed epithelial thymic tumors. Some of these rapidly growing tumors were mucoid on cutting. In many of the early tumors, the thymus showed hyperplasia of Hassall's corpuscles.

Mammary Carcinomas and Hair Follicle Epidermoid Carcinomas. Mammary carcinomas developed in about 25 per cent of the inoculated Swiss mice and also in some of the inoculated mice of other strains. These tumors developed not only in females, but occasionally also in males. About 40 per cent of mice with mammary carcinomas developed also tumors of hair follicles; some of these tumors were epidermoid carcinomas.

Bone Tumors. About 22 per cent of the Swiss mice inoculated with the tissue-culture-grown polyoma virus developed bone tumors in the skull, mandibles, scapula, vertebrae, and also in the long bones of the femur and humerus. The bone tumors were frequently multiple. Histologically, they ranged from those benign in appearance to malignant. Metastases to liver and lungs were observed in several mice.

Subcutaneous Sarcomas. Some of the mice that lived for several months or longer developed subcutaneous sarcomas, often associated with salivary gland neoplasms.

Other Tumors. Among other tumors observed were hemangio-endotheliomas, visceral hemangiomas, sweat gland adenocarcinomas, and medullary adrenal carcinomas.

Induction of Cysts in Mice. Rowson and his colleagues (1961) observed the development of multiple cysts, either in the subcutaneous tissues or arising in the lymph nodes, following inoculation of newborn mice with the tissue-culture-grown polyoma virus. Some cysts were multilobular; they were filled with lymph, or with a thin, blood stained fluid.

* * *

This impressive variety of tumors could be induced in mice with a single oncogenic virus, i.e., the tissue-culture-grown polyoma virus.

In the initial studies the possibility could not be excluded that the polyoma virus induced actually only some of the tumors observed in the inoculated mice, and that it might have activated other latent oncogenic viruses which could have been responsible for the development of some of the other tumors. However, repeated attempts, employing tissue culture plaque methods, to isolate the causative viral agent, or agents, resulted in the recovery of only the polyoma virus from the different primary neoplasms (Stewart, 1960).

It must be emphasized that parotid tumors and other salivary gland tumors as well as mammary carcinomas, subcutaneous sarcomas, and medullary adrenal carcinomas had been observed previously in earlier experiments in which extracts prepared from leukemic mouse tissues which contained the parotid tumor virus were inoculated into newborn C3H mice (Gross, 1953). Such tumors, however, were induced only occasionally with extracts prepared from leukemic mouse tissues, since these extracts contained a parotid tumor virus of only a relatively low potency. The tissue-culture-grown virus was considerably more potent and induced much more frequently a great variety of tumors.

INDUCTION OF TUMORS IN OTHER SPECIES WITH THE TISSUE-CULTURE-GROWN PAROTID TUMOR (POLYOMA) VIRUS

Induction of Tumors in Hamsters

Surprisingly, the tissue-culture-grown virus was also found to be oncogenic when inoculated into newborn hamsters.

In 1930, Aharoni captured 8 hamsters (*Cricetus auratus*) in Syria and brought them to Jerusalem. From an initial nucleus consisting of 1 male and 2 female litter-mates, Ben Menachem developed a colony of Syrian golden hamsters

> for experimental purposes in Prof. Saul Adler's Department of Parasitology in Hebrew University, Hadassah Medical School, in Jerusalem. All Syrian hamsters used for experimental research throughout the world are descendants of this initial breeding nucleus. This genealogical closeness is of importance for the comparison of studies from different laboratories. Among the pertinent attributes of the hamster are the ease with which it breeds under laboratory conditions, its relative freedom from spontaneous disease, and its high susceptibility to certain pathogenic viruses, such as poliomyelitis, foot-and-mouth disease, West Nile virus disease, influenza, mumps, psittacosis, etc. (Ashbel, 1956).

In a series of experiments carried out at the National Institute of Health in Bethesda, Md. (Eddy *et al.*, 1958), the parotid tumor virus was grown on mouse embryo cells with medium 199 containing 1 per cent inactivated calf serum. The nutrient fluid was removed and replaced at weekly intervals. The tissue culture fluid was harvested after an incubation, at 36°C, for at least 2 weeks or longer.

Newborn, less than one-day-old, Syrian golden hamsters (*Cricetus auratus*) were inoculated subcutaneously with the supernate from the harvested tissue culture fluid containing the parotid tumor virus. Of 61 inoculated hamsters, 34 (56 per cent) developed tumors, mostly sarcomas. Some of the tumors appeared as early as 2 to 3 weeks after inoculation. Most of the tumors developed within 4 to 8 weeks.

Development of Diffuse Renal Sarcomas, and also of Small Sarcomatous Nodules in the Heart Muscle

Most of the tumors induced in hamsters with the polyoma virus were found in the kidneys. In many of the inoculated hamsters both kidneys were massively and symmetrically enlarged because of diffuse and rapidly growing sarcomas. Multiple small nodular sarcomas were found in the myocardium in both auricles and in the ventricles. Multiple metastatic tumors

---

FIG. 56a. VIRUS-INDUCED SUBCUTANEOUS SARCOMA IN A C3H MOUSE.

This C3H(f) male was inoculated when less than 12 hours old with a cell-free centrifuged extract prepared from a mouse parotid tumor, and developed after 14 months a slowly growing spindle-cell fibrosarcoma under the skin of the back. The tumor grew progressively, infiltrating gradually also the peritoneal lining.

FIG. 56b. PHOTOMICROGRAPH OF A VIRUS-INDUCED SUBCUTANEOUS SARCOMA.

Subcutaneous spindle-cell fibrosarcoma in a C3H female. This mouse was inoculated when less than 15 hours old with a cell-free centrifuged extract prepared from a mouse parotid gland tumor, and developed $10\frac{1}{2}$ months later a slowly growing, hard and fibrous subcutaneous tumor on the back, in the vicinity of left groin. Magnification 310 × (H. & E.).

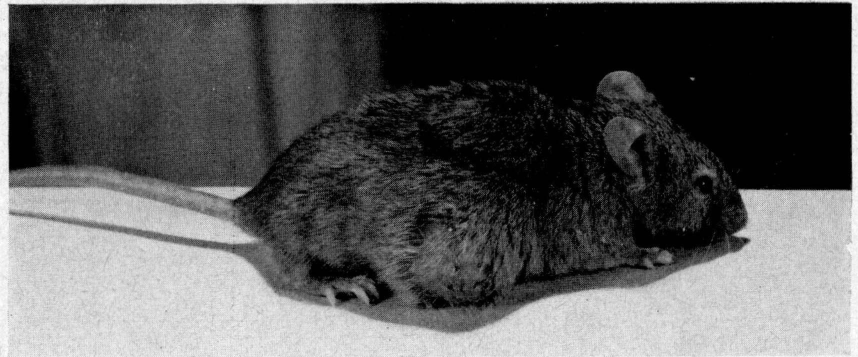

FIG. 56a. VIRUS-INDUCED SUBCUTANEOUS SARCOMA IN A C3H MOUSE.

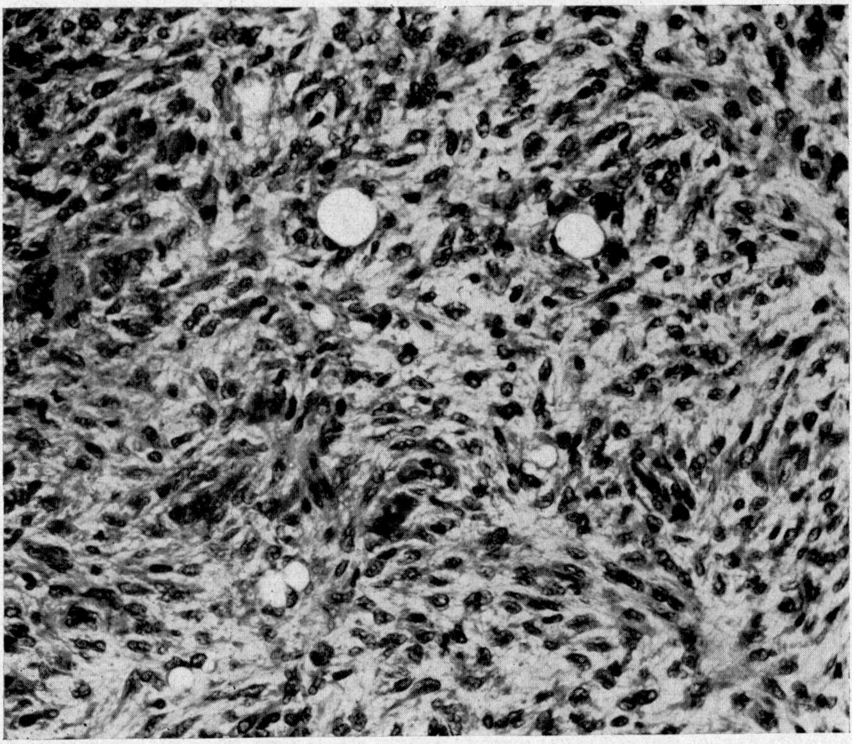

FIG. 56b. PHOTOMICROGRAPH OF A VIRUS-INDUCED SUBCUTANEOUS SARCOMA.

were observed in lungs and liver. Subcutaneous tumors, or small tumors of the organs of the gastrointestinal tract, on the serosal and mucosal surfaces, were also observed. Most of the tumors induced in hamsters were well differentiated spindle-cell sarcomas or anaplastic sarcomas of varying morphology; some contained multi-nucleated giant cells. Many animals also had lesions of the blood vessels. Angiomatous tumors and cavernous hemangiomas were common in the liver or lungs, and occasionally also in other organs. Many hamsters had multiple neoplasms.

Tissue culture fluid harvested from normal mouse embryo cells,* grown under similar conditions but not inoculated with the tumor virus, did not induce neoplasms when injected into 93 newborn hamsters (Eddy *et al.*, 1958).

No tumors were induced in 9 hamsters inoculated with extracts prepared directly from mouse leukemic tissues.

This fundamental observation was promptly confirmed and extended in several laboratories (Mirand *et al.*, 1958. Gimmy *et al.*, 1959. Negroni *et al.*, 1959. Rowe *et al.*, 1959. Axelrad *et al.*, 1960. Ham *et al.*, 1960. Chesterman and Negroni, 1961. McCulloch *et al.*, 1961). A few of these experiments were carried out with strains of polyoma virus isolated from different sources, such as the "Mill Hill" strain isolated from the spleen of a leukemic Ak mouse (Negroni *et al.*, 1959), or another strain isolated from a mammary carcinoma in a C3H mouse (McCulloch *et al.*, 1961).

Susceptibility of Suckling Hamsters. Two- to 4-day-old suckling hamsters were found to be most suitable for the inoculation of the tissue-culture-grown virus and were soon employed routinely for the bio-assay of the parotid tumor (polyoma) virus. The immediate mortality of such animals was lower than that which frequently followed the inoculation of the virus into newborn hosts; yet, they were found essentially as susceptible as newborn animals.

* Mirand and his associates (1958) observed the development of parotid tumors in 3 mice and multiple visceral tumors in 1 hamster, following inoculation of normal tissue culture fluid from a single batch of a control, non-seeded, mouse embryo cell-line.

We have also observed the development of parotid tumors in mice following inoculation of tissue culture fluid from normal mouse embryo cell cultures (Gross, unpublished, 1959). The possibility should be considered that either the parotid tumor virus contaminated the control tissue culture fluid, or that the normal mouse embryo cells harbor the virus in a low concentration; the titer of virus may then increase following cultivation of the embryo cells *in vitro.*

The latter possibility would be consistent with the results of our previous experiments in which normal healthy mice of several non-leukemic strains, such as C3H or C57 Brown/cd, were found to carry the parotid tumor virus in a latent form (Gross, 1955).

Nine- and even 24-day-old hamsters were found to be still susceptible when inoculated with the tissue-culture-grown virus (Eddy *et al.*, 1958). However, the susceptibility of older suckling animals, or weanlings, was lower than that of newborn or suckling, less than 4-day-old, hamsters.

Presence of Virus in Hamster Sarcomas

When extracts prepared from some of the virus-induced hamster sarcomas were passed through mouse-embryo tissue cultures, the harvested fluids again reproduced tumors on bio-assay in either hamsters or mice. This suggested that tumors induced in hamsters with the tissue culture fluid contained the oncogenic virus (Eddy *et al.*, 1958).

The virus could be passed without difficulty from one animal to another, and from one species to another, but always with tissue culture passage interposed between each animal passage.

> Rowe and his colleagues were able to transmit the virus directly from one hamster to another through several passages, without an interposed tissue-culture propagation of the virus. Tissue-culture-grown virus was inoculated into suckling hamsters, and the inoculated animals were sacrificed 3 to 7 days later, before they developed tumors. From organs (heart, livers, kidneys, and lungs) of such animals centrifuged extracts were again prepared and inoculated into newborn hamsters. This procedure was repeated several times. After 10 and even 17 successive hamster-to-hamster passages, the virus could still be demonstrated in the extracts. It induced tumors following inoculation into hamsters, and it could also be grown and identified in tissue-culture by serological methods. (Rowe, W. P. Personal communication to the author, 1960.)

It is apparent that the virus is present in a relatively low concentration in the induced hamster sarcomas; furthermore, antibodies or inhibitors may be also present in tumor cells. Tissue culture passage may not only increase the titer of the virus, but may release the virus from antibodies and inhibitors.

Transplantation, by Cell-Graft, of Hamster Sarcomas

Attempts to transplant the virus-induced tumors in hamsters failed in the initial experiments (Eddy *et al.*, 1958), but succeeded later in experiments carried out by Habel and Atanasiu (1959), in which a fibrosarcoma induced by inoculation of a tissue-culture-grown parotid tumor virus into a suckling hamster was transplanted through 8 successive cell-grafts in adult hamsters, preserving its original morphology. Axelrad and his co-workers (1960) transplanted, by cell-graft, virus-induced sarcomas from one hamster to another. Of 8 kidney tumors transplanted into adult hamsters, 5 grew progressively and killed their hosts in 3 to 10 weeks.

Negroni and his associates (1959) also transplanted, through several successive generations, the virus-induced kidney sarcomas in hamsters.

Suckling Hamster: the Animal of Choice for Bio-Assay of the Tissue-culture-grown Parotid Tumor (Polyoma) Virus. When, in the initial experiments performed by Eddy and her coworkers (1958), tumors were first induced in hamsters following inoculation of the tissue-culture-grown mouse parotid tumor (polyoma) virus, the susceptibility of the heterologous host might have been at first considered a curiosity, perhaps of theoretical interest, but of limited practical value. In the course of subsequent experiments, however, the suckling hamster gradually proved to be the animal of choice for the bio-assay of the tissue-culture-grown parotid tumor (polyoma) virus. When either unfiltered or filtered tissue culture extracts containing the virus were inoculated subcutaneously into newborn or suckling hamsters, multiple subcutaneous and visceral tumors, particularly those of heart and kidneys, were induced after a remarkably short incubation period of only 2 to 5 weeks.

Induction of Tumors in Rats

The rat was found to be the third mammalian species susceptible to the induction of tumors with the tissue-culture-grown mouse parotid tumor virus (Eddy *et al.*, 1959).

As in previous experiments, the virus cultures originally derived from leukemic tissues of an Ak mouse were first passed serially through monkey kidney cells, and later through mouse embryo cells, with intervening passages through newborn mice. The virus was then grown routinely on mouse embryo cells, with synthetic medium 199 and 1 per cent calf serum employed as nutrient. The tissue cultures were incubated at 36°C. The nutrient fluids were replaced at weekly intervals, but only fluids removed after 2 or more weeks were transferred to new cultures, or used for inoculation of animals.

Development of Kidney Sarcomas, Subcutaneous Sarcomas, and Hemangiomas of Liver

The tissue culture fluid containing the virus was inoculated into newborn, less than 24-hour-old, rats of the random-bred Sprague-Dawley stock.

Of a total of 65 newborn rats inoculated with tissue culture fluid, 7 developed subcutaneous sarcomas, and 18 developed sarcomas of the kidneys. Several of the kidney tumors were bilateral. Some of the kidney tumors measured over 5 cm in diameter. They infiltrated the surrounding tissues, growing progressively.

Many rats had multiple tumors. Three of the rats with renal tumors had also metastatic tumors in the lungs. A few rats had cavernous hemangiomas of liver (Eddy *et al.*, 1959).

These findings were promptly confirmed and extended in other laboratories (Mirand *et al.*, 1958. Negroni *et al.*, 1959. Fogel *et al.*, 1960).

The virus-induced tumors in rats could be readily transplanted by cell-graft through several successive generations (Mirand *et al.*, 1960).

Howatson and his colleagues (1960), working with a tissue-culture-grown oncogenic mouse virus closely related to, and considered to be a variant of, the parotid tumor (polyoma) virus, also observed the development of massive kidney sarcomas appearing within 3 to 6 weeks following inoculation of the virus into newborn rats of the Wistar stock.

In more recent studies, Flocks and his coworkers (1965) observed that the microscopic forms of tumors induced in rats varied with the concentration of the injected virus. Intravenous inoculations of highest (undiluted) virus doses into newborn W/Fu rats resulted in the formation of multiple, capillary, cystic or cavernous hemangiomas in the brain and spinal cord, which caused death within 2 to 4 weeks. Medium doses (10^{-1} to 10^{-2}) induced multiple tumors, including renal sarcomas, hemangiomas, osteogenic sarcomas, etc., after a slightly prolonged latency. Low virus doses (10^{-3}) caused a single tumor, usually a renal sarcoma, with a relatively long survival time of 2 to 4 months.

Attempt to Recover the Oncogenic Agent from Virus-induced Rat Sarcomas

An attempt was made to recover the virus from the renal sarcomas (Eddy *et al.*, 1959). An extract consisting of minced spleen and tumor tissue from a rat with a virus-induced renal sarcoma was used for inoculation of mouse embryo cells in tissue culture. The fluid was harvested after 2 weeks and passed serially. The fourth serial transfer was harvested and inoculated into a litter consisting of 7 suckling, 3-day-old hamsters; six of them developed visceral tumors not different from those previously induced with the tissue-culture-grown parotid tumor virus. The twelfth serial passage of the rat-derived virus was used for inoculation of a litter consisting of 11 rats less than one day old; as a result, 6 of them developed renal sarcomas at ages varying from 2 to $4\frac{1}{2}$ months; three of these animals had also subcutaneous sarcomas, and one had a liver hemangioma.

It was thus apparent that tumors induced with the tissue-culture-grown virus in rats also contained the virus, which multiplied in the rats and could later be harvested from these hosts.

The virus could be recovered from the induced kidney sarcomas, provided that a tissue culture passage was interposed. No experimental evidence has yet been reported suggesting that a filtrate prepared directly from a renal rat sarcoma reproduced this tumor following inoculation into newborn rats without an intermediary passage of the virus through tissue culture. It is quite probable, however, that a direct rat-to-rat filtrate transmission of the virus will also eventually be accomplished.

Induction of Tumors in Ferrets

Harris, Chesterman and Negroni (1961) described the induction of tumors in ferrets following inoculation of the Mill Hill strain of the polyoma virus. The tumors were induced by subcutaneous or intraperitoneal inoculation of the tissue-culture-grown polyoma virus or of phenol-treated virus (to obtain infective DNA) into newborn ferrets, and developed at the inoculation site in 6 of the 39 inoculated animals. The induction periods varied from 2 to 12 months. Five of the tumors were fibrosarcomas; three of these arose at the subcutaneous injection site, and 2 in the retroperitoneal tissues following intraperitoneal inoculation. The sixth tumor was an osteosarcoma which developed in the diaphragm with metastases in liver and lung. One subcutaneous fibrosarcoma was surgically excised and followed through five recurrencies (Pomerance and Chesterman, 1965).

Induction of Tumors in Guinea Pigs

Eddy and her coworkers reported (1960) that tumors having a microscopic character of undifferentiated sarcomas could be induced with the polyoma virus in guinea pigs. The tissue-culture-grown polyoma virus was inoculated into 94 newborn, less than 24-hour-old hybrid guinea pigs, and 28 of them developed tumors at the site of inoculation. The latency period varied from a few weeks to several months; in some instances the latency was prolonged and exceeded one year. The tumors were round and firm, usually adherent to the overlying skin; most of the tumor nodules were encapsulated, but in some areas there was invasion of the adjacent muscles and connective tissues. The tumors grew progressively and eventually killed the animals (personal communication to the author from Dr. B. E. Eddy). Microscopically these tumors had a character of spindle-cell, or pleomorphic, undifferentiated sarcomas. Small tumor nodules could also be found in the liver, kidney, spleen, or lungs of some of the tumor-bearing animals.

The larger tumors developed only at the site of inoculation. When tumors were present at other sites, they were very small macroscopically, or could be detected only on microscopic examination.

The virus could be isolated from one of the induced tumors by passage through tissue culture.

Induction of Tumors in Rabbits. Small tumor nodules having a character of fibromas could be induced with the tissue-culture-grown polyoma virus following inoculation of newborn rabbits (Eddy *et al.*, 1958). These tumors regressed spontaneously in all animals after one to four months.

Induction of Tumors in Mastomys

The polyoma virus was also found to be pathogenic for *Rattus* (*Mastomys*) *natalensis*, an African rodent intermediate in size between the rat and the mouse. In experiments carried out by Rabson and his colleagues (1960), the tissue-culture-grown polyoma virus was inoculated subcutaneously into 4 litters of newborn, less than 12-hour-old, *Mastomys*.

Six months after inoculation, 24 out of 30 inoculated animals were found dead; because of cannibalism, only 17 animals were autopsied and in 14 of them tumors were found; some had multiple tumors. Thirteen animals developed sarcomas of the kidneys, 2 animals had small sarcomatous tumors in the heart ventricle and atrium, and 2 had subcutaneous sarcomas. Four animals developed angiomatous tumors in the liver; three of these tumors were associated with rupture of the blood vessels resulting in accumulation of blood in peritoneal cavity.

The virus could be recovered from one of the renal sarcomas by passage through tissue culture.

The "Parotid Tumor Virus" and the "Polyoma Virus" Two Names for the Same Oncogenic Agent

When first isolated in our laboratory from Ak leukemic extracts, this oncogenic virus was designated the "parotid tumor agent" (Gross, 1953), because when inoculated into newborn C3H mice it induced as a primary neoplastic manifestation multicentric parotid gland tumors; in some mice, in addition to parotid tumors, development of other neoplasms followed, such as submaxillary gland carcinomas, subcutaneous fibromyxosarcomas, mammary gland carcinomas (Gross, 1953), and medullary adrenal tumors (Gross 1955a).

Stewart, Eddy, and their coworkers (1957, 1958) passed Ak leukemic extract through monkey kidney cells, and later through mouse embryo-cell tissue cultures, with intermediary passages through newborn mice. The virus passed under these conditions regularly induced in the inoculated mice parotid gland carcinomas, microscopically identical with those previously observed when Ak leukemic filtrates were used for bio-assay. Furthermore, some of the mice inoculated with the tissue-culture-grown agent developed a spectrum of tumors, essentially similar to that previously described in our studies. After several tissue-culture passages, the potency of the agent increased; the induced spectrum of tumors became broader; moreover, the agent now also induced sarcomas and other tumors in hamsters and rats.

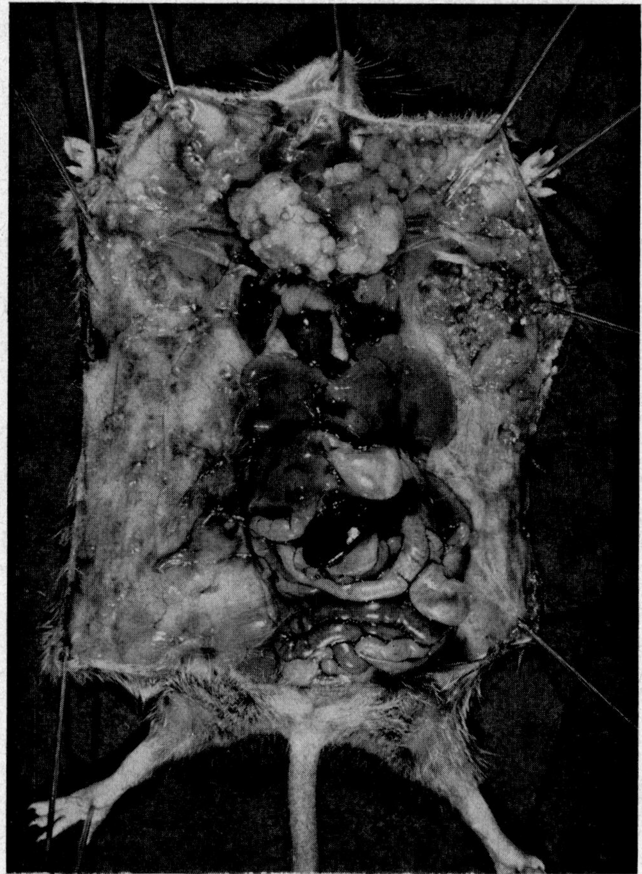

FIG. 57. SALIVARY GLAND TUMORS, MULTIPLE EPIDERMOID SKIN CARCINOMAS, AND OTHER NEOPLASMS INDUCED WITH A HEATED MOUSE LEUKEMIA EXTRACT.

This C3H(f) female was inoculated when less than 1-day-old with heated (56°C for ½ hour) passage A virus filtrate, and developed after 2½ months parotid and submaxillary gland carcinomas, multiple epidermoid skin carcinomas, a subcutaneous sarcoma in the vicinity of the left groin, and a subcutaneous carcinoma in the left axillary area. The development of these tumors was caused by the parotid tumor virus. The passage A virus extract prepared from organs of leukemic mouse donors frequently contains not only the mouse leukemia virus, but also the parotid tumor (polyoma) agent. Heating to 56°C for ½ hour inactivates the mouse leukemia virus, but does not affect the relatively more resistant parotid tumor virus.

Stewart and Eddy proposed to designate the tissue-culture-grown virus the "S.E. Polyoma virus" (1958). However, they were dealing with the same virus which had first been isolated and identified in our laboratory. It had the same origin, the same physical properties, and an essentially similar, though increased, pathogenic potential (Eddy *et al.*, 1958).

The Tissue-culture-grown Polyoma Virus is Immunologically Indistinguishable from the Parotid Tumor Virus. Immunologically, the tissue-culture-grown polyoma virus was found to be indistinguishable from the parotid tumor virus isolated directly from the leukemic extracts in our laboratory. The immunological hemagglutination-inhibiting cross neutralization tests were carried out by W. P. Rowe and J. W. Hartley (personal communication to the author, 1959).

Neutralization of the Parotid Tumor Virus Present as a Contaminant in Passage A Filtrates with Anti-Polyoma Immune Serum. Immune mouse serum prepared against the tissue-culture-grown polyoma virus did not affect the potency of the mouse leukemia virus; the same serum, however, neutralized the small amount of the parotid tumor virus present in passage A filtrates.

Passage A filtrates contain the leukemic virus but frequently also, as a contaminant, traces of the parotid tumor virus (Gross, 1957, 1958). When such filtrates are inoculated into newborn C3H mice, most of the animals develop leukemia, but some may develop parotid gland tumors.

In an experiment carried out by W. P. Rowe, L. Gross, J. W. Hartley, and R. J. Huebner (1959, unpublished) a 20 per cent passage A filtrate was mixed (1 : 1), prior to inoculation, with immune mouse serum (1 : 10 dil.) obtained from mice that had received inoculations of tissue-culture-grown parotid tumor (polyoma) virus. When such filtrates were subsequently inoculated into 50 newborn C3H mice, 47 of them, or 94 per cent, developed leukemia at 3 months average age; none, however, developed parotid tumors. In a control experiment, 32 newborn C3H mice were inoculated with passage A filtrate that had been mixed (1 : 1), prior to inoculation, with a serum (1 : 10 dil.) obtained from mice that had been treated with normal, unseeded, tissue culture fluid. Twenty-nine mice (91 per cent) in this control group developed leukemia at 3 months average age, and 2 mice developed parotid gland tumors. In another control series, 33 newborn C3H mice were inoculated with the same passage A filtrate mixed (1 : 1) with sterile physiological saline solution instead of serum. Thirty-one mice (94 per cent) in this group developed leukemia at 3 months average age, and one developed parotid gland tumors. In a third control group, the passage A filtrate was mixed (1 : 1) with normal mouse serum (1 : 10 dil.) and inoculated into 11 newborn C3H mice; 8 of them, or 73 per cent, developed leukemia (none parotid tumors) at 3 months average age.

The parotid tumor virus was originally isolated from a leukemic mouse of the Ak strain (Gross, 1953). It could be isolated later, almost at will, from leukemic Ak mice in several laboratories (Stewart, 1953, 1955. Law *et al.*, 1955. Woolley and Small, 1956. Dulaney, 1956. Dulaney *et al.*, 1957. Hays and Beck, 1958. Buffett *et al.*, 1958. Latarjet *et al.*, 1958). The parotid tumor virus could also be isolated from mice of Ak colonies that were removed from the United States several years ago and have been maintained in England (Salaman, 1959).

The parotid tumor virus is essentially a mouse virus. It has never been found to be carried naturally by either hamsters or rats. Neither the rat nor the hamster is the natural host of the parotid tumor virus, although both species were found to be susceptible to its pathogenic potential.

Affinity of the Parotid Tumor (Polyoma) Virus for Mouse Salivary Glands. In its natural mouse host, following inoculation into newborn animals, this virus exhibits a remarkable affinity for the salivary glands in general, and for the parotid glands in particular. Even after more than a score of tissue-culture passages, when inoculated into newborn mice, this virus still induces parotid gland tumors in practically all of them. Other tumors develop in the inoculated mice also, but are considerably less frequent. Some, such as medullary adrenal tumors, sweat gland tumors, intestinal carcinomas, etc., have been observed only exceptionally. The primary and consistent neoplastic manifestation induced in its natural host is, and has been, the parotid gland tumor.

After tissue culture passages, the polyoma virus can also induce a variety of subcutaneous and visceral tumors, mostly kidney and heart sarcomas, in hamsters and rats. However, when it is removed from rat or hamster tumors, and, after intermediary tissue culture passage, inoculated back into newborn mice, it still induces consistently parotid gland tumors in its natural mouse host.

The term "polyoma virus," originally suggested as designation of the tissue-culture-grown parotid tumor virus, has been generally accepted and used in many laboratories when referring to this oncogenic agent, irrespective of its source of isolation. We have employed in this monograph the term "polyoma virus" interchangeably with the term "parotid tumor virus." Both terms are synonymous. They represent the same virus.

Hemagglutination

Many viruses agglutinate red blood cells *in vitro*. This phenomenon was first discovered by Hirst (1941), and was reported only a few months later also by McClelland and Hare (1941) in studies dealing with culturing the influenza virus on chick embryos. When the infected allantoic fluid was accidentally mixed with chick embryo blood cells, clumping of erythrocytes resulted.

The importance of this phenomenon was rapidly recognized. Many other viruses were found to agglutinate red blood cells of one or several species.

Each virus has its own spectrum of red cell species with which it can combine. In a few cases the spectrum is narrow and may be largely limited to erythrocytes from species susceptible to infection with the virus employed for agglutination tests. In other instances the spectrum is broad. In general, the susceptibility of red blood cells from different species to the agglutinating action of viruses varies; erythrocytes of some species are more susceptible than others. Fowl erythrocytes are commonly used. Of the readily available mammalian types, human and guinea pig red blood cells are susceptible to the agglutinating action of a wide range of viruses.

In one group of viruses, which includes variola, vaccinia, and ectromelia, the hemagglutinins are separable from the virus particles. Another group consists of viruses, such as mumps, Newcastle disease, or influenza, which agglutinate by virtue of a specific adsorption of the virus particles by the red cells, the virus, as the smaller entity, forming a series of bridges holding the agglutinated red cells together. In this group there is considerable evidence that the hemagglutinin is a part of the virus particle.

Some viruses form a rather stable combination with susceptible erythrocytes, which can be dissociated only by changing the conditions under which adsorption took place, such as pH, salt concentration, etc. Another group of viruses, which includes influenza, Newcastle disease, and mumps, are characterized by the ability of the adsorbed virus particles to spontaneously elute from the red cells (Hirst, 1942). This phenomenon could readily be observed when the influenza virus was allowed to act in test tubes on chicken erythrocytes at refrigerator (+4°C) temperature. Agglutination resulted. When, however, the test tubes containing the agglutinated red blood cells with the adsorbed virus were placed in an incubator, at 37°C, or at room temperature, after a relatively short period of time the virus was liberated and eluted spontaneously. With the liberation of the virus, the red blood cells recovered their suspension stability. The agglutination phenomenon was thus abolished, the erythrocytes dispersed and settled normally. From then on, the red blood cells were insensitive to agglutination with the same virus, since they had lost their receptors.

The agglutinating property of the virus, as well as its infectivity, could be neutralized by a specific immune serum. This agglutination-inhibition test soon became a routine and rapid procedure in the identification of certain viruses in the laboratory.

It would be beyond the scope of this monograph to discuss in detail the important developments which followed these fundamental observations (for review see Hirst, 1950. Burnet, 1955. Anderson, 1959). These studies led to the development of standard diagnostic procedures in virus laboratories.

Hemagglutinating Action of the Tissue-culture-grown Parotid Tumor (Polyoma) Virus

The tissue-culture-grown parotid tumor virus was found to agglutinate red blood cells *in vitro* (Eddy *et al.*, 1958). Erythrocytes of hamsters, guinea pigs, or humans (group O) were found susceptible; in subsequent experiments (Hartley *et al.*, 1959), red blood cells from mice, chickens, rhesus and cynomolgus monkeys were found equally susceptible, whereas sheep and cat erythrocytes were relatively resistant. No agglutination occurred when horse, cow, or pigeon erythrocytes were employed. Sachs (1959), Fogel (1959), and their colleagues tested a large selection of red blood cells from different species in agglutination tests carried out with the tissue-culture-grown parotid tumor (polyoma) virus; in their studies, frog (*Hyla arborea*), guinea pig, and adult hen or turkey erythrocytes were found to be most susceptible. Mouse (Swiss), dog, and newborn chick erythrocytes were less susceptible. Horse, cow, and goat erythrocytes were completely resistant.

Rowe and his colleagues at the National Institutes of Health, in their extensive immunological and epidemiological studies of the parotid tumor (polyoma) virus, used guinea pig erythrocytes routinely for the agglutination tests. They found that with guinea pig red blood cells high agglutination titers could be consistently obtained; furthermore, there was relatively little variation among individual animals serving as donors for the erythrocytes (Rowe *et al.*, 1959. Hartley *et al.*, 1959).

The agglutination tests were carried out routinely in Kahn tubes by mixing the tissue culture fluid containing the virus (usually 0.2 or 0.5 cm^3 in each tube) with an equal amount of a 0.4 per cent suspension of freshly prepared and washed red blood cells. The mixture was then placed in a refrigerator at $+4$°C. This was important. Hemagglutination occurred at refrigerator temperature with dilutions of virus in titers 1 : 160 to 1 : 2560. When, however, the tubes were placed in an incubator at 37°C, or even at room temperature, the virus eluted. If, following agglutination at refrigerator temperature, the tubes were removed and placed in an incubator or at room temperature, the virus eluted promptly, and the red blood cells dispersed and settled normally.

Only tissue-culture-grown virus agglutinated. Extracts prepared from mouse parotid gland tumors did not agglutinate either mouse or guinea pig erythrocytes.

The agglutinating property of the tissue culture fluids containing the parotid tumor (polyoma) virus appeared to be correlated with the cytopathogenic effect produced by the agent on the mouse embryo cells on which it was grown, and also with the tumor-inducing property of the extracts (Eddy *et al.*, 1958. Rowe *et al.*, 1959). Tissue culture fluid harvested from tubes showing pronounced cytopathic effect of the agent on mouse embryo cells on which it had been grown had a high agglutinating titer and induced a high incidence of tumors on inoculation tests in hamsters or mice.

However, tumors could also be induced with tissue culture fluids having a relatively low agglutinating titer. It was quite apparent, therefore, that the bio-assay is a substantially more sensitive test for the presence of the oncogenic virus than the agglutinating property of the tissue culture fluid containing the agent.

The tumor inducing potency of different samples of tissue-culture-grown parotid tumor virus varied. Some were more active than others on inoculation tests. If a tissue culture fluid had a high agglutinating titer, it was then found to produce also a high incidence of tumors on inoculation tests carried out either on newborn mice or on newborn hamsters. If, on the other hand, the tissue culture fluid had a low agglutinating titer, or even none at all, it could still induce a relatively high incidence of tumors on bio-assay (Gross and Dreyfuss, 1960, unpublished); its tumor-inducing potency, however, was unknown, unless and until it was determined on animal tests.

The agglutinating potency of some of the weaker extracts could be increased by heating for 30 minutes at 37°C or 56°C (Hartley and Rowe, 1959).

Antigenic Properties of the Parotid Tumor (Polyoma) Virus

The tissue-culture-grown parotid tumor (polyoma) virus was found to have a considerable antigenic potency. When injected into guinea pigs, rabbits, or mice, it induced the development of specific antibodies. Serum from such animals (inactivated at 56°C for $\frac{1}{2}$ hour) neutralized, *in vitro*, the tumor-inducing potency of the virus, and also inhibited the cytopathogenic and agglutinating potency of the tissue culture fluid containing the agent.

High titers of humoral antibodies could be induced in heterologous hosts, such as guinea pigs or rabbits, by inoculating one dose of Freund's adjuvant mixed with tissue-culture-grown virus, followed by 2 or 3 doses of virus without adjuvant (Eddy *et al.*, 1958. Stewart *et al.*, 1959). Potent sera could also be obtained from young adult mice which received only one intraperitoneal injection of the tissue-culture-grown virus (Rowe *et al.*, 1959).

Antibodies could also be found in the sera of mice or hamsters which developed tumors as a result of virus inoculation.

The presence of antibodies could be detected either by serum-virus neutralization tests carried out by bio-assay, using hamsters or mice for inoculation tests, or by inhibition of hemagglutination *in vitro*. Normal rabbit or mouse serum, or serum from rabbits or mice that had been previously injected with normal mouse tissues, had no inhibiting effect on either the cytopathogenic, agglutinating, or tumor-inducing property of the tissue-culture-grown virus. Normal mouse sera contained only occasionally non-specific low-titer inhibitors.

It was also possible to immunize hamsters passively by injecting immune serum into such animals prior to the inoculation of the virus (Stewart *et al.*, 1959). However, injection of serum within only 60 minutes after the inoculation of the virus did not prevent the development of tumors.

The Hemagglutination-Inhibition (*HI*) *Test*

The addition of a few drops of highly diluted specific immune serum to the tissue-culture-grown virus neutralized its hemagglutinating potency. This inhibition of the agglutinating potency of the virus by a serum containing specific antibodies, a test routinely used in virus laboratories, became a useful tool also in immunological and epidemiological studies of the parotid tumor (polyoma) virus.

Hemagglutination-inhibiting (HI) antibodies in mouse serum, when present, are usually in high titers; this is true for spontaneously infected mice (Rowe *et al.*, 1959) and particularly for artificially infected animals; the titers are usually in thousands. The HI antibodies are durable, and could be detected in Rowe's experiments even 9 to 12 months after the infection of mice with large doses of virus. In tests of individual mouse sera, neutralizing or complement fixing antibodies have never been found in the absence of the HI antibody.

All strains of parotid tumor (polyoma) virus thus far studied were found to be serologically identical (Rowe *et al.*, 1960). This survey included tests on strains recovered from laboratory mice from four different cities, as well as on strains recovered from wild mice.

Non-specific heat-stable inhibitors of hemagglutination are very infrequent in mouse sera. RDE (receptor-destroying-enzyme)-sensitive inhibitor, at a level of 1 : 100 or 1 : 200, occurs in less than 0.5 per cent of mouse sera (Rowe *et al.*, 1959).

The neutralizing effect of the immune serum on the virus could also be tested using, as indicator, the cytopathogenic effect of the virus on the mouse embryo cells. The immune serum neutralized also this property of the virus. However, such tests required periods of time varying from 2 to 3 weeks; furthermore, the necessity of several nutrient-fluid changes in long observation tests made the possibility of cross-contamination a distinct risk.

The Mouse Antibody Production (*MAP*) *Test*. A very sensitive test for the detection of small quantities of the parotid tumor (polyoma) virus was

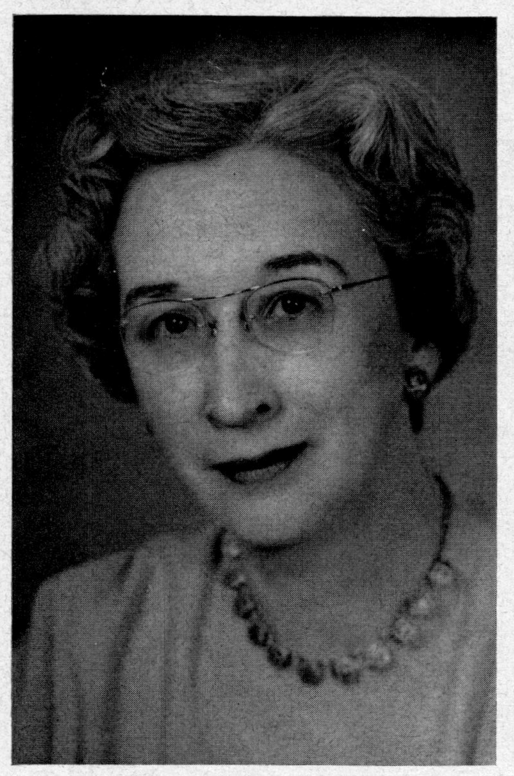

Sarah E. Stewart

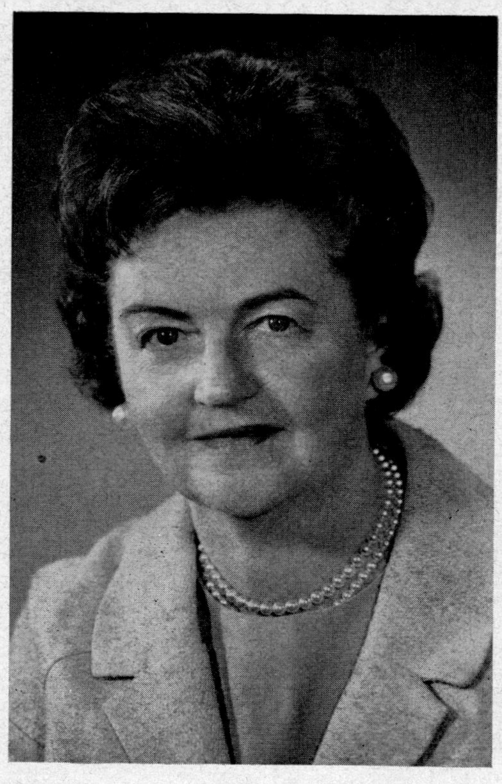

Bernice E. Eddy

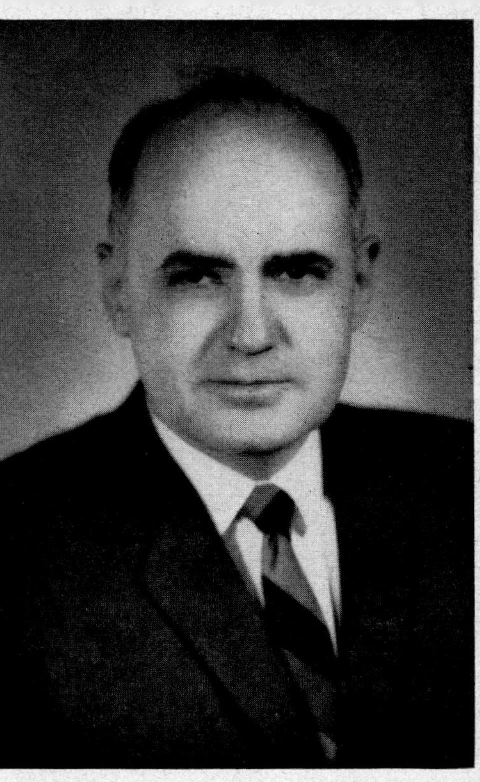

Maurice R. Hilleman

FIG. 58

developed by Rowe and his associates (1959). This test consisted of injecting a high dilution of a fluid containing the parotid tumor (polyoma) virus into young (weanling) Swiss mice. About 21 to 35 days later these mice were bled, and their serum was found to contain a high titer of hemagglutination-inhibiting antibodies which could then be demonstrated without difficulty. This test was found particularly useful in detecting the presence of virus in low titer in biological samples examined, such as in the blood of normal mice, etc.

Complement Fixation Test. Rowe and his associates (1958) carried out a series of experiments in which they demonstrated that complement fixation tests could be carried out with the parotid tumor (polyoma) virus, using tissue-culture-grown virus as antigen. Complement fixing antibodies developed regularly in newborn and adult Swiss mice given high dilutions of virus intraperitoneally, or low dilutions intranasally. Antibodies were also found in normal animals of several colonies of mice. In sera of individual mice from naturally infected stocks, the complement fixing antibodies were invariably accompanied by hemagglutination-inhibiting antibodies and hamster tumor neutralizing antibodies. However, the complement fixation test was somewhat less sensitive for the detection of antibodies, since sera from mice with low titers of hemagglutination-inhibiting and neutralizing antibodies often gave negative results in complement fixation tests.

Which Experimental Procedure Is Most Sensitive for the Detection of the Polyoma Virus? The following experimental procedures were compared (Rowe *et al.*, 1959b) in their sensitivity to detect the presence and the titer of the parotid tumor (polyoma) virus: (a) production of cytopathogenic effect (CPE) in mouse embryo tissue culture, (b) the production of hemagglutination-inhibiting (HI) antibodies after inoculation into weanling mice (mouse antibody production, or MAP test), and finally, (c) induction of tumors in suckling hamsters during a 3 to 5 week observation period. The conclusion was reached (Rowe *et al.*, 1959b) that the tissue culture and mouse antibody production tests were comparable in sensitivity, whereas the bio-assay on hamsters was not suitable for quantitative tests because of marked variations in susceptibility among the test animals.

Factors Influencing Variations in Potency of Tissue-culture-grown Virus

The potency of the tissue culture fluids containing the parotid tumor (polyoma) virus, as determined by their cytopathogenic or hemagglutinating effects, or their tumor-inducing potency, varied. Some of the factors influencing the potency of the virus could be determined; other factors remained unknown. The following observations were of interest and provided a partial explanation:

The virus grew better on mouse cells than on cells of certain other species, such as those of monkeys, rabbits, hamsters, or rats. The cytopathogenic effect could be observed only occasionally when the virus was cultured on monkey kidney cells, whereas it occurred quite regularly when mouse embryo cells were inoculated (Eddy *et al.*, 1958, 1959). Studies employing the plaque assay technique were also carried out in which the parotid tumor (polyoma) virus was grown in tissue culture in small foci under agar. The plaques induced with the virus appeared as small discrete foci of degenerated cells. Isolations from such plaques produced pure lines of virus and were then tested *in vitro* for cytopathic effect and hemagglutination, and *in vivo* for the type of tumors they induced (Sachs *et al.*, 1959a,b).

In animal experiments it has been observed by several investigators that the same stock of polyoma virus could induce the formation of various tumors in several species of animals, with different rate of release of virus, and in some instances no virus release at all. In tissue culture studies, a relatively high multiplication of the polyoma virus occurred in mouse cells, whereas very little or no multiplication of the same stock of virus was observed in hamster, rat, and rabbit cells.

The virus could be grown on normal mouse embryo, kidney or heart cells, producing a distinct cytopathogenic effect (Eddy *et al.*, 1959. Howatson *et al.*, 1960). Furthermore, the virus could also be cultured on neoplastic mouse cells, producing also a cytopathogenic effect. Rabson (1959), Banfield (1959) and their colleagues reported the propagation of the parotid tumor (polyoma) virus on transplantable mouse lymphoma cells; Howatson and his associates (1960) reported the propagation of the virus on mouse mammary carcinoma cells.

No cytopathogenic effect was noticed when the virus was cultured on either normal hamster, rat, or rabbit cells (Howatson *et al.*, 1960).

Among other factors of importance in determining the titer of the virus grown in tissue culture was the pH of the nutrient medium, the type of serum added, the length of time the virus was allowed to grow between individual passages, etc. Eddy and her associates observed (1959) that the addition of 2.5 to 3.5 cc. of a 5 per cent solution of sodium bicarbonate to each 100 cc. of nutrient medium, increased to a marked degree the cytopathogenic effect and the titer of the virus.

The importance of the serum added to the nutrient medium was also recognized (Eddy *et al.*, 1959). In the early experiments, calf serum was employed, but some of the stocks were found to contain inhibitors; accordingly, in subsequent experiments rabbit serum and later horse serum were substituted and were found more suitable.

Two Types of Virus-Cell Interaction Destruction of Cells with Virus Replication or Cell Transformation with No Virus Release

In experimental studies dealing with propagation of the parotid tumor (polyoma) virus in tissue culture two different types of virus-cell interaction could be observed. It became apparent that the virus could exert a cytocidal action leading to degeneration of cells which was accompanied by virus replication. This was observed most frequently when the virus was grown on mouse embryo cells. The cells were destroyed and large quantities of virus were released.

On the other hand, the polyoma virus could also exert a moderate stimulus on the infected cells leading to their transformation into neoplastic cells. This was observed most frequently in hamster cell cultures infected with the polyoma virus. Such transformed cells were usually unable to produce detectable virus, and were at the same time also resistant to reinfection with the same virus. Both mouse and hamster cells could be transformed into neoplastic cells as a result of infection with the polyoma virus; such transformation occurred, however, more frequently in hamster cells (Dawe and Law, 1959. Negroni *et al.*, 1959. Habel and Atanasiu, 1959. Sachs and Winocour, 1959. Vogt and Dulbecco, 1960, 1962. Dulbecco and Vogt, 1960. Eddy, 1960).

The virus-cell interaction observed in tissue culture studies is reflected also in the course of events observed in animals inoculated with the polyoma virus. Following inoculation into newborn mice, the virus produces extensive cell degeneration, which is followed only a few months later by the development of tumors. By contrast, in the newborn hamster the virus produces few degenerative manifestations, but within a short time of only a few weeks it leads to the formation of tumors.

This dual action of the virus is not an exclusive phenomenon. In hamster cells the virus usually produces neoplastic transformation, but may still undergo a limited multiplication. In some cases the transformed neoplastic hamster cell cultures may release the virus indefinitely, although in small quantities and without degenerative phenomena. This may be due to reinfection of a few cells possibly with a mutant of the polyoma virus (Dulbecco and Vogt, 1960. Sachs and Medina, 1960). Persistent virus release may be caused and maintained in mass culture by reinfection of a small proportion of cells.

Only very few virus-releasing cells occur in hamster cell cultures. In transformed mouse cell cultures this phenomenon occurs more frequently, and a small proportion of virus-releasing transformed cells is maintained. The virus may also produce a few degenerative phenomena and may be released slowly and in small quantities, insufficient to act as an effective antigenic stimulus.

On the other hand, in the mouse cells the virus induces in most instances degenerative manifestations which are accompanied by virus multiplication and release. However, some of the cells may become transformed, and these lead to a subsequent development of tumors. Among the transformed mouse cells, a few cells may also release small quantities of virus. This may be due to superinfection of some of the cells, or to a moderate virus replication accompanied by degenerative manifestations in some cells, or by virus release without any apparent degenerative phenomena occurring in other cells.

Titration of the Tissue-culture-grown Parotid Tumor Virus

The parotid tumor virus, cultured *in vitro*, multiplied actively and increased gradually in concentration. Titrations carried out with tissue culture fluid, harvested after an incubation of 2 weeks and inoculated into newborn mice, induced parotid tumors in up to 50 per cent of the inoculated animals when 10^{-3} or 10^{-4} dilutions were used for bio-assay. No tumors were induced with higher dilutions (Stewart *et al.*, 1958).

In titration experiments carried out with the tissue-culture-grown virus on suckling hamsters by Rowe and his associates (1959), tumors could be induced in 67 per cent of the inoculated hamsters with 10^{-2} dilutions, in 29 per cent of the animals with 10^{-3} dilutions, and in 16 per cent with 10^{-4} dilutions. Only one out of 35 hamsters developed tumors following inoculation with a 10^{-5} dilution, and one out of 14, following inoculation of a 10^{-6} dilution of virus. Rowe and his colleagues concluded that titrations on animals were unsatisfactory because of considerable variations in susceptibility among the inoculated hosts.

When tests were carried out *in vitro*, using, as indicator, the cytopathogenic effect of the virus on mouse embryo cells instead of animal bio-assay, dilutions as high as 10^{-6}, and even up to 10^{-7}, were found to be active on infectivity tests (Eddy *et al.*, 1959. Rowe *et al.*, 1959).

Stability of the Tissue-culture-grown Virus

The parotid tumor (polyoma) virus was found to be remarkably stable. This was determined in the experiments carried out with the parotid tumor virus isolated from Ak leukemic extracts. In these initial studies it was already recognized that the virus required heating to 70°C for 30 minutes for inactivation (Gross, 1953). Subsequent experiments demonstrated that the virus could be preserved in 50 per cent glycerin (Gross, 1956), by lyophilization (Gross, 1956), or by freezing at −70°C (Gross, 1957), and that it resisted *in vitro* exposure to ethyl ether (Gross, 1956).

These findings were confirmed and extended later on in experimental studies carried out with the tissue-culture-grown virus (Eddy *et al.*, 1958. Rowe *et al.*, 1959). Heating to 70°C for 30 minutes destroyed most of the tissue-culture-grown virus (Eddy *et al.*, 1958), usually producing complete inactivation of its infectivity and hemagglutinating potency (Brodsky *et al.*, 1959).

The virus resisted *in vitro* exposure to 2 per cent phenol, or to 50 per cent ethyl alcohol, but was destroyed by dehydrated (absolute) ethyl alcohol (Brodsky *et al.*, 1959). The tissue-culture-grown virus was sufficiently stable to retain full infective potency when preserved for at least 8 weeks at refrigerator (+4°C) temperature.

Gradocol Filtration and Ultracentrifugation Experiments. Attempts to Determine the Size of the Parotid Tumor (Polyoma) Virus

Initial experiments dealing with gradocol filtration of the parotid tumor virus were carried out with filtrates prepared from mouse leukemic extracts containing both the leukemic and the parotid tumor viruses. Extracts filtered through membranes of 340 or 200 mμ porosity induced typical generalized leukemia on bio-assay. On the other hand, extracts passed through membranes of 140 or 93 mμ porosity were still able to induce parotid gland tumors following inoculation into newborn C3H mice. No tumors were induced when filtrates passed through membranes of 60 mμ porosity were inoculated (Gross, 1957). The results of these preliminary experiments suggested that, according to the empiric formula of Elford (1931, 1933), the diameter of the parotid tumor virus particles was probably somewhere between 46 and 30 mμ (Gross, 1957).

Essentially similar results were obtained in subsequent gradocol filtration experiments carried out with the tissue-culture-grown parotid tumor virus (Eddy *et al.*, 1959). Tissue culture fluid, containing the virus and passed through either 200 mμ or 120 mμ porosity membranes, induced tumors in hamsters on bio-assay experiments. Fluids passed through membranes of 82 mμ porosity induced tumors in only 2 out of 17 inoculated hamsters. Membranes of 79 and 77 mμ porosity retained most of the virus, since only 2 out of 51 hamsters inoculated with such filtrates developed tumors. No tumors developed when fluids filtered through membranes of 43 mμ porosity were inoculated. These experiments suggested that the tissue-culture-grown virus had a diameter somewhere between 26 and 39 mμ, according to Elford's empiric formula (Eddy *et al.*, 1959).

Ultracentrifugation experiments carried out with the tissue-culture-grown parotid tumor (polyoma) virus suggested that the diameter of the virus is probably somewhere between 52 and 62 mμ (Kahler *et al.*, 1959).

Attempts to Determine the Size of the Parotid Tumor (Polyoma) Virus on the Basis of Electron Microscopic Studies

On ultrathin sections examined in the electron microscope, the size of the parotid tumor (polyoma) virus particles found in the nuclei of infected cells varied from 27 to 38 mμ in diameter.

The size of the virus particles was larger on measurement of dehydrated and chromium shadowed preparations (40 to 45 mμ), or when negative contrast preparations were examined (45 mμ).

In summary, the parotid tumor (polyoma) virus was found to be rather small, similar in size, morphology, and location in the cell nucleus to the Shope rabbit papilloma virus or to the human wart virus.

On dehydrated electron microscopic sections the polyoma virus particles have a diameter of approximately 30 to 40 mμ, whereas in solutions the size of the virus particles, determined by ultracentrifugation tests, should be placed probably somewhere between 50 to 60 mμ. These are only approximate estimates which may have to be adjusted when more exact measurements become available.

ELECTRON MICROSCOPIC STUDIES OF THE PAROTID TUMOR (POLYOMA) VIRUS

Studies of Shadowed Drop Preparations

Preliminary attempts to visualize the parotid tumor virus in the electron microscope met with difficulties. In the initial experiments, pure cultures of the parotid tumor virus were not yet available. Instead, filtrates prepared from leukemic mouse tissues, and containing not only the parotid tumor virus but also the leukemic agent, were employed. Drop preparations, deposited on collodion or formvar films, and shadowed with chromium, were examined in the electron microscope. Spherical particles varying in diameter from 30 to 70 mμ were observed (Gross, 1956). It is quite possible, indeed probable, that at least some of the smaller particles thus observed represented the parotid tumor virus; examination of drop preparations was not satisfactory, however, since other biological particles, unrelated to the parotid tumor virus but morphologically similar, could have been present in such filtrates. Furthermore, the preparations contained also the leukemic virus, presumably represented by the larger particles.

Kahler, Rowe and their associates (1959) examined in the electron microscope chromium-shadowed drop preparations of two different strains of tissue-culture-grown parotid tumor virus. Such preparations contained a relatively high concentration of the parotid tumor (polyoma) virus. Electron microscopic examination of chromium-shadowed drop preparations of such tissue culture fluids revealed the presence of spherical particles, some of them packed in crystalline arrays. These particles were remarkably uniform in size and morphology. The average diameter of particles measured in packed groups was approximately 40 to 45 mμ. The size of isolated particles was 59 mμ in length and 24 mμ in height. The determination of the size of particles by sedimentation method led to a diameter range of 52 mμ to 62 mμ. These data were consistent with the range of the size of the parotid tumor virus computed in our previous

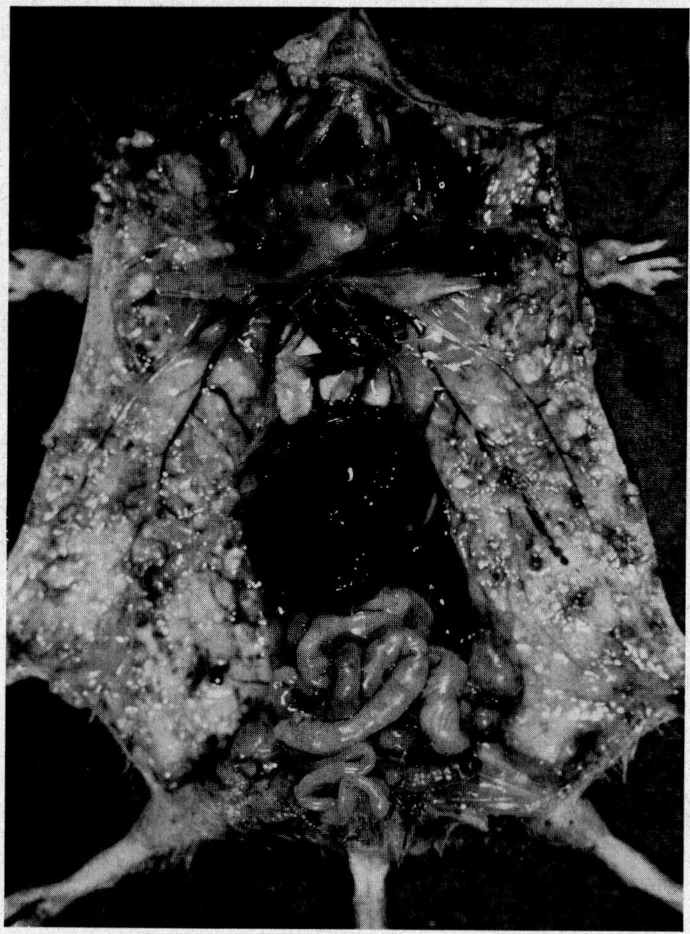

FIG. 59. SALIVARY GLAND TUMORS AND MULTIPLE NEOPLASMS INDUCED IN A MOUSE FOLLOWING ACTIVATION OF A LATENT PAROTID TUMOR VIRUS BY TOTAL-BODY X-RAY IRRADIATION.

This C3H female received 5 total-body X-ray irradiations (150 R each) at weekly intervals, starting at 4 weeks of age. When 6 months old, this mouse developed bilateral carcinomas of the parotid and submaxillary glands, multiple epidermoid skin carcinomas, and multiple liver hemangiomas. Similar tumors can be induced in mice with tissue-culture-grown parotid tumor (polyoma) virus. Normal C3H mice often carry a latent parotid tumor (polyoma) virus. Occasionally, this latent virus can be activated by fractionated total-body X-ray irradiation. More often, however, fractionated total-body X-ray irradiation induces in mice the development of leukemia resulting from activation of a latent leukemogenic virus.

studies on the basis of ultracentrifugation and gradocol filtration of tissue extracts containing the agent (Gross, 1957).

Identification of the Parotid Tumor (Polyoma) Virus on Ultrathin Sections

The introduction of ultrathin sections in electron microscopy of tumor viruses, discussed in more detail in previous chapters, made it possible to visualize the morphology of oncogenic viruses, and to differentiate virus particles from non-viral biological particles of similar size and shape.

The identification of the parotid tumor virus in electron microscopic studies of ultrathin sections of virus-infected cells was accomplished in 1959 independently, and almost simultaneously, in several laboratories (Bernhard *et al.*, 1959. Banfield *et al.*, 1959. Dmochowski *et al.*, 1959. Howatson *et al.*, 1960. Edwards *et al.*, 1960. Howatson and Almeida, 1960a,b).

The morphology of the parotid tumor (polyoma) virus and its location in cell components was revealed when ultrathin sections were examined from either: (a) virus-infected tissue culture cells or from (b) organs of virus-infected animals removed from the donors prior to the development of tumors. In some instances the virus particles could also be found on (c) examination of ultrathin sections prepared from parotid tumors or other neoplasms induced with the polyoma virus.

Intranuclear Particles and Filaments. Some Particles also Present in Cytoplasm

Bernhard and his coworkers (1959) examined ultrathin sections prepared from tissue culture preparations of the parotid tumor (polyoma) virus. Mouse embryo cells were infected with the virus. After 3 consecutive virus passages in tissue culture, the cytopathic effect resulting eventually in complete destruction of cells was produced regularly after 5 days. The virus-infected cells showing cytopathic and degenerative changes were removed, fixed with osmic acid, embedded in methacrylate, sectioned, and examined in the electron microscope. Innumerable small particles were found in the nuclei of infected cells. The particles were spherical, varying in diameter from 26 to 32 mμ, and averaging about 30 mμ. Frequently they were observed in strings or clusters, occasionally also densely packed in geometrical crystalline arrays. Often, in advanced phases, the entire nucleus was filled with the virus particles. The particles had no outer membrane, and no internal nucleoid, but rather a homogeneous density extending equally from periphery through the center.

In addition, filaments having the same diameter as the particles were found either isolated or grouped in bundles. These filaments, which were found only in the nucleus, appeared to disintegrate into individual spherical particles. It was noted in the same study that larger spherical particles varying in size from 40 to 60 mμ could also be found, although less frequently, in the cytoplasm; these larger particles were found agglomerated in certain areas within the cytoplasm. The nature and possible significance of these larger cytoplasmic particles remained undetermined.

Banfield and his coworkers (1959) used for their studies tissue culture preparations of parotid tumor (polyoma) virus grown on cell cultures of murine lymphoma strain P388 D_1. The parotid tumor virus was found to grow and multiply readily in the murine lymphoma strain, producing a cytopathic effect. After the cytopathic effect of the virus on the lymphoma cells grown in tissue culture became evident, the cells were removed, embedded in methacrylate, sectioned, and examined in the electron microscope. Intranuclear, intracytoplasmic, and extracellular spherical particles of relatively uniform size measuring approximately 27 to 35 mμ were found. Similar particles did not occur in non-infected control cultures.

Dmochowski and his associates (1959) used for their studies mouse embryo cells infected with the parotid tumor (polyoma) virus and showing cytopathic changes. Electron microscopic examination of ultrathin sections of the virus-infected cells again showed the presence of spherical particles about 27 mμ in diameter. These particles were found chiefly in the nuclei, but occasionally also in the cytoplasm and outside of cells.

Howatson and his associates (1960) used a different approach; they inoculated newborn hamsters with a virus which they considered to be a variant of the polyoma virus,* and removed the kidneys of the infected animals 5 to 7 days later, i.e. before the appearance of tumors. Light-microscope studies had shown previously that the necrotizing effect of the virus was at that time at its peak. Electron miscoscopic examination of ultrathin sections of such hamster kidneys revealed the presence of innumerable spherical particles, some of them packed densely in crystalline arrays in the nuclei of the infected cells. The diameter of individual particles was about 28 mμ, although in sections stained with lead hydroxide the particles appeared somewhat larger. Measurements made in crystalline arrays, however, gave minimum center to center separation of 38 mμ (Howatson and Almeida, 1960). The particles had no obvious limiting membrane, and they were of uniform density. These particles were located mainly in the nucleus, but some of them were found also in groups in inclusion bodies in the cytoplasm. In addition, filamentous structures with a diameter of 28 mμ often arranged in the form of bundles, similar to

* Howatson and his colleagues isolated their virus strain from a C3H mouse mammary tumor (McCulloch *et al.*, 1959). This agent was presumably a variant of the polyoma virus.

those described previously by Bernhard and his colleagues (1959), were also observed in the nuclei of infected cells (Howatson and Almeida, 1960).

A second type of particle, considerably larger than that previously described, was also observed, but only in the cytoplasm. These larger particles were less numerous than the smaller particles, and they were found only in some of the specimens examined. They had an overall diameter of about 60 mμ, and were surrounded by a single limiting membrane; they also had a centrally located nucleoid having a diameter of about 30 mμ, and surrounded by a clear zone. The larger particles were observed most frequently scattered among the smaller 28 mμ particles which greatly outnumbered them. In some instances, however, the 60 mμ particles were arranged in groups, and occasionally they were the most numerous constituents of inclusion bodies which were found in the cytoplasm. They were not observed in the nuclei (Howatson and Almeida, 1960). The role of these larger particles remained obscure, but their possible relationship to the smaller particles was considered.

The intranuclear particles, 28 to 32 mμ in diameter, were found by Howatson and his colleagues (1959) not only in the kidneys of hamsters that had been inoculated with the virus, but also in the nuclei of mouse embryo and kidney cells in which the polyoma virus was propagated in tissue culture. Occasionally a few particles were also seen in the nuclei of cells of parotid tumors that had been induced in Swiss mice with the same virus.

Edwards and his coworkers (1960) examined in the electron microscope ultrathin sections of a salivary gland tumor induced in a (Ak $\times$ C3H) F_1 hybrid female mouse by inoculation of an extract from Ak leukemic tissues containing the parotid tumor virus. Intranuclear virus particles having an average diameter of about 30 mμ were observed in the tumor cells examined. The particles were frequently associated with filaments which were also present in the nuclei. Similar small virus particles were also observed in crystalline aggregates in inclusion bodies located in the cytoplasm. Larger particles, ranging in size from 60 to 70 mμ, and surrounded by a single membrane, some of them with nucleoids, were also observed in the cytoplasm, but their possible relation to the parotid tumor virus or to other tumor viruses remained undetermined.

* * *

It was thus apparent that the electron microscopic identification of the parotid tumor (polyoma) virus was readily accomplished when ultrathin sections were examined from either virus-infected tissue culture cells, or from organs of virus-infected animals removed from the donors prior to the development of tumors. It was also possible, but more difficult, to find virus particles in the virus-induced tumors.

Types of Particles Found in Infected Cells

In summary, the following two types of virus particles and filamentous structures related to the formation of the virus particles can be seen in cells infected with the parotid tumor (polyoma) virus:

(a) *Small particles about 30 to 38 mμ in diameter* without an outer membrane. These particles are dense and spherical, often aggregated in geometrical crystalline arrays, and are present most often *in the nuclei* of infected cells. The particles have no limiting membrane and are usually of uniform density. In advanced phases the nucleus can be almost entirely replaced by arrays of closely packed particles. Particles of identical morphology can also be observed in the cytoplasm, frequently packed in crystalline arrays in what may appear as inclusion bodies. Some of these particles can also be found in groups outside of cells, occasionally arranged in rows on the outside of cellular membranes (Dourmashkin, 1962).

(b) Groups of *larger particles*, about *50 to 60 mμ in diameter*, can be found *in the cytoplasm* in what appear to be inclusion bodies. These particles have a single outer membrane, and a nucleoid having a diameter of about 30 mμ surrounded by a clear zone.

(c) *Filamentous structures* present *in the nuclei* of infected cells, having the same diameter as the smaller virus particles. The filaments are often present in bundles; some of them criss-cross at different angles and are frequently surrounded by the small particles scattered around the filaments. Apparently the filaments may break off into individual particles.

Electron Microscopic Studies of the Replication of the Polyoma Virus in Infected Cells

In more recent studies, Mattern and his coworkers at the National Institutes of Health (1966) studied step by step the replication of the polyoma virus in mouse embryo cell cultures. Fragments of infected tissues were removed at short consecutive time intervals for examination. Electron microscopic studies of ultrathin sections of the infected cells revealed invasion of the cells by the virus, the replication of the virus in the cell, and its release from the cell.

During the first 16 to 20 hours after initial infection small densely staining accumulations of material developed in the nucleus. Similar aggregates had been reported previously by Howatson and Almeida (1960) in polyoma-infected cells. In some regions, these dense bodies were resolved into bundles of filaments. Some of the bundles were surrounded by other bundles whose long axes were in slightly different directions. After 24 hours, some cells contained large numbers of filaments as well as large numbers of spherical particles. Individual filaments were of approximately the same diameter as those spherical particles which appeared frequently surrounding the bundles. It was often not possible to distinguish between individual filaments cut in cross-sections and spherical particles. Cell nuclei containing large numbers of spherical virus particles almost invariably also contained filaments in large numbers. Bernhard and his coworkers first suggested (1959) that these filaments might represent a developmental form of polyoma virus. Mattern and his coworkers (1966) offered strong support to this suggestion by the observation of a very early appearance of filaments in multiple bundles in the nucleus, their proximity to the spherical particles, and their absence in the cytoplasm.

As early as 24 hours after infection large numbers of filaments and non-arrayed particles, as well as small crystalline arrays of viruses, were observed. At later periods substantially larger nuclear crystals consisting of virus particles were encountered. Within 28 hours after infection virus particles were found not only in the nuclei but also in the cytoplasm. After this lapse of time the cell nuclei were usually filled with virus particles and were already degenerating. The virus particles were tightly packed in the nuclei and arranged in monolayers on nuclear, cytoplasmic, and on cell membranes. The particles were also observed packed between two membranes, or enclosed in spherical membranes 5 to 6 mμ in diameter as previously described by Bernhard and his coworkers (1959), Howatson and Almeida (1960), and Dourmashkin (1962). The filaments appeared to be restricted to the nucleus and were absent from the cytoplasm.

An additional feature, seen from 24 hours of infection on, was the occasional appearance of massive cytoplasmic inclusions filled with virus particles in cells which appeared to have normal nuclei. Occasionally these inclusions appeared indistinguishable from heavily infected nuclei.

The Fine Structure of Virus Particles

The negative staining method originally developed by Brenner and Horne (1959) was employed by Wildy and his colleagues (1960) for the study of the fine structure of the polyoma virus particles. Mouse-embryo cells grown in tissue culture were inoculated with a polyoma virus strain isolated in Toronto (McCulloch *et al.*, 1959). The virus was harvested from cells and employed for the preparation of specimens for electron microscopic studies. Crude suspensions of virus, or virus suspensions concentrated by centrifugation, or partially purified by extraction with fluorocarbon or chromatography, were treated with phosphotungstic acid, and then studied in the electron microscope. Spherical particles identified as viruses were found to have a mean diameter of 45 mμ. The diameter of the polyoma virus examined in specimens prepared with the negative staining method was therefore larger than that measured on ultrathin sections.

The particles showed a shell, or capsid, of regularly arranged, elongated, hollow subunits or capsomeres. In the majority of particles the capsomeres surrounded a central core; however, some particles appeared to be empty. Although there was no evidence of icosahedral shape, the capsomere arrangement showed 5 : 3 : 2 axial symmetry. It was deduced that the virus particle contains 42 capsomeres, each aligned radially along an axis of symmetry. Wildy and his colleagues concluded that even though the particle may be spherical, it nevertheless shows evidence of the 5 : 3 : 2 axial symmetry predicted by Crick and Watson (1956).

EPIDEMIOLOGY OF THE PAROTID TUMOR (POLYOMA) VIRUS

Spontaneous development of parotid gland tumors in untreated mice has been observed, but is exceedingly rare (Gross, 1955a. Rogel and Rudali, 1957. Law, 1957). Yet, the parotid tumor virus was found to be widely prevalent in normal, healthy mice of different strains (Gross, 1955a. Rowe *et al.*, 1959b, 1961. Rowe, 1961a,b).

Shortly after the isolation of the parotid tumor virus from leukemic Ak mice, it was realized that this virus is also carried by normal, healthy mice of strains C3H or C57 Brown/cd which are essentially free from spontaneous leukemia. Cell-free extracts made from normal C3H or C57 Brown mouse organs and injected into newborn C3H mice induced the development of parotid tumors in some of the inoculated animals (Gross, 1955).

Employing refined immunological methods, surveys of hundreds of mice of different strains could be carried out more recently with speed and efficiency. This survey consisted mostly of testing mice for the presence of specific antibodies, and less frequently for the actual presence of virus. Different procedures were employed, but most frequently the presence and titer of hemagglutinin antibodies (HI) were determined in the sera

Fig. 60. Polyoma Virus Grown in Mouse Embryo Cells. Intranuclear Virus Particles and Tubular Forms.

(a). Ultrathin section of a mouse embryo cell infected in tissue culture with the polyoma virus and harvested 4 days later. Nucleus of a degenerated cell packed with polyoma virus particles both in crystalline and random arrays. Magnification 50,000 ×. (b). Collection of tubular or filamentous viral forms in association with normal spherical virus particles in the nucleus of a mouse embryo cell cultivated *in vitro* for 4 days after infection with the polyoma virus. Virus particles 40 mμ in diameter. Filaments 30 mμ in diameter. Magnification 90,000 ×. Electron micrographs prepared by A. F. Howatson and M. Betlem, Ontario Cancer Institute, Toronto, Canada.

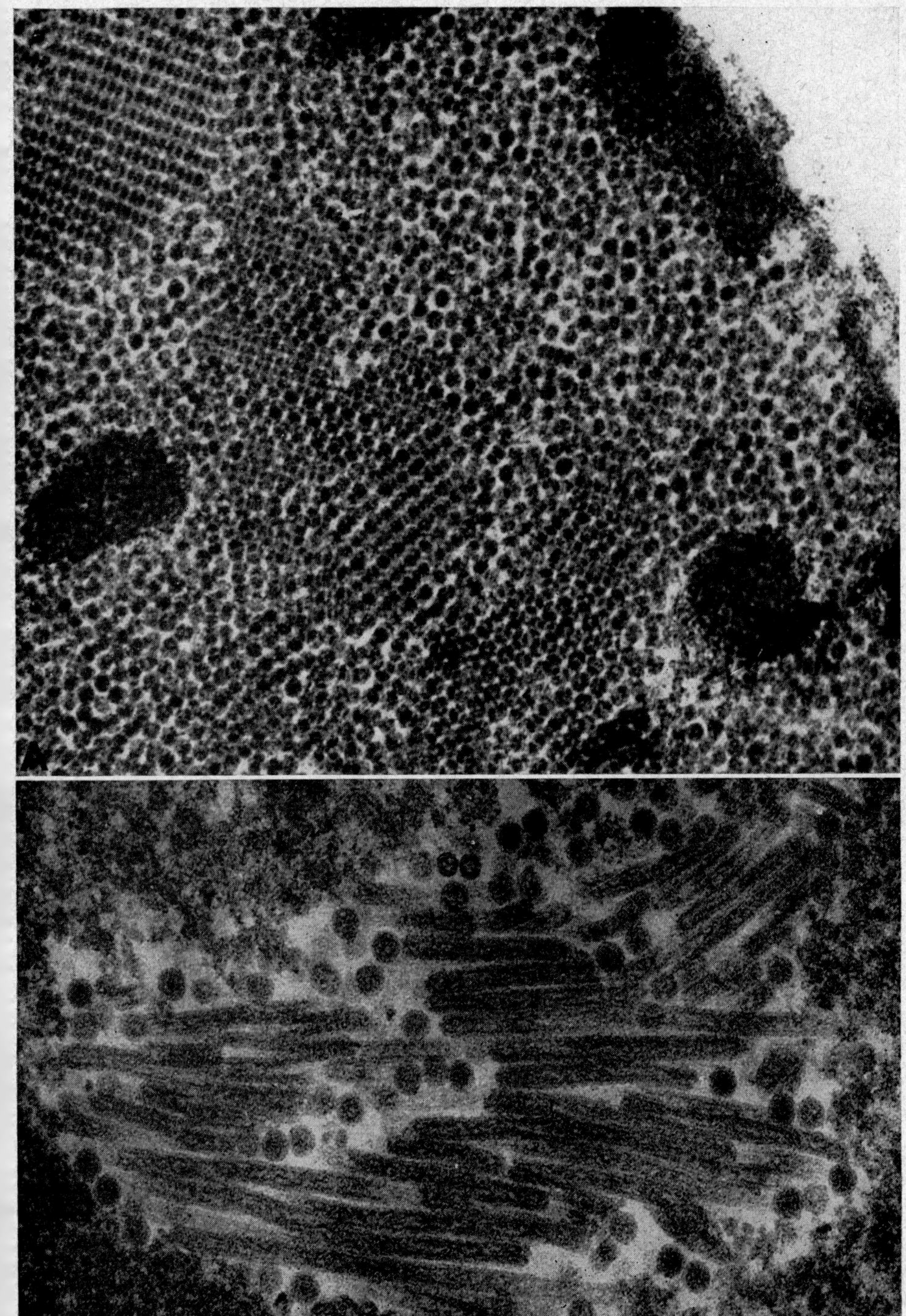

Fig. 60. Polyoma Virus Grown in Mouse Embryo Cells. Intranuclear Virus Particles and Tubular Forms.

of tested mice, or the mouse antibody production test (MAP) was employed; the latter consisted of inoculating intraperitoneally weanling mice with test material containing small quantities of virus, with the purpose of inducing specific antibody production in the injected mice; several weeks later the serum of such mice was then collected and tested for the presence of the specific antibodies. As already discussed in this chapter, this test was found to be very sensitive for the detection of small quantities of virus (Rowe *et al.*, 1959b). The complement fixation test was also employed.

The presence of specific antibodies was usually determined by inhibiting, with the serum tested, the hemagglutinating potency of the parotid tumor virus, or inhibiting the cytopathogenic effect of the virus on mouse embryo cells in tissue culture.

Over 50 per cent of mice in which specific HI antibodies were detected also carried the virus. On the other hand, only 10 per cent of mice that did not have specific antibodies carried the virus. Thus, the detection of a relatively high titer of specific antibodies in the serum of a mouse suggested that such an animal was, or had been in the past, a carrier of the parotid tumor (polyoma) virus. However, the occasional mice that did not have specific antibodies, but nevertheless carried the virus, were found only in colonies infected with the virus. Neither antibodies nor virus could be found in mice of colonies free from the parotid tumor (polyoma) virus.

The epidemiology of mouse polyoma virus infection was investigated extensively both in laboratory and field studies by Rowe, Huebner and their associates (Rowe, 1961a,b. Rowe *et al.*, 1959c, 1961. Huebner *et al.*, 1962). These studies suggested that the parotid tumor (polyoma) virus is widely prevalent in mice of different strains, and particularly in older animals. Quite frequently young adult mice, under 3 months of age, had no evidence of the presence of antibodies; in the breeding colonies, however, specific antibodies could be found in older mice. In infected colonies, mother-mice, which carried specific antibodies against polyoma virus, transmitted such antibodies to their offspring. Accordingly, newborn mice carried antibodies which they had received from their mothers. Such mice continued to carry antibodies while they were suckling their immune mothers, but lost their passive immunity after they were weaned from their mothers, i.e. when about 3 to 4 weeks old. As young adult mice, they were at first free from antibodies and presumably also from virus; however, later on many of them became infected; gradually many of the older animals in such colonies developed antibodies, indicating exposure to the virus and infection.

In another study, in a colony where mice were kept for breeding and for experiments, 19 per cent of 217 untreated mice of all ages had polyoma-virus-positive sera. However, sera from untreated mice younger than 6 months were free from polyoma virus antibodies (Yabe *et al.*, 1961).

The importance of contact infection, already suspected in previous studies (Gross, 1955), became quite apparent in subsequent experiments (Stewart *et al.*, 1958a. Rowe *et al.*, 1958–1960. Buffett *et al.*, 1958): female mice nursing inoculated litters became uniformly infected within a very short period of time, while mice kept in the same cages with the infected weanlings, or even in the same room, also acquired antibodies, but at a much slower rate.

After it was established that infection with the parotid tumor (polyoma) virus is highly prevalent in certain laboratory colonies (Rowe, 1959, 1960), serological tests were carried out on trapped wild house mice (*Mus musculus*) in tenement houses in Harlem, New York City (Rowe *et al.*, 1960. Rowe, Hartley, and Huebner, 1961). Mice from certain areas of densely populated low economic apartment house sections were found to carry specific antibodies, whereas other blocks of the same area were found relatively free from infection. Mice trapped in other boroughs were completely free from specific antibodies. The distribution of infection was thus suggestive for localized foci. Attempts were also made to recover the virus directly from trapped wild mice. The amount recovered was small but significant. Parotid tumor (polyoma) virus could be recovered particularly from mice with HI antibodies and only infrequently from mice without antibodies. The polyoma virus was found in focal areas in certain farms investigated in Maryland,* but always only in wild mice closely related to the house mouse (*Mus musculus*). When some of the field mice were examined, such as White-footed deer mice (*Peromyscus leucopus*) or Meadow voles (*Microtus pennsylvanicus*), they were found to be free from infection with the polyoma virus (Huebner *et al.*, 1962).

Other rodents and various mammals have also been tested and were found to be free from specific antibodies. Rats and cats from infected areas in New York City were also examined and found free from infection (Rowe *et al.*, 1961). Thus far, therefore, the natural infection was found to be limited to mice.

Presence of Virus in Organs and Tumors of Mice Harvested at Various Periods after Inoculation

Newborn mice were inoculated with the parotid tumor (polyoma) virus; at various periods after inoculation, several organs and also salivary glands of such animals were collected and tested for the presence of virus by the usual serological methods. In newborn mice the virus propagated in a wide variety of tissues. Virus infectivity titers reached their peak in 7 to 14 days after inoculation, particularly in kidneys and salivary glands, and gradually declined thereafter. Virus could be recovered from the tissues, and

* Rowe, W. P., and Huebner, R. J. Personal communication to the author (1960).

particularly from the parotid tumors, for at least 4 to 5 months after inoculation. By indirect immunological methods, and in a few instances also by direct tests, the virus was found in high titers in urine, and also in the saliva, but was also widely distributed in other organs. The duration of the excretion was prolonged; mice still had virus in the urine after 5 to 9 months. This applied to mice that had been infected, by inoculation, when newborn. Mice inoculated at the age of about 3 weeks, i.e. as weanlings, excreted the virus less frequently.

It was quite apparent that mice infected when newborn, or as young sucklings, were the most important carriers and donors of virus; such mice became highly infectious for their parents and cage-mates, and to some extent also for room contacts. Mice infected as weanlings or adults were much less efficient carriers of the virus. The infection pattern in such mice was characterized by lower titers of virus during the peak phase and prolonged persistence of very low quantities of virus.

Gradually, the infected mice also developed antibodies. Within 10 days after inoculation antibodies were present, and reached high levels by the 30th day. The high titers of antibodies interfered with the detection of virus in the parotid tumors by either tissue culture or mouse antibody production tests. At the time the tumors developed, such animals carried not only the virus, but also antibodies. Much of the virus was neutralized and was no longer detectable. Recovery of the virus from infected animals was thus more readily accomplished if the virus was harvested prior to the development of antibodies, i.e. prior to the development of tumors (Rowe *et al.*, 1960).

Presence of Virus Harvested from Organs and Tumors of Hamsters, at Various Periods after Inoculation

In suckling hamsters, the virus reached peak titers 4 to 6 days after inoculation, and declined rapidly thereafter. The tissues were generally non-infectious when they were tested by the third or fourth week after inoculation. Hamster tumors harvested during the third week of infection generally contained small amounts of virus, but tumors harvested at 6 to 11 weeks were generally non-infectious (Rowe *et al.*, 1960).

Routes of Natural Entry of the Virus

Infection could be accomplished by intranasal instillation of the virus, although this route was substantially less sensitive than intraperitoneal inoculation. It was quite apparent, however, that in nature mice could be readily infected by inhalation of the virus. On the other hand, only some of the mice developed antibodies when large amounts of virus were added to food or drinking water supply, suggesting thereby that, under the experimental conditions employed, the oral route was only relatively sensitive to infection with the polyoma virus. It is quite possible, however, that the digestive tract is more susceptible, as a port of entry, to polyoma virus infection in newborn and in few-day-old suckling mice.

These experiments, carried out by Rowe and his associates (1959, 1960), lead to the conclusion that the parotid tumor virus is widely prevalent among mouse populations in the laboratories, as well as among wild mice; the infection spreads and is maintained by carriers excreting the virus and infecting newborn and suckling mice. The chain of transmission may be broken when no suckling mice are infected, and when too few adult carriers excrete the virus.

Fundamental Importance of Antibodies Determining Susceptibility to the Development of Parotid Tumors, Following Inoculation of the Virus

The presence of specific antibodies in relatively high concentrations in animals belonging to particular litters born to parents that had been infected, and carried the virus, explained the curious phenomenon previously observed (Gross, 1953–1955, unpublished. Law *et al.*, 1955. Stewart, 1955. Dawe *et al.*, 1959) that some litters of newborn mice of an otherwise susceptible strain were resistant to the inoculation of the parotid tumor (polyoma) virus. Other litters of mice of the same inbred line, but free from antibodies, were highly susceptible to the inoculation of the same virus. Thus, following inoculation of either extracts from leukemic tissues containing the parotid tumor virus or of tissue-culture-grown virus into newborn mice, tumors developed in all mice of an entire litter, or in none at all, according to the presence or absence of antibodies (Law *et al.*, 1959). There was a striking correlation between the presence of hemagglutination-inhibiting antibodies carried by the mother and the susceptibility of the newborn offspring to tumor induction by tissue-culture-grown parotid tumor (polyoma) virus. Natural infection of the mother with the parotid tumor virus, apparently through contact, such as from nursing of an inoculated litter of newborn mice or by artificial exposure of mothers to the virus by inoculation, resulted in the building up of levels of specific antibodies in the mothers which were capable of protecting entire litters born to such mothers from infection with the parotid tumor virus (Law *et al.*, 1959).

The critical importance of specific antibodies in determining the susceptibility or resistance of litters employed for bio-assay thus became apparent. Inoculation of newborn mice of an otherwise susceptible strain with a potent tissue-culture-grown parotid tumor (polyoma) virus did not result in the development of tumors if the inoculated animals carried antibodies.

Infection with the Parotid Tumor (Polyoma) Virus Does Not Necessarily Lead to Subsequent Development of Tumors

These studies gradually led to the realization of the rather remote relationship between infection with a potentially pathogenic, oncogenic virus and the actual development of tumors in its natural carrier.

It has long been recognized that many potentially pathogenic viruses, such as those causing poliomyelitis or herpes, may cause symptoms of disease only in an occasional carrier. This rather remote relationship between the prevalence of infection with a given virus, and the relatively rare occurrence of disease caused by the same agent, may not have been sufficiently appreciated in the study of oncogenic viruses.

Actually, the parotid tumor virus represents an example of a "perfect parasite," a symbiont, essentially harmless for its carrier host; yet this relationship is not always harmonious. The "perfect" parasite has a formidable pathogenic potential. Under certain obscure conditions, the same virus may become pathogenic and cause the development of tumors in its carrier host. Under normal conditions of life, a spontaneous change of the virus in its natural carrier from a symbiont to a pathogen occurs only on very rare occasions.

The latent and hitherto harmless parotid tumor virus, however, can be activated in its natural carrier by certain inducing factors, such as cortisone (Woolley, 1954), "blind passage," consisting of inoculating cell-free extracts of normal mouse organs containing the agent from one host to another (Gross, 1955), or by fractionated total-body X-ray irradiation (Gross, 1958. Gross *et al.*, 1959).

One or Different Variants of the Parotid Tumor (Polyoma) Virus?

All strains of the parotid tumor (polyoma) virus thus far studied were found to be serologically identical; this included tests on strains of the virus recovered from laboratory mice from four different cities, as well as strains recovered from wild mice (Rowe *et al.*, 1961).

It is quite apparent, however, that variants of the parotid tumor (polyoma) virus exist, even though they have not been thus far differentiated serologically. Some of such variants are less carcinogenic for mice, but have a higher oncogenic potential for rats and hamsters (Howatson *et al.*, 1960). Other variants show a particular affinity for certain tissues, and induce a high incidence of thymic epithelial tumors, following inoculation into newborn mice of susceptible strains (Dawe *et al.*, 1959 b). Still other variants may retain their cytopathogenic effect on cells grown in tissue culture, yet show a reduced tumor-inducing potency (Sachs and Medina, 1960), or can be differentiated only on the basis of their agglutinating potency (Hartley *et al.*, 1959).

Isolation of an Oncogenic Agent Closely Related to the Polyoma Virus from Mouse Mammary Carcinoma. An oncogenic virus closely related to, if not identical with, the parotid tumor (polyoma) virus was recovered from a spontaneous C3H mouse mammary carcinoma (McCulloch *et al.*, 1959) at the Ontario Cancer Institute in Toronto, Canada. This virus was found to be cytopathogenic when grown on mouse embryo cells in tissue culture; it induced parotid tumors and other related neoplasms following inoculation into newborn mice, sarcomas of the kidneys and heart in hamsters, and rapidly growing kidney sarcomas in rats (Axelrad *et al.*, 1960. Howatson *et al.*, 1960. Ham *et al.*, 1960). The virus isolated by the Canadian investigators was indistinguishable serologically from the tissue-culture-grown parotid tumor (polyoma) virus maintained at the National Institute of Health by Stewart, Eddy, Rowe, and their associates. However, the virus isolated by the Canadian group was found to be less oncogenic for mice, and more pathogenic for rats and hamsters. Howatson and his colleagues concluded that the agent which they isolated was a variant of the polyoma virus (Howatson *et al.*, 1960).

The BB/T2-Polyoma Strain. From a lymph node of a mouse that had chloroleukemia, Graffi, Gimmy, and Krause (1959) isolated a virus strain closely related to the parotid tumor (polyoma) virus. This virus strain induced a variety of tumors following inoculation into newborn mice, rats, hamsters, and guinea pigs. The spectrum of the induced tumors was similar to that induced with the polyoma virus (Gimmy and Graffi, 1962).

It is conceivable that some of the variants of the polyoma virus may be so closely related that they cannot be differentiated by serological methods. Immune serum prepared against one of them may neutralize another close variant of the same virus. Such variants may, nevertheless, be sufficiently

---

FIG. 61. POLYOMA VIRUS GROWN IN HAMSTER KIDNEY CELLS. CYTOPLASMIC INCLUSION BODIES CONTAINING VIRUS PARTICLES.

Ultrathin section through a fragment of a hamster kidney cell infected with the parotid tumor (polyoma) virus. The tissue-culture-grown virus was inoculated into a newborn hamster, and 6 days later the kidney was removed. A small tissue fragment was fixed with osmic acid, embedded in methacrylate, treated with lead hydroxide, and sectioned. Two intracytoplasmic inclusion bodies are shown separated by a finger-like extension of the nucleus. The lower inclusion body (arrow) is filled with densely packed small virus particles about 30 to 40 mμ in diameter, i.e. of the size usually observed when the particles are located in the nucleus. The upper membrane-bound cytoplasmic inclusion vacuole (arrow) contains larger virus particles, most of them surrounded by a thin membrane; their average diameter is about 60 mμ. In addition there are also a few smaller virus particles about 30 mμ in diameter. Magnification 42,000 ×. Electron micrograph prepared by A. F. Howatson and J. D. Almeida, The Ontario Cancer Institute, Toronto, Canada. (From: *J. Biophys. & Biochem. Cytol.*, 7: 753, 1960.)

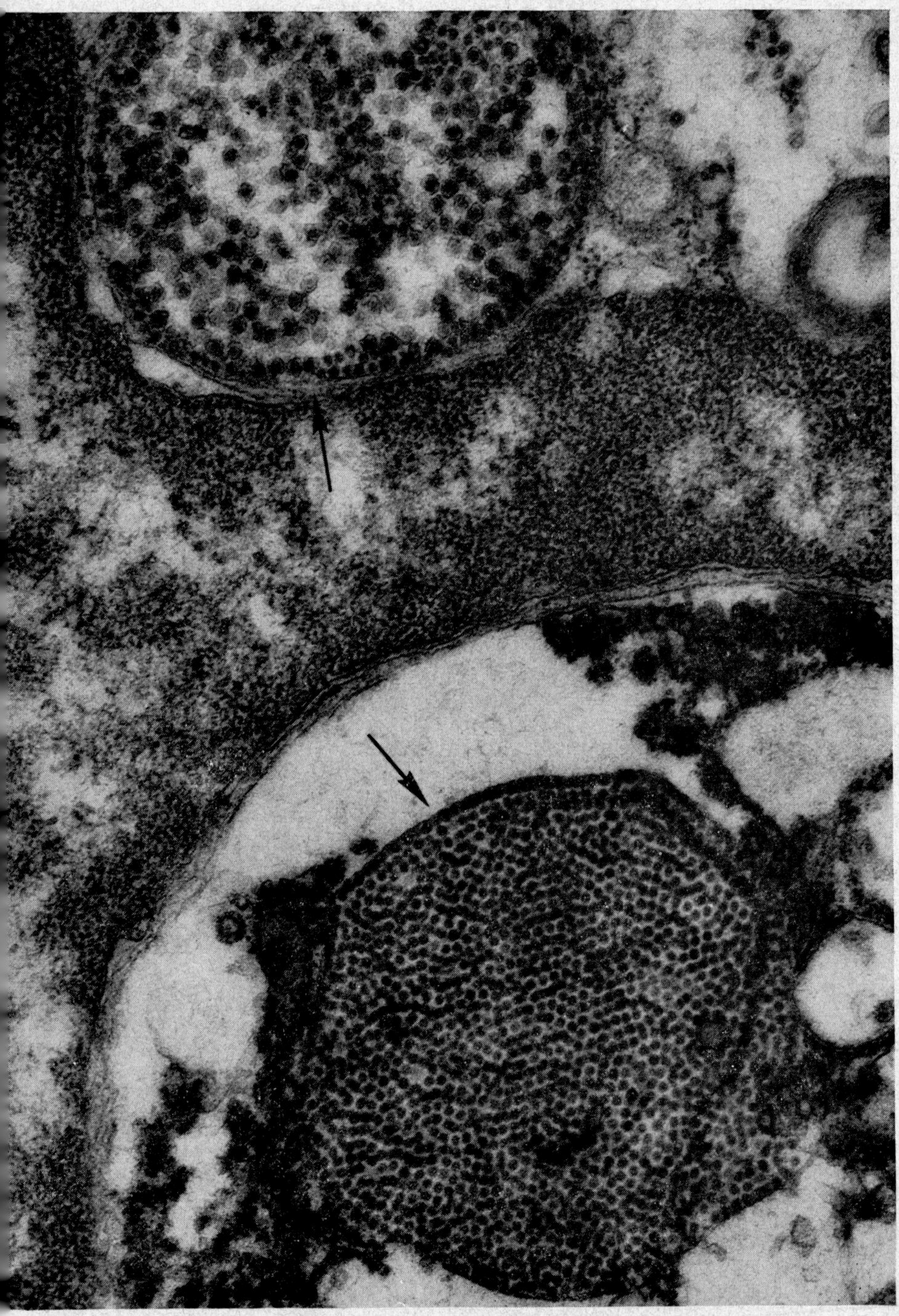

FIG. 61. POLYOMA VIRUS GROWN IN HAMSTER KIDNEY CELLS. CYTOPLASMIC INCLUSION BODIES CONTAINING VIRUS PARTICLES.

distinct to show differences in their affinity for certain species, or for certain tissues. Many viruses become gradually adapted to particular hosts, or to certain cells within a given host. This adaptation may reflect itself in the tendency of such virus types to induce a particular form of disease.

One Pluripotent, or Several Distinct Oncogenic Viruses?

The fundamental problem had to be faced whether we have been dealing with a single virus capable of inducing a spectrum of tumors, such as pleomorphic tumors of the salivary glands, subcutaneous sarcomas, mammary carcinomas, bone tumors, medullary adrenal tumors in mice, or renal and heart sarcomas in hamsters or rats, etc., or whether the polyoma virus represents a mixture of several distinct viruses of similar size and physical properties, but having a different oncogenic potential.

The general consensus of opinion among those who have been working with the parotid tumor (polyoma) virus now favors the view that we have been dealing with a single pluripotent virus which may induce a variety of neoplasms in hosts of susceptible species. Such an assumption would be consistent with the uniformity of size and morphology of virus particles observed in electron microscopic examinations of ultrathin sections prepared from polyoma virus-infected cells grown in tissue culture (Bernhard *et al.*, 1959. Dmochowski *et al.*, 1959. Banfield *et al.*, 1959), or from polyoma virus-induced tumors in mice (Edwards *et al.*, 1960) or hamsters (Howatson *et al.*, 1960). Furthermore, several attempts made to segregate this pluripotent virus into individual distinct component-viruses, by either physical and serological methods (Rowe *et al.*, 1958, 1959, 1960), or by plaque isolation technique (Sachs *et al.*, 1959. Stewart *et al.*, 1959. Dulbecco *et al.*, 1959. Vogt *et al.*, 1960. Winocour and Sachs, 1959), have thus far failed. It has not yet been possible to develop homogenous strains of polyoma virus capable of inducing a single form of tumors, such as only salivary gland tumors in mice, or only subcutaneous sarcomas in mice or rats, or only kidney sarcomas in hamsters and rats, etc. With only occasional exceptions (such as that reported by Howatson *et al.*, 1960), strains of parotid tumor (polyoma) virus isolated from various unrelated sources, including wild mice, were found to be capable of inducing, after tissue-culture passage, a very similar wide spectrum of different neoplasms in mice, hamsters, and rats.

Crawford and Crawford (1963) carried out a comparative study of polyoma and papilloma viruses. The polyoma virus was found to be different in size and in nucleic acid properties from the papilloma viruses. The Shope rabbit papilloma, bovine papilloma, canine papilloma and human papilloma viruses were similar in most respects, but differed significantly in the base composition of their nucleic acids.

ATTEMPTS TO RECOVER INFECTIOUS NUCLEIC ACID FROM LEUKEMIC EXTRACTS AND ALSO FROM TISSUE-CULTURE-GROWN PAROTID TUMOR (POLYOMA) VIRUS

Our knowledge of the physical structure and chemical composition of virus particles is only fragmentary. Very few viruses of a relatively simple structure have thus far been studied on the physical and chemical level. Perhaps the most important generalization that has emerged from these studies is that all virus particles contain nucleic acid and protein; in fact, the smaller animal and plant viruses consist probably only of these two principal components. Many animal viruses, however, range from this simplest composition to a considerably more complex structure which, in addition to nucleic acid and protein, may, among other components, also contain lipids. Larger viruses are clearly beyond the macromolecular level and can be regarded as primitive organisms. Nucleic acid is, however, the essential element which determines the reproduction of the virus particle. Infection and disease of the host are, in turn, associated with virus reproduction.

The nucleic acid, which may be either of the ribose or of the deoxyribose type, is generally centrally located and is surrounded by a protein coat. All known plant viruses contain only ribonucleic acid (RNA), while either deoxyribonucleic acid (DNA) or RNA may occur in animal and bacterial viruses.

When the virus particle enters a susceptible cell, it disintegrates into its component parts. The virus nucleic acid then initiates the production of necessary components which are later assembled into new virus particles. The newly formed particles subsequently leave the cell which may be either unharmed, partially damaged, or completely destroyed by this process. The damage to the cell, resulting from virus reproduction, is the fundamental basis for lesions due to virus diseases.

Fraenkel-Conrat (1956), and Gierer and Schramm (1956) made the remarkable observation that nucleic acid separated from the virus particles is itself infective and that it can initiate reproduction of new virus particles inducing at the same time symptoms of disease. Preliminary work on the smaller animal viruses, such as those of poliomyelitis, West Nile encephalitis, and Mengo encephalitis (Colter *et al.*, 1957), is pointing in the same direction. Ribonucleic acid preparations isolated from such viruses were infectious and induced symptoms of the corresponding diseases; they also initiated the growth of the respective viruses. One of the great difficulties in these studies, however, has been the fact that ribonucleic acid represents only a very small fraction of the dried weight of the infected particles.

In more recent experiments carried out by Holland, McLaren, and Syverton (1959), ribonucleic acid extracted with phenol from poliomyelitis virus (type I) and from certain types of Coxsackie and ECHO viruses proved infectious for animals insusceptible to complete virus. Viral ribonucleic acid proved also infectious for cells in tissue culture which were otherwise insusceptible to the virus from which the RNA had been extracted. These experiments are of considerable interest, since they suggest that, in some instances at least, the infectious ribonucleic acid extracted from certain viruses may have a wider spectrum of hosts susceptible to infection than the complete virus.

It is quite apparent that nucleic acid is the carrier of the genetic pattern of the virus and that it determines the reproduction of the newly formed particles and also the infectious process associated with the reproductive cycle of the viral agent. The important role of the protein coat of the virus cannot be minimized, however; it is directly related to the antigenic properties of the virus and also to the initiation of the infectious process, i.e. to the actual entrance of the virus particle into the susceptible cell.*

* * *

Preliminary attempts to isolate infectious nucleic acid from mouse leukemic extracts were reported by Hays and her associates (1957). The possibility was not ruled out, however, that in these studies the nucleic acid preparations, which were moderately leukemogenic, might have contained live virus particles; furthermore, the hybrid mice employed for bioassay had a relatively high incidence of spontaneous leukemia.

> In another similar study (Colter, Gross and Dreyfuss, 1959, unpublished)† RNA was prepared either from passage A leukemic filtrates or directly from leukemic tissues removed from C3H donors with passage A virus-induced leukemia. The RNA preparations were then inoculated into suckling C3H mice less than 8 days old. Out of 236 mice inoculated with the RNA preparations, only one mouse developed leukemia at $14\frac{1}{2}$ months of age.
>
> In another experiment, 113 suckling C3H mice were inoculated with DNA preparations extracted from leukemic tissues of C3H donors with passage A virus-induced leukemia. Two mice in this group developed parotid tumors at 9 months of age.

Isolation of Infectious Nucleic Acid from Leukemic Mouse Tissues. Latarjet and his associates (1958b) inoculated nucleic acid (RNA and DNA) extracted from AkR leukemic cells into newborn AkR and C3H mice. Out of 80 inoculated mice, 7 developed multiple tumors, including pleomorphic tumors of the parotid glands, subcutaneous sarcomas, and carcinomas.

* It would be beyond the scope of this monograph to review in more detail our present knowledge of the chemical architecture and physical properties of viruses. The interested reader is referred to volume I (General Virology) in *The Viruses* by Burnet and Stanley (1959), and to other more recent reviews of this subject.

† More detailed data of these experiments were summarized on pages 335 and 336 of the first edition of this monograph.

Ak leukemic cells frequently carry the parotid tumor virus; it is quite possible, therefore, that the extracts prepared by Latarjet and his coworkers contained traces of the polyoma virus, or its DNA, which could have been responsible for the induction of tumors in some of the inoculated animals. The assumption that these extracts contained infectious polyoma DNA was consistent with the information subsequently supplied by Dr. Latarjet (see DiMayorca *et al.*, 1959) that the preparations extracted from leukemic cells lost their ability to induce tumors in mice after treatment with the enzyme DNase.

Bielka and Graffi (1959) inoculated RNA prepared from mouse myeloid leukemia tissues into newborn mice. About 10 per cent of the inoculated mice developed leukemia. The leukemogenic activity of the RNA preparations was inactivated by treatment with the enzyme ribonuclease. In control experiments, the leukemogenic activity of untreated leukemic extracts was substantially higher, inducing an incidence of leukemia of 72.5 per cent.

In a more recent study, Schramm, Graffi and Förster (1965) extracted nucleic acid from lymph nodes, thymus, and spleen of mice with virus-induced myeloid leukemia. The extracts contained mostly RNA, but also some DNA. Inoculation of these nucleic acid extracts into newborn mice induced an incidence of about 9 per cent of leukemia and an incidence of 6.5 per cent of a variety of solid tumors, such as parotid tumors, fibrosarcomas, etc. It was apparent, therefore, that the nucleic acid extracts prepared by Schramm and his coworkers contained not only mouse leukemia virus or its infectious nucleic acid, but also the parotid tumor (polyoma) virus or its DNA.

The induction of anaplastic tumors in mice inoculated with ribonucleic acid preparations extracted by the phenol method from Ehrlich ascites mouse tumors was reported also by Huppert (1959), Lacour (1960), and their associates.

Isolation of Infectious Deoxyribonucleic Acid from Tissue-culture-grown Polyoma Virus*

DiMayorca and his colleagues reported (1959) the isolation of infectious DNA from mouse embryo cell cultures infected with the polyoma virus. The DNA isolated from such cultures induced cytopathic changes when introduced into normal mouse embryo cells in tissue culture. After one or two successive tissue culture passages, the polyoma virus could be recovered

* The nucleic acid of the polyoma virus was identified as DNA by the isolation of P^{32}-labeled deoxyribonucleotides from purified P^{32}-labeled polyoma virus (Smith *et al.*, 1960).

from such cultures and identified on bio-assay; it induced sarcomas following inoculation into suckling hamsters.

The infectivity of the isolated DNA could be neutralized by *in vitro* treatment of the infected tissue culture cells with the enzyme deoxyribonuclease.

The neutralization of DNA infectivity with the enzyme DNase was crucial, since it corroborated the assumption that the infective substance isolated from the polyoma virus was in fact the infectious deoxyribonucleic acid.

In a subsequent study the isolation by phenol extraction of a DNase-sensitive subviral infective agent related to polyoma virus was confirmed by Weil (1961); physical and chemical factors influencing the infectivity of the phenol extracts were described. Among the factors studied, addition of sodium versenate was found to increase and stabilize the infectivity of the phenol extracts tested by the production of plaques on mouse-embryo cell monolayers.

Similar studies were also performed with the BB-T_2 strain* of a tissue-culture-grown parotid tumor virus (Graffi and Fritz, 1960. Graffi, 1960). Nucleic acid preparations consisting of a mixture of DNA and RNA were extracted from the polyoma virus, employing the phenol method of Gierer and Schramm (1956). The neucleic acid preparations were then inoculated into normal mouse embryo cell cultures and induced a cytopathic effect. After a few passages, fluids collected from such tissue cultures were inoculated into newborn rats and induced kidney sarcomas and also bone tumors.

Atanasiu and his coworkers (1962) extracted DNA, using the phenol method, from mouse embryo cells in which the polyoma virus was propagated. The extract was inoculated in newborn hamsters. Anti-polyoma circulating antibodies could be demonstrated as early as 30 days after injection, and macroscopic subcutaneous angio-fibrosarcomas began to appear 2 months after inoculation. Similar tumors appeared in some of the animals in the livers, and in one case also in the lungs. The same extract was found to be infectious *in vitro*, inducing characteristic cytopathic changes in mouse kidney cell cultures. The infectious potency of the extracted DNA on mouse cells in tissue culture could be inhibited by the enzyme DNase.

In an extension of this study by the same group of investigators (Orth *et al.*, 1964), 35 newborn hamsters were injected subcutaneously or intracerebrally with DNA extracted from tissue-culture-grown polyoma virus. All inoculated animals showed circulating antibodies, and 26 of them

* This strain (BB-T_2) of parotid tumor (polyoma) virus was isolated from a leukemic lymph node of a mouse with virus-induced chloroleukemia (Graffi *et al.*, 1959, Gimmy and Graffi, 1962). See p. 728.

developed tumors, mostly subcutaneous fibrosarcomas, after a latency of 2 to 3 months. Adult hamsters were less susceptible to inoculation of the extracts; of 17 inoculated animals, 11 developed antibodies and only 5 developed sarcomas. The same DNA preparations were shown to be capable of infecting primary cultures of mouse kidney cells. In a control series, the extracted DNA treated with the enzyme DNase did not induce cytopathic changes in tissue culture or tumors in animals.

In an extensive study employing three different methods of DNA extraction (detergents, phenol, or papain), the following conclusions were reached by Paoletti and his colleagues (1963):

Infectious DNA can be readily extracted from polyoma virus grown in mouse embryo cells by either of the three methods employed. It is difficult, however, to eliminate with certainty any residual virus particles from the nucleic acid preparations. The best method seems to be the heating of cells at 75°C to 100°C prior to nucleic acid extraction. The polyoma DNA is heat resistant. It preserves its infectivity when the infected cells, from which it is extracted, are heated to 100°C for 30 minutes prior to the extraction procedure.

The cytopathic effect produced with polyoma DNA on mouse cells in tissue culture is in all respects comparable to that induced with the virus. However, it appears rather late, because of the low infectious titer of the extracts.

The authors suggest, as a method of choice, to extract the infectious DNA by the phenol method; furthermore, the cells from which the infectious nucleic acid is extracted should be heated to 80°C for 30 minutes prior to the extraction procedure in order to eliminate any residual virus particles (Paoletti *et al.*, 1963).

FIG. 62. POLYOMA VIRUS PARTICLES IN PAROTID TUMOR CELLS. LEUKEMIC VIRUS PARTICLES IN LYMPH NODE OF THE SAME MOUSE.

(A). Ultrathin section of a cell fragment from a parotid tumor. A group of parotid tumor, i.e. polyoma, virus particles in the nucleus of a tumor cell. The particles are spherical, and of uniform size, about 40mμ in diameter. Magnification 122,000×. (B). Section of a fragment of a lymph node from the same mouse. Budding (arrow) of a leukemic virus particle. Magnification 64,200×. (C). A group of characteristic, mature type C, leukemic virus particles (arrows), about 100 mμ in diameter, in the intercellular space in a lymph node from the same animal. Magnification 42,800×. Both sections from C3H(f) female #330, Exp. 6415C, inoculated when 6 days old with passage A mouse leukemia virus filtrate (dilution 10^{-4}) which also contained the parotid tumor (polyoma) virus. At the age of 4½ months this mouse developed a large mediastinal tumor and a generalized stem-cell leukemia; in addition, this mouse developed bilateral parotid gland tumors. Very few mice develop both leukemia and parotid tumors following inoculation of a mixture of both viruses; this is one of the few examples observed in our laboratory (L. Gross and D. G. Feldman, unpublished).

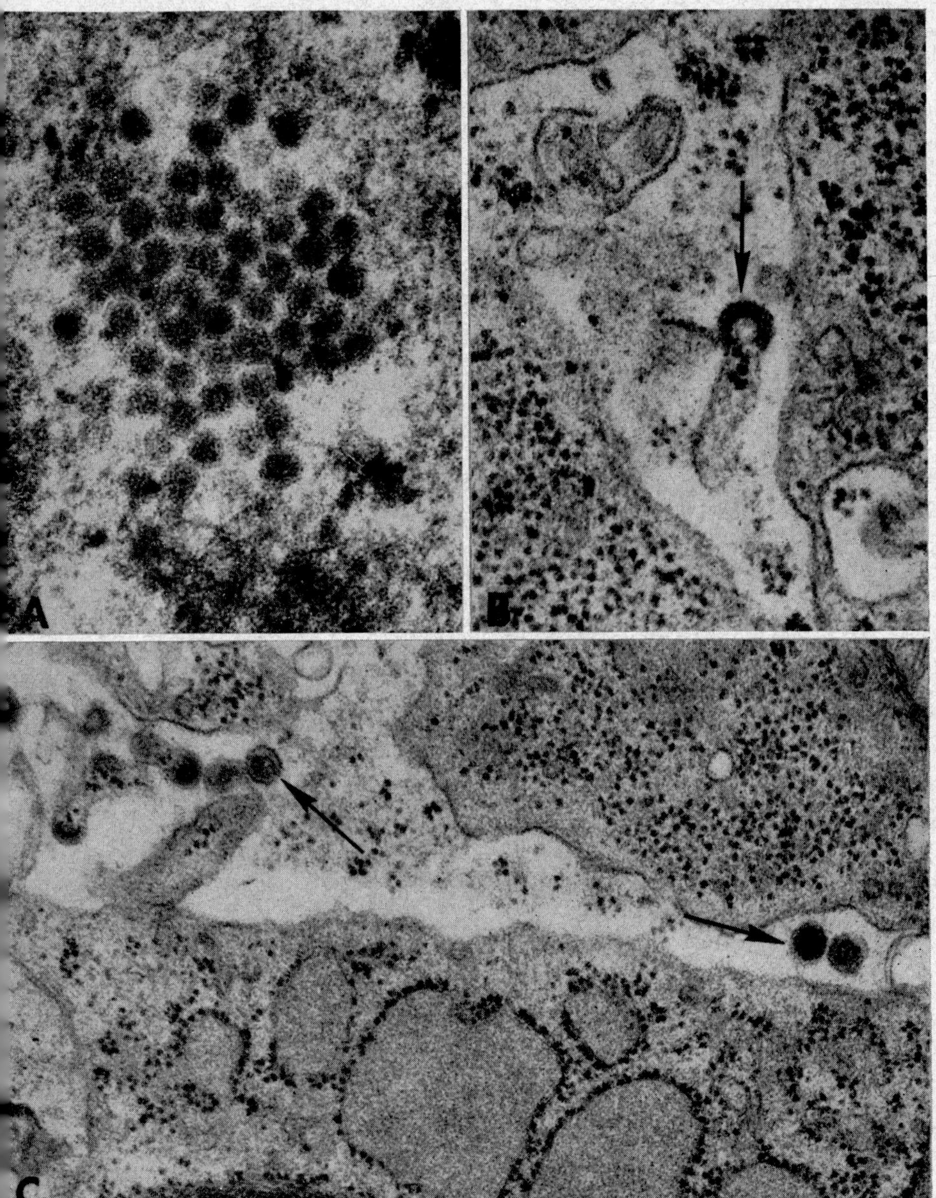

FIG. 62. POLYOMA VIRUS PARTICLES IN PAROTID TUMOR CELLS. LEUKEMIC VIRUS PARTICLES IN LYMPH NODE OF THE SAME MOUSE.

Isolation of Infectious DNA from Shope Rabbit Papilloma and from SV 40

Ito reported (1960) isolation of infectious DNA from Shope rabbit papilloma, a virus belonging to the same group as the parotid tumor, i.e. polyoma, virus. Furthermore, Ito also observed (1961) that the Shope rabbit papilloma DNA conserves its infectivity after heating to 100°C for 30 minutes. In this respect, therefore, the Shope papilloma DNA is also similar to the polyoma DNA. Isolation of infectious DNA from SV 40 has also been reported (Boiron *et al.*, 1962. Gerber, 1962).

* * *

Attempts to transmit neoplasms with nucleic acid preparations isolated from oncogenic viruses are obviously of considerable interest. They are still, however, in a preliminary phase. Additional studies are needed to clarify this fundamental problem. At least in some of the experiments thus far performed, the possible presence of live residual virus particles in presumably purified nucleic acid extracts has not yet been entirely eliminated. Furthermore, many of such purified nucleic acid extracts have at best only a very slight oncogenic potency.

REFERENCES

ANDERSON, S. G., Hemagglutination by animal viruses. Chapter III, pp. 21–50, in vol. 3 "Animal Viruses." *The Viruses.* Edited by F. M. Burnet and W. M. Stanley. Academic Press, New York and London, 1959.

ANDREWES, C. H., and HORSTMANN, D. M., The susceptibility of viruses to ethyl ether. *J. Gen. Microbiol.*, **3**: 290–297, 1949.

ASHBEL, R., Development of tumors in hamsters and rats following the injection of mycobacteria. *Pubbl. Staz. Zool. Napoli*, **28**: 12–31, 1956.

ATANASIU, P., A propos du virus du polyome. pp. 319–322 in: *Symposion über Fragen der Carcinogenese*, Berlin (December 11–16, 1959). Akademie-Verlag, Berlin, 1960.

ATANASIU, P., ORTH, G., REBIÈRE, J.-P., BOIRON, M., and PAOLETTI, C., Production de tumeurs chez le Hamster par inoculation d'acide désoxyribonucléique extrait de cultures de tissus infectées par le virus du polyome. *Compt. Rend. Acad. Sci.* (*Paris*), **254**: 4228–4230, 1962.

AXELRAD, A. A., McCULLOCH, E. A., HOWATSON, A. F., HAM, A. W., and SIMINOVITCH, L., Induction of tumors in Syrian hamsters by a cytopathogenic virus derived from a C3H mouse mammary tumor. *J. Nat. Cancer Inst.*, **24**: 1095–1111, 1960.

BANFIELD, W. G., DAWE, C. J., and BRINDLEY, D. C., Intracellular and extracellular particles in tissue cultures inoculated with parotid-tumor agent (polyoma virus). *J. Nat. Cancer Inst.*, **23**: 1123–1135, 1959.

BAUER, A., and CONSTANTIN, T., Multiplication du virus de Shope dans les cellules en culture. Étude au microscope électronique. *Compt. Rend. Soc. Biol.*, **150**: 246–249, 1956.

BERNHARD, W., and GROSS, L., Présence de particules d'aspect virusal dans les tissus tumoraux de souris atteintes de leucémies induites. *Compt. Rend. Acad. Sci.* (*Paris*), **248**: 160–163, 1959.

BERNHARD, W., FEBVRE, H. L., and CRAMER, R., Mise en évidence au microscope électronique d'un virus dans des cellules infectées *in vitro* par l'agent du Polyome. *Compt. Rend. Acad. Sci.* (*Paris*), **249**: 483–485, 1959.

BIELKA, H., and GRAFFI, A., Untersuchungen über die leukämogene Wirkung von Nukleinsäuren aus virusinduziertem Leukämiegewebe. *Acta Biologica et Medica Germanica*, **3**: 515–517, 1959.

BOIRON, M., PAOLETTI, C., THOMAS, M., REBIÈRE, J.-P., and BERNARD, J., Acide désoxyribonucléique infectieux extrait de cultures de cellules de rein de Singe Babouin infectées par le virus SV 40. *Compt. Rend. Acad. Sci.* (*Paris*), **254**: 2097–2099, 1962.

BRENNER, S., and HORNE, R. W., A negative staining method for high resolution electron microscopy of viruses. *Acta Biochim. and Biophys.*, **34**: 103–110, 1959.

BRODSKY, I., ROWE, W. P., HARTLEY, J. W., and LANE, W. T., Studies of mouse polyoma virus infection. II. Virus stability. *J. Exp. Med.*, **109**: 439–447, 1959.

BUFFETT, R. F., COMMERFORD, S. L., FURTH, J., and HUNTER, M. J., Agent in Ak leukemic tissues, not sedimented at 105,000 g causing neoplastic and non-neoplastic lesions. *Proc. Soc. Exp. Biol. & Med.*, **99**: 401–407, 1958.

BURNET, F. M., *Principles of Animal Virology*. p. 486, Academic Press, New York, 1955.

BURNET, F. M., and STANLEY, W. M., *The Viruses*, Vol. 1, General Virology, p. 609; Vol. 2, Plant and Bacterial Viruses, p. 408; Vol. 3, Animal Viruses, p. 428. Academic Press, New York, 1959.

BURTON, L., FRIEDMAN, F., KASSEL, R. KAPLAN, M. L., and ROTTINO, A., The purification and action of tumor factor extracted from mouse and human neoplastic tissue. *Trans. N.Y. Acad. Sci.*, **21**: 700–707, 1959.

CARREL, A., Some conditions of the reproduction *in vitro* of the Rous virus. *J. Exp. Med.*, **43**: 647–688, 1926.

CHESTERMAN, F. C., and NEGRONI, G., Tumours and other lesions induced in golden hamsters by a polyoma virus (Mill Hill strain): Induction time and dose response. *Brit. J. Cancer*, **15**: 790–797, 1961.

COLTER, J. S., BIRD, H. H., and BROWN, R. A., Infectivity of ribonucleic acid from Ehrlich ascites tumour cells infected with Mengo encephalitis. *Nature*, **179**: 859–860, 1957.

COLTER, J. S., BIRD, H. H., MOYER, A. W., and BROWN, R. A., Infectivity of ribonucleic acid isolated from virus-infected tissues. *Virology*, **4**: 522–532, 1957.

CONSTANTIN, T., and FEBVRE, H., Les corps d'inclusion observés dans les cultures de tissus infectées par le virus du fibrome de Shope du lapin. *Compt. Rend. Soc. Biol.*, **150**: 114–116, 1956.

CRAWFORD, L. V., and CRAWFORD, E. M., A comparative study of polyoma and papilloma viruses. *Virology*, **21**: 258–263, 1963.

CRICK, F. H. C., and WATSON, J. D., Structure of small viruses. *Nature*, **177**: 473–475, 1956.

DAWE, C. J., and LAW, L. W., Morphologic changes in salivary-gland tissue of the newborn mouse exposed to parotid-tumor agent *in vitro*. *J. Nat. Cancer Inst.*, **23**: 1157–1177, 1959a.

DAWE, C. J., LAW, L. W., and DUNN, T. B., Studies of parotid-tumor agent in cultures of leukemic tissues of mice. *J. Nat. Cancer Inst.*, **23**: 717–797, 1959b.

DiMayorca, G. A., Eddy, B. E., Stewart, S. E., Hunter, W. S., Friend, C., and Bendich, A., Isolation of infectious deoxyribonucleic acid from SE polyoma-infected tissue cultures. *Proc. Nat. Acad. Sci., USA*, **45**: 1805–1808, 1959.

Dmochowski, L., and Grey, C. E., Subcellular structures of possible viral origin in some mammalian tumors. *Ann. N. Y. Acad. Sci.*, **68**: 559–615, 1957.

Dmochowski, L., and Grey, C. E., Electron microscopy of tumors of known and suspected viral etiology. *Texas Rep. Biol. & Med.*, **15**: 704–756, 1957.

Dmochowski, L., Grey, C. E., and Magee, L. A., Studies on a virus ("polyoma") inducing multiple tumors in animals. *Proc. Soc. Exp. Biol. & Med.*, **102**: 575–579, 1959.

Doljanski, L., and Pikovski, M., Cultures *in vitro* of blood cells, bone marrow, and myocardium from leukotic fowls. *Cancer Research*, **1**: 205–216, 1941.

Doljanski, L., and Pikovski, M., Agent of fowl leukosis in tissue cultures. *Cancer Research*, **2**: 626–631, 1942.

Dourmashkin, R. R., Electron microscopy of polyoma virus: A review. pp. 151–182 in: *Tumors Induced by Viruses: Ultrastructural Studies*. Academic Press, New York and London, 1962.

Dourmashkin, R. R., and Negroni, G., Identification with the electron microscope of particles associated with polyoma virus in induced parotid gland tumours of C3H mice. *Exp. Cell Research*, **18**: 573–576, 1959.

Dulaney, A. D., Parotid gland tumor in AKR mice inoculated when newborn with cell-free AK leukemic extracts. *Cancer Research*, **16**: 877–879, 1956.

Dulaney, A. D., and Goss, M. F., Serial passage of the parotid gland tumor agent in mice. The activity of such tumor extracts for several strains of mice. *Cancer Research*, **20**: 887–890, 1960.

Dulaney, A. D., Maxey, M., Schillig, M. G., and Goss, M. F., Neoplasms in C3H mice which received Ak-leukemic extracts when newborn. *Cancer Research*, **17**: 809–814, 1957.

Dulbecco, R., and Freeman, G., Plaque production by the polyoma virus. *Virology*, **8**: 396–397, 1959.

Dulbecco, R., and Vogt, M., Significance of continued virus production in tissue cultures rendered neoplastic by polyoma virus. *Proc. Nat. Acad. Sci., USA*, **46**: 1617–1623, 1960.

Dunn, T. B., Heston, W. E., and Deringer, M. K., Subcutaneous fibrosarcomas in strains C3H and C57BL female mice, and F_1 and backcross hybrids of these strains. *J. Nat. Cancer Inst.*, **17**: 639–655, 1956.

Eddy, B. E., The polyoma virus. Section B. *Advances in Virus Research*, **7**: 91–102, 1960. Academic Press, New York.

Eddy, B. E., Borman, G. S., Kirschstein, R. L., and Touchette, R. H., Neoplasms in guinea pigs infected with SE polyoma virus. *J. Infect. Dis.*, **107**: 361–368, 1960.

Eddy, B. E., Rowe, W. P., Hartley, J. W., Stewart, S. E., and Huebner, R. J., Hemagglutination with the SE polyoma virus. *Virology*, **6**: 290–291, 1958a.

Eddy, B. E., Stewart, S. E., and Berkeley, W., Cytopathogenicity in tissue cultures by a tumor virus from mice. *Proc. Soc. Exp. Biol. & Med.*, **98**: 848–851, 1958b.

Eddy, B. E., Stewart, S. E., and Grubbs, G. E., Influence of tissue culture passage, storage, temperature and drying on viability of SE polyoma virus. *Proc. Soc. Exp. Biol. & Med.*, **99**: 289–292, 1958c.

Eddy, B. E., Stewart, S. E., Young, R., and Mider, G. B., Neoplasms in hamsters induced by mouse tumor agent passed in tissue culture. *J. Nat. Cancer Inst.*, **20**: 747–761, 1958d.

Eddy, B. E., and Stewart, S. E., Physical properties, and hemagglutinating and cytopathogenic effects of the SE polyoma virus. pp. 307–324 in: *Proc. Third Canadian Cancer Conference, Honey Harbour, Ontario* (June 17–21, 1958). Academic Press, New York, 1959a.

Eddy, B. E., and Stewart, S. E., Characteristics of the SE polyoma virus. *Am. J. Pub. Health*, **49**: 1486–1492, 1959b.

Eddy, B. E., Stewart, S. E., Kirschstein, R. L., and Young, R. D., Induction of subcutaneous nodules in rabbits with the SE polyoma virus. *Nature*, **183**: 766–767, 1959.

Eddy, B. E., Stewart, S. E., Stanton, M. F., and Marcotte, J. M., Induction of tumors in rats by tissue-culture preparations of SE polyoma virus. *J. Nat. Cancer Inst.*, **22**: 161–171, 1959.

Editorial. Filtrable agent causing mouse salivary gland carcinoma. *J. Am. Med. Assoc.*, **153**: 150, 1953.

Edwards, G. A., Buffett, R. F., and Furth, J., The micromorphology of a salivary gland tumor of a mouse infected with polyoma virus. *J. Nat. Cancer Inst.*, **25**: 25–51, 1960.

Elford, W. J., A new series of graded collodion membranes suitable for general bacteriological use, especially in filterable virus studies. *J. Path. & Bact.*, **34**: 505–521, 1931.

Elford, W. J., The principles of ultrafiltration as applied in biological studies. *Proc. Royal Soc. London, Series B.* (*Biol. Sci.*), **112**: 384–406, 1933.

Flocks, J. S., Weis, T. P., Kleinman, D. C., and Kirsten, W. H., Dose-response studies to polyoma virus in rats. *J. Nat. Cancer Inst.*, **35**: 259–284, 1965.

Fogel, M., and Sachs, L., The *in vitro* and *in vivo* analysis of mammalian tumour viruses. II. The haemagglutinating system of the polyoma virus. *Brit. J. Cancer*, **13**: 266–281, 1959.

Fogel, M., and Sachs, L., The *in vitro* and *in vivo* analysis of mammalian tumor viruses. IV. Antibody response and tumor induction with polyoma virus in different species. *J. Nat. Cancer Inst.*, **24**: 839–857, 1960.

Fraenkel-Conrat, H., The role of the nucleic acid in the reconstitution of active tobacco mosaic virus. *J. Am. Chem. Soc.*, **78**: 882–883, 1956.

Fraser, K. B., and Crawford, E. M., Immunofluorescent and electron-microscopic studies of polyoma virus in transformation reactions with BHK21 cells. *Exp. Mol. Path.*, **4**: 51–65, 1965.

Furth, J., and Breedis, C., Attempts at cultivation of viruses producing leukosis in fowls. *Arch Path.*, **24**: 281–302, 1937.

Furth, J., and Stubbs, E. L., Tissue culture studies on relation of sarcoma to leukosis of chickens. *Proc. Soc. Exp. Biol. & Med.*, **32**: 318–383, 1934.

Furth, J., Buffett, R. F., Banasiewicz-Rodriguez, M., and Upton, A. C., Character of agent inducing leukemia in newborn mice. *Proc. Soc. Exp. Biol. & Med.*, **93**: 165–172, 1956.

Gerber, P., An infectious deoxyribonucleic acid derived from vacuolating virus (SV 40). *Virology*, **16**: 96–98, 1962.

Gierer, A., and Schramm, G., Infectivity of ribonucleic acid from tobacco mosaic virus. *Nature*, **177**: 702–703, 1956.

Gimmy, J., Graffi, A., and Krause, L., Über die Wirkung des polyvalenten Sarkom-Virus beim Goldhamster. *Acta Biologica et Medica Germanica*, **3**: 509–510, 1959.

GIMMY, J., and GRAFFI, A., Zur Transplantabilität der durch den BB/T2-Polyoma-Virusstamm induzierten Tumoren. *Arch. f. Geschwulstforsch.*, **20**: 1–21, 1962.

GRAFFI, A., Über einen neuen Polyoma-Virusstamm und einige biologische Eigenschaften desselben. Angemeldeter Diskussionsbeitrag über das Polyoma-Virus. pp. 323–325 in: *Symposion über Fragen der Carcinogenese*, Berlin (December 11–16, 1959). Akademie-Verlag, Berlin, 1960.

GRAFFI, A., BIELKA, H., FEY, F., SCHARSACH, F., and WEISS, R., Gehäuftes Auftreten von Leukämien nach Injektion von Sarkom-Filtraten. *Wiener Med. Wochenschr.*, **105**: 61–64, 1955.

GRAFFI, A., BIELKA, H., and FEY, F., Leukämieerzeugung durch ein filtrierbares Agens aus malignen Tumoren. *Acta Haemat.*, **15**: 145–174, 1956.

GRAFFI, A., GIMMY, J., and KRAUSE, L., Über ein polyvalentes Sarkomvirus der Ratte. *Naturwissenschaften*, **46**: 330, 1959.

GRAFFI, A., and FRITZ, D., Essais de transmission par acides nucléiques extraits de la souche BB-T_2 du virus de la tumeur parotidienne polyome. *Revue Française d'Études Cliniques et Biologiques*, **5**: 388–390, 1960.

GROSS, L., Hemolytic action of mouse mammary carcinoma filtrate on mouse erythrocytes *in vitro*. *Proc. Soc. Exp. Biol. & Med.*, **65**: 292–293, 1947.

GROSS, L., Increased hemolytic potency of mouse mammary carcinoma extracts following incubation with tumor cells. *Proc. Soc. Exp. Biol. & Med.*, **67**: 341–343, 1948a.

GROSS, L., Destructive action of mouse and rat tumor extracts on red blood cells *in vitro*. *J. Immunol.*, **59**: 173–188, 1948b.

GROSS, L., "Spontaneous" leukemia developing in C3H mice following inoculation, in infancy, with Ak-leukemic extracts, or Ak-embryos. *Proc. Soc. Exp. Biol. & Med.*, **76**: 27–32, 1951a.

GROSS, L., Pathogenic properties, and "vertical" transmission of the mouse leukemia agent. *Proc. Soc. Exp. Biol. & Med.*, **78**: 342–348, 1951b.

GROSS, L., A filterable agent, recovered from Ak leukemic extracts, causing salivary gland carcinomas in C3H mice. *Proc. Soc. Exp. Biol. & Med.*, **83**: 414–421, 1953a.

GROSS, L., Neck tumors, or leukemia, developing in adult C3H mice following inoculation, in early infancy, with filtered (Berkefeld N), or centrifuged (144,000 × g), Ak-leukemic extracts. *Cancer*, **6**: 948–957, 1953b.

GROSS, L., Filterable agents in Ak and C58 mouse leukemia. (Abstract.) *Proc. Am. Assoc. Cancer Research*, **1**: 17, 1954a.

GROSS, L., Transmissible mouse leukaemia: Biological properties of the mouse leukaemia agent. pp. 76–95 in: *CIBA Foundation Symposium on Leukaemia Research*. J. & A. Churchill Ltd., London, 1954b.

GROSS, L., Induction of parotid carcinomas and/or subcutaneous sarcomas in C3H mice with normal C3H organ extracts. *Proc. Soc. Exp. Biol. & Med.*, **88**: 362–368, 1955a.

GROSS, L., Mouse leukemia: An egg-borne virus disease (with a note on mouse salivary gland carcinoma). *Acta Haemat.*, **13**: 13–29, 1955b.

GROSS, L., Influence of ether, *in vitro*, on pathogenic properties of mouse leukemia extracts. *Acta Haemat.*, **15**: 273–277, 1956a.

GROSS, L., Viral (egg-borne) etiology of mouse leukemia. Filtered extracts from leukemic C58 mice, causing leukemia (or parotid tumors) after inoculation into newborn C57 Brown or C3H mice. *Cancer*, **9**: 778–791, 1956b.

GROSS, L., Development and cell-free transmission of a highly potent strain of mouse leukemia virus. *Proc. Soc. Exp. Biol. & Med.*, **94**: 767–771, 1957a.

GROSS, L., Studies on the nature and biological properties of a transmissible agent causing leukemia following inoculation into newborn mice. *Ann. N.Y. Acad. Sci.*, **68**: 501–521, 1957b.

GROSS, L., High susceptibility of 1 to 14-day-old C3H mice to "passage A" leukemic filtrates. *Proc. Soc. Exp. Biol. & Med.*, **97**: 300–304, 1958a.

GROSS, L., Attempt to recover filterable agent from X-ray-induced leukemia. *Acta Haemat.*, **19**: 353–361, 1958b.

GROSS, L., Agglutinating action of heat-inactivated passage A mouse leukemia filtrates on mouse red blood cells. *Proc. Soc. Exp. Biol. & Med.*, **101**: 113–117, 1959.

GROSS, L., Biological and pathogenic properties of a mouse leukemia virus. *Acta Haemat.*, **23**: 259–275, 1960.

GROSS, L., ROSWIT, B., MADA, E. R., DREYFUSS, Y., and MOORE, L. A., Studies on radiation-induced leukemia in mice. *Cancer Research*, **19**: 316–320, 1959.

GUÉRIN, M., *Tumeurs spontanées des animaux de laboratoire* (*Souris-Rat-Poule*). p. 215. Amédée Legrand & Cie., Paris, 1954.

HABEL, K., Immunological determinants of polyoma virus oncogenesis. *J. Exp. Med.*, **115**: 181–193, 1962.

HABEL, K., Polyoma tumor antigen in cells transformed *in vitro* by polyoma virus. *Virology*, **18**: 553–558, 1962.

HABEL, K., and ATANASIU, P., Transplantation of polyoma virus induced tumor in the hamster. *Proc. Soc. Exp. Biol. & Med.*, **102**: 99–102, 1959.

HALBERSTAEDTER, L., DOLJANSKI, L., and TENENBAUM, E., Experiments on the cancerization of cells *in vitro* by means of Rous sarcoma agent. *Brit. J. Exp. Path.*, **22**: 179–187, 1941.

HAM, A. W., MCCULLOCH, E. A., AXELRAD, A. A., SIMINOVITCH, L., and HOWATSON, A. F., The histopathological sequence in viral carcinogenesis in the hamster kidney. *J. Nat. Cancer Inst.*, **24**: 1113–1129, 1960.

HARE, J. D., Transplant immunity to polyoma virus induced tumors. I. Correlations with biological properties of virus strains. *Proc. Soc. Exp. Biol. & Med.*, **115**: 805–810, 1964.

HAREL, J., HUPPERT, J., LACOUR, F., and LACOUR, J., Induction de tumeurs malignes chez le souriceau nouveau-né, par injection d'une préparation d'acide ribonucléique extrait de ganglions leucémiques humains. *Compt. Rend. Acad. Sci.* (*Paris*), **247**: 795–796, 1958.

HAREL, J., HUPPERT, J., LACOUR, F., and LACOUR, J., Tumeurs malignes transmissibles de la souris, provoquées par injection de préparations contenant de l'acide ribonucléique. Étude biologique et histologique. *Bull. du Cancer*, **46**: 75–91, 1959.

HARRIS, R. J. C., CHESTERMAN, F. C., and NEGRONI, G., Induction of tumours in newborn ferrets with Mill Hill polyoma virus. *Lancet*, **1**: 788–791, 1961.

HARTLEY, J. W., and ROWE, W. P., "Unmasking" of mouse polyoma virus hemagglutinin by heat and RDE. *Virology*, **7**: 249–250, 1959.

HARTLEY, J. W., ROWE, W. P., CHANOCK, R. M., and ANDREWS, B. E., Studies of mouse polyoma virus infection. IV. Evidence for mucoprotein erythrocyte receptors in polyoma virus hemagglutination. *J. Exp. Med.*, **110**: 81–91, 1959.

HAYS, E. F., and BECK, W. S., The development of leukemia and other neoplasms in mice receiving cell-free extracts from a high leukemia (AKR) strain. *Cancer Research*, **18**: 676–681, 1958.

HAYS, E. F., SIMMONS, N. S., and BECK, W. S., Induction of mouse leukaemia with purified nucleic acid preparations. *Nature*, **180**: 1419–1420, 1957.

Hirst, G. K., The agglutination of red cells by allantoic fluid of chick embryo infected with influenza virus. *Science*, **94**: 22–23, 1941.

Hirst, G. K., Adsorption of influenza hemagglutinins and virus by red blood cells. *J. Exp. Med.*, **76**: 195–209, 1942.

Hirst, G. K., Hemagglutination as applied to the study of virus infections. pp. 44–51 in: *Viruses*, 1950. Calif. Inst. Techn., Publ., 1950.

Holland, J. J., McLaren, L. C., and Syverton, J. T., Mammalian cell-virus relationship. III. Poliovirus production by non-primate cells exposed to poliovirus ribonucleic acid. *Proc. Soc. Exp. Biol. & Med.*, **100**: 843–845, 1959.

Holland, J. J., McLaren, L. C., and Syverton, J. T., The mammalian cell virus relationship. IV. Infection of naturally insusceptible cells with enterovirus ribonucleic acid. *J. Exp. Med.*, **110**: 65–80, 1959.

Howatson, A. F., and Almeida, J. D., An electron microscope study of polyoma virus in hamster kidney. *J. Biophys. and Biochem. Cytol.*, **7**: 753–760, 1960a.

Howatson, A. F., and Almeida, J. D., Observations on the fine structure of polyoma virus. *J. Biophys. and Biochem. Cytol.*, **8**: 828–834, 1960b.

Howatson, A. F., and Almeida, J. D., Studies of polyoma virus in hamster kidney. *Proc. European Regional Conference on Electron Microscopy*, **2**: 986–989, 1960c.

Howatson, A. F., and Almeida, J. D., An electron microscope study of polyoma virus in hamster kidney. *J. Biophys. and Biochem. Cytol.*, **7**: 753–760, 1960d.

Howatson, A. F., McCulloch, E. A., Almeida, J. D., Siminovitch, L., Axelrad, A. A., and Ham, A. W., Studies *in vitro*, *in vivo* and by electron microscope of a virus recovered from a C3H mouse mammary tumor: Relationship to polyoma virus. *J. Nat. Cancer Inst.*, **24**: 1131–1151, 1960.

Huebner, R. J., Rowe, W. P., Hartley, J. W., and Lane, W. T., Mouse polyoma virus in a rural ecology. pp. 314–328 in: *CIBA Foundation Symposium on Tumour Viruses of Murine Origin*. J. & A. Churchill Ltd., London, 1962.

Huppert, J., Lacour, F., Lacour, J., and Harel, J., Cancérisation précoce chez la souris par injection de préparations contenant l'acide ribonucléique de tumeurs homologues. *Compt. Rend. Acad. Sci.* (*Paris*), **248**: 1590–1592, 1959.

Ito, Y., A tumor-producing factor extracted by phenol from papillomatous tissue (Shope) of cottontail rabbits. *Virology*, **12**: 596–601, 1960.

Ito, Y., Heat-resistance of the tumorigenic nucleic acid of Shope papillomatosis. *Proc. Nat. Acad. Sci., USA*, **47**: 1897–1900, 1961.

Kahler, H., Rowe, W. P., Lloyd, B. J., and Hartley, J. W., Electron microscopy of mouse parotid tumor (polyoma) virus. *J. Nat. Cancer Inst.*, **22**: 647–657, 1959.

Kassel, R., and Rottino, A., Problems in the production of leukemia with cell-free extracts. *Cancer Research*, **19**: 155–158, 1959.

Kassel, R., Burton, L., Friedman, F., and Rottino, A., Carcinogenic action of refined tumor factor isolated from mouse leukemia tissue. *Proc. Soc. Exp. Biol. & Med.*, **101**: 201–204, 1959.

Kilham, L., Propagation of fibroma virus in tissue cultures of cottontail testes. *Proc. Soc. Exp. Biol. & Med.*, **92**: 739–742, 1956.

Kilham, L., Fibroma-myxoma virus transformation in different types of tissue culture. *J. Nat. Cancer Inst.*, **20**: 729–739, 1958.

Kimura, R., Züchtung von Hühnermyxosarkom *in vitro*. 2. Mitteilung. *Arch. f. exper. Zellforsch.*, **10**: 174–177, 1930.

Lacour, F., Lacour, J., Harel, J., and Huppert, J., Transplantable malignant tumors in mice induced by preparations containing ribonucleic acid extracted from human and mouse tumors. *J. Nat. Cancer Inst.*, **24**: 301–328, 1960.

LASFARGUES, E. Y., MOORE, D. H., and MURRAY, M. R., Maintenance of the milk factor in cultures of mouse mammary epithelium. *Cancer Research*, **18**: 1281–1285, 1958.

LATARJET, R., and DE JACO, M., Production de cancers multiples chez des souris AkR ayant reçu un extrait leucémique a-cellulaire isologue. *Compt. Rend. Acad. Sci. (Paris)*, **246**: 499–501, 1958a.

LATARJET, R., REBEYROTTE, N., and MOUSTACCHI, E., Production de cancers multiples chez des souris ayant reçu de l'acide nucléique extrait de tissus leucémiques isologues ou homologues. *Compt. Rend. Acad. Sci. (Paris)*, **246**: 853–855, 1958b.

LAW, L. W., Discussion, pp. 102–103 in: General Discussion (pp. 95–104) following presentation of paper by L. Gross, in *CIBA Foundation Symposium on Leukaemia Research*. J. & A. Churchill Ltd., London, 1954.

LAW, L. W., Present status of nonviral factors in the etiology of reticular neoplasms of the mouse. *Ann. N.Y. Acad. Sci.*, **68**: 616–635, 1957.

LAW, L. W., Thymus: Role in resistance to polyoma virus oncogenesis. *Science*, **147**: 164–165, 1965.

LAW, L. W., Studies of thymic function with emphasis on the role of the thymus in oncogenesis. *Cancer Research*, **26**: 551–574, 1966.

LAW, L. W., and DAWE, C. J., Influence of total body X-irradiation on tumor induction by parotid tumor agent in adult mice. *Proc. Soc. Exp. Biol. & Med.*, **105**: 414–419, 1960.

LAW, L. W., DUNN, T. B., and BOYLE, P. J., Neoplasms in the C3H strain and in F_1 hybrid mice of two crosses following introduction of extracts and filtrates of leukemic tissues. *J. Nat. Cancer Inst.*, **16**: 495–539, 1955.

LAW, L. W., DAWE, C. J., ROWE, W. P., and HARTLEY, J. W., Antibody status of mice and response of their litters to parotid tumour virus (polyoma virus). *Nature*, **184**: 1420–1421, 1959.

LAW, L. W., ROWE, W. P., and HARTLEY, J. W., Studies on mouse polyoma virus infection. V. Relation of virus infection to lymphocytic neoplasms of the mouse. *J. Exp. Med.*, **111**: 517–523, 1960.

LIPPINCOTT, S. W., EDWARDS, J. E., GRADY, H. G., and STEWART, H. L., A review of some spontaneous neoplasms in mice. *J. Nat. Cancer Inst.*, **3**: 199–210, 1942.

LUDFORD, R. J., The production of tumours by cultures of normal cells treated with filtrates of filterable fowl tumours. *Am. J. Cancer*, **31**: 414–429, 1937.

MACPHERSON, I., and STOKER, M., Polyoma transformation of hamster cell clones—An investigation of genetic factors affecting cell competence. *Virology*, **16**: 147–151, 1962.

MALMGREN, R. A., RABSON, A. S., and CARNEY, P. G., Immunity and viral carcinogenesis. Effect of thymectomy on polyoma virus carcinogenesis in mice. *J. Nat. Cancer Inst.*, **33**: 101–104, 1964.

MANAKER, R. A., STROTHER, P. C., MILLER, A. A., and PICZAK, C. V., Behavior *in vitro* of a mouse lymphoid-leukemia virus. *J. Nat Cancer. Inst.*, **25**: 1411–1419, 1960.

MATTERN, C. F. T., Polyoma and papilloma viruses: Do they have 42 or 92 subunits? *Science*, **137**: 612–613, 1962.

MATTERN, C. F. T., TAKEMOTO, K. K., and DANIEL, W. A., Replication of polyoma virus in mouse embryo cells: Electron microscopic observations. *Virology*, **30**: 242–256, 1966.

MCCLELLAND, L., and HARE, R., The adsorption of influenza virus by red cells and a new method *in vitro* of measuring antibodies for influenza virus. *Canad. J. Publ. Health (Lab. Suppl.)*, **32**: 530–538, 1941.

McCulloch, E. A., Howatson, A. F., Siminovitch, L., Axelrad, A. A., and Ham, A. W., A cytopathogenic agent from a mammary tumour in a C3H mouse that produces tumours in Swiss mice and hamsters. *Nature*, **183**: 1535–1536, 1959.

McCulloch, E. A., Siminovitch, L., Ham, A. W., Axelrad, A. A., and Howatson, A. F., Carcinogenesis *in vivo* by polyoma virus. *Canadian Cancer Conference*, **4**: 253–270. Academic Press, New York, 1961.

Miller, J. F. A. P., Ting, R. C., and Law, L. W., Influence of thymectomy on tumor induction by polyoma virus in C57BL mice. *Proc. Soc. Exp. Biol. & Med.*, **116**: 323–327, 1964.

Mirand, E. A., Grace, J. T., Moore, G. E., and Mount, D., Relationship of viruses to malignant disease. Part I. Tumor induction by SE polyoma virus. *Arch. Intern. Med.*, **105**: 469–481, 1960.

Mirand, E. A., Mount, D. T., Moore, G. E., Grace, J. T., Jr., and Sokal, J. E., Induction of tumors by a virus-like agent(s) released by tissue culture. *Proc. Soc. Exp. Biol. & Med.*, **99**: 1–5, 1958.

Negroni, G., Dourmashkin, R., and Chesterman, F. C., A "polyoma" virus derived from a mouse leukemia. *Brit. Med. J.*, **2**: 1359–1360, 1959.

Orth, G., Atanasiu, P., Boiron, M., Rebière, J. P., Paoletti, C., Infectious and oncogenic effect of DNA extracted from cells infected with polyoma virus. *Proc. Soc. Exp. Biol. & Med.*, **115**: 1090–1095, 1964.

Paoletti, C., Orth, G., Boiron, M., Lamonthezie, N., and Atanasiu, P., Étude sur l'extraction et le pouvoir infectieux *in vitro* de l'acide désoxyribonucléique du virus du polyome. *Ann. Inst. Pasteur*, **104**: 717–733, 1963.

Pikovski, M. A., The survival of the mammary tumor milk agent in cultures of heterologous cells. *J. Nat. Cancer Inst.*, **13**: 1275–1282, 1953.

Pomerance, A., and Chesterman, F. C., The pathology of polyoma induced tumours in ferrets. *Brit. J. Cancer*, **19**: 211–215, 1965.

Rabson, A. S., and Legallais, F. Y., Cytopathogenic effect produced by polyoma virus in cultures of milk-adapted murine lymphoma cells (strain P388 D_1). *Proc. Soc. Exp. Biol. & Med.*, **100**: 229–233, 1959.

Rabson, A. S., Branigan, W. J., and Legallais, F. Y., Production of tumours in *Rattus* (*Mastomys*) *natalensis* by polyoma virus. *Nature*, **187**: 423–425, 1960.

Rogel, R., and Rudali, G., Production de tumeurs épithéliales chez les souris à l'aide d'extraits a-cellulaires saccharosiques de lymphosarcomes. *Bull. du Cancer*, **44**: 483–492, 1957.

Rogel, R., Jullien, P., Rudali, G., and Stern, G., Étude de corpuscules contenant des acides nucléiques, dans les tissus leucosiques de souris AKR. *Le Sang*, **29**: 292–297, 1958.

Rowe, W. P., The epidemiology of mouse polyoma virus infection. *Bacteriol. Rev.*, **25**: 18–31, 1961a.

Rowe, W. P., Mouse polyoma virus infection. *Trans. & Studies Coll. Physicians of Philadelphia*, 4 Ser., **29**: 66–70, 1961b.

Rowe, W. P., Gross, L., Hartley, J. W., and Huebner, R. J., Failure of antiserum to mouse polyoma virus to neutralize mouse leukemia virus (Gross). Unpublished, 1959a.

Rowe, W. P., Hartley, J. W., Brodsky, I., and Huebner, R. J., Complement fixation with mouse tumor virus (SE polyoma). *Science*, **128**: 1339–1340, 1958a.

Rowe, W. P., Hartley, J. W., Brodsky, I., and Huebner, R. J., Observations on the spread of mouse polyoma virus infection. *Nature*, **182**: 1617, 1958b.

Rowe, W. P., Hartley, J. W., Estes, J. D., and Huebner, R. J., Studies of mouse polyoma virus infection. I. Procedures for quantitation and detection of virus. *J. Exp. Med.*, **109**: 379–391, 1959b.

Rowe, W. P., Hartley, J. W., Law, L. W., and Huebner, R. J., Studies of mouse polyoma virus infection. III. Distribution of antibodies in laboratory mouse colonies. *J. Exp. Med.*, **109**: 449–462, 1959c.

Rowe, W. P., Hartley, J. W., Estes, J. D., and Huebner, R. J., Growth curves of polyoma virus in mice and hamsters. pp. 189–209 in: *Symposium. Phenomena of the Tumor Viruses, Nat. Cancer Inst. Monograph No. 4*, 1960. U.S. Publ. Health Service, Bethesda, Md.

Rowe, W. P., Huebner, R. J., and Hartley, J. W., An approach to the study of tumor viruses. B. Ecology of a mouse tumor virus. Chapter 14, pp. 177–194 in: *Perspectives in Virology*, vol. 2. Burgess Publishing Co., Minneapolis, Minn., 1961.

Rowson, K. E. K., Roe, F. J. C., Ball, J. K., and Salaman, M. H., Induction of tumours by polyoma virus: Enhancement by chemical agents. *Nature*, **191**: 893–895, 1961.

Ruffilli, D., Coltivazione di tessuti di pollo eritroleucemico. *Boll. Lega Ital. p. lotta contro tumori*, **11**: 3–26, 1937.

Ruffilli, D., Azione del plasma di pollo eritroleacemico su tessuti cultivati *in vitro* *Boll. Lega Ital. p. lotta coutro tumori*, **12**: 3–16, 1938.

Sachs, L., and Medina, D., Polyoma virus mutant with a reduction in tumour formation. *Nature*, **187**: 715–716, 1960.

Sachs, L., and Winocour, E., Formation of different cell-virus relationships in tumour cells induced by polyoma. *Nature*, **184**: 1702–1704, 1959.

Sachs, L., Fogel, M., and Winocour, E., *In vitro* analysis of a mammalian tumour virus. *Nature*, **183**: 663–664, 1959a.

Sachs, L., Fogel, M., Winocour, E., Heller, E., Medina, D., and Krim, M., The *in vitro* and *in vivo* analysis of mammalian tumour viruses. *Brit. J. Cancer*, **13**: 251–265, 1959b.

Salaman, M. H., The early development of tumours in mice inoculated with a cell-free filtrate of mouse leukaemic tissue. *Brit. J. Cancer*, **13**: 76–86, 1959.

Schmidt, F., Über das Auftreten verschiedenartiger Tumoren bei Mäusen nach Injektion einer Zytoplasmafraktion aus Ehrlich-Ca-Zellen. *Zeitschr. f. ges. Inn. Med. & Grenzgeb.*, **11**: 640–644, 1956.

Schmidt, F., Das Polyomavirus. *Zeitschr. f. ges. Inn. Med. & Grenzgeb.*, **18**: 586–597, 1963.

Schramm, T., Graffi, A., and Förster, W., Weitere Versuche zum Nachweis einer infektiösen RNS aus virusinduzierten Mäuseleukämien. *Arch. Geschwulstforsch.*, **25**: 212–214, 1965.

Sjögren, H. O., Further studies on the induced resistance against isotransplantation of polyoma tumors. *Virology*, **15**: 214–219, 1961.

Smith, J. D., Freeman, G., Vogt, M., and Dulbecco, R., The nucleic acid of polyoma virus. *Virology*, **12**: 185–196, 1960.

Stanton, M. F., Stewart, S. E., Eddy, B. E., and Blackwell, R. H., Oncogenic effect of tissue-culture preparations of polyoma virus on fetal mice. *J. Nat. Cancer Inst.*, **23**: 1441–1475, 1959.

Stewart, H. L., Snell, K. C., Dunham, L. D., and Schylen, S. M., Transplantable and transmissible tumors of animals. *Atlas of Tumor Pathology*. Sect. 12. Fasc. 40, pp. 378. Am. Reg. Path., Armed Forces Inst. of Path., Washington, D.C., 1959.

STEWART, S. E., Leukemia in mice produced by a filterable agent present in AKR leukemic tissues with notes on a sarcoma produced by the same agent. (Abstract). *Anat. Rec.*, **117**: 532, 1953.

STEWART, S. E., Neoplasms in mice inoculated with cell-free extracts or filtrates of leukemic mouse tissues. I. Neoplasms of the parotid and adrenal glands. *J. Nat. Cancer Inst.*, **15**: 1391–1415, 1955.

STEWART, S. E., The polyoma virus. Section A. *Advances in Virus Research*, 7: 61–90, 1960. Academic Press, New York.

STEWART, S. E., EDDY, B. E., GOCHENOUR, A. M., BORGESE, N. G., and GRUBBS, G., Parotid gland tumors and other neoplasms in Swiss mice inoculated with a tumor agent carried in tissue culture. (Abstract). *Proc. Am. Assoc. Cancer Research*, **2**: 253, 1957a.

STEWART, S. E., EDDY, B. E., GOCHENOUR, A. M., BORGESE, N. G., and GRUBBS, G. E., The induction of neoplasms with a substance released from mouse tumors by tissue culture. *Virology*, **3**: 380–400, 1957b.

STEWART, S. E., EDDY, B. E., and BORGESE, N., Neoplasms in mice inoculated with a tumor agent carried in tissue culture. *J. Nat. Cancer Inst.*, **20**: 1223–1243, 1958a.

STEWART, S. E., EDDY, B. E., STANTON, M. F., and BERKELEY, W. H., Influence of age on tumor induction in mice and hamsters injected with tumor agent carried in tissue culture. (Abstract). *Proc. Am. Assoc. Cancer Research*, **2**: 348–349, 1958b.

STEWART, S. E., and EDDY, B. E., Tumor induction by SE polyoma virus and the inhibition of tumors by specific neutralizing antibodies. *Am. J. Pub. Health*, **49**: 1493–1496, 1959a.

STEWART, S. E., EDDY, B. E., STANTON, M. F., and LEE, S. L., Tissue culture plaques of SE polyoma virus. (Abstract). *Proc. Am. Assoc. Cancer Research*, **3**: 67, 1959b.

STEWART, S. E., EDDY, B. E., IRWIN, M., and LEE, S., Development of resistance in mice to tumour induction by SE polyoma virus. *Nature*, **186**: 615–617, 1960.

STOKER, M., Mechanisms of viral carcinogenesis. *Proc. Sixth Canadian Cancer Research Conference, Honey Harbour, Ontario, 1964*, pp. 357–368. Pergamon Press, Oxford and New York, 1965.

STOKER, M., and MACPHERSON, I., Studies on transformation of hamster cells by polyoma virus *in vitro*. *Virology*, **14**: 359–370, 1961.

VANDEPUTTE, M., DENYS, P., LEYTEN, R., and DE SOMER, P., The oncogenic activity of the polyoma virus in thymectomized rats. *Life Sci.*, **7**: 475–478, Pergamon Press, Oxford, 1963.

VANDEPUTTE, M., and DE SOMER, P., Influence of thymectomy on viral oncogenesis in rats. *Nature*, **206**: 520–521, 1965.

VERNE, J., OBERLING, C., and GUÉRIN, M., Tentatives de culture in vitro de l'agent de la leucémie transmissible des poules. *Compt. Rend. Soc. Biol.*, **121**: 403–405, 1936.

VINOGRAD, J., LEBOWITZ, J., RADLOFF, R., WATSON, R., and LAIPIS, P., The twisted circular form of polyoma virus DNA. *Proc. Nat. Acad. Sci., USA*, **53**: 1104–1111, 1965.

VOGT, M., and DULBECCO, R., Virus-cell interaction with a tumor-producing virus. *Proc. Nat. Acad. Sci., USA*, **46**: 365–370, 1960.

VOGT, M., and DULBECCO, R., Studies on cells rendered neoplastic by polyoma virus: The problem of the presence of virus-related materials. *Virology*, **16**: 41–51, 1962.

WATSON, M. L., Staining of tissue sections for electron microscopy with heavy metals. II. Application of solutions containing lead and barium. *J. Biophys. and Biochem. Cytol.*, **4**: 727–729, 1958.

WEIL, R., A quantitative assay for a subviral infective agent related to polyoma virus. *Virology*, **14**: 46–53, 1961.

WEIL, R., PÉTURSSON, G., KÁRA, J., and DIGGELMANN, H., On the interaction of polyoma virus with the genetic apparatus of host cells. pp. 593–626 in: *The Molecular Biology of Viruses*. Academic Press, New York and London, 1967.

WILDY, P., STOKER, M. G. P., MACPHERSON, I. A., and HORNE, R. W., The fine structure of polyoma virus. *Virology*, **11**: 444–457, 1960.

WILLIAMS, M. G., and SHEININ, R., Cytological studies of mouse embryo cells infected with polyoma virus, using acridine orange fluorescent antibody. *Virology*, **13**: 368–370, 1961.

WINOCOUR, E., Purification of polyoma virus. *Virology*, **19**: 158–168, 1963.

WINOCOUR, E., and SACHS, L., A plaque assay for the polyoma virus. *Virology*, **8**: 397–400, 1959.

WOOLLEY, G. W., Occurrence of "neck tumors" in cortisone-treated leukemic-strain mice. (Abstract). *Proc. Am. Assoc. Cancer Research*, **1**: 53, 1954.

WOOLLEY, G. W., and SMALL, M. C., Filterable agent prepared from leukemic tissue causing cancer in mice. (Abstract). *Proc. Am. Assoc. Cancer Research*, **2**: 158, 1956a.

WOOLLEY, G. W., and SMALL, M. C., Experiments on cell-free transmission of mouse leukemia. *Cancer*, **9**: 1102–1106, 1956b.

YABE, Y., NERIISHI, S., SATO, Y., LIEBELT, A., TAYLOR, H. G., and TRENTIN, J. J., Distribution of hemagglutination-inhibiting antibodies against polyoma virus in laboratory mice. *J. Nat. Cancer Inst.*, **26**: 621–628, 1961.

ADDENDUM: SKIN TUMORS AND LYMPHOMAS IN HAMSTERS

Graffi and his coworkers inoculated newborn hamsters with normal hamster embryo cell cultures and observed the development in 80 hamsters of multiple wart-like skin tumors originating from hair follicles. Electron microscopic examination revealed in the nuclei of the tumor cells the presence of crystalline arrays of virus particles about 35 mμ in diameter; occasionally, particles were also found in the cytoplasm and in intercellular spaces (GRAFFI, A., SCHRAMM, T., BENDER, E., BIERWOLF, D., and GRAFFI, I., Über einen virushaltigen Hauttumor beim Goldhamster. *Arch. Geschwulstforsch.*, **30**: 277–283, 1967). When an attempt was made to transmit these skin tumors by filtrates to newborn hamsters, lymphomas developed in 45 per cent of the inoculated animals; reticulum-cell sarcomas were also induced when centrifuged skin tumor extracts were inoculated into newborn Wistar rats. Electron microscopic examination of the hamster lymphomas revealed in the cytoplasm a small number of spherical virus particles, about 90 to 100 mμ in diameter; some particles were budding from the membrane of the endoplasmic reticulum. The lymphomas induced either in hamsters or in rats could be transmitted by filtrates to newborn hamsters, reproducing the same disease (GRAFFI, A., SCHRAMM, T., BENDER, E., GRAFFI, I., HORN, K.-H., and BIERWOLF, D., Cell-free transmissible leukoses in Syrian hamsters, probably of viral aetiology. *Brit. J. Cancer*, **22**: 577–581, 1968).

CHAPTER 19

Oncogenic Potency of Simian Virus 40 (SV 40)

Monkey kidney cell cultures have been used extensively in recent years for the propagation of certain viruses, such as poliomyelitis or adenoviruses, particularly for the preparation of vaccines. Cell cultures prepared from kidneys of thousands of monkeys have been employed by pharmaceutical companies engaged in the production of such vaccines.

Ideally, a cell culture employed for the propagation and subsequent harvesting of a virus should be free from other bacterial or viral agents; this is particularly imperative in case such cultures are to be used for the preparation of live vaccines, such as the Sabin oral poliomyelitis vaccine. This condition, however, is difficult to fulfill; no cell cultures are entirely free from indigenous viruses, particularly if these agents are latent and not detectable under the usual laboratory conditions. Certain viruses may multiply in a cell and yet may not cause any degenerative changes in cell morphology; such viral agents are obviously very difficult to detect. Other viruses are cytopathogenic and cause characteristic degenerative changes in the cells in which they are propagated.

Attempts to Detect Latent Viruses in Tissue Culture. Several methods are employed in order to detect latent viruses. To begin with, a virus which is initially latent may become cytopathogenic following serial passage in the same type of cells. In another attempt to detect a latent virus, the fluid collected from tissue culture in which a latent virus is presumably present can be transferred to a cell culture of another type. This is done in order to determine whether a virus latent in one type of cells may not induce degenerative changes in another cell variety, perhaps in a cell culture from another organ of the same species, or in a cell line from another animal species. In some instances, electron microscopic study of cell cultures in which the virus is grown may reveal the presence of characteristic virus particles. One of the most important methods employed in an attempt to detect a virus is that of bio-assay; under proper experimental conditions, a virus which either does or does not cause a cytopathic effect in tissue culture may still induce characteristic disease symptoms following inoculation into susceptible animals.

All these experimental tools directed at the detection of latent viruses have, however, considerable limitations; in spite of all attempts at its detection a virus may remain latent in cell cultures, and its presence may remain unrecognized. It may be very difficult to find the proper cell line in which such a latent virus may induce a cytopathic effect. The same applies to the bio-assay method; a virus may not necessarily be pathogenic for the animal species employed for the bio-assay tests, and yet it may remain fully pathogenic for another animal species not yet tested, and also for humans.

Early Isolation of Viruses from Normal Monkey Kidney Cells. Viral agents have long been isolated from normal monkey kidney cells. In 1933 Gay and Holden isolated the W virus; in 1934 Sabin and Wright recovered the B virus from a young physician who was bitten on the hand by an apparently healthy rhesus monkey in the laboratory and, as a result, developed an ascending myelitis which terminated fatally. Both viruses were related to the herpes virus; it is generally believed that W and B viruses are identical. Six strains of virus B were recently isolated from pools of poliomyelitis virus which had been grown on rhesus monkey kidney cells; out of 650 pools examined, six were found contaminated with the B virus (Wood and Shimada, 1954).

In recent years it has been gradually recognized that monkey kidney cell cultures which have been so extensively employed in the preparation of vaccines contain a large number of latent indigenous viruses most of which defy detection under the usual laboratory conditions.

How Many Latent Viruses in Normal Rhesus Monkey Kidney Cells? It has been noticed repeatedly that degenerative changes occur in the monkey kidney cells grown in tissue culture, even if they have not been seeded with any extraneous viruses. At first it was thought that such degenerative changes were due to a possible toxic effect of some substances present either in cells or in the media, or to some extraneous factors; however, it was realized later that these degenerative changes were frequently caused by cytopathic action of a latent virus or viruses present in such cells. At least some of these viruses were eventually isolated and the cytopathic effect they cause was reproduced by transferring such viruses from one culture to another. Other viruses present in monkey kidney cells did not cause degenerative changes in cells in which they were naturally harbored, and their presence had to be determined by other methods; among such viruses many remained unidentified.

Rustigian and his colleagues (1955) reported that normal monkey kidney cells harbor several latent viruses which under certain conditions, such as serial passage in tissue culture, may become cytopathogenic. Among the isolated viruses one was designated as the "foamy virus" because of characteristic cytopathic changes it induces on passage in rhesus monkey kidney cells. During production and testing of poliomyelitis vaccines in which many thousands of monkey kidney cell cultures were prepared, many latent viruses were recovered from normal monkey kidney cells.

Hull and his colleagues (1956, 1957, 1958) at the Lilly Research Laboratories in Indianapolis, Indiana, described and classified a considerable number of simian viruses recovered from rhesus and cynomolgus monkey kidney cell cultures. At least some of these viruses caused distinct cytopathic changes on passage in rhesus monkey kidney cells. On the basis of cytopathic changes induced, Hull and his coworkers classified these simian viruses into 4 groups. Other viruses, also present in normal monkey kidney cells, could not be properly identified. There were so many of these agents that Hull and his colleagues suggested (1956) the designation of these viruses as "Simian Viruses" (S.V.) with added numbers, such as SV 1, SV 2, SV 3, etc. Viruses were also recovered from patas (*Erythrocebus patas*) monkey kidney cells by Hsiung and Gaylord (1961). At least 6 different viruses were recovered by Malherbe and Harwin (1957) from *Cercopithecus aethiops* monkey kidney cells; these viral agents caused characteristic cytopathic effect with formation of nuclear inclusion bodies and were designated as "Simian Agents" (S.A.) with added numbers, such as SA 1, SA 2, SA 3, etc.

The latent viruses of monkey kidney origin presented a real problem in the cell culture technique and in the preparation of vaccines. Such indigenous simian viruses contaminated, or in some instances even inhibited, the inoculated virus which was to be propagated in monkey kidney cultures. Most important of all, such viruses had to be excluded from any live virus vaccines prepared in monkey kidney cells and intended for use in man, since it was immediately realized that the long-term effect of human infection with such agents was unknown and had to be considered.

Isolation of the "Vacuolating Agent" from Normal Rhesus Monkey Kidney Cells

Most of the simian viruses derived from monkey kidney cell cultures could be detected in kidney cell cultures of the same monkey species, either in primary cultures or in further passages, because of the cytopathic effect they eventually exerted on the cells in which they were grown. This cytopathic effect could be recognized by a characteristic destruction of the cells in which such viruses were propagated, and frequently also by the formation of nuclear inclusion bodies. However, the question has often been raised whether there could also exist in monkey kidney cells latent viruses which may be present in such cells, but which could not be detected by current procedures because of their failure to induce degenerative changes in the cell cultures in which they were naturally harbored.

Formation of Characteristic Vacuoles in the Cytoplasm of Cercopithecus Monkey Kidney Cells Infected with the Newly Isolated Virus. Sweet and Hilleman at the Merck Institute for Therapeutic Research in West Point, Pennsylvania, reported in 1960 that in their tissue culture studies they observed what appeared to be a new simian virus of either rhesus or cynomolgus monkey kidney origin which did not cause any significant cytopathic changes in kidney cell cultures of the same species, and which was therefore undetectable when grown in its natural host cells; the same virus, however, caused very marked and distinctive cytopathic changes in kidney cell cultures of the African green monkey, *Cercopithecus aethiops*, i.e. grivet, according to Sanderson (1957), obtained from Equatorial East Africa. Sweet and Hilleman referred to this newly isolated virus as the "*vacuolating agent*" because of the prominent development of vacuoles in the cytoplasm of cells infected with this virus. This cytopathic effect on the morphology of grivet kidney cells was very characteristic and appeared to be specific for this particular viral agent.

Formation of Intranuclear Inclusion Bodies. A few days prior to the development of the cytoplasmic vacuoles, formation of intranuclear inclusion bodies in cells infected with this virus could frequently be observed, particularly in patas monkey kidney cells in which the vacuolating agent was propagated (Hsiung and Gaylord, 1961. Gaylord and Hsiung, 1961), but also in vervet monkey kidney cells, and at least in some instances in rhesus kidney cells (Pay, 1961) as well. However, intranuclear inclusions were also produced by other simian viruses, and an attempt to identify the vacuolating agent on the basis of nuclear chromatin alterations could have presented serious difficulties.

Sweet and Hilleman noted in their report (1960) that even though the vacuolating agent which they had just isolated caused the characteristic cytopathic changes when grown in kidney cell cultures of the African green monkey, *Cercopithecus aethiops*, yet *Cercopithecus* monkey kidney cells were found to be remarkably free from contamination with this agent. In the course of more than 1000 lots of individual monkey kidney cell cultures examined, the presence of the vacuolating agent was detected only in one lot. On the other hand, this agent is very common, and essentially ubiquitous, in rhesus monkey kidney cell cultures, and is also a common contaminant of cynomolgus kidney cell cultures.

The "Vacuolating Agent" is Designated "Simian Virus 40" i.e. "S.V. 40"

In an attempt to classify this virus Hull suggested (Sweet and Hilleman, 1960) that the vacuolating virus be included in his group 4 of simian viruses causing cytopathic effect in tissue culture, and that it be designated "Simian Virus 40," i.e., "S.V. 40," or simply SV 40.

In their initial report, Sweet and Hilleman concluded that the vacuolating agent "appears to be just one more of the troublesome simian agents to be screened and then eliminated from virus seed stocks and from live virus vaccines." They stressed at the same time, however, that the demonstration of the vacuolating agent as a common contaminant of rhesus and cynomolgus monkey kidney cells also raised the question of the possible presence of other indigenous and inapparent monkey kidney agents which might be detected under different methods of testing. The possible long range pathogenic effects of either the SV 40 virus, or some other indigenous agents present in such cells, on their natural hosts, and particularly on humans, had to be considered.

The vacuolating agent was first isolated and recognized in Dr. Hilleman's Virus and Tissue Culture Laboratories at the Merck Institute by L. McClelland in the course of safety testing of vaccines (Sweet and Hilleman, 1960).

The presence of a previously undescribed latent simian virus in either rhesus (Pay, 1961) or patas (Hsiung and Gaylord, 1961) monkey kidney cells had been previously suspected. Sweet and Hilleman were the first, however, to identify, isolate, and pass this virus in different cell lines, to describe its physical and biological properties, and to recognize its ability to induce consistently the characteristic vacuolating degenerative changes in *Cercopithecus* monkey kidney cells, in contrast to its latency in rhesus monkey kidney cells, and thus to provide a test for the recognition and identification of this virus.

Induction of Tumors in Hamsters with Normal Monkey Kidney Cell Culture Extracts

The possible pathogenic potential of some of the latent viruses present in normal monkey kidney cell cultures employed extensively in recent years for the preparation of vaccines has long been considered by virologists and public health officials, and particularly by those concerned with the investigation of the safety of biological products prepared for use in humans.

The possibility that some of the latent viruses present in normal rhesus monkey kidney cell cultures may be potentially oncogenic was also considered. In order to test such a possibility, Dr. Bernice E. Eddy and her coworkers, Borman, Berkeley, and Young, at the Division of Biologics Standards of the National Institute of Health in Bethesda, Md., carried out an experimental study (1961) in which tissue culture fluid collected from normal monkey kidney cell cultures was inoculated into newborn hamsters. Since the number of viruses present in monkey kidney cells was very large, it was impractical to test each virus individually; for that reason, two lots of rhesus monkey kidney cells taken from kidneys of 8 to 10 monkeys were incubated for 14 days, and the tissue culture fluids were then pooled and inoculated into 23 newborn hamsters.

The high susceptibility of newborn animals in bio-assay experiments dealing with the study of oncogenic viruses in mammals had been recognized since the early studies dealing with the isolation of the mouse leukemia and the parotid tumor viruses (Gross, 1951, 1953). Newborn hamsters proved even more susceptible than newborn mice to the induction of the polyoma virus (Eddy *et al.*, 1958). Accordingly, newborn hamsters were selected by Eddy as test animals for the determination of the possible oncogenic potential of latent viruses present in normal monkey kidney cell cultures.

In the initial experiment, 20 out of 23 injected hamsters developed tumors. The first tumor appeared after about 4 months, other tumors gradually later, some as late as 15 months after inoculation. The tumors, undifferentiated sarcomas, developed at the site of inoculation; they increased rapidly in size, some of them eventually becoming as large as the rest of the animal (Eddy *et al.*, 1961).

The experiment was repeated. Fluid collected from normal monkey kidney cell cultures was inoculated into 154 newborn hamsters, and as a result, 109 of them (70 per cent) developed tumors. The extract could be passed through a bacterial Selas 03 filter candle and still retained its oncogenic potential; out of 14 newborn hamsters inoculated with such a filtered extract, 13 developed tumors. The earliest tumor was detected after 3 months, but most of the tumors developed after 9 months. All tumors developed at the site of inoculation as single, occasionally multiple, subcutaneous sarcomas. Some hamsters had tumors in the lungs or kidneys as well.

The tumors could be transplanted without difficulty by cell-graft to newborn hamsters; they developed in the inoculated animals after two to three weeks and grew progressively.

An Unidentified Oncogenic "Substance" in Normal Monkey Kidney Cells Posing a Serious Safety Problem. The observation that extracts prepared from normal rhesus kidney cell cultures induced malignant tumors following inoculation into newborn hamsters posed a serious problem, since such cultures were used routinely to propagate poliovirus and adenoviruses for the production of vaccines. It was imperative to determine the source of the oncogenic material in normal monkey kidney cell cultures. However, in the initial experiments carried out by Eddy and her coworkers (1961), no virus could be recovered from the tumors which had been induced in hamsters with normal monkey cell extracts. Several attempts were made to recover a virus; extracts made from the induced tumors were inoculated into newborn hamsters, but no tumors developed in the injected animals; in another experiment tumor extracts were

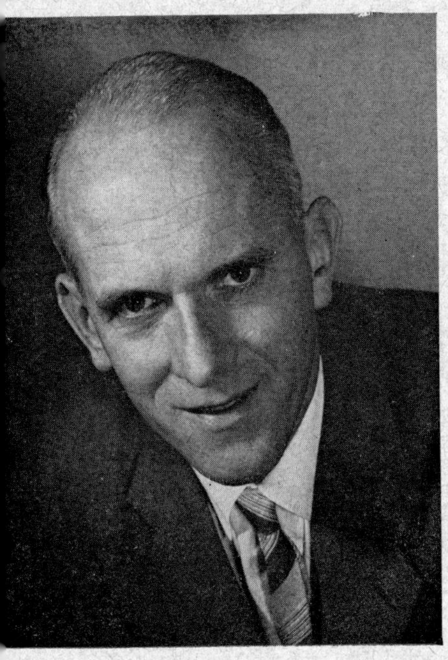

Allan F. Howatson

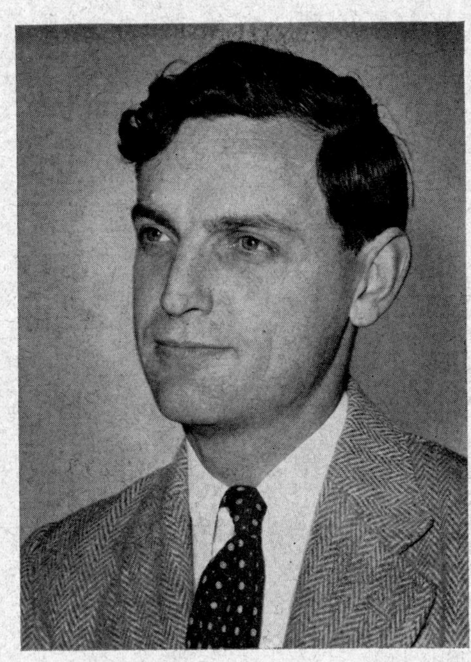

R. W. Horne

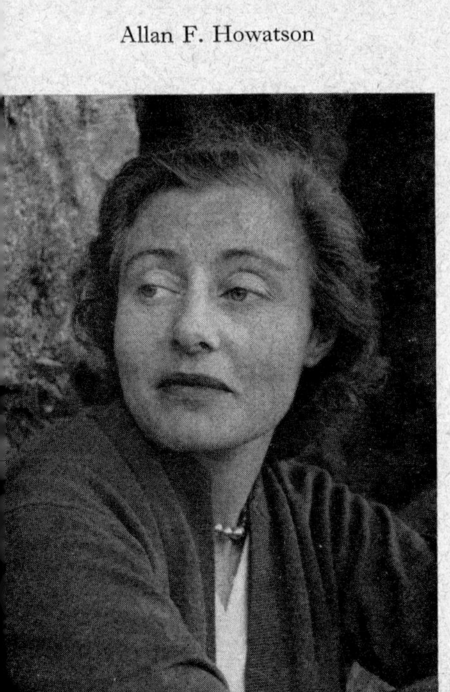

Françoise Haguenau

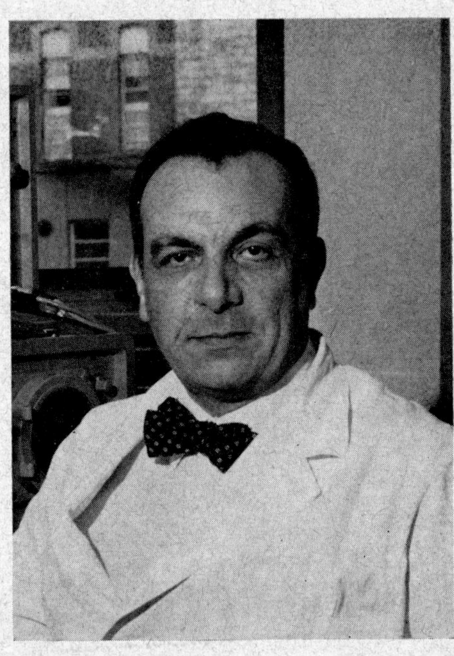

Marcel Bessis

Fig. 63

inoculated into several cell lines, such as mouse embryo, rhesus monkey, and vervet monkey kidney cells, but no definite evidence of virus growth could be obtained in tissue culture. Failure to recover a virus from the induced tumors led Dr. Eddy and her coworkers (1961) to designate the tumor-inducing material present in normal rhesus monkey kidney cells as a "substance."

Tumors Induced in Hamsters with Normal Monkey Kidney Cell Extracts Were Not Caused by Polyoma Virus. It was necessary to exclude the possibility that the inoculated extracts contained the polyoma virus, since it is known that the parotid tumor, i.e. polyoma, virus is also capable of inducing subcutaneous sarcomas following inoculation into newborn hamsters. However, although there were similarities in microscopic morphology between the tumors induced in hamsters by monkey kidney cell extracts and those induced by the polyoma virus, there was a striking difference in the distribution of the tumors. The monkey kidney cell extracts consistently induced subcutaneous sarcomas, and in a few instances also tumors in the lungs and kidneys. On the other hand, if a sufficient dose of polyoma virus was inoculated into newborn hamsters, not only subcutaneous sarcomas were induced, but also tumors or hemangiomas in the heart muscle, in the liver, stomach, intestines, and other internal organs. No such tumors, and particularly no hemangiomas, were induced with the monkey kidney cell extracts.

The polyoma virus causes hemagglutination of red blood cells which can be inhibited by a specific immune serum collected from animals infected with this virus. However, extracts of either tumors or organs of hamsters which developed sarcomas as a result of inoculation of normal monkey kidney cell extracts did not agglutinate erythrocytes; furthermore, the serum from such animals did not inhibit the agglutinating ability of the polyoma virus.

It was quite apparent, therefore, that the oncogenic potency of normal rhesus monkey kidney cell extracts for hamsters was not due to the presence in such extracts of the polyoma virus (Eddy *et al.*, 1961).

IDENTIFICATION OF THE TUMOR-INDUCING "SUBSTANCE" PRESENT IN MONKEY KIDNEY CELL EXTRACTS AS SIMIAN VIRUS 40 AND INDEPENDENT DEMONSTRATION IN ANOTHER LABORATORY THAT SV 40 IS ONCOGENIC FOR HAMSTERS

Isolation of the vacuolating agent (SV 40) by Sweet and Hilleman marked a significant development in the study of indigenous simian viruses; such latent, and often difficult to detect, viruses had been frequently referred to as nothing more than troublesome agents interfering with normal production of commercial vaccines; however, the possible pathogenic potential of such viruses has long been considered. The newly isolated virus was latent in rhesus monkey kidney cell cultures, even though it multiplied in such cells to a considerable degree; the same virus, however, was consistently cytopathogenic for kidney cells of another, i.e. *Cercopithecus aethiops*, monkey species. This virus could now be readily identified, and it became immediately apparent that it is a very common contaminant of most of the rhesus monkey kidney cell cultures, and that most of the commercially available lots of polio and adenovirus vaccines employed for humans, including young children and in some instances also newborn human infants, contained traces of this virus. Unfortunately, this virus was found to have considerable resistance to heating and to formaldehyde, and for that reason not only live virus vaccines but also some of the formalin-inactivated vaccines were found to contain viable simian virus 40.

Accordingly, the question of the possible long-term pathogenic, and particularly oncogenic potential of this newly discovered and ubiquitous contaminant had to be seriously considered.

Identification of the Tumor-inducing "Substance" Present in Normal Rhesus Monkey Kidney Cells as Simian Virus 40

The striking oncogenic potential of the vacuolating agent was discovered simultaneously in two laboratories. Eddy and her coworkers, who only one year earlier (1961) had observed that normal rhesus monkey kidney cell extracts induced malignant tumors following inoculation into newborn hamsters, were now able to identify the oncogenic "substance" present in such extracts as the vacuolating agent, i.e. the SV 40 virus. After initial unsuccessful attempts (1961), Eddy and her coworkers now succeeded (1962) in recovering, by intermediate passage through tissue culture, the simian virus 40 from tumors which they had induced in hamsters with normal rhesus monkey kidney cell extracts. Furthermore, they reported at the same time that an anti-SV 40 immune serum neutralized the oncogenic action of such extracts (Eddy *et al.*, May, 1962a).

Induction of Tumors in Hamsters with Cultures of Simian Virus 40. At about the same time, Girardi, Sweet, Slotnick, and Hilleman reported on April 13, 1962, at the Annual Meeting of the American Association for Cancer Research in Atlantic City, N.J., that inoculation of SV 40 virus cultures into newborn hamsters resulted in the development of subcutaneous progressively growing malignant sarcomas in most of the inoculated animals.

It was therefore recognized independently in two different laboratories that the SV 40 virus has a considerable oncogenic potential for hamsters. The possible oncogenic potential of this common contaminant of normal monkey kidney cell cultures for other animal species, including humans, raised a serious problem concerning the safety of many lots of vaccines prepared in monkey kidney cells for use in human patients.

Properties of the Simian Virus 40

The vacuolating agent, also designated the SV 40 virus, a small spherical particle about 30 to 40 mμ in diameter, is a common contaminant of normal Asian rhesus (*Macaca mulatta*), and less frequently also of cynomolgus monkey kidney cell cultures. The SV 40 virus is essentially ubiquitous in various virus seed stocks and vaccines, suggesting a high infection rate with this virus among normal monkey kidney cell cultures.

The SV 40 virus can readily be propagated in rhesus and cynomolgus monkey kidney cells, and attains a high titer in such cultures without inducing any of the destructive changes in the morphology of infected cells which would indicate the presence of the virus. The virus can also be propagated in grivet, i.e., *Cercopithecus* monkey kidney cells; however, in the grivet kidney cells the virus induces a characteristic cytopathic effect. In addition to being cytopathic for the grivet monkey, it was also found to be cytopathic for the vervet monkey kidney cells.

> There are now some 20 subspecies of the *Cercopithecus* group of monkeys recognized, but the differences between many of them are very slight. They are spread around Africa from Senegambia to Abyssinia (Ethiopia) and thence south to the Cape. They are known as vervets in South Africa, as grivets in northern areas, and as green monkeys in West Africa (Sanderson, 1957).

The SV 40 virus was also cytopathogenic for the closely to the grivet related patas (*Erythrocebus patas*) monkey kidney cells, and for rhesus monkey testicle cells; however, these cells were about 30 to 300 times less sensitive than grivet kidney cells to the cytopathic effect of the vacuolating agent.

Cytopathic Changes Induced with SV 40 Virus in Cercopithecus Aethiops Kidney Cells. The cytopathic changes induced with the SV 40 virus in green monkey, i.e. *Cercopithecus aethiops*, kidney cells are very characteristic for this particular virus and quite different from those induced by other monkey kidney cell viruses previously described. Following inoculation of the grivet kidney cell cultures with a sufficient dose of the virus, the first morphological changes in the cell morphology begin to appear 3 to 4 days later; some of the cells appear rounded or shrunken, and a few may show a beginning vacuolation of the cytoplasm. Soon typical changes develop, consisting predominantly of ballooning of cells and intense vacuolation of the cytoplasm of such cells. These vacuoles are highly characteristic, particularly in wet preparations; in hematoxylin and eosin stained material they appear as "holes" with intensely stained boundaries. Five to 10 days after inoculation of the virus the cells aggregate together and detach from the glass. These cytopathic changes are very specific and can be recognized at once. Intense vacuolation of the infected cells led to the initial designation of this virus as the "vacuolating agent," later changed to "simian virus 40."

Resistance to Heat, Ether, and Formaldehyde. The SV 40 virus is remarkably resistant to heat. There is only a moderate loss of viral activity after heating the virus to 60°C for 30 minutes; in certain experiments the presence of some infectivity could still be demonstrated after heating the virus to 70°C for 30 minutes.

The virus is resistant to treatment for 18 hours with an equal amount of ethyl ether.

It is of considerable practical importance that the SV 40 virus is also relatively resistant to formaldehyde; it is not inactivated by a concentration of formaldehyde which is sufficiently strong to inactivate polio or adenoviruses; viable SV 40 virus could be recovered from certain lots of formalin-inactivated adenovirus, or from Salk polio vaccines. Most of the SV 40 virus present in tissue culture fluid could be inactivated with 1 : 4000 formaldehyde at 37°C, but less rapidly than the poliomyelitis virus.

No Hemagglutinating Activity. Culture fluid containing the virus does not cause hemagglutination of guinea pig, chicken, or human "O" erythrocytes, at 4°C, or at 25°C. Furthermore, the virus is not adsorbed by red blood cells.

Electron Microscopic Studies

Tournier, Granboulan and Bernhard (1961) examined in the electron microscope ultrathin sections of *Cercopithecus aethiops* kidney cells infected with the SV 40 virus. Beginning with the second day after virus inoculation, and more extensively a day or two later, characteristic changes could be observed in the nuclei of the infected cells, consisting of margination and development of irregularly-shaped dense areas in the chromatin with a simultaneous striking appearance of innumerable small spherical virus particles; these particles were homogenous, and had no external membranes. The medium diameter of individual particles was 33 mμ; the center-to-center distance of packed particles within the crystalline arrays was 40 to 42 mμ. The regularity of the size of the individual particles was striking (Granboulan *et al.*, 1963).

At the same time characteristic lesions could be observed in the nucleoli, consisting of development of very dense areas containing granules and also filaments. With each advancing day the number of virus particles in the cell nuclei increased, until they formed crystalline arrays of packed virus particles which practically filled out the entire nucleus. Between the fifth and tenth day after infection, most of the cell nuclei were found to be filled with virus particles. At this phase, virus particles appeared also in the cytoplasm, and the cells began to disintegrate.

In the cytoplasm the number, and particularly the size, of the vacuoles increased considerably following infection with the virus; this observation corresponded closely to the cytopathic effect of the virus on the cells, described in the studies with the light microscope. Virus particles could be found in the cytoplasm in general after 6 days following infection, and in some cases earlier (Granboulan *et al.*, 1963).

Gaylord and Hsiung (1961) studied the SV 40 virus propagated on *Erythrocebus patas* kidney cells. They observed formation in the infected cells of nuclear inclusion bodies which contained virus particles. In advanced phases the nuclei were almost entirely filled with virus particles. The particles were spherical, homogenous, of moderate electron density, and about 30 mμ in diameter.

Melnick (1962), Bernhard and his coworkers (1962), and also Horne (1963a) studied the SV 40 particles by the negative staining method and found that these particles are made up of 42 capsomeres in a 5 : 3 : 2 (icosahedral) pattern, the same as the polyoma virus. The electron microscopic studies of the structure and symmetry of virus particles were reviewed by Horne (1963b).

Papova Virus Group. Melnick observed (1962) that the papilloma, polyoma, and SV 40 viruses seem to form a natural group with certain common properties for which he suggested the name "*papova virus group*". Members of this group have the following properties: 45 mμ diameter, deoxyribonucleic acid core, 42 capsomeres, absence of essential lipids, thermal resistance, slow growth cycle with multiplication within the cell nucleus, and oncogenic potential. For additional information see page 890.

It is of interest that SV 40 virus particles could be detected with the electron microscope without difficulty in infected monkey kidney cells in tissue culture, but not in tumors induced in hamsters with the same virus. This interesting observation will be discussed in more detail on subsequent pages of this chapter.

Chemical Nature of the SV 40 Virus. Because virus-containing inclusions in the cytoplasm were found to be Feulgen positive (Gaylord and Hsiung, 1961), it may be assumed that SV 40 is a DNA virus.

Antigenic Properties of the Simian Virus 40. The SV 40 virus is strongly antigenic. A specific immune serum could be obtained from rabbits that had been immunized with several injections of this virus. The antibodies could be detected either by direct virus neutralization tests, or by complement fixation. In the virus neutralization tests the oncogenic potency of tissue culture fluid containing simian virus 40 could be completely neutralized by a specific anti-SV 40 immune rabbit serum. In a more rapid test, the cytopathic effect of the virus, i.e. the formation of characteristic vacuoles in the cytoplasm of *Cercopithecus* monkey kidney cells in tissue culture, could be inhibited following neutralization of the virus *in vitro* by a specific immune serum.

Antigenically, the SV 40 virus is distinct from any other known viruses; no antigenic variants of the simian virus 40 have yet been described. All strains of vacuolating virus studied until now have been of the same single immunologic group.

Specific antibodies directed against the simian virus 40 could be detected in monkeys carrying this virus as a latent contaminant, and also in hosts of different species, including monkeys and humans, which had received this virus by inoculation.

Routes of Natural Transmission of the SV 40 Virus

The spread of the virus under natural life conditions in its simian hosts has not yet been sufficiently clarified and the information thus far available is limited. One of the difficulties in determining experimentally the manner of natural transmission of the SV 40 virus is caused by the fact that this virus does not seem to induce definite symptoms of disease in its rhesus carrier, or in other related monkey species, and the presence of infection can be determined only by isolation of the virus from either nasopharyngeal swabs or from feces of such hosts, or on the basis of development of specific humoral antibodies in the infected animals. Information thus far accumulated suggests that the virus can be transmitted by respiratory route, by intimate contact of susceptible hosts exposed to animals which excrete the virus, and possibly to some limited extent also by oral route. The route of natural transmission may be influenced by the susceptibility of the host species in which it is studied. There was no evidence of virus transmission by contact among newborn hamsters (Girardi *et al.*, 1963), but contact infection did occur in green monkeys caged with virus-carrying animals (Meyer *et al.*, 1962).

In his experiments, Girardi and his colleagues inoculated one half of each of four litters of newborn hamsters with the SV 40 virus. The inoculated and the control animals of each litter were housed together in the same cages. No tumors developed in any of the uninoculated control animals. However, Girardi and his colleagues were looking for tumor development as evidence of virus infection. On the other hand, in experiments performed on monkeys by Meyer and his coworkers the appearance of specific antibodies in the blood of animals exposed to contact infection was considered as evidence of virus infection; the latter may be a much more sensitive test.

Induction of Tumors in Hamsters Following Inoculation of Simian Virus 40

Following inoculation of the SV 40 virus into newborn hamsters, most of the inoculated animals developed either single or multiple tumors at the site of inoculation after a latency varying from $2\frac{1}{2}$ to 3 months. In addition, some animals developed similar tumors also in lungs and kidneys. If a sufficient dose of the virus was inoculated, practically all animals developed tumors. The induced subcutaneous tumors consisted of hard masses which infiltrated the skin and subcutaneous tissues, and invaded the adjacent muscles. The tumors grew progressively, and never regressed; in some instances they eventually became larger than the rest of the animal.

Influence of Age at Inoculation. Newborn and less than 2-day-old suckling hamsters were uniformly susceptible to the oncogenic potency of the SV 40 virus; over 95 per cent of such animals developed tumors following inoculation of a sufficient dose of virus. The susceptibility of hamsters decreased rapidly with increasing age. When hamsters were inoculated at 7 to 8 days of age, about 60 per cent still developed tumors, but the latency was prolonged. The animals remained relatively susceptible to inoculation up to about 3 weeks of age, but the incidence of induced tumors was substantially lower in the older group, and the latency considerably prolonged. Girardi and his coworkers (1963) observed a few tumors in hamsters that had been inoculated at one month of age; tumors appeared in such animals after a latency of about one year. No tumors could be induced when older animals were inoculated. Eddy and her coworkers (1962b) did not observe development of tumors when hamsters more than three weeks old were inoculated.

The susceptibility of the newborn hamsters to the oncogenic potency of the SV 40 virus, and the rapid development of relative resistance with increasing age, bore a striking resemblance to earlier observations recorded in the study of mouse leukemia. In these experiments (Gross, 1951), newborn mice were found susceptible to the leukemogenic action of the mouse leukemia virus; gradually, however, with increasing age, the animals became relatively resistant to the induction of disease following inoculation of the virus; this was apparent from the lower incidence of induced disease, and longer latency elapsing between the inoculation of the virus and development of leukemia in such animals.

Route of Inoculation, and Dose of the Injected Virus. Several routes of inoculation were tested, such as subcutaneous, intraperitoneal, intrathoracic, and intracerebral; tumors could be induced by any of these routes, but the subcutaneous route of virus inoculation was found to be most suitable for the induction of tumors (Eddy *et al.*, 1961, 1962b). As a rule tumors were induced at the site of inoculation; following intraperitoneal or intrathoracic inoculation, tumors could be induced in the peritoneal or in the chest cavity, but frequently in such animals subcutaneous tumors developed also at the site where the virus was introduced through the skin puncture. In some experiments, only subcutaneous tumors developed even following intraperitoneal or intrathoracic inoculation (Girardi *et al.*, 1962). All these tumors, including neoplasms developing in the abdominal and chest cavities, had a similar microscopic morphology, i.e. that of undifferentiated sarcomas.

Intracerebral inoculation of the SV 40 virus into newborn hamsters resulted in the development of ependymomas (Kirschstein and Gerber, 1962. Eddy, 1962).

There was a correlation between the injected doses and the incidence and time of development of tumors. A higher incidence of tumors developing after a shorter latency was observed after inoculation of higher doses of the virus.

Morphology of the Induced Tumors. All tumors developing in hamsters following either subcutaneous, intraperitoneal, or intrathoracic inoculation of the virus were sarcomas. These tumors grew progressively, infiltrating the adjacent tissues. Microscopic examination revealed that these tumors were undifferentiated sarcomas, frequently containing multinucleated giant cells. Parts of some of the subcutaneous tumors had the morphology of fibrosarcomas. The ependymomas developing in the brain as a result of intracerebral inoculation of simian virus 40 were gliomas, brain tumors, arising from the ependymal lining of the ventricles, and consisting of papillary masses of cuboidal cells with darkly stained nuclei and scant cytoplasm.

Transplantation of the Induced Tumors. The induced tumors could be transplanted without difficulty from one hamster to another either in newborn or young adult animals. Following transplantation by cell-graft, tumors developed in the inoculated animals after a latency of 2 to 3 weeks; the transplanted tumors grew progressively.

Difficulty in Recovering Virus from the Induced Tumors

No virus could be recovered from the tumors in sufficient quantity in order to pass the virus directly from one animal to another. However, the virus could be recovered by intermediary passage through tissue culture. Following inoculation of *Cercopithecus* kidney cell cultures with tumor extracts, a characteristic cytopathic effect consisting of the formation of vacuoles in the cytoplasm of infected cells could be detected in most

---

FIG. 64. SV 40 VIRUS PARTICLES.

(A). Section of *Cercopithecus* kidney cell 10 days after infection with SV 40 virus. Intranuclear virus particles. Magnification 30,000 ×. (B). Section of *Cercopithecus* kidney cell 10 days after infection with SV 40 virus. Intranuclear crystalline array of small uniform virus particles. The particles have no external membrane, but present a clear zone on their periphery, which may correspond to the capsid. Magnification 70,000 ×. Photomicrographs prepared by N. Granboulan, Institut de Recherches Scientifiques sur le Cancer, Villejuif (Seine), France.

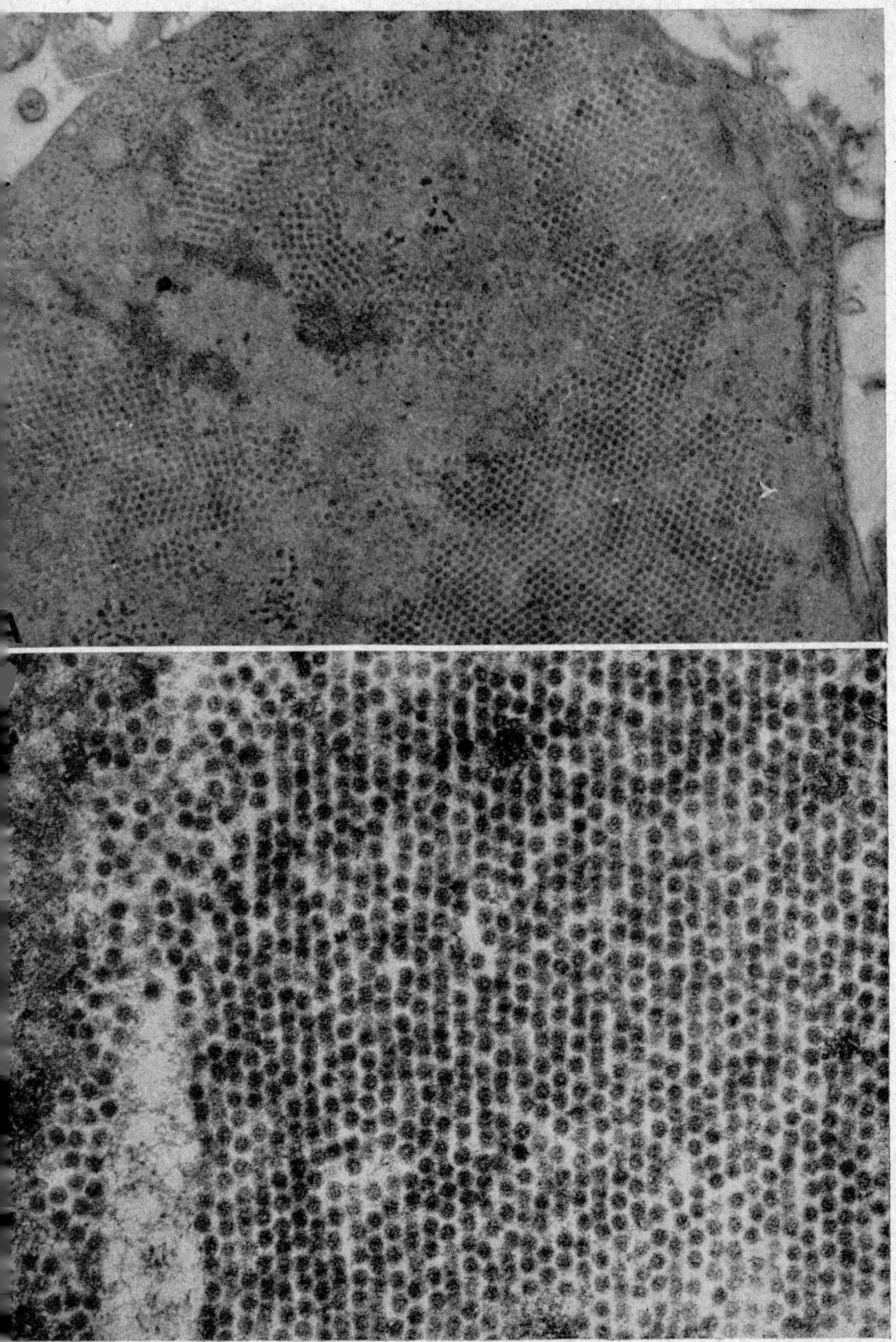

Fig. 64. SV 40 Virus Particles.

of the infected cultures; frequently, however, this occurred only after a prolonged incubation, or after a preliminary blind passage made in order to increase the titer of the isolated virus. More virus was present in large than in small tumors. However, often many difficulties were encountered in recovering the virus from the induced tumors (Girardi *et al.*, 1962. Eddy, 1962. Sabin and Koch, 1963. Ashkenazi and Melnick, 1963). In general, only very small quantities of virus could be recovered from the induced primary or transplanted tumors, and frequently no virus at all could be recovered from some of the tumors.

Failure to Detect Virus Particles on Electron Microscopic Examination of Tumor Cells. Electron microscopic examination did not reveal the presence of virus particles in the induced tumors, in contrast to the commonly accomplished demonstration of the presence of such particles in infected tissue culture cells.

* * *

The failure to detect virus particles in the induced tumors on electron microscopic examination recalled similar difficulties encountered in experiments dealing with tumors induced by either adenoviruses or by the polyoma virus. In these experiments, discussed in separate chapters of this monograph, there were also difficulties in recovering the virus directly from tumors that had been induced by either of these viruses; furthermore, no virus particles could be detected on electron microscopic examination of such tumors. As in the case of experiments dealing with simian virus 40, these difficulties contrasted sharply with the successful isolation of adenoviruses or polyoma virus from the induced tumors following an intermediary tissue culture passage, and also with the ready detection of characteristic virus particles on electron microscopic examination of infected cells in which either of these two viruses had been grown in tissue culture.

Induction of Brain Tumors (Ependymomas) in Mastomys with the Simian Virus 40

Rabson and his coworkers (1962) at the Department of Pathology of the National Cancer Institute in Bethesda, Md., reported that subcutaneous inoculation of newborn *Mastomys* (*Rattus Mastomys natalensis*), an African rodent, with simian virus 40 (SV 40) resulted in the development of brain tumors having histopathologic characteristics of papillary ependymomas. These tumors have been found in 8 out of 10 animals that survived the inoculation trauma. The development of tumors became apparent after periods varying from 111 to 225 days.

Rattus (*Mastomys*) *natalensis* is an African rodent, intermediate in size between the rat and mouse; it has been employed in cancer research in recent years because of the high incidence of spontaneous adenocarcinoma of the stomach observed in these animals by Oettlé (1959) and because of the susceptibility of *Mastomys* to tumor induction by polyoma virus (Rabson *et al.*, 1960) and adenoviruses (Rabson *et al.*, 1964).

These experiments were of considerable interest; they demonstrated that the simian virus 40 could induce tumors not only in hamsters, but also in another animal species; moreover, it was of particular interest that subcutaneous inoculation of an oncogenic virus could induce brain tumors without the development of either subcutaneous or visceral neoplasms resulting from such inoculation.

Papillary ependymomas could be induced also in hamsters following direct intracerebral inoculation of simian virus 40 into newborn hamsters (Kirschstein and Gerber, 1962. Eddy, 1962).

Effect of Virus Infection on its Natural Carrier Host and Related Species

It appears that monkeys which are natural carriers of simian virus 40 do not develop symptoms of disease resulting from a latent infection with this virus. Experimental inoculation of simian virus 40 into monkeys did not induce any apparent illness in such animals and did not lead, thus far at least, to the formation of tumors. It must be stressed, nevertheless, that in order to obtain a more definite information on the possible oncogenic effect of simian virus 40 on its natural host, or on related species, newborn monkeys of a species or subspecies which is not a natural carrier of this virus, but is susceptible to virus propagation, would have to be inoculated. Furthermore, as an equally important condition, the observation time of the inoculated animals would have to be extended until they reach old age. It is known that some of the hamsters that had been inoculated with simian virus 40 when newborn did not develop tumors until almost at the end of their life span (Eddy, 1964).

Even though in studies thus far performed, no definite symptoms of disease could be induced following inoculation of the SV 40 virus into monkeys that were not natural carriers of this virus, the inoculated virus persisted and multiplied in the inoculated animals inducing an inapparent infection; the virus was excreted from such carriers in nasopharyngeal secretions, stools, and urine.

Ashkenazi and Melnick (1962), at Baylor University in Houston, inoculated the vacuolating SV 40 virus into seven baboons (*Papio doguera*) about 6 months old, and 12 green monkeys (*Cercopithecus aethiops*); the latter included eight young one-year-old animals and four infant seven-day-old monkeys. Both the green monkeys and the baboons are usually free from the SV 40 virus unless they are placed in contact with the infected Asian animals (Sweet and Hilleman, 1960. Meyer *et al.*, 1962. Ashkenazi and Melnick, 1962). The inoculations were made mostly by subcutaneous route; some of the animals received the virus intracutaneously or intracranially, and in a few instances by intranasal instillation or by oral route. No symptoms of illness were induced in any of the inoculated animals, but there was evidence that the virus persisted and multiplied more abundantly in the green monkeys than in the baboons. The SV 40 virus was found to be excreted in the urine collected from green monkeys during the first four weeks after infection. Virus was also recovered from the urine of all four baboons inoculated parenterally, but not from three baboons infected by intranasal or oral administration of virus. Later, in the course of infection, neutralizing antibodies appeared in blood and also in urine of these animals.

In another study, experimental infection of *Cercopithecus* monkeys with simian virus 40 by intranasal instillation resulted in viremia; again no illness resulted from the administration of the virus. However, a transient presence of the virus in the pharyngeal secretions and in the stools of the inoculated monkeys could be revealed in such animals during the first two weeks after inoculation; later on neutralizing antibodies appeared in the serum of the inoculated monkeys reaching a maximum titer by the seventh week (Meyer *et al.*, 1962). The virus was transmitted by contact infection to another uninoculated *Cercopithecus* monkey which was placed in the same cage; this was evident by the appearance of specific antibodies in that animal.

What is the Effect of Simian Virus 40 on Humans?

Only limited information is available concerning infection of humans with simian virus 40. No disease symptoms could be induced in humans following infection with this virus; however, observations thus far reported suggest that SV 40 virus can multiply in human hosts to some degree, and that at least a transient inapparent infection with this virus can be induced. The fact that a low grade latent infection with simian virus 40 could be established in humans following inoculation of this virus became evident after it was demonstrated that specific antibodies directed against the SV 40 virus appeared in subjects which had received this virus inadvertently in small quantities during parenteral administration of poliomyelitis or adenovirus vaccines. Live SV 40 virus in traces, or sometimes in moderate quantities, was present as a contaminant of vaccines prepared from virus pools grown in rhesus and cynomolgus kidney cell cultures (Sweet and Hilleman, 1960. Gerber *et al.*, 1961. Goffe *et al.*, 1961. Magrath *et al.*, 1961. Melnick, 1962). The monkey kidney cell cultures employed for the propagation of virus pools frequently contained the vacuolating agent, and for that reason vaccines prepared from such cultures also contained this virus. Not only live polio vaccines, but formalin-inactivated vaccines frequently contained viable SV 40 virus, since the vacuolating agent is relatively resistant to formalin.

The simian virus 40 could also infect humans, without causing symptoms of disease, following administration by the respiratory route. This became evident when the respiratory syncytial virus vaccine, which also contained as a contaminant the SV 40 virus, was given by intranasal route, by nebulization, and also by instillation of the virus into the nostrils (Morris *et al.*, 1961). Out of 35 inoculated volunteers, 3 showed presence of the vacuolating agent in throat swabs taken 7 to 11 days after inoculation; specific neutralizing antibodies appeared in the blood serum of 22 individuals.

Infection with simian virus 40 by oral route also occurred in certain instances. Most of the Sabin live poliomyelitis vaccines employed contained only trace amounts of infectious simian virus 40; a few, however, contained relatively larger amounts, and some among them even close to 10^5 TCD_{50} (Melnick and Stinebaugh, 1962). In several studies no evidence of infection was found in human subjects following ingestion of the oral, live, poliomyelitis vaccine which contained traces of simian virus 40 as a contaminant (Sweet and Hilleman, 1960. Magrath *et al.*, 1961. Goffe *et al.*, 1961). However, in the study reported by Melnick and Stinebaugh (1962), some of the children who ingested the vacuolating virus present in oral poliomyelitis vaccine later on excreted in their stools very small amounts of live SV 40 for as long as 4 to 5 weeks. This was true when 3 to 6 months old children and when newborn infants received the vacuolating agent with the oral vaccine. Similar observations were reported more recently by Horváth and Fornosi (1964).

The following personal communication was received by the author (1967) from Dr. Albert B. Sabin:

"With regard to excretion of SV 40 virus by children who ingested oral polio vaccine, Melnick and Stinebaugh (1962) reported only the occasional isolation of small traces of virus in a few children after relatively large amounts were ingested. In our own laboratory, tests were carried out on a total of 149 stool specimens from 45 persons who had ingested about 10^3 to $10^{4.5}$ TCD_{50} of SV 40 virus. No virus was isolated in any instance but it must be said that since the cultures were observed for only a period of two weeks the excretion of small traces of virus could have been missed (Pelon, W., and Sabin, A. B., unpublished data)."

Low Grade Inapparent Infection, but No Symptoms of Disease. These studies established therefore the fact that a low grade infection with the simian virus 40 may occur in humans following introduction of this virus, particularly by parenteral route, but occasionally also by ingestion. However, no symptoms of disease have been observed in hundreds of thousands of persons who either had been injected with, or were fed, this agent (Fraumeni *et al.*, 1963). Most important of all, there is no evidence available, thus far at least, that this virus could be oncogenic for man. However, it must be emphasized that the period of observation of humans that received this virus is still relatively short, and does not allow a definite answer to this important question.

Because of the considerable influence of age on the susceptibility of the host to the oncogenic action of the vacuolating agent, it would appear that any oncogenic effect that could be anticipated in humans, or in other animal species, following introduction of the SV 40 virus, could be expected, if at all, only following the introduction of virus into newborn infants, and not into adult individuals. It is true that in a few instances newborn human infants did receive small quantities of live SV 40 virus, inadvertently present in either Salk or Sabin polio vaccine. This occurred prior to the isolation of the SV 40 virus, and the recognition of its oncogenic potential; in the early years the presence of the simian virus 40 contaminant in such vaccines had not yet been recognized. Thus far, however, no untoward effects in any of these or other individuals who received the SV 40 virus have been observed.

Propagation of Simian Virus 40 in Human Cells in Tissue Culture and Induction of Abnormal Cells and Chromosomal Aberrations

Several successful attempts have been made to propagate simian virus 40 in human cells in tissue culture (Sweet and Hilleman, 1960. Hsiung and Gaylord, 1961. Eddy *et al.*, 1962). At the Children's Hospital Medical Center in Boston, Shein and Enders (1962c) observed that simian virus 40 could be propagated in human cell lines, inducing no cytopathic effect on first passages; after subsequent passages, when it was transferred into human kidney cell cultures, proliferating foci were induced which became progressively large. Eventually, epithelioid transformation of primary cultures of human renal cells was observed in such infected cultures.

The fact that human cell cultures could be infected with simian virus 40, and that such cultures could carry the virus in continuous passage, was of considerable interest. The viral infectivity attained maximum titers by the 25th to 41st day after inoculation and remained constant during several weeks. Most striking, however, was the appearance of epithelioid cell forms, with abnormal growth pattern and chromosomal aberrations.

In a similar study, Koprowski and his colleagues (1962), at the Wistar Institute in Philadelphia, inoculated organ cultures, prepared from human skin and buccal mucosa, with the SV 40 virus. A transformation could be observed in the infected cell cultures 8 to 14 weeks after exposure to the virus. This transformation was characterized by the appearance of colonies of morphologically abnormal cells of an irregular epithelial-like growth pattern; these cells eventually spread and overgrew the normal cell population. Distinct chromosomal abnormalities accompanied this cell transformation.

The alterations in the morphology of human cells grown in tissue culture, as well as chromosomal abnormalities observed after introduction of simian virus 40, raise the serious problem of a possible long term oncogenic potential of this virus on humans.

Enhancement of Adenovirus Growth in Rhesus Monkey Kidney Cells by Presence of SV 40 Virus. The demonstration of oncogenic potency of simian virus 40 led to numerous efforts directed at removing any traces of the vacuolating agent from pools of poliomyelitis virus or adenoviruses which were to be used for the preparation of vaccines. Among the methods employed, treatment with appropriate immune serum directed against the SV 40 virus was successfully used. However, in the course of these studies it was found that this treatment could not be applied to adenoviruses. It appeared that cultures of certain types of adenoviruses containing a slight contamination with the SV 40 virus could not readily be freed from SV 40 virus, without at the same time impairing the propagation of the adenoviruses grown in such cell cultures. This applied particularly to type 4 adenovirus. It appeared that adenovirus type 4 did not propagate in grivet monkey kidney cells in the absence of SV 40 virus. Very small amount of residual infections with SV 40 virus was required, but it appeared to be necessary for adenovirus replication (Rowe and Baum, 1964, 1965. Huebner *et al.*, 1964. Rowe *et al.*, 1965).

Similar observations were later made with adenovirus types 5 and 12 (Rabson *et al.*, 1964) showing that an enhancement of growth of adenovirus types 5 and 12 in African green monkey kidney cells was noticed if such cell cultures were preinfected with the SV 40 virus. The presence of SV 40 antigen was demonstrated in cell cultures infected with type 7 adenovirus that had been contaminated with, but subsequently freed from, detectable SV 40 virus (Rapp *et al.*, 1964. Huebner *et al.*, 1964. Rowe *et al.*, 1965). It is possible that there may occur some linkage, or other association, of the SV 40 virus with adenovirus type 7, whether by genetic mixing or perhaps by hybridization.

The problem of vaccine safety became more complex when it was

---

Fig. 65. SV 40 Virus Particles in Negatively Stained Preparations.

(A). SV 40 virus particles in negatively stained preparations treated with phosphotungstic acid. Magnification 280,000 ×. (B). SV 40 virus particles in negatively stained preparations treated with phosphotungstic acid. Each virus particle has probably 42 capsomeres. Magnification 400,000 ×. Electron micrographs prepared (A) by C. Vasquez and (B) by N. Granboulan, W. Bernhard and P. Tournier, Institut de Recherches Scientifiques sur le Cancer, Villejuif (Seine), France.

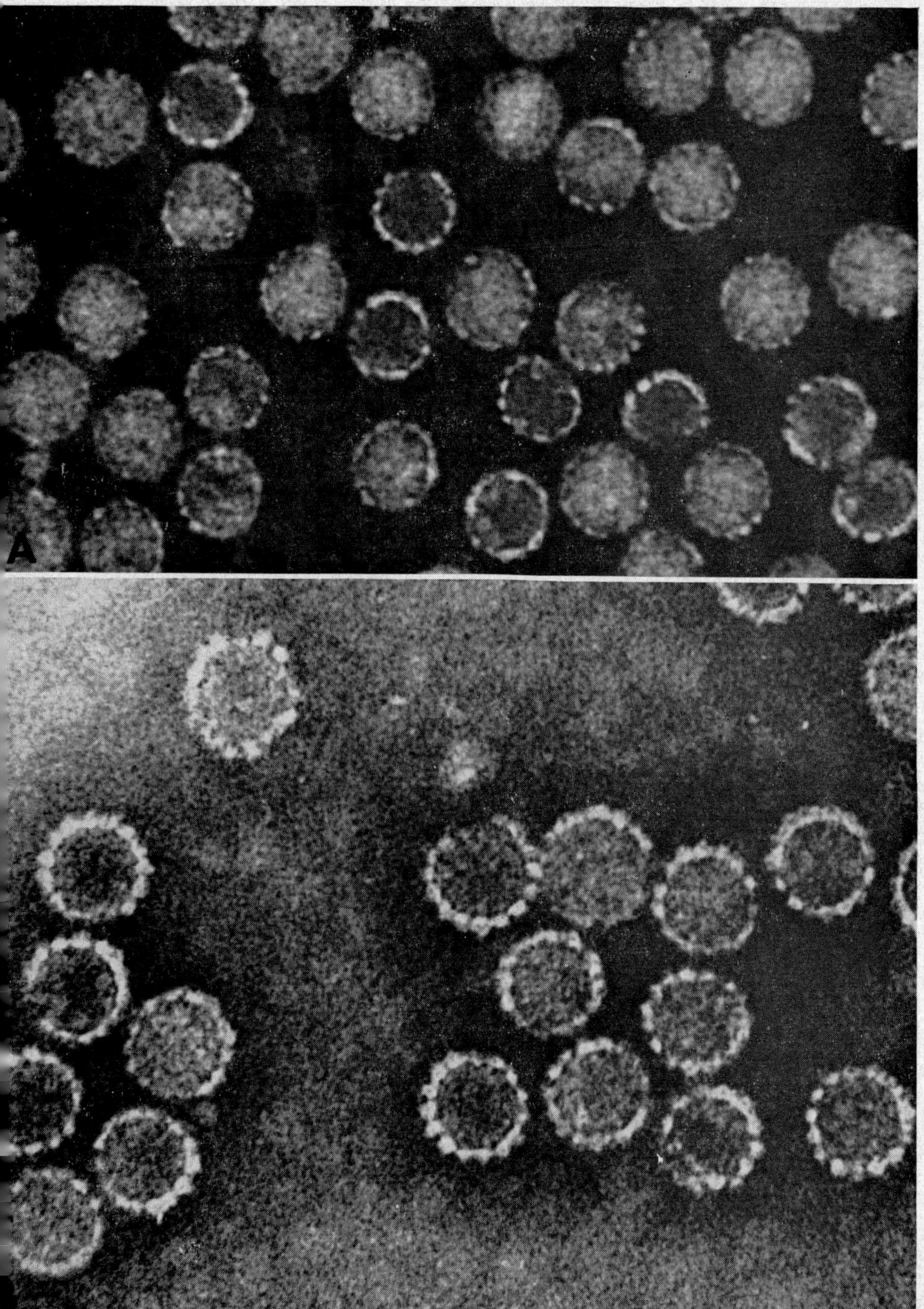

Fig. 65. SV 40 Virus Particles in Negatively Stained Preparations.

discovered that a portion of the SV 40 virus could become incorporated into the type 7 adenovirus resulting in the formation of a "virus hybrid" which possessed the oncogenic potential of the SV 40 virus (Huebner *et al.*, 1964. Rowe and Baum, 1965).

Elimination of the SV 40 Virus from Vaccines

Following the isolation of the simian virus 40, and the recognition of its oncogenic potential, it became of utmost importance to test vaccines produced for human use for presence of the vacuolating agent, and to free such vaccines from any traces of live SV 40 virus. A provision of U.S. Federal regulations governing the preparation of poliomyelitis virus and adenovirus vaccines excludes from sale all vaccines containing an adventitious agent of unknown pathogenicity. Upon discovery of the SV 40 virus in killed poliovirus and adenovirus vaccines, the elimination of this contaminating virus became imperative, and several methods have been described for either selectively destroying the SV 40 virus, or for employing for the preparation of vaccines cell cultures free from the vacuolating agent. The SV 40 virus is relatively resistant to amounts of formaldehyde sufficient to inactivate either poliovirus or adenoviruses (Sweet and Hilleman, 1960b. Gerber *et al.*, 1961. Eddy, 1964. Girardi, 1965). However, the SV 40 virus is susceptible to inactivation by visible light in the presence of toluidine blue (Hiatt *et al.*, 1962), or by heating at 50°C for one hour in the presence of molar solution of magnesium or calcium salts (Wallis and Melnick, 1961). It was also observed (Hayashi and LoGrippo, 1962) that simian virus 40 is more susceptible to inactivation by beta-propiolactone than either the poliomyelitis virus or the adenoviruses, and that this chemical is effective in destroying SV 40 virus in poliomyelitis virus and adenovirus vaccines without impairing their potency.

Later it became mandatory that virus pools prepared for production of vaccines be tested and found free from SV 40 contamination prior to inactivation of such vaccines with formaldehyde. The method of choice, however, to prevent contamination of vaccines with simian virus 40 is to propagate the poliomyelitis virus, or another virus which is to be used for the preparation of vaccines, on cell cultures free from the vacuolating agent. Many rhesus monkey kidney cell cultures contain the vacuolating agent, but some are relatively, or even completely, free from such contamination. Traces of SV 40 virus, if present in such monkey kidney cell cultures, can be neutralized by specific anti-SV 40 immune serum. Careful tests are required to determine whether the cell cultures which are to be used for propagation of virus are free from contamination with the vacuolating agent. Such tests include incubation of fluid from the cultures on green monkey (*Cercopithecus*) kidney cells for prolonged periods of time, in order to determine whether the characteristic vacuolating effects of the simian virus 40 may not become apparent. Another measure consists of successive serological tests performed on monkeys serving as prospective donors for the preparation of monkey kidney cell cultures, in order to determine the possible presence of specific antibodies directed against simian virus 40. Animals with antibodies are likely to provide contaminated tissues. On the other hand, monkeys which remain free from antibodies for a number of weeks, while maintained under isolated conditions, should provide tissues which will not yield SV 40 in cell cultures.

Finally, it may also be possible to employ monkey cell cultures originating from species known to be free from the vacuolating agent for the propagation of poliomyelitis or other viruses.

Lépine and Sautter at the Pasteur Institute in Paris reported (1962) that for the preparation of polio vaccines they have propagated the poliomyelitis virus on kidney cells obtained from African monkeys (*Cynocephalus Papio papio*) which are not natural carriers of the vacuolating agent. Furthermore the vaccines prepared at the Pasteur Institute were carefully tested for absence of the SV 40 virus. In view of the fact that the vacuolating agent is relatively resistant to formol, the vaccines were inactivated by beta-propiolactone.

Oncogenic Potential of Simian Virus 40 Its Significance and Theoretical Implications

The significance of the oncogenic potential of the vacuolating virus (SV 40) is considerable. The observation that a latent virus indigenous in monkey kidney cells, and apparently harmless for its carrier host species, can induce a high incidence of malignant, progressively growing tumors when inoculated into newborn animals of another species is striking. Similar observations have been recorded in studies dealing with adenoviruses, a group of agents either remaining latent or producing only a mild and transient disease in their human carriers, but at the same time capable of inducing tumors in another species, i.e. in hamsters. This pattern of biological behavior of a potentially pathogenic agent does not seem to be an isolated phenomenon in nature. Many parasitic, bacterial, and viral agents may either remain latent and propagate without causing symptoms of disease, or cause only a transient, mild illness in one or more species of carrier hosts, whereas they may be capable of causing symptoms of serious, frequently fatal, disease in certain other animal species. Rocky Mountain spotted fever, certain forms of epidemic encephalitis, herpes, yellow fever, distemper, and many other transmissible diseases of animals and man can be quoted as examples. In this respect, therefore, oncogenic viruses do not fundamentally differ from other pathogenic agents.

The obvious question arises whether there exist viruses, other than simian virus 40 in monkeys, or adenoviruses in humans, which may belong to this group, i.e. which would be latent under natural life conditions, or cause only a transient disease in their natural carrier hosts, but could be potentially oncogenic for some other species? Are there perhaps some other as yet undetected, latent, but potentially oncogenic viruses in tissue culture cells, or in other live media, such as embryonated chicken eggs, now routinely employed for preparation of vaccines for animals or for humans?

REFERENCES

ASHKENAZI, A., and MELNICK, J. L., Induced latent infection of monkeys with vacuolating SV-40 papova virus. Virus in kidneys and urine. *Proc. Soc. Exp. Biol. & Med.*, **111**: 367–372, 1962.

ASHKENAZI, A., and MELNICK, J. L., Tumorigenicity of simian papovavirus SV40 and of virus-transformed cells. *J. Nat. Cancer Inst.*, **30**: 1227–1265, 1963.

BERNHARD, W., VASQUEZ, C., and TOURNIER, P., La structure du virus SV 40 étudiée par coloration négative en microscopie électronique. *J. Microscopie*, **1**: 343–350, 1962.

BLACK, P. H., and TODARO, G. J., *In vitro* transformation of hamster and human cells with the adeno 7-SV 40 hybrid virus. *Proc. Nat. Acad. Sci., USA*, **54**: 374–381, 1965.

EDDY, B. E., Tumors produced in hamsters by SV40. *Fed. Proc.*, **21**: 930–935, 1962.

EDDY, B. E., Simian virus 40 (SV-40): An oncogenic virus. pp. 1–26 in: *Progress Experimental Tumor Research*, vol. 4, S. Karger, Basel/New York, 1964.

EDDY, B. E., BORMAN, G. S., BERKELEY, W. H., and YOUNG, R. D., Tumors induced in hamsters by injection of rhesus monkey kidney cell extracts. *Proc. Soc. Exp. Biol. & Med.*, **107**: 191–197, 1961.

EDDY, B. E., BORMAN, G. S., GRUBBS, G. E., and YOUNG, R. D., Identification of the oncogenic substance in rhesus monkey kidney cell cultures as Simian Virus 40. *Virology*, **17**: 65–75, 1962a.

EDDY, B. E., BORMAN, G. S., YOUNG, R. D., and GRUBBS, G. E., Influence of route of injection, age and animal passage on induction of neoplasms in hamsters by Simian Virus 40. (Abstract). *Proc. Internat. Congress Microbiol., Montreal*, **8**: 89, 1962b.

EDDY, B. E., GRUBBS, G. E., and YOUNG, R. D., Persistent infection of human carcinoma and primary chick embryo cell cultures with Simian Virus 40. *Proc. Soc. Exp. Biol. & Med.*, **111**: 718–722, 1962c.

EDDY, B. E., STEWART, S. E., YOUNG, R., and MIDER, G. B., Neoplasms in hamsters induced by mouse tumor agent passed in tissue culture. *J. Nat. Cancer Inst.*, **20**: 747–761, 1958.

FRAUMENI, J. F., JR., EDERER, F., and MILLER, R. W., An evaluation of the carcinogenicity of Simian Virus 40 in man. *J. Am. Med. Assoc.*, **185**: 713–718, 1963.

GAY, F. P., and HOLDEN, M., The herpes encephalitis problem II. *J. Infect. Dis.*, **53**: 287–303, 1933.

GAYLORD, W. H., JR., and HSIUNG, G.-D., The vacuolating virus of monkeys. II. Virus morphology and intranuclear distribution with some histochemical observations. *J. Exp. Med.*, **114**: 987–996, 1961.

GERBER, P., An infectious deoxyribonucleic acid derived from vacuolating virus (SV40). *Virology*, **16**: 96–98, 1962.

GERBER, P., HOTTLE, G. A., and GRUBBS, R. E., Inactivation of vacuolating virus (SV40) by formaldehyde. *Proc. Soc. Exp. Biol. & Med.*, **108**: 205–209, 1961.

GIRARDI, A. J., Prevention of SV 40 virus oncogenesis in hamsters, I. Tumor resistance induced by human cells transformed by SV 40. *Proc. Nat. Acad. Sci., USA*, **54**: 445–451, 1965.

GIRARDI, A. J., and HILLEMAN, M. R., Host-virus relationships in hamsters inoculated with SV40 virus during the neonatal period. *Proc. Soc. Exp. Biol. & Med.*, **116**: 723–728, 1964.

GIRARDI, A. J., SWEET, B. H., and HILLEMAN, M. R., Factors influencing tumor induction in hamsters by vacuolating virus, SV40. *Proc. Soc. Exp. Biol. & Med.*, **112**: 662–667, 1963.

GIRARDI, A. J., LARSON, V. M., and HILLEMAN, M. R., Further tests in hamsters for oncogenic quality of ordinary viruses and *Mycoplasma*, with correlative review. *Proc. Soc. Exp. Biol. & Med.*, **118**: 173–179, 1965.

GIRARDI, A. J., SWEET, B. H., SLOTNICK, V. B., and HILLEMAN, M. R., Development of tumors in hamsters inoculated in the neonatal period with vacuolating virus, SV 40. *Proc. Soc. Exp. Biol. & Med.*, **109**: 649–660, 1962.

GIRARDI, A. J., SWEET, B. H., SLOTNICK, V. B., and HILLEMAN, M. R., Tumors in hamsters inoculated with vacuolating virus, SV40. (Abstract). *Proc. Am. Assoc. Cancer Research*, **3**: 322, 1962.

GOFFE, A. P., HALE, J., and GARDNER, P. S., Poliomyelitis vaccines. Letter to the Editor. *Lancet*, **1**: 612, 1961.

GRANBOULAN, N., TOURNIER, P., WICKER, R., and BERNHARD, W., An electron microscopic study of the development of SV40 virus. *J. Cell Biol.*, **17**: 423–441, 1963.

GROSS, L., Pathogenic properties, and "vertical" transmission of the mouse leukemia agent. *Proc. Soc. Exp. Biol. & Med.*, **78**: 342–348, 1951.

GROSS, L., A filterable agent, recovered from Ak leukemic extracts, causing salivary gland carcinomas in C3H mice. *Proc. Soc. Exp. Biol. & Med.*, **83**: 414–421, 1953.

HABEL, K., Immunological determinants of polyoma virus oncogenesis. *J. Exp. Med.*, **115**: 181–193, 1962.

HABEL, K., and EDDY, B. E., Specificity of resistance to tumor challenge of polyoma and SV 40 virus-immune hamsters. *Proc. Soc. Exp. Biol. & Med.*, **113**: 1–4, 1963.

HAYASHI, H., and LOGRIPPO, G. A., Inactivation of vacuolating virus (SV-40) by beta-propiolactone. I. Evaluation in tissue culture. *Henry Ford Hosp. Med. Bull.*, **10**: 463–470, 1962.

HIATT, C. W., GERBER, P., and FRIEDMAN, R. M., Photodynamic inactivation of the vacuolating virus, SV_{40}. *Proc. Soc. Exp. Biol. & Med.*, **109**: 230–232, 1962.

HILLEMAN, M. R., Adenovirus: History and future of a vaccine. pp. 377–402 in: *Viruses Inducing Cancer*. Univ. of Utah Press, Salt Lake City, Utah, 1966.

HORNE, R. W., Architectural symmetry in viruses and their components. Chapter 4, pp. 43–57 in: *Perspectives in Virology III* (1962). Harper & Row, Publ., Hoeber Medical Division, New York, 1963a.

HORNE, R. W., Electron microscope studies on the structure and symmetry of virus particles. pp. 40–62 in: Viruses, Nucleic Acids, and Cancer. *17th Ann. Symposium on Fundamental Cancer Research. Univ. of Texas*, M. D. Anderson Hospital and Tumor Inst. Williams & Wilkins Co., Baltimore, Md., 1963b.

HORVÁTH, B. L., and FORNOSI, F., Excretion of SV-40 virus after oral administration of contaminated polio vaccine. *Acta Microbiol. Acad. Sci. Hung.*, **11**: 271–275, 1964.

HSIUNG, G.-D., and GAYLORD, W. H., JR., The vacuolating virus of monkeys. I. Isolation, growth characteristics, and inclusion body formation. *J. Exp. Med.*, **114**: 975–986, 1961.

HUEBNER, R. J., CHANOCK, R. M., RUBIN, B. A., and CASEY, M. J., Induction by adenovirus type 7 of tumors in hamsters having the antigenic characteristics of SV 40 virus. *Proc. Nat. Acad. Sci., USA*, **52**: 1333–1340, 1964.

HULL, R. N., and MINNER, J. R., New viral agents recovered from tissue cultures of monkey kidney cells. II. Problems of isolation and identification. *Ann. N.Y. Acad. Sci.*, **67**: 413–423, 1957.

HULL, R. N., MINNER, J. R., and SMITH, J. W., New viral agents recovered from tissue cultures of monkey kidney cells. I. Origin and properties of cytopathic agents S.V.$_{\cdot 1}$, S.V.$_{\cdot 2}$, S.V.$_{\cdot 4}$, S.V.$_{\cdot 5}$, S.V.$_{\cdot 6}$, S.V.$_{\cdot 11}$, S.V.$_{\cdot 12}$, and S.V.$_{\cdot 15}$. *Am. J. Hyg.*, **63**: 204–215, 1956.

HULL, R. N., MINNER, J. R., and MASCOLI, C. C., New viral agents recovered from tissue cultures of monkey kidney cells. III. Recovery of additional agents both from cultures of monkey tissues and directly from tissues and excreta. *Am. J. Hyg.*, **68**: 31–44, 1958.

KIRSCHSTEIN, R. L., and GERBER, P., Ependymomas produced after intracerebral inoculation of SV40 into newborn hamsters. *Nature*, **195**: 299–300, 1962.

KOPROWSKI, H., PONTEN, J. A., JENSEN, F., RAVDIN, R. G., MOORHEAD, P., and SAKSELA, E., Transformation of cultures of human tissue infected with simian virus SV 40. *J. Cell. and Comp. Physiol.*, **59**: 281–292, 1962.

LÉPINE, P., and SAUTTER, V., Sur l'absence dans le vaccin français de l'agent vacuolant (virus SV40). *Bull. Acad. Nat. Méd. (Paris)*, **146**: 112–115, 1962.

MAGRATH, D. I., RUSSELL, K., and TOBIN, J. O'H., Vacuolating agent. *Brit. Med. J.*, **2**: 287–288, 1961.

MALHERBE, H., and HARWIN, R., Seven viruses isolated from the vervet monkey. *Brit. J. Exp. Path.*, **38**: 539–541, 1957.

MAYOR, H. D., JAMISON, R. M., and JORDAN, L. E., Biophysical studies on the nature of the simian papova virus particle (vacuolating SV 40 virus). *Virology*, **19**: 359–366, 1963.

MELNICK, J. L., Papova virus group. *Science*, **135**: 1128–1130, 1962.

MELNICK, J. L., and STINEBAUGH, S., Excretion of vacuolating SV-40 virus (papova virus group) after ingestion as a contaminant of oral poliovaccine. *Proc. Soc. Exp. Biol. & Med.*, **109**: 965–968, 1962.

MEYER, H. M., JR., HOPPS, H. E., ROGERS, N. G., BROOKS, B. E., BERNHEIM, B. C., JONES, W. P., NISALAK, A., and DOUGLAS, R. D., Studies on Simian Virus 40. *J. Immunol.*, **88**: 796–806, 1962.

MILLER, G. S., JR., The groups and names of macaques. Chapter 1, pp. 1–9 in: *The Anatomy of the Rhesus Monkey*. Hafner Publ. Co., New York, 1961.

MORRIS, J. A., JOHNSON, K. M., AULISIO, C. G., CHANOCK, R. M., and KNIGHT, V., Clinical and serologic responses in volunteers given vacuolating virus (SV40) by respiratory route. *Proc. Soc. Exp. Biol. & Med.*, **108**: 56–59, 1961.

O'CONOR, G. T., RABSON, A. S., BEREZESKY, I. K., and PAUL, F. J., Mixed infection with simian virus 40 and adenovirus 12. *J. Nat. Cancer Inst.*, **31**: 903–917, 1963.

OETTLÉ, A. G., DEMEILLON, B., and LAZER, B., Carcinomas of the glandular stomach and hepatoma in *Rattus (Mastomys) natalensis* infected with *Bilharzia mansoni*. *Acta Internat. Union Against Cancer*, **15**: 200–202, 1959.

Pay, T. W. F., Some observations on vacuolating agent virus (SV40). pp. 132–137 in: *Proc. 7th Internat. Congress Microbiol. Stand., London*, 1961.

Rabson, A. S., Branigan, W. J., and Legallais, F. Y., Production of tumours in *Rattus* (*Mastomys*) *natalensis* by polyoma virus. *Nature*, **187**: 423–425, 1960.

Rabson, A. S., Kirschstein, R. L., and Paul, F. J., Tumors produced by adenovirus 12 in *Mastomys* and mice. *J. Nat. Cancer Inst.*, **32**: 77–87, 1964.

Rabson, A. S., O'Conor, G. T., Kirschstein, R. L., and Branigan, W. J., Papillary ependymomas produced in *Rattus* (*Mastomys*) *natalensis* inoculated with vacuolating virus (SV40). *J. Nat. Cancer Inst.*, **29**: 765–787, 1962.

Rabson, A. S., O'Conor, G. T., Berezesky, I. K., and Paul, F. J., Enhancement of adenovirus growth in African green monkey kidney cell cultures by SV40. *Proc. Soc. Exp. Biol. & Med.*, **116**: 187–190, 1964.

Rapp, F., Melnick, J. L., Butel, J. S., and Kitahara, T., The incorporation of SV 40 genetic material into adenovirus 7 as measured by intranuclear synthesis of SV 40 tumor antigen. *Proc. Nat. Acad. Sci., USA*, **52**: 1348–1352, 1964.

Rowe, W. P., Studies of adenovirus-SV 40 hybrid viruses, III. Transfer of SV 40 gene between adenovirus types. *Proc. Nat. Acad. Sci., USA*, **54**: 711–717, 1965.

Rowe, W. P., and Baum, S. G., Evidence for a possible genetic hybrid between adenovirus type 7 and SV 40 viruses. *Proc. Nat. Acad. Sci., USA*, **52**: 1340–1347, 1964.

Rowe, W. P., and Baum, S. G., Studies of adenovirus SV40 hybrid viruses. II. Defectiveness of the hybrid particles. *J. Exp. Med.*, **122**: 955–966, 1965.

Rowe, W. P., Baum, S. G., Pugh, W. E., and Hoggan, M. D., Studies of adenovirus SV40 hybrid viruses. I. Assay system and further evidence for hybridization. *J. Exp. Med.*, **122**: 943–954, 1965.

Rustigian, R., Johnston, P., and Reihart, H., Infection of monkey kidney tissue cultures with virus-like agents. *Proc. Soc. Exp. Biol. & Med.*, **88**: 8–16, 1955.

Sabin, A. B., and Koch, M. A., Evidence of continuous transmission of noninfectious SV 40 viral genome in most or all SV 40 hamster tumor cells. *Proc. Nat. Acad. Sci., USA*, **49**: 304–311, 1963.

Sabin, A. B., and Wright, A. M., Acute ascending myelitis following a monkey bite, with isolation of a virus capable of reproducing the disease. *J. Exp. Med.*, **59**: 115–136, 1934.

Sanderson, I. T., *The Monkey Kingdom. An Introduction to the Primates*. p. 200. Doubleday & Co., Garden City, N.Y., 1957.

Shein, H. M., and Enders, J. F., Multiplication and cytopathogenicity of Simian Vacuolating Virus 40 in cultures of human tissues. *Proc. Soc. Exp. Biol. & Med.*, **109**: 495–500, 1962.

Shein, H. M., and Enders, J. F., Transformation induced by Simian Virus 40 in human renal cell cultures, I. Morphology and growth characteristics. *Proc. Nat. Acad. Sci., USA*, **48**: 1164–1172, 1962.

Shein, H. M., Enders, J. F., and Levinthal, J. D., Transformation induced by Simian Virus 40 in human renal cell cultures, II. Cell-virus relationships. *Proc. Nat. Acad. Sci., USA*, **48**: 1350–1357, 1962.

Sweet, B. H., and Hilleman, M. R., Detection of a "non-detectable" simian virus (vacuolating agent) present in rhesus and cynomolgus monkey-kidney cell culture material. *Second Internat. Conference on Live Poliovirus Vaccines, Pan American Health Organization and the World Health Organization, Washington, D.C.* pp. 79–85, June, 1960a.

Sweet, B. H., and Hilleman, M. R., The vacuolating virus, S.V. 40. *Proc. Soc. Exp. Biol. & Med.* **105**: 420–427, 1960b.

Tournier, P., Granboulan, N., and Bernhard, W., Examen au microscope électronique des cellules de rein de Cercopithèque infectées *in vitro* par le virus SV 40. *Compt. Rend. Acad. Sci.* (*Paris*), **253**: 2283–2285, 1961.

Wallis, C., and Melnick, J. L., Cationic inactivation of vacuolating virus (SV_{40}) in poliovirus suspensions. *Texas Rep. Biol. & Med.*, **19**: 701–705, 1961.

Wood, W., and Shimada, F. T., Isolation of strains of virus B from tissue cultures of cynomolgus and rhesus kidney. *Canadian J. Public Health*, **45**: 509–518, 1954.

CHAPTER 20

Oncogenic Potency of Adenoviruses

One of the most surprising and, in its significance, far reaching observations was made in 1962 by John Trentin and his colleagues at Baylor University in Houston. They reported that human adenovirus type 12 induced malignant tumors following inoculation into newborn hamsters.

This rather startling observation was at first received with considerable surprise and also with certain reservations. In particular, the question was raised whether the adenovirus strain harvested from tissue culture, and inoculated by Trentin and his coworkers into hamsters, did not contain as a contaminant either the polyoma virus or the SV 40 virus, both known for their oncogenic activity. As discussed later in this chapter, this possibility could be excluded; the oncogenic potency of certain types of adenoviruses was soon confirmed and extended, and gradually the new and unexpected fact had to be accepted that a virus belonging to a common group of human viral agents responsible for mild and usually inconsequential upper respiratory infections may under certain experimental conditions induce progressively growing, malignant tumors in animals.

Initial Isolation and Identification of Adenoviruses

The adenoviruses form a group of closely related virus strains which may remain latent or may cause a variety of febrile upper respiratory infections, conjunctivitis, or transient intestinal tract infections. This interesting and important group of viruses was discovered only very recently, and soon became the subject of intensive laboratory and clinical studies.

Isolation of the "AD Agent." In an attempt to study the etiology of common cold and other similar diseases of the upper respiratory tract associated with inflammatory changes of pharynx, tonsils, and adenoids, Wallace P. Rowe, Robert J. Huebner, and their colleagues (1953) in the Laboratory of Infectious Diseases at the National Institutes of Health, in Bethesda, Md., placed in tissue culture fragments of adenoids obtained from operations on young children during the winter and spring of 1952 and 1953. The tissue fragments were minced with scissors, washed, then cultured in test tubes in nutrient media. In the course of these studies a characteristic degeneration of the cultured cells was noticed, apparently caused by a hitherto unrecognized virus present in the adenoid tissue. This cytopathogenic effect could be serially transmitted by removing a few drops of the fluid from the infected cultures and inoculating this fluid into new cell cultures. The very characteristic cytopathogenic effect became apparent after one to 3 weeks; it was most pronounced when the virus was propagated in certain human epithelial cell cultures, such as HeLa cells, also in certain human embryonic cell cultures, and in monkey kidney cells. The virus could be passed serially, and eventually produced degenerative cell changes after shorter periods of time varying from 3 to 8 days.

The authors concluded that they had recovered a new agent from human adenoids, and suggested the term *adenoid degeneration agent*, or the *AD agent*, for this newly isolated virus.

Isolation of the "RI Agent." Shortly thereafter Hilleman and Werner (1954) working at that time at the Army Medical Service Graduate School in Washington, D.C., recovered a similar agent from throat washings of a young military recruit suffering from atypical pneumonia during an epidemic of acute respiratory illnesses in winter, 1952–1953, at Fort Leonard Wood; they designated this virus the *respiratory illness agent*, *i.e.* the *RI agent* (Hilleman *et al.*, 1955).

Within the next few years additional isolations of similar virus strains belonging to the same general group of viral agents were made in several laboratories, and at least 18 distinct serologic virus types were recognized in the early studies (Huebner *et al.*, 1954). Later on additional serological types were isolated bringing the total number of distinct types recognized in humans to at least 31.

The APC Virus Group. It soon became apparent that viruses belonging to this group could be isolated in tissue culture from adenoids and tonsils removed at surgery from nasopharyngeal and conjunctival secretions, and in some instances also from feces of young adults and children with a variety of respiratory illnesses, or from persons in apparently good health. All these virus strains had essentially the same properties and were designated by the *adenoidal-pharyngeal-conjunctival* group symbol *APC*.

A few similar virus strains belonging to the same general APC group were isolated from other animal species, such as monkeys, chickens, cattle, dogs, and mice.

The "APC" Viruses Change their Name to "Adenoviruses"

The group symbol APC was soon replaced by another term. The problem of nomenclature of this group of viruses was discussed by investigators and others interested in this field at the National Institute of Health in Bethesda, Md., at Walter Reed Army Institute of Research in Washington, D.C., and at several universities, both in the United States and abroad. At a meeting held in New York City on May 25, 1956, attended by leading investigators in this field, and by several prominent virologists, an agreement was reached on the term *adenovirus group* (Enders *et al.*, 1956) which suggested a characteristic involvement of lymphadenoid tissue. It was also agreed that viruses included in this group have the following characteristics: (a) they produce acute infections of respiratory and ocular mucous membranes, associated with enlargement of submucous lymphadenoid tissues in these areas, and that of regional lymph nodes; however, it was stressed that virus strains belonging to this group have been also frequently isolated from adenoid and tonsillar tissues of persons having no clinical symptoms of acute disease; (b) viruses in this group multiply readily in tissue culture in certain types of human and simian cells, leading to distinctive cytopathic changes; (c) electron microscopic studies reveal presence of symmetrical arrays of virus particles in nuclei of cells infected with these virus strains; (d) an antigen demonstrable by complement fixation test is shared by members of this group; antigenic specificity of individual virus types may be demonstrated by serum neutralization tests; (e) no virus strain of this group had yet produced (up to the time of that meeting) manifest disease following inoculation into commonly used laboratory animals.

General Properties of Adenoviruses

Cytopathogenic Effect. The many virus strains belonging to this group have certain common properties. They can be propagated in epithelial human cell lines, such as HeLa or KB cell cultures, and in primary human embryo kidney cells, inducing a characteristic degeneration of the cells in which they are grown; the cytopathogenic effect can also be observed when growing the virus in monkey kidney cells, and to a lesser extent also in certain other animal cell lines; however, the multiplication of the virus is less pronounced under such conditions, although gradually a certain degree of virus adaptation could be obtained with serial passage.

Resistance to Ether. Inactivation by Heat. Virus strains belonging to this group are resistant to treatment *in vitro* with ether and are generally quite stable; most of them can withstand room temperature for about 3 weeks with no apparent decrease in infectivity. They are inactivated after heating to 56°C for 30 minutes.

Common Complement Fixation Antigen. Of considerable practical importance is the fact that virus strains belonging to this group have a common complement fixation antigen; accordingly, a single complement fixation test may detect the presence of antibodies directed against any of the members of the human adenovirus group. However, in order to determine the specific adenovirus type, such as, for example, type 4, 12,

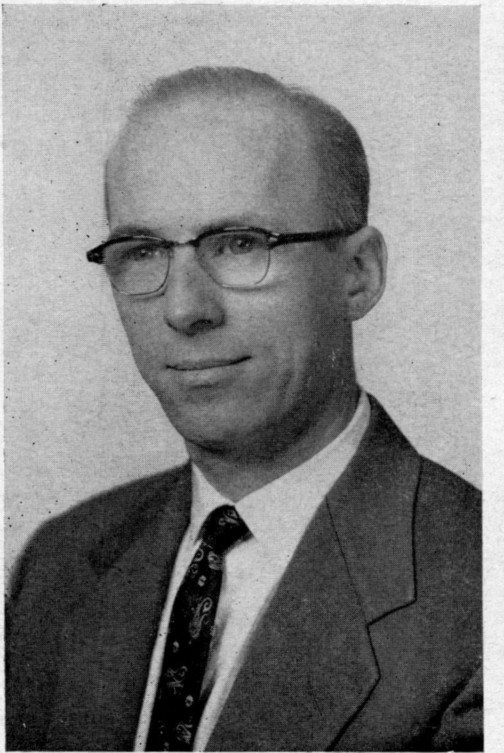
John J. Trentin

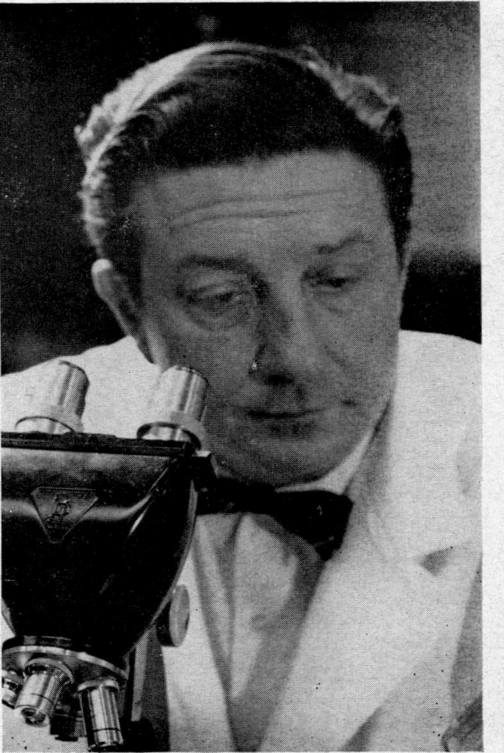
Robert J. Huebner

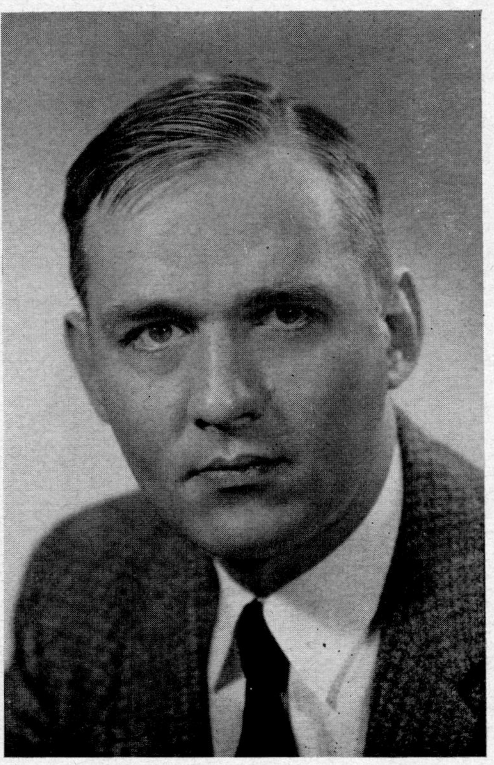
Wallace P. Rowe

Fig. 66

or 18, it is necessary to employ specific serum neutralization tests directed against the individual virus types, i.e. inhibition of the cytopathogenic effect of the virus on cells in tissue culture by neutralization with a type-specific immune serum.

Hemagglutination. Most of the adenovirus types, with the exception of types 12 and 18, and also type 31 (which is closely related in all its properties to type 12) have the ability to agglutinate *in vitro* rhesus monkey, or rat erythrocytes (Rosen, 1958, 1960). The agglutinating potency varies among the different types of adenoviruses; furthermore, there are characteristic differences among adenovirus types in regard to their ability to hemagglutinate red blood cells from different animal species.

The hemagglutinating ability of adenoviruses can be inhibited by a type-specific immune serum. This may provide a basis for a prompt diagnostic test determining the type of adenovirus; however, the serum neutralization test inhibiting the cytopathogenic effect of the adenovirus is more reliable and more sensitive.

Pathogenic Potency for Laboratory Animals. A characteristic feature of the adenoviruses was thought to be their lack of pathogenic potency for common laboratory animals; this was considered to be true until the experiments performed by Trentin and his coworkers (1962), described in this chapter, determined that at least certain types of this group of viruses have a marked oncogenic effect following inoculation into newborn hamsters.

Electron Microscopic Studies

Uniform particles associated with the infective properties of adenoviruses were demonstrated by electron microscopy in tissue culture cells in which the virus was grown (Hilleman *et al.*, 1955. Kjellén *et al.*, 1955. Morgan *et al.*, 1956, 1957, 1960. Tousimis and Hilleman, 1956, 1957. Bloch *et al.*, 1957). Most of these studies were carried out on HeLa cells infected with one of the adenovirus strains, such as type 4 (Tousimis and Hilleman, 1957), or type 5 (Morgan *et al.*, 1956, 1960. Godman *et al.*, 1960). On electron microscopic examination of ultrathin sections of tissue fragments, characteristic crystalline arrays of densely packed virus particles of uniform size and shape could be found in the nuclei of infected cells. The particles were found to have a crystal-like geometrical structure and an average diameter of approximately 70 mμ.

The development of virus particles seems to be confined to the nucleus where most of the characteristic agglomerations of virus particles were found. However, occasionally crystal-like aggregations of virus particles could also be found in the cytoplasm of infected cells (Tousimis and Hilleman, 1956). Subsequent studies demonstrated that the virus particles have a symmetrical, polyhedral, hexagonal shape (Valentine and Hopper,

1957), a configuration already suspected in previous electron microscopic studies.

The structure of adenovirus particles was further clarified in an impressive manner by Horne and his coworkers in Cambridge (Horne *et al.*, 1959. Brenner and Horne, 1959. Horne, 1962, 1963). Employing a purified type 5 adenovirus treated with phosphotungstic acid (PTA), Horne and his coworkers confirmed the hexagonal outline of this virus, and showed that the particle is an icosahedron with 20 triangular faces. In addition to proving the characteristic shape of the adenovirus particle, this technique also demonstrated that the outer layer of the particle, the capsid, is arranged in a definite pattern consisting of a total of 252 capsid units, i.e. capsomeres, on the virus surface. The capsomeres could be considered as finger-like, dense, often hollow, extensions which form the outer shell of the virus. The phosphotungstic acid is capable of penetrating into extremely small areas between, and even within, the capsomeres.

Virus Particles in Virus-infected Tissue Culture Cells, but Not in Virus-induced Tumors. On electron microscopic examination of ultrathin sections, virus particles could be found regularly in the virus-infected tissue culture cells, such as HeLa cells, or in some of the other susceptible cell lines carried in tissue culture and infected with one of the adenovirus types. However, no virus particles could be found in cells of tumors that had been induced in hamsters with one of the oncogenic adenovirus types; this will be discussed in more detail later on in this chapter.

The Different Types of Adenoviruses and the Variety of Common Respiratory and Other Illnesses They Cause in Humans

At least 31 distinct serologic types of this group of viruses have been recognized in humans. Many of these virus types cause frequent infections in man; other types are latent and cause no apparent disease. Infections with these viral agents are widely prevalent, since specific antibodies to several adenovirus types can be found in many humans. Serologic surveys indicated that about 50 per cent of infants 6 months to one year of age have been infected with at least one adenovirus type. Upon reaching the age of 15 years, the average person usually has had infections with several types of adenoviruses.

The various types of adenoviruses have been associated with a variety of clinical diseases, chiefly fever, pharyngitis, conjunctivitis, other febrile respiratory illnesses, and occasionally diarrhea; in many instances, however, these viruses could also be isolated from apparently normal subjects. Adenovirus type 3 has been associated with a distinct clinical disease (Huebner *et al.*, 1954. Parrott *et al.*, 1954) characterized by fever and pharyngitis, also with sporadic cases of catarrhal conjunctivitis or of acute follicular conjunctivitis and cervical lymph nodes enlargement; the same virus has also been associated with mild epidemics of acute febrile respiratory illnesses in military recruits and in children. Adenovirus types 1 and 5 have also been found in cases of acute pharyngitis (Huebner *et al.*, 1954). Type 4 was recovered from acute phases in febrile respiratory illnesses including atypical pneumonia (Hilleman and Werner, 1954. Rowe and Huebner, 1956). Adenovirus types 1 and 2 were present in throat washings of young children, and types 4, 5, 6 and 7 in adults. Types 3, 4 and 7 were recovered repeatedly from respiratory illnesses, including atypical pneumonia in children and in young military recruits (Berge *et al.*, 1955. Rowe and Huebner, 1956. Kjellén *et al.*, 1957). Adenovirus type 7 has been isolated repeatedly from epidemics of acute febrile respiratory illnesses in populations of military recruits. Type 8 was found associated with epidemic kerato-conjunctivitis. Other types, such as types 1, 6, 8 through 12, etc., have been isolated occasionally, chiefly in cases of ocular infections, or in the course of stool surveys made for presence of other viruses, such as poliomyelitis. There is some evidence that infection with certain types of adenoviruses may lead to abdominal pain and diarrhea; this was described by some authors, particularly with types 3 and 7 adenovirus infections.

To summarize, the various adenovirus types could be classified, according to the clinical symptoms of disease they may cause in humans, into three groups:

The first category would include types 3, 4, 7 and 14; these occur in epidemics and are frequently associated with acute respiratory infections. They are not commonly found to be latent in human tonsils and adenoid tissues.

The second category would at present consist of type 8 which causes a rather specific syndrome of epidemic kerato-conjunctivitis.

The third clinical group would be represented by serologic types 1, 2, 5 and 6. In contrast to the other groups, the adenovirus types in this group may often be found to be latent in lymphoid tissues. Their ability to cause latent infections may well account for the relatively high incidence of antibodies to these types in the general population.

Most of the other types of human adenoviruses, including types 12 and 18, have not been found frequently in association with clinical symptoms of disease, even though their infection rate appears to be high, as indicated by presence of antibodies in epidemiological surveys (personal communication to the author from Dr. W. P. Rowe, 1968).

* * *

It would be beyond the scope of this monograph to discuss in more detail the properties and characteristics of the very important group of human adenoviruses. The interested reader is referred to the original publications, and also to several excellent reviews of this subject (Huebner *et al.*, 1954. Rowe and Huebner, 1956. Rowe *et al.*, 1957. Ginsberg, 1957, 1962. Ginsberg and Dingle, 1965. Pereira, 1959. Rowe and Hartley, 1962. Brandon and McLean, 1962. McLeod and Ham, 1963. Thomas, 1964. Hilleman 1957, 1966).

INDUCTION OF MALIGNANT TUMORS FOLLOWING INOCULATION OF CERTAIN TYPES OF ADENOVIRUSES INTO NEWBORN HAMSTERS

In 1962 the surprising report was made by John J. Trentin and his colleagues that human adenovirus type 12 could induce a high incidence of malignant tumors following inoculation into newborn hamsters.

In a brief preliminary communication presented on April 13, 1962, at the Annual Meeting of the American Association for Cancer Research in Atlantic City, John J. Trentin, Y. Yabe and G. Taylor reported that 8 of 10 hamsters injected into the chest cavity with type 12 adenovirus culture developed tumors at the site of inoculation, i.e. in the thorax. In another experiment, 33 out of 35 hamsters injected with tissue culture fluid filtrate containing adenovirus type 12 developed tumors in the thorax, and 4 of these developed tumors in the liver also. All six tumors tested, including one from the liver, were successfully transplanted into young adult hamsters.

No animals injected with control tissue culture fluids developed tumors. The experiments performed by Trentin and his colleagues were carried out under careful conditions in an isolated building designed and constructed for that particular study to prevent cross contamination. The incidence of spontaneous tumors in untreated hamsters was negligible; only one hamster developed a spontaneous tumor among several hundred observed.

Why were Adenoviruses Tested for Their Possible Oncogenic Potential?

The report made by Trentin and his colleagues on the oncogenic potential of adenoviruses was so unexpected and surprising that a comment is justified on the reasons which apparently led to this important and successful study.

The demonstration that mouse leukemia is caused by a transmissible virus, and the unexpected isolation of the parotid tumor virus following inoculation of newborn mice with leukemic filtrates (Gross, 1951, 1953), gave a renewed impetus to the study of the role of viruses in the etiology of cancer. In particular, new efforts were made to reopen experimental studies on the possible viral etiology of human cancer.

There seemed to be considerable difficulty, however, in either transmitting the hypothetical cancer virus directly from human tumors into animals, or in demonstrating by electron microscopy the presence of specific virus particles in human neoplasms. An indirect approach was therefore chosen by Trentin and his coworkers. A search was made for the possible oncogenic potential of human viruses causing forms of common diseases unrelated to cancer in humans, and to test such viruses for their possible oncogenic potential in animals. This approach was based on the previous demonstration by F. Duran-Reynals (1940, 1959) that under certain experimental conditions animal tumor viruses, such as the Rous sarcoma virus in chickens, could induce acute non-cancerous inflammatory or hemorrhagic disease.

Among the viruses to be tested by Trentin, the adenoviruses were chosen for extensive studies because of the prevalence of certain adenovirus types among human infants. Furthermore, there seemed to be a morphologic resemblance of adenoviruses to certain animal tumor viruses, such as the polyoma or papilloma virus, the former highly oncogenic for newborn hamsters. On electron microscopic examination, the adenoviruses can be detected in the nuclei of infected cells in characteristic crystalline aggregates consisting of homogeneous virus particles of uniform size, larger than, but quite similar to, those observed in the nuclei of cells infected with the polyoma or papilloma virus.

In studies planned by Trentin and his coworkers, newborn hamsters were to be used for inoculation of human adenoviruses in order to test these viruses for their possible oncogenic potential.

The high susceptibility of newborn mice revealed in the initial studies dealing with the isolation of the mouse leukemia and the parotid tumor viruses (Gross, 1951, 1953) led to the recognition of the importance of using newborn hosts in bio-assay experiments dealing with the study of oncogenic viruses in mammals. Newborn hamsters proved even more susceptible than newborn mice to the oncogenic action of the polyoma virus (Eddy *et al.*, 1958).

Development of Tumors in Hamsters following Inoculation of Type 12 Adenovirus

In Trentin's study, types 2, 3, 7, 9, 10, 11, 12, and 14 of human adenoviruses, obtained from the American Type Culture Collection, National Institute of Health, Bethesda, Md., were diluted to a concentration of 1 : 10 and inoculated into newborn hamsters. In these initial experiments, of the several types of human adenoviruses tested, only type 12 revealed an oncogenic potential.

In the initial study of 10 hamsters injected directly into the chest cavity with type 12 adenovirus, and surviving longer than 3 weeks, 8 developed tumors after a latency varying from 1 to 3 months following inoculation of the virus. The tumors developed in the mediastinum, on the internal wall of the chest, or on the diaphragm. No tumors developed in the control group injected with tissue culture fluid collected from non-inoculated, free from adenovirus 12, HeLa cells.

A second shipment of human adenovirus type 12, obtained 5 months later from the American Type Culture Collection, was used again for inoculation of newborn hamsters, and again similar tumors were induced. In 3 successive experimental series, a total of 40 out of 42 injected hamsters developed tumors following inoculation of the virus.

Origin of the Type 12 Adenovirus. The original prototype 12 adenovirus was isolated by Kibrick and his colleagues (1955) from a stool of a child in Boston in which the diagnosis of non-paralytic poliomyelitis was considered; this virus strain was later identified by its properties as belonging to the adenovirus group (Kibrick *et al.*, 1957), and classified as serotype No. 12 by Rowe and his colleagues (1958).

Development of Undifferentiated Sarcomas at the Site of Inoculation. Some tumors appeared as early as 30 days after injection of the virus; others developed after a latency varying from 2 to 3 months following inoculation. The induced tumors developed at the site of virus injection, infiltrating surrounding tissues. Four pathologists examined histological sections of several tumors and agreed that these tumors were undifferentiated sarcomas (Trentin *et al.*, 1962b).

The Virus Could be Injected by Different Routes, i.e. directly into the chest cavity, intraperitoneally, or subcutaneously. When higher doses of the virus were injected, the subcutaneous route appeared as effective as other routes; at lower doses of virus, however, the subcutaneous route appeared less effective (Yabe *et al.*, 1963).

Importance of Age at Inoculation. Of primary importance was the age of the animals at the time of virus inoculation. When less than 24-hour-old hamsters were inoculated with a sufficient dose of the virus, practically all of them developed tumors. However, the susceptibility of hamsters to the

---

FIG. 67a. SUBCUTANEOUS SARCOMA INDUCED IN A HAMSTER WITH HUMAN ADENOVIRUS TYPE 12.

This Syrian hamster was inoculated subcutaneously when newborn with human adenovirus type 12 and developed a palpable tumor at the site of inoculation after 2 months. The tumor grew progressively. Photograph taken 5 months after inoculation. Photograph received from John J. Trentin, Baylor University, Texas Medical Center, Houston.

FIG. 67b. PHOTOMICROGRAPH OF A SARCOMA INDUCED IN A HAMSTER WITH HUMAN ADENOVIRUS TYPE 12.

Intrathoracic sarcoma adhering to the diaphragm which developed, after a latency of 45 days, at the site of intrapulmonary inoculation of type 12 human adenovirus into a newborn hamster. Magnification 175 × (H. & E.). Photomicrograph received from J. J. Trentin, Y. Yabe and G. Taylor, Baylor University, Texas Medical Center, Houston. (From: *Science*, **137**: 835, 1962.)

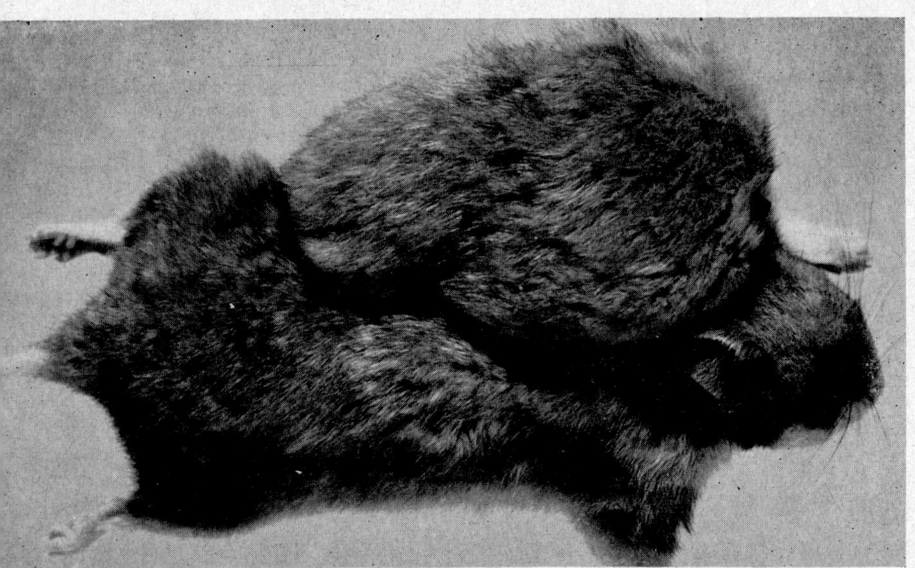

Fig. 67a. Subcutaneous Sarcoma Induced in a Hamster with Human Adenovirus Type 12.

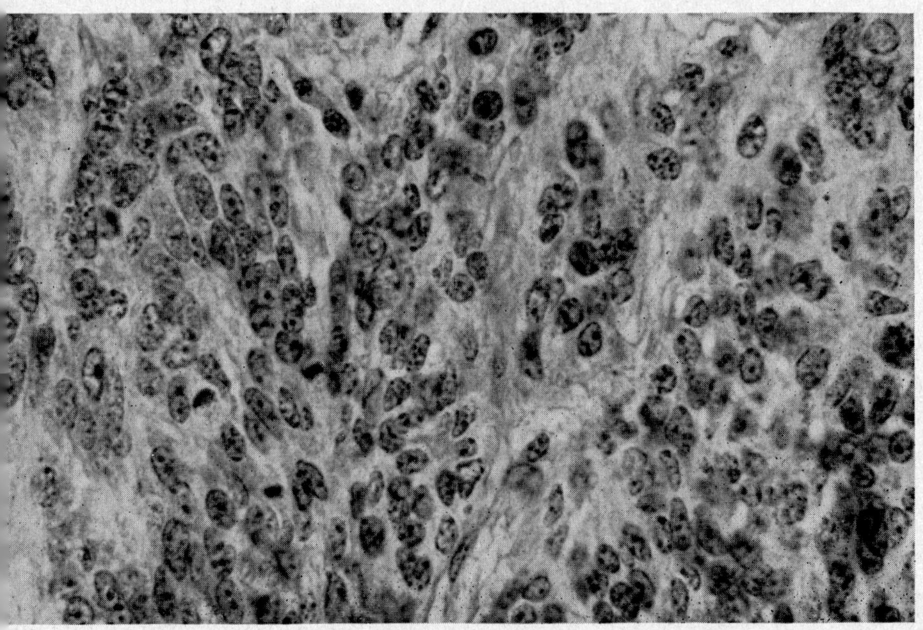

Fig. 67b. Photomicrograph of a Sarcoma Induced in a Hamster with Human Adenovirus Type 12.

oncogenic potency of the inoculated virus decreased rapidly with increasing age. When two-week-old hamsters were inoculated with the same virus, only 1 out of 8 injected animals developed a tumor. Older hamsters seemed to be completely resistant to inoculation of type 12 adenovirus; when three-week-old hamsters were inoculated, none of them developed tumors (Yabe *et al.*, 1962).

Initial Difficulties in Determining the Exclusive Role of Adenovirus Type 12 in the Induction of Tumors. Following the first report of Trentin and his colleagues on the induction of tumors following inoculation of adenovirus type 12 into newborn hamsters, the immediate question was raised whether these tumors were actually induced by the injected adenovirus, or whether there was perhaps another oncogenic virus present in the fluid employed for inoculation. In particular, the question was considered whether the tissue culture fluid harvested from adenovirus cultures and employed for inoculation was contaminated either by the polyoma or by the SV 40 virus, both known to be highly oncogenic for newborn hamsters. However, both possibilities could be eliminated in a series of experiments (Trentin *et al.*, 1962b, 1963) described below:

Experiments Designed to Eliminate the Possible Role of the Polyoma Virus in the Induction of Tumors Presumably Caused by Type 12 Adenovirus. The polyoma virus is very antigenic and its presence in an animal can be determined by a sensitive serological test, i.e. inhibition of the agglutinating potency of the polyoma virus by a specific antibody present in the serum of animals infected with this virus. Such tests were carried out in Trentin's laboratory and the results were clear: sera of 30 untreated hamsters, as well as those of 14 hamsters which developed tumors after injection of type 12 adenovirus, were tested for polyoma hemagglutinating antibodies; the results of all these tests were negative.

As another point of differentiation, Trentin and his colleagues also emphasized that following inoculation of the type 12 adenovirus into newborn hamsters, tumors usually develop after a short latency at the site of inoculation. On the other hand, inoculation of the polyoma virus into newborn hamsters usually results in the development of kidney sarcomas.

These observations and the serological tests just described were consistent with the assumption that tumors which developed in hamsters following inoculation of adenovirus type 12 were not caused by contamination of the injected fluid with the polyoma virus.

Experiments Designed to Eliminate the Possible Role of the SV 40 Virus in the Induction of Tumors Presumably Caused by Type 12 Adenovirus. Another problem, however, remained to be solved. Hamsters develop tumors at the site of inoculation following injection of the simian virus 40 (SV 40). Thus, the possibility of the presence of the SV 40 virus in the fluid employed for inoculation had to be excluded. This possibility could also be eliminated on the basis of the following experimental data: neither the polyoma virus nor the SV 40 virus can be propagated in HeLa cells; however, adenovirus type 12, with its characteristic oncogenic potential, could be readily propagated in HeLa cells in tissue culture. Furthermore, following inoculation of adenovirus type 12 into newborn hamsters, tumors began to appear as early as one month after inoculation, and almost all inoculated animals developed tumors when they reached, or shortly after they passed the age of 3 months. On the other hand, it is known that following inoculation of the SV 40 virus, tumors do not usually begin to appear until later, i.e. after about $3\frac{1}{2}$ months.

In another experiment the type 12 adenovirus culture was heated to 60°C for 30 minutes; this treatment is known to inactivate the adenovirus, but not the SV 40 virus, the latter being more resistant to heat. The heated adenovirus cultures were inactive when they were tested in several tissue culture cell lines. As expected, they did not induce degenerative changes in epithelial human cell lines which are sensitive to the cytopathogenic action of adenovirus strains. Moreover, the presence of the relatively heat-resistant SV 40 virus in these extracts could also be excluded on the basis of the observation that the heat-inactivated adenovirus cultures did not induce the characteristic vacuolating effect on *Cercopithecus aethiops* monkey kidney cells; the latter are particularly sensitive to the cytopathogenic action of the SV 40 agent.

Serum Neutralization Tests Carried Out in an Attempt to Exclude the Possibility of Contamination of the Adenovirus Strain with SV 40 Virus. In another experiment (Trentin *et al.*, 1962b) serological tests were performed in order to determine whether the adenovirus strain employed for inoculation was contaminated with the SV 40 virus. Rabbit anti-SV 40 serum did not inactivate the cytopathic effect of the type 12 adenovirus in tissue culture cells, nor did it inactivate its tumor-inducing potency. On the other hand, rabbit anti-serum directed against type 12 adenovirus inactivated not only the cytopathic property of the adenovirus in tissue culture, but also its tumor-inducing property in newborn hamsters.

Electron microscopic studies of ultrathin sections of HeLa cells infected with the adenovirus strain employed in Trentin's experiments (1962) revealed in the nuclei of infected cells the presence of considerable numbers of virus particles arranged in crystalline arrays and having the characteristic morphology of adenoviruses.

In another series of similar serum neutralization experiments carried out independently by Huebner and his colleagues (1962) the presence of neither the polyoma nor the SV 40 virus could be demonstrated in the adenovirus 12 prototype material employed for the induction of tumors in newborn hamsters.

Thus, the possible presence of either the polyoma or SV 40 virus as a contaminant of adenovirus type 12 cultures could be excluded. The induction of tumors with adenovirus type 12 cultures was apparently the result of the direct oncogenic action of this particular virus and not that of a fortuitous contaminant.

No Infective Virus could be Recovered from Adenovirus-induced Tumors and No Virus Particles could be Detected on Electron Microscopic Examination of the Tumor Sections

It is of considerable importance that in experiments thus far performed, no infective virus could be recovered from the adenovirus-induced tumors. All attempts thus far made to recover adenovirus type 12 from tumors induced by inoculation of this virus into hamsters have been unsuccessful. However, it is quite possible that under favorable experimental conditions, isolation of the virus from hamster tumors may succeed, particularly after intermediary passage through tissue culture. Connor and Marti reported recently (1966) isolation of adenovirus 12 from two tissue culture cell lines derived from adenovirus 12-induced hamster tumors.

Furthermore, electron microscopic studies did not reveal the presence of virus particles in the induced tumors. This was in striking contrast to electron microscopic examination of HeLa cells or of other susceptible tissue culture cells in which the adenovirus type 12 was grown. As discussed in the preceding part of this chapter, electron microscopic examination of tissue culture cells in which the adenovirus was grown usually revealed the presence of considerable numbers of characteristic virus particles in the nuclei of the infected cells.

In this respect the adenovirus-induced tumors proved to be similar to tumors induced by the SV 40 or by the polyoma virus. As discussed in more detail in the chapters of this monograph dealing with the SV 40 or the polyoma virus, electron microscopic studies revealed presence of either SV 40 or polyoma virus particles in tissue culture cells in which these viruses were propagated, but not in either SV 40 or polyoma-induced tumors. Furthermore, no infective virus could usually be recovered from such tumors.

Transplantation of the Induced Tumors. Tumors induced with adenovirus type 12 could readily be transplanted by cell-graft into young adult hamsters (Trentin *et al.*, 1962); they grew progressively, and killed the inoculated animals. The morphology of the transplanted tumors remained similar to that of the primary neoplasms (Trentin *et al.*, 1962. Huebner *et al.*, 1962).

Confirmation of Trentin's Initial Experiments, and Induction of Tumors in Hamsters with Adenovirus Type 18

The initial experiments of Trentin and his colleagues (1962a,b) were soon confirmed and extended by Huebner and his coworkers (1962) at the

Laboratory of Infectious Diseases, National Institutes of Health, Bethesda, Md. Following inoculation of newborn hamsters with the prototype 12 adenovirus strain, tumors similar to those described by Trentin developed in 51 out of 65 inoculated animals. In another experiment Huebner and his colleagues employed type 12 adenovirus strains freshly isolated from anal swabs of children in Washington, D.C. Following inoculation of these newly isolated adenovirus strains into newborn hamsters, 10 out of 42 inoculated animals developed undifferentiated sarcomas at the site of inoculation. This experiment demonstrated that the oncogenic potency of certain adenoviruses, such as type 12, is the property present in naturally occurring strains of adenoviruses, and is not necessarily limited to virus strains carried through serial passages and exposed to laboratory manipulation.

In an extension of this study, Huebner and his coworkers (1962) injected adenovirus type 18 into newborn hamsters, and observed that 4 out of 14 animals developed subcutaneous tumors after a latency varying from 2 to 4 months. On microscopic examination the induced tumors had a similar morphology to that observed in tumors resulting from inoculation of adenovirus type 12. This experiment demonstrated that adenovirus type 18 has also an oncogenic potential, although apparently less pronounced than that of type 12.

Tumors induced by either type 12 or type 18 adenovirus were examined in Huebner's laboratory by Dr. L. Berman, and were diagnosed as "primitive undifferentiated mesenchymal neoplasms with some definite epithelioid characteristics."

Huebner and his coworkers (1962) also reported that the oncogenic potency of either type 12 or type 18 adenovirus could be neutralized by a specific immune serum.

Induction of Tumors in Hamsters with Adenovirus Types 7 and 31

Girardi (1964), Larson (1965), and their colleagues observed recently that a low, but significant, incidence of tumors could be induced in hamsters with human adenovirus type 7. Following either subcutaneous or intrathoracic inoculation of type 7 adenovirus into 51 newborn hamsters, 4 of

---

Fig. 68. Human Adenovirus Type 12 Virus Particles.

Ultrathin section of a fragment of HeLa cell propagated in tissue culture and infected with type 12 human adenovirus. Intranuclear array of crystalline virus particles. Magnification 57,000×. Electron micrograph prepared at Baylor University College of Medicine, Texas Medical Center, Houston, by J. J. Trentin, Y. Yabe and G. Taylor. (From: *Science*, **137**: 835, 1962.)

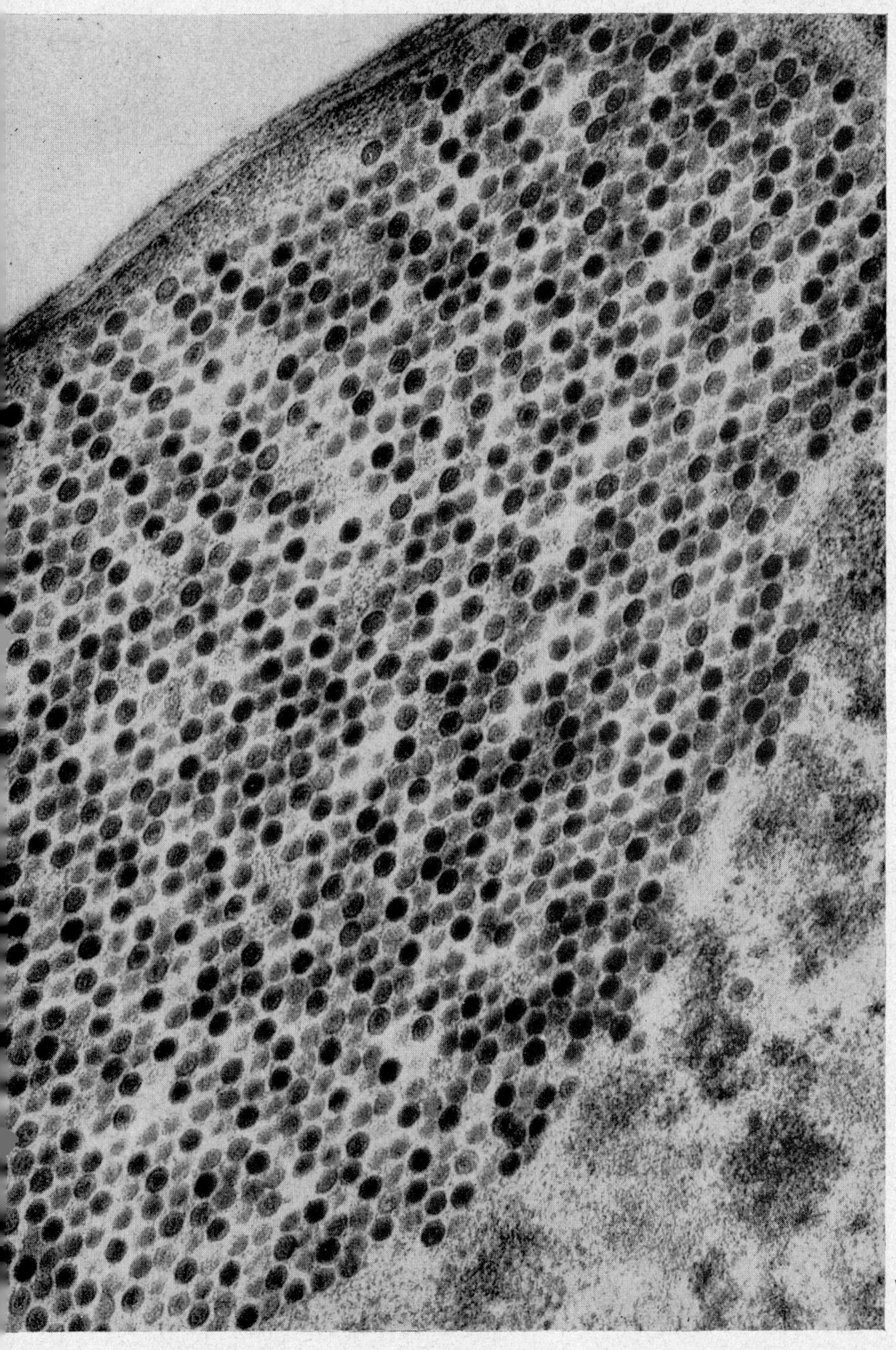

Fig. 68. Human Adenovirus Type 12
Virus Particles.

the injected animals developed subcutaneous undifferentiated sarcomas. The induction of tumors with type 7 adenovirus was of particular interest, since this virus has been known to induce acute epidemic respiratory illnesses in military recruits.

More recently it was observed that human adenovirus type 31 could also induce tumors in a small percentage of animals following inoculation into newborn hamsters (Pereira *et al.*, 1965). Two newborn hamster litters were inoculated with type 31 adenovirus strain, and in one animal out of each of the two injected litters an undifferentiated sarcoma developed at the site of inoculation. Adenovirus type 31 is very closely related in most of its properties to type 12 (personal communication to the author from Dr. W. P. Rowe).

Induction of Tumors in Hamsters with Adenovirus Type 3

Huebner and his colleagues reported (1965) that adenovirus type 3 is oncogenic for newborn hamsters. A subcutaneous tumor developed after 9 months at the site of inoculation in one of 8 hamsters injected with this virus; in another experiment, a tumor appeared after 5 months in one out of 17 inoculated hamsters. It is of interest that adenovirus type 3 is one of the most frequent causative agents responsible for febrile respiratory illnesses and pharyngo-conjunctival fever due to adenovirus infection in the United States and abroad.

Induction of Tumors in Rats with Type 12 Adenovirus

Huebner and his colleagues observed (1963) that adenovirus type 12 can also induce tumors in rats. Following subcutaneous or intraperitoneal inoculation in 10 newborn Sprague-Dawley rats with undiluted adenovirus 12 prototype, 3 rats developed tumors in the peritoneal cavity after a latency of 130 to 140 days. These tumors were massive, arising from the peritoneal surface; they had the same histological structure as those induced under similar experimental conditions in hamsters. The virus-induced tumors could be transplanted by cell-graft from rat to rat, employing suckling rats for inoculation.

This experiment demonstrated that newborn rats are also susceptible to the oncogenic potential of type 12 adenovirus, although to a lesser degree than newborn hamsters.

Induction of Tumors in Mice with Type 12 Adenovirus

Newborn mice were also found to be susceptible to the tumor-inducing potency of type 12 adenovirus, as explained in more detail in the following experiments:

Yabe and his colleagues in Trentin's laboratory (1964) injected type 12 adenovirus into newborn mice of strains A, DBA, and C3H/Gs. They observed that 4 out of 13 C3H/Gs mice developed tumors at the site of injection; histologically these undifferentiated tumors were very similar to those induced with the same virus in hamsters. In a subsequent experiment, 12 out of 17 C3H/Gs mice developed tumors after a latency varying from 2 to 5 months, following intraperitoneal inoculation, when newborn, with adenovirus type 12.

In a similar experiment, Rabson and his colleagues at the National Cancer Institute in Bethesda, Md. (1964), inoculated human adenovirus type 12 into newborn C3H/Bi mice. As a result, 7 out of the 29 injected mice developed tumors after a latency varying from $2\frac{1}{2}$ to 6 months.

However, not all strains of mice were susceptible to the oncogenic action of adenoviruses. Susceptibility of some of the otherwise resistant strains could be increased by thymectomy (Kirschstein *et al.*, 1964).

Induction of Tumors in Mastomys (Rattus natalensis) with Type 12 Adenovirus

Rattus (*Mastomys*) *natalensis* is an African rodent intermediate in size between the rat and the mouse. These animals have been used in microbiological studies because they are highly susceptible to infection with certain bacteria and protozoa. They have recently been used in cancer research laboratories following Oettlé's report (1957) of a high incidence of spontaneous adenocarcinoma of the stomach in a *Mastomys* colony in Johannesburg, South Africa (see also p. 769 in preceding chapter).

In view of the susceptibility of the *Mastomys* to the polyoma virus (Rabson *et al.*, 1960) and to the simian virus 40 (Rabson *et al.*, 1962), these animals were also tested for their possible susceptibility to the oncogenic action of adenoviruses.

Two newborn *Mastomys* litters were inoculated with Type 12 adenovirus, and one animal in each of the two litters developed a small tumor at the site of inoculation after a latency of 5 to 6 months (Rabson *et al.*, 1964).

Effect of Thymectomy

Thymectomy performed in newborn mice or in less than 8-day-old hamsters increased their susceptibility to the oncogenic action of adenoviruses.

Newborn BALB/c and C3H/HeN mice inoculated subcutaneously with human adenovirus 12 developed tumors only when thymectomized at birth. Tumors developed after a latency of 2 to 4 months in 5 out of 30 BALB/c, and in 3 out of 18 C3H/HeN, thymectomized mice. No tumors developed in any of the 28 and 25 mice of the corresponding control groups which also received the virus but were not thymectomized (Kirschstein *et al.*, 1964).

In a similar experiment, 6 to 8-day-old hamsters were thymectomized, and were then inoculated with either adenovirus type 7 or 21 (Van Hoosier *et al.*, 1967). Eleven out of 39 thymectomized hamsters inoculated with adenovirus type 7 developed tumors, as compared with only one among 23 non-thymectomized controls. In another series, 4 out of 26 thymectomized animals inoculated with adenovirus type 21 developed tumors, as compared with none out of 12 controls.

Oncogenic Potency of the Various Types of Human Adenoviruses

At least 31 distinct types of human adenoviruses have been recognized. They all have the same morphology and similar physical properties. Their classification as to type is based on serum neutralization tests; differences in their hemagglutination pattern (Rosen, 1960) and their nucleic acid composition (Piña and Green, 1965) may also be helpful in the identification of the individual types.

The different adenovirus types vary in their epidemiology, and in their ability to induce symptoms of disease in man. Only some of the human adenovirus types have been found to be oncogenic.

The oncogenic potential of the individual virus types may vary. Only a few, i.e. 12 and 18, perhaps also 31 which is closely related to type 12, are strongly oncogenic. Among the remaining potentially oncogenic types, most have a low tumor-inducing potential; they induce tumors only occasionally following inoculation into newborn hamsters.

Trentin and his colleagues recently tested (1968) human adenovirus types 1 through 30 (with the exception of types 2, 10, and 11 which were found to be non-oncogenic in earlier studies). The bio-assay experiments were carried out on newborn hamsters. The results of this extensive experimental survey revealed the oncogenic potential of types 1, 7, 8, 12, 14, 18, 21, and 24. However, with the exception of types 12 and 18, the incidence of induced tumors was relatively small in actual figures representing the numbers of inoculated animals and of those developing tumors.

The following is a summary of the results obtained following inoculation of the different types of human adenoviruses into newborn hamsters:

Type 1 induced tumors in 4 out of 60 hamsters; type 7 in 1 out of 23; type 8 in 1 out of 9; type 12 in 100 out of 183; type 14 in 1 out of 15; type 18 in 15 out of 97; type 21 in 2 out of 13; and type 24 in 1 out of 11 hamsters. It is apparent that with the exception of types 12 and 18, other "oncogenic" adenovirus types have only a very low tumor-inducing potential. Furthermore, whereas tumors induced with type 12 developed after a short latency of 3 months, those which developed after inoculation of other oncogenic adenovirus types appeared after a more prolonged average latency varying from 9 to 23 months.

Most of the tumors induced in hamsters with adenovirus types 12 and 18 were undifferentiated sarcomas; however, some of the tumors induced with adenovirus types 1, 7, 8, 14, 21, or 24 were neoplasms which were diagnosed microscopically as malignant lymphomas, some of them originating in the mesenteric lymphoid tissue.

Further studies are needed, however, in order to determine whether these tumors actually represent lymphosarcomas; blood and bone marrow studies are also needed to clarify this important question.

* * *

It is quite possible to speculate that in additional bio-assay studies employing adequate doses of high-titer virus strains, tumors may eventually also be induced with other types of human adenoviruses; the list of oncogenic adenovirus types, which was at first limited principally to types 12 and 18, seems to be growing, and now includes a considerable number of other adenovirus types; most of the additional types, however, were found to have only a very low oncogenic potential.

Induction of Tumors with Adenoviruses of Simian Origin in Hamsters, Rats, and Mice

Oncogenic potential of adenoviruses does not seem to be limited to virus strains isolated from humans. Hull and his coworkers demonstrated recently (1965) that 5 out of 17 simian adenoviruses of rhesus or cynomolgus origin induced tumors following inoculation into newborn hamsters. An additional simian adenovirus, SA7, isolated from an African *Cercopithecus aethiops* monkey, had a particularly high oncogenic potential. When 23 newborn hamsters were inoculated with this virus strain, all developed tumors after a short latency of only 20 to 40 days. The SA7 adenovirus type also induced tumors in 3 out of 21 rats, and in 1 out of 15 newborn C3H mice, after a latency period of 3 months. All animals were inoculated when newborn.

FIG. 69. HUMAN ADENOVIRUS TYPE 12 VIRUS PARTICLES.

(A). Adenovirus type 12 in human KB cells after 3 days of culture. Virus particles in a crystalline array in the nucleus. Magnification about 33,000 ×. Electron micrograph prepared by W. Bernhard, Institut de Recherches Scientifiques sur le Cancer, Villejuif (Seine), France. (B). Negatively stained preparation of human adenovirus type 12 treated with phosphotungstic acid. Magnification 200,000 ×. Electron micrograph prepared at Baylor University College of Medicine, Texas Medical Center, Houston, by H. D. Mayor, B. Powell and J. J. Trentin. (From: *Virology*, **23**: 614, 1964.)

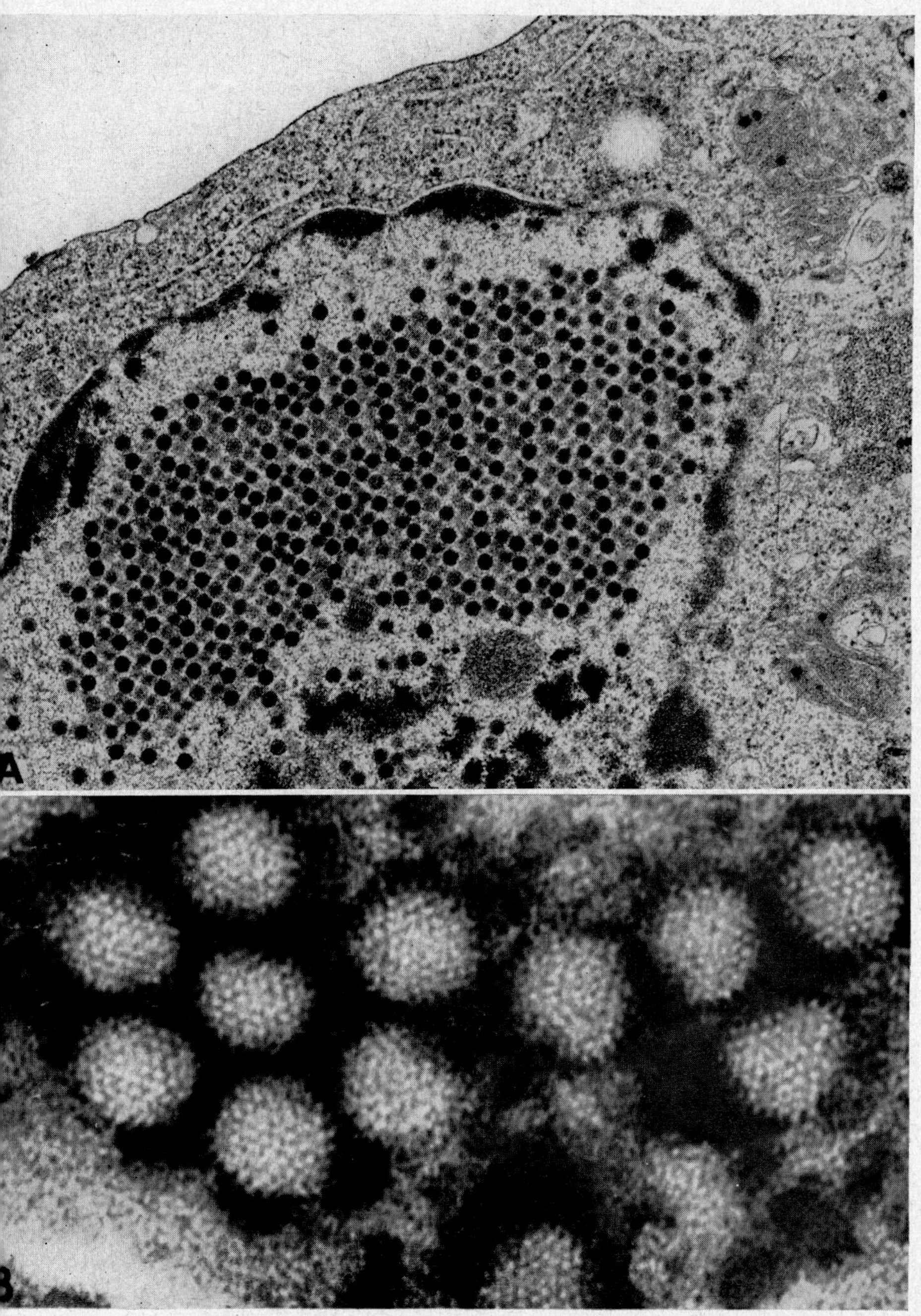

FIG. 69. HUMAN ADENOVIRUS TYPE 12
VIRUS PARTICLES.

The tumors were "undifferentiated neoplasms with some characteristics of lymphomas."

Oncogenic Potency of an Avian Adenovirus for Hamsters

The "chicken-embryo lethal orphan virus" (CELO) is responsible for inapparent or mild infections of the respiratory tract of chickens, and belongs to the group of adenoviruses. Sarma and his coworkers observed (1965) that this avian adenovirus is highly oncogenic for newborn hamsters. Twenty-three out of 69 hamsters inoculated with this virus developed progressively growing fibrosarcomas at the site of inoculation after a latency varying from 3 to 6½ months.

Oncogenic Potency of Bovine Adenovirus 3 for Hamsters

Darbyshire reported recently (1966) that bovine adenovirus type 3 can induce a high incidence of undifferentiated sarcomas in hamsters. Out of 45 hamsters inoculated when newborn with this virus, 22 developed subcutaneous sarcomas at the site of inoculation, after a short latency of 1 to 2 months; most of the sarcomas were firm, but some were cystic. Primary tumors of the firm type were transplanted to weanling and newborn hamsters, and induced progressively growing sarcomas.

Enhancement of the Growth of Certain Types of Adenoviruses in Tissue Culture by Presence of the SV 40 Virus. Under certain experimental conditions, mixed infection of simian virus 40 (SV 40) and adenovirus 12 can occur in African green monkey kidney cells grown in tissue culture, and electron micrographs may demonstrate in such cases the presence of both viruses in the nuclei of some of the infected cells (O'Conor *et al.*, 1963). More recently Rabson and his colleagues (1964) observed that the growth of type 12 adenovirus in African green monkey kidney cells was enhanced by the presence of the SV 40 virus in such cultures. In absence of the SV 40 virus, the presence of adenovirus 12 grown in such cells for 72 hours was evident on electron microscopic examination in only one per cent of the cells examined, and titration showed no increase in virus content. On the other hand, when similar cell cultures were inoculated with both viruses, after 72 hours of incubation 75 per cent of the cells contained adenovirus particles, and there was also an increase in the titer of the virus, evident at titration. A similar enhancement of adenovirus growth by presence of the SV 40 virus was observed when adenovirus type 5 was substituted for type 12 previously tested.

In a similar study, Huebner and his colleagues (1964) observed that the oncogenic potential of either the SV 40 virus or of adenovirus type 7 was enhanced following propagation of both viruses together in tissue culture. Furthermore, tumors induced in hamsters with adenovirus type 7 grown in mixed cultures with the SV 40 virus acquired virus-specific antigen for the SV 40 virus. In other studies Huebner and his associates observed that the combination of adenovirus 7 and SV 40 grown in tissue culture had an enhanced oncogenic potential on bio-assay; following inoculation of tissue culture fluid harvested from such mixed virus cultures into newborn hamsters, tumors could be induced after a shorter latency than those induced with either SV 40 or adenovirus 7 alone. The authors raised the interesting possibility that one animal virus might serve as a vector of the antigenic and/or oncogenic potential of a second unrelated virus grown in a mixed culture.

The possibility of a genetic hybrid between adenovirus type 7 and SV 40 virus was further explored in experiments performed by Rowe and Baum (1964). The *in vitro* transformation of hamster cells by the adenovirus-SV 40 hybrid viruses was studied by Black and White (1967).

THEORETICAL IMPLICATIONS OF THE ONCOGENIC POTENTIAL OF HUMAN ADENOVIRUSES

Several important implications must be considered in view of the unexpected discovery of the oncogenic potency of adenoviruses.

First of all, it is now quite apparent that certain viruses can either remain latent or cause an inconsequential and transient disease in one species, i.e. in the case of adenoviruses in humans, and at the same time be capable of inducing progressively growing, malignant tumors in other animal species, such as hamsters, and to a lesser extent also in rats and mice.

Similar considerations refer to the recently isolated simian virus 40 (SV 40), discussed in the preceding chapter of this monograph. This virus is commonly carried by the Asian rhesus monkey (*Macaca mulatta*) in which it causes no symptoms of disease; the same virus, however, can induce a high incidence of progressively growing undifferentiated sarcomas following inoculation into newborn hamsters.

It is, therefore, entirely possible to speculate that there may exist other viruses which may remain latent, or may cause only a transient, self-limited disease in certain animal species, but may be potentially oncogenic for humans.

The fundamental question remains to be answered whether the oncogenic potential of certain types of human adenoviruses is limited to hamsters, rats, and mice only, or whether viruses belonging to this group may also induce malignant tumors in other species, particularly in their natural carrier host, i.e. in humans. This question has not yet been adequately answered. Several reports referring to isolation of adenovirus strains from human neoplasms (Sohier *et al.*, 1963. Bronitki *et al.*, 1964. McAllister *et al.*, 1964) are interesting, but far from convincing. The observation that an adenovirus strain could be isolated from malignant tumors in humans does not necessarily suggest that there is a causal relationship between the etiology of such tumors and the isolated agents. However, the possibility that certain types of adenoviruses may represent one of the causative factors in the etiology of human cancer is of considerable interest and should be carefully explored in further studies.

The crucial question also remains to be answered whether in addition to the adenovirus group there exist other human viruses which may usually remain latent, or cause only a transient and non-neoplastic disease, but which may also have an as yet unrecognized oncogenic potential for other animal species, or for humans. Experiments thus far performed have not revealed a definite oncogenic potential of other human viruses tested to date. However, it should be emphasized that there are many unknown factors which increase the difficulty in answering this important question. A bio-assay method, employing for inoculation newborn hamsters, or newborn mice or rats, may not necessarily reveal a latent oncogenic potential of the virus strains tested. Another animal species may be needed for the bio-assay tests, or another bio-assay method altogether may be required. Furthermore, only a limited number of viruses has been thus far isolated from humans and tested for their pathogenic, and in particular for their oncogenic potential. Even among the viruses and virus strains known to exist in humans, not all have yet been tested adequately for their possible oncogenic potency. In addition, it is quite apparent that there may exist other as yet unrecognized viruses, or virus strains, carried by humans, which remain to be isolated and tested for their possible oncogenic potential.

REFERENCES

BERGE, T. O., ENGLAND, B., MAURIS, C., SHUEY, H. E., and LENNETTE, E. H., Etiology of acute respiratory disease among service personnel at Fort Ord, California. *Am. J. Hygiene*, **62**: 283–294, 1955.

BLACK, P. H., and WHITE, B. J., In vitro transformation by the adenovirus-SV 40 hybrid viruses. II. Characteristics of the transformation of hamster cells by the adeno 2-, adeno 3-, and adeno 12-SV40 viruses. *J. Exp. Med.*, **125**: 629–646, 1967.

BLOCH, D. P., MORGAN, C., GODMAN, G. C., HOWE, C., and ROSE, H. M., A correlated histochemical and electron microscopic study of the intranuclear crystalline aggregates of adenovirus (RI-APC virus) in HeLa cells. *J. Biophys. and Biochem. Cytol.*, **3**: 1, 1957.

BRANDON, F. B., and MCLEAN, I. W., JR., Adenovirus. *Advances in Virus Research*, **9**: 157–193, Academic Press, New York, 1962.

BRENNER, S., and HORNE, R. W., A negative staining method for high resolution electron microscopy of viruses. *Acta Biochim. and Biophys.*, **34**: 103–110, 1959.

BRONITKI, A., DEMETRESCU, R., POPESCU, G., and MALIAN, A., Isolation of adenovirus from a human case of pulmonary carcinoma. *Acta Virologica*, **8**: 472, 1964.

CONNOR, J. D., and MARTI, A., Isolation of adenoviruses from tissue cultures of adenovirus type 12 induced hamster tumors. (Abstract.) *Proc. Am. Assoc. Cancer Res.*, **7**: 14, 1966.

DARBYSHIRE, J. H., Oncogenicity of bovine adenovirus type 3 in hamsters. *Nature,* **211**: 102, 1966.

DURAN-REYNALS, F., A hemorrhagic disease occurring in chicks inoculated with the Rous and Fuginami viruses. *Yale J. Biol. and Med.*, **13**: 77–98, 1940.

Duran-Reynals, F., Virus-induced tumors and the virus theory of cancer. pp. 238–292, in: *The Physiopathology of Cancer*. Second edition. Hoeber-Harper, New York, 1959.

Eddy, B. E., Stewart, S. E., Young, R., and Mider, G. B., Neoplasms in hamsters induced by mouse tumor agent passed in tissue culture. *J. Nat. Cancer Inst.*, **20**: 747–761, 1958.

Enders, J. F., Bell, J. A., Dingle, J. H., Francis, T., Jr., Hilleman, M. R., Huebner, R. J., and Payne, A. M.-M., "Adenoviruses": Group name proposed for new respiratory-tract viruses. *Science*, **124**: 119–120, 1956.

Ginsberg, H. S., Biological and physical properties of the adenoviruses. *Ann. N.Y. Acad. Sci.*, **67**: 383–391, 1957.

Ginsberg, H. S., Identification and classification of adenoviruses. *Virology*, **18**: 312–319, 1962.

Ginsberg, H. S., and Dingle, J. H., The adenovirus group. pp. 860–891, in: *Viral and Rickettsial Infections of Man*. (F. L. Horsfall and I. Tamm, Edit.). Fourth edition. J. B. Lippincott, Philadelphia, 1965.

Girardi, A. J., Hilleman, M. R., and Zwickey, R. E., Tests in hamsters for oncogenic quality of ordinary viruses including adenovirus type 7. *Proc. Soc. Exp. Biol. & Med.*, **115**: 1141–1150, 1964.

Girardi, A. J., Larson, V. M., and Hilleman, M. R., Further tests in hamsters for oncogenic quality of ordinary viruses and *Mycoplasma*, with correlative review. *Proc. Soc. Exp. Biol. & Med.*, **118**: 173–179, 1965.

Godman, G. C., Morgan, C., Breitenfeld, P. M., and Rose, H. M., A correlative study by electron and light microscopy of the development of type 5 adenovirus. II. Light microscopy. *J. Exp. Med.*, **112**: 383–402, 1960.

Gross, L., Pathogenic properties, and "vertical" transmission of the mouse leukemia agent. *Proc. Soc. Exp. Biol. & Med.*, **78**: 342–348, 1951.

Gross, L., A filterable agent, recovered from Ak leukemic extracts, causing salivary gland carcinomas in C3H mice. *Proc. Soc. Exp. Biol. & Med.*, **83**: 414–421, 1953.

Hilleman, M. R., Epidemiology of adenovirus respiratory infections in military recruit populations. *Ann. N.Y. Acad. Sci.*, **67**: 262–272, 1957.

Hilleman, M. R., Adenovirus: History and future of a vaccine. pp. 377–402 in: *Viruses inducing cancer*. Univ. of Utah Press, Salt Lake City, 1966.

Hilleman, M. R., and Werner, J. H., Recovery of new agent from patients with acute respiratory illness. *Proc. Soc. Exp. Biol. & Med.*, **85**: 183–188, 1954.

Hilleman, M. R., Tousimis, A. J., and Werner, J. H., Biophysical characterization of the RI (RI-67) viruses. *Proc. Soc. Exp. Biol. & Med.*, **89**: 587–593, 1955.

Horne, R. W., The comparative structure of adenoviruses. *Ann. N.Y. Acad. Sci.*, **101**: 475–484, 1962.

Horne, R. W., The structure of viruses. *Scientific Am.*, **208**: 48–56, 1963.

Horne, R. W., and Wildy, P., Symmetry in virus architecture. *Virology*, **15**: 348–373, 1961.

Horne, R. W., Brenner, S., Waterson, A. P., and Wildy, P., The icosahedral form of an adenovirus. *J. Molec. Biol.*, **1**: 84–86, 1959.

Huebner, R. J., Casey, M. J., Chanock, R. M., and Schell, K., Tumors induced in hamsters by a strain of adenovirus type 3: sharing of tumor antigens and "neoantigens" with those produced by adenovirus type 7 tumors. *Proc. Nat. Acid. Sci., USA*, **54**: 381–388, 1965.

Huebner, R. J., Chanock, R. M., Rubin, B. A., and Casey, M. J., Induction by adenovirus type 7 of tumors in hamsters having the antigenic characteristics of SV 40 virus. *Proc. Nat. Acad. Sci., USA*, **52**: 1333–1340, 1964.

Huebner, R. J., Rowe, W. P., Ward, T. G., Parrott, R. H., and Bell, J. A., Adenoidal-Pharyngeal-Conjunctival agents. A newly recognized group of common viruses of the respiratory system. *New Eng. J. Med.*, **251**: 1077–1086, 1954.

Huebner, R. J., Rowe, W. P., and Lane, W. T., Oncogenic effects in hamsters of human adenovirus types 12 and 18. *Proc. Nat. Acad. Sci., USA*, **48**: 2051–2058, 1962.

Huebner, R. J., Rowe, W. P., Turner, H. C., and Lane, W. T., Specific adenovirus complement-fixing antigens in virus-free hamster and rat tumors. *Proc. Nat. Acad. Sci., USA*, **50**: 379–389, 1963.

Hull, R. N., Johnson, I. S., Culbertson, C. G., Reimer, C. B., and Wright, H. F., Oncogenicity of the simian adenoviruses. *Science*, **150**: 1044–1046, 1965.

Kibrick, S., Enders, J. F., and Robbins, F. C., An evaluation of the roller-type tissue culture for the isolation of poliomyelitis viruses from feces. *J. Immunology*, **75**: 391–409, 1955.

Kibrick, S., Meléndez, L., and Enders, J. F., Clinical associations of enteric viruses with particular reference to agents exhibiting properties of the echo group. *Ann. N.Y. Acad. Sci.*, **67**: 311–325, 1957.

Kirschstein, R. L., Rabson, A. S., and Peters, E. A., Oncogenic activity of adenovirus 12 in thymectomized BALB/c and C3H/HeN mice. *Proc. Soc. Exp. Biol. & Med.*, **117**: 198–200, 1964.

Kjellén, L., Lagermalm, G., Svedmyr, A., and Thorsson, K.-G., Crystalline-like patterns in the nuclei of cells infected with an animal virus. *Nature*, **175**: 505–506, 1955.

Kjellén, L., Zetterberg, B., and Svedmyr, A., An epidemic among Swedish children caused by adenovirus type 3. *Acta Paediatrica*, **46**: 561–568, 1957.

Larson, V. M., Girardi, A. J., Hilleman, M. R., and Zwickey, R. E., Studies of oncogenicity of adenovirus type 7 viruses in hamsters. *Proc. Soc. Exp. Biol. & Med.*, **118**: 15–24, 1965.

McAllister, R. M., Landing, B. H., and Goodheart, C. R., Isolation of adenoviruses from neoplastic and non-neoplastic tissues of children. *Lab. Invest.*, **13**: 894–901, 1964.

McCormick, K. J., Van Hoosier, G. L., Jr., and Trentin, J. J., Attempts to find human adenovirus type-12 tumor antigens in human tumors. *J. Nat. Cancer Inst.*, **40**: 255–261, 1968.

McLeod, D. L., and Ham, A. W., Search for oncogenic properties in various viruses found in man: Positive results with adenovirus types 12 and 18. *J. Canadian Med. Assoc.*, **89**: 799–805, 1963.

Morgan, C., Godman, G. C., Rose, H. M., Howe, C., and Huang, J. S., Electron microscopic and histochemical studies of an unusual crystalline protein occurring in cells infected by type 5 adenovirus. Preliminary observations. *J. Biophys. and Biochem. Cytol.*, **3**: 505–508, 1957.

Morgan, C., Godman, G. C., Breitenfeld, P. M., and Rose, H. M., A correlative study by electron and light microscopy of the development of type 5 adenovirus. I. Electron microscopy. *J. Exp. Med.*, **112**: 373–382, 1960.

Morgan, C., Howe, C., Rose, H. M., and Moore, D. H., Structure and development of viruses observed in the electron microscope. IV. Viruses of the RI-APC group. *J. Biophys. and Biochem. Cytol.*, **2**: 351–360, 1956.

O'Conor, G. T., Rabson, A. S., Berezesky, I. K., and Paul, F. J., Mixed infection with simian virus 40 and adenovirus 12. *J. Nat. Cancer Inst.*, **31**: 903–917, 1963.

Oettlé, A. G., Spontaneous carcinoma of the glandular stomach in *Rattus* (*Mastomys*) *natalensis*, an African rodent. *Brit. J. Cancer*, **11**: 415–433, 1957.

Parrott, R. H., Rowe, W. P., Huebner, R. J., Bernton, H. W., and McCullough, N. B., Outbreak of febrile pharyngitis and conjunctivitis associated with type 3 Adenoidal-Pharyngeal-Conjunctival virus infection. *New Eng. J. Med.*, **251**: 1087–1090, 1954.

Pereira, H. G., Adenoviruses. *Brit. Med. Bull.*, **15**: 225–230, 1959.

Pereira, M. S., Pereira, H. G., and Clarke, S. K. R., Human adenovirus type 31. A new serotype with oncogenic properties. *Lancet*, **1**: 21–23, 1965.

Piña, M., and Green, N., Biochemical studies on adenovirus multiplication, IX. Chemical and base composition analysis of 28 human adenoviruses. *Proc. Nat. Acad. Sci., USA*, **54**: 547–551, 1965.

Rabson, A. S., Branigan, W. J., and Legallais, F. Y., Production of tumours in *Rattus* (*Mastomys*) *natalensis* by polyoma virus. *Nature*, **187**: 423–425, 1960.

Rabson, A. S., O'Conor, G. T., Kirschstein, R. L., and Branigan, W. J., Papillary ependymomas produced in *Rattus* (*Mastomys*) *natalensis* inoculated with vacuolating virus (SV 40). *J. Nat. Cancer Inst.*, **29**: 765–787, 1962.

Rabson, A. S., Kirschstein, R. L., and Paul, F. J., Tumors produced by adenovirus 12 in *Mastomys* and mice. *J. Nat. Cancer Inst.*, **32**: 77–87, 1964.

Rabson, A. S., O'Conor, G. T., Berezesky, I. K., and Paul, F. J., Enhancement of adenovirus growth in African green monkey kidney cell cultures by SV 40. *Proc. Soc. Exp. Biol. & Med.*, **116**: 187–190, 1964.

Rosen, L., Hemagglutination by adenoviruses. Letter to the Editor. *Virology*, **5**: 574–577, 1958.

Rosen, L., A hemagglutination-inhibition technique for typing adenoviruses. *Am. J. Hygiene*, **71**: 120–128, 1960.

Rowe, W. P., and Baum, S. G., Evidence for a possible genetic hybrid between adenovirus type 7 and SV 40 viruses. *Proc. Nat. Acad. Sci., USA*, **52**: 1340–1347, 1964.

Rowe, W. P., and Hartley, J. W., A general review of the adenoviruses. *Ann. N.Y. Acad. Sci.*, **101**: 466–474, 1962.

Rowe, W. P., and Huebner, R. J., Present knowledge of the clinical significance of the Adenoidal-Pharyngeal-Conjunctival group of viruses. *Am. J. Tropical Med. and Hygiene*, **5**: 453–460, 1956.

Rowe, W. P., Hartley, J. W., and Huebner, R. J., Serotype composition of the adenovirus group. *Proc. Soc. Exp. Biol. & Med.*, **97**: 465–470, 1958.

Rowe, W. P., Huebner, R. J., Gilmore, L. K., Parrott, R. H., and Ward, T. G., Isolation of a cytopathogenic agent from human adenoids undergoing spontaneous degeneration in tissue culture. *Proc. Soc. Exp. Biol. & Med.*, **84**: 570–573, 1953.

Rowe, W. P., Huebner, R. J., and Bell, J. A., Definition and outline of contemporary information on the adenovirus group. *Ann. N.Y. Acad. Sci.*, **67**: 255–261, 1957.

Sarma, P. S., Huebner, R. J., and Lane, W. T., Induction of tumors in hamsters with an avian adenovirus (CELO). *Science*, **149**: 1108, 1965.

Sohier, R., Chardonnet, Y., and Prunieras, M., Isolement d'un adénovirus type I à partir d'une adénopathie cervicale maligne. *Press Méd.*, **71**: 1733–1734, 1963.

THOMAS, M., Les adénovirus cancérigènes. *Pathologie et Biologie*, **12**: 330, 1964.

TOUSIMIS, A. J., and HILLEMAN, M. R., Size and shape of adenovirus (RI-APC-ARD) type 4. Electron microscopy of purified and intracellular virus. (Abstract.) *J. Applied Physics*, **27**: 1392, 1956.

TOUSIMIS, A. J., and HILLEMAN, M. R., Electron microscopy of type 4 adenovirus strain RI-67. *Virology*, **4**: 499–508, 1957.

TRENTIN, J. J., VAN HOOSIER, G. L., JR., and SAMPER, L., The oncogenicity of human adenoviruses in hamsters. *Proc. Soc. Exp. Biol. & Med.*, **127**: 683–689, 1968.

TRENTIN, J. J., YABE, Y., and TAYLOR, G., Tumor induction in hamsters by human adenovirus. (Abstract.) *Proc. Am. Assoc. Cancer Research*, **3**: 369, 1962a.

TRENTIN, J. J., YABE, Y., and TAYLOR, G., The quest for human cancer viruses. *Science*, **137**: 835–841, 1962b.

TRENTIN, J. J., YABE, Y., and TAYLOR, G., Studies on the oncogenicity of human adenovirus. pp. 559–563 in: Viruses, Nucleic Acids, and Cancer. *17th Ann. Symp. on Fundamental Cancer Research, Univ. of Texas*, M. D. Anderson Hosp. and Tumor Inst., Williams & Wilkins, Baltimore, Md., 1963.

VALENTINE, R. C., and HOPPER, P. K., Polyhedral shape of adenovirus particles as shown by electron microscopy. *Nature*, **180**: 928, 1957.

VAN HOOSIER, G. L., JR., GIST, C., and TRENTIN, J. J., Facilitation, by thymectomy, of tumor formation by weakly oncogenic adenoviruses. (Abstract.) *Proc. Am. Assoc. Cancer Res.*, **8**: 70, 1967.

YABE, Y., SAMPER, L., TAYLOR, G., and TRENTIN, J. J., Cancer induction in hamsters by human type 12 adenovirus. Effect of route of injection. *Proc. Soc. Exp. Biol. & Med.*, **113**: 221–224, 1963.

YABE, Y., SAMPER, L., BRYAN, E., TAYLOR, G., and TRENTIN, J. J., Oncogenic effect of human adenovirus type 12, in mice. *Science*, **143**: 46–47, 1964.

YABE, Y., TRENTIN, J. J., and TAYLOR, G., Cancer induction in hamsters by human type 12 adenovirus. Effect of age and of virus dose. *Proc. Soc. Exp. Biol. & Med.*, **111**: 343–344, 1962.

CHAPTER 21

The Burkitt Lymphoma Syndrome in African Children

A brief description of the curious lymphoma syndrome in African children, recently described by Burkitt, is included in this monograph, even though no definite experimental evidence has yet been furnished to prove that this tumor is actually caused by a transmissible virus. There is, nevertheless, sufficient circumstantial evidence to suggest that an oncogenic virus may be responsible for the induction of this neoplastic disease which has attracted much attention during the last decade.

Denis Burkitt, a British surgeon at Makerere University Medical School and Mulago Hospital, in Kampala, Uganda, described a curious tumor syndrome occurring commonly in children in certain parts of Africa (Burkitt, 1958, 1961, 1962a,b,c,d. Burkitt and Davies, 1961).

The age at which most of these tumors develop is striking. Nearly all cases recorded have occurred between the ages of 2 to 14 years, with a peak incidence at 5 years of age. The tumors develop in approximately the same frequency in both sexes.

The most characteristic feature of this syndrome is the remarkable tendency of the tumors to develop in the mandibular and maxillary bones. The tumors grow rapidly and cause disfigurement. The maxillary tumors commonly invade the orbit. Bilateral ovarian tumors are present in more than 70 per cent of female patients. Thyroid tumors and bilateral renal tumors are also very common. The adrenals, heart, and stomach are frequently involved, and lesions in the spinal column may cause paraplegia.

This curious tumor syndrome accounts for more than 50 per cent of children's cancers seen in Uganda.* Burkitt reported (1958, 1962b) that more than 200 cases had been recorded during the 8 years preceding his publications.

* The tumor is not new in East Africa. Dr. Albert Cook, who founded the first hospital in Uganda, described a case in detail in 1904 and, according to information supplied by Burkitt (1964), these records still exist. That this was an observation of a common childhood malignancy with widespread distribution in large areas of Africa was not appreciated initially. Thijs (1957) first reported the frequent occurrence of malignancies in the jaw in children in the Congo, with involvement of from one to all 4 quadrants of the mandible and maxilla.

This tumor was histologically identified as a malignant lymphoma (O'Conor and Davies, 1960. O'Conor, 1961. O'Conor *et al.*, 1965); however, this neoplasm is recognized rather as a clinical syndrome and is in many respects different from the usually observed malignant lymphomas. Thus, in the neoplastic syndrome described by Burkitt, tumors of the jaw, frequently involving more than one quadrant, and also bilateral ovarian neoplasms and renal tumors, are common, whereas enlargement of peripheral lymph nodes and spleen does not occur, and there is no peripheral blood involvement. On the other hand, in the usual malignant lymphomas observed in humans or in animals, enlargement of peripheral lymph nodes and spleen is common, and leukemic blood and bone marrow manifestations are frequently observed, particularly in terminal phases of the disease.

Geographical Distribution and Occurrence of the Tumor Syndrome

In view of the fact that the characteristic mandibular and maxillary tumors could not be easily mistaken for any other condition, they were used as a recognizable symptom in a survey initiated by Burkitt (1962a,b,c). Leaflets, accompanied by questionnaires, containing pictures of typical jaw tumors in children, were circulated in order to determine the geographical distribution of this tumor syndrome. These leaflets were sent out to doctors and hospitals in areas across tropical and Central Africa.

After prolonged postal preparation to alert doctors to be watchful for these lesions, a 10,000 mile road safari was undertaken by Dr. Denis Burkitt with his two colleagues, Dr. Ted Williams and Dr. Clifton Nelson. Over 50 hospitals were visited, and additional information was obtained through doctors who had served in several stations. The strikingly characteristic jaw tumors were used as an index for the existence or absence of the syndrome in any area (Burkitt, 1962a,b,c).

From this survey, information became available which made it possible to determine that this tumor syndrome occurred right across tropical Africa from the coast of East Africa to Dakar in the extreme West.

In the West and in Central Africa the northern limit of the tumor belt was found to be at about 15° latitude. This line fell below 10° in the East. The condition was found to be common in West Africa as far south as the sea coast and has been recognized as far south as the middle of Angola.

Geographical plotting of all cases observed in Uganda showed that the only factor, other than population, affecting tumor distribution was altitude. Near the equator the tumor does not appear to exist above an altitude of about 5,000 feet.

East and Central Africa with its varying mountain ranges and the two limbs of the Great Rift Valley were examined in some detail to determine the areas of tumor distribution. The findings of this survey could be summarized as follows (Burkitt, 1962b):

(1) Throughout Uganda, Kenya, and Tanganyika the tumor can occur anywhere except at altitudes of more than about 5,000 feet, with the possible exception of the southern part of Tanganyika.

(2) The off-shore islands of Zanzibar and Pemba are a notable and significant exception.* No case of this syndrome has been observed in these islands with a population of more than a quarter of a million.

(3) Throughout the Federation of Nyasaland and southern and northern Rhodesia, the syndrome was found only in or near the great river valleys, and on the shores of Lake Nyasa.

(4) The tumor was found to be common throughout the coastal plain of Mozambique.

(5) The tumor was thought to be virtually unknown in South Africa.*

It thus became evident that the critical altitude above which the tumor is not observed falls progressively as the distance from the equator increases. Altitude is therefore only a limiting factor in so far as it reflects temperature. The actual limiting factor appears to be a minimum temperature of about 60°F in the coldest season of the year (July).

The fact that the tumor distribution appears to be dependent on climatic factors is consistent with the theoretical assumption advanced by Burkitt (1962a,b,c,d) that some vector, perhaps a mosquito, may be responsible for the transmission of a causative agent. This has led, furthermore, to the speculation that an oncogenic virus may actually be responsible for the induction of this tumor syndrome.

Occurrence of Neoplastic Disease Syndrome Similar to Burkitt Lymphoma in New Guinea, and in Other Parts of the World, Beyond the "Lymphoma Belt"

Following the description of the lymphoma syndrome in African children by Burkitt, several reports appeared indicating that this tumor syndrome is not limited in its appearance to the "lymphoma belt" in Central Africa, but also occurs, although with lesser frequency, in other parts of the African continent and in different parts of the world, beyond the geographic and climatic limitations described by Burkitt.

Ten Seldam, Cooke, and Atkinson (1966) reported that a childhood lymphoma syndrome very similar to the Burkitt tumor was diagnosed in 35 cases during 6 years (1958 to 1963) in the territories of Papua and

* More recently, cases of the characteristic lymphoma syndrome in children similar to those described by Burkitt have also been reported from South Africa (Gluckman, 1963. Chapman and Jenkins, 1963), and from the island of Zanzibar (Khan, 1964).

New Guinea (which have a population of about 2,000,000), and was the most commonly reported childhood malignancy. The clinical and pathological features of these cases followed closely the description of similar tumors described by Burkitt in African children, but distinct geographical and climatic limitations were not observed; jaw tumors were observed only in one third of the cases.

Khan (1964) described a case of multifocal malignant lymphoma syndrome in an Arab child from the island of Zanzibar. Gluckman (1963) described 3 cases of the Burkitt tumor syndrome occurring in white European children 3 to 10 years old, in Johannesburg, South Africa. Chapman and Jenkins (1963) described 5 cases of the same tumor syndrome occurring in children in Natal, South Africa. All these cases were observed therefore in geographical areas previously thought to be exempt from this tumor syndrome, i.e. beyond the "lymphoma belt" described by Burkitt.

Beltrán and his coworkers (1966) described 6 cases of Burkitt lymphoma occurring in children 4 to 5 years old in Colombia. A case of African lymphoma which developed in a $5\frac{1}{2}$-year-old boy of Lebanese parents in Sierra Leone was discussed at a clinicopathological conference at the Postgraduate Medical School of London (Booth *et al.*, 1964).

Reports of Lymphoma Cases Very Similar to Burkitt Lymphoma Syndrome Occurring in the United States and in Canada

Dorfman (1965) reviewed 16 autopsy records of lymphosarcoma in children at the Institute of Pathology, Washington University School of Medicine in St. Louis, Missouri, and reported that several of these cases had features considered unique for the Burkitt tumor syndrome, such as bilateral ovarian tumors, tumors of the bones, etc. At a clinicopathological conference at Washington University School of Medicine (1965) a typical case reported in 1928 by Brown and O'Keefe was reviewed; this case concerned a 16-year-old girl from St. Louis who developed lymphosarcoma of all 4 quadrants of the jaws, and in both ovaries; the histological appearance of the tumor was the same as that of the Burkitt tumor.

Another case of a lymphosarcoma resembling the Burkitt tumor was described by Ziegler and Miller (1966) in a 16-year-old girl from New Britain, Connecticut. This tumor invaded mandibular bone and both ovaries. In the terminal phase, the patient developed paraplegia due to tumor infiltration of the spinal cord; bone marrow was also infiltrated with tumor cells.

O'Conor, Rappaport, and Smith (1965) reviewed 148 cases recorded in the pediatric file of the Armed Forces Institute of Pathology in Washington,

D.C., as lymphoma or reticulum-cell sarcoma in children under 14 years of age. Of the 148 cases reviewed, 20 were selected on the basis of histological appearance and clinical presentation similar to those reported in the majority of cases of the lymphoma syndrome described by Burkitt in African children. Among the 20 selected examples of lymphoma cases observed in children in the United States, 16 had abdominal tumors, 2 had bone lesions, 1 had involvement of the orbital contents, and another a spinal cord compression by tumor infiltration. Microscopic examination of the tumors occurring in the American children revealed a morphology similar to that of the Burkitt tumor syndrome in equatorial Africa. The authors concluded that the "Burkitt tumor" is not a disease entity peculiar to Africa, and that this eponym actually represents an expression of an incidence phenomenon in a section of Africa where this type of lymphoma is rather common. The two principal ways wherein the disease differs in the two geographical areas is the frequency of the syndrome in Africa, contrasted with the comparatively rare occurrence in the United States, and a common development of tumors in the jaw and facial bones in African cases, contrasted with very rare facial tumors reported in the United States.

A case of a massive ovarian tumor resembling clinically, and also in microscopic morphology, the Burkitt lymphoma was observed in a 15-year-old English girl (Epstein *et al.*, 1966. Seed, 1966).

Hoogstraten (1967), at the Children's Hospital in Winnipeg, Manitoba, observed 12 cases of lymphosarcoma occurring in children 9 months to 16 years old in Central Canada. Most of these tumors were observed in children 2 to 4 years old. Jaw tumors, orbital tumors, ovarian tumors in girls, and other multifocal tumors very similar to those described in African children were observed. On microscopic examination these tumors were indistinguishable from the Burkitt tumor. The occurrence in Central Canada of several cases of the lymphoma syndrome similar to the Burkitt tumor was of interest since it obviously had no relation to the geographic distribution of this tumor in Africa and its presumable dependence on tropical climatic conditions. A recent example of this tumor syndrome observed by Hoogstraten (1967) occurred in an Eskimo from the North West Territories.

It is thus quite apparent that the childhood lymphoma syndrome described by Burkitt is not limited to the "lymphoma belt" in Equatorial Africa, but occurs in different parts of the world. However, the disease is common in Central Africa, perhaps also quite frequent in New Guinea, but occurs only occasionally in other parts of the world. In Equatorial Africa this tumor is more common than the total of all other tumors occurring in children, whereas in Great Britain and in the United States this tumor syndrome is exceptionally rare.

Pathological Manifestations of the Lymphoma Syndrome in African Children

Clinical Syndrome. The neoplastic disease observed by Burkitt in African children has a special predilection for the bones of the jaw; maxillary or mandibular tumors are characteristic and very common in the young patients afflicted with this disease. The reports indicate that in East African patients, jaw and facial tumor involvement occurs in about 50 per cent of cases, whereas in West Africa it is found only in 20 to 30 per cent of cases (Edington *et al.*, 1964. O'Conor, 1961). Furthermore, there is a common involvement of visceral organs, frequently bilateral, such as kidneys, adrenals, ovaries, and testes; there are also frequently tumors in the thyroid, liver, stomach, intestines, etc. A characteristic feature of this syndrome is multifocal development of tumors, manifested by apparently simultaneous appearance of tumors in several quadrants of bones of the jaw, in both ovaries, both kidneys, etc. Paraplegia may be observed caused by infiltration of the vertebral column with tumor cells.

The peripheral lymph nodes and spleen are usually spared, except for microscopic involvement; this is in striking contrast to the frequent involvement of abdominal nodes, and massive tumor development in visceral organs, such as kidneys or ovaries.

Lack of leukemic manifestations in peripheral blood is a striking and rather consistent feature of the tumor syndrome observed in African children.

The report of Clift and his colleagues (1963) of terminal leukemia in Burkitt's lymphoma is not convincing, and represents at best an isolated occurrence, subject to reservations (Lambert, 1964). The 4 patients studied by Clift and his colleagues had leukemic bone marrow, but only one had a small proportion of neoplastic cells in peripheral blood.

O'Conor (1961) analyzed the pathological features of 106 cases of malignant lymphomas in African children. The development of these neoplasms, predominantly in the bones of the jaw, as well as the development of tumors, frequently bilateral, in kidneys, ovaries, and other visceral organs, was a characteristic feature of this syndrome. No patients had leukemic manifestations in peripheral blood morphology at any time during the rapidly progressive course of the disease.

Microscopic Morphology

O'Conor and Davies (1960) in a review of all malignant tumors of children recorded in the Kampala Cancer Registry, Uganda, confirmed that all the jaw and abdominal tumors were histologically identical, and concluded, on the basis of microscopic studies, that they were malignant lymphomas. These tumors constituted about 50 per cent of all malignant tumors observed in African children.

On microscopic examination these tumors have a surprising cytological uniformity, and, according to O'Conor (1961), there seems little doubt that they take their origin from the mesenchymal or stem cells of the reticulo-endothelial system, and therefore fall into the broad general category of malignant lymphomas.

The microscopic morphology of the tumors was remarkably uniform; the predominant cell in 83 per cent of cases in O'Conor's series (1961) was smaller than a stem cell, and structurally similar to a primitive lymphoid type.

According to the studies of Wright (1963), the Burkitt tumor consists of masses of poorly differentiated malignant lymphocytes resembling those of lymphoblastic leukemia, together with a varying number of non-malignant histiocytes.

Some Characteristic Differences Between the Lymphoma Syndrome in African Children and the Common Conventional Forms of Lymphoma in Humans. We have already discussed on the preceding pages of this chapter some of the characteristic features of the Burkitt lymphoma syndrome observed in African children. Although it is generally accepted that the Burkitt tumor can be classified as a form of "malignant lymphoma," there are certain important differences between this characteristic disease syndrome and a typical lymphoma.

In the lymphoma syndrome described in African children there is a distinct predilection for primary and secondary tumor development in the jaw and facial bones; furthermore, the peripheral lymph nodes are not enlarged, and there is usually no spleen enlargement, whereas massive tumors may develop in abdominal nodes and in the viscera, particularly in kidneys and ovaries. The histological pattern is characterized by uniformity and "starry-sky" appearance (O'Conor *et al.*, 1965) and features massive proliferation of primitive cells of lymphoreticular tissue, and phagocytic activity by neoplastic or non-neoplastic histiocytes. Finally, lack of blood involvement is also characteristic; true leukemia is rare, if it occurs at all.

On the other hand, in the common human lymphomas usually observed in children and in adults, there is often an enlargement of peripheral lymph nodes and of the spleen due to tumor growth and tumor cell infiltration. Lymphoid tumors develop as a rule in organs of the hematopoietic system, predominantly in the lymph nodes and in the spleen, but much less frequently in the bones in general, and very rarely in facial bones and in the jaw in particular. The microscopic features are varied and are represented by lymphosarcomas, reticulum-cell sarcomas, Hodgkin's-like lesions, etc. Finally, generalized leukemia with peripheral blood involvement occurs quite frequently, particularly in terminal phases of the disease.

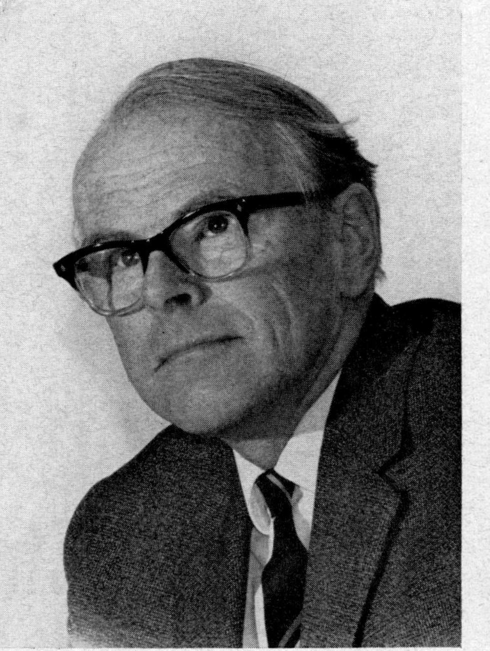
Denis P. Burkitt

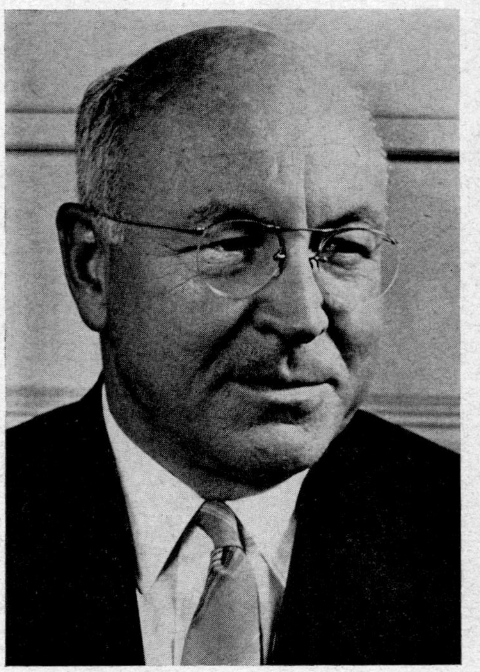
Wendell M. Stanley

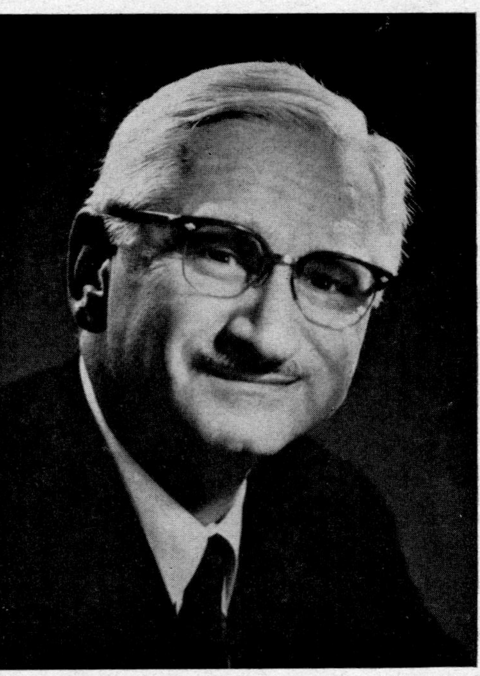
Albert B. Sabin

Fig. 70

Electron Microscopic Studies

Epstein and Herdson (1963) studied ultrathin sections of biopsy fragments from jaw tumors removed from 2 boys, 5 and 6 years old, suffering from Burkitt lymphoma. The tumors were composed of typical small cells with large nuclei and relatively little cytoplasm; there was much evidence of degeneration among the cells examined; the most characteristic features, such as marginated chromatin masses, spherical granular bodies 1.5 μ in diameter, and aggregations of very small dense particles about 15 mμ in diameter, were observed in the nuclei.

Bernhard and Lambert (1964) examined ultrathin sections prepared from biopsy fragments of jaw tumors from 5 cases of Burkitt lymphoma which developed in children 7 to 11 years old in Dakar. These tumors were diagnosed in the optical microscope as either "stem-cell" or reticulum-cell sarcoma (Camain *et al.*, 1964). No virus particles were observed in the examined material. The cellular structure was that of undifferentiated or differentiated reticulum cells, less frequently also lymphoblasts. In two cases unusual alterations were observed in the nucleus which were characterized by a pronounced margination of the chromatin, the appearance of dense granular masses, and of discrete clusters of very small granular particles.

Similar nuclear alterations had been observed in previous electron microscopic studies also in human lymphosarcoma and in Hodgkin's disease (Shipkey and Tandler, 1962. Leplus *et al.*, 1961).

In a continuation of this study ultrathin sections were prepared from tumor cells grown *in vitro* in an established tissue culture strain (EBI) derived from a Burkitt lymphoma. These sections were then examined in the electron microscope (Epstein and Achong, 1965). Among the most striking features observed were peculiar cytoplasmic projections of the nuclear envelope; the nature and significance of these structures were obscure. In addition, some of the cells showed in their cytoplasm the presence of striking, parallel arrays of annulate longitudinal lamellae. The annuli measured about 100 mμ in diameter and their profuse, closely packed, arrangement was especially well seen when they were cut tangentially to include a sufficient area within the thickness of the section. Annulate lamellae have been previously observed in malignant as well as in normal cells (Swift, 1956. Wessel and Bernhard, 1957. Ross, 1962. Chambers and Weiser, 1964).

In further electron microscopic studies, biopsy fragments of tumors from 6 patients from Uganda with Burkitt lymphomas were examined (Achong and Epstein, 1966). The tumors were found to be composed of large numbers of lymphoblasts, with some macrophages, and occasional plasma cells. Characteristic projections of the nuclear envelope were again observed in the tumor cells, similar to those previously observed in Burkitt tumor cells grown in tissue culture; the material enclosed by these projections was cytoplasmic, since it contained mitochondria and centrioles.

Propagation of African Lymphoma in Tissue Culture

Pulvertaft (1964) examined over 50 cases of Burkitt African lymphoma by tissue culture technique at the University of Ibadan in Western Nigeria. Fragments of tumors collected directly in the operating room from patients were placed in tissue culture. The tumor cells were then grown *in vitro*. They survived only when human serum was added. The cells were found to be uniform spheres about 10 μ in diameter and markedly granular. They were characterized by non-motility, and non-adhesion to glass; the cytoplasmic granularity was also very characteristic. The cells remained at first floating as single spheres, but after some weeks they aggregated into masses of several hundreds; even then, however, they did not adhere to glass. At the time this report was published, one strain of tumor cells had been maintained *in vitro* in subcultures for 10 weeks, and a second for 5 weeks, without change of characteristics. The second strain of tumor cells differed from the first in being slightly motile and loosely adherent to glass; in this respect the second strain was different from most of the other cultures observed.

At about the same time Epstein and Barr (1964) also reported cultivation *in vitro* of tumor cells from Burkitt lymphoma; biopsy fragments taken from a child with a typical maxillary tumor in Kampala, Uganda, were placed in a sterile bottle and flown to London. On arrival, the biopsy fragments were distributed in several sterile containers, with tissue culture fluid and human serum added, and were then incubated. The cells were cultured for 8 weeks in 4 serial passages. Again, as in Pulvertaft's study, it was observed that the cells did not adhere to the glass of the containers in which they were propagated, but remained free floating.

In a subsequent study Epstein and Barr (1965) attempted to culture tumor cells from biopsy specimens of 22 patients with Burkitt lymphoma. After some preliminary trials it was possible to propagate a strain of tumor cells by serial passages for more than 10 months in a continuous culture. This cell strain, designated EB1, originated from a biopsy specimen taken from a 9-year-old girl with a typical tumor of the right upper maxilla. In a more recent publication Epstein reported (1967) that this cell line has now been passaged in continuous culture *in vitro* for 25 months. The cells grew as free floating single or double spheres; the cells were usually round, sometimes pear-shaped, and measured 5 to 8 μ in diameter. Occasionally there were multinucleated round cells. Because of their manner of growth and uniform morphology when stained, these cells were identified as altered primitive lymphoblasts. A second, similar tumor cell strain of human lymphoblasts, designated EB2, was established in a continuous cell culture and was maintained in serial passage for 6 months (Epstein *et al.*, 1964b). This strain originated from a biopsy sample taken in Kampala, Uganda, from a massive ovarian tumor in a 7-year-old girl who had a short history of abdominal and left facial swelling.

A similar long-term tumor cell line, designated the "Raji strain," which originated in Pulvertaft's studies (1964) from a biopsy taken from an 11-year-old Yoruba boy in Nigeria, was maintained and studied between the 16th and 28th months of culture by Epstein and his colleagues (1966). Judged by their appearance, fine structural organization, and manner of growth, the cells were considered undifferentiated lymphoblasts. Characteristics suggesting a lack of differentiation were the formation of large aggregations containing many hundreds of individual cells, a relatively large diameter of the cells, and the presence of irregularly indented nuclei. Other long-term lymphoblast cell lines from Burkitt tumors were also established and studied in tissue culture (Epstein *et al.*, 1966).

Stewart and her coworkers (1965) propagated in tissue culture tumor cells taken from a biopsy specimen removed from a mandibular tumor in a 7-year-old African boy. The patient was flown from Nigeria to the Clinical Center, National Institutes of Health, Bethesda, Md., for treatment. The tumor cells grew in suspensions, usually in clumps varying from a few to several hundred cells, in a free floating mass. The cells retained their original microscopic morphology. A similar continuous cell line of human lymphoblasts derived from the same tumor case was established in a separate study by Rabson and his coworkers (1966).

O'Conor and Rabson (1965) established a continuous line of tumor cells from a lymphoma which developed in a 27-year-old white American female born in the United States. This patient had bilateral ovarian tumors followed by a generalized lymphoma. Microscopically, the lymphoma was of a poorly differentiated lymphocytic type, similar to that seen frequently in children in Equatorial Africa.

In summary, it is quite apparent that Burkitt tumor cells can be propagated in tissue culture in primary cultures, as well as in long-term cell lines.

In previous studies, under proper experimental conditions, human leukemic lymphocytic cells could also be propagated in long-term cultures *in vitro* (Brooke and Osgood, 1959).

* * *

Attempts to Transmit Burkitt Lymphoma to Monkeys. Epstein and his colleagues attempted to transmit Burkitt lymphoma to suckling African green monkeys (*Cercopithecus aethiops*).

In the first experiment (Epstein *et al.*, 1964c) a centrifuged extract prepared from fresh biopsy material of a maxillary tumor removed from a 5-year-old girl was inoculated into 4 suckling African green monkeys. One monkey died shortly afterwards. Of the three which survived for more than 2 years, two were found to have gross lesions of long bones. These lesions consisted of bone destruction by excess fibrous tissue and formation of cystic spaces, and by expansion of bone marrow cavity by what appeared as sheets of lymphoblastic tumor cells.

In a subsequent experiment (Epstein *et al.*, 1966) frozen tumor material from typical Burkitt jaw and ovarian tumors was employed. The tumor samples were thawed, minced, and then inoculated into suckling African green monkeys. Three out of 7 inoculated monkeys which survived for more than 2 years developed cystic bone changes. Some of the cysts contained normal marrow, or increased fibrous or fatty tissue, but no evidence of tumor formation was found in this second group of animals.

Wright and Bell (1964) pointed out, however, that similar bone lesions occur spontaneously in African monkeys. It is questionable, therefore, whether the lesions observed in the inoculated monkeys were related to the tumor extracts which these monkeys received. Further studies are needed to determine whether Burkitt lymphoma can be transmitted, by experimental inoculation, to monkeys, or to other animal species. In this respect the problem of experimental transmission of Burkitt lymphoma syndrome to animals is not different from the more general problem of experimental transmission of human neoplasms to other animal species.

THE SEARCH FOR A CAUSATIVE VIRUS IN AFRICAN LYMPHOMAS

There have been numerous attempts to isolate viruses from Burkitt lymphomas, or to identify in electron microscopic studies a presumably causative viral agent in either biopsy tissue fragments or in cultured tumor cells.

Isolation of Herpes Virus from Tumor Biopsies

In December, 1961, a unit from the Imperial Cancer Research Fund of London joined the staff of the East African Virus Research Institute in Entebbe, Uganda, in an attempt to isolate a causative virus from African lymphomas.

In the first series of experiments (Simons and Ross, 1965) fresh tumor material was collected in the operating room. Fragments from 50 biopsies were finely minced, washed, and then inoculated into tubes containing primary hamster kidney cells, or early passage human fetal lung cells. The inoculated cells were then observed for morphological changes. Forty-eight hours after inoculation of the extracts into primary hamster kidney cells, groups of round refractile cells could be seen in some of the inoculated cultures. Passage of medium from infected to fresh cultures produced similar changes after 24 hours. The altered cells were examined in the electron microscope by Dr. R. R. Dourmashkin of the Imperial Cancer Research Fund, and showed the presence of an agent which resembled the herpes virus. The infective passage material from such tubes was then inoculated into the scarified cornea of two rabbits, and induced after 3 days a marked kerato-conjunctivitis. Eight days later one of the rabbits was found moribund. The same virus was isolated from the rabbit lesions. It became apparent that the isolated agent was the herpes virus. This was confirmed by serum cross neutralization tests.

A total of 5 virus isolates was obtained, each identified as herpes simplex virus; all these isolates were obtained from biopsy fragments of jaw tumors. Throat swabs were also taken from 3 of the 5 patients whose tumors contained herpes simplex virus. Two of these 3 throat swabs revealed presence of herpes simplex virus, indicating that at least 2 of the patients were actively releasing herpes virus at the time the biopsies were taken. Four throat swabs from other lymphoma cases did not yield any virus isolates.

It has been shown that young children can discharge herpes virus into the mouth or stools, without showing signs of disease (Buddingh *et al.*, 1953). This observation was confirmed in Uganda (Simons and Ross, 1965). Throat swabs were collected from 104 normal healthy African children 1 to 4 years old, and inoculated into primary hamster kidney cells grown in tissue culture. Herpes simplex virus was recovered from 8 of the 104 samples tested. It was therefore apparent that herpes simplex virus is carried by normal, healthy African children, as it is also ubiquitous in healthy carriers in the United States and in other parts of the world. The authors concluded, therefore, that the herpes virus which they isolated from the tumor biopsies was probably not involved in the etiology of African lymphoma.

In another related study, carried out at the same Institute (Woodall *et al.*, 1965), biopsy material was collected from 76 biopsies of African lymphomas. From this material 6 isolations of herpes virus were made. In this study the virus isolations were performed by inoculating newborn mice with extracts prepared from the biopsy material. In positive cases the inoculated mice died with characteristic symptoms of encephalitis. The virus was then recovered from the inoculated mice, and identified as herpes virus by serum neutralization tests, and in some instances also by complement fixation tests. With only one questionable exception, all the biopsies yielding virus were from jaw tumors connected with the oral cavity of the patients. This made it rather apparent that the herpes virus could have gained its entry into the tumor cells from the oral cavity of the patients, who were probably natural carriers of the herpes virus. The authors concluded that the herpes virus was present in these tumors only as a passenger, although an etiological connection with the tumor origin was not entirely excluded.

Electron Microscopic Studies Reveal the Presence of Herpes, or "Herpes-like," Virus Particles in Cultured Burkitt Lymphoma Cells

Attempts have also been made to identify a causative virus, by electron microscopic studies, in cultured tumor cells from Burkitt lymphoma (Epstein *et al.*, 1964a). Virus particles were found in a small fraction of the tumor cells examined. The particles were observed in both the nucleus and in the cytoplasm. They were spherical; some of them had nucleoids. In their appearance these virus particles resembled the herpes virus, but in the opinion of the authors the agent which they observed was smaller by about 20 per cent. In a continuation of this study, Epstein and his colleagues (1964b, 1965) found similar virus particles in the tumor cells of two tissue culture lines (EB1 and EB2) of the Burkitt lymphoma and subsequently also in cultured lymphoblasts derived from a New Guinea case of this tumor syndrome (Epstein *et al.*, 1967). The virus particles were present only in about 1 to 2 per cent of the cells examined. The immature particles were seen in both the nucleus and in the cytoplasm; they had a diameter of approximately 75 to 80 mμ, and were either "empty" or contained a central, electron-dense nucleoid. These particles matured by budding at cellular membranes, acquiring thereby an additional membrane. The mature particles with this additional membrane measured 115 to 120 mμ in diameter, and their nucleoids about 45 mμ. These mature particles were present in cytoplasmic vacuoles, in the perinuclear space, or just outside the cell surface. Attempts to isolate and identify the virus were not successful.

In their overall morphology, and also in location in relation to cell structures, i.e., presence in the cytoplasm and also in the nucleus, these particles were very similar to the herpes simplex virus, and, in fact, could have been readily identified as the herpes virus. However, Epstein and his colleagues felt that the virus which they observed in the Burkitt lymphoma cells was in certain respects different from the herpes simplex virus, even though they acknowledged that it probably belongs to the herpes group. The differences were based not only on the slightly smaller size of this virus as compared with the herpes simplex virus (Epstein *et al.*, 1964a, 1967), but also on certain biological and immunological data (Epstein *et al.*, 1965. Henle and Henle, 1966. Henle *et al.*, 1966). This differentiation, however, can be accepted only with reservations and requires further documentation.

Stewart and her colleagues (1965) also observed herpes-like virus particles in some of the cells of a tumor cell line derived from a Nigerian case of Burkitt lymphoma; the cells from both the 20 and 34-day-old cultures were examined by Dr. A. J. Dalton.

Rabson and his coworkers (1966) established a similar cell line of human lymphoblasts (AL1) derived from a malignant lymphoma involving the jaw in a Nigerian boy. On microscopic examination, less than 1 per cent of the cells studied during the first 4 months of the culture were found to contain herpes-like virus particles; subsequently no cells containing virus particles were seen. The particles were usually found in the nucleus. They had a diameter of about 90 mμ, and had a single outer membrane; many of them had a centrally located nucleoid. Attempts to isolate a virus from the cells were unsuccessful.

O'Conor and Rabson (1965) established a continuous line of tumor cells from a 27-year-old white American woman born in the United States, who developed bilateral ovarian tumors histologically similar to the type frequently observed in children in Equatorial Africa. Herpes-like virus particles were found in about one in 300 cells examined. The intranuclear immature particles measured approximately 90 mμ in diameter, and the cytoplasmic particles had a diameter of about 145 to 150 mμ. Attempts to isolate this virus were not successful. The possible significance of these particles and their role as causative agents or as etiologically unrelated passengers remained to be determined.

No Virus Particles could be Observed on Electron Microscopic Examination of Biopsy Fragments from Primary Burkitt Lymphomas

It is of interest that although the herpes-like virus particles could be observed in some of the cells propagated in tissue culture and derived from Burkitt lymphomas, no virus particles of any kind could be observed thus far in tissue sections prepared directly from biopsy fragments of primary Burkitt tumors.

Bernhard and Lambert (1964) examined biopsy specimens from 5 Burkitt lymphomas with negative results. More recently Bernhard (personal communication to the author, 1968) examined in the electron microscope ultrathin sections from 47 cases of Burkitt lymphomas, but failed to detect the presence of virus particles in any of these specimens.

Isolation of Unidentified Cytopathogenic Agents, and of Mycoplasma (PPLO)

Dalldorf and Bergamini (1964) isolated unidentified filterable agents from African children with malignant lymphomas. These agents induced a peculiar twisting and spindling of primary human amnion cells in cultures into which they were inoculated. Fluid collected from such cultures and inoculated into embryonic human kidney cells induced destructive changes in the cells. However, direct inoculation of embryonic kidney cells with extracts from tumors, or from bone marrow, did not cause a cytopathogenic effect. These agents were later cultivated on protein-rich media and were found to have the characteristics of mycoplasma (PPLO).

In a continuation of this study (Dalldorf *et al.*, 1966) 5 additional patients from East Africa with Burkitt lymphomas were studied. A bone marrow aspirate, and a tumor extract from another case, induced the characteristic changes in the amnion cells. Other samples were negative. Five additional patients from South Africa were also studied. Again the characteristic changes in the human amnion cell cultures were induced with either tumor extracts or with bone marrow aspirates, and in some instances also with blood clots; however, none of the fluids collected from the altered amnion cell cultures was cytopathogenic for embryonic kidney cells. Mycoplasma was not isolated from these patients.

The nature of the cytopathogenic agents isolated by Dalldorf and his coworkers was not clarified, and their relation, if any, to the tumors remained obscure. The source of the mycoplasma (PPLO) recovered in some of the patients in Dalldorf's studies also remained unknown.

All patients from whom mycoplasma was isolated had tumors of the jaw. It is well known that mycoplasma can frequently be recovered from oral and genital tissues (Hayflick and Chanock, 1965).

Isolation of Reovirus

Bell and his coworkers (1964) isolated a reovirus,* probably related to type 3, from a Burkitt tumor biopsy of a tumor which developed in the left cheek of a 5-year-old African boy observed at Mulago Hospital, in Kampala, Uganda. Following inoculation of extracts prepared from this tumor into hamster kidney and human amnion cells, a cytopathogenic effect was produced similar to that observed in tissue culture cells in which the reovirus is propagated. Further passage in hamster kidney cells and also in vervet monkey kidney cells was performed, and the virus thus isolated was studied. When the cells infected with the passaged virus were examined in the electron microscope by Dr. R. R. Dourmashkin, they were found

* The name "reovirus" was coined from the initials for respiratory, enteric, and orphan viruses. These are medium-sized, ether-resistant viruses. The members of this group occur widely in the respiratory and the enteric tracts of man and animals and were originally called echovirus 10, before being grouped separately on the basis of their biophysical properties. Three antigenic types have been recovered from humans, mice and cattle (Melnick and McCombs, 1966).

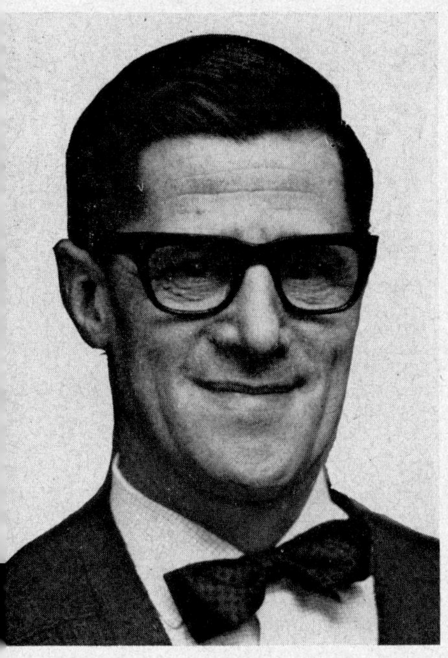

Michael Stoker

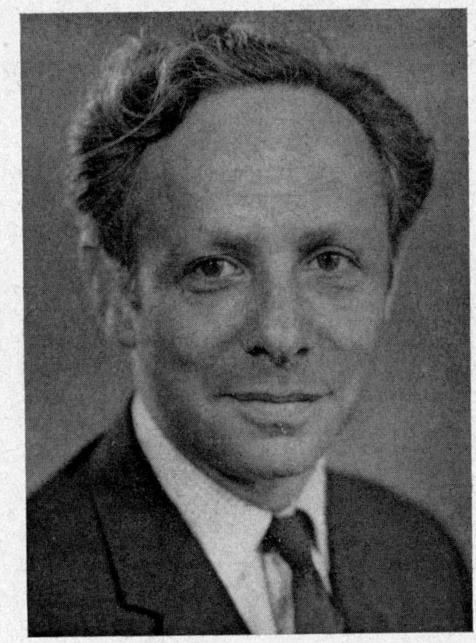

M. A. Epstein

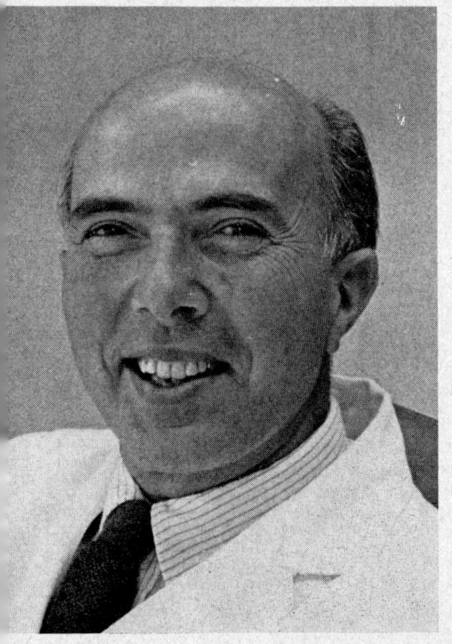

Renato Dulbecco

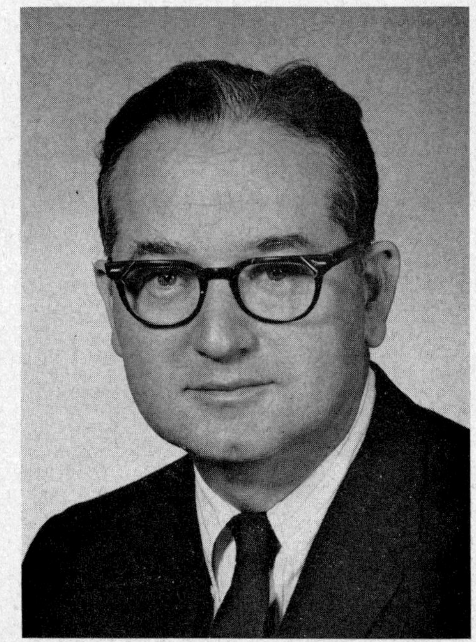

Joseph L. Melnick

FIG. 71

to be packed with reovirus-like particles. The virus was found to be ether-resistant. Antiserum to reovirus type 3 neutralized the isolated agent. Intracerebral inoculation into newborn mice was rapidly fatal. The virus could be again recovered from the brains of the inoculated mice.

Reoviruses are common, and are carried by different animal species and also by humans. Strains related to those reoviruses which can infect man have been isolated from monkeys, dogs, cats, cattle, mice, and insects.

In a continuation of this study, Bell and his coworkers reported (1966) the isolation of 12 virus strains from 9 cases of Burkitt lymphoma. Ten of these virus strains, isolated from 7 cases, were identified as reovirus type 3. One of the others appeared to be herpes simplex, and one has not yet been identified. The appearance of the isolated reoviruses in electron micrographs, and their pathogenic effect on mice, were characteristic and led to their identification. The authors concluded that reovirus is associated with at least some of the cases of Burkitt lymphoma. However, whether this association is incidental, or causative, remains to be determined.

The fact that certain viruses, such as herpes simplex, or reovirus type 3, could be isolated from some of the biopsy fragments of Burkitt lymphomas, does not necessarily suggest that any of these virus strain isolations was etiologically related to the development of tumors. The same refers to the herpes, or "herpes-like," virus particles detected on electron microscopic examination in tumor cell lines derived from Burkitt lymphomas. It has long been known that tumor cells form a favorable environment in which a variety of viruses may propagate as passengers (Levaditi and Nicolau, 1922. Levaditi *et al.*, 1937). More recently it has been amply documented that transplanted tumor cells in mice may carry as a passenger the virus of mouse leukemia (Graffi *et al.*, 1956).*

The Isolated Viruses: Causative Agents or Passengers?

Until proof to the contrary it appears reasonable to assume that the herpes virus strains isolated from Burkitt's lymphomas represent most probably passenger viruses unrelated to the tumor etiology. Whether the herpes-like virus observed by Epstein is actually a different virus from the common herpes group still remains to be determined. Its possible relation to the etiology of lymphomas has not been documented.

The reovirus which was isolated by Bell and his coworkers from the tumor cells (1964, 1966) is probably also unrelated to the etiology of Burkitt tumor syndrome; at least no evidence has yet been furnished to support a different assumption.

* The isolation of mouse leukemia virus strains from transplanted mouse tumors is discussed in chapter 12 of this monograph.

Mycoplasma (PPLO) which has been isolated from some cases of Burkitt lymphoma seems to be unrelated etiologically to the tumors from which it was recovered; it also appears to be unrelated to other neoplasms, including leukemia, from which similar isolations have been reported.

General Considerations and Some Tentative Conclusions

The curious lymphoma syndrome described by Burkitt in African children and later also observed in other parts of the world, attracted considerable attention of clinicians, pathologists, oncologists, and virologists during the past decade. The extensive bibliography which the reader will find at the end of this chapter will attest to the widespread interest in this disease syndrome. Yet many questions have not yet been answered. Is the Burkitt leukemia syndrome a disease entity? It is quite apparent that this tumor syndrome is not limited to the "lymphoma belt" in tropical Africa described by Burkitt, but can be observed also in other parts of Africa and on other continents, including North America. The fact that this tumor syndrome with its characteristic involvement of facial bones is rather common in Central Africa remains unchanged, nevertheless, and requires further studies.

The dependence of this tumor syndrome on climatic conditions may be authentic, at least under the tropical African conditions, but has not been sufficiently documented and could certainly not explain the occurrence of this tumor in certain other parts of the world, including North America and Canada. The possibility should be considered, however, that this tumor may be transmitted under certain conditions by mosquitoes or other vectors, and under other conditions by different means which may not necessarily require an intermediary insect vector.

It is now generally suspected that this tumor syndrome is caused by a transmissible oncogenic virus, even though the presence of such a virus has not yet been documented. It seems reasonable to assume, however, that the viral causation of the tumor syndrome occurring in African children is not more probable for this particular tumor than it is for other malignant neoplasms, including leukemia and lymphomas, in humans. From the point of view of presumable viral etiology, the tumor syndrome described in African children does not seem to stand apart from other malignant neoplasms in man.

REFERENCES

Achong, B. G., and Epstein, M. A., Fine structure of the Burkitt tumor. *J. Nat. Cancer Inst.*, **26**: 877–897, 1966.

Bell, T. M., Massie, A., Ross, M. G. R., and Williams, M. C., Isolation of a reovirus from a case of Burkitt's lymphoma. *Brit. Med. J.*, **1**: 1212–1213, 1964.

Bell, T. M., Massie, A., Ross, M. G. R., Simpson, D. I. H., and Griffin, E., Further isolations of reovirus type 3 from cases of Burkitt's lymphoma. *Brit. Med. J.*, **1**: 1514–1517, 1966.

Beltrán, G., Baez, A., and Correa, P., Burkitt's lymphoma in Colombia. *Am. J. Med.*, **40**: 211–216, 1966.

Bernhard, W., and Lambert, D., Ultrastructure des tumeurs de Burkitt de l'enfant africain. pp. 270–284 in: *Symp. Lymph. Tumours in Africa* (Paris, 1963). S. Karger, Basel and New York, 1964.

Booth, C. C., Davies, J. N. P., *et al.*, Clinicopathological Conference. A case of African lymphoma demonstrated at the Postgraduate Medical School of London. *Brit. Med. J.*, **1**: 296–299, 1964.

Brooke, J. H., and Osgood, E. E., Long-term mixed cultures of human hemic cells, with granulocytic, lymphocytic, plasmocytic and erythrocytic series represented. *Blood*, **14**: 803–815, 1959.

Brown, J. B., and O'Keefe, C. D., Sarcoma of the ovary with unusual oral metastases. *Ann. Surg.*, **87**: 467–471, 1928.

Buddingh, G. J., Schrum, D. I., Lanier, J. C., and Guidry, D. J., Studies of the natural history of herpes simplex infections. *Pediatrics*, **11**: 595–610, 1953.

Burkitt, D., A sarcoma involving the jaws in African children. *Brit. J. Surg.*, **46**: 218–223, 1958.

Burkitt, D., A lymphoma syndrome in African children. *Ann. Royal Coll. Surg. Eng.*, **30**: 211–219, 1962a.

Burkitt, D., A children's cancer dependent on climatic factors. *Nature*, **194**: 232–234, 1962b.

Burkitt, D., Determining the climatic limitations of a children's cancer common in Africa. *Brit. Med. J.*, **2**: 1019–1023, 1962c.

Burkitt, D., A tumour syndrome affecting children in tropical Africa. *Postgrad. Med. J.*, **38**: 71–79, 1962d.

Burkitt, D., A lymphoma syndrome dependent on environment. Part I. Clinical aspects. pp. 80–93 in: *Symp. Lymph. Tumours in Africa* (Paris, 1963). S. Karger, Basel and New York, 1964.

Burkitt, D., and Davies, J. N. P., Lymphoma syndrome in Uganda and tropical Africa. *Med. Press*, **245**: 367–369, 1961.

Burkitt, D., and O'Conor, G. T., Malignant lymphoma in African children. I. A clinical syndrome. *Cancer*, **14**: 258–269, 1961.

Camain, R., Baylet, R., Bres, P., and Lambert, D., Les hématosarcomes de la face chez l'enfant en Afrique occidentale et centrale fracophone. III. Histopathologie, tentatives de culture et autres examens biologiques. pp. 256–269 in: *Symp. Lymph. Tumours in Africa* (Paris, 1963). S. Karger, Basel and New York, 1964.

Chambers, V. C., and Weiser, R. S., Annulate lamellae in sarcoma I cells. *J. Cell Biol.*, **21**: 133–139, 1964.

Chapman, D. S., and Jenkins, T., The Burkitt lymphoma in Natal. A significant medical tail. *Med. Proc. (Johannesburg)*, **9**: 320–331, 1963.

Clifford, P., Malignant disease of the nose, paranasal sinuses and post-nasal space in East Africa. *J. Laryng. (London)*, **75**: 707–733, 1961.

Clift, R. A., Wright, D. H., and Clifford, P., Leukemia in Burkitt's lymphoma. *Blood*, **22**: 243–251, 1963.

Dalldorf, G., Lymphomas of African children. With different forms or environmental influences. *J. Am. Med. Assoc.*, **181**: 1026–1028, 1962.

DALLDORF, G., and BERGAMINI, F., Unidentified, filtrable agents isolated from African children with malignant lymphomas. *Proc. Nat. Acad. Sci., USA,* **51**: 263–265, 1964.

DALLDORF, G., BERGAMINI, F., and FROST, P., Further observations of the lymphomas of African children. *Proc. Nat. Acad. Sci., USA,* **55**: 297–302, 1966.

DAVIES, J. N. P., WILSON, B. A., and KNOWELDEN, J., Cancer in Kampala: A survey in an underdeveloped country. *Brit. Med. J.*, **2**: 439–443, 1958.

DAVIES, J. N. P., WILSON, B. A., and KNOWELDEN, J., Cancer incidence of the African population of Kyandondo (Uganda). *Lancet,* **2**: 328–330, 1962.

DORFMAN, R. F., Childhood lymphosarcoma in St. Louis, Missouri, clinically and histologically resembling Burkitt's tumor. *Cancer,* **18**: 418–430, 1965.

EDINGTON, G. M., MACLEAN, C. M. U., and OKUBADEJO, O. A., 101 necropsies on tumours of reticulo-endothelial system in Ibadan, Nigeria, with special reference to childhood lymphoma. pp. 236–252 in: *Symp. Lymph. Tumours in Africa* (Paris, 1963). S. Karger, Basel and New York, 1964.

EPSTEIN, M. A., Histogenesis of the Burkitt lymphoma. pp. 29–33 in: UICC Monograph Series, vol. 8: *Treatment of Burkitt's Tumour.* Springer-Verlag, Berlin, Heidelberg, New York, 1967.

EPSTEIN, M. A., Viruses in Burkitt's Tumour. pp. 64–68 in: UICC Monograph Series, vol. 8: *Treatment of Burkitt's Tumour.* Springer-Verlag, Berlin, Heidelberg, New York, 1967.

EPSTEIN, M. A., ACHONG, B. G., and BARR, Y. M., Virus particles in cultured lymphoblasts from Burkitt's lymphoma. *Lancet,* **1**: 702–703, 1964a.

EPSTEIN, M. A., and ACHONG, B. G., Fine structural organization of human lymphoblasts of a tissue culture strain (EB1) from Burkitt's lymphoma. *J. Nat. Cancer Inst.*, **34**: 241–253, 1965.

EPSTEIN, M. A., ACHONG, B. G., BARR, Y. M., ZAJAC, B., HENLE, G., and HENLE, W., Morphological and virological investigations on cultured Burkitt tumor lymphoblasts (strain Raji), *J. Nat. Cancer Inst.*, **37**: 547–559, 1966.

EPSTEIN, M. A., ACHONG, B. G., and POPE, J. H., Virus in cultured lymphoblasts from a New Guinea Burkitt lymphoma. *Brit. Med. J.*, **2**: 290–291, 1967.

EPSTEIN, M. A., and BARR, Y. M., Cultivation *in vitro* of human lymphoblasts from Burkitt's malignant lymphoma. *Lancet,* **1**: 252–253, 1964.

EPSTEIN, M. A., BARR, Y. M., and ACHONG, B. G., A second virus-carrying tissue culture strain (EB2) of lymphoblasts from Burkitt's lymphoma. *Path. Biol. (Paris),* **12**: 1233–1234, 1964b.

EPSTEIN, M. A., and BARR, Y. M., Characteristics and mode of growth of a tissue culture strain (EB1) of human lymphoblasts from Burkitt's lymphoma. *J. Nat. Cancer Inst.*, **34**: 231–240, 1965.

EPSTEIN, M. A., BARR, Y. M., and ACHONG, B. G., Preliminary observations on new lymphoblast strains (EB4, EB5) from Burkitt tumours in a British and a Ugandan patient. *Brit. J. Cancer,* **20**: 475–479, 1966.

EPSTEIN, M. A., and HERDSON, P. B., Cellular degeneration associated with characteristic nuclear fine structural changes in the cells from two cases of Burkitt's malignant lymphoma syndrome. *Brit. J. Cancer,* **17**: 56–58, 1963.

EPSTEIN, M. A., HENLE, G., ACHONG, B. G., and BARR, Y. M., Morphological and biological studies on a virus in cultured lymphoblasts from Burkitt's lymphoma, *J. Exp. Med.*, **121**: 761–770, 1965.

Epstein, M. A., Thomson, A. D., and Woodall, J. P., Experiments with Burkitt's lymphoma: Attempted transmission to monkeys in relation to virological findings. pp. 323–335 in: *Some Recent Developments in Comparative Medicine*. Symposia of The Zoological Society of London, No. 17. Academic Press, London and New York, 1966.

Epstein, M. A., Woodall, J. P., and Thomson, A. D., Lymphoblastic lymphoma in bone-marrow of African green monkeys (*Cercopithecus aethiops*) inoculated with biopsy material from a child with Burkitt's lymphoma. *Lancet*, **2**: 288–290, 1964c.

Feldman, D. G., and Gross, L., Electron-microscopic study of the mouse leukemia virus (Gross), and of tissues from mice with virus-induced leukemia. *Cancer Research*, **24**: 1760–1783, 1964.

Foley, G. E., Lazarus, H., Farber, S., Uzman, B. G., Boone, B. A., and McCarthy, R. E., Continuous culture of human lymphoblasts from peripheral blood of a child with acute leukemia. *Cancer*, **18**: 522–529, 1965.

Gluckman, J., Multifocal lymphoma in South Africa. Its first observation in South Africa and in white children. *South African Cancer Bull.*, **7**: 7–12, 1963.

Graffi, A., Bielka, H., and Fey, F., Leukämieerzeugung durch ein filtrierbares Agens aus malignen Tumoren. *Acta Haemat.*, **15**: 145–174, 1956.

Griffin, E. R., Wright, D. H., Bell, T. M., and Ross, M. G. R., Demonstration of virus particles in biopsy material from cases of Burkitt's tumour. *European J. Cancer*, **2**: 353–358, 1966.

Haguenau, F., Significance of ultrastructure in virus-induced tumors. pp. 211–249 in: Symposium, Phenomena of the Tumor Viruses. *Nat. Cancer Inst. Monograph No. 4*. U.S. Publ. Health Service, Bethesda, Md., 1960.

Harris, R. J. C., Aetiology of Central African lymphomata. *Brit. Med. Bull.*, **20**: 149–153, 1964.

Hayflick, L., and Chanock, R. M., *Mycoplasma* species of man. *Bact. Rev.*, **29**: 185–221, 1965.

Henle, G., and Henle, W., Immunofluorescence in cells derived from Burkitt's lymphoma. *J. Bact.*, **91**: 1248–1256, 1966.

Henle, W., Hummeler, K., and Henle, G., Antibody coating and agglutination of virus particles separated from the EB3 line of Burkitt lymphoma cells. *J. Bact.*, **92**: 269–271, 1966.

Higginson, J., and Oettlé, A. G., Cancer incidence in the Bantu and "Cape Colored" races of South Africa: Report of a cancer survey in the Transvaal (1953–55). *J. Nat. Cancer Inst.*, **24**: 589–671, 1960.

Hoogstraten, J., Observations on Burkitt's tumour in Central and Northern Canada. *Internat. J. Cancer*, **2**: 566–575, 1967.

Iwakata, S., and Grace, J. T., Jr., Cultivation *in vitro* of myeloblasts from human leukemia. *New York J. Med.*, **64**: 2279–2282, 1964.

Khan, A. G., The multifocal lymphoma syndrome in African children in Kenya. *J. Laryng.* (*London*), **78**: 480–498, 1964.

Lambert, D., Les hématosarcomes de la face chez l'enfant en Afrique. *Thèse pour le Doctorat en Médecine, No. 212*, Faculté de Médecine de Paris. p. 194, Grande Imprimerie Africaine, Dakar, 1964.

Leading Article. Virus and Burkitt's lymphoma. *Lancet*, **2**: 872–873, 1967.

Leplus, R., Debray, J., Pinet, J., and Bernhard, W., Lésions nucléaires decelées au microscope électronique dans des cellules de *Lymphomes malins* chez l'homme. *Compt. Rend. Acad. Sci.* (*Paris*), **253**: 2788–2790, 1961.

LEVADITI, C., and NICOLAU, S., Vaccine et néoplasmes. *Compt. Rend. Acad. Sci. (Paris)*, **174**: 1649–1652, 1922.

LEVADITI, C., SCHOEN, R., and REINIÉ, L., Virus rabique et cellules néoplasiques. *Ann. Inst. Pasteur*, **58**: 353–376, 1937.

MELNICK, J. L., and MCCOMBS, R. M., Classification and nomenclature of animal viruses, 1966. *Progr. Med. Virol.*, **8**: 400–409, 1966.

MOORE, A. E., Consideration of means for determining if viruses are causally related to cancer in man. *Progr. Med. Virol.*, **5**: 295–306, 1963.

O'CONOR, G. T., Malignant lymphoma in African children. II. A pathological entity. *Cancer*, **14**: 270–283, 1961.

O'CONOR, G. T., and DAVIES, J. N. P., Malignant tumors in African children with special reference to malignant lymphoma. *J. Pediat.*, **56**: 526–535, 1960.

O'CONOR, G. T., and RABSON, A. S., Herpes-like particles in an American lymphoma: Preliminary note. *J. Nat. Cancer Inst.*, **35**: 899–903, 1965.

O'CONOR, G. T., RAPPAPORT, H., and SMITH, E. B., Childhood lymphoma resembling "Burkitt tumor" in the United States. *Cancer*, **18**: 411–417, 1965.

OETTGEN, H. F., BURKITT, D., and BURCHENAL, J. H., Malignant lymphoma involving the jaw in African children: Treatment with methotrexate. *Cancer*, **16**: 616–623, 1963.

PULVERTAFT, R. J. V., Cytology of Burkitt's tumour (African lymphoma). *Lancet*, **1**: 238–240, 1964.

RABSON, A. S., O'CONOR, G. T., BARON, S., WHANG, J. J., and LEGALLAIS, F. Y., Morphologic, cytogenetic and virologic studies *in vitro* of a malignant lymphoma from an African child. *Internat. J. Cancer*, **1**: 89–106, 1966.

ROSS, M. H., Annulate lamellae in the adrenal cortex of the fetal rat. *J. Ultrastructure Research*, **7**: 373–382, 1962.

ROWE, N. H., and JOHNSON, C. M., A search for Burkitt lymphoma in tropical Central America. *Brit. J. Cancer*, **18**: 228–232, 1964.

SEED, P. G., Burkitt's tumour in Britain. *J. Obstet. Gynaec. Brit. Comm.*, **73**: 808–811, 1966.

SHIPKEY, F. H., and TANDLER, B., Observations on human malignant lymphoma cells. page PP-9 in: *Electron Microscopy*, vol. 2. Proc. 5th Internat. Congress for Electron Microscopy, Philadelphia, Pa. (Aug. 29–Sept. 5, 1962). Academic Press, New York and London, 1962.

SIMONS, P. J., and ROSS, M. G. R., The isolation of herpes virus from Burkitt tumours. *European J. Cancer*, **1**: 135–136, 1965.

STANSFIELD, D., Haematological findings in African children in Uganda with malignant lymphoma. *Brit. J. Cancer*, **15**: 41–44, 1961.

STEWART, S. E., LOVELACE, E., WHANG, J. J., and NGU, V. A., Burkitt tumor: Tissue culture, cytogenetic and virus studies. *J. Nat. Cancer Inst.*, **34**: 319–327, 1965.

SWIFT, H., The fine structure of annulate lamellae. *J. Biophys. and Biochem. Cytol.*, vol. **2** (No. 4, Suppl.): 415–418, 1956.

TEN SELDAM, R. E. J., COOKE, R., and ATKINSON, L., Childhood lymphoma in the territories of Papua and New Guinea. *Cancer*, **19**: 437–446, 1966.

THIJS, A., Considérations sur les tumeurs malignes des indigènes du Congo belge et du Ruanda-Urundi. À propos de 2.536 cas. *Ann. Soc. Belge Méd. Trop.*, **37**: 483–514, 1957.

TOSHIMA, S., TAKAGI, N., MINOWADA, J., MOORE, G. E., and SANDBERG, A. A., Electron microscope and cytogenetic studies of cells derived from Burkitt's lymphoma. *Cancer Research*, **27**: 753–771, 1967.

WESSEL, W., and BERNHARD, W., Vergleichende elecktronenmikroskopische untersuchung von Ehrlich-und Yoshida-ascitestumorzellen. *Zeitschr. f. Krebsforsch.*, **62**: 140–162, 1957.

WOODALL, J. P., WILLIAMS, M. C., SIMPSON, D. I. H., and HADDOW, A. J., The isolation in mice of strains of herpes virus from Burkitt tumours. *European J. Cancer*, **1**: 137–140, 1965.

WRIGHT, D. H., Cytology and histochemistry of the Burkitt lymphoma. *Brit. J. Cancer*, **17**: 50–55, 1963.

WRIGHT, D. H., Malignant lymphoma. *42nd Ann. Rep. Brit. Empire Cancer Campaign for Research*, **42** (part II): 535, 1964.

WRIGHT, D. H., Burkitt's tumour. A post-mortem study of 50 cases. *Brit. J. Surg.*, **51**: 245–251, 1964.

WRIGHT, D. H., and BELL, T. M., Bone disease in African green monkeys. Letter to the Editor. *Lancet*, **2**: 969–970, 1964.

ZEVE, V. H., LUCAS, L. S., and MANAKER, R. A., Continuous cell culture from a patient with chronic myelogenous leukemia. II. Detection of a herpes-like virus by electron microscopy. *J. Nat. Cancer Inst.*, **37**: 761–773, 1966.

ZIEGLER, J. L., and MILLER, D. G., Lymphosarcoma resembling the Burkitt tumor in a Connecticut girl. *J. Am. Med. Assoc.*, **198**: 1071–1073, 1966.

CHAPTER 22

The Search for Oncogenic Viruses in Human Tumors

The problem of the possible role of oncogenic viruses as causative factors in the development of human tumors is one of the most difficult in experimental medicine. The investigator has very few experimental tools at his disposal. How to approach such a problem in humans? How can we determine whether malignant tumors, including leukemia and allied diseases, are actually caused by transmissible viruses in man?

Let us briefly consider the following principal approaches to the problem of the hypothetical oncogenic viruses in humans: (a) epidemiology; (b) experimental transmission; (c) tissue culture; (d) electron microscopy.

DEVELOPMENT OF CANCER IN FAMILIES AND SUCCESSIVE GENERATIONS IN MAN

Although cancer is a comparatively common disease, and an accidental occurrence of tumors in more than one member of the same family must be considered, numerous "cancer families" have been reported with such a striking incidence of tumors (Paulsen, 1924. Warthin, 1928), that mere chance could be reasonably excluded.

Broca (1866, 1869) observed breast cancer in a woman whose 4 daughters had cancerous tumors; of the 16 grandchildren, 8 died with neoplasms. Finney (1932) reported a family in which the mother, 4 daughters, and 3 nieces had all been operated upon for cancer at the Mayo Clinic; all but one had cancer of the breast. Graham (1936) reported the case of a woman with cancer of the rectum; her 3 daughters and a son all died from cancer of the rectum. Handley (1938) reported 4 sisters with breast cancer; their mother and grandmother also died from tumors. In a case reported by Körbler (1934) both parents and their 3 children died from cancer; in another case a mother, 4 daughters, and a son died from tumors. In a third case described by the same author, 5 out of 7 children of apparently healthy parents developed tumors. One of the daughters with a tumor had 3 daughters, all of whom developed cancer of the breast. Two granddaughters of this patient also developed breast carcinomas. Cancer appeared therefore in members of 3 successive generations of this family. Wood and Darling (1943) reported a family in which bilateral carcinoma of the breast, or other tumors, developed in several members of 4 successive generations. Three sisters of the third generation developed cancer of the breast. Williams (1898) treated a woman with uterine cancer whose maternal grandmother, mother, and mother's sister all died of cancer of the uterus; 2 sisters of the patient also had cancer of the uterus. Manson (1913) treated a 27-year-old woman who developed a fatal sarcoma on the left side of her neck; two of her 3 sons died of identical sarcomas at the same site.

Power described in 1898 the following extraordinary cancer family: Dr. Kirkwood, in the infirmary at Peterborough, treated a patient who had his right breast removed because of scirrhus carcinoma with metastatic axillary glands. The patient's father died of cancer of the left breast at age 46. First brother died at age 65 of cancer of the throat. Second brother died at age 24 of cancer under the left arm. First sister died at age 63 of cancer of the right breast. Second sister died at age 46 of cancer of both breasts. Third sister died at age 40 of cancer of both breasts. Fourth sister died at age 54 of cancer of the breast. Fifth and sixth sisters, still alive at the time of Power's report, also had cancer of the breast.

Heinzelmann (1964) described a remarkable cancer family. A male patient had, over a period of 30 years, 3 primary carcinomas of the colon. In 5 generations of the same family 13 members, including the patient's brother, developed carcinomas; 10 of these tumors were carcinomas of the colon.

Silcock (1892) reported melanosarcoma of the eyeball in 3 successive generations. Retinoblastoma, a highly malignant tumor of the eye that affects infants, is a very rare disease, one case being observed in 34,000 births; in many families, however, half of all the children are afflicted. "Only recently," stated Weller (1941), "has it been appreciated that the disease may exhibit also a vertical familial distribution appearing in successive generations, or in collateral lines." Records of 30 families giving evidence of the appearance of retinoblastoma in successive generations have been collected (Weller, 1937, 1941).

Instances of concurrent development of cancer of the stomach in brothers (Pack, 1934) or twins (Militzer, 1935), or of the appearance of tumors of the breast (Burkard, 1922) or ovaries (Twinem, 1927) in twin sisters, or the concurrent development of osteogenic sarcoma in brother and sisters (Roberts and Roberts, 1935), or in sisters (Pohle, 1936), have been compiled (McFarland and Meade, 1932).

Liber (1950) reported a family in which the mother and 5 of her 7 daughters died of a highly malignant papillary adenocarcinoma of the ovary.

More recently Brisman and his coworkers (1967) described a Negro family in which 4 out of 8 siblings, 3 men and 1 woman, developed carcinoma of the lung when they were 50 to 59 years old. They all had been smoking one-half to one pack of cigarettes a day since they were 16 years old. The remaining 4 other siblings, all men, 40 to 48 years old, were well at the time this report was published.

Numerous statistical studies on familial incidence of cancer in humans have been conducted, leaving little doubt that cancer is more frequent in families of cancer patients than in the average population (Franck, 1904. Paulsen, 1924. Warthin, 1928. Deelman, 1931. McFarland and Meade, 1932. Körbler, 1934. Graham, 1936. Hauser and Weller, 1936. Martynova, 1937. Waaler, 1931. Pass, 1938. Weller, 1937, 1941. Bargen *et al.*, 1941. Grossman and Kesert, 1944. Macklin, 1932, 1955, 1959. Morse, 1951. Videbaek and Mosbech, 1954, etc.).

Although most cancer patients seem to represent sporadic cases, the number of cancer families is considerable. Studies on cancer families have been limited, with only few exceptions, to 2 or 3 successive generations; it has been established that the disease can follow members of certain families for the number of generations observed. There is no reason to doubt that a similar high incidence of tumors may occur in either preceding or succeeding generations. Other families, on the contrary, have very few tumors or practically no record of cancer through several successive generations.

DEVELOPMENT OF LEUKEMIA IN FAMILIES AND SUCCESSIVE GENERATIONS IN MAN

Clinical observations suggesting that in some instances leukemia in humans may appear more frequently in certain families than in the average population are of considerable interest, particularly in view of the fact that this disease is relatively rare in man.

It is true that in most instances leukemia occurs in man sporadically with no records of other cases of leukemia among other members of the same family. And yet, numerous instances have been recorded in which leukemia developed in two or more members of the same family, either within the same or in successive generations (Videbaek, 1947). Among the families described by Videbaek, one involved 4 cases of leukemia in three successive generations. In the study reported by Rigby and his colleagues (1966), 92 families whose probands had leukemia or lymphoma, and 16 control families, have been investigated. Twenty-one families with multiple cases of leukemia and lymphomas have been recorded with an impressive aggregation of other forms of cancer as well. The occurrence of leukemia and lymphomas was $2\frac{1}{2}$ times more frequent in family members of the leukemia-lymphoma proband group than in the control group. In a continuation of this study (Rigby *et al.*, 1968) 39 families have been identified with multiple cases of leukemia or lymphoma.

Cases of leukemia developing in brothers, brothers and sisters, or in a child and in one of its parents, have been recorded and reviewed by numerous observers (Steiner, 1933. Videbaek, 1947. Thiersch, 1947. Guasch, 1954. Kaliampetsos, 1954). Some of the authors, such as Cameron (1888), were able to trace leukemia in members of up to four successive generations of the same family. We have observed two cases of familial incidence of leukemia. In one case a patient and his mother both died from leukemia. In another case the patient suffered from Hodgkin's disease; his mother and maternal grandmother both died from leukemia; in addition, one of his mother's sisters also had leukemia (Gross and Matte, 1948). Hornbaker (1942) reported leukemia in three sisters. Ioachim reported (1962) acute leukemia in two uniovular twin sisters aged 7 and 9 months; numerous cases of leukemia in uniovular twins occurring frequently almost at the same time have been reported.* Multiple myeloma in 2 siblings, aged 53 and 55, was reported by Herrell and his colleagues (1958). Decastello (1939) described a family in which six members of two successive generations developed leukemia. Mazar and Straus (1951) reported a family in which 3 persons had Hodgkin's disease and 2 others died from leukemia. Gunz and Dameshek (1957) described chronic lymphocytic leukemia in a 53-year-old man 27 years after his father and the father's identical twin died of the same disease, both at the age of 56. Gordon (1963) described 4 cases of leukemia occurring in a family during 2 generations. The most striking familial incidence was reported by Anderson (1951); in family "S," examined and treated at the University of Minnesota Hospital, 5 out of 8 siblings developed leukemia when 4 to 8 years old. Steinberg and his colleagues (1953) observed a family in which, among 7 children, 3 had acute leukemia and a fourth had a lymphosarcoma; in addition, 8 of the 22 individuals comprising this family's second and third generations had cancer. In another family (Steinberg, 1960), 3 adults in 2 generations died from acute leukemia; a fourth case had occurred in this family several years earlier. Johnson and Peters (1957) described 3 adult cases of acute leukemia and one of lymphosarcoma among 12 siblings.

More recently Weiner (1965) observed a family in which the father had lymphatic leukemia, and 3 out of his 4 children (2 males and 1 female) developed chronic myelogenous leukemia; in addition, one of the patient's grandsons developed a thymic tumor.

* * *

* For additional review and references see Guasch (1954) and Ioachim (1962).

The occurrence of a rare disease in man in two or more members of the same family, such as in brothers and/or sisters, or in a child and in one or both parents, or an uncle or aunt, or perhaps a cousin, may not be due to mere coincidence, and is obviously of considerable interest.

The development of tumors or leukemia in several members of a family, possibly in several successive generations, may be interpreted by a working hypothesis explaining the induction of such tumors by latent oncogenic agents transmitted naturally from one generation to another within certain families (Gross, 1951, 1954). This approach to the problem of cancer in humans has, however, considerable limitations as a method of study. The heterogeneity of human families, the relatively long life span of man, the lack of adequate family records, and the difficulty in tracing ancestors, make the task of tracing the host-to-host transmission of the hypothetical oncogenic virus extremely difficult, if not impossible, at the present time.

Congenital Leukemia. Leukemia in the newborn is very rare, and almost invariably of the myelogenous form. Four cases of congenital leukemia were reported by Bernhard and his coworkers (1951), and one case by Taylor and Geppert (1950). The mothers of the five leukemic infants were apparently in good health. Additional cases of congenital leukemia were reviewed in both publications.

Epidemiological Studies

During the past few years reports have appeared describing cases of leukemia occurring in "clusters" among children attending a certain school, or living in a certain limited neighborhood area.

Heath and Hasterlik reported (1963) that between 1957 and 1960 eight cases of leukemia occurred in children living in Niles, Illinois. According to the authors, these cases constituted a significantly increased incidence of leukemia in children for this town, and their association with a single school exceeded chance expectation.

The hypothesis that cases of childhood leukemia may occur grouped together in space and in time has been tested also by examining the distribution of the disease in Greater London in a study carried out by Till and her colleagues (1967). No evidence was found to suggest that the disease had been unusually common in any one year, or at any one season. However, a "weak evidence of clustering" was found for cases of lymphoblastic leukemia with regard to the date and place of onset.

In another similar study (Lock and Merrington, 1967) statistical criteria for testing the association of cases of leukemia in place and time were calculated for 115 patients in the London borough of Lewisham from

1957 to 1963. The analysis gave no evidence for any clustering of these cases.

The study of Milham (1965) is of interest and should be mentioned at this point. Review of death certificates of 876 spouses of widows and widowers who died of leukemia revealed that seven of the spouses also died of leukemia. However, five cases of leukemia were identified among matched controls of the spouses. Accordingly, it appears from this study that the incidence of leukemia in husbands and wives of individuals who die of leukemia is not significantly greater than that in a control group. This is consistent with the hypothesis that adult leukemia is not contagious in the usual sense.

* * *

On the basis of information thus far available it can only be stated that it is very difficult to evaluate at the present time reports of a possible contact transmission of cancer or leukemia in humans. It appears highly improbable that leukemia or cancer is transmitted from one host to another "horizontally" within the same generation by contact, or otherwise, in a manner similar to other infectious diseases. Even under more favorable experimental conditions, in studies carried out on chickens and mice, in which a highly potent passage virus was employed, transmission of the leukemogenic virus from host to host within the same generation occurred only to a limited degree, and presumably only among newborn hosts, i.e. among newly hatched chicks, or among newborn mice exposed to contact infection. If contact infection occurred under such experimental conditions, it was usually latent, and led only occasionally to the development of disease.

Horizontal transmission of a "wild" or "street" virus of a limited potency, such as that which is presumably responsible for the development of spontaneous or field cases of leukemia and lymphomas in mice and chickens, and which may be comparable to the hypothetical leukemogenic virus in humans, appears therefore improbable. The fact that such an infection would have to be transmitted among genetically unrelated individuals, beyond newborn or earliest childhood age, adds considerably to the difficulty of contact infection and suggests that horizontal transmission of a hypothetical leukemic virus in humans occurs only exceptionally, if it occurs at all. Development of leukemia in several children or adults living within a limited geographical area, such as among children attending certain schools, or among inhabitants of a group of adjoining homes, etc., could be explained more reasonably by chance coincidence than by "horizontal" host-to-host transmission of an oncogenic virus.

ACCIDENTAL AND EXPERIMENTAL TRANSMISSION OF HUMAN CANCER

It is common knowledge that tumors, which are treated and dissected daily by physicians and other hospital personnel without particular precaution, are not transmissible from one person to another by contact infection. However, under certain experimental conditions cancer can be transmitted from man to man.

Accidental Auto-Inoculation of Cancer in Man

Accidental contact transplantations of tumors in the same patient, such as from one lip to another, from tongue to gum, from one vocal cord to another, from breast to the adjacent chest skin, etc., have long been observed (Hahn, 1888. Brand, 1902. Levesque, 1903).

Accidental transplantations of tumors in the operating room during laparotomy, abdominal paracentesis, or debridement of a tumor through the vagina, have also been described by numerous surgeons (Levesque, 1903). An accidental transplantation of an adenocarcinoma from the breast to the skin of the thigh in a 43-year-old white female was observed by Spies and his colleagues (1934); two months after the plastic transplantation of Reverdin grafts from the patient's right thigh to the granulating wound surface of the left chest wall, a nodule developed in the skin of the right thigh where the autografts had been excised. The microscopic report on this nodule (Ewing) was "a very cellular infiltrating carcinoma of mammary gland type." A similar case of accidental transplantation of a breast tumor to the skin of the arm was observed by Hubard (1926).

Brandes and his colleagues (1946) removed a breast carcinoma in a 47-year-old female. A skin graft was then removed from her left side to cover the wound. After 4 months the patient died and multiple skin recurrences were noted along the mastectomy scar. Tumors were also noted on the skin of the thigh where the graft was removed. The largest nodule on the skin of the thigh was 0.5 inch in diameter; microscopic examination revealed a tumor structure similar to that of the primary tumor removed at operation.

Accidental Transmission of Cancer from Man to Man

Only very few reliable cases have been reported of actual person-to-person transmission of human cancer by accidental inoculation. A few examples follow:

According to Tross (1902), a man developed a carcinoma of the glans penis presenting a structure histologically identical with the cervical carcinoma from which his wife suffered. Weber and his associates (1930) reported the case of a melanosarcoma most probably transmitted from a 27-year-old mother to her child. The full term child had been delivered by Caesarean section in apparently good health 3 months before the woman died of generalized melanosarcoma; the physician (E. Holland) who delivered the child remarked that "the lower uterine segment of the mother was occupied by a huge black placenta proved to be infiltrated with masses of tumor." He thought it probable that tumor cells might have been carried in the placental blood stream from the mother to the liver of the fetus. The child died after 8 months from generalized melanosarcoma with large tumors in the liver.

Balacesco and Tovaru (1936) reported the case of a young woman who had a small nodule in her right breast. The woman delivered her child, and at this time the nodule in her breast ulcerated. Nevertheless, she nursed her baby. After 11 months the child developed a tumor on its lower lip. Both mother and child were then submitted to surgery, and the breast tumor as well as the lip tumor were excised. The mother proved to have an adenocarcinoma of the breast, the child had a spindle-cell sarcoma of the lip. In spite of the microscopic difference in the appearance of these tumors, there is a strong possibility that the tumor was transmitted from mother to child by contact inoculation.

Accidental Transmission of Cancer from Patient to a Medical Student. One of the most interesting and tragic cases was reported from Paris some forty years ago: Lecène and Lacassagne (1926), and later Katz (1930), described the dramatic case of a fatal accidental inoculation of human cancer into the hand of a medical student, Henri Vadon. The unfortunate Vadon aspirated serum from a wound following radical mastectomy in a woman suffering from an adenocarcinoma of the breast. The syringe slipped, however, and, while falling, accidentally punctured his left hand, injecting some of the fluid deep into the tissues of the palm. This happened on the 13th of February, 1923, in a ward of the Cochon Hospital in Paris. In February, 1925, i.e. 2 years later, an irregular induration appeared at the site, with a distinct prolongation toward the old scar remaining after the original puncture, and tuberculous synovitis was suspected by the attending physician who examined Vadon. The induration increased slowly in size. It was removed in August, 1925, and sent for histological examination. This revealed a fusiform sarcoma. The tumor recurred in the scar, and metastasis rapidly appeared under the skin of the internal surface of the arm. On September 23rd the whole arm was disarticulated by Lecène; 2 months later, however, metastasis appeared above the clavicle and in the neck. Vadon died on December 12, 1926, one year after the metastasis appeared. Thus, he inoculated himself, accidentally, with a mammary carcinoma, and developed a sarcoma at the site of inoculation,

There had been no tumors in Vadon's family for 3 preceding generations on his paternal side; on the maternal side, one grandfather died of a suspected tumor of the kidney.

Experimental Auto-Inoculation of Human Cancer

Cornil reported (1891) that an "anonymous surgeon" transplanted in 1887 a breast sarcoma and a breast carcinoma, each into the patient from whom it had been excised. The implants grew after incubation periods of 2 months and a few weeks, respectively. The sarcomatous implant was excised and found to be histologically identical with the original breast sarcoma. The carcinomatous implant grew, but was not excised, since the second patient disappeared from the surgeon's observation.*

Cases of successful, intentional auto-transplantation of human cancer were also reported by Delbet (see Kurtzahn, 1926) and Hahn (1888). Auto-inoculation of human cancer can be readily explained by cell-graft.

De Martel (1934) transplanted carcinoma of the breast in three patients, and carcinoma of the bowel in one patient, under the skin of the abdomen, and each into the patient in whom the tumor had originated. A latent period of approximately five months was observed in all four instances; after that time had elapsed, however, the implants began to grow very rapidly, so that they had to be destroyed by Roentgen rays. No evidence of a spontaneous regression of either the implanted tumors, or of the primary neoplasms, could be observed in these cases.

In another study (Gross, 1944, 1947) two patients with advanced metastatic cancer were inoculated intradermally, with their consent, with very small doses of cell suspensions prepared from their own tumors. This experiment was carried out in an attempt to produce a small and superficial neoplastic growth which would eventually regress spontaneously

* See Editorial: "Grafting Cancer in Human Subject" (*J. Am. Med. Assoc.*, **17**: 233–234, Aug. 1, 1891), and also a recent reprint of this Editorial in the Aug. 8, 1966, issue of the same journal (*J. Am. Med. Assoc.*, **197**: adv. p. 13, 1966).

FIG. 72. VIRUS-LIKE PARTICLES IN HUMAN LEUKEMIA.

Ultrathin section of a fragment of lymph node biopsy from a 28-year-old male patient with acute lymphatic leukemia. Virus-like spherical particles in the intercellular space; most of the particles have internal electron-dense nucleoids. Magnification 29,000×. Electron micrograph prepared by L. Dmochowski, Department of Virology, University of Texas, M. D. Anderson Hospital and Tumor Institute, Houston.

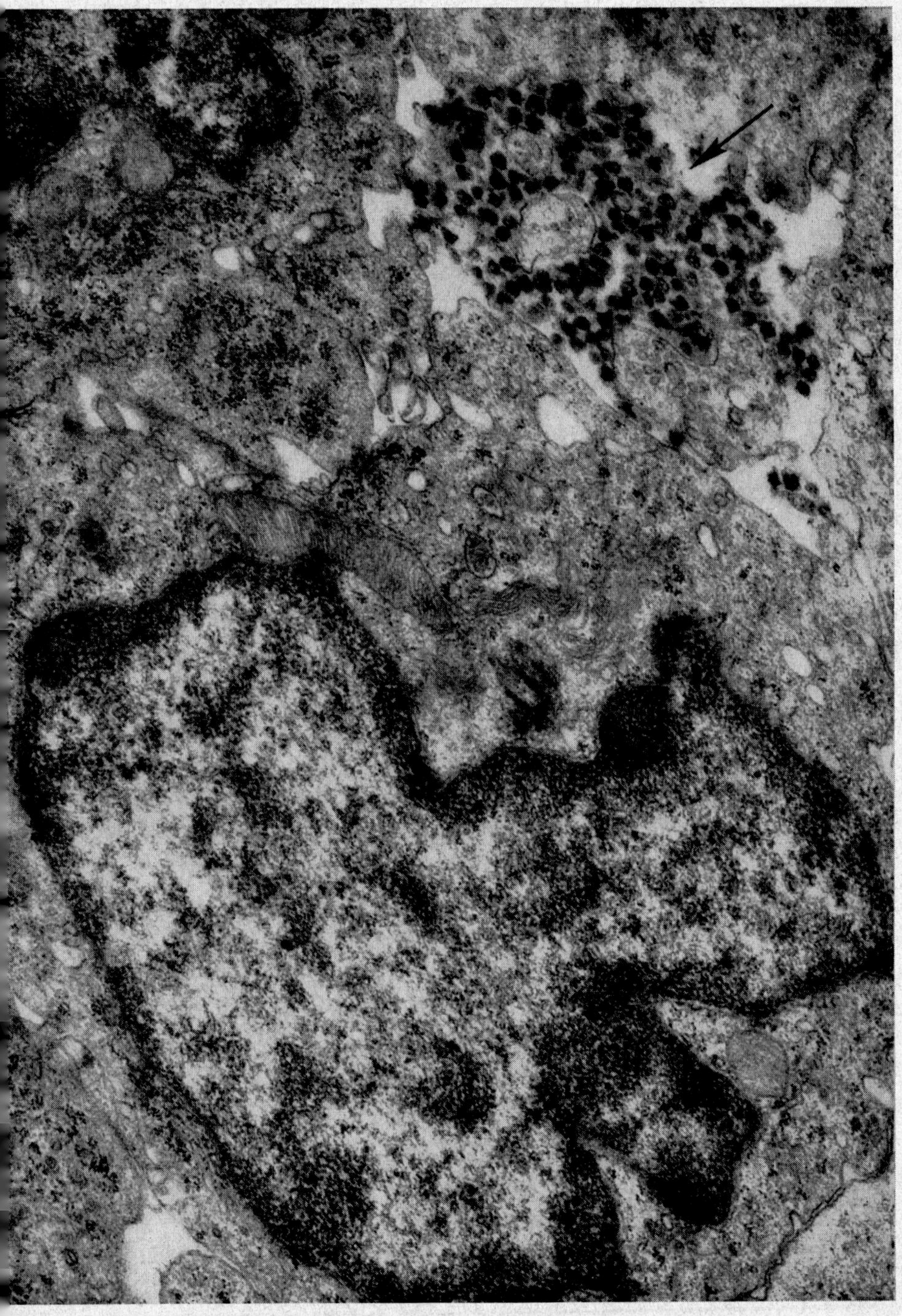

FIG. 72. VIRUS-LIKE PARTICLES IN HUMAN LEUKEMIA.

rendering the host immune to that particular tumor.* However, the small tumor nodules which developed at the site of inoculation, after latency periods varying from 6 weeks to several months, grew progressively so that they had to be promptly removed. There was no evidence whatever of a spontaneous regression of either the implants or of the primary tumors. We concluded (Gross, 1947, 1952) that auto-inoculation of a malignant tumor in man may be highly dangerous, since it may lead to the establishment of an artificial metastasis.

Inoculation of Tissue-culture-grown Human Cancer Cells into Cancer Patients and into Normal Volunteers. Southam and his coworkers (1957) inoculated tissue-culture-grown human cancer cell lines into either cancer patients or into healthy human volunteers. The cancer cells employed in this study were established cell lines originally isolated from human cancer tissues and maintained for at least 3 years in serial passages in tissue culture or in chick embryos, in cortisone-treated rats or hamsters, or in various alternating combinations of these. Fourteen cancer patients were inoculated; as a result, small nodules appeared in most of the recipients after 5 to 10 days at the implantation sites, reaching a maximum diameter in 1 to 2 weeks. If not immediately excised, the implants usually regressed in 4 to 6 weeks. However, in 4 patients there was recurrence of cancer growth after biopsy at several implantation sites; in 2 patients some of the recurrent nodules grew progressively. In one of these patients the implanted tumor cells metastasized to the axillary nodes; this patient's own cancer was uterine adenocarcinoma readily distinguished from the implanted cells and at autopsy found to be confined to the abdomen and perineum.

In a continuation of this study, Southam and Moore (1958) inoculated tissue-culture-grown human cancer cell lines into 14 healthy volunteers at the Ohio State Penitentiary in Columbus. The implantations resulted in the formation of sterile abscesses, or small nodules, after a short latency of 1 to 3 weeks. One or two nodules were then excised from each volunteer for electron microscopic study; the remaining implants regressed spontaneously after 3 to 4 weeks. There was no recurrence noted during the subsequent 5 months of observation. The authors concluded that normal healthy recipients responded to implanted human cells with a marked inflammatory reaction and a rapid regression of the implants. In contrast, recipients that had advanced cancer showed little or no inflammatory

* This experiment was based on previous observations which suggested that intradermal inoculation of very small doses of certain transplantable malignant tumors in mice may result in the development of tumors which in some instances may grow only temporarily, and later spontaneously regress, rendering such animals immune to reinoculation of the same neoplasms (Besredka and Gross, 1935. Gross, 1943).

response; in some of the cancer patients the implanted cancer cells grew progressively.

The experiments were continued at the Jewish Chronic Disease Hospital in Brooklyn, where several patients with chronic debilitating diseases were inoculated with tissue-culture-grown human cancer cells prepared by Dr. Southam and his associates. It was reported that the inoculated patients rejected the implanted cancer cells as promptly as did the healthy subjects. However, these experiments attracted the attention of newspapers and magazines, and the question of adequate ethical guideposts for medical research on human subjects was raised (Langer 1964).

> It should be emphasized, however, that these, and a few other similar studies, were relatively short-term experiments; a much longer observation period may be required to determine the ultimate fate of implantation of cancer cells into humans. It is apparent that the authors observed only the immediate reaction to the implantation of tumor cells. Such a reaction does not necessarily have to be complete and final. Other experiments performed on humans suggest that a latency of several, and even up to 18 months may elapse before a tumor may develop after a homologous implantation of cancer cells. Furthermore, the possibility of a delayed development of a tumor, possibly after several years, or even after a decade or two, in some of the inoculated subjects, or possibly in their offspring, should also be taken into consideration. This is discussed again, and in more detail, on subsequent pages of this chapter.

Further Studies on Auto- or Homologous Transplantation of Human Cancer. Southam and Brunschwig (1961) studied the effect of subcutaneous auto-transplantation of human cancer cell suspensions on patients with advanced cancer. Among 27 patients observed for 3 weeks or longer, only 6 had evidence of growth of the implanted tumors. In another series of similar experiments carried out by Howard (1963), fragments of tumors excised from patients with incurable cancer were reinoculated into the same individuals. At least 17 of the implants grew. One of the most significant observations was the fact that a transplanted squamous cell carcinoma first became clinically detectable as late as 18 months after implantation.

Grace and Kondo (1958) inoculated a variety of malignant tumors into volunteer cancer patients with advanced disease. The implants produced varying degrees of inflammatory reaction followed by the appearance of small nodules which later regressed, usually after a short period of 2 to 4 weeks.

Koike and his colleagues (1963) inoculated 6 tissue-culture-grown human cancer cell lines into volunteer cancer patients, in some instances into the same patients from whom the tumors had been removed. The implants produced small nodules in at least some of the inoculated patients in both groups. All nodules disappeared after several weeks.

In a continuation of this study (Nadler and Moore, 1965), 82 volunteer cancer patients with incurable disease received subcutaneous implants of small fragments of their own tumors. Only 11 out of the 82 implanted tumor fragments showed growth at the implantation site. The shortest period of time from implantation to positive biopsy was 10 days, and the longest was 3 months.

INADVERTENT TRANSMISSION OF CANCER FROM MAN TO MAN INCIDENT TO KIDNEY TRANSPLANTATION

Induction of a Fatal Generalized Carcinomatosis in a Patient Who Received a Renal Graft. Martin and his coworkers (1965) reported inadvertent transmission of cancer from man to man incident to homotransplantation of a kidney. The recipient was a 46-year-old male patient with a severe renal deficiency. The donor was a 29-year-old man who died from bronchogenic carcinoma with metastatic tumors to regional lymph nodes, pleura, left adrenal gland, and to the brain. Within less than 2 hours after the donor died, his left kidney, which had no macroscopic evidence of a metastatic tumor, was removed, and was transplanted into the iliac fossa of the recipient patient.

Four months after the kidney transplantation, because of a swelling and a tenderness over the grafted kidney, a needle biopsy of the transplanted kidney was performed and revealed the presence of neoplastic cells identical with those found in the lung tumor of the donor. A few weeks later the recipient patient died with widespread generalized carcinomatosis; large tumor masses surrounded the grafted kidney; there were numerous tumors replacing the retroperitoneal lymph nodes, and metastatic tumors were also present in the omentum, in the liver, lungs, and in the brain.

Development of Cancer in the Recipient, and Subsequent Disappearance of the Tumor, Following Removal of Grafted Kidney, and Discontinuance of Administration of Immunosuppressive Drugs. Another case of an inadvertent transmission of human cancer incident to kidney transplantation was reported by Wilson and his colleagues (1968). A kidney removed from the cadaver of a man who died of bronchogenic carcinoma with cerebral metastases was transplanted to a 34-year-old man in renal failure from glomerulonephritis. Eighteen months later a tumor mass appeared over the lower pole of the transplanted kidney. A biopsy of the tumor revealed metastatic epidermoid carcinoma histologically indistinguishable from the original primary bronchogenic carcinoma of the donor; a metastatic tumor was also noticed in the femoral lymph node. Irradiation treatment was applied to the tumor, but had no apparent success.

The administration of immunosuppressive drugs was discontinued; as a result, the previously functioning kidney was rejected, and was subsequently removed; however, the renal capsule was already invaded by the tumor mass and could not be completely excised; some lymph nodes that appeared to contain metastatic tumors were also left behind.

During the next month the painful swelling remaining in the former graft area in the right lower quadrant, and the enlarged lymph nodes, slowly regressed. Six months after removal of the transplanted kidney an exploratory laparotomy was performed, but no evidence of a tumor was found. Two months later the administration of immunosuppressive drugs was resumed and shortly thereafter a kidney from the patient's mother was transplanted into the patient's left groin. At the time the report was published, 10 months after the second kidney implantation, the patient appeared well, and had no evidence of a tumor.

Induction of Disseminated Cancer in the Recipient Following Renal Graft. A case of transmission of human cancer incident to kidney transplantation was reported by McPhaul (1965), McIntosh (1965), and their colleagues. A young woman moribund from chronic uremia received a kidney from the cadaver of a patient who died of squamous-cell carcinoma of the pyriform sinus. The left kidney was removed from the cadaver within 30 minutes after the donor died. The kidney which appeared normal was immediately implanted in the right iliac fossa of the recipient. Eight months later a liver disease in the patient became manifest; liver biopsy was performed and demonstrated the presence of carcinoma. A few weeks later the patient died and a postmortem examination revealed the presence of multiple carcinomatous nodules in the grafted kidney and also widely disseminated in the liver. Microscopic examination revealed an anaplastic undifferentiated carcinoma indistinguishable from that observed in the donor.

Other Cases. Several additional cases of transmission of human cancer in the course of kidney transplantations have been observed (see also Murray *et al.*, 1965); not all of them have been published. In the case reported by Dossetor (1965) the presence of metastatic breast cancer was revealed in a renal graft only 2 weeks after transplantation, when the patient died of postoperative hemorrhage.

Zukoski* observed a 27-year-old patient who had received previously, in another hospital in Texas, a renal transplant from a donor who had died from hepatoma with pulmonary metastases. The implanted kidney functioned well for 3 years; after this lapse of time the recipient developed pulmonary metastases. Biopsy of the kidney revealed the presence of hepatoma. Administration of immunosuppressive drugs was then discontinued; as a result, the implanted kidney was rejected within 6 weeks.

* Personal communication to the author from Dr. C. F. Zukoski, Nashville, Tenn., 1968.

The grafted kidney and its intrinsic hepatoma were then excised. The pulmonary metastases disappeared within 6 weeks. The patient has been carried on hemodialysis since the transplanted kidney was removed, and was apparently well at the time this information was received, about 5 months after the operation.

These case reports constitute a warning for those who plan to use kidneys, or in the future perhaps also hearts, or other human organs, or parts of organs, for homotransplantation to other human subjects. Obviously, no organs from donors having a history of any form of cancer or lymphoma should be employed for homotransplantation, even if the tumor in the donor is only localized, and the organ which is to be used for transplantation appears "normal" and apparently suitable for the graft. It would require microscopic examination of sections from different parts of the kidney, or other organs, in order to have a reasonable assurance that such an organ is free from metastatic tumor cells.*

Fatal Transplantation of Human Melanoma from a Cancer Patient to Her Healthy Mother

Scanlon and his coworkers (1965) reported a tragic case of fatal homotransplantation of human melanoma. The original tumor was a melanoma which appeared on the midback in a 50-year-old woman. The lesion was treated by excision; however, 3 years later generalized metastatic tumors appeared. The authors reported that the 80-year-old mother of the patient "volunteered" to have the tumor transplanted from her daughter to herself, in spite of a warning that the tumor might grow and metastasize.

The transplantation was performed on August 15, 1961. Under local anesthesia a small piece of subcutaneous melanoma was removed from the daughter and transplanted as a single piece into the right rectus muscle of the mother. Three weeks later a biopsy was taken and melanoma was found in the rectus muscle; a few days later a wide excision was made at the site of tumor implantation. However, it was too late; tumor development and generalization in different organs followed. Disseminated metastatic melanoma was found in the critically ill patient on the 86th day following the implantation of the tumor. The patient died several months later due to diffusely widespread metastatic melanoma.

* Whether the recently reported cases of lymphomas developing in patients who received renal transplants (Penn *et al.*, 1968) were coincidental, or were related to the prolonged administration of immunosuppressive drugs incident to organ transplantation, or whether they were caused by inadvertent transmission with the transplanted organ of leukemic cells or of a leukemogenic virus, remains to be determined and requires further study.

THE IMPLICATIONS OF THE STUDIES ON EXPERIMENTAL OR ACCIDENTAL TRANSMISSION OF HUMAN CANCER, AND SOME TENTATIVE CONCLUSIONS

On the basis of experimental data collected in extensive animal experimentation, and supplemented by observations made on humans, it is possible to form the following tentative conclusions referring to the possible effect of homologous cancer cell implantations in man.

Auto-Inoculation of Human Cancer. A cancer-bearing human or animal host is, as a rule, highly susceptible to the growth of its own tumor. This can be demonstrated experimentally by removing a fragment of the tumor and reinoculating this tumor into the same host (auto-inoculation). In most instances, if a sufficient number of viable cancer cells is implanted, the tumor will "take" and grow progressively. The result of such an auto-inoculation of cancer cells can be compared with an experimental establishment of an artificial metastasis.

Transplantation of Human Cancer to Healthy Family Members of the Cancer Patient. It is safe to assume that, as is the case in chickens and mice, in man also, close family members of a cancer patient may be highly susceptible to the implantation of tumor cells prepared from the cancer donor. Inoculation of viable tumor cells prepared from a cancer patient into his or her own children, parents, siblings, or other close family members, may readily result in the establishment of a progressively growing tumor in the recipient host, and may lead to a secondary establishment of metastatic tumors, and to eventual generalization of the disease. This has been convincingly established in animal experiments, and most probably also applies to humans. A tragic example of a fatal, experimental transmission, by the surgeon, of human melanoma from a woman patient to her mother, was described on the preceding page of this chapter.

Homologous Transplantation of Human Cancer to Unrelated Individuals. The results of implantation of viable cancer cells, or inoculation of cancer extracts from human patients to unrelated healthy human recipients are unpredictable. In most instances, the implanted tumor cells will not grow, and the implant will be rejected. In rare, unforeseeable instances, however, the implanted tumor may unexpectedly "take," grow progressively, and eventually lead to a generalization of the disease. A few examples of such a tragic outcome, usually accidental, have been recorded and were quoted on the preceding pages. This point is of particular importance at the present time, since transplantations of human organs, such as kidneys, have been introduced in clinical medicine, and have gradually gained general acceptance. It is obvious that in the future human donors will have to be carefully screened in order to avoid inadvertent transmission of cancer cells which may be present in the transplanted organs. Donors suffering from any form of cancer or other neoplastic disease should not be used.

Finally, an additional word of caution, based entirely on animal experiments but possibly applicable also to humans, appears necessary. In mice, at least, inoculation of tumor cells or of cell-free tumor extracts into relatively susceptible hosts may leave the inoculated recipient host at first apparently unharmed. However, such inoculation, even though not followed by the immediate development of a tumor, may, nevertheless, cause a delayed appearance of a progressively growing neoplasm in the inoculated host (Gross, 1952a), perhaps after several years or even after one or two decades in humans; it may possibly cause the development of a tumor in one of the children, or grandchildren, of the inoculated host. This has been observed in experimental studies on mouse leukemia and mouse mammary carcinoma; it is conceivable that it may also apply to humans.*

Spontaneous Regression of Human Cancer — A Rare Phenomenon

Spontaneous regression of naturally occurring malignant tumors, such as human cancer, should be clearly differentiated from regression of *implanted* tumors. It has been observed repeatedly in the laboratory that implantation of malignant tumor cells may not necessarily result in the development of a progressively growing tumor; quite frequently tumor cell transplantation from one animal to another may not cause the development of a tumor in the inoculated animal at all, or it may induce a tumor which will grow only temporarily and which may later spontaneously regress. This is true particularly when tumors are transplanted in heterogenous animals, such as non-inbred mice, rats, chickens, rabbits, and other species.

Spontaneous regression of implanted tumors has been observed since the early years of experimental cancer research in mice (Clowes and Baeslack, 1905. Gaylord and Clowes, 1906) and also in other animal species.†

On the other hand, regression and complete disappearance of naturally occurring malignant tumors, i.e. tumors developing spontaneously, without experimental manipulation, in animals or man, is rare but has been recorded occasionally. This refers to cancer and other malignant tumors, but does not include warts, papillomas, and certain other benign neoplasms which often regress spontaneously.

Cases of spontaneous regression of human cancer, although extremely rare, have been recorded (Lomer, 1903. Rohdenburg, 1918. Dunphy, 1950. Stewart, 1952. Morton and Morton, 1953. Nelson, 1962. Smithers, 1962. Brunschwig, 1963. Margolis and West, 1967). Everson and Cole (1959) reviewed cases of spontaneous regression of cancer reported in the world

* For additional information see chapters on Mouse Leukemia and Mouse Mammary Carcinoma in this monograph.

† For additional references and a discussion of the implications of these observations, see Gross, 1943 and 1952a.

literature since 1900, including unpublished reports from medical and surgical colleagues. Of the entire group, 112 cases which appeared to have adequate documentation were classified. Spontaneous regression of human cancer was reported most commonly in neuroblastoma (25 cases), choriocarcinoma (14 cases), carcinoma of the kidney (11 cases), malignant melanoma (10 cases), and soft tissue sarcoma (9 cases). Tumor regression was more rarely reported in cases of carcinoma of the bladder (7 cases), breast (5 cases), stomach, colon, rectum, and uterus (3 cases each). The remaining 19 tumors represented a variety of either primary or metastatic neoplasms.

Spontaneous regression of choriocarcinoma was recently reviewed by Bardawil and Toy (1959).

ATTEMPTS TO TRANSMIT ONCOGENIC AGENTS FROM HUMAN TUMORS TO ANIMALS*

Attempts to transmit cancer from man to animals by inoculation of tumor extracts, or attempts to detect, on microscopic examination, microorganisms causing cancer, have been reported by numerous investigators.

B. Peyrilhe, professor at the Royal College of Surgeons in Paris, received on December 8, 1773, the prize of the Academy of Sciences in Lyon, France, for his dissertation on the cause of cancer. Peyrilhe considered cancer to be caused by a contagious virus. In an attempt to transmit human cancer to animals, Peyrilhe collected a few drops of fluid from a cancerous breast of one of his woman patients, and inoculated it with a syringe under the skin of a dog. A swelling and discoloration of the wound appeared, and progressed considerably during the next 5 days. However, the suffering dog was drowned by Peyrilhe's servant. The animal had obviously developed an abscess. This experiment, and Peyrilhe's dissertation, indicate, nevertheless, the early interest in the infectious nature of cancer.

During the 19th century, the microscopic diagnosis of tumors, and the classification of tumors on the basis of their microscopic structure, gradually became established. Experimental studies of neoplasms could now be conducted on a more solid basis.

Attempts to transmit human tumors to animals and the search for cancer microorganisms continued.

Jürgens reported in 1896 successful transmission of a human sarcoma,

* Attempts to transmit a cancer-inducing microorganism, or an oncogenic virus, from humans to animals should be clearly differentiated from transplantation of human cancer cells into animals. Heterologous graft of human cancer cells into rabbits, guinea pigs, rats, or hamsters, is readily accomplished, employing either a particular route of inoculation (such as the anterior chamber of the eye) or implanting tumor cells into conditioned animals, i.e. animals pretreated with cortisone, or treated, prior to tumor inoculation, by total-body X-ray irradiation. These experiments were briefly discussed in the first chapter of this monograph.

and also of a human melanoma, to rabbits; the same author also described a "coccidium oviforme" as the causative cancer organism. Mayet, professor at the Medical Faculty in Lyon, reported in 1902 the induction of malignant tumors in 4, and possibly in 8, out of 53 white rats inoculated with cancer extracts, some of them filtrates, prepared from human tumors.

It would be beyond the scope of this monograph to enter into a detailed historical study of attempts to transmit human tumors to animals and to review the claims of many physicians and surgeons, such as Scheuerlen (1887), Queyrat (1893), Doyen (1904), Rappin (1890, 1934), Kritschewski and Rubinstein (1929), Blumenthal (1926), and others. Some of them thought that they had discovered in human tumors the causative cancer microorganism. Others reported successful transmission of human cancer organisms, or "agents," to animals, and the induction of tumors in animals, and even in plants (Bra, 1899), with such microorganisms, or with human tumor extracts.*

Gradually it became apparent, however, that the various microbes, cocci (such as the famous "micrococcus neoformans" of Doyen, 1904), and fungi had no causal relationship to the tumors from which they had been isolated. Similarly, tumors that developed in animals following inoculation of the various extracts prepared from human neoplasms were in all probability of dubious neoplastic nature, or were spontaneous tumors which developed in the inoculated animals incidentally, but had no causal relation to the human tumors from which such extracts were prepared for inoculation.

After the turn of the century it was realized that many diseases of infectious origin are caused by filterable pathogenic agents too small to be seen in an optical microscope. Attempts to transmit human tumors to animals continued. The search for microorganisms visible under the optical microscope, such as bacteria, fungi, or cocci, possibly causing cancer, was gradually abandoned. Attempts were made, instead, to induce with human tumor extracts the development of tumors, or to reproduce in the inoculated animals a specific syndrome presumably caused by an oncogenic virus.

Thus far, at least, attempts to transmit a hypothetical oncogenic agent from human malignant tumors or leukemia to animals have not succeeded. In spite of the numerous observations reporting apparent success, none of the positive findings thus far reported could be consistently reproduced, and none resisted rigorous control tests. It would be beyond the scope of this chapter to review all these reports. We will review only some of these studies, without entering into a specific criticism or evaluation of the reported experiments.

* The interested reader will find more detailed information in the reviews of Velich (1898), Brand (1902), Borrel (1907), Wolff (1907), Woglom (1913), Blumenthal (1926, 1932), Ewing (1940), in the monograph on cancer by Oberling (1954), and also in other sources dealing with the history of cancer research.

Heidenhain (1932) inoculated autolysates from human tumors into 2029 mice; in this group 6.7 per cent of animals developed tumors, as compared with only 1.6 per cent observed among 2128 control mice.

In more recent studies, Thiersch (1944, 1947) inoculated blood from human patients suffering from myeloid leukemia into 11-day-old chick embryos. Only a small percentage of the injected chicks survived; of 12 chickens hatched from the inoculated embryos, 5 developed osteopetrosis. Similar lesions were obtained by injecting one-day-old chicks. Osteopetrosis could be induced with blood from 3 different patients with chronic myeloid leukemia. Injection of blood from human subjects with chronic lymphoid leukemia did not induce osteopetrosis.

In another study guinea pigs were inoculated with human leukemic extracts, and were reported to have developed, as a result, a transmissible disease characterized by a severe anemia and extensive degenerative changes (Magrassi, 1951. Magrassi *et al.*, 1951). Similar results were reported by Mas y Magro (1954).

Schwartz and his associates reported (1956, 1957) that the development of leukemia in mice of high-leukemic strain AKR was accelerated following inoculation of filtrates prepared from brains of human patients that died from leukemia. More recently, these authors reported (Schwartz *et al.*, 1960) the induction of a high incidence of leukemia in Swiss mice within only a few weeks after inoculation of filtrates prepared from brains of human donors that died from leukemia. However, these results could not be confirmed in other laboratories.

DeLong (1960) inoculated filtrates prepared from human leukemic bone marrow cultures into Swiss mice and reported the induction of a high incidence of leukemia. Katzman (1962) attempted to reproduce this study under apparently similar experimental conditions; his results, however, were negative.

Purified extracts prepared from human tumor tissues (lymphosarcoma and myeloid leukemia) were inoculated into newborn mice by Burton and his associates (1959); the injection of such refined extracts induced the development of parotid tumors, mammary carcinomas, soft tissue sarcomas, and leukemia. It is questionable, however, whether these tumors were actually induced by a human oncogenic agent; they could have been prompted by the activation of a latent virus carried by the mice employed for inoculation. It is probable that the positive results of experiments carried out by Harel (1958), Lacour (1960), and their associates belong in the same category; in these studies extracts containing ribonucleic acid recovered from human leukemic nodes by the phenol method were inoculated into newborn mice, and were reported to have induced, after a relatively short latency period, rapidly growing malignant tumors.

Caution Needed in Evaluating Results of Injection of Human Tumor Extracts into Newborn Mice. In one of our earlier experiments (Gross, 1956, also unpublished data), we inoculated newborn C3H mice with cell-free extracts prepared from normal guinea pig organs. To our surprise, some of the inoculated mice developed parotid tumors and subcutaneous sarcomas. At that time, mice bred in our laboratory, and used for experimental purposes, often carried a latent parotid tumor, i.e. polyoma, virus. Apparently, the injection of guinea pig extracts into newborn mice occasionally prompted the activation of the latent polyoma virus present in such animals, and led to a subsequent development of tumors in some of the inoculated mice.*

Parotid tumors could also be induced in either C58 mice, or in (C58 × AKR) F_1 hybrids following application of cortisone (Woolley, 1954), or in C3H and C3H(f) mice following fractionated total-body X-ray irradiation (Gross, 1958).

It appears therefore that inoculation of foreign protein extracts into newborn mice may occasionally prompt the activation of a latent oncogenic virus; a similar activating effect of foreign protein injections on latent viruses causing certain neurotropic diseases in mice has also been observed.

Accordingly, when human tumor extracts are injected into newborn mice in an attempt to detect their possible oncogenic potential, the development of tumors in some of the inoculated animals should be interpreted with caution. The appearance of tumors, or leukemia, in such animals may not necessarily represent evidence of transmission of a hypothetical human oncogenic virus; it could be caused by activation of a latent indigenous virus carried in mice.

In order to avoid erroneous interpretations of bio-assay experiments dealing with injection of human or other animal tumor extracts into newborn mice, the following basic rules should be observed: (a) mice used for the bio-assay experiments should be free from a latent polyoma virus infection; (b) an adequate number of mice should be inoculated in each test; (c) an equal number of control animals, consisting preferably of littermates, or at least of animals of similar age and sex from the same breeding stock, should be injected with inactivated extracts; (d) in a separate control group, non-inoculated animals should also be observed for a sufficient length of time in each experiment.

Renewed Attempts to Isolate Oncogenic Viruses by Inoculation of Cell-free Extracts from Human Cancer and Leukemia into Newborn Mice and Rats

The interest in viral etiology of cancer and leukemia received a new impetus following the isolation of the mouse leukemia virus; the success

* Most of the mice of a variety of strains used for experimental purposes in laboratories also carry a latent leukemogenic virus; this virus can be activated by several inducing factors, such as certain carcinogenic chemicals or hormones, and particularly by ionizing radiation. This was reviewed in more detail in the chapters on Mouse Leukemia and on Radiation-induced Leukemia in Mice.

of these experiments was based on the use of newborn mice for bio-assay of mouse leukemia filtrates (Gross, 1951). Renewed attempts were then made to transfer human tumors and leukemia by cell-free extracts using newborn mice, rats, and hamsters, as test animals. Again, in some of these experiments, as in earlier studies, claims were made suggesting the induction of tumors or leukemia in animals inoculated with human tumor extracts. These claims, however, could not be substantiated, or reproduced, in experiments in which adequate controls were employed.

Bergoltz and his coworkers (Bergoltz, 1957, 1960. Nemenova and Bergoltz, 1959), in the U.S.S.R., reported transmission of human leukemia to mice by means of cell-free extracts. Newborn mice of strains CC57, CC3HA, and also albino non-inbred mice, were given either subcutaneous or intrasplenic inoculations of cell-free protein or lipoprotein fractions prepared from spleens and lymph nodes of persons who died from leukemia. Among 108 mice that survived the minimum latency period (elapsing between the inoculation and the earliest development of leukemia), 29 developed leukemia after an average latency of 6.2 months. In similar experiments (Bergoltz, 1958), filtrates prepared from either human leukemic brains, lymph nodes, or lymphoid tumors, or blood extracts from leukemic patients, inoculated either subcutaneously into newborn mice, or intrasplenically into adult mice, induced leukemia in about 18 per cent of mice that survived the minimum latency period. The average latency was about 4 months. Extracts from normal human tissues did not induce leukemia.

Ageenko (1962) inoculated extracts prepared from human leukemic organs into newborn rats and observed the development of leukemia in about 11 per cent of the inoculated animals.

Grace and his associates at the Roswell Park Memorial Institute in Buffalo (1960a,b) inoculated over 1300 newborn Swiss/Ha mice with cell-free extracts prepared from a variety of human malignant tumors and leukemias. About 5 per cent of the inoculated mice developed tumors, mostly mammary carcinomas, less frequently leukemia, sarcomas, or pulmonary tumors, after a latency varying from 3 to 9 months. There were no tumors at the time the report was prepared for publication (the mice were then 7 to 9 months old) among control animals inoculated with

---

Fig. 73. Virus-like Particles in Human Lymphosarcoma.

(a). Ultrathin section of a lymph node biopsy specimen from a 58-year-old patient with lymphosarcoma. Spherical virus-like particles varying in diameter from 90 to 160 mμ in an intercellular space. Most of the particles have internal electron-dense nucleoids. Magnification 60,000×. (b). (Inset). Budding particle (arrow) in a lymph node biopsy specimen from a 58-year-old patient with lymphosarcoma. Magnification 68,000×. Electron micrographs prepared by L. Dmochowski, Department of Virology, University of Texas, M. D. Anderson Hospital and Tumor Institute, Houston.

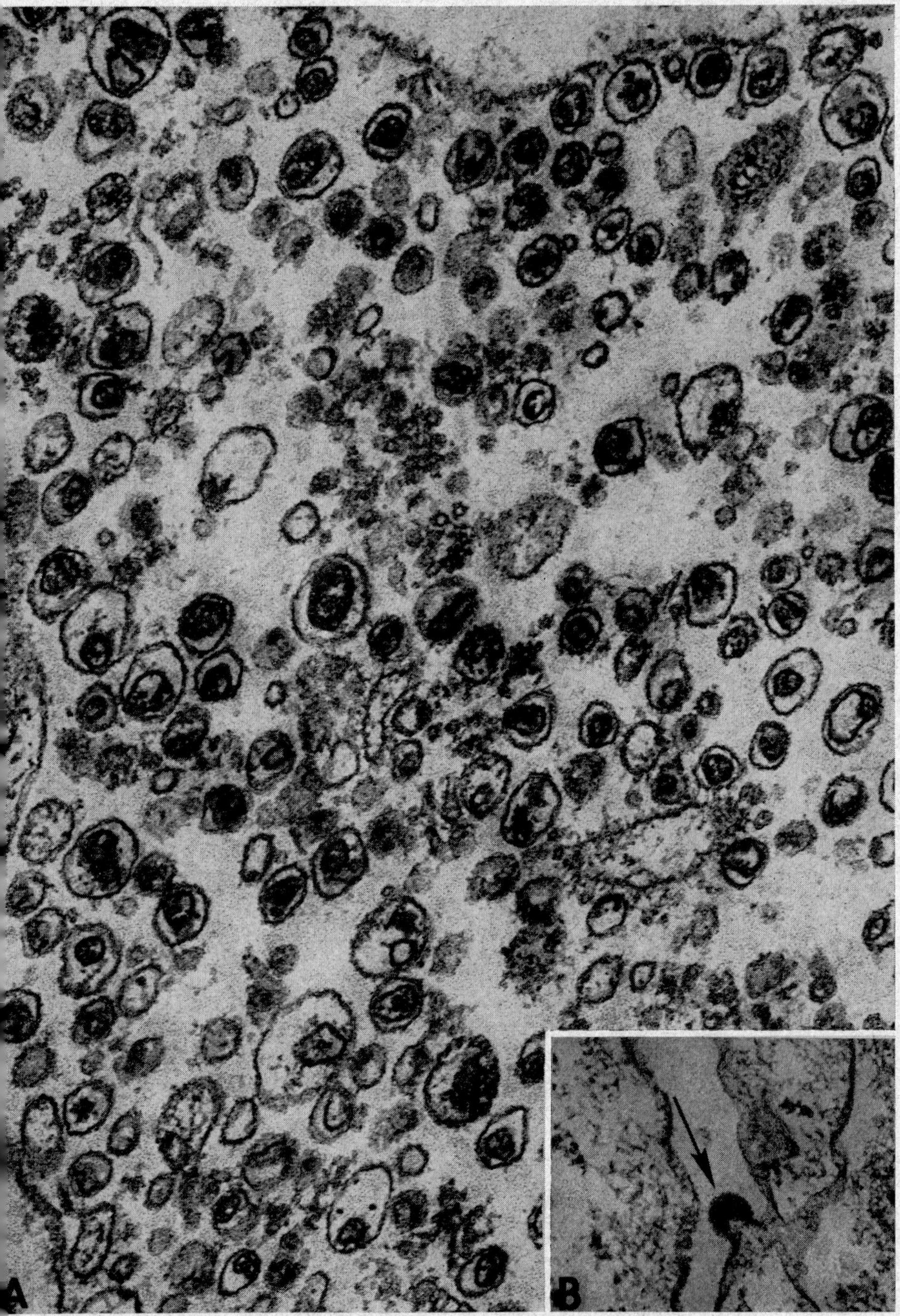

FIG. 73. VIRUS-LIKE PARTICLES IN HUMAN LYMPHOSARCOMA.

normal tissue culture preparations from patients hospitalized for conditions unrelated to cancer. In another experiment, human tumor extracts were inoculated into a variety of established tissue culture cell lines. Fluids from these tissue cultures were then injected into newborn Swiss mice and into newborn hamsters. No tumors developed in the inoculated animals.

Herbut (1967) inoculated 1229 Swiss and BALB/c mice with cell-free preparations from human leukemic blood, or with extracts from human leukemic spleen. The experimental animals were divided into 5 groups. A very low incidence of leukemia was observed in 4 of these groups; only one mouse in each group developed leukemia, apparently spontaneous, at 5 to 12 months of age. In the fifth group, which consisted of 24 mice, 6 mice inoculated with a cell-free extract from a human leukemic spleen developed leukemia when they were 4 to 13 months old. It is difficult to evaluate the relatively high incidence of leukemia in a single, small group of mice, since no simultaneous controls were performed with either heated preparations, or with normal blood or normal spleen extracts; furthermore, no uninoculated litter-mates, or other closely related control mice were observed.

Negative Results of Attempts to Transmit Human Tumors or Leukemia to Newborn Mice, Rats, or Hamsters

The following is a review of extensive experimental studies, carried out in several laboratories, in which attempts have been made to transmit cell-free extracts from human cancer and leukemia to newborn mice, rats, and hamsters, and which gave essentially negative results. The incidence of tumors or leukemia developing in the inoculated animals was in all these studies very similar to that observed in the control groups.

Alice E. Moore (1960), at the Sloan-Kettering Institute in New York, injected 1034 newborn Swiss mice with cell-free extracts prepared from human tumors and lymphomas from over 200 Memorial Hospital patients. A total incidence of 2.8 per cent of tumors, mostly mammary carcinomas and lymphosarcomas, was observed among the inoculated animals; this incidence varied from 0.9 to 5.5 per cent among the individual groups injected with different tumor extracts. No tumors developed in any of the 86 mice inoculated with extracts from non-malignant tissues of cancer patients. One mouse out of 179 control mice (0.6 per cent) inoculated with normal tissue extracts developed a tumor. Although more tumors occurred in mice given extracts from tumors than in the control animals, the difference was not significant statistically.

In a more recent study (1964), Moore and Caparó inoculated filtrates and tissue culture preparations made from 208 specimens obtained from patients with cancer, benign lesions, and normal tissues, into a total of

3990 newborn random-bred Swiss-Webster mice obtained from commercial dealers.* A relatively large number of the inoculated mice, but also of uninoculated controls, developed tumors, mostly mammary adenocarcinomas, and thymic or generalized lymphosarcomas.

> The incidence of tumors that developed in mice of the experimental group which received extracts of human neoplasms varied from 3.3 to 10.2 per cent. The lowest incidence (3.3 per cent) was observed among 210 mice which received extracts from sarcomas; the incidence of tumors was 5.7 per cent among 1165 mice which received extracts from adenocarcinomas, and 7.3 per cent among 426 mice which received extracts from epidermoid carcinomas. The highest incidence of tumors, i.e. 10.2 per cent, was observed among 774 mice which received extracts from human lymphomas; in this group 43 mice (5.5 per cent) developed lymphomas, and 36 mice (4.7 per cent) developed mammary carcinomas. However, among 182 mice which received extracts from benign human tumors, 5.5 per cent developed lymphomas, and an additional 2.2 per cent developed mammary carcinomas, a total of 7.7 per cent. Furthermore, among 258 mice which received extracts from normal human tissues, 5 per cent developed lymphomas, and 1.6 per cent mammary carcinomas, a total of 6.6 per cent. Finally, among 784 non-inoculated controls, 23 developed lymphosarcomas (2.9 per cent) and 11 developed mammary carcinomas (1.4 per cent), a total of 4.3 per cent. The authors concluded that the increased number of tumors in the inoculated animals was due to an activation of tumor viruses already present in these mice.

In a similar, extensive, and carefully controlled study, Girardi, Hilleman, and Zwickey (1962a) at the Merck Institute for Therapeutic Research in West Point, Pa., inoculated newborn, random-bred mice of the ICR/Ha Swiss strain with 84 preparations from human tumors and leukemia; the preparations employed for inoculation were in the form of crude or filtered extracts prepared from human specimens, or fluids from cell cultures of human malignant tissues, or from grivet monkey kidney cultures inoculated with human tumor extracts.

A total of 1976 mice was observed, and 908 of them were in the control

* There exist several substrains of mice of the Swiss stock. Only some of them are inbred, or partially inbred. When Swiss mice are furnished from commercial dealers, no accurate records are usually available concerning the incidence of spontaneous tumors and leukemia in such mice through a number of successive generations. In experiments performed on such mice it is therefore imperative to have an adequate number of simultaneous controls. Spontaneous tumors are not uncommon in Swiss mice, particularly in certain substrains. An incidence of about 19 per cent of spontaneous mammary carcinomas, and about 44 per cent of pulmonary tumors, was reported by the Committee on Standardized Genetic Nomenclature for Mice (1960). An incidence of spontaneous lymphatic leukemia, or lymphosarcomas, varying from 5 to 11 per cent, was also observed in certain substrains of the Swiss stock in our laboratory (Gross, unpublished), and elsewhere (Friend, C., personal communication to the author, 1960). The reader is referred to Table 2, on page 234,

group. The control animals received extracts prepared from tissues of patients who had no gross evidence of malignant disease, or extracts from cell cultures prepared from such normal human tissues, or normal tissue culture fluid; some of the control animals were left uninoculated.

There was a considerable incidence of spontaneous tumors, particularly of mammary carcinoma, in mice of both groups. However, there was no statistically significant difference in tumor incidence among the experimental animals inoculated with specimens derived from human malignant tissues compared with the control animals, except for a few cases of leukemia which occurred in the experimental group and a slightly more frequent occurrence of hepatomas and pulmonary adenocarcinomas among these animals. Among 580 survivors in the inoculated group, 120 developed tumors (21 per cent), as compared with 127 among the 503 control animals (25 per cent).

In another part of this study, newborn hamsters were also inoculated with human tumors and human lymphoma extracts. Among the 871 hamsters in the experimental group which received human tumor preparations, 2 hamsters developed hemangiomas, 1 developed a lymphoma, and 1 an adrenal medullary tumor, at ages varying from 18 to 21 months. In the control group consisting of 122 hamsters which received inoculation of normal tissue extracts, 1 animal developed an adrenal cortical adenoma at the age of 20 months; among 277 uninoculated hamsters, 1 animal developed a renal adenocarcinoma at the age of 2 years.

Kirsten and his coworkers (1967) prepared extracts from human leukemic tissues. The human material was obtained at autopsy or by biopsy from 24 children with acute, undifferentiated, or stem-cell leukemia. Cell-free filtrates of the spleen, liver, brain, or lymph nodes were inoculated by various routes into newborn C3H(f) mice. Control mice received similarly prepared tissue extracts from children who had died from congenital heart disease, neuroblastoma, or non-leukemic hematologic disorders. Untreated litter-mate and non-litter-mate control mice were also observed for the development of tumors. More than 2500 mice were used in this study. The overall tumor incidence in experimental and control mice was not significantly different after 18 to 26 months of observation. The authors concluded that their findings agreed with those of others who failed to observe carcinogenic or leukemogenic effects in mice following inoculation of extracts prepared from human leukemia or from other neoplasms.

Negative results were also reported by several other investigators. Dmochowski and his colleagues (1959) inoculated cell-free extracts prepared from human leukemia and lymphomas into newborn C3H and Swiss mice. In the first experimental series, extracts prepared from acute human lymphatic or myeloid leukemia were inoculated into 352 mice, and

52 of them (14.8 per cent) developed leukemia; among 103 uninoculated control animals, 8 mice (7.8 per cent) developed leukemia. In a second series, extracts prepared from human lymphosarcoma and chronic lymphocytic leukemia were inoculated into 237 mice, and 13 of them (5.5 per cent) developed leukemia; among 129 uninoculated control animals in this group, 6 mice (4.7 per cent) developed leukemia. In a third series, fluid harvested from tissue cultures that had been treated with extracts of human leukemic organs was inoculated into 453 mice, and 28 of them (6.2 per cent) developed leukemia; among 246 control mice which received fluid from untreated monkey kidney cultures, 15 animals (6.1 per cent) developed leukemia.

Katzman (1962) inoculated 6 to 7-week-old Swiss mice with filtrates prepared from leukemic human bone marrow cultures. The control group received filtrates from non-leukemic and apparently normal bone marrow cultures. Three successive groups of experimental and control mice were inoculated.

Out of a total of 63 mice in all 3 groups that had been inoculated with human leukemic extracts, only one animal (1.6 per cent) developed leukemia. In the control groups, 5 out of 43 mice (11.6 per cent) developed leukemia in the first group, none out of 13 in the second, and 3 out of 61 mice (4.9 per cent) in the third group; a total of 8 mice developed leukemia spontaneously among 117 control animals (6.8 per cent). The experiment was terminated when the inoculated mice were 10 months old, i.e. at a relatively early age; however, the data obtained appeared sufficient to conclude that under the experimental conditions employed it was not possible to induce leukemia in Swiss mice with cell-free extracts prepared from human leukemia.

In a similar study Schmidt (1960) inoculated human leukemic blood cells into newborn mice, rats, and guinea pigs. The results were negative.

Tentative Conclusions

No attempt is made to evaluate critically the results of experiments thus far reported, in which oncogenic viruses, presumably recovered from human malignant tumors or leukemia, induced malignant tumors or leukemia following inoculation into animals. These experiments are presented here at their face value.

The critical reader will notice, however, that unquestionable and consistently reproducible evidence has not yet been furnished. Additional and confirmatory data are needed. The induction of neoplasms, including leukemia, with filtrates presumably containing human oncogenic viruses would be far more convincing if mice of established inbred strains, bred under careful supervision, and known for their low incidence of spontaneous tumors, were employed for bio-assay, instead of using non-pedigreed mice with unknown incidence of spontaneous tumors, purchased from commercial dealers. Adequate litter-mate controls, inoculated simultaneously with heated, or otherwise inactivated, human tumor extracts would be essential. Commercially available mice of non-inbred, or partially inbred strains would be acceptable only if experimental conditions were determined with sufficient precision to assure the experimental induction in the inoculated animals of a significant incidence of tumors with human tumor extracts, and the reproduction, at will, of similar results not only by the original observers, but also in other laboratories.

Difficulties Facing Those Who May Try to Transmit Human Tumor Agents to Animals

The difficulties encountered in attempts to transmit a hypothetical human cancer virus to animals are considerable. Let us assume, as a working hypothesis, that human tumors are caused by oncogenic viruses. Could such viruses be readily extracted from tumors? Even in animals, such as chickens or mice, known to carry virus-caused neoplasms, it is frequently very difficult to extract infective virus from spontaneous tumors. Let us assume, however, that some of the human tumors employed as donors would yield active filtrates containing infectious virus particles. Which species of animals would be suitable for bio-assay? Most probably newborn hosts would have to be employed. The latency may be considerable, extending over a period of many months or possibly even years. For obvious reasons, inoculation of human hosts could not be considered. What other species would be susceptible?

Would we expect the inoculated hosts to develop the same forms of neoplasms which were employed for the preparation of extracts? Any other neoplasms? Another form of disease, perhaps of a non-neoplastic nature? What assurance would we have that the disease observed in some of the inoculated hosts was actually induced by the hypothetical oncogenic virus?*

ATTEMPTS TO ISOLATE ONCOGENIC VIRUSES FROM HUMAN TUMORS AND LYMPHOMAS IN TISSUE CULTURE STUDIES

It has been amply demonstrated that certain oncogenic viruses isolated from mice, rats, and other animal species can be grown in tissue culture, and that at least some of them can induce a characteristic cytopathic effect

* The reader is also referred to the editorial by R. E. Shope entitled "Koch's postulates and a viral cause of human cancer" (*Cancer Research*, **20**: 1119–1120, 1960).

in cells in which they are propagated. On the basis of these observations, in several laboratories extracts prepared from a variety of human tumors and lymphomas were inoculated into different cell lines propagated in tissue culture, in an attempt to isolate oncogenic viruses from human neoplasms.

The difficulties of this approach are immediately apparent to anyone familiar with the study of human viruses. Our tools for working with human viruses are quite limited. Cytopathogenic effect of the hypothetical oncogenic virus on tissue-culture-grown cells would be the obvious goal to look for, but would actually be a very unreliable guide, unless the virus could later be recovered from the infected tissue culture cells or fluid, and would prove to be consistently oncogenic on animal bio-assay.

Cytopathogenic effect alone would be of interest, but could not serve as identification of the virus, unless specific serological neutralization tests were available in which a serum recovered from human cancer patients would neutralize such a virus, whereas no neutralization would be obtained with a serum from appropriate normal controls. There exist several scores of cytopathogenic human viruses that have been recovered from healthy human carriers. The possibly pathogenic role of most of these viruses still remains obscure.*

It would be beyond the scope of this monograph to review in detail all studies dealing with attempts to recover a hypothetical oncogenic virus from human malignant tumors, or human leukemia, by passage of extracts prepared from human tumors into cells grown in tissue culture. It can be stated briefly that the results of all these attempts were essentially negative, or, if positive results were claimed, they could not be confirmed or reproduced.

No evidence was obtained in these studies which would suggest the isolation of an oncogenic virus etiologically related to human cancer or leukemia.

Girardi and his coworkers (1962b) carried out a well controlled study in which they inoculated extracts prepared from a large number of human tumors and leukemias into human and animal cell lines propagated in tissue culture. Among the many tests performed, extracts from a variety of human malignant tumors and human lymphomas were inoculated into primary human amnion cell cultures and also into grivet monkey kidney cells. Other clinical material, such as bone marrow aspirates, organ extracts, etc., were also tested. In the study of human leukemia, 105 clinical specimens from 23 cases were employed. In addition, 150 extracts from human malignant tumors were also tested in tissue culture. No detectable virus, or virus-like agent, of human malignant tumor origin, was recovered.

* The reader is referred to the conference on "Viruses in Search of Disease," *Ann. N.Y. Acad. Sci.*, vol 67, pp. 209–445, 1957.

Cytopathic Effect of Human Tumor or Leukemic Extracts in Tissue Culture. The Possible Role of Mycoplasma (PPLO) in these Experiments.* Quite frequently inoculation of tissue culture cells with extracts prepared from human tumors or leukemia resulted in morphological changes in the inoculated cells, which in some instances led to eventual destruction of such cell cultures; in certain experiments, this cytopathic effect could be reproduced on several subsequent tissue culture passages.

Dmochowski and his colleagues (1959) reported that cell-free extracts of lymph nodes from leukemic patients induced morphologic changes in monkey kidney cell cultures; this cytopathic effect could be serially transmitted. The agent presumably responsible for this cytopathic effect was not identified.

In most of the other, similar experiments, in which extracts from human leukemia induced a cytopathic effect in cell cultures, mycoplasma (PPLO) could eventually be recovered from such cultures.

Various strains of mycoplasma species of man have been isolated from human blood, and from human lymphomas, leukemia, and from malignant as well as from benign human neoplasms (Grist and Fallon, 1964. Girardi *et al.*, 1965. Fallon *et al.*, 1965. Armstrong *et al.*, 1965. Hummeler *et al.*, 1965. Murphy *et al.*, 1963, 1965a,b. Hayflick and Koprowski, 1965. Grace *et al.*, 1965).

Some of the mycoplasma (PPLO) strains are cytopathogenic when propagated in tissue culture. This could explain the fact that some of the human leukemia isolates, made from blood (Negroni, 1964) or from urine (Ames *et al.*, 1966) of leukemic patients had a cytopathic effect when introduced into tissue culture cell lines. Such isolates contain the rather ubiquitous PPLO organisms. However, a causal relationship between mycoplasma and leukemia or malignant tumors has never been established. The same is true for the many other microorganisms or submicroscopic agents which have been isolated from human tumors.

"Herpes-like" Virus in Burkitt Lymphoma Cell Lines. The presence of a virus belonging to the herpes simplex group in human Burkitt lymphoma cell lines was reported by Epstein and his colleagues (1964, 1967).† The possible causative relationship of this "herpes-like" virus to the etiology of Burkitt lymphoma has not yet been sufficiently documented. The herpes virus is rather ubiquitous in humans, and the presence of a virus belonging

*Mycoplasma or pleuropneumonia-like organisms (PPLO). The interested reader is referred for further information on these very small microorganisms to the recent review by Hayflick and Chanock (1965) and also to the monograph consisting of papers dealing with the *Biology of the Mycoplasma* presented at a conference held by the New York Academy of Sciences on May 10–13, 1966 in New York City (Hayflick, Editor, 1967).

† For more detailed information the reader is referred to the chapter on Burkitt Lymphoma in this monograph.

to the herpes group in human lymphoma cell lines may be accidental. Further studies are needed.

The isolations of unidentified cytopathic agents and mycoplasma (Dalldorf and Bergamini, 1964. Dalldorf *et al.*, 1966), as well as that of a reovirus (Bell *et al.*, 1964, 1966), from Burkitt childhood lymphoma most probably belong in the same category.

Oncogenic Potency of Adenoviruses. The oncogenic potency of certain types of human adenoviruses was recognized a few years ago.* These viruses can be grown in tissue culture; they exert a characteristic cytopathic effect on certain cell lines in which they are propagated; furthermore, they can be detected on electron microscopic examination of infected tissue culture cells in which they are grown. The adenoviruses induce tumors when inoculated into newborn hamsters, or to a lesser extent also when injected into certain other animal species; however, their possible role in the induction of human tumors has not yet been demonstrated. Several isolations of adenoviruses from a handful of human tumors have been reported;* however, the causative relationship of the isolated adenovirus strains to the neoplasms from which they were recovered has not been documented; their presence in the tumor cells was most probably accidental.

ELECTRON MICROSCOPIC STUDIES OF HUMAN CANCER AND LEUKEMIA

The Search for Virus Particles

It is apparent from studies reviewed in the preceding chapters of this monograph that virus particles could be found in a variety of tumors observed in animals. It was not difficult to determine the presence of virus particles in the cell nuclei of papillomas and warts not only in animals but also in man. Virus particles were readily observed in rabbit myxoma and fibroma, in frog kidney carcinoma, in chicken sarcoma, in mouse mammary carcinoma, etc. Characteristic virus particles could also be observed in lymphoid tumors in chickens, mice, and rats.

It should be stressed, nevertheless, that, with only occasional exceptions, virus particles could not be observed in certain other tumors, also known to be caused by oncogenic viruses, and readily induced by inoculation of filtrates containing the respective submicroscopic agents. This rather unexpected observation was made when sarcomas and related tumors, induced with the polyoma virus, and particularly those induced with the SV 40 virus and with certain types of human adenoviruses, were examined in the electron microscope. In most instances it has been extremely diffi-

* For more detailed information see chapter on the Oncogenic Potency of Adenoviruses in this monograph.

cult, if at all possible, to find virus particles on electron microscopic examination of such tumors. Yet the presence of virus particles could be readily demonstrated when susceptible cells grown in tissue culture and infected with these viruses were examined in the electron microscope.

It is understandable, nevertheless, that after the presence of virus particles was revealed without too much difficulty in mouse mammary carcinomas, and also in chicken, mouse, and rat leukemia, it appeared reasonable to anticipate that similar virus particles might also be present in human breast cancer and in human leukemia.

THE SEARCH FOR VIRUS PARTICLES IN HUMAN BREAST CANCER

Electron Microscopic Examinations of Human Milk Samples. In the early electron microscopic studies (Gross *et al.*, 1950), spherical particles were observed in milk samples obtained from women with a family history of breast cancer. At that time the technique of ultrathin sections had not yet been developed; accordingly, after differential centrifugation, the milk specimens were deposited on collodion-coated grids, air dried, lightly shadowed with chromium, and then examined in the electron microscope. The internal structure of the observed particles could not be revealed under such conditions. It is doubtful whether the spherical particles found in the milk samples, which varied in their diameters from 20 to 200 mμ, actually represented a virus.

In a similar more recent study (Lunger *et al.*, 1964), milk sample preparations obtained from 4 women patients with breast cancer were centrifuged; the resulting pellets were deposited on formvar-coated grids, treated with phosphotungstic acid, and examined in the electron microscope. Presence of spherical particles, 60 to 90 mμ in diameter, some of them with characteristic "tails," was observed in these preparations; again, the internal structure of the particles observed could not be revealed in these negatively stained preparations. Milk samples from normal women were also studied, but similar structures were not found in the control specimens. However, it is doubtful whether the structures found in the samples examined represented an oncogenic virus; it appears more probable that the particles observed represented either normal milk or cell components, or accidental contaminants, such as mycoplasma (PPLO). Similar problems were encountered in electron microscopic studies of negatively stained cow milk preparations recently reported, and discussed in more detail in the chapter on Bovine Leukosis.

Electron Microscopic Studies of Ultrathin Sections of Human Breast Cancer. Françoise Haguenau, at the College de France in Paris (1959, 1960a,b), examined ultrathin sections of fragments of breast cancer from 91 women patients, and compared the ultramicroscopic structure of human breast cancer with that of mammary carcinoma in mice. There were certain differences in general morphology between these two groups of specimens examined; the human breast cancer cells showed considerable variations in ultrastructure; their cell membranes appeared more intricate and had numerous protrusions; furthermore, there often were characteristic changes in the cell nuclei which included areas of densification of chromatin. The most striking difference, however, was the fact that no virus particles could be detected on electron microscopic examination of ultrathin sections prepared from human breast cancer in any of the specimens examined, whereas in mouse mammary carcinoma virus particles could be found consistently either in cell cytoplasm, or in extracellular spaces.*

In some of the sections of human breast cancer cells Haguenau observed in the cytoplasm, in the vicinity of the Golgi apparatus, the presence of vacuoles which contained small vesicular bodies about 40 mμ in diameter. However, similar structures have also been observed in frogs, mice, and in other animal species, in tumor cells as well as in normal tissues; it is now generally accepted that these "multivesicular bodies" represent normal components of cellular structure.

In a similar more recent study, Sykes and his coworkers (1968) examined in the electron microscope ultrathin sections prepared from 22 human breast cancers and 2 benign breast tumors. No structures resembling any oncogenic viruses were observed in the human tumor sections examined.

Virus-like Particles in Human Breast Cancer. Dmochowski and his coworkers (1968) examined ultrathin sections prepared from human breast tumors. In 3 out of 13 breast cancer biopsies, and in one fibroadenoma, spherical virus-like particles, about 120 mμ in diameter, with double membranes and eccentrically located electron-dense nucleoids were found in cytoplasmic vacuoles and in intercellular spaces. These particles resembled type B virus particles observed in mouse mammary carcinoma. In addition, smaller particles, 30 to 50 mμ in diameter, similar to those found by Feller and Chopra (1968) in 9 of 24 human breast cancer biopsies, were also observed. Further studies are needed to evaluate the possible significance of these observations.

THE SEARCH FOR VIRUS PARTICLES IN HUMAN LEUKEMIA AND LYMPHOMAS

Following the demonstration of characteristic and readily recognizable

* The morphology of mouse mammary carcinoma virus particles was described in the chapter on Mouse Mammary Carcinoma; the reader is referred to that chapter for additional information and pertinent references.

virus particles in mouse leukemia* (Dmochowski and Grey, 1957. Bernhard and Guérin, 1958. Bernhard and Gross, 1959), it was only logical to look for similar particles in human leukemia and lymphomas. Accordingly, ultrathin sections of lymph nodes, of blood plasma pellets, and in a few instances also of bone marrow fragments from patients with leukemia and lymphosarcomas were examined in the electron microscope. Specimens prepared from human leukemic blood plasma and centrifuged plasma pellets, treated with phosphotungstic acid, were also studied.

It was reported by several investigators that virus-like particles could be found in tissue and blood specimens from some of the leukemic patients examined. Other reports were essentially negative.

It must be stated immediately that, with very few exceptions, the reports describing the presence of virus-like particles in human leukemic specimens were not convincing. Most of these reports represented studies of pellets obtained by ultracentrifugation of leukemic blood plasma. However, identification of a few isolated particles detected among a mass of debris in plasma pellets is very difficult; the interpretation of the nature of such particles often presents insurmountable difficulties. In most instances such isolated particles cannot be differentiated from cellular debris, or from normal cell components. This is particularly true when negatively stained preparations are examined.

Although the interpretation of electron microscopic studies of ultrathin sections of lymph nodes from leukemic patients was more reliable, the results of these studies were in most instances not convincing, or essentially negative. The recent reports of Dmochowski and his colleagues (1965, 1967), which will be discussed in more detail on subsequent pages, are very interesting, but require confirmation.

Most of the other reports, including those describing the presence of virus-like particles in human leukemic cells grown in tissue culture, were also far from convincing. The differences in size, location, and morphology of the particles found by different observers in human lymphomas or leukemia, and the failure of other investigators to find similar particles, add to the confusion, and make it even more difficult to determine the validity of the scattered positive reports.

Electron Microscopic Studies of Ultrathin Sections

Virus-like Particles in Human Leukemic Lymph Nodes, Plasma Pellets, and Bone Marrow Fragments. The Studies of Dmochowski and his Coworkers. Several investigators reported the presence of virus-like particles observed on electron microscopic examination of ultrathin sections prepared from

* For detailed description of the morphology of the mouse leukemia virus, and pertinent references, the reader is referred to the chapter on Mouse Leukemia.

human leukemic lymph nodes and blood pellets (Dmochowski and Grey, 1957, 1958. Dmochowski *et al.*, 1959, 1965, 1967. Dalton *et al.*, 1964. Porter *et al.*, 1964). Virus-like particles observed in these studies were spherical and had an average diameter of about 90 mμ.

Most convincing among the observations thus far reported were the recent studies carried out by Leon Dmochowski and his colleagues (1965, 1967) at the M. D. Anderson Hospital and Tumor Institute in Houston, Texas. In these studies a relatively large number of specimens prepared from human leukemia and lymphomas revealed the presence of virus-like particles having a striking similarity to those observed in tissues of leukemic mice and rats. Some of the virus-like particles observed in human leukemic tissues were found budding from external cell membranes; other particles were observed in cytoplasmic vacuoles, or in intercellular spaces. The budding of particles from the cell membranes, and the location of groups of particles in cytoplasmic vacuoles and in intercellular spaces, represent important characteristic features which provide a basis for their identification and comparison with similar particles observed in leukemia in certain animal species, such as chickens, mice, or cats.

Electron microscopic examination of ultrathin sections of lymph node biopsy specimens from 16 patients with acute lymphatic leukemia revealed the presence of virus-like particles in 8 of the 16 specimens examined. Only 1 out of 10 biopsy specimens from patients with chronic lymphatic leukemia, and 2 out of 7 specimens from patients with monocytic leukemia, contained similar particles. Lymph node specimens from 38 patients with lymphosarcomas, or reticulum-cell sarcomas, revealed the presence of virus-like particles in 11 specimens examined. Sections of bone marrow aspirates were also examined from 7 patients with leukemia, and from 1 patient with reticulum-cell sarcoma; virus-like particles were found in 2 of the 8 specimens examined. When ultrathin sections of blood pellets from 16 patients with different forms of leukemia were examined, virus-like particles were found in 3 of 16 specimens examined (see Figures 72 and 73 on pages 851 and 865).

In their size, morphology, and their location in relation to cell components, the particles observed in human leukemia and lymphomas had a remarkable similarity to the mouse leukemia virus particles. It would be tempting to speculate on the basis of these reports, that the virus-like particles observed by Dmochowski and his colleagues in human leukemia and lymphomas actually represent a human leukemia virus, very similar in its morphology to the mouse leukemia virus. However, further studies and confirmatory observations are needed to substantiate such an assumption.

In most of the other similar electron microscopic studies of human leukemia and lymphomas thus far performed, which will be reviewed on subsequent pages of this chapter, no virus-like particles at all were found.

In the few experiments in which particles were observed, they had a different size, morphology, and location in relation to cell components.

Viola and his coworkers (1967) observed virus-like spherical particles having a diameter of 38 to 40 mμ in blood plasma pellets from a patient with granulocytic leukemia. The possible relation of these virus-like particles to the patient's disease remains to be determined.

Intracytoplasmic, Spherical Particles Observed by Seman in Human Leukemia. In a recent report Seman (1968), at the Paul-Brousse Hospital's Cancer Institute in Paris, described the presence of spherical, doughnut-like particles in several cases of human leukemia and lymphomas. However, these particles were different from those previously reported by Dmochowski and his colleagues. In Seman's studies electron microscopic examination of ultrathin sections prepared from human leukemic lymph nodes, and also from peripheral white blood cells studied in buffy coat preparations, revealed the presence of unusual spherical structures often found in groups in the cytoplasmic matrix. Significantly, these particles were not found in intercellular spaces; moreover, they were not found budding from the external cell membranes. The particles had a diameter varying from 70 to 100 mμ; they had 2 concentric membranes, and a central core of varying density.

In one series in which peripheral blood cells in buffy coat specimens were examined, 25 out of 80 preparations (31 per cent) revealed the presence of particles in the cytoplasm of leukemic cells. In another series in which ultrathin sections of biopsy fragments from leukemic lymph nodes were examined, 12 out of 24 specimens (50 per cent) revealed the presence of similar particles. However, the particles observed were not numerous, except in a few cases.

The nature of the particles observed by Seman remains obscure at the present time. His observation does not represent a confirmation of the results of previous electron microscopic studies of human leukemia reported by Dmochowski and other investigators. The morphology of the particles observed by Seman, and particularly their characteristic location in the cytoplasmic matrix, but not in intercellular spaces, places them in a different category from virus particles observed in mouse or chicken leukemia. In their general morphology, and particularly in their location within the cytoplasmic matrix, these particles may in certain features resemble the intracytoplasmic type A virus particles observed commonly in mouse mammary carcinoma.

However, this resemblance is at best incomplete. Type A particles observed in mouse mammary carcinoma have considerably less variation in size and usually a uniform, regularly spherical shape; they also have electron-lucent centers. On the other hand, the particles observed by Seman in human leukemic cells have an irregularly spherical shape; their outer membranes lack the circular uniformity so characteristic for the type A particles; furthermore, there are considerable variations in the density of their inner cores.*

It is difficult to evaluate at this point the significance of the particles observed by Seman in human leukemic cells. Further studies and confirmatory observations from other laboratories are needed in order to determine whether these spherical structures have any causal relation to human leukemia, and whether they actually represent a viral agent. The question whether they may represent cell components, or possibly some extraneous submicroscopic organisms only incidentally present in leukemic cells, must also be considered and requires further studies.

Similar spherical doughnut-like particles located directly in the cytoplasmic matrix were also observed in plasma-cell tumors in mice (Dalton *et al.*, 1961), and more recently in a transplanted mouse lymphoma (de Harven, 1964). However, it should be pointed out that the observation of type A particles in mouse lymphoma was rather unusual. In our extensive studies carried out with D. G. Feldman in our laboratory we have never observed intracytoplasmic type A particles in mouse leukemia. It is quite possible that an occasional presence of such particles in mouse lymphoma, or other related neoplasms, was only coincidental.

Essentially Negative Reports. Failure to Detect Virus-like Particles in Human Leukemic Lymph Nodes, Plasma Pellets, or Bone Marrow. Braunsteiner and his colleagues (1960) examined ultrathin sections prepared from lymph nodes and bone marrow from 16 patients with acute leukemia and from 27 additional patients with chronic leukemia, lymphosarcoma, and Hodgkin's disease. Virus-like particles were found only in one of the 16 patients with acute leukemia, and in none of the other specimens examined. The particles observed were spherical and had a diameter of 75 to 95 mμ; however, the authors stressed that they found similar particles in normal cells of the Chang cell line propagated in tissue culture and derived from an explant of human liver. Accordingly, the overall results of this study could be considered as negative, since, with only one question-

* In mouse mammary carcinoma, doughnut-like particles with double membranes, 60 to 75 mμ in diameter, can be observed directly in the cytoplasmic matrix, in addition to virus particles observed in the cytoplasmic vacuoles and in intercellular spaces.

According to the original classification, doughnut-like spherical particles with double membranes without electron-dense nucleoids would fall into the category designated "type A" (Bernhard and Guérin, 1958). According to a more recent classification (*J. Nat. Cancer Inst.*, **37**: 395–397, 1966), the location of such particles directly in the cytoplasmic matrix would more specifically place them in the subdivision designated "intracytoplasmic type A" particles. For additional information the reader is referred to the chapter on Mouse Mammary Carcinoma.

able exception, none of the specimens from 43 patients with leukemia, lymphoma, or related disease showed the presence of virus particles.

Leplus and his coworkers (1961) examined ultrathin sections from tumor specimens obtained from 26 patients with Hodgkin's disease and 10 patients with lymphomas or reticulum-cell sarcomas. In addition, they also examined ultrathin sections from 20 different metastatic tumors and 13 non-malignant human tumors. In none of the human tumors examined did they find any evidence of virus or virus-like particles.

Nuclear Lesions in Human Lymphomas. In 9 cases of Hodgkin's disease and in one case of lymphosarcoma, Leplus and his coworkers (1961) described nuclear changes in the form of margination of chromatin. In addition, in the center of the nucleus, presence of 1 or 2 very dense inclusions with irregular margins and varying in diameter from 0.15 to 0.3 μ was also observed; these inclusions were either opaque or consisted of very fine granules. In a few cases some of the cells contained nuclei with one or more hypertrophic nucleoli. Similar nuclear lesions have been observed by Shipkey and Tandler (1962) in human lymphosarcoma and by Haguenau (1960b) in human breast carcinoma and Rous chicken sarcoma. Nuclear changes of similar morphology were also reported in adenovirus infection (Morgan *et al.*, 1960), in *Molluscum contagiosum* (Dourmashkin and Bernhard, 1959), and in polyoma virus-infected cells (Bernhard *et al.*, 1959). However, the significance of these nuclear changes and their possible relation to a viral agent remains to be determined.

In an extensive and well documented study, Bessis and Thiéry (1961, 1962a,b) examined ultrathin sections prepared from peripheral white blood cells, bone marrow, lymph nodes, and lymphoid tumors, from 40 patients with myelogenous, stem-cell, lymphatic, and erythroblastic leukemia, as well as lymphosarcomas, reticulum-cell sarcomas, and Hodgkin's disease. Among the 40 cases examined,* in only 3 specimens, in a limited number of sections, a few single particles were found in intercellular spaces, in the vacuoles of young megakaryocytes, and in the cytoplasm of leukemic cells; however, the spherical structures observed could not be definitely identified as virus particles. In another case, smaller particles, resembling the polyoma virus, were observed in the nuclei of cells from a lymphosarcoma. None of the structures observed in these 4 specimens had a convincing viral morphology, and the overall result of this study could be classified as essentially negative.

In a recent study, still in progress (Gross and Feldman, 1969, to be published), ultrathin sections were prepared mostly from lymph nodes, bone marrow fragments, and buffy coats from patients with different forms of leukemia and lymphomas. Out of specimens from 18 patients thus far examined only two "questionable" cases were recorded; in one case, we

* This number has now been increased to 50, with no change in the overall evaluation of the results observed. (Personal communication to the author from Dr. M. Bessis, 1968.)

observed on ultrathin sections of a buffy coat preparation from a patient with chronic lymphatic leukemia, a characteristic thickening of the cell membrane, suggesting possibly an early budding of a virus particle; this was observed in several white blood cells. In another case of lymphatic leukemia, two virus-like spherical particles 100 to 110 mμ in diameter, with electron-dense centers, similar to type C particles, were found at the edge of two lymphocytes from a 2-day-old buffy coat culture. However, neither of these two observations was convincing. The results of examination of the remaining specimens were negative.

The Burkitt lymphoma belongs in a different category, at least for classification purposes, and was discussed in a separate chapter. It can be restated briefly that no virus particles could be observed on electron microscopic examination of ultrathin sections prepared from biopsy fragments.* Bernhard and Lambert (1964) examined biopsy specimens from 5 Burkitt lymphomas with negative results. More recently Bernhard (personal communication to the author, 1968) examined in the electron microscope ultrathin sections from 47 cases of Burkitt lymphomas, but failed to detect the presence of virus particles in any of these specimens.

Virus-like Particles in Cultured Leukemic Cells. Graffi and his coworkers (1964) observed in tissue-culture-grown leukemic cells from 4 patients with myelogenous leukemia the presence of virus-like particles varying in diameter from 40 to 70 mμ, located in the nucleus and in the cytoplasm.

Beard and Parsons observed virus-like particles in one out of 15 cases of human leukemia. Leukemic cells from lymph node of a patient who had lymphatic leukemia were placed in tissue culture; after several days the cells were sectioned and examined in the electron microscope. Spherical particles, 80 to 100 mμ in diameter, with electron-dense nucleoids, were found in the cytoplasm (personal communication to the author from Dr. J. W. Beard, 1960).

Stewart and her coworkers also reported (1963, 1964) presence of spherical virus-like particles, about 100 mμ in diameter, in cytoplasmic vacuoles, in cultured cells derived from human leukemic bone marrow cells or blood leukocytes.

Zeve and his colleagues (1966) observed herpes-like virus particles in cultured leukemic cells derived from a patient with chronic myelogenous leukemia.

Virus Particles in Cultured Burkitt Lymphoma Cells. In Burkitt lymphoma cells propagated in tissue culture, particles having the morphology of a viral agent of the herpes group were detected by Epstein and his coworkers

* However, herpes-like virus particles could be found in a small fraction of lymphoblasts derived from Burkitt lymphomas and propagated in tissue culture. This is discussed in more detail in the preceding chapter of this monograph.

(1964, 1967), and later also by other investigators. This was discussed in the preceding chapter of this monograph. The herpes-like virus particles could be detected at best only in a very small fraction (1 to 2 per cent) of the tissue-culture-grown lymphoblasts. No evidence of the presence of any virus particles could be detected on electron microscopic examination of ultrathin sections prepared from the original tumor biopsy material.

Other Cell Culture Studies. In studies carried out by Inman and his colleagues (1964), cell cultures inoculated with passage fluid derived from human leukemic bone marrow were examined in the electron microscope. The presence of virus-like particles was observed in the cell cytoplasm and in ultracentrifuged culture fluid pellets. These particles had an average diameter of about 73 mμ. Smaller particles, about 40 mμ in diameter, were also found in the nuclei of some of the infected cells.

The nature of these particles and their possible relation to human leukemia have not been determined.

Observation of Virus-like Particles in Leukemic Blood Preparations in which the Negative Staining Technique was Employed

In a separate category can be listed the many electron microscopic studies of human leukemic blood plasma and ultracentrifuged plasma pellets in which the negative staining technique was employed. In these studies, virus particles, some of them with "tails," were described in specimens prepared from leukemic blood plasma and plasma pellets, and stained with phosphotungstic acid (Almeida *et al.*, 1963. Benyesh-Melnick *et al.*, 1964a,b. Dalton *et al.*, 1964. Smith *et al.*, 1964. Porter *et al.*, 1964. Burger *et al.*, 1964. Murphy and Furtado, 1963. Murphy *et al.*, 1965a,b). However, these preparations did not reveal the internal structure of the particles; as a result, the identification of the virus-like particles observed in these studies encountered considerable difficulties.

Normal Cell Components May be Mistaken for Virus Particles

The validity of the initial observations reporting the presence of virus-like particles in human leukemia was impaired by subsequent reports pointing out that particles of similar size and morphology could be detected in blood and tissues from normal healthy human donors, particularly in preparations in which the negative staining method was employed. Evidence has been provided suggesting that these or similar particles may represent submicroscopic organisms unrelated to viral agents, such as mycoplasma (PPLO), only incidentally present in the samples examined. They may also represent either normal or disintegrating cell components; the latter may become more apparent after prolonged storage of blood samples at room temperature or in the cold (Prince and Adams, 1965, 1966. Dmochowski *et al.*, 1964. Dalton *et al.*, 1964. Smith *et al.*, 1964. Arnoult and Haguenau, 1966).

The specific granules from blood platelets and megakaryocytes, as well as secretion granules, all of them normal cell components, have the same size as certain viruses. The difficulty in identification is increased by the regularity of their dimensions, their spherical shape, the presence of a well defined external membrane, and the frequent appearance of a dense internal core which may be separated from the external envelope, giving an illusion of a central nucleoid (Arnoult and Haguenau, 1966). These structures can be readily mistaken for viruses, particularly when ultrathin sections of centrifuged blood pellets are examined. Prince and Adams demonstrated (1966) that virus-like particles released into blood serum or plasma during storage in the cold are actually specific platelet granules, probably lysosomal in nature. This conclusion was consistent with the report of Firkin and his associates (1965) who examined in the electron microscope ultrathin sections of platelets during blood storage, and observed release of intact granule content of platelets by a process resembling reverse phagocytosis.

Presence of Mycoplasma (PPLO) Organisms in Human Leukemia. The Problem of Differentiation from Viral Agents*

Electron micrographs of ultrathin sections of lymph nodes or blood pellets, or of negatively stained plasma pellet preparations from leukemic patients often revealed the presence of mycoplasma (PPLO).

On ultrathin sections the PPLO particles can usually be identified without much difficulty, and differentiated from virus particles. Although the mycoplasma particles may be of similar size, they have a different morphology; the individual mycoplasma elementary bodies have an external limiting membrane which is often found to be composed of two electron-dense layers separated by a clear intermediate zone; most characteristically, however, the entire particle is generally completely filled with an electron-dense material. Larger mycoplasma cells may have extensive internal areas of lesser density; delicate filaments similar to those found in the nuclear region of other bacteria may be located in areas of lesser density, usually in the center of the cell. The overall morphologic picture is therefore quite different from that of a virus; on electron micrographs of ultrathin sections there is usually little difficulty in differentiating myco-

* The reader interested in more information on the mycoplasma species, i.e. pleuropneumonia-like organisms (PPLO) of man, is referred to the recent review by Hayflick and Chanock (1965), and also to the monograph on the *Biology of the Mycoplasma* (Hayflick, Editor, 1967).

plasma from oncogenic viruses (Domermuth *et al.*, 1964. Dmochowski *et al.*, 1964. Anderson and Barile, 1965. Hummeler *et al.*, 1965).

However, in specimens prepared with the negative staining technique in which phosphotungstic acid is employed, and in which the specimens are not sectioned, the mycoplasma elementary bodies can be readily confused with virus particles of similar size. In such preparations only outside contours of the particulate elements are outlined, and the differentiation and identification of individual particles of similar size and of a similar overall appearance may be practically impossible.

Tentative Conclusions

Upon reviewing the available data it appears that no convincing evidence has yet been furnished to indicate the presence of virus particles in human leukemia or lymphomas.

The recent studies of Dmochowski and his colleagues (1965, 1967) are of considerable interest, since the virus particles which they observed in human leukemia have a striking similarity, in their morphology and location in relation to cell components, to the mouse leukemia virus; however, these studies require extensive and independent confirmation.

The recent report of Seman (1968) is also interesting, but requires confirmation and further studies; the particles which he observed were very different from those described in other similar studies; whether they actually represent a viral agent remains to be determined.

In most of the other electron microscopic studies of human leukemia and lymphomas the few isolated virus-like particles observed on ultrathin sections of human leukemic blood pellets or in other leukemic tissues, such as lymph nodes or fragments of bone marrow, are not convincing. In the same category can be classified the reports describing the presence of a variety of virus-like particles observed on negatively stained preparations.

In conclusion, it can only be emphasized that at the present time the question concerning the presence of virus particles in human leukemia and lymphomas has not yet been answered in a satisfactory manner.* Further studies are needed in order to clarify this important problem.

* * *

We have already mentioned in the introductory remarks preceding the review of electron microscopic studies of human cancer and leukemia that, with only occasional exceptions, virus particles could not be found in tumors induced by certain oncogenic agents, such as the polyoma virus, the

* The interested reader is referred for additional information on this subject to the recent review by Lévy and Oppenheim (1966).

SV 40 agent, or adenoviruses, even though, under proper experimental conditions, i.e., in infected cells grown in tissue culture, these agents can be readily detected with the electron microscope.

It is therefore apparent that the presence of causative viral agents cannot always be demonstrated in tumors known to be of viral origin. Accordingly, failure to detect the presence of virus particles in human tumors may not necessarily be inconsistent with the concept of viral origin of human neoplasms.

POLYOMA-LIKE VIRUS PARTICLES IN HUMAN DEMYELINATING BRAIN DISEASE, i.e., PROGRESSIVE MULTIFOCAL LEUKOENCEPHALOPATHY*

Observation of a New Disease Syndrome. In the course of post-mortem examination of brains of patients at the Massachusetts General Hospital in Boston, Åström, Mancall, and Richardson (1958) observed cases of an unusual demyelinating disease of the cerebral white matter; the lesions were characterized by widely disseminated, generally oval, small perivascular foci of destruction of myelin sheaths with relative sparing of axis cylinders. Three such cases were reported and recognized as a syndrome, and designated "progressive multifocal leukoencephalopathy." Two of these cases were observed in patients with chronic lymphatic leukemia and the third case in a patient with Hodgkin's disease. Shortly thereafter additional cases of a similar disease syndrome were reported by Cavanagh and his coworkers (1959), Lloyd and Urich (1959), Sibley and Weisberger (1961), and Richardson (1961).

Neurological symptoms in afflicted persons were progressive over an average period of three to four months and included hemiparesis, visual disturbances, aphasia, mental changes, and deterioration of intellect.

Most of Progressive Multifocal Leukoencephalopathy Cases were Observed in Patients with Leukemia. The majority of cases of progressive multifocal leukoencephalopathy occurred in middle aged or in older individuals, who at the same time also had leukemia or lymphomas, or less frequently another neoplastic disease; in some instances this syndrome occurred in patients who had generalized tuberculosis or sarcoidosis. Only rarely did this syndrome occur in advanced age without a concurrent or previous neoplastic or other chronic and debilitating disease.

Richardson (1961) reviewed 22 cases of progressive multifocal leukoencephalopathy; Weinstein and his associates (1963) tabulated 31 cases, and

* Observations concerning the presence of virus particles in the nuclei of glial cells in patients with multifocal leukoencephalopathy have been reviewed in this chapter because of their striking similarity to those observed in certain neoplastic diseases in animals, and because of a speculative possibility that these particles may be closely related to, if not identical with, the polyoma virus, the SV 40 virus, or the human wart virus; they probably belong to the papova group (see p. 890).

emphasized that most of these patients had a prior disease of the reticulo-endothelial system. Additional cases have been reported more recently by Silverman and Rubinstein (1965), Vanderhaeghen and Perier (1965), Zu Rhein and Chou (1965), Dolman and his coworkers (1967), Muller and Watanabe (1967), and others.

Presence of Virus Particles in the Nuclei of Glial Cells in Degenerated Cerebral White Matter Areas

Gabriele Zu Rhein and S.-M. Chou at the Department of Pathology and Neurology, University of Wisconsin Medical Center, Madison, reported (1964, 1965) that small virus particles, resembling in morphology the polyoma virus, were found on electron microscopic examination of ultrathin sections in the nuclei of glial cells of a patient who died from progressive multifocal leukoencephalopathy. The autopsy material was obtained from a 67-year-old woman who had a progressive paralysis of her left limbs, mental deterioration, and blurred speech for the last 7 months of life. At the time of death from pulmonary complications, multiple small and large areas of cerebral white matter were degenerated. Prior to electron microscopy, the brain slices had been kept for 2 years in 10 per cent formalin.* Discrete fragments of demyelinated gray areas, about 1 mm in diameter, located beyond the periphery, were selected for study. The tissue fragments were fixed in osmic acid, dehydrated, and embedded in Epon. Ultrathin sections were prepared, stained with lead citrate or uranyl acetate, and examined in the electron microscope.

Small virus particles were detected in the majority of the glial nuclei. Most of these particles were spherical and of a rather uniform size, 33 to 36 mμ in diameter, and had a medium electron opacity. They filled large parts of the nuclei; the residual chromatin was mostly marginated along the nuclear membrane. Crystalloid arrays of particles were also observed; in some instances the centrally located crystalloid arrangements occupied one-half to two-thirds of the sections of the nuclei. Filamentous structures about one-half to two-thirds the diameter of the spherical particles were also found in combination with the crystalline arrays of particles in the cell nuclei. Both the spherical particles and the characteristic filamentous

* It was rather surprising to find relatively well preserved virus particles in tissue specimens that had been kept in 10 per cent formalin for 2 years. This is obviously not a good method for preservation of tissue specimens for electron microscopy; it is quite apparent, nevertheless, that some cell components and certain more resistant virus particles can withstand such treatment, except for shrinkage and some deformation in morphology. The effect of immersion of polyoma virus in 10 per cent formalin for 10 days was studied in negatively stained preparations (Howatson *et al.*, 1965); there was some distortion of the capsomere arrangement and a slight diminution in particle size, due to shrinkage.

forms were similar to those observed in electron microscopic studies of the polyoma virus (Bernhard *et al.*, 1959. Howatson and Almeida, 1960).

Subsequent electron microscopic studies performed on grossly non-degenerated cerebral white matter of this patient, and another study performed on white matter of another elderly woman's brain, did not reveal presence of similar particles in the glial nuclei.

A similar observation was reported at about the same time in an independent study carried out by Silverman and Rubinstein (1965) at the Department of Pathology, Stanford University School of Medicine in Palo Alto, California. In this study the brain specimen was obtained, approximately 12 hours after death, from a 64-year-old white female who had characteristic symptoms of progressive multifocal leukoencephalopathy not associated with either leukemia or lymphoma. Electron microscopic examination of ultrathin sections of brain tissues from this case demonstrated in the nuclei of glial cells the presence of small virus particles about 35 to 40 mμ in diameter, very similar in their morphology to the polyoma virus, or to the SV 40 agent; in addition, the characteristic filamentous forms were also observed.

The initial observation of the presence of virus-like particles in glial cells of human demyelinating brain disease was presented by Dr. Zu Rhein in a brief communication at the Annual Meeting of the Association for Research in Nervous and Mental Diseases, which was held in December, 1964, in New York (Zu Rhein and Chou, 1964). In a discussion which followed this presentation, Dr. Rubinstein (1964) reported that a similar observation was made in an independent study which he carried out with Dr. L. Silverman. This is an interesting example of a concurrent and independent scientific observation made by different investigators working in separate laboratories.

The following personal communication received by the author in March, 1968, from Dr. L. J. Rubinstein, is an interesting illustration of this point: "We had completed our electron microscopic observations in September, 1964, in ignorance of Dr. Zu Rhein's findings. In November, 1964, I received the advance program of the December meeting in New York of the Association for Research in Nervous and Mental Diseases, in which Dr. Zu Rhein's paper entitled 'Papova Virus in Progressive Multifocal Leukoencephalopathy' was mentioned. I then communicated at once with Dr. Zu Rhein and also with Dr. Harry Zimmerman who was in charge of the program, and who kindly invited me to attend the meeting and present our findings in support of those of Dr. Zu Rhein."

Prompt Confirmation of the Original Observations in Other Laboratories. The initial observations were promptly confirmed by several observers. That same year Vanderhaeghen and Perier (1965) reported the presence of the characteristic virus particles in another case of this rare brain disease. Howatson and his coworkers (1965) examined specimens of brain tissues obtained at autopsy from 3 patients suffering from progressive multifocal leukoencephalopathy. One of these 3 specimens was the same that had been previously examined by Zu Rhein and Chou (1965); the two additional specimens were from new cases, one from a man who also had lymphatic leukemia, and the other from a patient with Hodgkin's disease. In all 3 specimens the characteristic virus particles were found in the nuclei of glial cells.

In other similar studies, a case of typical, progressive multifocal leukoencephalopathy was described by Muller and Watanabe (1967) in a 54-year-old patient with Hodgkin's disease; another case in a 69-year-old woman who also had chronic lymphatic leukemia was described by Zu Rhein (1967). Electron microscopic studies of ultrathin sections of brain specimens from both patients revealed the presence of virus particles in the nuclei of the abnormal glial cells. A similar observation was also reported by Dolman and his colleagues (1967).

By this time (Zu Rhein, 1967) 18 cases of progressive multifocal leukoencephalopathy had been observed in which the presence of the characteristic virus particles could be demonstrated; it now appeared that in practically all cases of progressive multifocal leukoencephalopathy the characteristic small virus particles could be found in the nuclei of the affected glial cells.

The Morphology of Virus Particles Observed in Human Demyelinating Brain Disease

Electron Microscopic Studies Employing the Negative Staining Method. Howatson, Nagai and Zu Rhein (1965) employed the negative staining method in their electron microscopic study of virus particles in 3 cases of human demyelinating brain disease. Using this method it was possible to reveal in more detail the morphology of the virus particles; it was determined on the basis of these studies that the virus particles observed in progressive multifocal leukoencephalopathy are similar in their ultrastructure to the polyoma virus, and to the SV 40 agent.

Similar conclusions were reached in a subsequent study by Schwerdt and his coworkers (1966) who also employed the negative staining method for electron microscopic examination of virus particles found in a case of human demyelinating brain disease.

The Possible Relation of the Particles Observed in Human Demyelinating Brain Disease to the Viruses of the "Papova Group." The virus particles observed in the nuclei of the glial cells in human demyelinating brain disease were found to be very similar in their size, morphology, and intranuclear locations, to the viruses observed in cells infected with the polyoma virus of mice, the papilloma virus of rabbits, cattle, and other species, including the wart virus of man, and the vacuolating virus (SV 40) of monkeys. This group of viruses was designated by Melnick (1962) the "*papova group.*" This term was derived from the first two letters of each virus name, i.e. *pa*pilloma, *po*lyoma, and *va*cuolating virus.

Later on the K virus (Kilham, 1952), causing pneumonitis in mice (Kilham and Murphy, 1953) was also added to this group. The K virus is similar in its morphology, and location in the cell nucleus, to other members of the papova group (Dalton *et al.*, 1963. Parsons, 1963).

Some General Properties of the Viruses of the Papova Group

According to Melnick (1962), viruses belonging to the papova group have certain common properties: (a) approximate average diameter of 45 mμ, (b) deoxyribonucleic acid core, (c) 42 capsomeres, and (d) relative resistance to heat; furthermore, (e) they multiply in the nuclei of susceptible cells, and (f) most of them have an oncogenic potential.

Members of this group are small spherical particles, about 38 to 55 mμ in diameter, present usually in the nuclei of the infected cells, often in striking crystalloid arrays; some of them also form characteristic filamentous structures. Occasionally they may also be present in closely packed groups in the cytoplasm. These viruses are characterized by the type of symmetry they possess. The viral protein coats, or capsids, are round or polyhedral, and are composed of projecting capsomeres arranged in accordance with icosahedral or 5 : 3 : 2 type of cubic symmetry. Although all of them have the same general structure, some of the members of this group have larger capsids than others (Howatson *et al.*, 1965).

The first subgroup consists of the polyoma virus and the SV 40 virus (i.e. vacuolating agent); the mouse pneumonitis K virus also belongs to this subgroup. These viruses are indistinguishable from one another on ultrathin sections or when examined on negatively stained preparations; they have a mean diameter of about 40 to 45 mμ in unfixed preparations (Crawford *et al.*, 1963. Bernhard *et al.*, 1962. Parsons, 1963).

The second subgroup includes the papilloma virus of rabbits, dogs, and cattle, and also the human wart virus. These viruses are morphologically identical and slightly larger than those of the first subgroup; their mean diameter ranges from 52 to 55 mμ.

Man is considered the natural host of only one of the members of this group, namely the human wart virus. The mouse is the natural host of the polyoma virus and of the K virus. The rabbit and certain other species, such as dogs and cattle, are natural hosts of the papilloma virus, and the monkey is the natural host of the SV 40 virus.

Particles Observed in Human Demyelinating Brain Disease Resemble Polyoma Rather than Papilloma or Wart Virus

The resemblance of the virus particles observed in progressive multifocal leukoencephalopathy to the particles of the papova group is striking. The mean diameter of unfixed particles observed in human brain tissues was 42.5 mμ, and particles found in tissues that had been kept in formalin was 40.5 mμ, due presumably to shrinkage (Howatson *et al.*, 1965); on the basis of these measurements the virus observed in progressive multifocal leukoencephalopathy resembles the polyoma virus rather than the papilloma or wart virus. In further agreement with this classification are certain morphological characteristics, such as the size and spacing of the surface projections, i.e. capsomeres, similar in both the progressive multifocal leukoencephalopathy particles and the polyoma virus particles observed on negatively stained preparations (Howatson *et al.*, 1965). Such classification would also be consistent with the presence of cylindrical or filamentous structures in the vicinity of crystalloid aggregates of spherical virus particles observed on electron microscopic examination of ultrathin sections in the nuclei of glial cells in human demyelinating brain disease. Similar structures have been observed in sections of nuclei of kidney cells infected with the polyoma virus (Howatson and Almeida, 1960), but have not been reported in cells infected with the papilloma virus.

What is the Nature of Virus Particles Observed in Progressive Multifocal Leukoencephalopathy?

Difficulties in Identification. The nature of the virus particles observed in progressive multifocal leukoencephalopathy cannot be determined in a satisfactory manner at the present time. Electron microscopic studies revealed in sufficient detail the morphology of these particles and their location in reference to cell components, to allow a presumptive classification in general terms. There is little doubt that these particles belong to the papova group and presumably rather to the polyoma, or SV 40 subgroup (Howatson *et al.*, 1965). The question, however, whether these particles are related to, or identical with, the polyoma virus or the SV 40 agent remains to be determined. Their possible relation to the papilloma or human wart virus also requires further studies. Serological tests and efforts to demonstrate specific antigens, as well as attempts to isolate and identify the causative virus in tissue culture and in bio-assay experiments on newborn mice, rats, and hamsters, are urgently needed.

Most of the electron microscopic examinations have been performed on autopsy specimens fixed in formalin. Such specimens have not been suitable for serological studies. Progressive multifocal leukoencephalopathy is a rare disease, often recognized only at the post-mortem brain examination. With the increasing interest in this disease it may be possible to recognize this unusual syndrome more often during the lifetime of the patients, and carry out appropriate serological tests. It may also be possible to obtain more often fresh brain specimens shortly after autopsy in order to carry out tissue culture studies and bio-assay experiments on animals, such as those already initiated by Schwerdt and his coworkers (1966), and more recently also carried out by Zu Rhein (personal communication to the author, 1968), and others. Such studies may eventually provide the necessary information leading to the identification of the causative virus.

What is the Relation of Progressive Multifocal Leukoencephalopathy to Leukemia? On the basis of electron microscopic examinations thus far performed there appears little doubt that the clinical manifestations of progressive multifocal leukoencephalopathy are caused by a submicroscopic agent closely related to the polyoma, SV 40, or papilloma virus, which produces degenerative changes in some of the glial cells in the brains of such patients. It is rather doubtful, however, whether these virus particles have any causal relation to leukemia, lymphomas, or cancer, concurrently present in the majority of patients suffering from this rare demyelinating brain disease.

Activation of a Latent Virus? Although purely speculative, a more probable explanation would be that some of the patients who develop progressive multifocal leukoencephalopathy were carrying a latent polyoma-like virus prior to the onset of the terminal brain disease, and that in the course of a progressive neoplastic disease, such as leukemia, lymphoma, or cancer, or after another chronic and debilitating disease, their resistance was lowered; the hitherto latent virus, presumably carried by such patients, could then have changed into a pathogenic agent causing the development of a demyelinating brain disease.

Exacerbation of Latent Herpes Simplex and Herpes Zoster Infection in Leukemic Patients. The development of acute eruptions of herpes simplex, or herpes zoster, in patients who have leukemia, and the increased susceptibility of such patients to common staphylococcal or streptococcal infections, have long been observed. The presumptive lowering of a natural resistance of the human host to a polyoma-like latent virus infection, leading eventually to the development of a fatal demyelinating brain disease, could be interpreted as a similar phenomenon.

Speculation on a Possible Oncogenic Potential of Virus Particles Observed in Progressive Multifocal Leukoencephalopathy. The striking morphologic similarity of the virus particles consistently found in human demyelinating brain disease to certain viruses of the papova group is of particular interest since these animal viruses have a striking oncogenic potential. Should it be established that the virus particles observed in progressive multifocal leukoencephalopathy in man are not only morphologically, but also biologically closely related to the polyoma virus, the SV 40 virus, or to the papilloma virus, it would be possible to speculate that they have a latent oncogenic potential not only, or necessarily, for man, but possibly for other animal species. There is no evidence at the present time to suggest that such a relationship actually exists; however, this possibility has to be considered, and requires further studies.

Some interesting implications could be anticipated if it is established that progressive multifocal leukoencephalopathy is actually caused by a potentially oncogenic virus. Should such a relationship be established, it would represent another example of an oncogenic virus capable of inducing a non-neoplastic disease in man. In this respect this would be similar to observations made on adenoviruses and described in a separate chapter of this monograph. Certain types of human adenoviruses can be either latent, or may induce only a transient infectious disease in humans, such as conjunctivitis, enteritis, or pharyngitis; yet, the same viruses can induce progressively growing tumors in hamsters and in certain other animal species.

The Parotid Tumor (Polyoma) Virus and Leukemia in Mice. The occurrence of polyoma-like virus particles in individuals who often present also symptoms of leukemia or lymphomas is of particular interest to those who have worked in the laboratory with mouse leukemia, and also with the parotid tumor, i.e. polyoma, virus. The parotid tumor virus was originally isolated from mouse leukemic tissues (Gross, 1953); since that time, repeated isolations of this virus from mouse leukemic tissues have been made, suggesting thereby some possible relationship between the mouse leukemia and the parotid tumor viruses. On the other hand, there appears to exist an interference phenomenon between these two viruses. When filtrates containing both viruses are injected into newborn mice, most of them develop manifestations of only one of the two diseases; occurrence of both leukemia and parotid tumors in the same animal has been observed, but is very rare (see p. 675, and also Fig. 62 on p. 737).

Summary and Tentative Conclusions

It now is apparent that small virus-like particles strikingly similar to the viruses of the papova group can be found consistently in the nuclei of glial cells of the cerebral white matter of patients who died from progressive multifocal leukoencephalopathy. This rare demyelinating brain disease occurs most frequently in individuals who at the same time have leukemia, lymphomas, or another neoplastic disease. There is little doubt that these virus particles are actually responsible for the development of progressive multifocal leukoencephalopathy in man. The possibility that this virus may also carry a latent oncogenic potential for man, or for other animal species, is purely speculative at the present time, but should be considered in view of the striking similarity of these particles to the polyoma virus in mice, the SV 40 virus in monkeys, or the papilloma virus of rabbits, cattle, or other animal species, including the wart virus of man.

Whether the small particles observed in progressive multifocal leukoencephalopathy have any relation to leukemia or other malignant tumors, which are common in patients with this rare brain disease, is doubtful; however, this question requires further studies.

REFERENCES

AGEENKO, A. I., Leukemias induced in rats with extracts from human leukaemic tissue. *Acta Internat. Union Against Cancer*, **18**: 140–142, 1962.

ALMEIDA, J. D., HASSELBACK, R. C., and HAM, A. W., Virus-like particles in blood of two acute leukemia patients. *Science*, **142**: 1487–1489, 1963.

AMES, R. P., SOBOTA, J. T., REAGAN, R. L., and KARON, M., Virus-like particles and cytopathic activity in urine of patients with leukemia. *Blood*, **28**: 465–478, 1966.

ANDERSON, D. R., and BARILE, M. F., Ultrastructure of mycoplasma hominis. *J. Bact.*, **90**: 180–192, 1965.

ANDERSON, R. C., Familial leukemia. *Am. J. Dis. Child.*, **81**: 313–322, 1951.

ARMSTRONG, D., HENLE, G., SOMERSON, N. L., and HAYFLICK, L., Cytopathogenic mycoplasmas associated with two human tumours. I. Isolation and biological aspects. *J. Bact.*, **90**: 418–424, 1965.

ARNOULT, J., and HAGUENAU, F., Problems raised by the search for virus particles in human leukemia. A study with the electron microscope of blood plasma, cerebrospinal fluid, and megakaryocytes from bone marrow. *J. Nat. Cancer Inst.*, **36**: 1089–1109, 1966.

FIG. 74. INTRANUCLEAR VIRUS PARTICLES AND FILAMENTS IN HUMAN DEMYELINATING BRAIN DISEASE (PROGRESSIVE MULTIFOCAL LEUKOENCEPHALOPATHY).

(A). Ultrathin section of a portion of glial nucleus from demyelinated cerebral white matter of a case of demyelinating brain disease (progressive multifocal leukoencephalopathy) in a 67-year-old female. Crystalloid arrangement of spherical virus particles with a center-to-center distance of 40 mμ. Single virus particles and chromatin fragments between aggregates. These particles are very similar in their location, size, and morphology to the polyoma virus particles. Magnification 58,000×. Electron micrograph prepared by Gabriele M. Zu Rhein, Department of Pathology, University of Wisconsin Medical School, Madison. (B). Ultrathin section of a portion of glial nucleus from demyelinated cerebellar white matter from a case of demyelinating brain disease in a 33-year-old female. Filamentous viral forms arranged in twisting and whirling bundles. Marked electron opacity of cross sectioned filaments; filament diameters from 16 to 24 mμ. A few normal spherical virus particles similar in size and morphology to those reproduced in the upper part (A) of this electron micrograph are also present and are scattered among the bundles of filaments and on their periphery. Magnification 46,000×. Electron micrograph prepared by Shi-Ming Chou, Department of Pathology, University of Wisconsin Medical School, Madison.

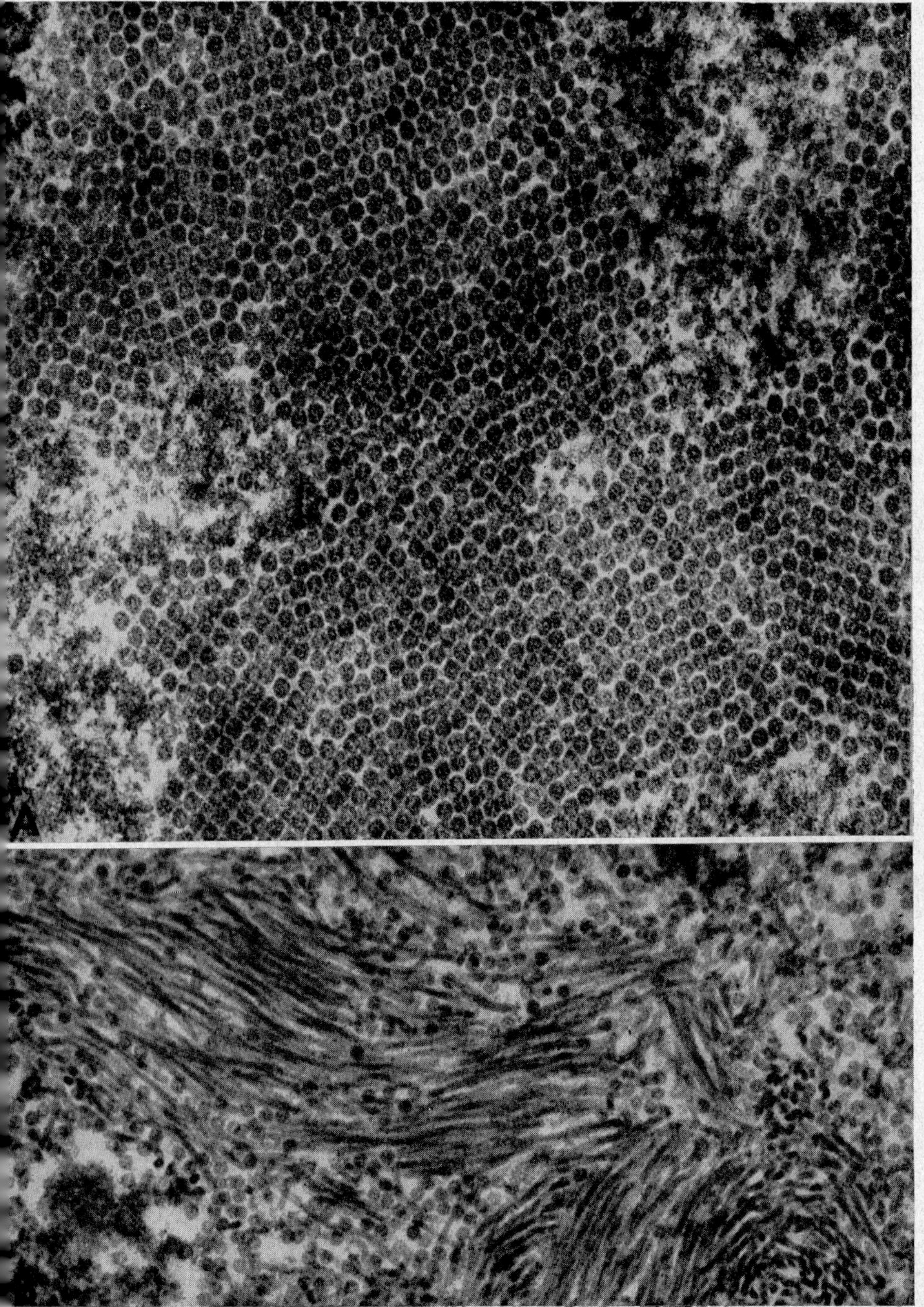

FIG. 74. INTRANUCLEAR VIRUS PARTICLES AND FILAMENTS IN HUMAN DEMYELINATING BRAIN DISEASE (PROGRESSIVE MULTIFOCAL LEUKOENCEPHALOPATHY).

ASHBEL, R., Development of tumors in hamsters and rats following the injection of mycobacteria. *Pubbl. Staz. Zool. Napoli*, **28**: 12–31, 1956.

ÅSTRÖM, K.-E., MANCALL, E. L., and RICHARDSON, E. P., JR., Progressive multifocal leuko-encephalopathy. A hitherto unrecognized complication of chronic lymphatic leukaemia and Hodgkin's disease. *Brain*, **81**: 93–111, 1958.

BALACESCO, I., and TOVARU, S., Une observation authentique de transmission spontanée du cancer d'homme à homme. *Bull. du Cancer*, **25**: 655–667, 1936.

BARDAWIL, W. A., and TOY, B. L., The natural history of choriocarcinoma: Problems of immunity and spontaneous regression. *Ann. N.Y. Acad. Sci.*, **80**: 197–261, 1959.

BARGEN, J. A., MAYO, C. W., and GIFFIN, L. A., Familial trends in human cancer. *J. Hered.*, **32**: 7–10, 1941.

BEHLA, R., Über "Cancer à deux" und Infektion des Krebses. *Deutsche med. Wochenschr.*, **1**: 427–431, 1901.

BELL, T. M., MASSIE, A., ROSS, M. G. R., and WILLIAMS, M. C., Isolation of a reovirus from a case of Burkitt's lymphoma. *Brit. Med. J.*, **1**: 1212–1213, 1964.

BELL, T. M., MASSIE, A., ROSS, M. G. R., SIMPSON, D. I. H., and GRIFFIN, E., Further isolations of reovirus type 3 from cases of Burkitt's lymphoma. *Brit. Med. J.*, **1**: 1514–1517, 1966.

BENEDICT, W. L., Retinoblastoma in homologous eyes of identical twins. *Arch. Ophthal.*, **2**: 545–548, 1929.

BENYESH-MELNICK, M., DESSY, S. I., and FERNBACH, D. J., Cytomegaloviruria in children with acute leukemia and in other children. *Proc. Soc. Exp. Biol. & Med.*, **117**: 624–630, 1964.

BENYESH-MELNICK, M., SMITH, K. O., and FERNBACH, D. J., Association of myxovirus-like particles with acute leukaemia of childhood. *Nature*, **202**: 1129–1130, 1964a.

BENYESH-MELNICK, M., SMITH, K. O., and FERNBACH, D. J., Studies on human leukemia. III. Electron microscopic findings in children with acute leukemia and in children with infectious mononucleosis. *J. Nat. Cancer Inst.*, **33**: 571–579, 1964b.

BERGOLTZ,* V. M., The leukemia-producing activity of cell-free filtrates of human leukemic tissue. *Bull. Exp. Biol. and Med.*, **45**: 731–734, 1958. (Transl. from Russian). Consultants Bureau, Inc., Am. Inst. Biol. Sci., Washington, D.C.

BERGOLZ, V. M., Experimental studies of the aetiology of leucosis in man. I. Cellfree factor obtained from the leukaemic tissue of man which induces leukaemia in mice (Russian text). *Probl. Gematol. Perel. Krovi*, **1**: 11–17, 1957. Abstract in *Excerpta Med., Sect. XVI*, (*Cancer*), **6**: (I): 8–9, 1958.

BERGOLZ, V. M., Transmission of human leukemia to mice. pp. 86–111, in vol. **1**, *Progress in Experimental Tumor Research*. S. Karger, Basel and New York, 1960.

BERNHARD, W., Electron microscopy of tumor cells and tumor viruses. *Cancer Research*, **18**: 491–509, 1958.

BERNHARD, W., and GROSS, L., Présence de particules d'aspect virusal dans les tissus tumoraux de souris atteintes de leucémies induites. *Compt. Rend. Acad. Sci.* (*Paris*), **248**: 160–163, 1959.

* Name spelled erroneously "Bergol'ts" in translated publication. Spelled also "Bergolz" elsewhere.

BERNHARD, W., and GUÉRIN, M., Présence de particules d'aspect virusal dans les tissus tumoraux de souris atteintes de leucémie spontanée. *Compt. Rend. Acad. Sci.* (*Paris*), **247**: 1802–1805, 1958.

BERNHARD, W., and LAMBERT, D., Ultrastructure des tumeurs de Burkitt de l'enfant africain. pp. 270–284 in: *Symp. Lymph. Tumours in Africa* (*Paris*, 1963). S. Karger, Basel and New York, 1964.

BERNHARD, W., FEBVRE, H. L., and CRAMER, R., Mise en évidence au microscope électronique d'un virus dans des cellules infectées *in vitro* par l'agent du Polyome. *Compt. Rend. Acad. Sci.* (*Paris*), **249**: 483–485, 1959.

BERNHARD, W., VASQUEZ, C., and TOURNIER, P., La structure du virus SV 40 étudiée par coloration négative en microscopie électronique. *J. Microscopie*, **1**: 343–350, 1962.

BERNHARD, W. G., GORE, I., and KILBY, R. A., Congenital leukemia. *Blood*, **6**: 990–1001, 1951.

BESREDKA, A., and GROSS, L., De l'immunisation contre le sarcome de la souris par voie intracutanée. *Ann. Inst. Pasteur*, **55**: 491–500, 1935.

BESSIS, M., and THIÉRY, J.-P., Études au microscope électronique sur les leucémies humaines. I. Les leucémies granulocytaires. *Nouv. Rev. Franç. Hématol.*, **1**: 703–728, 1961.

BESSIS, M., and THIÉRY, J.-P., Études au microscope électronique sur les leucémies humaines. II. Les leucémies lymphocytaires. Comparaison avec la leucémie de la souris de souche AK. *Nouv. Rev. Franç. Hématol.*, **2**: 387–414, 1962a.

BESSIS, M., and THIÉRY, J.-P., Étude au microscope électronique des hémosarcomes humains. III. Leucémies à cellules-souches, erythrémies, réticulo-lymphosarcomes, maladie de Hodgkin, plasmocytomes. *Nouv. Rev. Franç. Hématol.*, **2**: 577–601, 1962b.

BLUMENTHAL, F., Die neueren Arbeiten über parasitäre Entstehung bösartiger Tumoren. *Deutsche med. Wochenschr.*, **52**: 389–391, 1926, and **52**: 435–438, 1926.

BLUMENTHAL, F., Beitrage zur Frage der Entstehung bösartiger Tumoren. *Deutsche med. Wochenschr.*, **52**: 1283–1286, 1926.

BLUMENTHAL, F., Zur Frage der parasitären Krebsentstehung. Zum 100. Geburtstage Ernst v. Leydens. *Zeitschr. f. Krebsforsch.*, **36**: 130–144, 1932.

BORREL, A., Le problème du cancer. Revue. *Bull. Inst. Pasteur*, **5**: 497–512, 1907. **5**: 593–608, 1907. **5**: 641–662, 1907.

BOSTICK, W., The status of the search for a virus in Hodgkin's disease. *Ann. N.Y. Acad. Sci.*, **54**: 1162–1176, 1952.

BRA,* Übertragbarkeit des Krebsparasiten auf Bäume. *Deutsche Medizinal Zeitung*, No. 80, p. 910, 1899.

BRAND, A. T., The etiology of cancer. *Brit. Med. J.*, **2**: 238–242, 1902.

BRANDES, W. W., WHITE, W. C., and SUTTON, J. B., Accidental transplantation of cancer in the operating room. With a case report. *Surg., Gynec. and Obst.*, **82**: 212–214, 1946.

BRAUNSTEINER, H., FELLINGER, K., and PAKESCH, F., On the occurrence of virus-like bodies in human leukemia. *Blood*, **15**: 476–479, 1960.

BRISMAN, R., BAKER, R. R., ELKINS, R., and HARTMANN, W. H., Carcinoma of lung in four siblings. *Cancer*, **20**: 2048–2053, 1967.

BROCA, P., Traité des tumeurs. vol. **1**: Des tumeurs en general. p. 595. Paris, P. Asselin, 1866. vol. **2**: Des tumeurs en particulier. p. 540. Paris, P. Asselin, 1869.

* No first name in the original paper.

Brunschwig, A., Spontaneous regression of cancer. *Surgery*, **53**: 423–431, 1963.

Brunschwig, A., Southam, C. M., and Levin, A. G., Host resistance to cancer: Clinical experiments by homotransplants, autotransplants and admixture of autologous leucocytes. *Ann. Surg.*, **162**: 416–423, 1965.

Burger, C. L., Harris, W. W., Anderson, N. G., Bartlett, T. W., and Kinseley, R. M., Virus-like particles in human leukemic plasma. *Proc. Soc. Exp. Biol. & Med.*, **115**: 151–156, 1964.

Burkard, H., Gleichzeitige und gleichartige Geschwulstbildung in der linken Brustdrüse bei Zwillingschwestern. *Deutsche Zeitschr. f. Chir.*, **169**: 166–174, 1922.

Burton, L., Friedman, F., Kassel, R., Kaplan, M. L., and Rottino, A., The purification and action of tumor factor extracted from mouse and human neoplastic tissue. *Trans. N.Y. Acad. Sci.*, **21**: 700–707, 1959.

Cameron, J. C., The influence of leukemia upon pregnancy and labor. *Am. J. Med. Sci.*, **95**: 28–34, 1888.

Caspar, D. L. D., Dulbecco, R., Klug, A., Lwoff, A., Stoker, M. G. P., Tournier, P., and Wildy, P., Proposals. *Cold Spring Harbor Symposium on Quantitative Biology*, **27**: 49, 1962.

Cavanagh, J. B., Greenbaum, D., Marshall, A. H. E., and Rubinstein, L. J., Cerebral demyelination associated with disorders of reticuloendothelial system. *Lancet*, **2**: 524–529, 1959.

Champlin, H. W., Similar tumors of testis occurring in identical twins. *J. Am. Med. Assoc.*, **95**: 96–97, 1930.

Chowdhury, J. R., Tumor formation in Swiss mice with human cancer filtrate. *Ann. N.Y. Acad. Sci.*, **136**: 261–271, 1966.

Clowes, G. H. A., and Baeslack, F. W., Further evidence of immunity against cancer in mice after spontaneous recovery. *Med. News*, **87**: 968–971, 1905.

Committee on Standardized Genetic Nomenclature for Mice. Standardized nomenclature for inbred strains of mice. Second listing. *Cancer Research*, **20**: 145–169, 1960.

Cornil, V., Sur les greffes et inoculations de cancer. *Bull Acad. Méd.* (*Paris*), **25**: 906–909, 1891.

Crawford, L. V., and Crawford, E. M., A comparative study of polyoma and papilloma viruses. *Virology*, **21**: 258–263, 1963.

Dalldorf, G., and Bergamini, F., Unidentified, filtrable agents isolated from African children with malignant lymphomas. *Proc. Nat. Acad. Sci., USA*, **51**: 263–265, 1964.

Dalldorf, G., Bergamini, F., and Frost, P., Further observations of the lymphomas of African children. *Proc. Nat. Acad. Sci., USA*, **55**: 297–302, 1966.

Dalton, A. J., Kilham, L., and Zeigel, R. F., A comparison of polyoma, "K," and Kilham rat viruses with the electron microscope. *Virology*, **20**: 391–398, 1963.

Dalton, A. J., Moloney, J. B., Porter, G. H., Frei, E., and Mitchell, E., Studies on murine and human leukemia. *Trans. Assoc. Am. Physicians*, **77**: 52–63, 1964.

Dalton, A. J., Potter, M., and Merwin, R. M., Some ultrastructural characteristics of a series of primary and transplanted plasma-cell tumors of the mouse. *J. Nat. Cancer Inst.*, **26**: 1221–1267, 1961.

Dameshek, W., Savitz, H. A., and Arbor, B., Chronic lymphatic leukemia in twin brothers aged fifty-six. *J. Am. Med. Assoc.*, **92**: 1348–1349, 1929.

Decastello, A., Beitrag zur Kenntnis der familiären Leukämie. *Med. Klin.*, **35**: 1255–1257, 1939.

Deelman, H. T., Heredity and cancer. *Ann. Surg.*, **93**: 30–34, 1931.

de Harven, E., Virus particles in the thymus of conventional and germ-free mice. *J. Exp. Med.*, **120**: 857–868, 1964.

Delbet. (Cited by H. Kurtzahn. *Klin. Wochenschr.*, **1**: 1166–1168, 1926).

DeLong, R., Production of leukemia in mice with cell-free filtrates from human leukemias. *J. Lab. & Clin. Med.*, **56**: 891–893, 1960.

de Martel, T., À propos de l'évolution du cancer. *Bull. Soc. nat. Chir.*, **60**: 1390–1394, 1934.

de Pasqualini, C. D., Pavlovsky, A., Vasquez, C., Holmberg, E. A. D., and Rabasa, S. L., Leukemia of short latency in mice injected with human malignant tissue by intrasplenic route. *Cancer Research*, **25**: 565–574, 1965.

Dmochowski, L., and Grey, C. E., Subcellular structures of possible viral origin in some mammalian tumors. *Ann. N.Y. Acad. Sci.*, **68**: 559–615, 1957.

Dmochowski, L., and Grey, C. E., Studies on submicroscopic structure of leukemias of known or suspected viral origin: A review. *Blood*, **13**: 1017–1042, 1958.

Dmochowski, L., Grey, C. E., Sykes, J. A., Shullenberger, C. C., and Howe, C. D., Studies on human leukemia. *Proc. Soc. Exp. Biol. & Med.*, **101**: 686–690, 1959.

Dmochowski, L., Grey, C. E., Dreyer, D. A., Sykes, J. A., Langford, P. L., and Taylor, H. G., Mycoplasma (Pleuropneumonia-like Organisms [PPLO]) and human leukemia. *Med. Rec. and Ann.*, **57**: 563–568, 1964.

Dmochowski, L., Seman, G., Myers, B., and Gallager, H. S., Relationship of viruses to the origin of human breast cancer. An exploratory study of the submicroscopic appearance of human breast cancer. *Med. Rec. and Ann.*, **61**: 384–411, 1968.

Dmochowski, L., Taylor, H. G., Grey, C. E., Dreyer, D. A., Sykes, J. A., Langford, P. L., Rogers, T., Shullenberger, C. C., and Howe, C. D., Viruses and mycoplasma (PPLO) in human leukemia. *Cancer*, **18**: 1345–1368, 1965.

Dmochowski, L., Yumoto, T., Grey, C. E., Hales, R. L., Langford, P. L., Taylor, H. G., Freireich, E. J., Shullenberger, C. C., Shively, J. A., and Howe, C. D., Electron microscopic studies of human leukemia and lymphoma. *Cancer*, **20**: 760–777, 1967.

Dolman, C. L., Furesz, J., and Mackay, B., Progressive multifocal leukoencephalopathy: Two cases with electron microscopic and viral studies. *Canad. Med. Assoc. J.*, **97**: 8–12, 1967.

Domermuth, C. H., Nielsen, M. H., Freundt, E. A., and Birch-Andersen, A., Ultrastructure of *mycoplasma* species. *J. Bact.*, **88**: 727–744, 1964.

Dossetor, J. B., Unpublished data presented at Washington Conference on Human Kidney Transplants. Washington, D.C., May, 1965. (Cited by R. E. Wilson *et al.*, *New Eng. J. Med.*, **278**: 479–483, 1968).

Dourmashkin, R., and Bernhard, W., A study with the electron microscope of the skin tumour of molluscum contagiosum. *J. Ultrastructure Research*, **3**: 11–38, 1959.

Dourmashkin, R., and Duperrat, B., Observation au microscope électronique du virus du *Molluscum contagiosum*. *Compt. Rend. Acad. Sci.* (*Paris*), **246**: 3133–3136, 1958.

DOURMASHKIN, R., and FEBVRE, H. L., Culture *in vitro* sur des cellules de la souche HéLa et identification au microscope électronique du virus du *Molluscum contagiosum. Compt. Rend. Acad. Sci.* (*Paris*), **246**: 2308–2310, 1958.

DOYEN, E., Étiologie et traitement du cancer. p. 169. A. Maloine, Paris, 1904.

DUFFELL, D., HINZ, R., and NELSON, E., Neoplasms in hamsters induced by simian virus 40. Light and electron microscopic observations. *Am. J. Path.*, **45**: 59–73, 1964.

DUNPHY, J. E., Some observations on the natural behavior of cancer in man. *New Eng. J. Med.*, **242**: 167–172, 1950.

EPSTEIN, M. A., ACHONG, B. G., and BARR, Y. M., Virus particles in cultured lymphoblasts from Burkitt's lymphoma. *Lancet*, **1**: 702–703, 1964.

EPSTEIN, M. A., ACHONG, B. G., and POPE, J. H., Virus in cultured lymphoblasts from a New Guinea Burkitt lymphoma. *Brit. Med. J.*, **2**: 290–291, 1967.

EVERSON, T. C., and COLE, W. H., Spontaneous regression of cancer: Preliminary report. *Ann. Surg.*, **144**: 366–383, 1956.

EVERSON, T. C., and COLE, W. H., Spontaneous regression of malignant disease. Guest editorial. *J. Am. Med. Assoc.*, **159**: 1758–1759, 1959.

EWING, J., Neoplastic diseases. A treatise on tumors. 4th Edition. p. 1160. W. B. Saunders, Co., Philadelphia and London, 1940.

FALLON, R. J., GRIST, N. R., INMAN, D. R., LEMCKE, R. M., NEGRONI, G., and WOODS, D. A., Further studies of agents isolated from tissue cultures inoculated with human leukaemic bone-marrow. *Brit. Med. J.*, **2**: 388–391, 1965.

FALLS, H. F., Inheritance of retinoblastoma. Two families supplying evidence. *J. Am. Med. Assoc.*, **133**: 171–174, 1947.

FELLER, W. F., and CHOPRA, H. C., A small virus-like particle observed in human breast cancer by means of electron microscopy. *J. Nat. Cancer Inst.*, **40**: 1359–1373, 1968.

FINNEY, W. P., A cancer family. *Proc. Staff Meet. Mayo Clin.*, **7**: 383–384, 1932.

FIRKIN, B. G., O'NEILL, B. J., DUNSTAN, B., and OLDFIELD, R., Effect of incubation and storage on human platelet structure as studied by electron microscopy. *Blood*, **25**: 345–355, 1965.

FLOCKS, J. S., WEIS, T. P., KLEINMAN, D. C., and KIRSTEN, W. H., Dose-response studies to polyoma virus in rats. *J. Nat. Cancer Inst.*, **35**: 259–284, 1965.

FORKNER, C. E., Leukemia and allied disorders. p. 333. MacMillan Co., New York, 1938.

FRANCK, E., Napoleon's family (Ca). *Berl. Med. Wochenschr.*, **110**: 119–131, 1904.

GAYLORD, H. R., and CLOWES, G. H. A., On spontaneous cure of cancer. *Surg., Gynec. and Obst.*, **2**: 633–658, 1906.

GIRARDI, A. J., HAYFLICK, L., LEWIS, A. M., and SOMERSON, N. L., Recovery of mycoplasmas in the study of human leukaemia and other malignancies. *Nature*, **205**: 188–189, 1965.

GIRARDI, A. J., HILLEMAN, M. R., and ZWICKEY, R. E., Search for virus in human malignancies. 2. *In vivo* studies. *Proc. Soc. Exp. Biol. & Med.*, **111**: 84–93, 1962a.

GIRARDI, A. J., SLOTNICK, V. B., and HILLEMAN, M. R., Search for virus in human malignancies. 1. *In vitro* studies. *Proc. Soc. Exp. Biol. & Med.*, **110**: 776–785, 1962b.

GORDON, R. D., Hereditary factors in human leukaemia: A report of four cases of leukaemia in a family. *Austral. Ann. Med.*, **12**: 202–207, 1963.

GRACE, J. T., JR., and KONDO, T., Investigations of host resistance in cancer patients. *Ann. Surg.*, **148**: 633–641, 1958.

Grace, J. T., Jr., Horoszewicz, J. S., Stim, T. B., Mirand, E. A., and James, C., Mycoplasmas (PPLO) and human leukemia and lymphoma. *Cancer*, **18**: 1369–1376, 1965.

Grace, J. T., Mirand, E. A., Mount, D. T., and Metzgar, R., Oncogenic properties of extracts of human tumors. (Abstract). *Proc. Am. Assoc. Cancer Research*, **3**: 115, 1960a.

Grace, J. T., Jr., Mirand, E. A., and Mount, D. T., Relationship of viruses to malignant disease. Part II. Oncogenic properties of cell-free filtrates of human tumors. *Arch. Intern. Med.*, **105**: 482–491, 1960b.

Graffi, A., Bierwolf, D., Baumbach, L., Blankenhagel, H., Widmaier, R., and Randt, A., Viruspartikel in Zellen myeloischer Leukämien des Menschen. *Deutsche Gesundheitswesen*, **19**: 1576–1580, 1964.

Graham, H. F., The influence of heredity in cancer. *Ann. Surg.*, **104**: 952–956, 1936.

Grist, N. R., and Fallon, R. J., Isolation of viruses from leukaemic patients. Letter to the Editor. *Brit. Med. J.*, **2**: 1263, 1964.

Gross, L., Intradermal immunization of C3H mice against a sarcoma that originated in an animal of the same line. *Cancer Research*, **3**: 326–333, 1943.

Gross, L., Is cancer a communicable disease? *Cancer Research*, **4**: 293–303, 1944.

Gross, L., Cancer treatment by autovaccination. *J. Am. Med. Assoc.*, **133**: 800, 1947.

Gross, L., Pathogenic properties and "vertical" transmission of the mouse leukemia agent. *Proc. Soc. Exp. Biol. & Med.*, **78**: 342–348, 1951.

Gross, L., Danger of implanting tumor cells in human beings for the purpose of "immunization." Letter to the Editor. *Ann. Surg.*, **135**: 751–753, 1952a.

Gross, L., Delayed effects of inoculation of Ak-leukemic cells in mice of the C3H line. A working hypothesis on the etiology of mouse leukemia. *Cancer*, **5**: 620–624, 1952b.

Gross, L., A filterable agent, recovered from Ak leukemic extracts, causing salivary gland carcinomas in C3H mice. *Proc. Soc. Exp. Biol. & Med.*, **83**: 414–421, 1953.

Gross, L., Is leukemia caused by a transmissible virus? A working hypothesis. *Blood*, **9**: 557–573, 1954.

Gross, L., Viral (egg-borne) etiology of mouse leukemia. Filtered extracts from leukemic C58 mice, causing leukemia (or parotid tumors) following inoculation into newborn C57 Brown or C3H mice. *Cancer*, **9**: 778–791, 1956.

Gross, L., Attempt to recover filterable agent from X-ray-induced leukemia. *Acta Haemat.*, **19**: 353–361, 1958.

Gross, L., and Matte, M. L., Occurrence of tumors and leukemia in members of families of patients suffering from leukemia. *New York J. Med.*, **48**: 1283–1284, 1948.

Gross, L., Gessler, A. E., and McCarthy, K. S., Electron-microscopic examination of human milk particularly from women having family record of breast cancer. *Proc. Soc. Exp. Biol. & Med.*, **75**: 270–276, 1950.

Grossman, M. O., and Kesert, B. H., Familial incidence of tumors of the brain. Cerebellar hemangioblastoma. *Arch. Neurol. and Psychiat.*, **52**: 327–328, 1944.

Guasch, J., Hérédité des leucémies. *Le Sang*, **25**: 384–421, 1954.

Guelliot, O., La contagion du cancer. Revue générale. *Gazette des Hôpitaux*, **65**: 1209–1217, 1892.

Gunz, F., and Dameshek, W., Chronic lymphocytic leukemia in a family, including twin brothers and a son. *J. Am. Med. Assoc.*, **164**: 1323–1325, 1957.

Haguenau, F., Le cancer mammaire de la souris et de la femme. Étude comparative au microscope électronique. *Path. Biol.* (*Paris*), **7**: 989–1015, 1959.

HAGUENAU, F., Structure fine de cancers de la glande mammaire chez la femme. pp. 462–466 in: vol. II, *Proc. Fourth Internat. Conf. on Electron Microscopy* (Berlin, Sept. 10–17, 1958). Springer-Verlag, Berlin, 1960a.

HAGUENAU, F., Significance of ultrastructure in virus-induced tumors. pp. 211–249 in: *Symposium, Phenomena of the Tumor Viruses. Nat. Cancer Inst. Monograph No. 4,* U.S. Publ. Health Service, Bethesda, Md., 1960b.

HAGUENAU, F., and HOLLMANN, K. H., Diagnostic différentiel entre virus et particules cytoplasmiques d'autre nature. Le problème au cours de l'étude des tumeurs au microscope électronique. *Bull. du Cancer,* **50**: 29–48, 1963.

HAGUENAU, F., HOLLMANN, K. H., LÉVY, J.-P., and BOIRON, M., Étude au microscope électronique des plaquettes sanguines dans les leucémies humaines. *J. Microscopie,* **2**: 529–538, 1963.

HAHN, E., Über transplantation von carcinomatöser Haut. *Berliner klin. Wochenschr.,* **25**: 413–415, 1888.

HAMAZAKI, Y., Experimental induction of leukosis following ingestion of human neoplasms. *J. Karyopath.* (*Okayama*), **11**: 1–4, 1966.

HANDLEY, W. S., Chronic mastitis and breast cancer. A family history of five sisters. *Brit. Med. J.,* **2**: 113–116, 1938.

HAREL, J., HUPPERT, J., LACOUR, F., and LACOUR, J., Induction de tumeurs malignes chez le souriceau nouveau-né, par injection d'une préparation d'acide ribonucléique extrait de ganglions leucémiques humains. *Compt. Rend. Acad. Sci.* (*Paris*), **247**: 795–796, 1958.

HAREL, J., HUPPERT, J., LACOUR, F., and LACOUR, J., Tumeurs malignes transmissibles de la souris, provoquées par injection de préparations contenant de l'acide ribonucléique. Étude biologique et histologique. *Bull. du Cancer,* **46**: 75–91, 1959.

HAUSER, I. J., and WELLER, C. V., A further report on the cancer family of Warthin. *Am. J. Cancer,* **27**: 434–449, 1936.

HAYFLICK, L., Editor. Conference on the Biology of the mycoplasma. *Ann. N.Y. Acad. Sci.,* **143**: 1–824, 1967.

HAYFLICK, L., and CHANOCK, R. M., *Mycoplasma* species of man. *Bact. Reviews,* **29**: 185–221, 1965.

HAYFLICK, L., and KOPROWSKI, H., Direct agar isolation of mycoplasmas from human leukaemic bone marrow. *Nature,* **205**: 713–714, 1965.

HEATH, C. W., JR., and HASTERLIK, R. J., Leukemia among children in a suburban community. *Am. J. Med.,* **34**: 796–812, 1963.

HEATH, C. W., JR., and MOLONEY, W. C., Familial leukemia. Five cases of acute leukemia in three generations. *New Eng. J. Med.,* **272**: 882–887, 1965.

HEIDENHAIN, L., Ist Krebs durch Zerfallsprodukte übertragbar? *Zeitschr. f. Krebsforsch.,* **36**: 360–364, 1932.

HEINZELMANN, F., A cancer prone family. Discussion of the question of inheritability of colonic carcinoma. *Helv. Chir. Acta,* **31**: 316–324, 1964.

HERBUT, P. A., Human leukemia virus in mice. *Arch. Path.,* **83**: 123–131, 1967.

HERRELL, W. E., RUFF, J. D., and BAYRD, E. D., Multiple myeloma in siblings. *J. Am. Med. Assoc.,* **167**: 1485–1486, 1958.

HORNBAKER, J. H., Chronic leukemia in three sisters. *Am. J. Med. Sci.,* **203**: 322–325, 1942.

HOWARD, J. M., Studies of autotransplantation of incurable cancer. *Surg., Gynec. and Obst.,* **117**: 567–572, 1963.

HOWATSON, A. F., and ALMEIDA, J. D., An electron microscope study of polyoma virus in hamster kidney. *J. Biophys. and Biochem. Cytol.,* **7**: 753–760, 1960.

HOWATSON, A. F., NAGAI, M., and ZU RHEIN, G. M., Polyoma-like virions in human demyelinating brain disease. *Canad. Med. Assoc. J.,* **93**: 379–386, 1965.

HUBARD, 1926. (Cited by H. Kurtzahn. *Klin. Wochenschr.*, **1**: 1166–1168, 1926).

HUMMELER, K., TOMASSINI, N., and HAYFLICK, L., Ultrastructure of a mycoplasma (Negroni) isolated from human leukemia. *J. Bact.*, **90**: 517–523, 1965.

INMAN, D. R., WOODS, D. A., and NEGRONI, G., Electron microscopy of virus particles in cell cultures inoculated with passage fluid from human leukaemic bone-marrow. *Brit. Med. J.*, **1**: 929–931, 1964.

IOACHIM, H., Acute leukemia in uniovular twins. Review of genetic aspects of human leukemia. *Cancer*, **15**: 539–545, 1962.

JOHNSON, M. J. E., and PETERS, C. H., Lymphomas in four siblings. *J. Am. Med. Assoc.*, **163**: 20–25, 1957.

JÜRGENS,* Recherches expérimentales sur l'étiologie des sarcomes. *Semaine Médicale*, **16**: 229, 1896.

KALIAMPETSOS, G., Kommen Blutkrankheiten und Karzinome unter den Verwandten von Leukämiekranken gehäuft vor? *Deutsche med. Wochenschr.*, **79**: 1783–1785, 1954.

KATZ, S.,† Henri Vadon. Vadon et le problème de la transmission du cancer. p. 106. *Thèse de Paris.* Les Presses Universitaires de France, Paris, 1930.

KATZMAN, R. A., Studies on the induction of leukemia in Swiss mice by cell-free filtrates from human tissues. *J. Lab. and Clin. Med.*, **60**: 579–588, 1962.

KILHAM, L., Isolation in suckling mice of a virus from C3H mice harboring Bittner milk agent. *Science*, **116**: 391–392, 1952.

KILHAM, L., and MURPHY, H. W., A pneumotropic virus isolated from C3H mice carrying the Bittner milk agent. *Proc. Soc. Exp. Biol. & Med.*, **82**: 133–137, 1953.

KIRSTEN, W. H., MAYER, L. A., WOLLMANN, R. L., and PIERCE, M. I., Studies on a murine erythroblastosis virus. *J. Nat. Cancer Inst.*, **38**: 117–139, 1967.

KOIKE, A., MOORE, G. E., MENDOZA, C. B., JR., and WATNE, A. L., Heterologous, homologous, and autologous transplantation of human tumors. *Cancer*, **16**: 1065–1071, 1963.

KÖRBLER, J., Vererbung der Krebskrankheit. *Zeitschr. f. Krebsforsch.*, **40**: 271–279, 1934.

KRITSCHEWSKI, I. L., and RUBINSTEIN, P. L., Das durch Filtrate überimpfbare polymorphzellige Angiosarkom der Säugetiere. I. Die antigenen Eigenschaften der Geschwulst und die Fähigkeit ihres Filtrats, eine Geschwulst hervorzurufen. *Zeitschr. f. Krebsforsch.*, **28**: 96–105, 1929.

KURTZAHN, H., Über die transplantation menschlichen Carcinoms. *Klin. Wochenschr.*, **1**: 1166–1168, 1926.

LACOUR, F., LACOUR, J., HAREL, J., and HUPPERT, J., Transplantable malignant tumors in mice induced by preparations containing ribonucleic acid extracted from human and mouse tumors. *J. Nat. Cancer Inst.*, **24**: 301–328, 1960.

LANGER, E., Human experimentation: Cancer studies at Sloan-Kettering stir public debate on medical ethics. *Science*, **143**: 551–553, 1964.

LECÈNE, P., and LACASSAGNE, A., Une observation d'inoculation accidentelle d'une tumeur maligne chez l'homme. *Ann. Anat. Path.*, **3**: 97–112, 1926.

LEGG, M. A., and BRADY, W. J., Pathology and clinical behavior of thymomas. A survey of 51 cases. *Cancer*, **18**: 1131–1144, 1965.

LEPLUS, R., BERNHARD, W., and OBERLING, C., Mise en évidence au microscope électronique d'inclusions cytoplasmiques particulières dans un cas de myxosarcome humain. *Compt. Rend. Acad. Sci.* (*Paris*), **244**: 2110–2113, 1957.

* No first name in the original paper.

† The name of the author is Katz, S. The title of the paper is: "Henri Vadon. Vadon et le problème de la transmission du cancer."

LEPLUS, R., DEBRAY, J., PINET, J., and BERNHARD, W., Lésions nucléaires décelées au microscope électronique dans des cellules de "lymphomes malins" chez l'homme. *Compt. Rend. Acad. Sci.* (*Paris*), **253**: 2788–2790, 1961.

LEVESQUE, G., Contribution à l'étude des inoculations opératoires du cancer. p. 182. *Thèse de Paris No. 287.* G. Steinheil, Paris, 1903.

LÉVY, J.-P., and OPPENHEIM, E., Virus et leucémies humaines. *Path. Biol.* (*Paris*), **14**: 966–975, 1966.

LIBER, A. F., Ovarian cancer in mother and five daughters. *Arch. Path.*, **49**: 280–290, 1950.

LLOYD, O. C., and URICH, H., Acute disseminated demyelination of brain associated with lymphosarcoma. *Lancet*, **2**: 529–530, 1959.

LOCK, S. P., and MERRINGTON, M., Leukaemia in Lewisham (1957–63). *Brit. Med. J.*, **3**: 759–760, 1967.

LOMER, R., Zur Frage der Heilbarkeit des Carcinoms. *Zeitschr. f. Geburtsh. u. Gynäk.*, **50**: 305–384, 1903.

LUNGER, P. D., LUCAS, J. C., and SHIPKEY, F. H., The ultramorphology of milk fractions from normal and breast cancer patients. *Cancer*, **17**: 549–557, 1964.

MACKLIN, M. T., Human tumours and their inheritance. *Canad. Med. Assoc. J.*, **27**: 182–187, 1932.

MACKLIN, M. T., The role of heredity in gastric and intestinal cancer. *Gastroenterology*, **29**: 507–511, 1955.

MACKLIN, M. T., Comparison of the number of breast-cancer deaths observed in relatives of breast-cancer patients, and the number expected on the basis of mortality rates. *J. Nat. Cancer Inst.*, **22**: 927–951, 1959.

MAGRASSI, F., Human leukaemia as "conditional disease" related to a viral etiology. pp. 418–483, in: *Compt. Rend. 3rd Congress Internat. European Soc. Hemat.*, Rome, October 3–6, 1951.

MAGRASSI, F., LEONARDI, G., NEGRONI, G., and TOLU, A., Experimental studies on the aetiology of human leukaemias. *Acta Haemat.*, **6**: 38–50, 1951.

MANSON, J. S. Hereditary transmission of sarcoma. *Brit. Med. J.*, **2**: 1135–1137, 1913.

MARGOLIS, J., and WEST, D., Spontaneous regression of malignant disease: Report of three cases. *J. Am. Geriatrics Soc.*, **15**: 251–253, 1967.

MARTIN, A. J., Cancer *à deux*. *Brit. Med. J.*, **2**: 427, 1902.

MARTIN, D. C., RUBINI, M., and ROSEN, V. J., Cadaveric renal homotransplantation with inadvertent transplantation of carcinoma. *J. Am. Med. Assoc.*, **192**: 752–754, 1965.

MARTYNOVA, R. P., Studies in the genetics of human neoplasms. Cancer of the breast. Based upon 201 family histories. *Am. J. Cancer*, **29**: 530–540, 1937.

MAS Y MAGRO, F., Recherches morphologiques et expérimentales sur l'étiopathogenie de la leucémie humaine. IV. Expériences de transmission de la leucémie myéloïde chronique humaine chez le cobaye. *Le Sang*, **25**: 166–171, 1954.

MATHÉ, G., Virus et leucémies humaines. *Presse Méd.*, **72**: 2831–2832, 1964.

MAYET*, Production du cancer chez les rats blancs par introduction dans leur économie des substances constituantes des tumeurs malignes de l'homme. *Gazette Hebdomadaire de Médecine et de Chirurgie*, **7** (n.s.): 64–68, 1902.

MAZAR, S. A., and STRAUS, B., Marital Hodgkin's disease. A review of the familial incidence and of etiological factors. *Arch. Intern. Med.*, **88**: 819–830, 1951.

MCFARLAND, J., and MEADE, T. S., The genetic origin of tumors supported by their simultaneous and symmetrical occurrence in homologous twins. *Am. J. Med. Sci.*, **184**: 66–80, 1932.

* No first name in the original paper.

McIntosh, D. A., McPhaul, J. J., Peterson, E. W., Harvin, J. S., Smith, J. R., Cook, F. E., and Humphreys, J. W., Jr., Homotransplantation of a cadaver neoplasm and a renal homograft. *J. Am. Med. Assoc.*, **192**: 1171–1173, 1965.

McPhaul, J. J., Jr., and McIntosh, D. A., Tissue transplantation still vexes. Letter to the Editor. *New Eng. J. Med.*, **272**: 105, 1965.

Melnick, J. L., Papova virus group. *Science*, **135**: 1128–1130, 1962.

Milham, S., Jr., Leukemia in husbands and wives. *Science*, **148**: 98–100, 1965.

Militzer, R. E., Carcinoma of the stomach in identical twins. *Am. J. Cancer*, **25**: 544–550, 1935.

Moore, A. E., Induction of tumors in newborn mice by inoculation of preparations of human tissues. (Abstract). *Proc. Am. Assoc. Cancer Research*, **3**: 135, 1960.

Moore, A. E., and Caparó, A. C., Tumors occurring in newborn mice after inoculation of human cancer material. *Cancer Research*, **24**: 765–769, 1964.

Morgan, C., Godman, G. C., Breitenfeld, P. M., and Rose, H. M., A correlative study by electron and light microscopy of the development of type 5 adenovirus. I. Electron microscopy. *J. Exp. Med.*, **112**: 373–382, 1960.

Morse, D. P., The hereditary aspect of breast cancer in mother and daughter. *Cancer*, **4**: 745–748, 1951.

Morton, J. J., and Morton, J. H., Cancer as a chronic disease. *Ann. Surg.*, **137**: 683–703, 1953.

Muller, J., and Watanabe, I., Progressive multifocal leukoencephalopathy. A virus disease? *Am. J. Clin. Path.*, **47**: 114–123, 1967.

Murphy, W. H., and Furtado, D., Isolation of viruses from children with acute leukemia. *Univ. of Michigan Med. Bull.*, **29**: 201–228, 1963.

Murphy, W. H., Ertel, I. J., and Zarafonetis, C. J. D., Virus studies of human leukemia. *Cancer*, **18**: 1329–1344, 1965a.

Murphy, W. H., Furtado, D., and Plata, E., Possible association between leukemia in children and virus-like agents. *J. Am. Med. Assoc.*, **191**: 110–115, 1965b.

Murray, J. E., Gleason, R., and Bartholomay, A., Fourth Report of the Human Kidney Transplant Registry: 16 September 1964 to 15 March 1965. *Transplantation*, **3**: 684–699, 1965.

Nadler, S. H., and Moore, G. E., Autotransplantation of human cancer. *J. Am. Med. Assoc.*, **191**: 105–106, 1965.

Negroni, G., Isolation of viruses from leukaemic patients. *Brit. Med. J.*, **1**: 927–929, 1964.

Nelson, D. H., Spontaneous regression of cancer. *Clin. Radiology*, **13**: 138–140, 1962.

Nemenova, N. M., and Bergoltz*, V. M., Morphological analysis of systemic disease caused in mice by injection of acellular extracts of human tissue. (Russian text). *Probl. Gematol., Perel Krovi*, **4**/**1**: 28–33, 1959. Abstract in *Excerpta Med., Sect. XVI* (*Cancer*), **7** (2): 1143–1144, 1959.

Nilsson, O., Ultrastructure of mouse uterine surface epithelium under different estrogenic influences. 2. Early effect of estrogen administered to spayed animals. *J. Ultrastructure Research*, **2**: 73–95, 1958.

Oberling, C., *Le Cancer*. 7th Edition. p. 381. Gallimard, Publ., Paris, 1954.

* See different spelling (Bergolz) in other publications of same author.

PACK, G. T., Cancer of the stomach in brothers. *Ann. Surg.*, **100**: 1016–1018, 1934.

PARNES, V. A., and SUNTSOVA, V. V., Induction of leukemia in mice by administration of material from leukemic subjects. *Pat. Fiziol. Eksp. Ter.*, **3**: 14–20, 1959.

PARSONS, D. F., Morphology of K virus and its relation to the papova group of viruses. *Virology*, **20**: 385–387, 1963.

PASS, K. E., Erbpathologische Untersuchungen in Familien von Hirntumoren. *Zeitschr. f. d. ges. Neurol. u. Psychiat.*, **161**: 204–211, 1938.

PAULSEN, J., Konstitution und Krebs. *Zeitschr. f. Krebsforsch.*, **21**: 119–130, 1924.

PENN, I., HAMMOND, W., BRETTSCHNEIDER, L., and STARZL, T. E., Malignant lymphomas in transplantation patients. *Second Internat. Congress of Transplantation Soc., Sept. 4–11, 1968, New York.* Proceedings to be published by Grune and Stratton, Inc., New York.

PEYRILHE, B., Dissertation académique sur le cancer qui a remporté le prix double de l'Académie des Sciences, Arts & Belles Lettres de Lyon, le 8 Décembre 1773, pp. 135. Chez Ruault, Paris.

POHLE, E. A., Concurrence of osteogenic sarcoma in two sisters. *Radiology*, **27**: 545–548, 1936.

PORTER, G. H., III, DALTON, A. J., MOLONEY, J. B., and MITCHELL, E. Z., Association of electron-dense particles with human acute leukemia. *J. Nat. Cancer Inst.*, **33**: 547–556, 1964.

POWER, J. H., The history of a cancerous family. *Brit. Med. J.*, **2**: 154, 1898.

PRINCE, A. M., and ADAMS, W. R., Virus-like particles in human plasma and serum from leukemic, hepatitic, and control patients. (Abstract). *Fed. Proc.*, **24**: 175, 1965.

PRINCE, A. M., and ADAMS, W. R., Virus-like particles in human plasma and serum: Role of platelet lysosomes. *J. Nat. Cancer Inst.*, **37**: 153–166, 1966.

QUEYRAT, 1893. (Cited by A. Velich. *Wiener Med. Blätter*, **21**: 711–712, 1898, and **21**: 729–731, 1898.)

RABSON, A. S., O'CONOR, G. T., BARON, S., WHANG, J. J., and LEGALLAIS, F. Y., Morphologic, cytogenic and virologic studies *in vitro* of a malignant lymphoma from an African child. *Internat. J. Cancer*, **1**: 89–106, 1966.

RAPPIN, G., Recherches sur l'inoculabilité du cancer. pp. 15. Imprimerie Moderne, Nantes, 1890.

RAPPIN, G., Sur l'étiologie microbienne du cancer. *Compt. Rend. Acad. Sci. (Paris)*, **198**: 2030–2031, 1934.

RICHARDSON, E. P., JR., Progressive multifocal leukoencephalopathy. *New Eng. J. Med.*, **265**: 815–823, 1961.

RIGBY, P. G., PRATT, P. T., ROSENLOF, R. C., and LEMON, H. M., Genetic relationships in familial leukemia and lymphoma. *Arch. Intern. Med.*, **121**: 67–70, 1968.

RIGBY, P. G., ROSENLOF, R. C., PRATT, P. T., and LEMON, H. M., Leukemia and lymphoma. *J. Am. Med. Assoc.*, **197**: 25–30, 1966.

ROBERTS, C. W., and ROBERTS, C. P., Concurrent osteogenic sarcoma in brother and sisters. *J. Am. Med. Assoc.*, **105**: 181–185, 1935.

ROHDENBURG, G. L., Fluctuations in the growth energy of malignant tumors in man, with especial reference to spontaneous recession. *J. Cancer Research*, **3**: 193–225, 1918.

RUBINSTEIN, L. J., Discussion of paper by Zu Rhein and Chou. *44th Ann. Meeting of the Assoc. for Research in Nervous and Mental Disease, New York, December 4–5, 1964.* pp. 359–362 (vol. **44**), in: *Infections of the Nervous System.* Williams & Wilkins Co., Baltimore, Md., 1968.

Scanlon, E. F., Hawkins, R. A., Fox, W. W., and Smith, W. S., Fatal homotransplanted melanoma. A case report. *Cancer*, **18**: 782–789, 1965.

Scheuerlen*, Die Aetiologie des Carcinoms. *Berliner klin. Wochenschr.*, **24**: 935–936, 1887.

Schmidt, F., Zur heterologen Übertragung von Krebs- und Leukämiematerial des Menschen auf Laboratoriumstiere. *Zeitschr. f. Krebsforsch.*, **63**: 532–539, 1960.

Schmidt, P. J., Barile, M. F., and McGinniss, M. H., Mycoplasma (pleuropneumonia-like organisms) and blood group I; associations with neoplastic disease. *Nature*, **205**: 371–372, 1965.

Schwartz, S. O., Schoolman, H. M., and Szanto, P. B., Studies in leukemia. IV. The acceleration of the development of AKR lymphoma by means of cell-free filtrates. *Cancer Research*, **16**: 559–564, 1956.

Schwartz, S. O., Schoolman, H. M., Szanto, P. B., and Spurrier, W., Studies in leukemia. VI. The induction of leukemia in AKR mice by means of cell-free brain filtrates of humans who died of leukemia. *Cancer Research*, **17**: 218–221, 1957.

Schwartz, S. O., Spurrier, W., Yates, L., and Maduros, B. P., The induction of leukemia in Swiss mice with human leukemic brain extracts. (Abstract). *Proc. Am. Assoc. Cancer Research*, **3**: 149, 1960.

Schwerdt, P. R., Schwerdt, C. E., Silverman, L., and Rubinstein, L. J., Virions associated with progressive multifocal leukoencephalopathy. *Virology*, **29**: 511–514, 1966.

Seman, G., and Seman, C., Electron-microscopic search for virus particles in patients with leukemia and lymphoma. *Cancer*, **22**: 1033–1045, 1968.

Shipkey, F. H., and Tandler, B., Observations on human malignant lymphoma cells. page PP-9 in: *Electron Microscopy*, vol. 2. *Proc. 5th Internat. Congress for Electron Microscopy, Philadelphia, Pa.* (August 29–September 5, 1962). Academic Press, New York and London, 1962.

Shope, R. E., Koch's postulates and a viral cause of human cancer. Guest editorial. *Cancer Research*, **20**: 1119–1120, 1960.

Sibley, W. A., and Weisberger, A. S., Demyelinating disease of the brain in chronic lymphatic leukemia. Occurrence of a case in the husband of a patient with multiple sclerosis. *Arch. Neurol.*, **5**: 300–307, 1961.

Silcock, A. Q., Hereditary sarcoma of the eyeball in three generations. *Brit. Med. J.*, **1**: 1079, 1892.

Silverman, L., and Rubinstein, L. J., Electron microscopic observations on a case of progressive multifocal leukoencephalopathy. *Acta Neuropath.*, **5**: 215–224, 1965.

Smith, K. O., Benyesh-Melnick, M., and Fernbach, D. J., Studies on human leukemia. II. Structure and quantitation of myxovirus-like particles associated with human leukemia. *J. Nat. Cancer Inst.*, **33**: 557–570, 1964.

Smithers, D. W., Spontaneous regression of tumours. *Clin. Radiology*, **13**: 132–137, 1962.

Sorenson, G. D., Virus-like particles in myeloma cells of man. *Proc. Soc. Exp. Biol. & Med.*, **118**: 250–252, 1965.

Southam, C. M., and Brunschwig, A., Quantitative studies of autotransplantation of human cancer. Preliminary report. *Cancer*, **14**: 971–978, 1961.

Southam, C. M., Moore, A. E., and Rhoads, C. P., Homotransplantation of human cell lines. *Science*, **125**: 158–160, 1957.

* No first name in the original paper.

SOUTHAM, C. M., and MOORE, A. E., Induced immunity to cancer cell homografts in man. *Ann. N.Y. Acad. Sci.*, **73**: 635–653, 1958.

SPIES, J. W., ADAIR, F. E., and JOBE, M. C., An accidental autogenous transplantation of a mammary carcinoma to the thigh during a skin graft operation: A case report. *Am. J. Cancer*, **20**: 606–609, 1934.

STEINBERG, A. G., The genetics of acute leukemia in children. *Cancer*, **13**: 985–999, 1960.

STEINBERG, A. G., FARBER, S., and DOWNING, V., Case report. Personal communication to the author (unpublished), 1953.

STEINER, F., Familiäre Leukämie. *München. med. Wochenschr.*, **80**: 1822–1823, 1933.

STEWART, F. W., Experiences in spontaneous regression of neoplastic disease in man. *Texas Rep. Biol. & Med.*, **10**: 239–253, 1952.

STEWART, S. E., LANDON, J., LOVELACE, E., and MCBRIDE, J., Viruses in cultures of human leukemia cells. *Lavori Ist Anat. Univ. Perugia*, **23**: 153–166, 1963.

STEWART, S. E., LANDON, J., LOVELACE, E., and MCBRIDE, J., Viruses in cultures of human leukemia cells. pp. 271–282 in: *Internat. Symp.* (June 16–17, 1963, Rome). *Virus Nelle Leucemie dei Mammiferi*, vol. 361 (No. 65). Accademia Nazionale dei Lincei, Roma, 1964.

SYKES, J. A., DMOCHOWSKI, L., SHULLENBERGER, C. C., and HOWE, C. D., Tissue culture studies on human leukemia and malignant lymphoma. *Cancer Research*, **22**: 21–26, 1962.

SYKES, J. A., RECHER, L., JERNSTROM, P. H., and WHITESCARVER, J., Morphological investigation of human breast cancer. *J. Nat. Cancer Inst.*, **40**: 195–223, 1968.

TAYLOR, F. M., and GEPPERT, L. J., Congenital myelogenous leukemia. *Am. J. Dis. Child.*, **80**: 417–422, 1950.

THIERSCH, J. B., Attempts to transmit leucaemia of man and of mice to the chick embryo and to the young chick by the amniotic and intravenous routes. *Austral. J. Exp. Biol. & Med. Sci.*, **22**: 57–61, 1944.

THIERSCH, J. B., Attempted transmission of human leukemia in man. *J. Lab. & Clin. Med.*, **30**: 866–874, 1945.

THIERSCH, J. B., Aspects of leuchaemia. *Proc. Royal Austral. College of Physicians*, **2**: 31–47, 1947.

TILL, M. M., HARDISTY, R. M., PIKE, M. C., and DOLL, R., Childhood leukaemia in greater London: A search for evidence of clustering. *Brit. Med. J.*, **3**: 755–758, 1967.

TROSS, 1902. (Cited by A. T. Brand. *Brit. Med. J.*, **2**: 238–242, 1902).

TWINEM, F. P., Identical twins and the problem of heredity. *New York J. Med.*, **27**: 1192–1193, 1927.

VANDERHAEGHEN, J.-J., and PERIER, O., Leuco-encéphalite multifocale progressive. Mise en évidence de particules virales par la microscopie électronique. *Acta Neurol. Belg.*, **65**: 816–837, 1965.

VELICH, A., Beitrag zur Frage nach der Uebertragbarkeit des Sarcoms. *Wiener med. Blätter*, **21**: 711–712, and **21**: 729–731, 1898.

VIDEBAEK, A., Heredity in human leukemia and its relation to cancer. A genetic and clinical study of 209 probands. pp. 279. H. K. Lewis & Co., Ltd., London, 1947.

VIDEBAEK, A., and MOSBECH, J., The aetiology of gastric carcinoma elucidated by a study of 302 pedigrees. *Acta Medica Scandinavica*, **149**: 137–159, 1954.

VIOLA, M. V., DALTON, A. J., MITCHELL, E., and MOLONEY, J. B., Virus-like particles in a patient with chronic lymphocytic leukemia. *New Eng. J. Med.*, **277**: 503–506, 1967.

Waaler, G. H. M., Ueber die Erblichkeit des Krebses, Skrifter Utgitt av Det Norske Videnskaps-Akademi i Oslo. 1. Mat.-Naturv. Klasse No. 2, 1931. (Cited by C. V. Weller, *Am. J. Cancer*, **30**: 39–46, 1937).

Warthin, A. S., President's Address. The nature of cancer. Susceptibility in human families. *J. Cancer Research*, **12**: 249–258, 1928.

Weber, F. P., Schwartz, E., and Hellenschmied, R., Spontaneous inoculation of melanotic sarcoma from mother to foetus. *Brit. Med. J.*, **1**: 537–539, 1930.

Wehr, W., Demonstration der durch Impfung von Hund auf Hund erzeugten Carcinomknötchen. *Centralbl. f. Chir., Suppl. 24*, **15**: 8–9, 1888.

Weiner, L., A family with high incidence leukemia and unique Ph chromosome findings. (Abstract). *8th Ann. Meeting Am. Soc. Hemat., Philadelphia, Pa.* (December 4–7, 1965). *Blood*, **26**: 871, 1965.

Weinstein, V. F., Woolf, A. K., and Meynell, M. J., Progressive multifocal leucoencephalopathy and primary hypersplenism. With a note on the association between disease of the reticuloendothelial system and progressive multifocal leucoencephalopathy. *J. Clin. Path.*, **26**: 405–418, 1963.

Weller, C. V., Intrinsic factors in the etiology of neoplasms. *Am. J. Cancer*, **30**: 39–46, 1937.

Weller, C. V., The inheritance of retinoblastoma and its relationship to practical eugenics. *Cancer Research*, **1**: 517–535, 1941.

Whitaker, J. A., Bovis, R., Andrews, S. L., and Sulkin, S. E., Focal cellular alteration in stable amnion cells produced by inoculation with human leukemia brain extracts. *Cancer Research*, **23**: 519–522, 1963.

Williams, W. R., Note on multiple family cancer. *Brit. Med. J.*, **2**: 1612–1613, 1898.

Wilson, R. E., Hager, E. B., Hampers, C. L., Corson, J. M., Merrill, J. P., and Murray, J. E., Immunologic rejection of human cancer transplanted with a renal allograft. *New Eng. J. Med.*, **278**: 479–483, 1968.

Woglom, W. H., The study of experimental cancer. A review. *Studies in Cancer and Allied Subjects*, vol. 1, pp. 288. Columbia Univ. Press, New York, 1913.

Wolff, J., Die Lehre von der Krebskrankheit von den ältesten Zeiten bis zur Gegenwart. pp. 747. G. Fischer, Jena, 1907.

Wood, D. A., and Darling, H. H., A cancer family manifesting multiple occurrences of bilateral carcinoma of the breast. *Cancer Research*, **3**: 509–514, 1943.

Woolley, G. W., Occurrence of "neck tumors" in cortisone-treated leukemic-strain mice. (Abstract). *Proc. Am. Assoc. Cancer Research*, **1**: 53, 1954.

Zeve, V. H., Lucas, L. S., and Manaker, R. A., Continuous cell culture from a patient with chronic myelogenous leukemia. II. Detection of a herpes-like virus by electron microscopy. *J. Nat. Cancer Inst.*, **37**: 761–773, 1966.

Zu Rhein, G. M., Polyoma-like virions in a human demyelinating disease. *Acta Neuropath.* (*Berlin*), **8**: 57–68, 1967.

Zu Rhein, G. M., Association of papova virions with a human demyelinating disease (*progressive multifocal leukoencephalopathy*). *Progress in Medical Virology*, vol. **11**: 185–247. S. Karger, Publ., Basel and New York, 1969.

Zu Rhein, G. M., and Chou, S.-M., Papova virus in progressive multifocal leukoencephalopathy. *44th Ann. Meeting of the Assoc. for Research in Nervous and Mental Disease, New York, December 4–5, 1964*. pp. 307–359 (vol. **44**), in: *Infections of the Nervous System.* Williams & Wilkins Co., Baltimore, Md., 1968.

Zu Rhein, G. M., and Chou, S.-M., Particles resembling papova viruses in human cerebral demyelinating disease. *Science*, **148**: 1477–1479, 1965.

CHAPTER 23

The Etiology of Cancer and Allied Diseases Development of a Concept

We have reviewed in this monograph some of the principal oncogenic viruses recognized in experimental cancer research, and known to cause tumors in various species of animals. If a total list could be compiled of all tumors proved to be caused by filterable viruses, including also those for which only circumstantial evidence as to their viral origin is available, the results would be rather impressive.

The list of malignant tumors caused, or presumably caused, by oncogenic viruses would include most of the malignant tumors, including leukemia and lymphomas, in chickens, mice, and rats. Virus-induced tumors have also been described in rabbits, dogs, cats, hamsters, frogs, and other species. A virus-induced tumor in fish (Wessing and v. Bargen, 1959) and a lymphosarcoma transmissible by filtrates in the South African toad (Balls, 1965; Balls and Ruben, 1967) have been reported recently.

Oncogenic Viruses: Their Role in the Induction of Tumors

The number of tumors which can be transmitted by filtrates has been growing rapidly; it now appears that under proper experimental conditions most of the tumors observed in animals can be transmitted by filtered extracts, and are caused by oncogenic viruses. It is conceivable, and indeed probable, that virus-induced, malignant tumors in chickens, mice, rats, hamsters, and other animal species are essentially not different in their origin from those occurring in humans. Should this assumption, purely speculative at this time, prove to be true, it would then follow that all malignant tumors and lymphomas, including those occurring in man, are caused by oncogenic viruses.

Many questions remain unanswered, nevertheless. Are *all* malignant tumors caused by viruses? Are viruses necessary and indispensable to induce tumors, or do they represent only some of the many different factors which may be individually responsible for the development of tumors? Once an oncogenic virus has induced a tumor, is its presence required for the continuous growth of the neoplasm, or is the virus needed only to initiate the development of a tumor?

Data thus far available are insufficient to answer these fundamental questions. It is possible to assume, however, as a working hypothesis at least, that all malignant tumors are caused by viruses, and that the continuous presence of an oncogenic virus is necessary to assure progressive growth of the neoplasm. It is also possible to assume that oncogenic viruses enter the host's cells from without, or initially had entered the host's ancestors' cells from outside, i.e. are essentially of exogenous origin, although they might have been transmitted from host to host through many successive generations.

Is Cancer of Infectious Origin? Old and New Theories

The assumption that malignant tumors and related neoplastic diseases, such as leukemia and lymphomas, are caused by transmissible agents is not new. In the past, the theory of the infectious origin of cancer has been advanced and then abandoned many times. The belief that cancer is an infectious disease can be traced for several centuries. According to Brand (1902) and Ewing (1940), in the middle of the seventeenth century Sennert in Prague and Zacutus Lusitanus in Lisbon believed that cancer was contagious. In 1773 the Academy of Sciences at Lyon awarded a prize to Dr. B. Peyrilhe for his dissertation on the infectious origin of cancer (see also page 860 in the preceding chapter).

At first, when many communicable diseases were found to be caused by microbes or other relatively large microorganisms, attempts were made to detect similar causative microorganisms in malignant tumors. It soon became evident, however, that the various microbes, cocci, or other microorganisms readily visible in the light microscope and found in various human and animal tumors, were only accidentally present in such neoplasms, and that they actually had no causative relation to the etiology of cancer.*

At the turn of the century it became apparent that some of the diseases of infectious origin, for which no visible microbes could be detected under the microscope, were caused by submicroscopic, filterable viruses. The cause of cancer remained obscure, but its possibly infectious nature was considered.

In 1905, at the invitation of the editors of *Medizinische Klinik* (Berlin), some of the leading contemporary, mostly German, pathologists expressed their opinions as to the possibility of infectious origin of cancer (Umfrage über die Aetiologie des Krebses, *Med. Klin.*, **1**: 409–412, 496–499, and 544–547, 1905).

* For pertinent references the reader is referred to the preceding chapter.

The interested reader will find some of the data referring to the early theories of the infectious origin of cancer in the reviews of Guelliot (1892), Brand (1902), Borrel (1903, 1907), Blumenthal (1905), Wolff (1907), Woglom (1913), Gye (1925), Blumenthal (1926, 1932), Gye and Purdy (1931), and others.

Early Studies Suggesting that at Least Some Tumors May be Caused by Viruses

Some investigators began to suspect that after all cancer may also belong to the group of diseases caused by invisible, submicroscopic agents. The French bacteriologist, A. Borrel (1903, 1907), is credited with being one of the first to advance in an extensive study the concept of viral etiology of cancer. However, in these early years the assumption that cancer might be of viral origin was purely speculative, subject to strong criticism, and for all practical purposes in striking contrast to available experimental and clinical observations. Attempts to transmit by filtrates malignant tumors, such as sarcomas or carcinomas, in mice and rats, animals commonly employed at that time for experimental cancer research in all leading laboratories, failed consistently. In addition to rabbit myxomatosis (Sanarelli, 1898), only chicken leukemia (Ellermann and Bang, 1908) and chicken sarcoma (Rous, 1911) could be transmitted by filtrates in these early studies. Gradually, experimental data became available suggesting that a few additional tumors, such as papillomas and fibromas in rabbits (Shope, 1932, 1933), as well as warts in cattle, horses, and other species, including humans, could be transmitted by filtrates;* later, the frog kidney carcinoma (Lucké, 1934) and the mouse mammary carcinoma (Bittner, 1936) were also added to the growing list of tumors that could be transmitted by filtrates.

Even then, however, it was difficult to reconcile the concept of viral etiology of tumors with available experimental and clinical observations. At that time, in the early 1940's, only a few tumors could be transmitted by filtrates. Attempts to transmit other tumors by filtrates failed, and the theory of viral etiology of cancer could at best be applied to only a few tumors in rabbits, chickens, frogs, and mice.

Some of the Reasons Responsible for the Difficulties in Accepting the Concept of Infectious Origin of Cancer

One of the main difficulties in accepting in general terms the concept of infectious origin of cancer was the well established observation that malignant tumors, as well as leukemia, in animals and in humans are not transmissible by contact infection under natural life conditions.

* For additional information and bibliography referring to cell-free transmission of warts and papillomas the reader is referred to chapter 3 in this monograph.

Cancer and Leukemia are not Contagious. It has been known for many years that tumors, as well as leukemia, are not transmitted among family members, or in hospital wards from patients to other patients, to nurses or to physicians, from patients to surgeons in the operating room, or to pathologists in the dissecting room. Similar observations have been made in the laboratory. Mice or chickens having cancer or leukemia can be placed for the balance of their lives in the same cages with groups of healthy young, adult mice or chickens, respectively; yet, no transmission of the disease results in either case under usual experimental conditions.

Occasional transmission of leukemia among newly hatched chicks has been reported under certain experimental conditions employing a potent, passaged virus and newborn chicks of a highly susceptible inbred line. Usually, however, no significant contact transmission from one host to another occurs under natural life conditions. The occasional contact transmission of tumors or leukemia among animals within the same generation is unusual and contrasts sharply with the ready and prompt transmission of a variety of common infectious diseases in animals and in man.

Only recently it was recognized that certain oncogenic viruses may also spread among newborn or very young animals from one host to another within the same generation. However, such contact infection usually is latent, and remains undetected, since it only rarely leads to the development of tumors.

This apparent lack of transmissibility of tumors among individuals within the same generation has presented one of the principal difficulties in the acceptance of a theory of infectious origin of cancer.

Tumors and Leukemia can be Induced by a Variety of Physical and Chemical Factors. Another difficulty in accepting the concept of infectious origin of cancer has been directly related to the well documented observations suggesting that tumors can be induced in animals, and in man, by different physical factors, such as heat, chronic irritation, ultraviolet rays and particularly ionizing radiation, and also by carcinogenic chemicals and hormones. Leukemia and lymphomas can also be induced with a variety of nonspecific factors, such as ionizing radiation, hormones, carcinogenic chemicals, or certain chemical poisons.

Familial Incidence of Cancer: The Inherited, Genetic Susceptibility. Leukemia and malignant tumors have long been observed to occur with higher frequency in certain families than in the average population. This observation has been made repeatedly not only in animals but also in humans. However, the familial incidence of tumors and leukemia has been interpreted in terms suggesting an inherited genetic susceptibility rather than induction by a transmissible viral agent.

Only some 30 or 40 years ago it was generally assumed that cancer was a "spontaneous" disease, presumably due to "somatic mutation," and that it might be caused by various internal and external factors. Mutation could occur in an unpredictable manner, and with a higher frequency in certain predisposed families. This theory appeared to be consistent with clinical and experimental observations, such as experimental induction of tumors with a variety of physical and chemical factors, familial incidence of tumors due to inherited susceptibility, etc.

Actually, however, the theory of "spontaneous" origin of cancer, presumably due to "somatic mutation," was not unlike the ancient concept of "spontaneous tuberculous degeneration" advocated by Pidoux and other believers in "morbid diathesis;" at the time of Villemin, tuberculosis was thought to be a common result of a variety of external and internal causes.* It is worth emphasis that as late as 1885 typhoid fever and diphtheria were believed to originate *de novo* in filthy surroundings (Rivers, 1938). It took many years to demonstrate that the law of obligate communicability still prevails for all infectious diseases; the same is probably true also for cancer and leukemia.

As a result of these and similar considerations, and also in view of rather scarce experimental evidence of actual filtrate transmission of only a few tumors in animals, the concept of viral etiology of cancer was not generally favored. In the 1930's and 1940's a young scientist applying for a grant to carry out a research project in the field of tumor-inducing viruses was faced with considerable difficulties in obtaining a place to work, or sufficient funds to carry out his studies. The search for viruses as causative agents in cancer was considered to be rather fruitless. Theories based on genetic inheritance and mutation as a cause, or causes, of cancer were preferred by the majority of workers in the field of experimental cancer and pathology.

DEVELOPMENT OF THE CONCEPT OF VERTICAL TRANSMISSION OF ONCOGENIC VIRUSES

It was quite apparent that a concept of infectious origin of cancer, based on the conventional ways and means of natural transmission of bacterial and viral agents observed in common communicable diseases, could not be applied to cancer. However, the problem of viral etiology of cancer and other neoplastic diseases could be approached in a different manner. Since cancer and allied diseases, such as leukemia, have been observed in several animal species to develop in successive generations, it appeared possible to speculate that such tumors are caused by oncogenic viruses transmitted in certain families from parents to offspring. A working hypothesis was advanced (Gross, 1944) suggesting that malignant tumors are caused by oncogenic viruses transmitted directly from one generation to another. The terms "vertical" and "horizontal" transmission were coined and

* Reviewed by Vallery-Radot in *La vie de Pasteur*, 1931.

suggested to designate the transmission of potentially pathogenic viruses from one generation to another, or within the same generation, respectively (Gross, 1944, 1949).

The concept of vertical transmission of oncogenic viruses was consistent with experimental observations dealing with the natural spread of chicken lymphomatosis, a disease caused by a leukemogenic virus transmitted through the embryos in certain flocks of chickens. The transmission of the mouse mammary carcinoma virus in the milk of nursing females from one generation to another in certain strains of mice was also consistent with this hypothesis.

The Concept of "Vertical" Transmission of Oncogenic Agents Leads to the Isolation of the Mouse Leukemia Virus

The introduction of the concept of vertical transmission of oncogenic agents (Gross, 1944) actually formed the basis for the design of subsequent experiments leading to the isolation of the mouse leukemia virus, and to experimental documentation of the transmission of the mouse leukemia virus from one generation to another through the embryos (Gross, 1951).

It appeared only logical to employ mouse leukemia as an experimental tool to determine the validity of the concept of vertical transmission of oncogenic viruses. In certain high-leukemic inbred strains, such as Ak and C58, leukemia had been observed to appear consistently in mice of successive generations; previous studies failed to detect the presence of a causative leukemogenic agent in the milk of nursing female mice of the high-leukemic inbred lines (Richter and MacDowell, 1935. Barnes and Cole, 1941). However, according to the more recently developed concept of vertical transmission of oncogenic viruses, the presence of a latent leukemogenic agent in Ak or C58 embryos and a direct transmission of this agent through the embryos from one generation to another had to be considered.

A series of experiments carried out on the basis of this working hypothesis led to the isolation of the mouse leukemia virus (Gross, 1951a,b) and to the demonstration of the presence of the mouse leukemia virus in Ak and C58 embryos (Gross, 1951a,b. Gross, 1956).

A General Outline of the Concept of "Horizontal" and "Vertical" Transmission of Pathogenic Agents

"Horizontal" Transmission of Common Communicable Diseases. When speaking of a contagious disease, we are conditioned to think automatically of a disease spreading from one host to another within the same generation: by contact (chickenpox), through infected food or carriers (typhoid fever), or through insect hosts (malaria). In each case, both the infecting and the

infected hosts belong to the same generation; a very brief interval of time, frequently not exceeding a few days or weeks, elapses between the individual cases forming successive links in the chain of a horizontal transmission of a conventional communicable disease. The human observer can therefore actually follow the spread of the communicable disease, tracing it in either direction, back to the infecting carrier, or ahead to the newly infected host.

The "Vertical" Transmission of Pathogenic Agents in Nature. It is apparent, however, that the transmission of a parasitic agent may also take place in a different manner: instead of spreading rapidly among hosts of the same generation, a pathogenic agent may be transmitted from a carrier host to the host's offspring, thence to the offspring's offspring, thence, in turn, to the next generation, and so forth. Such a transmission would obviously require much more time than that observed in those communicable diseases which spread in the conventional manner within the same generation.

There exist in nature numerous examples of transmission of pathogenic agents from one generation to another. Pasteur (1865, 1866a,b, 1867) was first to observe that pébrine, a virus disease of the silkworm, is transmitted in these insects through the eggs. Certain diseases of plants, such as the mosaic disease of lettuce, tomatoes, or potatoes, are caused by extraneous filterable viruses. The infected plant may grow next to a healthy one, yet no transmission of the agent will occur among hosts of the same generation, unless an intermediary carrier, such as a certain insect vector, is interposed (Kunkel, 1928, 1943). The natural transmission of the mosaic virus occurs, however, through the seeds, or, in the case of the mosaic disease of potatoes, through the tubers, to the next generation of hosts. These viruses may remain dormant, causing no harm to their carrier hosts, unless activated.

The Rocky Mountain spotted fever rickettsiae (Spencer and Parker, 1924), or the tularemia organisms (Parker and Spencer, 1926), and other infectious agents (Davis *et al.*, 1938) are transmitted in the tick, through the eggs of these insects, from one generation to another, causing no apparent harm to their own insect-hosts. They are highly pathogenic, however, when transmitted to several other species, including humans. This is an interesting example of vertically transmitted agents which may be so adapted to their own hosts that they will not cause harm to their own carriers, but may become pathogenic when transmitted to other strains or species.

The bacteriophage may also be transmitted from one generation to another in certain strains of lysogenic bacteria (Lwoff, 1953b). The phage usually remains inactive. When activated, however, the phage becomes pathogenic and destroys its own host by lysis (Lwoff *et al.*, 1950. Lwoff, 1953). The bacteriophage may be pathogenic for certain strains of bacteria only, and not necessarily for those in which it is carried.

It is obvious that the vertically transmitted pathogenic agents can readily escape detection, particularly when such agents are submicroscopic, and therefore invisible, since they do not always cause symptoms of disease. The study of vertically transmitted infectious agents is difficult; experiments must be conducted on animals having a relatively short life span and a rapid reproductive cycle, thus permitting the human observer to follow several successive generations of the carrier hosts.

Vertical Transmission of Pathogenic Agents Should Not be Confused with Inheritance

When observing a disease appearing in successive generations of descendants of the same family, a casual observer may be tempted to consider such cases to be caused by some inherited, genetic factors; and yet, inheritance and vertical transmission of pathogenic agents are fundamentally different phenomena.

Inheritance is conditioned by genetic factors, and is never acquired. On the other hand, the vertically transmitted diseases, such as lymphomatosis in chickens, leukemia or mammary carcinoma in mice, pébrine in the silkworm, or mosaic disease in plants, are actually caused by viral agents which are transmitted from host to host. The same is true for the bacteriophage which is transmitted "vertically" in a lysogenic bacterial clone. These agents may appear to form an integral part of the host's cells; actually, however, they are foreign to the host. They were at one time acquired, and since that time have been transmitted from one generation to another. This is not inheritance. Vertical transmission is a form of infection.

"VERTICAL" TRANSMISSION OF ONCOGENIC VIRUSES

The virus theory of cancer and allied diseases can be approached, therefore, from a point of view different from that employed in reference to common communicable diseases. There may exist a group of submicroscopic, cell-free oncogenic agents, individually distinct, though possibly related, which may be transmitted "vertically," i.e. from one generation to another.

According to this concept, some, perhaps most, oncogenic viruses would be transmitted from one generation to another through the germinal cells. It is possible to speculate that certain oncogenic viruses would be transmitted as integral parts of the germinal cells, like the bacteriophage in a lysogenic bacterial clone; as an alternate possibility, the sperm or the ovum could pick up an oncogenic virus in the course of its passage through virus-infected ducts of the male or female genital organs (Feldman and

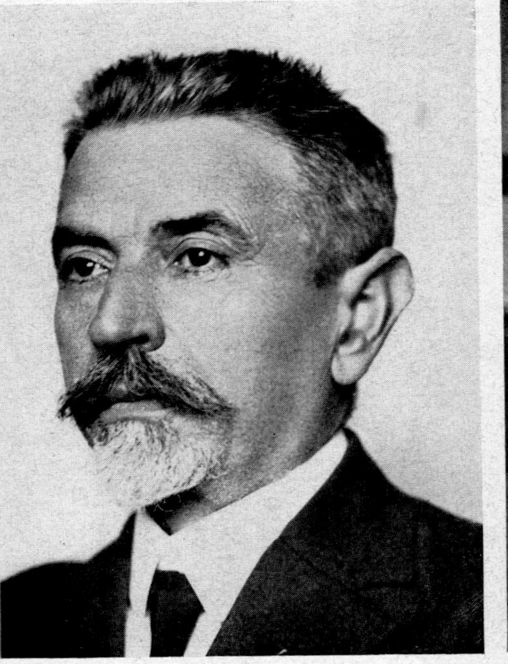

Amédée Borrel

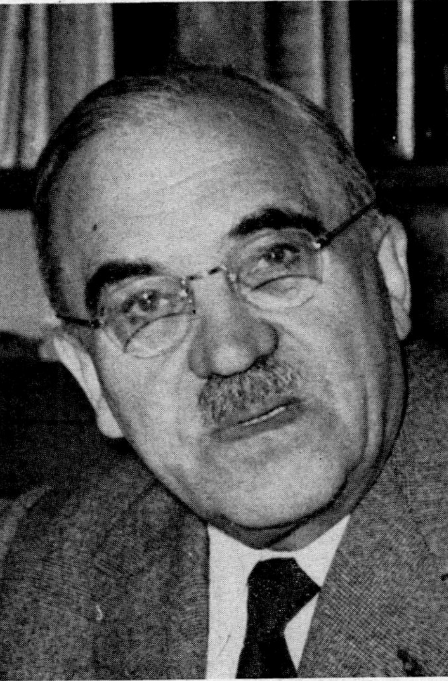

Charles Oberling

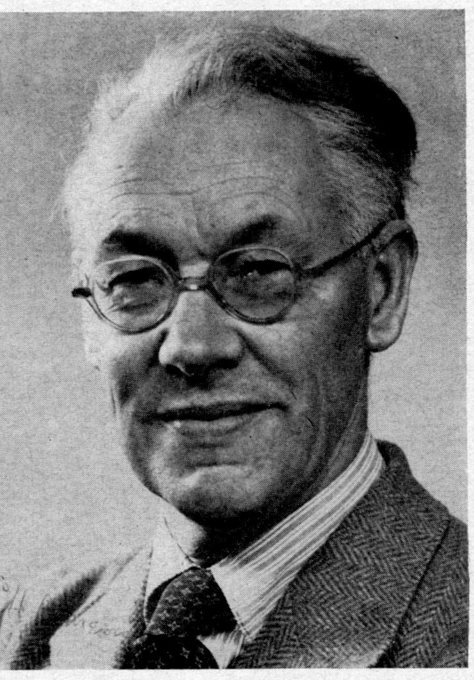

Christopher H. Andrewes

FIG. 75

Gross, 1967). Furthermore, it is also possible to assume that infection with an oncogenic virus could occur in some instances after fertilization, *in utero*.

Transmission of oncogenic viruses through the milk of nursing mothers, or by contact infection from parents to newborn offspring, would also be included in this general pattern.

According to this concept, each tumor case could be traced to another case caused by the same transmissible virus. Thus, the law of obligate communicability would apply not only to common infectious diseases, but also to cancer. However, since oncogenic viruses would usually be transmitted from one generation to another, a considerable period of time would elapse between two successive cases of neoplasms caused by the same causative agent. Furthermore, at the time of actual transmission of the virus, the infecting carriers would be in perfect health, even though they would spread the disease.

Such a concept would be consistent with the observations of familial occurrence of cancer and allied diseases, including leukemia, in several species, such as mice, chickens, cattle, and also in man.

The Epidemiology of Mouse Leukemia, Chicken Lymphomatosis and Mouse Mammary Carcinoma. The transmission of oncogenic viruses from one generation to another can be followed in mice or chickens of certain inbred lines in which the potency of the virus and the susceptibility of the hosts have been increased by selective inbreeding.

Let us consider as an example the mouse leukemia virus and its natural transmission in an inbred strain of mice, such as Ak or C58, with a high incidence of spontaneous leukemia. The potentially leukemogenic virus is transmitted in such mice from one generation to another. The transmission occurs most probably directly through the germinal cells of both parents, i.e. through the mother and also through the father. Even though the mouse is infected prior to its birth (since the embryo also carries the virus), it remains in good health until middle age.

The same is true for chicken lymphomatosis, which is also transmitted from one generation to another directly, though not exclusively, through the embryos; the virus of chicken lymphomatosis can also be transmitted by contact among newly hatched chicks.

The virus of certain forms of mouse mammary carcinoma is transmitted from one generation to another through the milk of nursing females.

"Horizontal" Transmission of Oncogenic Viruses

Although oncogenic viruses presumably follow in most instances the "vertical" pattern of transmission from one generation to another, it is quite apparent that some of them may also be transmitted from one host to another within the same generation. "Horizontal" transmission of oncogenic viruses may take place usually among newborn or very young hosts, either directly by contact infection, or in certain instances through intermediary carriers.

The parotid tumor (polyoma) virus can spread "horizontally" among newborn or suckling mice. The virus of chicken lymphomatosis is transmitted by contact among newly hatched chicks. The possibility of contact transmission of the Rous sarcoma virus among very young chicks of a susceptible breed should also be considered (Burmester *et al.*, 1960). Under certain experimental conditions, the mouse leukemia virus can also be transmitted horizontally among very young animals.* However, it appears that under natural life conditions, horizontal contact transmission of these or other oncogenic viruses usually leads only to the acquisition of a latent infection; this infection remains in most instances inapparent, and only rarely causes the development of leukemia or a tumor.

Experiments dealing with rabbit myxomatosis, or with rabbit and squirrel fibroma, have demonstrated that viruses which cause the development of these neoplasms can be transmitted by mosquitoes.*

In more recent experiments, transmission of a virus which causes lymphosarcoma in the South African Clawed Toad through water in which these amphibians have been maintained was observed by Balls and Ruben (1967).

Difficulties in Tracing Vertically Transmitted Oncogenic Viruses

It should be stressed that the tracing of pathogenic agents transmitted in an inactive, masked form from one generation to another is possible only when several successive generations of carrier-hosts are followed by the investigator. Activation of the virus, resulting in the development of symptoms of disease, may occur only occasionally, perhaps once every few generations. Should the theory of viral origin of cancer prove to be correct not only for animals, but also for humans, it would then be necessary to assume that, as in the case of chicken and mouse leukemia or mouse mammary carcinoma, the hypothetical oncogenic viruses causing human tumors, including leukemia and lymphomas, may be able to pass through several successive generations without causing any symptoms of disease.

According to this concept, oncogenic viruses would usually exist in an inactive form; in such a form, these agents would be frugal and moderate in their requirements, causing no apparent harm to their carrier hosts. Occasionally, however, prompted by as yet obscure but presumably varied trigger stimuli, the hitherto masked agents could change into formidable pathogens. Activated oncogenic agents would cause rapid multiplication of the cells harboring them, leading to the development of leukemia,

* For additional information and pertinent refererences the reader is referred to the respective chapters in this monograph.

lymphomas, or other malignant tumors, and usually sealing the fate of their carrier hosts. However, since the activation of an oncogenic agent would usually occur in middle-aged hosts, the survival of the virus would already have been assured. As a rule, transmission of the virus to the host's offspring would occur prior to its activation.

The Time Factor

The long interval of time intervening between the development of the initially observed and the transmitted neoplasms contributes considerably to the difficulty in understanding the nature of cancer as a "communicable" disease. The individual instances of the development of tumors should be viewed in their proper perspective, i.e., as single links only in a continuous chain of transmission of oncogenic viruses which pass from one generation to another. In order to appreciate the epidemiology of oncogenic viruses, the time factor should be disregarded. The "vertical," i.e. generation-to-generation, transmission of oncogenic viruses may then be compared, in principle, to that of various infections, except that diseases thus far recognized as being contagious spread, as a rule, among members of the same generation.

One could imagine that a hypothetical oncogenic agent might have caused a tumor in a distant ancestor, perhaps two or three centuries ago; the virus could then have passed, without causing any harm, through the great-grandfather, then through the grandfather, and might have caused a tumor in the father. The same oncogenic virus could then have become latent, and could have passed, unnoticed, through the children and grandchildren. After a considerable interval of time, the same hypothetical agent could then again cause another neoplasm in one of the distant descendants of the same family.

Accordingly, in the human host, one century, or even two, may conceivably elapse between successive cases of tumors or leukemia due to the same viral agent transmitted from one generation to another. The task of tracing the host-to-host transmission of hypothetical oncogenic viruses in human hosts would therefore be extremely difficult, if at all possible, at the present time. Adequate records concerning the cause of death are not always available for individuals who died only forty or fifty years ago. Leukemia, for instance, was first recognized as a distinct disease in humans only about one century ago (Craigie, 1845. Bennett, 1845, 1851. Virchow, 1847); it is probable that the identification of this disease has been missed quite frequently in earlier years, especially before the development of our basic knowledge in hematology and before the advent of modern diagnostic methods. Similarly, microscopic diagnosis of tumors was developed only during the last century.

Unfortunately, with only occasional exceptions, human records cannot be followed for more than two or three generations at the utmost. Thus, the time factor may prove to be one of the most formidable obstacles in further research on the epidemiology of tumors in humans.

Human life may well be too short to permit any one investigator to follow the host-to-host transmission of an oncogenic virus in man.

Infection with an Oncogenic Virus is Not Necessarily Followed by the Development of a Tumor

It is of the utmost importance to make a distinction between infection with a potentially oncogenic virus and the actual development of disease. This is true not only for the conventional viruses causing a variety of transmissible infectious diseases, but also for the tumor-inducing viruses. It is now quite apparent that oncogenic viruses are widely prevalent in the animal kingdom and that they are carried by innumerable hosts, which, nevertheless, in most instances may live out their life span without developing tumors. Under natural life conditions oncogenic viruses usually remain latent, but may occasionally induce tumors in their carrier hosts.

The very high incidence of leukemia or mammary carcinoma in certain inbred lines of mice, or visceral lymphomatosis in certain strains of chickens, reflects special experimental conditions resulting from selective inbreeding of susceptible animals carrying a particularly potent virus; such conditions do not occur in nature under normal circumstances. It seems that under natural life conditions, oncogenic viruses remain in most instances latent, causing only occasionally the development of tumors or leukemia in their carrier hosts.

The Development of Cancer or Leukemia — Only an "Accident" in the Chain of Natural Transmission of Oncogenic Viruses

On the basis of this working hypothesis, one could therefore regard the development of cancer, leukemia, lymphomas, or of other malignant tumors, as the result of an activation, frequently merely accidental, of an oncogenic agent, hitherto masked, and carried by the host since birth. Oncogenic agents carried in descendants of certain families, in humans as well as in other species, may have a higher pathogenic potential and be more readily activated than those carried in other families. Furthermore, members of certain families may have a higher inherited susceptibility to the development of tumors or leukemia, since genetic and other, such as hormonal or metabolic conditions favoring the activation of a latent oncogenic virus may be more prevalent in certain individuals than in others. As a result, cancer, leukemia, or other malignant tumors would develop more frequently in members of certain families than in others. However, in many, perhaps in most, instances the oncogenic agents would not become activated, even though they would continue being transmitted from one generation to another. The great majority of virus-carriers may never develop tumors. Even in families carrying oncogenic agents of a relatively high pathogenic potential, cases of leukemia or other malignant tumors may be separated by two or three generations of healthy individuals.

It is evident that, should this working hypothesis prove to be correct, it would logically follow that individuals with symptoms of tumors or leukemia would represent only a very small fraction of those actually carrying the seeds of either disease. This would apply to humans as well as to various species of animals.

Some of the Factors which May Trigger or Prompt the Activation of Latent Oncogenic Viruses

Our present knowledge concerning the nature and mechanism of action of the many factors capable of activating latent oncogenic viruses, and prompting such viruses into pathogenic action, is very limited. It is known, however, that the activation of oncogenic agents can be triggered by a variety of generally non-specific factors. Such factors can be: (a) external, such as ionizing radiation or certain chemical cell poisons, or (b) internal, i.e. metabolic or hormonal. Only some of the activating, inducing factors are known; most are still obscure.

Induction of Leukemia in Mice, or Tumors in Rats, Following Total-Body X-Ray Irradiation. Mice of certain low-leukemic strains, such as C3H, C57 Brown, or C57 Black, carry a potentially leukemogenic virus, although only very few of these animals, if left undisturbed, would develop leukemia or lymphosarcomas spontaneously. However, total-body X-ray irradiation, or treatment with hormones or certain carcinogenic chemicals, may prompt the development of leukemia or lymphosarcomas in such animals. A leukemogenic virus was recovered from organs of mice with radiation-induced leukemia (Gross, 1958a. Lieberman and Kaplan, 1959. Latarjet and Duplan, 1962).

In the same category probably belong experiments in which a variety of carcinomas and sarcomas were induced in rats following total-body X-ray irradiation. Although no evidence has yet been furnished suggesting that these tumors are caused by oncogenic viruses, it is possible to speculate that, not unlike the induction of leukemia in mice, the development of solid tumors in rats following total-body X-ray irradiation is also caused by activation of a latent oncogenic virus carried in such animals.*

* For more detailed information and pertinent references the interested reader is referred to the chapter on Radiation-induced Leukemia in Mice.

Factors which May Delay or Prevent the Activation of Latent Oncogenic Viruses

It was observed in earlier experiments that the development of spontaneous mammary carcinoma in C3H female mice carrying the mammary carcinoma virus could be significantly inhibited by low caloric food intake (Sivertsen and Hastings, 1938. Tannenbaum, 1940). Similarly, it was also observed in subsequent studies that the development of spontaneous leukemia in mice of certain high-leukemic inbred strains, such as Ak, could be significantly reduced by reduction of food intake* (Saxton *et al.*, 1944).

The mechanism of this inhibiting effect on the obscure process of activation of an oncogenic agent has not been clarified. Should this inhibiting effect of caloric food reduction on activation of oncogenic viruses represent a more general phenomenon, not necessarily limited to mouse leukemia and mouse mammary carcinoma, it would be possible to speculate that a general and prolonged shortage of food, quite prevalent in nature during certain seasonal periods of time, leading to a reduced food intake, may inhibit in wild animals the activation of latent oncogenic agents, and may thereby considerably decrease the incidence of spontaneous tumors occurring under natural life conditions in such hosts. Other factors may condition the host, increasing or decreasing its susceptibility to activation of latent oncogenic viruses. Most of these factors are unknown and require further studies. Whether such factors as emotional or physical stress, prolonged fatigue, exposure to intercurrent infections, etc., play a role in increasing the susceptibility to activation of latent oncogenic viruses remains to be determined.

In another category belongs the presence of specific antibodies due to latent, intercurrent, or previous infections with certain oncogenic viruses, such as the polyoma virus, the SV 40 virus, or certain types of adenoviruses. The presence of antibodies may prevent reinfection with these viruses or their multiplication, and it may preclude the development of tumors in the infected carriers.

Some Examples of Activation of Latent Viruses in Nature

Activation of latent viral infections in animals and in man is a rather common phenomenon.† A good example is presented by the *herpes simplex*

* For further information on the effect of caloric food restriction on the development of spontaneous mammary carcinoma and leukemia in mice, the interested reader is referred to pages 256 and 419 in the chapters on Mouse Mammary Carcinoma and Mouse Leukemia.

† The reader is referred to the excellent review on "Latent virus infections and their possible relevance to the cancer problem" by C. H. Andrewes (1939).

virus. This particular virus is carried in a latent form by many persons since early childhood; it can be triggered by a variety of non-specific conditions, such as prolonged exposure to sun, acute infection with fever, extreme fatigue, menstruation, and many other inducing factors. The activated virus induces a characteristic eruption on the skin and mucous membranes, which later subsides. The virus continues to be carried, however, and is frequently reactivated in the same individual either by the same or by another trigger factor.

Dr. P. Lépine in Paris (personal communication to the author, 1968) observed for over 20 years a man who was athletic, generally in good health, and had no allergy; however, each time this patient consumed even only a trace of Gruyère cheese he developed within 48 hours a typical herpetic eruption on the lips; curiously, other varieties of cheese did not have a similar effect. All attempts to desensitize the patient were unsuccessful. This case presented an unusual example of activation of a latent virus by a very precise stimulus.

The development of the painful shingles syndrome, i.e. appearance of crops of vesicles, identical with those observed in chickenpox but developing only in areas supplied by affected sensory nerves, caused by *herpes zoster virus*, has been observed in patients suffering from leukemia, or Hodgkin's disease; such patients apparently carry a latent herpes zoster virus infection which becomes activated following the development of leukemia or lymphomas.

*Activation of Latent Virus Infections Following Prolonged Muscular Exertion and Fatigue.** Physical factors, such as very prolonged muscular exertion and fatigue, may also activate latent infections in humans, and may lead to an unexpected dramatic appearance of paralysis of one or more limbs caused by the virus of poliomyelitis that was carried by such individuals in a latent form. Cases of sudden development of paralysis have been observed in rare instances after prolonged and exhausting competitions in swimming, racing, or dancing.

Prolonged muscular exertion, such as may occur in dogs as a result of an extensive chase, may activate a latent virus causing hepatitis in these animals.

A long transport in crowded cars of large numbers of cattle exposed to prolonged effects of heat, immobilization, and fatigue, without proper nourishment and fresh water, may activate latent infections in such animals; once activated the infections may spread, causing considerable mortality.

* These illustrative examples of activation of latent non-oncogenic viral infections in humans and in animals have been brought to the attention of the author by Dr. Pierre Lépine, Chief of the Virus Service at the Pasteur Institute in Paris (1968).

Activation of Lymphocytic Choriomeningitis Virus in Guinea Pigs. The virus of lymphocytic choriomeningitis is frequently carried in a latent form in many animal species, particularly in mice, guinea pigs, monkeys, and occasionally also in humans. Following inoculation, preferably by the intracerebral route, of a sufficient dose of the virus into mice or guinea pigs, tremor, convulsions, and other symptoms of choriomeningitis develop within one to two weeks, and the animals die a few days after the onset of illness. However, many mice and guinea pigs carry the virus as a latent infection. An entire colony of guinea pigs or mice in a laboratory may be infected without showing any symptoms of disease; the virus is propagated in such colonies by normal appearing carriers. It is possible, however, to activate the virus and produce symptoms of disease; when sterile broth, or another similar apparently harmless solution, is injected intraperitoneally into guinea pigs carrying such a latent infection, the inoculated animals develop fever and die from pneumonia within one week (personal communication to the author from Dr. P. Lépine, 1968). Activation of a latent lymphocytic choriomeningitis virus may also occur, or be induced, by non-specific factors, in mice and in other species.

Activation of Bacteriophage. The activation of bacteriophage in lysogenic bacterial strains should also be mentioned at this point, although it may represent a different phenomenon. The bacteriophage remains latent when carried under normal life conditions by certain strains of lysogenic bacteria. However, under the influence of ultraviolet light rays (Lwoff *et al.*, 1950), exposure to X-rays (Latarjet, 1951), or following exposure to certain inducing agents (Lwoff, 1953a), the latent form of bacteriophage becomes activated, and destroys its own bacterial host by lysis.

Many other examples of activation of viruses in man and in animals could be quoted. These observations only emphasize the fact that activation of latent oncogenic viruses is not an isolated phenomenon, and that similar activations of latent viruses have been observed in infections caused by non-oncogenic viral agents.

Oncogenic Viruses which Usually Remain Latent in Their Natural Carriers

There exist certain potentially oncogenic viruses which remain in most instances harmless for their natural carrier hosts; however, under certain conditions these viruses may induce tumors in their own natural hosts or in other species. The parotid, i.e. polyoma, virus belongs to this group. It is now realized that a latent infection with the polyoma virus is very common in mice. However, as a general rule, this virus is harmless for its natural host; spontaneous development of tumors caused by this virus in mice is exceedingly rare. And yet the same virus is known to possess a formidable oncogenic potential. Under certain experimental conditions it can induce a spectrum of some of the most malignant, progressively growing, and uniformly fatal neoplasms. The activation of the virus may be prompted in the natural carrier by prolonged treatment with cortisone or by total-body X-ray irradiation. The method of choice, however, leading to the unmasking of the tumor-inducing potential of the polyoma virus is its passage through tissue culture, followed by inoculation into newborn mice (Stewart *et al.*, 1958), hamsters (Eddy *et al.*, 1958), or rats (Eddy *et al.*, 1959).

Viruses which May Become Oncogenic when Transferred to Other Species

A new chapter in the field of oncogenic viruses has been added as a result of recent studies on adenoviruses (Trentin *et al.*, 1962, 1963) and on the SV 40 agent (Sweet and Hilleman, 1960. Eddy *et al.*, 1961, 1962. Girardi *et al.*, 1962). There exist viruses which may remain latent in their natural carriers, or which induce in such species only a transient non-neoplastic disease; the same viruses, however, may induce malignant tumors in other species.

Certain types of human adenoviruses remain latent, or induce only a transient infectious disease, such as pharyngitis, conjunctivitis, or enteritis, in their human carriers; however, the same viruses can induce progressively growing sarcomas following inoculation into newborn hamsters. Similarly, the SV 40 virus remains latent in its natural carrier, the Asian rhesus monkey (*Macaca mulatta*), but can induce a high incidence of sarcomas following inoculation into newborn hamsters.

It has long been observed that many infectious agents may remain latent in their natural carrier hosts, to which they might have become adapted in the course of years. However, some of these latent agents may become pathogenic when transferred to other species. This is true for a variety of infectious agents, and may also be true for certain oncogenic viruses.

Humans do not lead an isolated existence; man lives in continuous contact with animals and parasites. Humans contract infections from animals, as animals contract infections from man. Frequently humans or animals may become infected without showing symptoms of disease; the infection may persist, however, and either humans or animals may become reservoirs of potentially pathogenic bacterial or viral agents.

Nicolle (1931) demonstrated that distemper, a common and frequently fatal disease in the dog, may be carried by man, and that the causative agent of this disease induces in man only an asymptomatic, latent infection. There are many other bacterial or viral agents which frequently induce only a transient or asymptomatic infection in humans, but may be pathogenic for animals. The reverse is also true; some of the bacterial or viral agents carried by animals, and latent for their carrier hosts, may be pathogenic for humans.

Would it be possible to speculate that some of the domestic animals may be carriers of pathogenic agents which under certain conditions may induce tumors in humans? This is obviously only a remote possibility which does not appear to be very realistic at present; however, the induction of tumors in humans with a virus carried in a latent form in animals would not be more surprising than the recently reported observations which demonstrated that human adenoviruses may induce sarcomas in hamsters (Trentin *et al.*, 1962, 1963).

THE TURN OF THE TIDE

The Viral Theory of Cancer Gains Acceptance and Gradually Becomes the Favored Approach to the Problem of Cancer and Leukemia

The initial experimental basis for the development of the concept of viral etiology of cancer was provided by the early fundamental studies which demonstrated transmission by filtered extracts of leukemia and sarcomas in chickens, and more recently also that of kidney carcinoma in frogs, and mammary carcinoma in mice. However, these observations were at first accepted with certain reservations, and at best only as isolated demonstrations of a presumably viral etiology of a few individual tumors in certain animal species; they were not interpreted as an early documentation of a general concept of viral etiology of cancer. Several decades elapsed, until new and fundamental observations provided the necessary additional evidence which turned the tide.

Gradually, in the span of less than two decades the concept of viral etiology of cancer and leukemia has gained momentum. The isolation of the mouse leukemia virus, and shortly thereafter the discovery of the parotid tumor, i.e. polyoma, virus, and the subsequent observation demonstrating that a variety of tumors, including sarcomas and carcinomas, could be induced with the tissue-culture-grown polyoma virus in mice, rats, and hamsters represented significant progress in the study of viral etiology of cancer. Other fundamental advances in the field of oncogenic viruses included the discovery of the oncogenic action of human adenoviruses and of the simian virus 40. The introduction of tissue culture techniques in cancer research and the technical improvements in the use of the electron microscope contributed substantially to the rapid progress in this field.

The viral theory of cancer slowly gained acceptance and gradually became the favored approach to the problem of etiology of cancer and leukemia (Andrewes, 1939. Oberling, 1954. Duran-Reynals, 1953, 1956. Gross, 1944, 1954, 1958b. Stanley, 1958).

The relatively high incidence of tumors and leukemia observed in certain families in animals and in man could now be explained by an assumption consistent with the concept of viral etiology of cancer. If oncogenic viruses are transmitted "vertically" from one generation to another, the development of tumors or leukemia in family members of successive generations could be interpreted by an assumption that such neoplasms are caused by oncogenic viruses transmitted in certain families from one generation to another, rather than by genetic transmission of an obscure inherited susceptibility.

During the past decade, the concepts of "vertical" and "horizontal" transmission of oncogenic viruses have gradually gained acceptance and have been generally employed in studies and reviews dealing with the epidemiology of tumor-inducing viruses.

Viral Etiology of Human Cancer?

The viral origin of the majority of all malignant tumors, including leukemia and lymphomas, in chickens, mice, rats, and several other species, has now been documented beyond any reasonable doubt. It has already been pointed out elsewhere in this chapter that it would be rather difficult to assume a fundamentally different etiology for human tumors. The various sarcomas, carcinomas, leukemia, and related neoplasms in man are so similar in their morphology and clinical course to those observed in lower species of animals that it would appear only logical to assume that they represent the same disease, and that they are also caused by oncogenic viruses.

The assumption that human tumors are of viral origin is also consistent with several direct observations on humans, such as: (a) the numerous, some of them striking, cases of familial incidence of tumors and leukemia; (b) the induction of leukemia with ionizing radiation (known to be caused by activation of a latent leukemogenic virus in mice); (c) the clinical course of leukemia and lymphomas with periods of fever and exacerbations, alternating with remissions; (d) recent electron microscopic studies which revealed the presence of virus-like particles in some human lymphomas, and more recently also in a few biopsy fragments of human breast cancer.

The assumption that human malignant tumors, leukemia and lymphomas are caused by oncogenic viruses is nevertheless based at the present time on circumstantial evidence only. The concept of viral etiology of tumors and leukemia has not yet been conclusively documented in humans; however, it has proven to be one of the most productive and fruitful approaches to the problem of cancer in animals; it also represents the most logical explanation of the origin of cancer and allied diseases in man.

REFERENCES

ANDREWES, C. H., Latent virus infections and their possible relevance to the cancer problem: President's Address. *Proc. Royal Soc. Med.*, **33**: 75–86, 1939.

BALLS, M., Lymphosarcoma in the South African Clawed Toad, *Xenopus laevis*: A virus tumor. *Ann. N.Y. Acad. Sci.*, **126**: 256–273, 1965.

BALLS, M., and RUBEN, L. N., The transmission of lymphosarcoma in *Xenopus laevis*, the South African Clawed Toad. *Cancer Research*, **27**: 654–659, 1967.

BARNES, W. A., and COLE, R. K., The effect of nursing on the incidence of spontaneous leukemia and tumors in mice. *Cancer Research*, **1**: 99–101, 1941.

BENNETT, J. H., Case of hypertrophy of the spleen and liver, in which death took place from suppuration of the blood. *Edinburgh Med. and Surg. J.*, **64**: 413-423, 1845.

BENNETT, J. H., On leucocythemia, or white cell blood. *Monthly J. Med. Sci.*, **12**: 312–326, 1851.

BITTNER, J. J., Some possible effects of nursing on the mammary gland tumor incidence in mice. *Science*, **84**: 162, 1936.

BLUMENTHAL, F., Zur Infektiosität des Krebses. *Med. Klin.*, **1**: 532–533, 1905.

BLUMENTHAL, F., Beiträge zur Frage der Entstehung bösartigen Tumoren. *Deutsche Med. Wochenschr.*, **52**: 1283–1286, 1926.

BLUMENTHAL, F., Zur Frage der parasitären Krebsentstehung. Zum 100. Geburtstage Ernst V. Leydens. *Zeitschr. f. Krebsforsch.*, **36**: 130–144, 1932.

BORREL, A., Epithélioses infectieuses et epithéliomas. *Ann. Inst. Pasteur*, **17**: 81–122, 1903.

BORREL, A., Le problème du cancer. Revue. *Bull. Inst. Pasteur*, **5**: 497–512, 593–608, and 641–662, 1907.

BRAND, A. T., The etiology of cancer. *Brit. Med. J.*, **2**: 238–242, 1902.

BURMESTER, B. R., FONTES, A. K., and WALTER, W. G., Contact transmission of Rous sarcoma. *J. Nat. Cancer Inst.*, **25**: 307–313, 1960.

Committee on Standardized Genetic Nomenclature for Mice. Standardized nomenclature for inbred strains of mice. Second listing. *Cancer Research*, **20**: 145–169, 1960.

CRAIGIE, D., Case of disease of the spleen, in which death took place in consequence of the presence of purulent matter in the blood. *Edinburgh Med. and Surg. J.*, **64**: 400–413, 1845.

DAVIS, G. E., COX, H. R., PARKER, R. R., and DYER, R. E., A filter-passing infectious agent isolated from ticks. *Public Health Reports*, **53**: 2259–2282, 1938.

DURAN-REYNALS, F., Virus-induced tumors and the virus theory of cancer. Chapter 13, pp. 298–337 in: *The Physiopathology of Cancer*. P. B. Hoeber, Inc., Harper Bros., New York, 1953.

DURAN-REYNALS, F., Realities and hypotheses of viral infection as a cause of cancer. *Revue Canadienne de Biologie*, **14**: 411–428, 1956.

EDDY, B. E., BORMAN, G. S., BERKELEY, W. H., and YOUNG, R. D., Tumors induced in hamsters by injection of rhesus monkey kidney cell extracts. *Proc. Soc. Exp. Biol. & Med.*, **107**: 191–197, 1961.

EDDY, B. E., BORMAN, G. S., GRUBBS, G. E., and YOUNG, R. D., Identification of oncogenic substance in rhesus monkey kidney cell cultures as simian virus 40. *Virology*, **17**: 65–75, 1962.

EDDY, B. E., STEWART, S. E., YOUNG, R., and MIDER, G. B., Neoplasms in hamsters induced by mouse tumor agent passed in tissue culture. *J. Nat. Cancer Inst.*, **20**: 747–761, 1958.

EDDY, B. E., STEWART, S. E., STANTON, M. F., and MARCOTTE, J. M., Induction of tumors in rats by tissue-culture preparations of SE polyoma virus. *J. Nat. Cancer Inst.*, **22**: 161–171, 1959.

ELLERMANN, V., and BANG, O., Experimentelle Leukämie bei Hühnern. *Centralbl. f. Bakt., Abt. I, (Orig.)*, **46**: 595–609, 1908.

EWING, J., Neoplastic diseases. *A Treatise on Tumors*. 4th Edition. Revised and enlarged. pp. 1160. W. B. Saunders, Co., Philadelphia and London, 1940.

FELDMAN, D. G., and GROSS, L., Electron microscopic study of the distribution of the mouse leukemia virus (Gross) in genital organs of virus-injected C3Hf mice and Ak mice. *Cancer Research*, **27**: 1513–1527, 1967.

GIRARDI, A. J., SWEET, B. H., SLOTNICK, V. B., and HILLEMAN, M. R., Development of tumors in hamsters inoculated in the neonatal period with vacuolating virus SV 40. *Proc. Soc. Exp. Biol. & Med.*, **109**: 649–660, 1962.

GROSS, L., Is cancer a communicable disease? *Cancer Research*, **4**: 293–303, 1944.

GROSS, L., The "vertical epidemic" of mammary carcinoma in mice. Its possible implications for the problem of cancer in general. *Surg. Gynec. and Obstet.*, **88**: 295–308, 1949.

GROSS, L., "Spontaneous" leukemia developing in C3H mice following inoculation, in infancy, with Ak-leukemic extracts, or Ak-embryos. *Proc. Soc. Exp. Biol. & Med.*, **76**: 27–32, 1951a.

GROSS, L., Pathogenic properties, and "vertical" transmission of the mouse leukemia agent. *Proc. Soc. Exp. Biol. & Med.*, **78**: 342–348, 1951b.

GROSS, L., A filterable agent, recovered from Ak leukemic extracts, causing salivary gland carcinomas in C3H mice. *Proc. Soc. Exp. Biol. & Med.*, **83**: 414–421, 1953.

GROSS, L., Is leukemia caused by a transmissible virus? A working hypothesis. *Blood*, **9**: 557–573, 1954.

GROSS, L., Viral (egg-borne) etiology of mouse leukemia. Filtered extracts from leukemic C58 mice, causing leukemia (or parotid tumors) following inoculation into newborn C57 Brown, or C3H mice. *Cancer*, **9**: 778–791, 1956.

GROSS, L., Attempt to recover filterable agent from X-ray-induced leukemia. *Acta Haemat.*, **19**: 353–361, 1958a.

GROSS, L., The aetiology of cancer and allied diseases. Development of a concept based on recent experiments dealing with a cell-free transmission of mouse leukaemia. *Brit. Med. J.*, **2**: 1–5, 1958b.

GUELLIOT, O., La contagion du cancer. Revue générale. *Gazette des Hôpitaux*, **65**: 1209–1217, 1892.

GYE, W. E., The etiology of malignant new growths. *Lancet*, **2**: 109–117, 1925.

GYE, W. E., and PURDY, W. J., *The Cause of Cancer*. pp. 515. Cassel & Co., Publ., London, 1931.

KUNKEL, L. O., Virus diseases of plants. Chapter IX, pp. 325–364 in: *Filterable Viruses*, edited by T. M. Rivers, pp. 428. Williams & Wilkins Co., Baltimore, Md., 1928.

KUNKEL, L. O., New hosts as a key to progress in plant virus disease research. pp. 63–82 in: *Virus Diseases*. Cornell Univ. Press, Ithaca, N.Y., 1943.

LATARJET, R., Induction, par les rayons X, de la production d'un bactériophage chez *B. Megatherium* lysogène. *Ann. Inst. Pasteur*, **81**: 389–393, 1951.

LATARJET, R., and DUPLAN, J.-F., Experiment and discussion on leukaemogenesis by cell-free extracts of radiation-induced leukaemia in mice. *Internat. J. Radiation Biol.*, **5**: 339–344, 1962.

LIEBERMAN, M., and KAPLAN, H. S., Leukemogenic activity of filtrates from radiation-induced lymphoid tumors of mice. *Science*, **130**: 387 388, 1959.

LUCKÉ, B., A neoplastic disease of the kidney of the frog, *Rana pipiens*. *Am. J. Cancer*, **20**: 352–379, 1934.

LWOFF, A., Le bactériophage: L'induction. *Ann. Inst. Pasteur*, **84**: 225–241, 1953a.

LWOFF, A., Lysogeny. *Bacteriol. Reviews*, **17**: 269–337, 1953b.

LWOFF, A., SIMINOVITCH, L., and KJELDGAARD, N., Induction de la production de bactériophages chez une bactérie lysogène. *Ann. Inst. Pasteur*, **79**: 815–859, 1950.

NICOLLE, C., La maladie du jeune âge des chiens est transmissible expérimentalement à l'homme sous forme inapparente. Portée de cette constatation. *Compt. Rend. Acad. Sci.* (*Paris*), **192**: 1069–1071, 1931.

OBERLING, C., *Le Cancer*. pp. 381. 7th Edition. Gallimard, Paris, 1954.

PARKER, R. R., and SPENCER, R. R., Hereditary transmission of tularemia infection by wood tick *Dermacentor andersoni* Stiles. *Public Health Reports*, **41**: 1403–1407, 1926.

PASTEUR, L., Observations sur la maladie des vers à soie. *Compt. Rend. Acad. Sci.* (*Paris*), **61**: 506–512, 1865.

PASTEUR, L., Nouvelles études sur la maladie des vers à soie. *Compt. Rend. Acad. Sci.* (*Paris*), **63**: 126–142, 1866.

PASTEUR, L., Nouvelles études expérimentales sur la maladie des vers à soie. *Compt. Rend. Acad. Sci.* (*Paris*), **63**: 897–903, 1866.

PASTEUR, L., Sur la maladie des vers à soie. (Lettre de L. Pasteur à M. Dumas). *Compt Rend. Acad. Sci.* (*Paris*), **64**: 1109–1113, and **64**: 1113–1120, 1867.

PEYRILHE, B., Dissertation académique sur le cancer qui a remporté le prix double de l'Académie des Sciences, *Arts & Belles Lettres de Lyon*, le 8 Décembre 1773. pp. 135. Chez Ruault, Paris.

RICHTER, M. N., MACDOWELL, E. C., Experiments with mammalian leukemia. *Physiological Reviews*, **15**: 509–524, 1935.

RIVERS, T. M., Viruses and virus diseases. Twentieth century version of *de novo* origin of infectious agents and its significance in relation to the control of disease. *Bull. N.Y. Acad. Med.*, **14**: 383–397, 1938.

ROUS, P., Transmission of a malignant new growth by means of a cell-free filtrate. *J. Am. Med. Assoc.*, **56**: 198, 1911.

SANARELLI, G., Das myxomatogene Virus. Beitrag zum Studium der Krankheitserreger ausserhalb des Sichtbaren. *Centralb. f. Bakt., Abt. I*, **23**: 865–873, 1898.

SAXTON, J. A., JR., BOON, M. C., and FURTH, J., Observations on the inhibition of development of spontaneous leukemia in mice by underfeeding. *Cancer Research*, **4**: 401–409, 1944.

SHOPE, R. E., A filterable virus causing tumor-like condition in rabbits and its relationship to virus myxomatosum. *J. Exp. Med.*, **56**: 803–822, 1932.

SHOPE, R. E., Infectious papillomatosis of rabbits. *J. Exp. Med.*, **58**: 607–624, 1933.

SIVERTSEN, I., and HASTINGS, W. H., A preliminary report on the influence of food and function on the incidence of mammary gland tumor in "A" stock of albino mice. *Minnesota Med.*, **21**: 873–875, 1938.

SPENCER, R. R., and PARKER, R. R., Rocky Mountain spotted fever. Experimental studies on tick virus. *Public Health Reports*, **39**: 3027–3040, 1924.

STANLEY, W. M., Relationships, established and prospective, between viruses and cancer. *Ann. N.Y. Acad. Sci.*, **71**: 1100–1113, 1958.

STEWART, S. E., EDDY, B. E., and BORGESE, N., Neoplasms in mice inoculated with a tumor agent carried in tissue culture. *J. Nat. Cancer Inst.*, **20**: 1223–1243, 1958.

SWEET, B. H., and HILLEMAN, M. R., The vacuolating virus, S.V. 40. *Proc. Soc. Exp. Biol. & Med.*, **105**: 420–427, 1960.

TANNENBAUM, A., The initiation and growth of tumors. Introduction. I. Effects of underfeeding. *Am. J. Cancer*, **38**: 335–350, 1940.

TRENTIN, J. J., YABE, Y., and TAYLOR, G., Tumor induction in hamsters by human adenovirus. (Abstract). *Proc. Am. Assoc. Cancer Research*, **3**: 369, 1962.

TRENTIN, J. J., YABE, Y., and TAYLOR, G., The quest for human cancer viruses. *Science*, **137**: 835–841, 1962.

TRENTIN, J. J., YABE, Y., and TAYLOR, G., Studies on the oncogenicity of human adenovirus. pp. 559–563 in: *Viruses, Nucleic Acids, and Cancer*. 17th Ann. Symp. on Fundamental Cancer Research, Univ. of Texas, M. D. Anderson Hosp. and Tumor Inst., Williams & Wilkins, Baltimore, Md., 1963.

Umfrage über die Aetiologie des Krebses. ASCHOFF, L., ZIEGLER, E., MARCHAND,* RIBBERT, H., *Med. Klin.*, **1**: 409–412, 1905. CZERNY, V., HENKE, F., *Med. Klin.*, **1**: 496–499, 1905. BASHFORD, E. F., *Med. Klin.*, **1**: 544–547, 1905.

VALLERY-RADOT, R., *La vie de Pasteur*. 31st Edition. pp. 702. Librairie Hachette, Paris, 1931.

VIRCHOW, R., Zur pathologischen Physiologie des Blutes. II. Weisses Blut (Leukämie). *Virchow's Archiv. path. Anat.*, **1**: 547–583, 1847.

WELLER, C. V., Intrinsic factors in the etiology of neoplasms. *Am. J. Cancer*, **30**: 39–46, 1937.

WESSING, A., and v. BARGEN, G., Untersuchungen über einen virusbedingten Tumor bei Fischen. *Arch. f. Virusforsch.*, **9**: 521–536, 1959.

WOGLOM, W. H., Studies on cancer and allied subjects. The study of experimental cancer. A review. vol. **1**, pp. 288. Columbia Univ. Press, New York, 1913.

WOLFF, J., Die Lehre von der Krebskrankheit von den ältesten Zeiten bis zur Gegenwart. pp. 747. G. Fischer, Jena, 1907.

* No first name in the original paper.

Author Index

Numbers in italics refer to pages on which references are listed in bibliographies at end of each chapter.

* No initials appeared in the original paper.

* No initials in the original paper.

*No initials in the original paper.

*No first name appeared in the original paper.

*Also spelled Kryukova.

*No first name in the original paper.

*No first name in original paper.

*Spelled also Novinsky.

*No first name in the original paper.

Subject Index